MW01000248

IMMUNOLOGY

IMMUNOLOGY

Second Edition

JANIS KUBY

Professor of Biology,
San Francisco State University

Faculty,
Joint Medical Program,
University of California at Berkeley

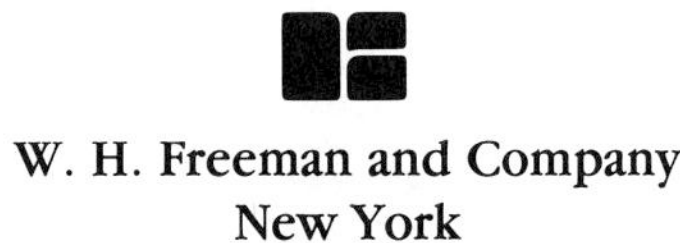

W. H. Freeman and Company
New York

Cover credits
Background: lymph node macrophage attached to an endothelial cell.

Inset: X-ray crystallography of a peptide bound to a human class II MHC molecule, DR1.
Courtesy of J. H. Brown, 1993, *Nature* **364**:33.

Library of Congress Cataloging-in-Publication Data

Kuby, Janis.
Immunology / Janis Kuby. — 2nd ed.
p. cm.
Includes bibliographical references and index.
ISBN 0-7167-2400-6
1. Immunology. I. Title.
[DNLM: 1. Immune System. 2. Immunity. QW 504 K951 1994]
QR181.K83 1994
616.07′9 — dc20
DNLM/DLC
for Library of Congress 93-46423
CIP

Printed in the United States of America

1 2 3 4 5 6 7 8 9 0 KP 9 9 8 7 6 5 4

To
My family, David, Rebecca, and Beth,
whose sacrifice and love has made it possible to complete this book.

And to
Violet Kiteley
who was an invaluable source of strength
and inspiration during the most difficult hours,
and Kim Clement for his vision and life-giving words.

And to
My mentor, Leon Wofsy,
who instilled in me a love for immunology and teaching
and who taught me, by his example, to always put people first.

And to
all the support from friends, extended family, and the grace of God
that has seen me through an earthquake, a fire, and cancer
during the writing of this book!

CONTENTS

PREFACE

The publication of the Second Edition of *Immunology* within just two years of the first edition testifies to the explosive development of the field of immunology. Despite economic restraints on research, the continued growth of immunology is inevitable and challenges both the medical and academic community to stay current. Like the middle-aged parents of young children, we are forced to keep growing and adapting to stay in tune with those entrusted to our care. Despite the growing pains, I am excited by the recent advances in immunology and find it rewarding to keep up with the growth spurts in this field.

Immunology has been successfully used in scores of introductory courses for undergraduates and students of clinical medicine alike. The book evolved from my sixteen years of teaching at San Francisco State University and, more recently, teaching in the joint medical school program at the University of California at Berkeley. As a teacher I became aware of the need for a textbook that first, and foremost, emphasizes that immunology is based solidly upon experimental results, and second, highlights the relationship between basic research and clinical applications. This second edition preserves these two goals.

The text's focus on the experimental process has proved popular with both students and instructors; it conveys much of the excitement of scientific discovery in the course of presenting the relevant facts. Exposure to the landmark experiments that underlay the theoretical framework of immunology enables students to appreciate how the current immunologic paradigms evolved. This approach also illustrates how experiments are designed and interpreted in order to test scientific hypotheses, thus encouraging students to develop the intellectual skills needed to critically read the current immunologic literature. Also crucial to a meaningful course in immunology is insight into the clinical applications of basic research. I have included discussions of important clinical applications throughout the text, and the last seven chapters are devoted to the most important clinically related subjects. As the AIDS epidemic highlights, these topics are not matters of abstract research interest but a question of life and death for ever increasing numbers of men, women, and children.

Although the objectives of the course served by this text have not changed in the last two years, the field itself is burgeoning with new information and methodology. The major goal of this second edition was therefore to update the text coverage of such topics as

- Apoptosis and its role in hematopoiesis, lymphocyte maturation, and AIDS
- Cell-adhesion molecules and their role in cell-to-cell interactions and lymphocyte recirculation
- Antigen processing and presentation including discussion of proteosomes and peptide transporters
- Signal transduction and the role of co-stimulatory signals in T-cell activation
- B-cell receptor complex and signal transduction
- Surrogate light chain expression in B cell maturation
- Recombination activating genes, RAG-1 and RAG-2 and their role in immunoglobulin and T-cell receptor gene rearrangement
- Positive and negative selection in the thymus with particular emphasis to the important contributions that transgenic systems have played in furthering our understanding of these processes

- Role of the CD28/B7 interaction as a co-stimulatory signal and its role in clonal anergy
- Cytokine receptor family
- Interleukins 12 and 13
- Putative role of CD26 as a coreceptor for HIV infection
- Structure of MHC molecules, including the newly crystallized class II MHC
- The relationship of MHC structure to peptide binding
- Generation of knock-out mice by homologous recombination and the usefulness of these mice to immunological research
- Cyclosporin A and FK 506
- Updated coverage on AIDS including changes in lymph node architecture, cytokine imbalance, apoptosis, and current vaccine trials
- Mucosal-associated lymphoid tissue

I am gratified by the wide use of the first edition of *Immunology* and have retained the organizational motifs that were enthusiastically received. Once again the book opens with a detailed overview of the immune system in Chapter 1 to provide a conceptual framework for the material presented in subsequent chapters. Chapter 2 again reviews some of the important experimental systems and techniques used in modern immunology; these are critical to the design of many of the most creative experiments in the field today. The book continues with a series of chapters (Chapters 3–18) that describe the components and functioning of the immune system. These chapters build on one another, with later chapters integrating key concepts from previous ones, so that underlying principles and recurring themes are reinforced. Readers familiar with the first edition will notice the addition of two new chapters in this section: Chapter 10 "Antigen Processing and Presentation" and Chapter 12 "T-Cell Maturation, Activation, and Differentiation." Chapter 19 begins a series of clinically oriented chapters on autoimmunity, vaccines, infectious diseases, immunodeficiency diseases, AIDS, transplantation immunology, and cancer. In these chapters the basic concepts discussed in the previous chapters are applied to topics of clinical interest.

Preparation of this second edition offered me the opportunity to improve both the prose and diagrams. With the help of my editors and colleagues, I have diligently tried to do just that: clarifying explanations of complicated topics and modifying many figures to better illustrate the topics depicted. Some of the more significant changes and additions to the text of the second editions include the following:

- Chapter 2 on experimental systems includes new material on the analysis of DNA regulatory sequences by DNA footprinting, gel-shift analysis, and the CAT assay. The production of "knock-out" mice is also described.
- Chapter 5 on immunoglobulin structure and function features additional material on the structural features of IgA. New data on the B-cell receptor complex allows students to make comparisons with the T-cell receptor.
- A new color insert, depicting the molecular structure of antibodies, T-cell receptors, and MHC molecules, vividly complements the text descriptions and schematic diagrams of these important proteins.
- Chapter 8 has been reorganized, updated, and clarified to more logically introduce students to the generation of antibody diversity. It features revised discussions of recombination signal sequences: recombination activating genes (RAG-1 and RAG-2); joining of V, D, and J gene segments; and the early stages in B-cell maturation within the bone marrow.
- Chapter 9 on the major histocompatibility complex has been reorganized so that the structure of each class of MHC molecule is presented early in the discussion. Techniques for mapping the MHC and a detailed, updated map are presented later in the chapter.
- Chapter 10, new in the second edition, provides a unified discussion of antigen processing and presentation, drawing on material that was spread over several chapters in the first edition. New information on proteosomes and peptide transporters is presented, and several relevant clinical applications are described.
- Coverage of T-cells was subdivided in this edition so that Chapter 11 covers the T-cell receptor while 12 covers the cellular aspects of T-cell activity: maturation, activation, and differentiation. These topics, which were treated in separate chapters in the first edition, are now presented in a coordinated fashion. The material on signal transduction and the role of co-stimulatory signals in T-cell activation has been updated and expanded considerably.
- Chapter 13 on cytokines has been extensively revised. The cytokines are presented in a comprehensive updated table followed by a discussion of the common structural and functional features of cytokines and cytokine receptors. The chapter features a great many new diagrams and concludes with a discussion of sev-

eral of the important biological effects of cytokine activity.

- Chapter 14 on the humoral response was reorganized and rewritten to update coverage of the complex interactions between APCs, B-cells, and T-cells, providing a comprehensive introduction to the events leading up to antibody synthesis. The chapter also includes a discussion of the events taking place within the lymph node during the induction of a humoral response. Included in this section is a discussion of somatic mutation, selection, apoptosis, and class switching during the in vivo response.

- Chapter 16 on immune regulation and tolerance has an expanded discussion of the CD28/B7 costimulatory signal and clonal anergy.

- Chapter 23 on AIDS has been rewritten to clarify the discussion and describes recent discoveries on changes in lymph-node architecture, cytokine imbalances, current vaccine trials, and other subjects.

Back by popular demand are the practical teaching aids at the end of each chapter: summaries, research references, and study questions. The chapter summaries highlight and review major concepts. The references enable students to sample the primary literature relating to various topics. The study questions are a useful teaching tool and provide a challenging review for students. Answers to the questions, as well as a glossary, are provided at the back of the book.

The second edition has benefitted from the feedback of its users and the suggestions of its many reviewers. I am especially grateful for the advice of John M. Lammert of Gustavus Adolphus College and Kathleen H. Lavoie of the University of Michigan-Flint who read the entire manuscript from the standpoint of teachers "in trenches" and added many insightful suggestions and clarifications. Their reviews were truly a labor of love and this book has benefitted tremendously from their contributions. I would also like to thank the following reviewers who read all or parts of this manuscript and have provided me with many helpful suggestions: Linda Bradley, University of California at San Diego; Mark M. Davis, Stanford University School of Medicine; Walter J. Esselman, Michigan State University; Bryan M. Gebhardt, Louisiana State University Medical Center; Kirk W. Johnson, Chiron Corporation; Robert I. Krasner, Providence College; Judy D. Marsh, Emporia State University; Allen Rosenspire, Wayne State University; Ellen Robey, University of California at Berkeley; Nilabh Shastri, University of California at Berkeley; Astar Winoto, University of California at Berkeley. The suggestions by Paul Knopf, Brown University, are thankfully acknowledged as well. Thanks are also due to reviewers of the first edition whose advice has had an ongoing influence: Allen T. Andrew, Indiana University of Pennsylvania; Diane D. Eardley, University of California at Santa Barbara; Robert P. Ellis, Colorado State University; Edgar G. Engleman, Stanford University Medical Center; Anne Good, University of California at Berkeley; Joseph Goodman, University of California at San Francisco; Wendy Havran, University of California at Berkeley; Andrea K. Hubbard, University of Arizona; Patricia P. Jones, Stanford University; Marian E. Koshland, University of California at Berkeley; David Lubaroff, University of Iowa; John G. Nedrud, Case Western Reserve University; David Raulet, MIT; Nora Sarvetnik, Scripps Research Institute; Eli Sercarz, University of California at Los Angeles; Lisa Steiner, MIT; Susan L. Swain, University of California at San Diego.

This book could not have been written without the help and encouragement of many relatives, friends, and colleagues. Special thanks to the students at San Francisco State University and the University of California at Berkeley who have been guinea pigs for much of the new material that appears in this second edition. I want to thank my former secretary and good friend Dotty Sims for her continued support and encouragement during those times when it was most needed. I also want to thank my relatives Jeanne and Dennis Kuby, Tom and Barbara Kuby, and Ray and Alma Kuby for their love and support. My colleagues at San Francisco State University deserve recognition for their support: my dean, James Kelley, and my colleagues, William Wu, Remo Morelli, Ruth Doell, Mary Luckey, Michael Goldman, Dean Kenyon, Crellin Pauling, Dick Davis, Ann and Leigh Auleb, Tony Catena, Rick Bernstein, John Stubbs, and Gregory Antipa.

I would also like to acknowledge my pleasure in working with the staff of W. H. Freeman and Company. Despite the pressures of never-ending publishing deadlines, I have truly enjoyed working with this group of people and feel that the publication of this book reflects a group effort. I would like to thank Deborah Allen for her direction of the early stages of the second edition and offer my sincere appreciation to Carol Pritchard-Martinez for her many invaluable suggestions as developmental editor and for helping me order my priorities to meet the various publishing deadlines. I would like to thank my project editor, Diane C. Maass, who has provided expert editorial direction of the production of both manuscript and illustrations and who has provided a warm and supportive friendship that has made the stressful stages of this process more bearable during both editions of this text. I am also very grateful for copy editor Ruth Steyn's dedication to this book and particularly for her improvement of both prose and diagrams, for catching the inconsistencies, and for paying attention to all the little details that my mind can so easily overlook. I am also appreciative of the design influence of Alice Fernandes-Brown. Thanks also to Larry Marcus and Travis Amos for photo research on the color insert. The book continues to benefit from the contribution of Armand Schwab as developmental editor of the first edition, and from the input of Patrick Fitzgerald and Kirk Jensen as acquisition editors of the first edition.

I welcome comments and suggestions from users of this text and will make every effort to incorporate these into the next edition. Please direct your letters to Dr. Janis Kuby, Department of Biology, San Francisco State University, 1600 Holloway, San Francisco, Ca. 94132 or to W. H. Freeman and Company, 41 Madison Avenue, New York, NY, 10010.

Janis Kuby
February 1994

OVERVIEW OF THE IMMUNE SYSTEM

The immune system is a remarkably adaptive defense system that has evolved in vertebrates to protect them from invading pathogenic microorganisms and cancer. It is able to generate an enormous variety of cells and molecules capable of specifically recognizing and eliminating an apparently limitless variety of foreign invaders. These cells and molecules act together in an exquisitely adaptable dynamic network whose complexity rivals that of the nervous system.

Functionally, an immune response can be divided into two interrelated activities—recognition and response. Immune recognition is remarkable for its specificity. The immune system is able to recognize subtle chemical differences that distinguish one foreign pathogen from another. At the same time, the system is able to discriminate between foreign molecules and the body's own cells and proteins. Once a foreign organism is recognized, the immune system enlists the participation of a variety of cells and molecules to mount an appropriate response, known as an effector function, to eliminate or neutralize the organism. In this way the system is able to convert the initial recognition event into different effector responses, each uniquely suited to eliminate a particular type of pathogen. Later exposure to the same foreign organism induces a memory response, characterized by a heightened immune reactivity, that serves to eliminate the pathogen and prevent disease.

This chapter presents a broad overview of the cells and molecules that compose the immune system and the mechanisms by which they protect the body against foreign invaders. As is always the case with an overview, the details have been simplified to reveal the essential structure of the immune system. Substantive discussions, experimental approaches, and in-depth definitions are left to the chapters that follow.

Historical Perspective

The discipline of immunology grew out of the observation that individuals who had recovered from certain infectious diseases were thereafter protected from the disease. The Latin term *immunis,* meaning exempt, is the source of the English word *immunity.* The concept of immunity can be traced back to 430 B.C. In describing a plague in Athens, Thucydides, the great historian of the Peloponnesian War, wrote that only those who had recovered from the plague could nurse the sick because they would not contract the disease a second time. Although the concept of immunity existed in folklore, it was almost two thousand years before the concept was successfully converted into a medically effective practice.

The first recorded crude attempts to induce immunity were performed by the Chinese and Turks in the fifteenth century. Various reports suggest that the dried crusts derived from smallpox pustules were either inhaled into the nostrils or inserted into small cuts in the skin (a technique called *variolation*). In 1718 Lady Mary Wortley Montagu, the wife of the British ambassador to Constantinople, observed the positive effects of variolation on the native population and had the technique applied to her own children. The technique was significantly improved by the English physician Edward Jenner in 1798. Jenner was intrigued by the fact that milkmaids who contracted cowpox (a mild disease) were subsequently immune to smallpox (a disfiguring and often fatal disease) and reasoned that it might be possible to protect people from smallpox by inoculating them with the fluid from a cowpox pustule. He tested his idea by inoculating an eight-year-old boy with fluid from a cowpox pustule and later intentionally infected the child with smallpox. The child did not develop smallpox. Nevertheless, one cannot help but question the ethical implications of such an experiment!

Jenner's technique of inoculating with cowpox to protect against smallpox spread quickly throughout Europe, but it was nearly 100 years before the technique was applied to other diseases by Louis Pasteur. As so often happens in science, serendipity combined with astute observation provided the next major advance in immunology. Pasteur had been studying the bacterium that causes fowl cholera. He had succeeded in growing the organism in culture and had shown that it could induce cholera when injected into chickens. His studies were interrupted by his summer vacation, and when he returned, he used an old culture of the bacterium to inject into the chickens. The chickens became ill but surprisingly they recovered. Pasteur then grew a fresh culture of the bacterium. He intended to inject it into some fresh chickens, the story goes, but was low on chickens and therefore used the previously injected chickens. Much to his surprise, the chickens survived and were completely protected from the disease. Pasteur recognized that aging had weakened the virulence of the pathogen and that such an attenuated strain might be administered to protect against disease. He called this attenuated strain a

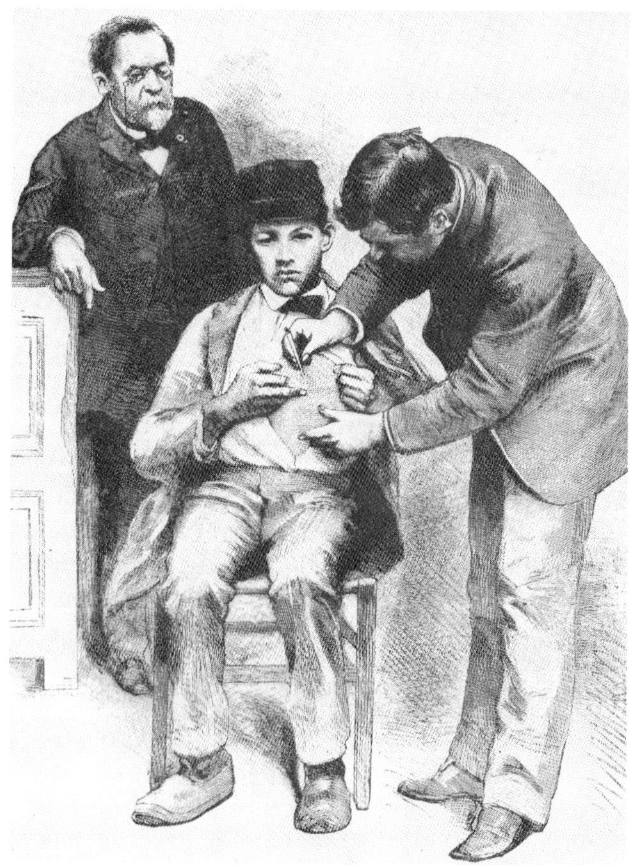

FIGURE 1-1 Wood engraving of Louis Pasteur watching Joseph Meister receive the rabies vaccine. [From *Harper's Weekly* **29**:836, 1885; courtesy of National Library of Medicine.]

vaccine (from Latin *vacca,* cow) in honor of Jenner's work with cowpox inoculation.

Pasteur extended these findings to other diseases, demonstrating that it was possible to attenuate, or weaken, a pathogen and administer the attenuated strain as a vaccine. In a now classical experiment at Pouilly-le-Fort in 1881, Pasteur vaccinated one group of sheep with heat-attenuated anthrax bacillus and then invited the public to watch as he challenged the sheep with a virulent culture of *Bacillus anthracis.* All the vaccinated sheep lived, whereas all unvaccinated animals died. These experiments marked the beginnings of the discipline of immunology. In 1885, Pasteur administered the first vaccine to a human, a young boy who had been bitten repeatedly by a rabid dog (Figure 1-1). The boy, Joseph Meister, lived and later became a custodian at the Pasteur Institute. In 1940, during the Nazi occupation of Paris, the Nazis asked Meister to give them the keys to Pasteur's crypt. Rather than surrender the keys to the Nazis, Meister took his own life.

Discovery of Humoral and Cellular Immunity

Although Pasteur proved that vaccination worked, he did not understand the mechanisms involved. The experimental work of Emil von Behring and Shibasaburo Kitasato in 1890 provided the first insights into the mechanism of immunity, earning von Behring the Nobel prize in medicine in 1901 (Table 1-1). Von Behring and Kitasato demonstrated that *serum* (the

TABLE 1-1 NOBEL PRIZES FOR IMMUNOLOGIC RESEARCH

Year	Recipient	Country	Research
1901	Emil von Behring	Germany	Serum antitoxins
1905	Robert Koch	Germany	Cellular immunity to tuberculosis
1908	Elie Metchnikoff Paul Ehrlich	Russia Germany	Role of phagocytosis (Metchnikoff) and antitoxins (Ehrlich) in immunity
1913	Charles Richet	France	Anaphylaxis
1919	Jules Bordet	Belgium	Complement-mediated bacteriolysis
1930	Karl Landsteiner	U.S.A.	Discovery of human blood groups
1951	Max Theiler	South Africa	Development of yellow fever vaccine
1957	Daniel Bovet	Switzerland	Antihistamines
1960	F. Macfarlane Burnet Peter Medawar	Australia Great Britain	Discovery of acquired immunological tolerance
1972	Gerald Edelman Rodney Porter	U.S.A. Great Britain	Chemical structure of antibodies
1977	Rosalyn Yalow	U.S.A.	Development of radioimmunoassay
1980	George Snell Jean Dausset Baruj Benacerraf	U.S.A. France U.S.A.	Major histocompatibility complex
1984	Georges Koehler Cesar Milstein Niels Jerne	Germany Great Britain Denmark	Monoclonal antibody Immune regulatory theories
1987	Susumu Tonegawa	Japan	Gene rearrangement in antibody production
1991	E. Donnall Thomas Joseph Murray	U.S.A. U.S.A.	Transplantation immunology

noncellular part of blood) from animals previously immunized to diphtheria could transfer the immune state to unimmunized animals. A serum antitoxin was suggested as the protective agent, and researchers spent the next decade characterizing the active component from immune serum. A serum component was shown to neutralize toxins, precipitate toxins, rupture (lyse) bacteria, and clump (agglutinate) bacteria and it was named for each of these activities: antitoxin, precipitin, bacterolysin, and agglutinin. For some time it seemed that each of these activities might be due to a different serum component, and it was not until the 1930s that a single substance, called an *antibody,* was shown to be responsible for all of these activities. Because immunity was mediated by antibodies contained in body fluids (known at the time as *humors*), it was called *humoral immunity.*

Paralleling the discovery of serum antibody was the discovery by Elie Metchnikoff, in 1883, that cells also contribute to the immune state of an animal. Metchnikoff had observed that certain white blood cells were able to engulf microorganisms. He named these cells *phagocytes* in reference to their ability to ingest foreign material. Metchnikoff observed that phagocytic cells were more active in immunized animals and hypothesized that cells, rather than antibodies, were the major effector of immunity. A controversy developed between those who held to the concept of humoral immunity and those who agreed with Metchnikoff's concept of *cell-mediated immunity.* The controversy foreshadowed the interrelated roles of humoral and cellular activities, both of which were later shown to be necessary for the immune response. In the 1950s the *lymphocyte* was identified as the cell responsible for both cellular and humoral immunity.

Early Theories of Immunity

One of the greatest enigmas about the antibody molecule facing early immunologists was its specificity for foreign material, or *antigen.* Two major theories were proposed to account for this specificity: the *selective* theory and the *instructional* theory. The earliest conception of the selective theory dates to Paul Ehrlich in 1900. In an attempt to explain the origin of serum antibody, Ehrlich proposed that cells expressed a variety of "side-chain" receptors that could react with infectious agents. Binding of an infectious agent to a side-chain receptor was envisioned as a complementary lock-and-key type of interaction. Ehrlich suggested that the interaction between an infectious agent and a cell's side-chain receptor would result in the release of the side chain and would induce the cell to produce and release more side-chain receptors with the same specificity. Ehrlich's theory was a selective theory: The side-chain specificity was determined prior to antigen exposure and antigen selected the appropriate side chain.

In the 1930s and 1940s the selective theory was replaced by various instructional theories. According to these theories, antigen played a central role in determining the specificity of the antibody molecule. The instructional theories suggested that a particular antigen would serve as a template around which antibody would fold. The antibody would thus assume a configuration complementary to that of the antigen template. Such concepts, first postulated by Friedrich Breinl and Felix Haurowitz and later popularized by Linus Pauling, made sense within the limitations of scientific knowledge at that time. But as new information emerged about the structure of DNA, RNA, and protein, the instructional theories were disproven.

In the 1950s, selection theories resurfaced and, through the insights of Niels Jerne, David Talmadge, and Macfarlane Burnet, were refined into a theory that came to be known as the *clonal-selection theory.* According to this theory, individual lymphocytes express membrane receptors that are specific for distinct antigens. Each lymphocyte expresses a unique receptor specificity, which is determined prior to the appearance of antigen. Binding of an antigen to a specific receptor activates the cell, resulting in its proliferation into a clone of cells, each with the same immunologic specificity as the original parent cell. The clonal-selection theory has been further refined and is now accepted as the underlying paradigm of modern immunology. This theory is examined in more depth later in the chapter.

Innate (Nonspecific) Immunity

Immunity—the state of protection from infectious disease— has both nonspecific and specific components. Innate, or nonspecific, immunity refers to the basic resistance to disease that a species possesses. Innate immunity can be envisioned as comprising four types of defensive barriers: anatomic, physiologic, endocytic and phagocytic, and inflammatory.

Anatomic Barriers

Physical and anatomic barriers that tend to prevent the entry of pathogens are an organism's first line of defense against infection. The skin and the surface of mucous membranes are included in this category because they provide an effective barrier to the entry of most microorganisms. The skin consists of two distinct layers: a relatively thin outer layer—the *epidermis*—and a thicker layer—the *dermis.* The epidermis contains several layers of tightly packed epithelial cells. The outer layer of cells is dead and is filled with a waterproofing protein called keratin. The epidermis is completely renewed every 15–30 days; old cells are sloughed off and new cells next to the dermis divide throughout life to replace the lost epidermal cells. The epidermis does not contain blood vessels, and epidermal cells are instead bathed in nutrients that diffuse from the underlying dermis. The dermis is composed of connective tissue and contains blood vessels, hair follicles, sebaceous glands, and sweat glands. The sebaceous glands, which are associated with the hair follicles, produce an oily secretion called *sebum.* Sebum consists of lactic and fatty acids, maintaining the pH of the skin between 3 and 5, which is inhibitory to the growth of most microorganisms. A few bacteria that metabolize sebum live as commensals on the skin and are responsible for a severe form of acne. One acne drug, Isotretinoin (Accutane), is a vitamin A derivative that prevents sebum formation.

Intact skin not only prevents the penetration of most pathogens but also inhibits most bacterial growth due to its low pH. Breaks in the skin, even small ones, resulting from wounds or abrasion are obvious routes of infection. The skin also is penetrated by biting insects (e.g., mosquitoes, mites, ticks, fleas, and sandflies); if these harbor pathogenic organisms, they can introduce the pathogen into the body as they feed. The protozoan that causes malaria, for example, is carried by mosquitoes who deposit it in humans when they take a blood meal. Similarly, bubonic plague is spread by the bite of fleas, and Lyme disease is spread by the bite of ticks.

The conjunctivae and the alimentary, respiratory, and urogenital tracts are not covered by dry, protective skin but by mucous membranes, which consist of an outer epithelial layer and an underlying connective tissue layer. Although most pathogens enter the body by binding to and penetrating mucous membranes, a number of nonspecific defense mechanisms serve to prevent this entry. For example, saliva, tears, and mucous secretions act to wash away potential invaders and also contain antibacterial or antiviral substances. The viscous fluid called *mucus,* which is secreted by epithelial cells of mucous membranes, entraps foreign microorganisms. In the lower respiratory tract and the gastrointestinal tract, the mucous membrane is covered by cilia, which move in a synchronous fashion to propel mucus-entrapped microorganisms from these tracts.

Some organisms have evolved ways to escape this defense mechanism and thus are likely to invade the body through mucous membranes. For example, influenza virus (the agent that causes flu) has a surface molecule that enables it to firmly attach to cells in the mucous membrane, preventing the virus from being swept out by the ciliated epithelial cells. Similarly, the organism causing gonorrhea has surface projections that allow it to bind to mucous membrane epithelia cells in the urogenital tract. Adherence of bacteria to mucous membranes involves interactions between hairlike protrusions on a bacterium, called *fimbriae* or *pili,* and certain glycoproteins or glycolipids that are only expressed by some mucous membrane epithelia cells (Figure 1-2). For this reason, some tissues are susceptible to bacterial invasion, while others are not.

The importance of anatomic barriers to host defense is vividly illustrated by a group of mice described in a report in *Nature.* These mice appeared to be immune to the parasitic helminth (worm) that causes schistosomiasis, a chronic and debilitating disease affecting more than 300 million people worldwide. After initial infection with this helminth, the mice initially developed portal hypertension similar to that observed in humans with the disease. However, when mice were reinfected with the helminth a second time, a very low yield of the helminth was recovered, and the mice appeared to be resistant to the infection. Because the mice apparently had developed immunity to the helminth, they were considered to be a potential animal model for the disease in humans. After considerable funding was poured into research on this mouse model, it turned out that the ability to clear the helminth had nothing to do with a specific immunologic response and was instead due to a complex anatomical reorganization in blood vessel architecture that occurred at the time of the second injection. The *Nature* article warned "not to postulate immunological mechanisms where simple anatomical or physiological explanations might suffice."

Even when a pathogen eludes the anatomic defenses provided by the skin and mucous membranes, it still faces other types of innate defenses including various physiologic, phagocytic, and inflammatory barriers. Only by successfully evading these barriers can a pathogen become established in a host.

Physiologic Barriers

Physiologic barriers include temperature, pH, oxygen tension, and various soluble factors. Many species are not susceptible to certain diseases simply because their body temperature inhibits pathogen growth. Chickens, for example, display innate immunity to anthrax because their high body temperature inhibits the growth of this pathogen. Gastric acidity also

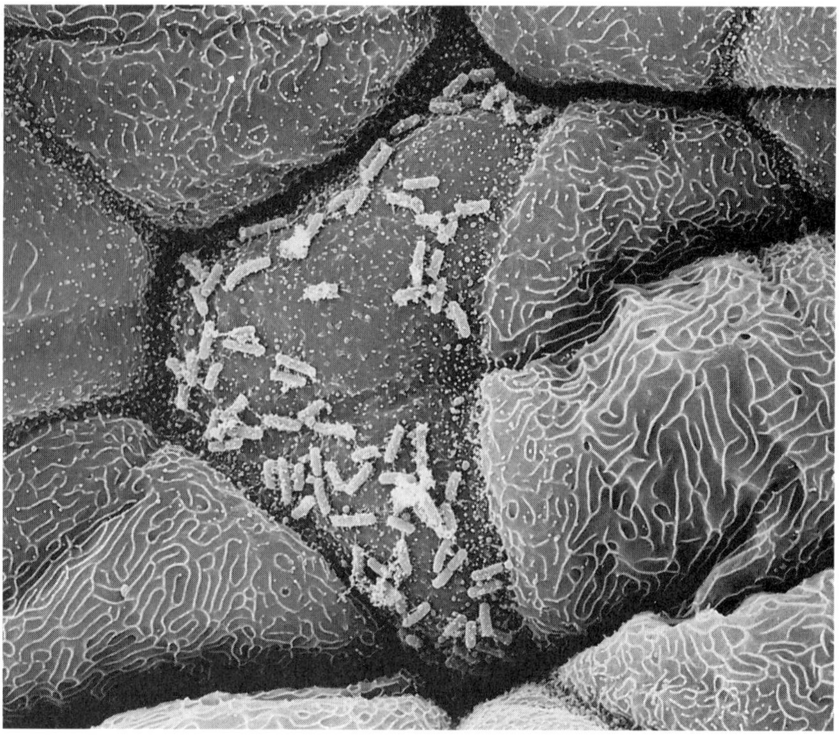

FIGURE 1-2 Electron micrograph of rod-shaped *Escherichia coli* bacteria adhering to surface of epithelial cells of the urinary tract. [From N. Sharon and H. Lis, 1993, *Sci. Am.* **268** (Jan.):85.]

provides an innate physiologic barrier to infection because very few ingested microorganisms can survive the low pH of the stomach. One reason newborns are susceptible to some diseases that do not afflict adults is that their stomach contents are less acid than that of adults.

A variety of soluble factors also contribute to nonspecific immunity. Among these soluble proteins are lysozyme, interferon, and complement. *Lysozyme*—a hydrolytic enzyme found in mucous secretions—is able to cleave the peptidoglycan layer of the bacterial cell wall. *Interferons* are a group of proteins produced by virus-infected cells. Among their many functions is the ability to bind to nearby cells and induce a generalized antiviral state. *Complement* is a group of serum proteins that circulate in an inactive proenzyme state. These proteins can be activated by a variety of specific and nonspecific immunologic mechanisms that convert the inactive proenzymes into active enzymes. The activated complement components participate in a controlled enzymatic cascade that results in membrane-damaging reactions, which destroy pathogenic organisms or facilitate their clearance.

Endocytic and Phagocytic Barriers

Another important innate defense mechanism is the ingestion of extracellular macromolecules and particles through *endocytosis* and *phagocytosis,* respectively. In endocytosis, the macromolecules contained within the extracellular tissue fluid are internalized by cells. This internalization occurs as small regions of the plasma membrane invaginate, or fold inward, forming small (approximately 0.1 μm) endocytic vesicles. Endocytosis occurs through one of two processes: *pinocytosis* or *receptor-mediated endocytosis* (Figure 1-3). In pinocytosis, macromolecules are internalized through nonspecific membrane invagination. Because pinocytosis is nonspecific, the internalization of macromolecules occurs in proportion to their concentration. In receptor-mediated endocytosis, macromolecules are selectively internalized after binding to specific membrane receptors.

Following internalization by either process, the endocytic vesicles fuse with each other and are delivered to *endosomes.* The endosomes, acidic compartments within the cell, serve a sorting function. Their acid environment facilitates dissociation of the receptor from its ligand. The remaining macromolecules contained within the endosome are routed along a different pathway, where they fuse with *primary lysosomes,* to form structures known as *secondary lysosomes.* Primary lysosomes are derived from the Golgi complex and contain large numbers of degradative enzymes, including proteases, nucleases, lipases, and other hydrolytic enzymes. Within secondary lysosomes, the ingested macromolecules are then digested into small

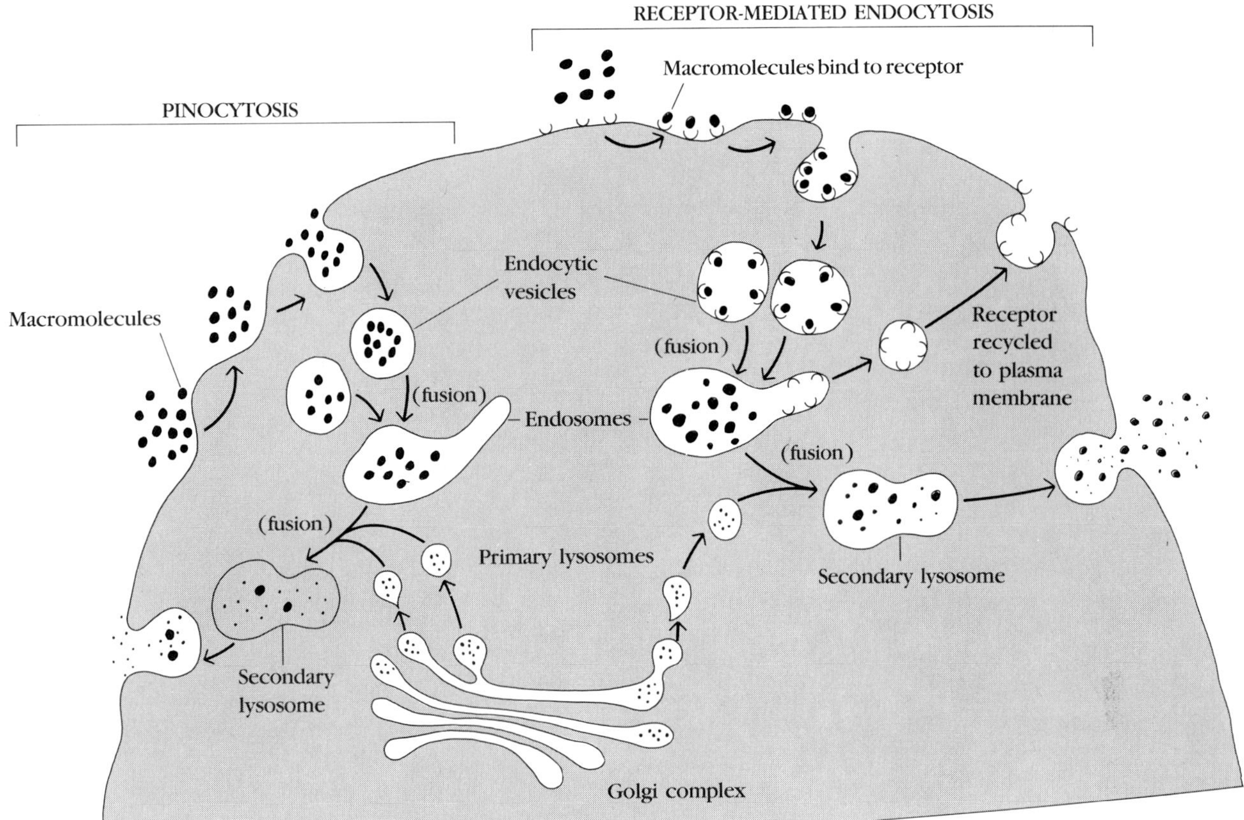

FIGURE 1-3 Endocytosis—the internalization of macromolecules within the extracellular fluid—occurs by pinocytosis or receptor-mediated endocytosis. In both processes, the ingested material is degraded via the endocytic processing pathway.

breakdown products (e.g., peptides, nucleotides, and sugars), which eventually are eliminated from the cell.

Phagocytosis involves the ingestion of particulate material, including whole pathogenic microorganisms (Figure 1-4). In phagocytosis, which differs from endocytosis in several ways, the plasma membrane expands around the particulate material to form large vesicles called *phagosomes.* These vesicles are roughly 10–20 times larger than endocytic vesicles. The expansion of the membrane in phagocytosis requires participation of microfilaments, which do not take part in endocytosis. Only specialized cells are capable of phagocytosis, whereas virtually all cells are capable of endocytosis. The specialized phagocytic cells include blood monocytes, neutrophils, and tissue macrophages (see Chapter 3). Once particulate material is ingested into phagosomes, the phagosomes fuse with lysosomes and the ingested material is then digested in the endocytic processing pathway by a process similar to that seen in endocytosis.

Barriers Created by the Inflammatory Response

Tissue damage caused by a wound or by invasion by a pathogenic microorganism induces a complex sequence of events collectively known as the *inflammatory response.* Many of the classic features of the inflammatory response were described as early as 1600 B.C. in Egyptian papyrus writings. In the first century A.D., the Roman physician Celsus described the "four cardinal signs of inflammation" as *rubor* (redness), *tumor* (swelling), *calor* (heat), and *dolor* (pain). In the second century A.D., another physician, Galen, added a fifth sign: *functio laesa* (loss of function).

The cardinal signs of inflammation reflect three major events that occur during an inflammatory response: (1) vasodilation, (2) increased capillary permeability, and (3) influx of phagocytic cells. Vasodilation—an increase in the diameter of blood vessels—occurs as the vessels that carry blood away

(a)

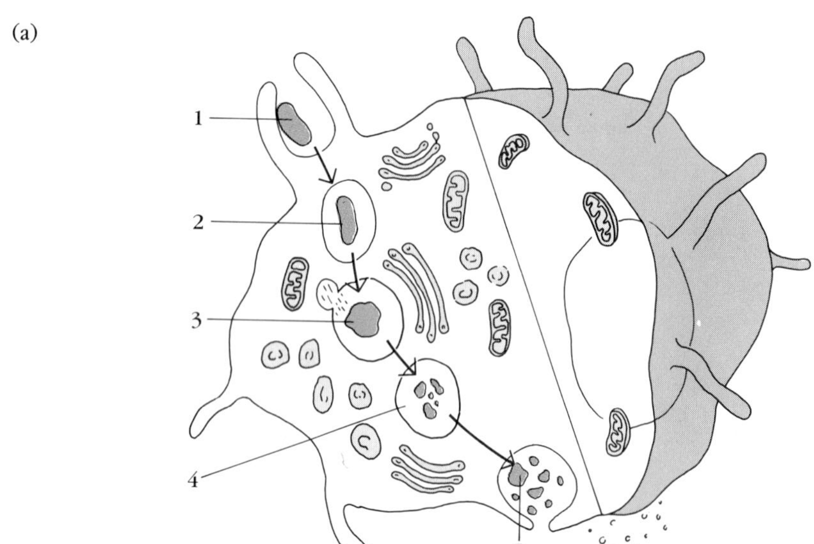

(b)

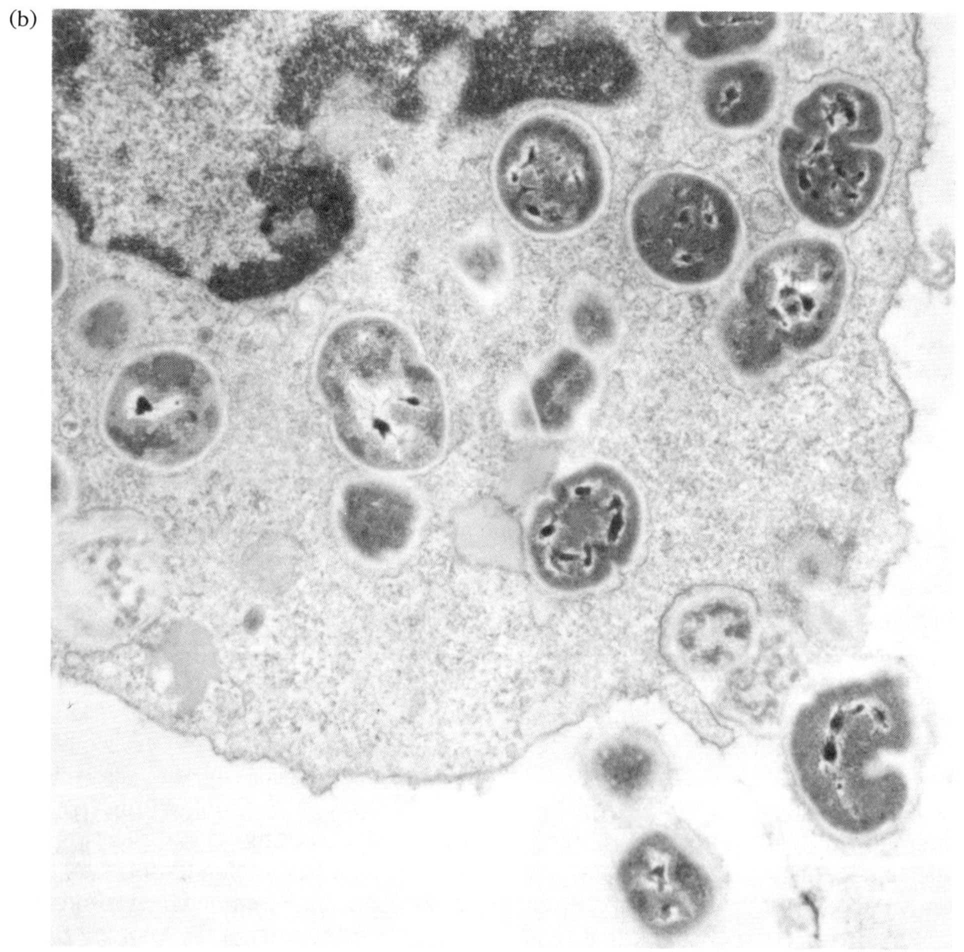

FIGURE 1-4 Phagocytosis of bacteria. (a) Schematic diagram of the steps in phagocytosis: 1) attachment of a bacterium (purple) to long membrane evaginations, called pseudopodia; 2) ingestion of bacterium forming a phagosome, which moves toward a lysosome; 3) fusion of the lysosome and phagosome, releasing lysosomal enzymes into the phagosome; 4) digestion of ingested material; and 5) release of digestion products from the cell. (b) Photomicrograph of a portion of a phagocytic cell. Note bacterium in process of being ingested in lower right and dark-colored phagosomes within the cytoplasm. [Part (b) from A. G. Macleod, 1973, *Aspects of Acute Inflammation,* Scope Monograph, p 27; courtesy of Dorothea Zucker-Franklin, Dept. of Medicine, New York University.]

from an affected area constrict, resulting in engorgement of the capillary network. The engorged capillaries are responsible for the tissue redness *(erythema)* and an increase in tissue temperature. An increase in capillary permeability facilitates an influx of fluid and cells from the engorged capillaries into the tissue. The fluid that accumulates *(exudate)* has a much higher protein content than fluid normally released from the vasculature. Accumulation of exudate contributes to the tissue swelling *(edema)*. The increased capillary permeability also facilitates the migration of various white blood cells from the capillaries into the tissues (Figure 1-5). Phagocytic cells are the major type of white blood cell to emigrate. The emigration of phagocytes involves a complex series of events including cellular adherence *(margination)* to the endothelial wall followed by emigration between the capillary endothelial cells into the tissue *(diapedesis* or *extravasation)* and, finally, migration through the tissue to the site of the inflammatory response *(chemotaxis)*. As the phagocytic cells accumulate at the site and begin to phagocytose bacteria, they release lytic enzymes, which can damage nearby healthy cells. The accumulation of dead cells, digested material, and fluid forms a substance called *pus*.

The events in the inflammatory response are initiated by a complex series of interactions involving a variety of chemical mediators, whose interactions are still only partially understood. Some of these mediators are derived from invading microorganisms, some are released from damaged cells in response to tissue injury, some are generated by several plasma enzyme systems and some are products of various white blood cells participating in the inflammatory response. Among the chemical mediators released in response to tissue damage are various serum proteins called *acute-phase proteins*. The concentrations of these proteins increase dramatically in tissue-damaging infections. *C-reactive protein*—a major acute-phase protein produced by the liver in response to tissue damage—binds to the C-polysaccharide cell-wall component found on a variety of bacteria and fungi.

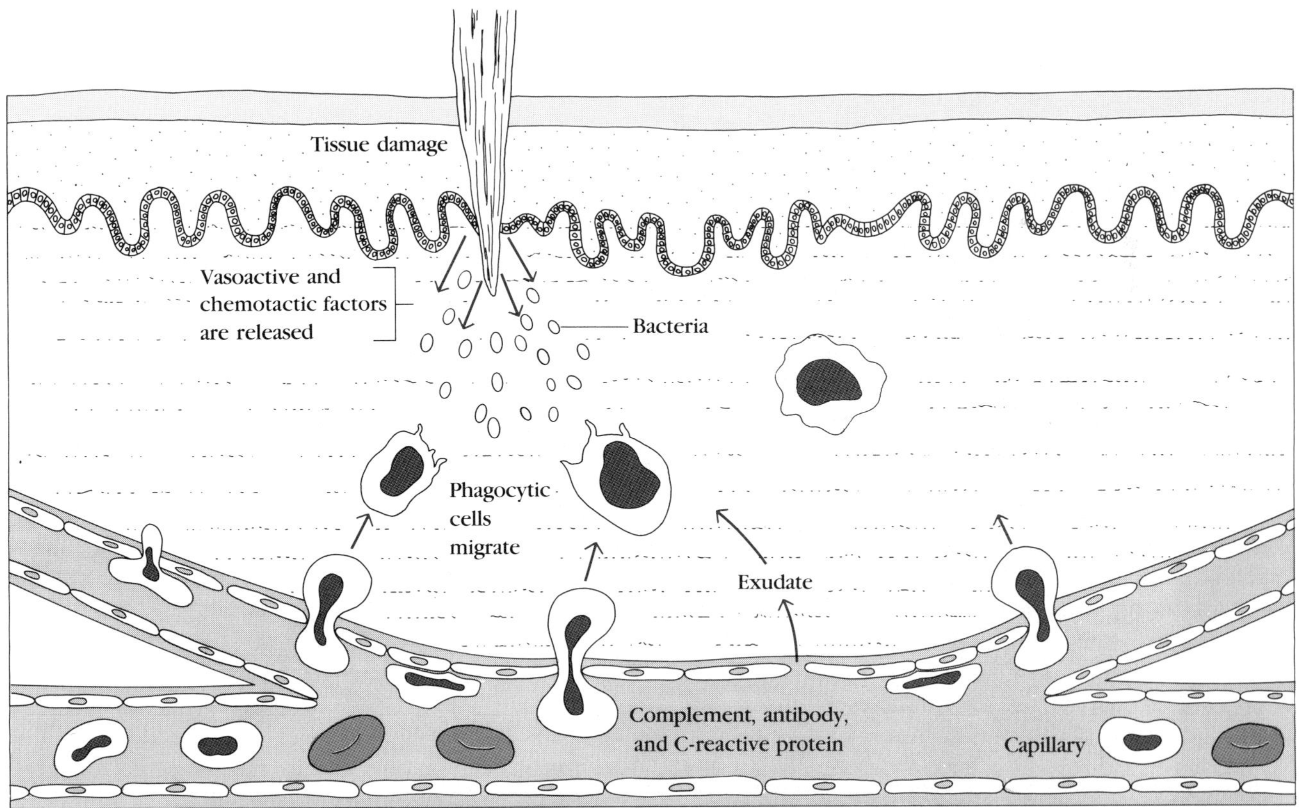

FIGURE 1-5 Major events in the inflammatory response. A bacterial infection causes tissue damage with release of various vasoactive and chemotactic factors. These factors induce increased blood flow to the area, increased capillary permeability, and influxes of white blood cells, including phagocytes and lymphocytes, from the blood into the tissues. The serum proteins contained in the exudate have antibacterial properties, and the phagocytes begin to engulf the bacteria.

This binding activates the complement system, resulting in increased clearance of the pathogen either by complement-mediated lysis of the pathogen or by complement-mediated increase in phagocytosis.

One of the principle mediators of the inflammatory response is *histamine,* a chemical released by a variety of cells (mast cells of the connective tissue, circulating blood basophils, and blood platelets) in response to tissue injury. Histamine binds to receptors on nearby capillaries and venules, causing vasodilation and increased permeability. Another important group of mediators that are present in blood plasma in an inactive form are small peptides called *kinins.* When tissue injury occurs, these peptides are activated and cause vasodilation and increased capillary permeability. A particular kinin, called *bradykinin,* also stimulates pain receptors in the skin. This effect probably serves a protective role since pain normally causes an individual to protect the injured area. Vasodilation and the increase in capillary permeability also enable enzymes of the blood-clotting system to enter the tissue where an enzyme cascade is activated resulting in the deposition of insoluble strands of fibrin that compose a blood clot. The fibrin clots wall off the injured area from the rest of the body and serve to prevent the spread of infection.

Once the inflammatory response has subsided and most of the debris has been cleared away by phagocytic cells, tissue repair and regeneration of new tissue occur. Tissue repair begins as capillaries grow into the fibrin of a blood clot. New connective tissue cells, called fibroblasts, replace the fibrin as the clot dissolves. As fibroblasts and capillaries accumulate, a scar tissue is formed. The inflammatory response is discussed in more detail in Chapter 13.

Acquired (Specific) Immunity

Acquired, or specific, immunity reflects the presence of a functional immune system that is capable of specifically recognizing and selectively eliminating foreign microorganisms and molecules. Unlike innate immunity, acquired immunity displays *specificity, diversity, memory,* and *self/nonself recognition.* These four features characterize all immune responses.

The specificity of the immune system can be seen in its capacity to distinguish subtle differences among antigens. In some cases a single mutation, resulting in a single amino acid substitution, is all that is necessary for an antigen to escape an effective immune response. The immune system is capable of generating tremendous diversity in its recognition molecules, allowing it to specifically recognize billions of uniquely different structures on foreign antigens. Once the immune system has responded to an antigen, it exhibits memory; that is, a second encounter with the same antigen induces a heightened state of immune reactivity. Because of this attribute, the immune system can confer life-long immunity to many infectious agents. Finally, the ability of the immune system to respond only to foreign antigens indicates that the immune system is capable of distinguishing self from nonself. It is essential that the immune response be limited to nonself-antigens, for the consequence of an inappropriate response to self-antigens can be a fatal autoimmune disease.

Acquired immunity does not occur independently of innate immunity. Cells of the phagocytic system, most notably macrophages, are intimately involved in activation of the specific immune response. At the same time, various soluble factors, produced during a specific immune response, have been shown to augment the activity of these phagocytic cells. As an inflammatory response develops, for example, soluble mediators are produced that attract cells of the immune system. The immune response will, in turn, serve to regulate the intensity of the inflammatory response. Through the carefully regulated interplay of acquired and innate immunity, the two systems work together to effectively eliminate a foreign invader.

The Cells of the Immune System

Generation of an effective immune response involves two major groups of cells: *lymphocytes* and *antigen-presenting cells.* Lymphocytes are one of many types of white blood cells produced in the bone marrow during the process of hematopoiesis (see Chapter 3). Lymphocytes leave the bone marrow, circulate in the blood and lymph system, and reside in various lymphoid organs. The attributes of specificity, diversity, memory, and self/nonself recognition are mediated by the lymphocytes. Lymphocytes are able to recognize antigens by means of membrane receptors specific for the foreign material. There are two major populations of lymphocytes: B lymphocytes (B cells) and T lymphocytes (T cells).

B Lymphocytes

B lymphocytes mature within the bone marrow and leave the marrow expressing a unique antigen-binding receptor on their membrane (Figure 1-6a). The B-cell receptor is an *antibody molecule,* a membrane-bound glycoprotein. The basic structure of the antibody molecule consists of two identical heavy polypeptide chains and two identical light polypeptide chains. The

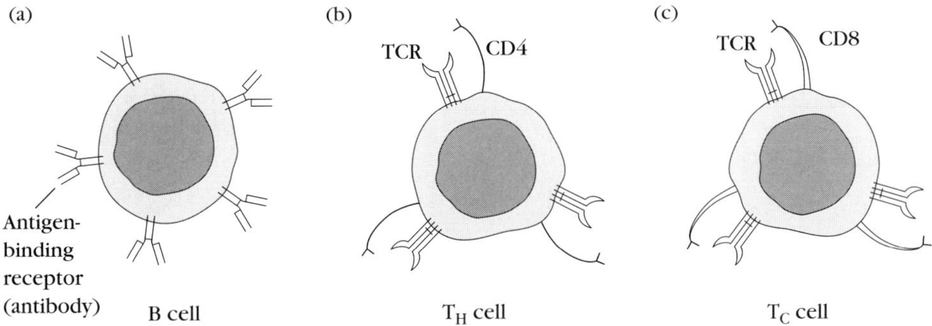

FIGURE 1-6 Distinctive membrane molecules on lymphocytes. (a) B cells have about 10^5 molecules of membrane-bound antibody per cell. All the antibody molecules on a given B cell exhibit the same antigenic specificity and can interact directly with antigen. (b) T cells bearing CD4 only recognize antigen associated with class II MHC molecules. (c) T cells bearing CD8 only recognize antigen associated with class I MHC molecules. In general, $CD4^+$ T cells function as helper cells and $CD8^+$ cells function as cytotoxic cells. Both types of T cells express about 10^5 identical molecules of the antigen-binding T-cell receptor (TCR) per cell, each with the same antigenic specificity.

chains are held together by disulfide bonds. The amino-terminal ends of each pair of heavy and light chains form a cleft within which antigen binds. When a *naive* B cell first encounters the antigen for which its membrane-bound antibody is specific, the cell begins to divide rapidly; its progeny differentiate into *memory B cells* and effector cells called *plasma cells.* Memory B cells have a longer life span and continue to express membrane-bound antibody with the same specificity as the original parent cell. Plasma cells do not produce membrane-bound antibody but instead produce the antibody in a form that can be secreted. Plasma cells live for only a few days but they secrete enormous amounts of antibody during this time. It has been estimated that a single plasma cell can secrete more than 2000 molecules of antibody per second. Secreted antibodies are the major effector molecule of humoral immunity.

T Lymphocytes

T lymphocytes also arise from hematopoietic stem cells in the bone marrow. Unlike B cells, which mature within the bone marrow, T cells migrate to the thymus gland to mature. During its maturation within the thymus, the T cell comes to express a unique antigen-binding receptor on its membrane, called the *T-cell receptor.* The receptor molecule is a heterodimer, composed of two protein chains, either alpha and beta ($\alpha\beta$) or gamma and delta ($\gamma\delta$), which are linked by disulfide bonds. The amino-terminal ends of the two chains fold together to form the antigen-binding cleft of the T-cell receptor. Unlike membrane-bound antibodies on B cells, which can recognize antigen alone, T-cell receptors can recognize antigen only in association with cell-membrane proteins known as *major histocompatibility complex (MHC) molecules.* When a naive T cell encounters antigen associated with an MHC molecule on a cell, the T cell proliferates and differentiates into *memory T cells* and various effector T cells.

There are two subpopulations of T cells: *T helper* (T_H) *cells* and *T cytotoxic* (T_C) *cells.* A third type of T cell, called a *T suppressor* (T_S) *cell* has been postulated, but recent evidence has led many researchers to question whether its lineage is distinct from the T_H and T_C subpopulations (see Chapter 16). The T helper and T cytotoxic cells can be distinguished by their display of one of two membrane glycoproteins, either CD4 or CD8 (Figure 1-6b,c). T cells displaying CD4 generally function as T_H cells, whereas those displaying CD8 generally function as T_C cells (see Chapter 3). In response to the recognition of an antigen-MHC complex, a T_H cell secretes various growth factors known collectively as *cytokines* or, more specifically, *lymphokines.* As a T_H cell is activated, it becomes an effector cell secreting various cytokines, which play an important role in activating B cells, T_C cells, macrophages, and various other cells that participate in the immune response. Differences in the pattern of cytokines produced by activated T_H cells results in qualitative differences in the type of immune response that develops. Under the influence of T_H-derived cytokines, a T_C cell that recognizes an antigen–MHC molecule complex proliferates and differentiates into an effector cell called a *cytotoxic T lymphocyte (CTL).* In contrast to the T_H cell, the CTL generally does not secrete many cytokines and instead exhibits cytotoxic activity. The CTL has a vital function in monitoring the cells of the body and eliminating any that display antigen, such as virus-infected cells, tumor cells, and cells of a foreign tissue graft.

Antigen-Presenting Cells

Activation of both the humoral and cell-mediated branches of the immune system requires cytokines produced by T_H cells. It is essential that activation of T_H cells be carefully regulated because an inappropriate T_H cell response to self-components can have fatal autoimmune consequences. To ensure careful regulation, the T_H cell can be activated following antigen recognition only when the antigen is displayed together with MHC molecules on the surface of specialized cells called *antigen-presenting cells (APCs).* Antigen-presenting cells, which include macrophages, B lymphocytes, and dendritic cells, are distinguished by their expression of a particular type of MHC molecule. These specialized cells internalize antigen, either by phagocytosis or by endocytosis, and then re-express a part of that antigen, together with the MHC molecule, on their membrane. The T_H cell then recognizes the antigen associated with the MHC molecule on the membrane of the antigen-presenting cell. (Figure 1-7).

Functions of Humoral and Cell-Mediated Immune Responses

As mentioned earlier, immune responses can be divided into humoral and cell-mediated responses. The term *humoral* is derived from the Latin *humor,* meaning body fluid; thus humoral immunity refers to immunity that can be conferred on a nonimmune individual by administration of serum antibodies from an immune individual. The humoral branch of the immune system involves interaction of B cells with antigen and their subsequent proliferation and differentiation into antibody-secreting plasma cells (Figure 1-8). Antibody functions as the effector of the humoral response by binding to antigen and neutralizing it or facilitating its elimination. When an antigen is coated with antibody, it can be eliminated in several ways. For example, antibody can cross-link the antigen, forming clusters that are more readily ingested by phagocytic cells. Binding of antibody to antigen on a microorganism also can activate the complement system, resulting in lysis of

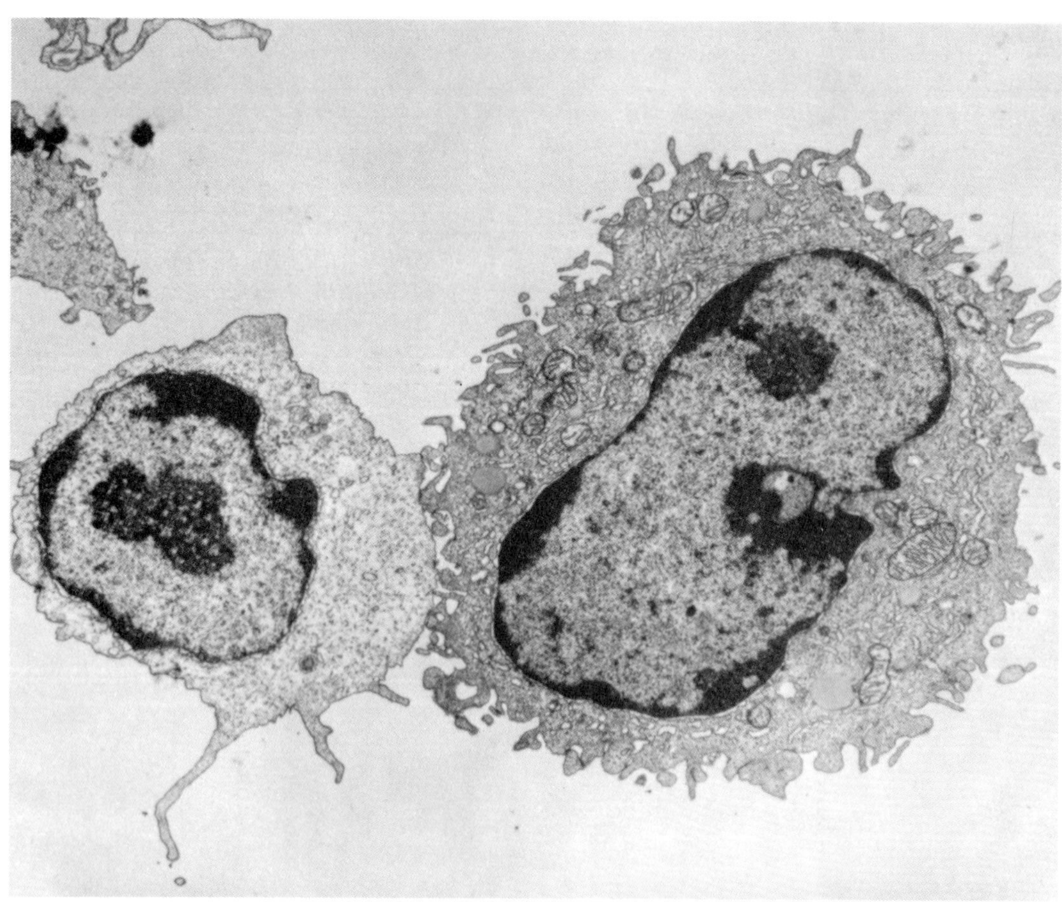

FIGURE 1-7 Electron micrograph of an antigen-presenting macrophage *(right)* associating with a T lymphocyte. [From A. S. Rosenthal et al., 1982, in *Phagocytosis—Past and Future,* Academic Press, p. 239.]

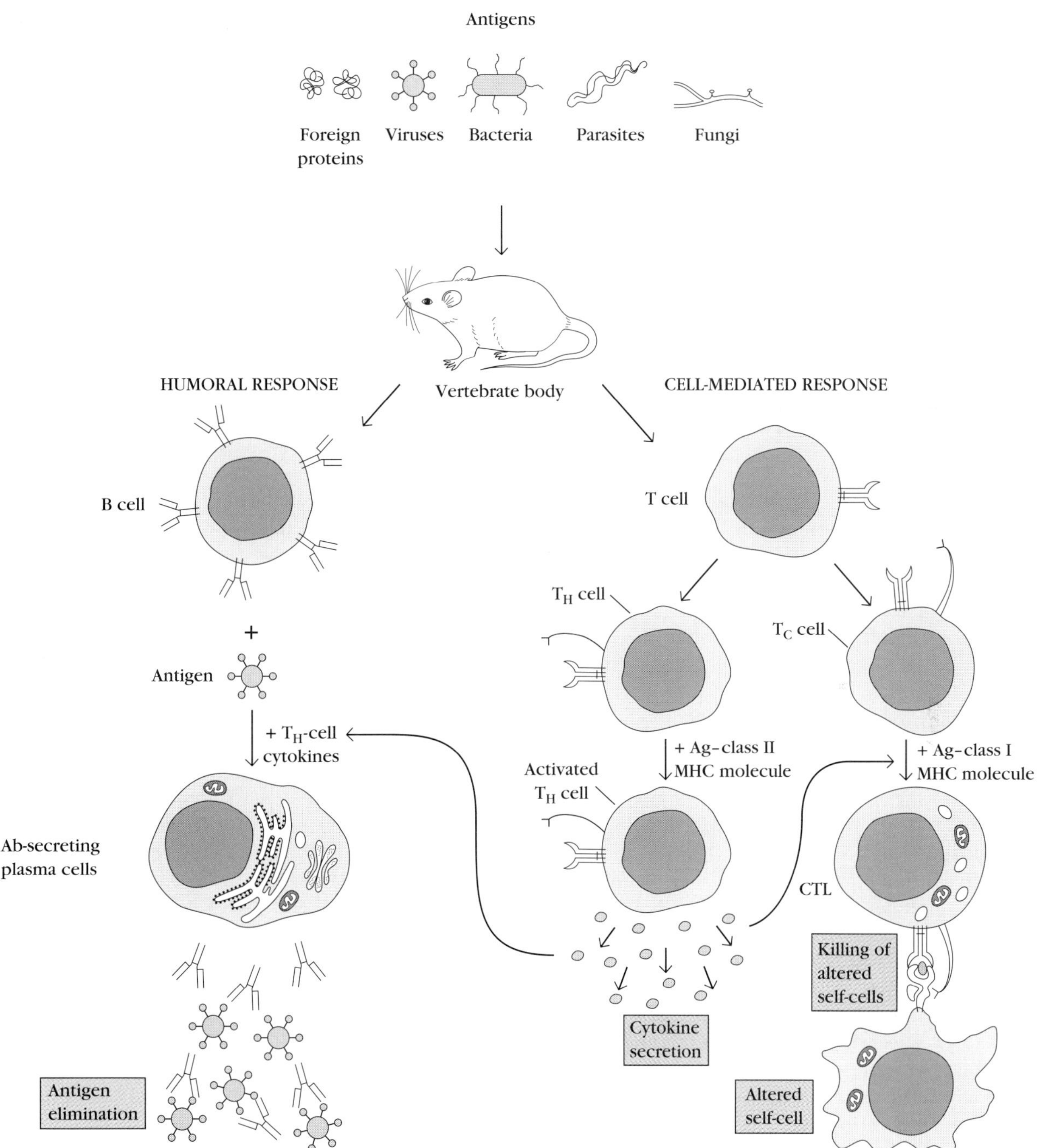

FIGURE 1-8 Overview of the humoral and cell-mediated branches of the immune system. The humoral response involves interaction of B cells with antigen (Ag) and their differentiation into antibody-secreting plasma cells. The secreted antibody (Ab) binds to the antigen and facilitates its clearance from the body. The cell-mediated response involves various subpopulations of T cells that recognize antigen presented on self-cells. T_H cells respond to antigen by producing cytokines. T_C cells respond to antigen by developing into cytotoxic T lymphocytes (CTLs), which mediate killing of altered self-cells (e.g., virus-infected cells).

the foreign organism. Antibody can also neutralize toxins or viral particles by coating them and preventing their subsequent binding to host cells.

Effector T cells generated in response to antigen are responsible for cell-mediated immunity (see Figure 1-8). Unlike humoral immunity, which can be transferred by serum antibody, cell-mediated immunity can only be transferred by immune T cells. Both activated T_H cells and CTLs serve as effector cells in cell-mediated immune reactions. Cytokines secreted by T_H cells can activate various phagocytic cells, enabling them to phagocytose and kill microorganisms more effectively. This type of cell-mediated immune response is especially important in host defense against intracellular bacteria. Cytotoxic T lymphocytes participate in cell-mediated immune reactions by killing altered self-cells; they play an important role in the killing of virus-infected cells and tumor cells.

Recognition of Antigen by B and T Lymphocytes

Antigens, which are generally very large and complex, are not recognized in their entirety by T or B lymphocytes. Instead, both T and B lymphocytes recognize discrete sites on the antigen called antigenic determinants, or *epitopes.* Epitopes are the immunologically active regions on a complex antigen, the regions that actually bind to a B- or T-cell's receptor. The most important difference in antigen recognition by T lymphocytes and B lymphocytes is that B cells can recognize an epitope alone, whereas T cells can recognize an epitope only when it is present on the surface of a self-cell in association with an MHC molecule. The two branches of the immune system are therefore uniquely suited to recognize antigen in different milieus. The humoral branch (B cells) recognizes an enormous variety of epitopes; those displayed on the surface of bacteria or viral particles, as well as those displayed on soluble proteins or glycoproteins that have been released from invading pathogens. The cell-mediated branch (T cells) recognizes epitopes displayed together with molecules of the major histocompatibility complex on self-cells. As noted previously, the cell-mediated branch of the immune response is uniquely suited to recognize altered self-cells, such as virus-infected self-cells and cancerous cells.

Four related but distinct cell-membrane molecules are responsible for antigen recognition by the immune system: membrane-bound antibodies on B cells; heterodimeric T-cell receptors (either $\alpha\beta$ or $\gamma\delta$); class I MHC molecules present on all nucleated cells; and class II MHC molecules present on antigen-presenting cells. Each of these molecules plays a unique role in antigen recognition, ensuring that the immune system can recognize and respond to the different types of antigen that it encounters.

Generation of Lymphocyte Specificity and Diversity

The antigenic specificity of each B cell is determined by the membrane-bound antigen-binding receptor (i.e., antibody) expressed by the cell. The antibody on a B cell can recognize different epitopes with incredible precision. Even protein antigens that differ by only a single amino acid often can be discriminated from each other. As a B cell matures in the bone marrow, its specificity is generated by random rearrangements of a series of gene segments encoding the antibody molecule (see Chapter 8). As a result of this process, each mature B cell possesses a single functional gene encoding the antibody heavy chain and a single functional gene encoding the antibody light chain. Thus the B lymphocyte synthesizes and displays antibody with one specificity on its membrane. All 10^5 antibody molecules on a given B lymphocyte have identical specificity, giving each B lymphocyte, and the clone of daughter cells to which it gives rise, a distinct specificity for antigen. The mature B lymphocyte is therefore said to be *antigenically committed.*

The fine specificity of the antibody molecule is coupled to an enormous diversity. The random gene rearrangements that occur during B-cell maturation generate an enormous number of antibody specificities. The resulting B-cell population consists of individual B cells, each exhibiting a distinct antibody specificity, that collectively exhibit enormous diversity estimated to exceed 10^8 different antibody specificities.

The attributes of specificity and diversity that characterize the antibody molecule of the B cell also apply to the $\alpha\beta$ or $\gamma\delta$ heterodimers of the T cell. As in B-cell maturation, the process of T-cell maturation also involves random rearrangements of a series of gene segments encoding the cell's antigen receptor (see Chapter 11). Each T lymphocyte expresses about 10^5 receptors per cell, and all 10^5 receptors on a cell and its clonal progeny have identical specificity for antigen. The process of random rearrangement of the genes encoding the T-cell receptor is capable of generating enormous diversity—on the order of 10^{15} unique receptor specificities. Unlike the antibody on the B cell, the enormous potential diversity of the T-cell receptor is later diminished through a process of selection in the thymus—a process ensuring that only T cells with receptors capable of recognizing antigen associated with MHC molecules will be able to mature (see Chapter 12).

Role of the Major Histocompatibility Complex

The major histocompatibility complex (MHC) is a large genetic complex with multiple loci. The MHC loci encode two major classes of membrane molecules—class I and class II MHC molecules. As noted previously, T_H cells generally recognize antigen associated with a class II molecule, whereas T_C cells generally recognize antigen associated with class I molecules (Figure 1-9).

Class I MHC molecules are glycoproteins found on the membrane of nearly all nucleated cells, always in association with a small protein called β_2-microglobulin. There are three class I loci in humans (*A, B,* and *C*) and two in mice (*K* and *D*). Each of the class I MHC loci has a large number of different *alleles,* that is, different forms of the same gene. A person inherits one allele from each parent for each locus and therefore expresses multiple class I MHC molecules on each of his or her nucleated cells. Class II MHC molecules are glycoproteins expressed by the various specialized cells that function as antigen-presenting cells. There are three class II loci in humans (*DR, DP,* and *DQ*) and two in mice (*IA* and *IE*). Each class II locus has two genes, an α gene and a β gene, which respectively encode the α and β chains of the class II MHC molecule. As in the case of the class I MHC, there are a large number of different alleles for each class II locus. Because a person inherits one allele from each parent for each locus, the surface of the antigen-presenting cell has multiple class II MHC molecules.

MHC molecules also function as antigen-recognition molecules, but unlike the B- and T-cell antigen-binding receptors, MHC molecules do not possess fine specificity for antigen; instead, MHC molecules bind to a broader spectrum of molecules than do antibodies and T-cell receptors. In both class I and class II MHC molecules the distal region (farthest from the membrane) of different alleles display wide variation in their amino acid sequences. These distal regions form a cleft within which the antigen sits. With the antigen thus bound, class I and class II MHC molecules present the foreign antigen to T lymphocytes. Because the structure of the antigen-binding cleft is determined by differences in the allelic form of the genes encoding class I and class II molecules, the ability to present an antigen to T lymphocytes is influenced by the particular set of alleles that an individual inherits.

Processing and Presentation of Antigens

In order for a foreign protein antigen to be recognized by a T cell it must be degraded into small peptides that form physical complexes with a class I or class II MHC molecule. This conversion of proteins into MHC-associated peptide fragments is called *antigen processing.* Whether an antigen will be processed and presented together with class I MHC or class II MHC molecules

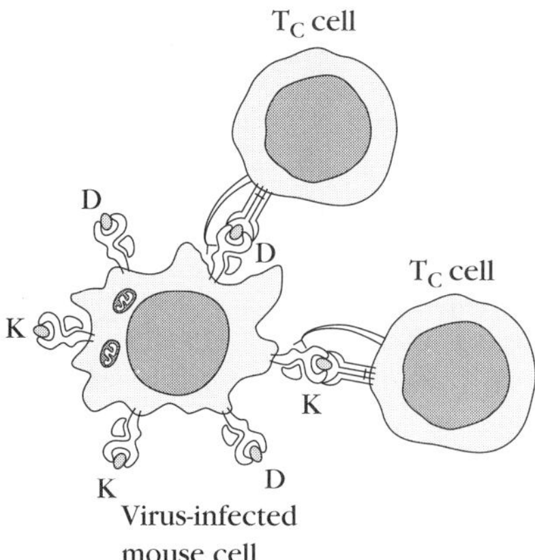

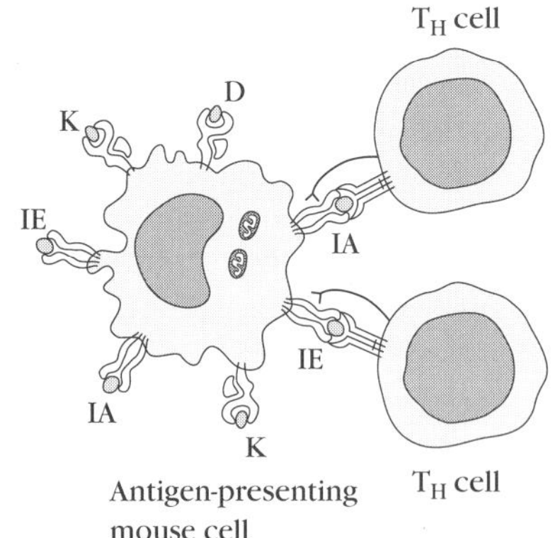

FIGURE 1-9 Role of MHC molecules in antigen recognition by T cells. Class I MHC molecules are encoded by the *K* and *D* loci in mice (*A, B,* and *C* loci in humans) and are expressed on nearly all nucleated cells. Class II MHC molecules are encoded by the *IA* and *IE* loci in mice (*DP, DQ,* and *DR* loci in humans) and are expressed only on antigen-presenting cells. $CD4^+$ T cells only recognize antigen displayed with a class II MHC molecule; they generally function as T helper (T_H) cells. $CD8^+$ T cells only recognize antigen displayed with a class I MHC molecule; they generally function as T cytotoxic (T_C) cells.

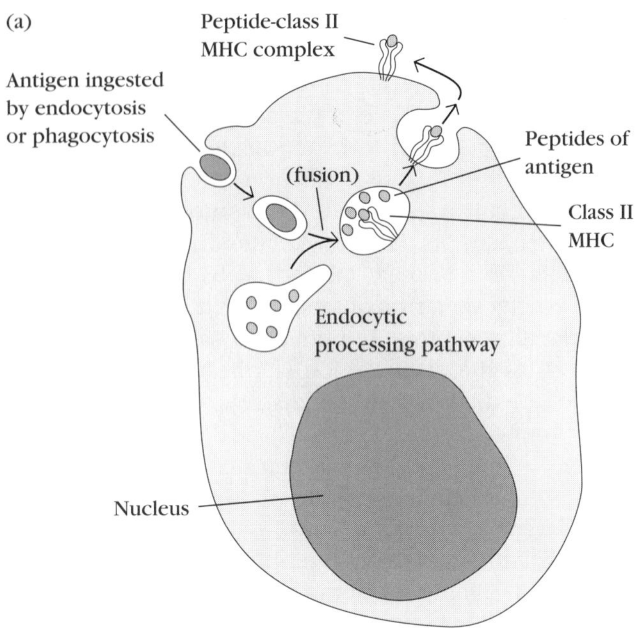

FIGURE 1-10 Processing and presentation of exogenous and endogenous antigens. (a) Exogenous antigen is ingested by endocytosis or phagocytosis and then enters the endocytic processing pathway. Here, within an acidic environment, the antigen is degraded into small peptides, which then are presented with class II MHC molecules on the membrane of the antigen-presenting cell. (b) Endogenous antigen, which is produced within the cell itself (e.g., in a virus-infected cell), is processed within the cytoplasm and presented with class I MHC molecules.

appears to be determined by the route that the antigen takes to enter a cell (Figure 1-10).

Exogenous antigen is produced outside of the host cell and enters the cell by endocytosis or phagocytosis. Antigen-presenting cells, such as macrophages and B cells, process the exogenous antigen into peptide fragments within the endocytic processing pathway. Experiments suggest that class II MHC molecules are expressed within the endocytic processing pathway and that peptides produced during antigen processing bind to the cleft within the class II MHC molecule. The MHC molecule bearing the peptide is then exported to the cell surface. Since class II MHC expression is limited to antigen-presenting cells, expression of exogenous peptide–class II MHC complexes is limited to these cells. T cells displaying CD4 only recognize antigen associated with class II MHC molecules and thus are said to be *class II MHC restricted.* These cells generally function as T helper cells.

Endogenous antigen is produced within the host cell itself. Two common examples are viral proteins synthesized within virus-infected host cells and unique proteins synthesized by cancerous cells. Endogenous antigens are thought to be degraded into peptide fragments that bind to class I MHC molecules within the endoplasmic reticulum. The peptide–class I MHC complex is then transported to the cell membrane. Since all nucleated cells express class I MHC molecules, all cells producing endogenous antigen use this route to process the antigen. T cells displaying CD8 only recognize antigen associated with class I MHC molecules and thus are said to be *class I MHC restricted.* These cells generally function as T cytotoxic cells.

Clonal Selection of Lymphocytes

A mature immunocompetent animal contains a large number of antigen-reactive clones of T and B lymphocytes; the specificity of each of these clones is determined by the specificity of the antigen-binding receptor on the membrane of the clone's lymphocytes. *The specificity of each T and B lymphocyte is determined prior to its contact with antigen* by random gene rearrangements in the bone marrow during maturation of lymphocytes. The role of antigen becomes critical when it interacts with and activates mature, antigenically committed T and B cells, bringing about the expansion of the population of cells with a given antigenic specificity. In this process of *clonal selection,* an antigen binds to and stimulates a particular cell to undergo mitosis and develop into a clone of cells with the same antigenic specificity as the original parent cell (Figure 1-11).

Clonal selection provides a framework for understanding three aspects of acquired immunity: specificity, memory, and self/nonself recognition. Specificity is shown because only lymphocytes whose receptors are specific for a given epitope on an antigen will be clonally expanded and thus mobilized for an immune response. Memory is displayed by the larger number of antigen-reactive lymphocytes present after clonal selection. Many of these lymphocytes appear to have a longer life span and are referred to as memory cells. The initial encounter of an antigen-specific lymphocyte with an antigen induces a *primary response;* a second contact with antigen will induce a more rapid and heightened *secondary response* (Figure 1-12). The amplified memory-cell population accounts for the more rapid and intense response that characterizes a secondary response and distinguishes it from the initial primary response. Self/nonself discrimination is accomplished by the clonal elimination, during development, of lymphocytes bearing self-reactive receptors or by the functional suppression of these cells in adults.

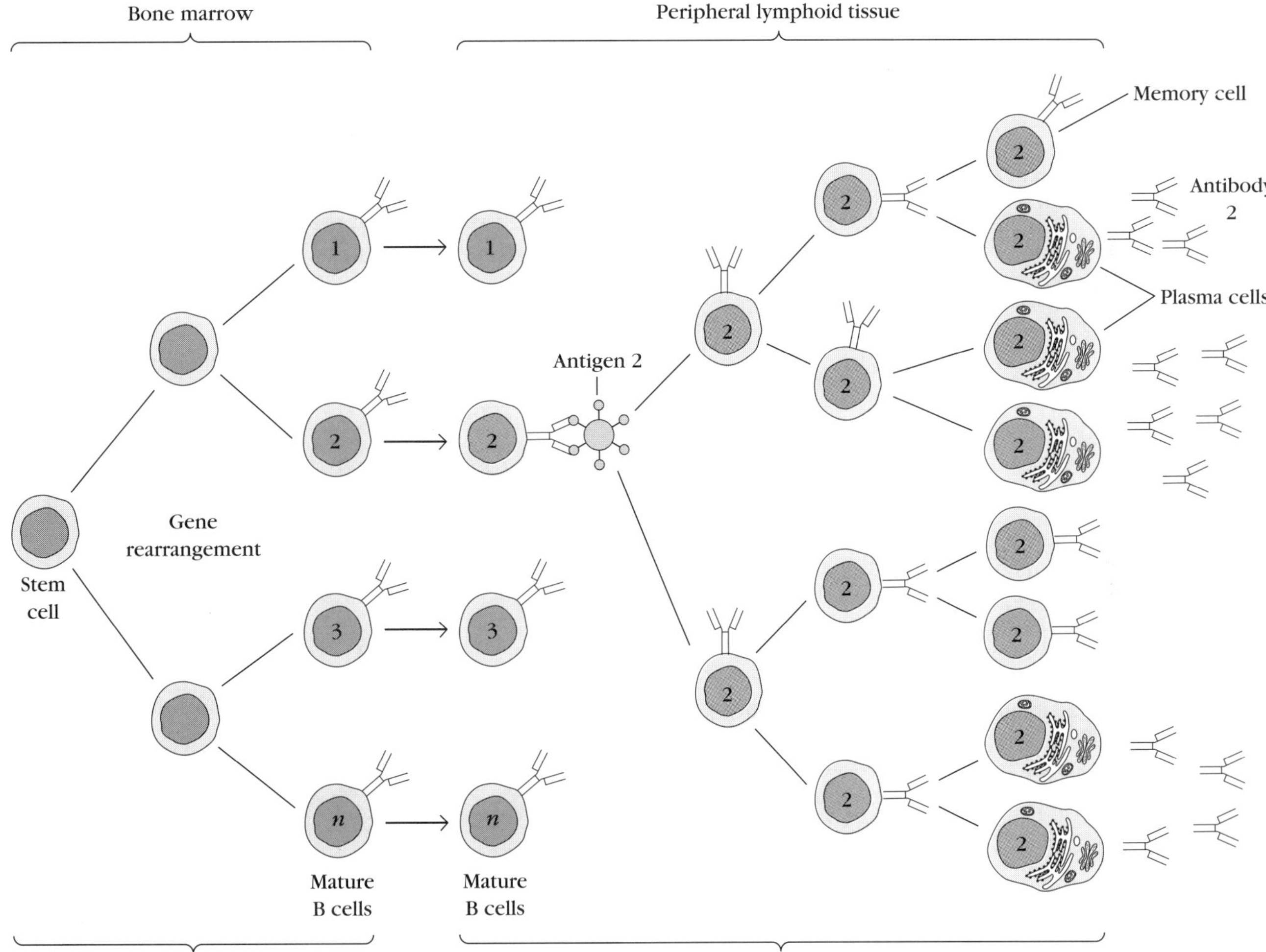

FIGURE 1-11 Maturation and clonal selection of B lymphocytes. Maturation, which occurs in the absence of antigen, produces antigenically committed B cells, each of which expresses antibody with a single antigenic specificity (indicated by 1, 2, 3, and *n*). Clonal selection occurs when a given antigen binds to a B cell whose membrane-bound antibody molecules are specific for epitopes on that antigen. Clonal expansion of the selected antigen-reactive B cells leads to a clone of memory B cells and effector cells, called plasma cells; all cells in the expanded clone are specific for the original antigen. The plasma cells secrete antibody reactive with the activating antigen. Similar processes occur in the T-lymphocyte population resulting in clones of T memory and effector cells; the latter include activated T_H cells, which secrete cytokines, and cytotoxic T lymphocytes (CTL).

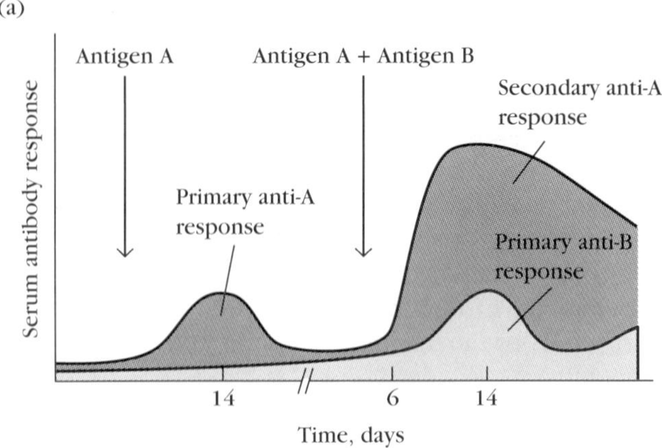

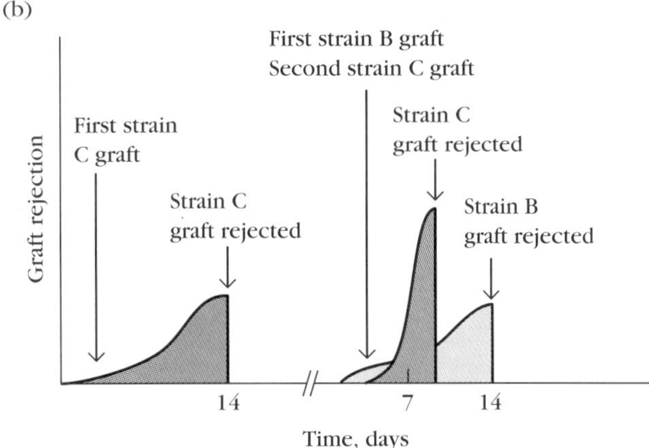

FIGURE 1-12 Differences in the primary and secondary response to injected antigen (humoral response) and to a skin graft (cell-mediated response) reflect the phenomenon of immunologic memory. (a) When an animal is injected with an antigen, it produces a primary serum antibody response of low magnitude and relatively short duration, peaking at about 10–17 days. A second immunization with the same antigen results in a secondary response that is greater in magnitude, peaks in less time (2–7 days), and lasts longer (months to years) than the primary response. (b) When skin from a strain C mouse is grafted onto a strain A mouse, the graft is rejected in about 10–14 days. If a second strain C graft is grafted onto the same mouse, it is rejected much more vigorously and rapidly than the first graft.

Clonal selection occurs within both the humoral and cell-mediated branches of the immune system. In the humoral branch, antigen induces the clonal proliferation of B lymphocytes into antibody-secreting plasma cells and B memory cells (see Figure 1-11). In the cell-mediated branch, the recognition of an antigen-MHC complex by a specific T lymphocyte induces clonal proliferation into various T cells with effector functions, such as T_H cells and CTLs, and into T memory cells.

Cellular Interactions Required for Generation of Immune Responses

Both the humoral and the cell-mediated branches of the immune system require interaction among several different types of cells to induce a specific immunologic response. These cells include various antigen-presenting cells, T_H cells, and either B cells for induction of humoral immunity or T_C cells for induction of cell-mediated immunity. Both branches require that antigen be processed and presented with a class II MHC molecule on the membrane of appropriate antigen-presenting cells.

Activation and Proliferation of T Helper Cells

The generation of both humoral and cell-mediated immune responses depends on the activation of T_H cells. This process begins when antigen receptors on T_H cells interact with antigenic peptide–class II MHC complexes on antigen-presenting cells (Figure 1-13). This interaction generates a signal that, together with a necessary co-stimulatory signal, leads to activation of

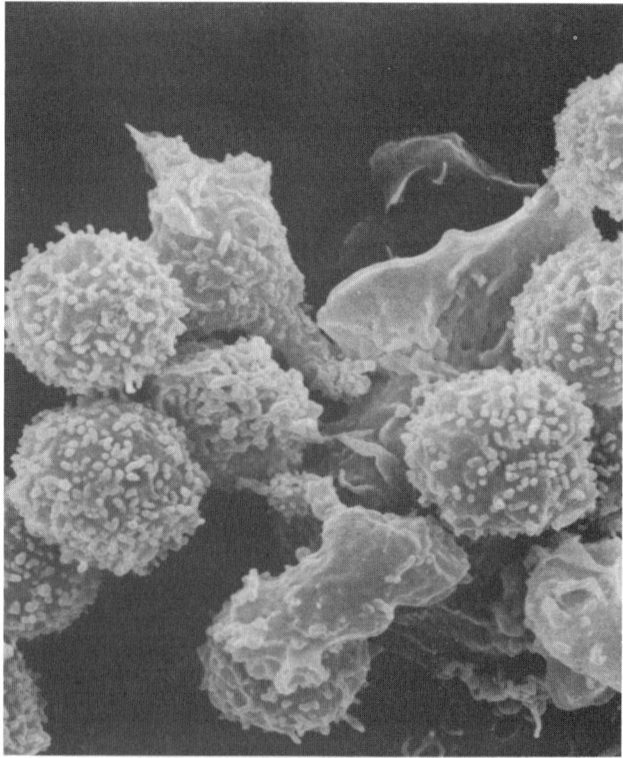

FIGURE 1-13 Scanning electron micrograph reveals numerous T lymphocytes interacting with a single macrophage. The macrophage presents processed antigen associated with class II MHC molecules to the T cells. [From William E. Paul (ed.), 1991, *Immunology: Recognition and Response,* W. H. Freeman and Company, New York; courtesy of Morten H. Nielsen and Ole Werdelin.]

the genes encoding interleukin 2 (IL-2) and the high-affinity receptor for IL-2. The secreted IL-2 then binds to the newly expressed receptor and autostimulates T_H-cell proliferation (Figure 1-14a). The clonally expanded population of antigen-specific T_H cells can now play a role in the activation of the B and T lymphocytes that generate the humoral and cell-mediated responses, respectively.

Generation of the Humoral Response

Mature antigen-committed B lymphocytes are seeded out from the bone marrow to circulate in the blood or lymph or to reside in various lymphoid organs. A mature B cell lives for only a few days unless it interacts with antigen, triggering its activation and further proliferation and differentiation. This process begins when antigen cross-links membrane-bound antibody molecules on a B cell and the B cell interacts with an antigen-specific T_H cell. The interaction with antigen-specific T_H cells is facilitated by the B cell itself, which internalizes some antigen bound to its surface antibody. After processing the antigen, the B cell presents it together with a class II MHC molecule on its membrane. The antigen-specific T_H cell binds to this antigen-MHC complex and thereupon secretes a number of cytokines, including interleukin 2 (IL-2), interleukin 4 (IL-4), interleukin 5 (IL-5), interleukin 6 (IL-6), and interferon gamma (IFN-γ), which serve to stimulate various stages of B-cell division and differentiation. Interleukin 1 (IL-1) secreted by macrophages also acts as a growth factor for the B lymphocyte. The activated B lymphocyte undergoes a series of cell divisions over approximately a 5-day period differentiating

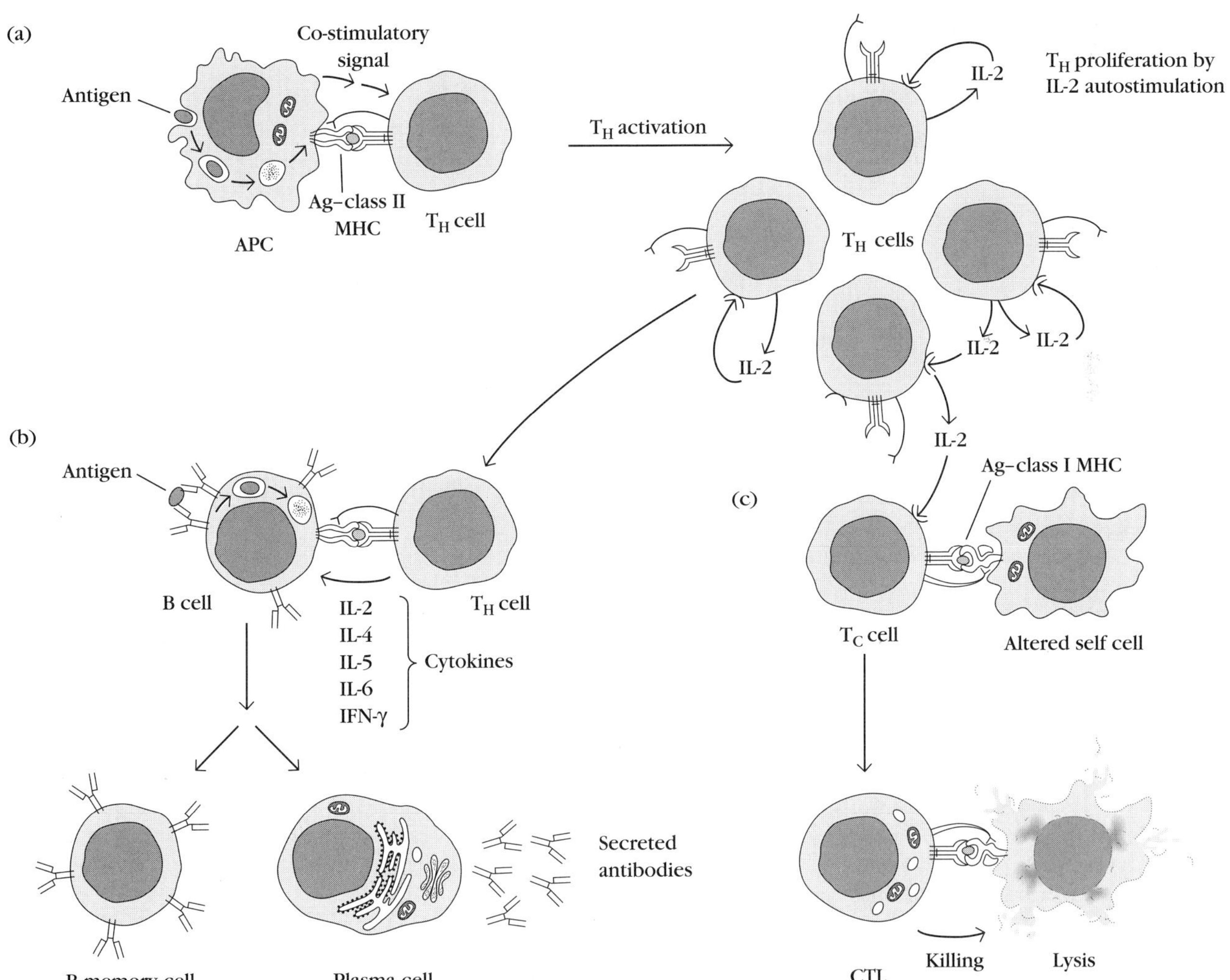

FIGURE 1-14 Cellular interactions involved in induction of immune responses. Activation and proliferation of T_H cells (a) is required for generation of a humoral response (b) and a cell-mediated response to altered self-cells (c). APC = antigen-presenting cell; Ag = antigen. See text for discussion.

into a population of both antibody-secreting plasma cells and memory cells (Figure 1-14b).

Generation of the Cell-Mediated Response

The cell-mediated response is generated by various subpopulations of T lymphocytes. As in the case of the humoral response, a clonally expanded population of antigen-specific activated T_H cells is required. These T_H cells serve to activate various T effector cells that generate cell-mediated responses. The T_C cell, for example, recognizes processed antigen associated with class I MHC molecules on the membrane of self-cells. In the presence of IL-2 secreted by the T_H cell, the T_C cell becomes a cytotoxic T lymphocyte (CTL), which mediates membrane damage to the altered self-cell leading to cell lysis (Figure 1-14c).

The cytokines secreted by activated T_H cells also regulate the proliferation and differentiation of a number of nonspecific effector cells that play various roles in cell-mediated immune responses. These nonspecific effector cells do not possess the immunologic attributes of specificity and memory, and so the regulation of their activity depends on the activity of the antigen-specific T_H cell. Various cytokines, such as interleukin 2 and interferon gamma, have been shown to activate macrophages, for example. These *activated macrophages* exhibit enhanced phagocytic activity and enhanced ability to kill ingested pathogens. In addition, activated macrophages have been shown to be capable of killing certain tumor cells and cells infected by parasites. The *natural killer (NK) cell* is another nonspecific effector cell whose activity is enhanced by interleukin 2 and interferon gamma produced by activated T_H cells. The NK cell is a large, granular lymphocyte that lacks the membrane markers of the T- and the B-cell lineages. NK cells have been shown to kill tumor cells; however, how these cells recognize a tumor cell is unclear, given that they lack the specific antigen-binding receptors of either B or T cells.

In some cases antibody molecules produced during the humoral response can influence the cell-mediated response to a foreign cell. Both macrophages and some NK cells, for example, have membrane receptors that can bind the carboxyl-terminal end of an antibody molecule. The amino-terminal end of an antibody molecule contains the antigen-binding site. Thus, an antibody may bind both to a foreign cell and to NK cells or macrophages, forming a bridge that allows these cells to interact with the foreign cell. In this process, referred to as *antibody-dependent cell-mediated cytotoxicity (ADCC),* antibody provides the specificity, but killing is mediated by the nonspecific macrophage or NK cell.

References

ADA, G. L., and G. NOSSAL. 1987. The clonal selection theory. *Sci. Am.* **257**(2):62.

GREY, H. M., A. SETTE, and S. BUUS. 1989. How T cells see antigen. *Sci. Am.* **261**(5):56.

MARRACK, P., and J. KAPPLER. 1986. The T cell and its receptor. *Sci. Am.* **254**(2):36.

Readings from Scientific American Magazine. 1994. Life, Death and the Immune System. W. H. Freeman and Company.

TONEGAWA, S. 1985. The molecules of the immune system. *Sci. Am.* **253**(4):122.

Study Questions

1. Indicate to which branch(es) of the immune system the following statements apply using H for the humoral branch and CM for the cell-mediated branch. Some statements may apply to both branches.
   a. _____ Involves class I MHC molecules
   b. _____ Most likely responds to viral infection
   c. _____ Involves T helper cells
   d. _____ Involves processed antigen
   e. _____ Most likely responds following an organ transplant
   f. _____ Involves T cytotoxic cells
   g. _____ Involves B cells
   h. _____ Involves $CD8^+$ cells
   i. _____ Most likely responds to bacterial infection
   j. _____ Involves secreted antibody

2. Name three features of a secondary immune response that make it different from a primary immune response.

3. How does clonal selection contribute to memory in the immune response?

4. Interleukin 2 is a nonspecific growth factor that stimulates growth of T_H cells during the immune response. In view of this nonspecificity of IL-2, what mechanism assures that only those T_H cells specific for a given antigen proliferate and that all other T_H cells do not proliferate.

5. Compare and contrast the four antigen-binding molecules utilized by the immune system—antibody, T-cell receptor, class I MHC molecule, and class I MHC molecule—in terms of the following characteristics:
   a. Specificity for antigen
   b. Cellular expression
   c. Types of antigen recognized

6. Antigen-presenting cells play a role in both humoral and cell-mediated immune responses.
   a. Name three types of antigen-presenting cells.
   b. Which class of MHC molecules are expressed on the membrane of antigen-presenting cells?
   c. Which lymphocytes interact with antigen-presenting cells?

7. The $CD8^+$ T cell is said to be class I restricted. What does this mean?

8. Match each term related to innate immunity (a–p) with the most appropriate description listed below (1–19). Each description may be used once, more than once, or not at all.
   a. _____ Fimbriae or pili
   b. _____ Exudate
   c. _____ Sebum
   d. _____ Margination
   e. _____ Dermis
   f. _____ Lysosome
   g. _____ Histamine
   h. _____ Macrophage
   i. _____ Lysozyme
   j. _____ Bradykinin
   k. _____ Interferon
   l. _____ Edema
   m. _____ Complement
   n. _____ Extravasation
   o. _____ C-reactive protein
   p. _____ Phagosome

1. Thin outer layer of skin
2. Layer of skin containing blood vessels and sebaceous glands
3. One of several acute-phase proteins
4. Hydrolytic enzyme found in mucous secretions
5. Migration of a phagocyte through the endothelial wall into the tissues
6. Acidic antibacterial secretion found in the skin
7. Has antiviral activity
8. Induces vasodilation
9. Accumulation of an exudate resulting in swelling
10. Large vesicle containing ingested particulate material
11. Accumulation of dead cells, digested material, and fluid
12. Adherence of phagocytic cells to the endothelial wall
13. Structures involved in microbial adherence to mucous membranes
14. Stimulates pain receptors in the skin
15. Phagocytic cell found in the tissues
16. Phagocytic cell found in the blood
17. Group of serum proteins involved in cell lysis and clearance of antigen
18. Cytoplasmic vesicle containing degradative enzymes
19. Protein-rich fluid that leaks from the capillaries into the tissue

EXPERIMENTAL SYSTEMS

Experimental systems of various types are used to unravel the complex cellular interactions involved in the immune response. The choice of experimental system influences the kinds of data that can be generated and places certain limitations on the interpretation of those data. In vivo systems, which involve the whole animal, provide the most natural experimental conditions. However, due to their complexity, in vivo systems have a myriad of unknown and uncontrollable cellular interactions that add ambiguity to the interpretation of data. At the other extreme are in vitro systems in which defined populations of lymphocytes are studied under controlled and consequently repeatable conditions; in vitro systems can be simplified to the extent that individual cellular interactions can be studied effectively. Yet in vitro systems have their own limitations, the most notable of which is their artificiality. One must ask whether a cellular response observed in vitro reflects reality or is a product of the unique conditions generated by the in vitro system itself.

In this chapter some of the experimental systems routinely used by immunologists to study the immune system are described. The chapter also includes a discussion of some recombinant DNA techniques that have revolutionized the study of the immune system in the past decade or so.

Experimental Animal Models

The study of the immune system in vertebrates requires suitable animal models. The choice of an animal depends on its suitability for attaining a particular research goal. If large amounts of antiserum are sought, a rabbit, goat, sheep, or horse might be an appropriate experimental animal. If the goal is development of a protective vaccine, the animal chosen must be susceptible to the infectious agent so that the efficacy of the vaccine can be assessed. In many cases mice or rabbits will serve for vaccine development, but if growth of the infectious agent is limited to humans and primates, vaccine development may require the use of monkeys, chimpanzees, or baboons. The use of primates for research purposes must be carefully regulated to ensure that each species is protected from extinction.

For most basic research in immunology, mice have been the experimental animal of choice. They are easy to handle, are genetically well characterized, and have a rapid breeding cycle. The immune system of the mouse has been characterized more extensively than that of any other species. The value of basic research in the mouse system is highlighted by the enormous impact this research has had on clinical intervention in human disease.

Inbred Strains

To control experimental variation caused by differences in the genetic backgrounds of experimental

Table 2-1 Some inbred mouse strains commonly used in immunology

Strain	Common substrains	Characteristics
A	A/He A/J A/WySn	High incidence of mammary tumors in some substrains
AKR	AKR/J AKR/N AKR/Cum	High incidence of leukemia Thy 1.2 allele in AKR/Cum, and Thy 1.1 allele in other substrains (this gene encodes a T-cell surface protein)
BALB/c	BALB/c*j* BALB/c AnN BALB/cB*y*	Sensitivity to radiation Used in hybridoma technology
CBA	CBA/J CBA/H CBA/N	Gene *(rd)* causing retinal degeneration in CBA/J Gene *(xid)* causing X-linked immunodeficiency in CBA/N
C3H	C3H/He C3H/HeJ C3H/HeN	Gene *(rd)* causing retinal degeneration High incidence of mammary tumors in many substrains (these carry a mammary-tumor virus that is passed via maternal milk to offspring)
C57BL/6	C57BL/6J C57BL/6By C57BL/6N	High incidence of hepatomas after irradiation High complement activity
C57BL/10	C57BL/10J C57BL/10ScSn C57BL/10N	Very close relationship to C57BL/6 but differences in at least two loci Frequent partner in preparation of congenic mice
C57BR	C57BR/cd*j*	High frequency of pituitary and liver tumors Very resistant to x-irradiation

animals, immunologists often work with *inbred strains*—that is, genetically identical animals produced by inbreeding. The rapid breeding cycle of mice makes them particularly well suited for the production of inbred strains, which are developed by repeated inbreeding between brother and sister littermates. In this way the heterozygosity of alleles that is normally found in randomly outbred mice is replaced by homozygosity at all loci. Repeated inbreeding for 20 generations usually yields an inbred strain whose progeny are homozygous at more than 98% of all loci. More than 150 different inbred strains of mice are available; these are designated by a series of letters and/or numbers (Table 2-1). Most of these strains are purchased by immunologists from such suppliers as Jackson Laboratory in Bar Harbor, Maine. Inbred strains have also been produced in rats, guinea pigs, hamsters, rabbits, and domestic fowl.

Because inbred animals are genetically identical *(syngeneic),* their immune responses can be studied in the absence of variables introduced by genetic differences among individual animals. Inbred strains are invaluable in the study of immunology. With inbred strains, lymphocyte subpopulations isolated from one animal can be injected into another animal of the same strain without eliciting a rejection reaction. This type of experimental system permitted immunologists to first demonstrate that lymphocytes from an antigen-primed animal could transfer immunity to an unprimed syngeneic recipient.

TABLE 2-1 (CONTINUED) SOME INBRED MOUSE STRAINS COMMONLY USED IN IMMUNOLOGY

Strain	Common substrains	Characteristics
C57L	C57L/J C57L/N	Susceptibility to experimental autoimmune encephalomyelitis (EAE) High frequency of pituitary and reticular-cell tumors
C58	C58/J C58/LwN	High incidence of leukemia
DBA/1	DBA/1J DBA/1N	High level of activity High incidence of mammary tumors
DBA/2	DBA/2J DBA/2N	High level of activity Low response to pneumococcal polysaccharide type II
HRS	HRS/J	Hairless *(hr)* gene, usually in heterozygous state
NZB	NZB/BINJ NZB/N	High incidence of autoimmune hemolytic anemia and lupus-like nephritis Autoimmune disease similar to systemic lupus erythematosus (SLE) in F_1 progeny from crosses with NZW
NZW	NZW/N	SLE-type autoimmune disease in F_1 progeny from crosses with NZB
P	P/J	High incidence of leukemia
SJL	SJL/J	High level of aggression and severe fighting to the point of death, especially in males Tendency to develop certain autoimmune diseases
SWR	SWR/J	Tendency to develop several autoimmune diseases
129	129/J 129/SvJ	High incidence of spontaneous teratocarcinoma

SOURCE: Adapted from Federation of American Societies for Experimental Biology, 1979, *Biological Handbooks,* Vol. III: Inbred and Genetically Defined Strains of Laboratory Animals.

Adoptive-Transfer Systems

In some cases it is important to eliminate the immune responsiveness of the syngeneic host so that the response of only the transferred lymphocytes can be studied in isolation. In adoptive-transfer systems the immune cells of the syngeneic recipient are inactivated by exposing the host to x-rays. Subjecting a mouse that will serve as host to sublethal doses of x-rays (650–750 rads) can kill 99.99% of its lymphocytes, after which the lymphocytes from the spleen of a syngeneic donor can be studied without interference from host lymphocytes. If the host's hematopoietic cells might influence an adoptive-transfer experiment, then higher x-ray levels (900–1000 rads) are used to eliminate the entire hematopoietic system. Mice irradiated with such doses will die unless reconstituted with bone marrow from a syngeneic donor.

The adoptive-transfer system has enabled immunologists to study the development of injected lymphoid stem cells in various organs of the recipient. Adoptive-transfer experiments have also facilitated the study of various populations of lymphocytes and of the cellular interactions required to generate an immune response. For example, it was through such experiments that immunologists were first able to show that a T helper cell is necessary for B-cell activation in the humoral response.

Scid Mice and *Scid*-Human Mice

An autosomal recessive mutation resulting in severe combined immunodeficiency disease (scid) developed spontaneously in a strain of mice called CB-17. These CB-17 *scid* mice fail to develop mature T and B cells and consequently are severely compromised immunologically. The mechanism of the defect in these mice has been determined and is discussed in Chapter 8. *Scid* mice must be housed in a sterile (germfree) environment if they are to survive, since they cannot fight off microorganisms of even low pathogenicity. The absence of functional T and B cells enables these mice to accept foreign cells and grafts from other strains of mice or even from other species. Apart from their lack of functional T and B cells, *scid* mice appear to be normal in all respects. When normal bone marrow cells are injected into *scid* mice, normal T and B cells develop, and the mice are cured of their immunodeficiency. This finding has made *scid* mice a valuable model system for the study of immunodeficiency and the process of differentiation of bone-marrow stem cells into mature T or B cells.

Interest in *scid* mice has mushroomed recently with the development of a new way to utilize them to study the human immune system. Implantation in *scid* mice of portions of human fetal liver, thymus, and lymph nodes causes the mice to become populated with mature human T and B lymphocytes (Figure 2-1). Because the mice lack mature T and B cells of their own, they do not reject the transplanted human tissue. The fetal liver contains immature human blood cells, including lymphocytes, and these immature cells mature into T and B cells within the human tissue implants. Because the human lymphocytes are exposed to mouse antigens while they are still immature, they later recognize mouse cells as self and do not mount an immunologic response against the mouse host. The beauty of this system is that it enables one to study human lymphocytes within an animal model. As will become apparent in later chapters, the *scid*-human mouse has become a valuable animal model that has been used to study development of various lymphoid cells and has also served as an important animal model in AIDS research. There are, however, important ethical considerations that must be addressed concerning the use of human fetal tissue in research.

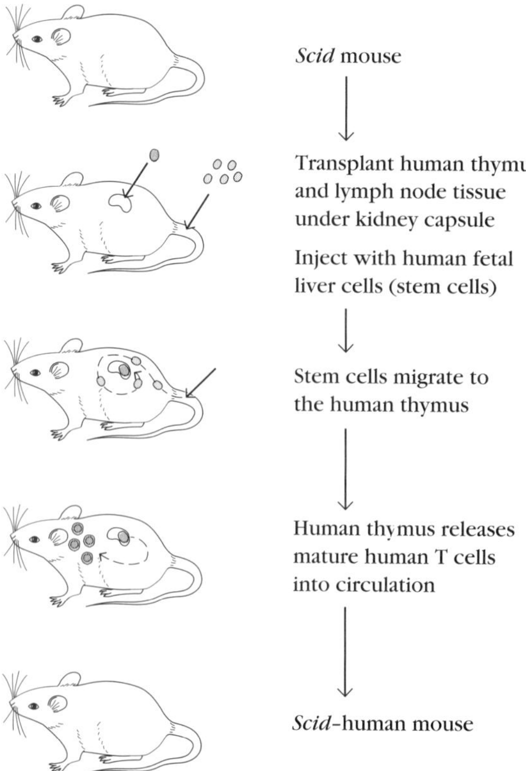

FIGURE 2-1 Production of *scid*-human mouse. This system permits study of human lymphocytes within an animal model.

Cell-Culture Systems

The complexity of the cellular interactions that generate an immune response has led immunologists to rely heavily on various types of in vitro cell-culture systems. A variety of cells can be cultured including primary lymphoid cells, cloned lymphoid cell lines, and hybrid cells.

Primary Lymphoid Cell Cultures

Primary lymphoid cell cultures can be obtained by isolating lymphocytes directly from blood or lymph or from various lymphoid organs by tissue dispersion. The lymphocytes can then be grown in a chemically defined basal medium (containing saline, sugars, amino acids, vitamins, trace elements, and other nutrients) to which various serum supplements are added. For some experiments serum-free culture conditions are employed. Because in vitro culture techniques require from 10- to 100-fold fewer lymphocytes than typical in vivo techniques, they have enabled immunologists to assess the functional properties of minor subpopulations of lymphocytes. It was by means of cell-culture techniques, for example, that immunologists were first able to define the functional differences between $CD4^+$ T helper cells and $CD8^+$ T cytotoxic cells.

Cell-culture techniques have also been used to identify various cytokines involved in the activation, growth, and differentiation of various cells involved in the immune response. Early experiments showed that media conditioned by the growth of various lymphocytes or antigen-presenting cells would support the growth of other lymphoid cells. Many of the individual cytokines that characterized various conditioned media have subsequently been identified and purified, and in many cases the genes encoding them have been cloned. The soluble growth factors elaborated by monocytes and macrophages are called *monokines,* and the ones elaborated by lymphocytes are called *lymphokines.* These cytokines, which play a central role in the activation and regulation of the immune response, are discussed more fully in Chapter 13.

Cloned Lymphoid Cell Lines

Primary lymphoid cell cultures comprise a heterogeneous group of cells that can be propagated only for a limited time. This heterogeneity complicates interpretation of experiments aimed at understanding the molecular and cellular mechanisms by which lymphocytes generate an immune response. To avoid these problems immunologists use cloned lymphoid cell lines and hybrid cells.

Normal mammalian cells generally have a finite life span in culture; that is, after a number of population doublings characteristic of the species and cell type, the cells stop dividing. Tumor cells or normal cells transformed with chemical carcinogens or viruses, however, can be propagated indefinitely in tissue culture (they are said to be immortal). Such cells are referred to as *cell lines.* The first cell line—the mouse fibroblast L cell—was derived in the 1940s from cultured mouse subcutaneous connective tissue by exposing the cultured cells to a chemical carcinogen, methylcholanthrene, over a 4-month period. In the 1950s another important cell line, the HeLa cell, was derived by culturing human cervical cancer cells. Since these early studies, hundreds of cell lines have been established. Various techniques can be used to ensure that a cell line is derived from a single parent cell. Such a cloned cell line consists of a population of genetically identical cells that can be grown indefinitely in culture.

A variety of cell lines are used in immunologic research. Table 2-2 lists some of these lines and describes some of the properties of the cells. (Many of the properties described will not have meaning for the reader at this stage, but later chapters refer to some of these lines, so the table can serve as a helpful summary.) Some of these cell lines were derived from spontaneously occurring tumors of lymphocytes, macrophages, or other accessory cells involved in the immune response. In other cases the cell line was induced by transformation of normal lymphoid cells with viruses such as Abelson's murine leukemia virus (A-MLV), simian virus 40 (SV40), Epstein-Barr virus (EBV), and human T-cell leukemia virus (HTLV-1). The lymphoid cell lines differ from primary lymphoid cell cultures in several important ways: They survive indefinitely in tissue culture, they show various abnormal growth properties, and they often have an abnormal number of chromosomes. Cells with more or less than the normal diploid number of chromosomes for a species are said to be *aneuploid.* The big advantage of cloned lymphoid cell lines is that they can be grown for extended periods in tissue culture, enabling immunologists to obtain large numbers of homogeneous cells in culture.

Until the late 1970s immunologists had not succeeded in maintaining normal T cells in tissue culture for extended periods. In 1978 a serendipitous finding led to the observation that conditioned medium containing a T-cell growth factor was required. The essential component of the conditioned medium turned out to be interleukin 2 (IL-2). By culturing normal T lymphocytes with antigen in the presence of IL-2, clones of antigen-specific T lymphocytes could be isolated.

TABLE 2-2 CELL LINES COMMONLY USED IN IMMUNOLOGIC RESEARCH

Cell line	Description
L-929	Mouse fibroblast cell line; often is used in DNA transfection studies and to assay tumor necrosis factor (TNF)
SP2/0	Nonsecreting mouse myeloma; often is used as a fusion partner for hybridoma secretion
P3X63-Ag8.653	Nonsecreting mouse myeloma; often is used as a fusion partner for hybridoma secretion
MPC 11	Mouse IgG2a-secreting myeloma
P3X63 Ag 8	Mouse IgG1-secreting myeloma
MOPC 315	Mouse IgA-secreting myeloma
J558	Mouse IgA-secreting myeloma
ABE-8.1/2	Mouse pre-B cell lymphoma
7OZ/3	Mouse pre-B lymphoma; used to study early events in B-cell differentiation
BCL 1	Mouse B-cell lymphoma that expresses membrane IgM and IgD and can be activated with mitogen to secrete IgM
LBRM-33	Mouse T-cell lymphoma that secretes high levels of IL-2 after mitogen activation
CTLL-2	Mouse T-cell line whose growth is dependent on IL-2; often is used to assay IL-2 production
C6VL	Mouse thymoma expressing CD3 and CD4
PU 5-1.8	Mouse monocyte-macrophage line
P338 D1	Mouse monocyte-macrophage line that secretes high levels of IL-1
WEHI 265.1	Mouse monocyte line
P815	Mouse mastocytoma cells; often is used as target to assess killing by cytotoxic T lymphocytes (CTLs)
YAC-1	Mouse lymphoma cells; often is used as target for NK cells
COS-1	African green monkey kidney cells transformed by SV40; often is used in DNA transfection studies

These individual clones could be propagated and studied in culture and even frozen for storage. After thawing, the clones continued to grow and express their original antigen-specific functions.

By using cloned lymphoid cell lines immunologists have been able to study a number of events that would have been impossible to examine without large numbers of homogeneous cells. For example, the study of the molecular events involved in lymphocyte activation by antigen was hampered by the low frequency of antigen-specific B and T lymphocytes because molecular changes occurring in one responding cell could not be detected against a background of 10^3-10^6 nonresponding cells. T- and B-cell lines with known antigenic specificity have provided immunologists with clonal populations in which to study the membrane and intracellular events involved in antigen recognition. Similarly, the molecular-level genetic changes corresponding to different maturational stages can be studied in cell lines that appear to be "frozen" at different stages of differentiation. Cell lines have also contributed to understanding of soluble factors produced by lymphoid cells. The value of some cell lines lies in their ability to secrete large quantities of various monokines or lymphokines; other lines have proved to be valuable because they express membrane receptors for particular monokines or lymphokines. These cell lines have been used by immunologists to purify and eventually to clone the genes of various lymphokines and their receptors.

There are, however, a number of limitations with lymphoid cell lines. Variants arise spontaneously in the course of prolonged culture, necessitating frequent subcloning to limit the cellular heterogeneity that can develop. If variants are selected in subcloning, it is possible that two subclones derived from the same parent clone may represent different subpopulations. Moreover, any cell line derived from tumor cells or transformed cells may have unknown genetic contributions characteristic of the tumor or of the transformed state, so that caution is called for when one extrapolates from results obtained with cell lines to the normal situation in vivo. Nevertheless, transformed cell lines have made a major contribution to the study of the immune response, and a number of molecular events discovered in experiments with transformed cell lines have later been shown to take place in normal lymphocytes.

Hybrid Lymphoid Cell Lines

In somatic-cell hybridization, immunologists fuse normal B or T lymphocytes with tumor cells, obtaining a heterokaryon; after random loss of some chromo-

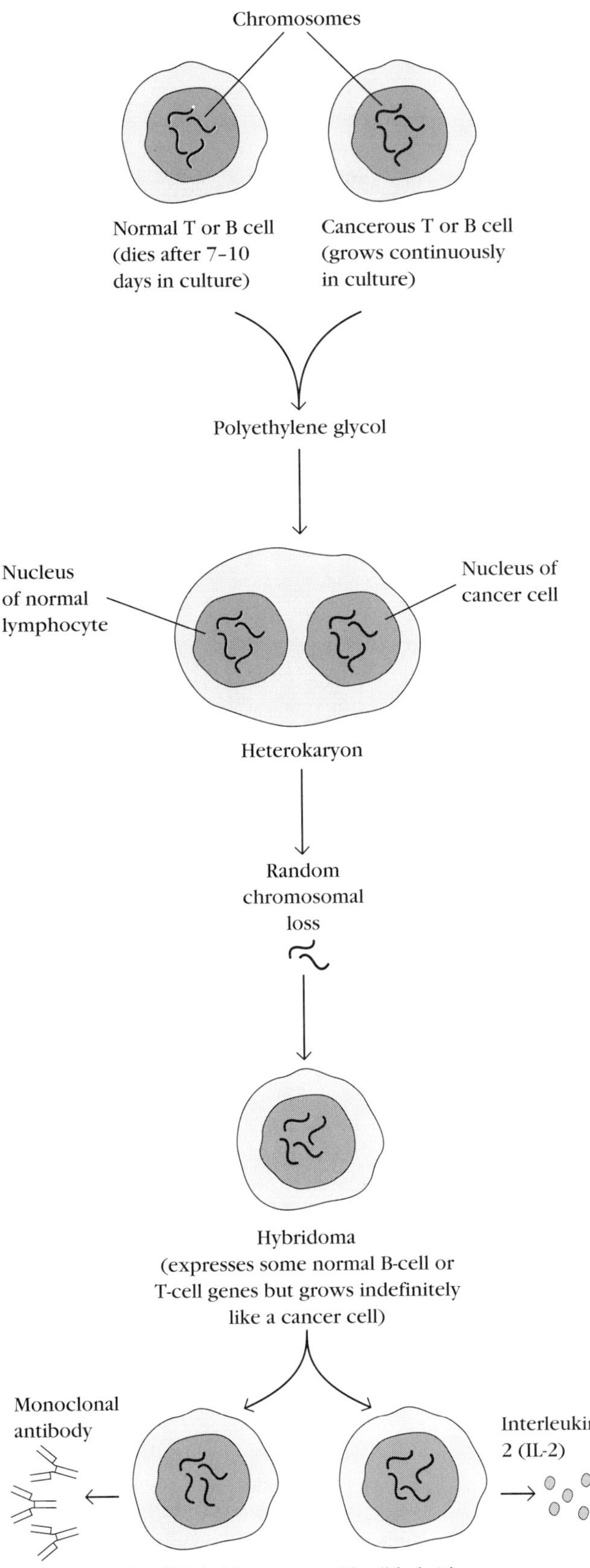

FIGURE 2-2 Production of B-cell or T-cell hybridomas by somatic-cell hybridization. The resulting hybridomas express some of the genes of the fused B or T cell but also exhibit the immortal-growth properties of the tumor cell. This procedure is used to produce B-cell hybridomas secreting monoclonal antibody or T-cell hybridomas secreting various growth factors.

somes, a *hybridoma* is formed containing a single nucleus with chromosomes from each of the fused cells. Historically, cell fusion was promoted with Sendai virus, but now it is generally done with polyethylene glycol. Normal antigen-primed B cells, for example, can be fused with cancerous plasma cells, called myeloma cells (Figure 2-2). The hybridoma thus formed continues to express the antibody genes of the normal B lymphocyte but is capable of unlimited growth, a characteristic of the myeloma cell. Such B-cell hybridomas have revolutionized immunology because hybridoma clones can be propagated that secrete antibody with a single antigenic specificity, called *monoclonal antibody* in reference to its derivation from a single clone. Chapter 7 discusses this process in detail.

T-cell hybridomas can also be obtained by fusing T lymphocytes with cancerous T-cell lymphomas. Again, the resulting hybridoma continues to express the genes of the normal T cell but acquires the immortal-growth properties of the cancerous T lymphoma cell. Immunologists have generated a number of stable hybridoma cell lines representing T helper and T cytotoxic lineages. These T-cell hybridomas have two major disadvantages: (1) The cells tend to be unstable, since they are aneuploid as a result of random chromosome loss and (2) the tumor-cell fusion partner contributes some unknown genetic components to the hybrid cells.

Recombinant DNA Technology

The techniques developed in recombinant DNA technology have had an impact on every area of immunologic research. Genes can be cloned, DNA can be sequenced, and recombinant protein products can be produced, providing immunologists with defined components with which to study the structure and function of the immune system. Some of the recombinant DNA techniques commonly employed in immunologic research are briefly described in this section; many of these techniques are referred to in subsequent chapters.

TABLE 2-3 SOME RESTRICTION ENZYMES AND THEIR RECOGNITION SEQUENCES

Microorganism source	Abbreviation	Sequence* 5′ → 3′ 3′ → 5′
Bacillus amyloliquefaciens H	*Bam*HI	G G A T C C C C T A G G
Escherichia coli RY13	*Eco*RI	G A A T T C C T T A A G
Haemophilus aegyptius	*Hae*III	G G C C C C G G
Haemophilus haemolyticus	*Hha*I	G C G C C G C G
Haemophilus influenzae Rd	*Hin*dIII	A A G C T T T T C G A A
Haemophilus parainfluenzae	*Hpa*I	G T T A A C C A A T T G
Providencia stuartii 164	*Pst*I	C T G C A G G A C G T C

* Purple lines indicate locations of single-strand cuts within the restriction site. Enzymes that make off-center cuts produce fragments with short, single-stranded extensions at their ends.

SOURCE: J. D. Watson et al., 1983, *Recombinant DNA: A Short Course*, W. H. Freeman and Company.

Restriction-Endonuclease Cleavage of DNA

A variety of bacteria produce enzymes, called *restriction endonucleases,* that degrade foreign DNA (e.g., bacteriophage DNA) but spare the bacterial cell DNA, which contains methylated residues. The discovery of these bacterial enzymes in the 1970s opened the way to a major technological advance in the field of molecular biology. Before the discovery of restriction endonucleases, double-stranded DNA (dsDNA) could be cut only with DNases. These enzymes do not recognize defined sites and therefore randomly cleave DNA into a variable series of small fragments, which are impossible to order. In contrast, restriction endonucleases recognize and cleave DNA at specific sites, called *restriction sites,* which are short double-stranded sequences containing four to eight nucleotides (Table 2-3).

A restriction endonuclease cuts both DNA strands at a specific point within its restriction site. Some enzymes, like *Hpa*I, cut on the central axis and thus generate blunt-ended fragments. Other enzymes, such as *Eco*RI, cut the DNA off-center from the central axis of the recognition site, producing staggered cleavage products. These staggered fragments have a short single-stranded DNA extension, called a *sticky end,* extending from one of the strands of the double-stranded fragment. When two DNA molecules are cut with the same restriction enzyme, the sticky ends will be complementary, so that the two molecules can be joined by base pairing to generate a recombinant DNA molecule (Figure 2-3). Several hundred different restriction endonucleases have been isolated and many are available commercially, allowing researchers to purchase enzymes that cut DNA at defined restriction sites.

FIGURE 2-3 Formation of recombinant DNA molecules. A ▶ restriction endonuclease that produces fragments with sticky ends is used to cleave two different DNA molecules (in this case, a circular plasmid DNA and a linear chromosomal DNA). The complementary sticky ends of the two different fragments anneal and can be joined permanently with DNA ligase. In this example a recombinant plasmid DNA molecule is formed.

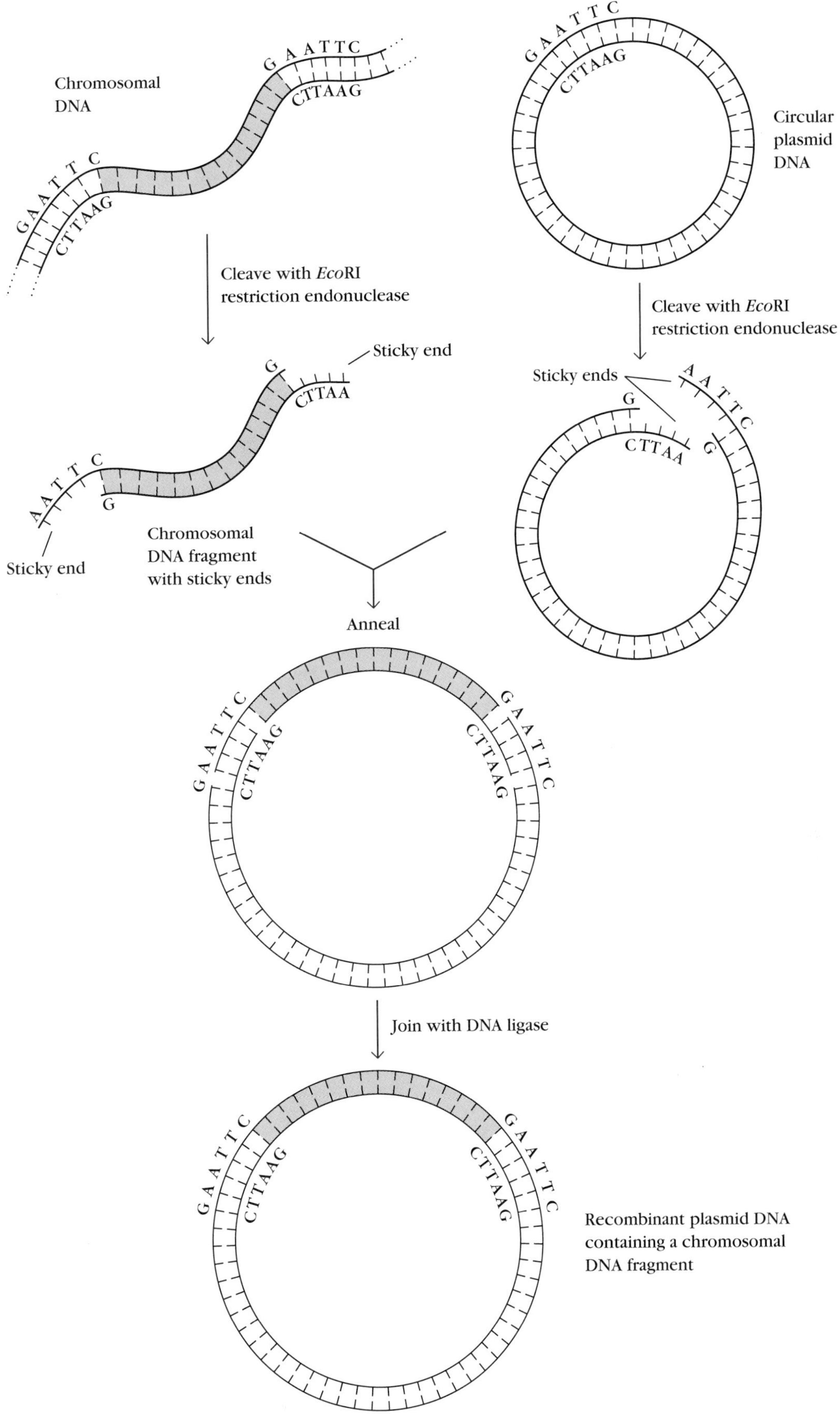
Chromosomal DNA
G A A T T C
CTTAAG
G A A T T C
CTTAAG
Circular plasmid DNA
G A A T T C
CTTAAG
Cleave with *Eco*RI restriction endonuclease
Cleave with *Eco*RI restriction endonuclease
Sticky end
G
CTTAA
A A T T C
G
Sticky end
Chromosomal DNA fragment with sticky ends
Sticky ends
G
CTTAA
A A T T C
G
Anneal
G A A T T C
CTTAAG
G A A T T C
CTTAAG
Join with DNA ligase
G A A T T C
CTTAAG
G A A T T C
CTTAAG
Recombinant plasmid DNA containing a chromosomal DNA fragment

Restriction Mapping of DNA

The DNA fragments generated with restriction endonucleases can be separated according to size by means of agarose gel electrophoresis. The smaller DNA fragments move faster than the larger fragments, generating a series of bands that can be detected with ethidium bromide dye, which binds to DNA. The molecular weight of each DNA fragment can be determined from standard curves obtained by electrophoresing DNA fragments of known size in parallel. By cleaving a DNA sample with two or more restriction endonucleases (alone and in combination), it is possible to determine the location of the restriction sites and the relative distances between them. This procedure is called *restriction mapping* (Figure 2-4).

Cloning of DNA Sequences

The development of DNA cloning technology in the 1970s provided a means of amplifying a given DNA fragment to such an extent that unlimited amounts of identical DNA fragments *(cloned DNA)* could be produced.

Cloning Vectors

In DNA cloning a given DNA fragment is inserted into an autonomously replicating DNA molecule, called a *cloning vector,* so that the inserted DNA is replicated with the vector. A number of different viruses have been used as vectors including bacterial viruses, insect viruses, and mammalian retroviruses. A common bacterial virus used as a vector is bacteriophage λ. If a gene is inserted into bacteriophage λ and the recombinant λ phage is used to infect *E. coli,* the inserted gene will be expressed by the bacteria.

Retroviruses, which can infect virtually any type of mammalian cell, are a common vector used to clone DNA in mammalian cells. Retroviruses are RNA viruses that contain *reverse transcriptase,* which catalyzes conversion of the viral RNA genome into DNA. The viral DNA then integrates into the host chromosomal DNA where it is retained as a *provirus,* replicating along with the host chromosomal DNA at each cell

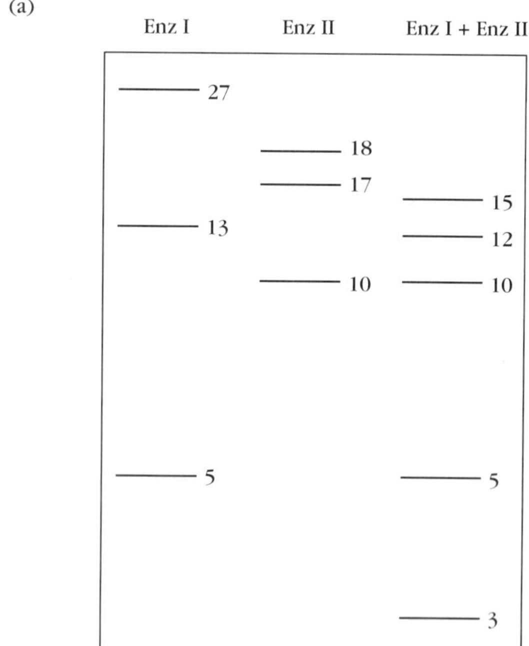

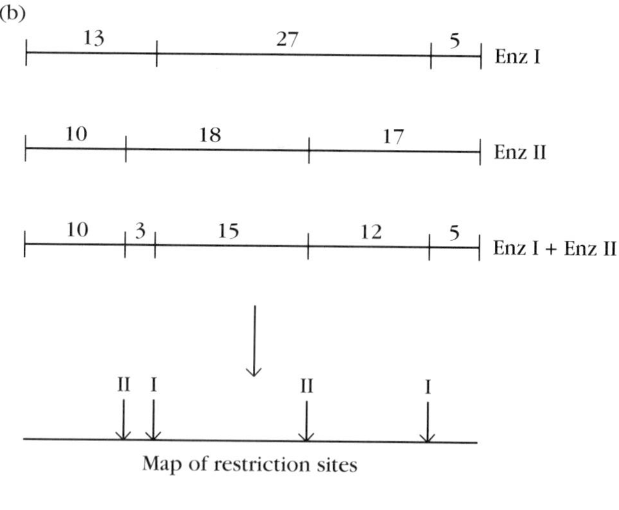

FIGURE 2-4 A simplified illustration of restriction-enzyme mapping. (a) Cloned DNA is digested with two restriction endonucleases (Enz I and Enz II) alone and in combination, and the resulting fragments are separated by gel electrophoresis. The numbers in the diagram refer to the length of each fragment in kilobases. (b) Comparison of the sizes of the fragments produced in the three digests permits ordering of the restriction sites relative to each other. In this example, the DNA sample contained two sites for Enz I and two sites for Enz II.

division. When a retrovirus is used as a vector, most of the retroviral genes are removed so that the vector cannot produce viral particles; the retroviral genes that are left include a strong promoter region, located at the 5′ end of the viral genome, in a sequence called the *long terminal repeat* (LTR). If a gene is cloned in such a retroviral vector and the vector is then used to infect mammalian cells, the gene will be expressed under the control of the retroviral promoter region.

A *plasmid vector* is a small circular, extrachromosomal DNA molecule that can replicate independently in a host cell; the most common host is *E. coli.* In general the DNA to be cloned is inserted into a plasmid that contains an antibiotic-resistance gene. After the recombinant plasmid is incubated with bacterial cells, the infected cells containing the recombinant plasmid can be selected by their ability to grow in the presence of the antibiotic. Another type of plasmid vector that is often used for cloning is called a *cosmid vector.* This type of vector is a plasmid that has been genetically engineered to contain the *cos* sites of λ-phage DNA, a drug-resistance gene, and a replication origin. *Cos* sites are DNA sequences that allow any DNA up to 50 kb in length to be packaged into the λ-phage head.

Cloning of Complementary DNA

Complementary DNA is prepared by isolating messenger RNA (mRNA) from cells and transcribing it into complementary DNA (cDNA) with the enzyme reverse transcriptase. This enzyme, which can be isolated from certain RNA viruses, copies mRNA by adding nucleotides to a primer, forming a mRNA-cDNA hybrid; in the production of cDNA, a poly-T primer is used, since most mRNAs have a poly-A tail. Double-stranded cDNA can be obtained from the mRNA-cDNA hybrid in a number of ways. In one method, the hybrid is treated with alkali, which destroys the RNA strand but not the DNA strand. The resulting single-stranded cDNA forms a small hairpin at its 3′ end, which serves as a primer for the synthesis by DNA polymerase of a complementary strand. After synthesis of the second strand, the hairpin is cleaved with S1 nuclease to generate a conventional double-stranded cDNA (Figure 2-5).

The cDNA can be cloned by inserting it into a plasmid vector carrying a selectable gene that confers resistance to the antibiotic ampicillin. The circular plasmid is cut with a restriction endonuclease that produces double-stranded blunt ends. The cDNA and the plasmid can be joined by several methods. In one method, called *tailing,* a terminal deoxynucleotidyl transferase enzyme adds short stretches of poly C to the 3′ ends of the cDNA molecule and short stretches of poly G to the 3′ ends of the plasmid DNA. When the plasmid DNA and cDNA are then mixed, the poly-G tail of the vector molecule anneals with the poly-C tail of the cDNA molecule. Following ligation, the recombinant plasmid DNA is subsequently transferred into specially treated *E. coli* cells by one of several possible techniques; this transfer process is called *transformation.* The ampicillin-resistance gene on the plasmid serves as a selectable marker for identifying bacterial cells containing the plasmid DNA because only those cells are able to grow in the presence of the antibiotic (see Figure 2-5). A collection of DNA sequences within plasmid vectors representing all the mRNA sequences derived from a cell or tissue is called a *cDNA library.*

Cloning of Genomic DNA

Genomic DNA fragments are obtained by cleaving chromosomal DNA with restriction endonucleases that produce sticky ends. The genomic DNA can be cloned using bacteriophage λ as the vector (Figure 2-6). Bacteriophage λ DNA is 48.5 kilobases (kb) long and contains a central section of about 15 kb that is not necessary for λ replication in *E. coli* and can therefore be replaced with foreign genomic DNA. Generally, the λ DNA is treated with a restriction endonuclease that cuts the DNA on both sides of the central 15-kb section, and this section is removed. Then the genomic DNA is cut with the same restriction enzyme. The single-stranded sticky ends of the λ DNA and the genomic DNA can be annealed and ligated to form a recombinant phage. Sometimes the genomic DNA is cut with another restriction endonuclease that does not produce sticky ends complementary to those on the λ-DNA fragments. In these cases, short DNA duplexes that include a restriction site, called linkers, are added to the genomic DNA fragments, enabling the fragments to anneal with the sticky ends on the λ fragments. As long as the recombinant DNA does not exceed the length of the original λ-phage DNA by more than 5%, it can be packaged into the λ-phage head and can be propagated in *E. coli.* This means that somewhat more than 1.5×10^4 base pairs can be cloned in one λ-phage particle. It has been calculated that about 1 million different recombinant λ-phage particles would be needed to form a complete *genomic DNA library* representing the entire haploid genome of a mammalian cell, which contains about 3×10^9 base pairs.

Often the 15- to 20-kb stretch of DNA that can be cloned in bacteriophage λ is not long enough to include the regulatory sequences that lie outside the 5′ and 3′ ends of the direct coding sequences of a gene. However, much larger genomic DNA fragments—between 30 and 50 kb in length—can be cloned in a

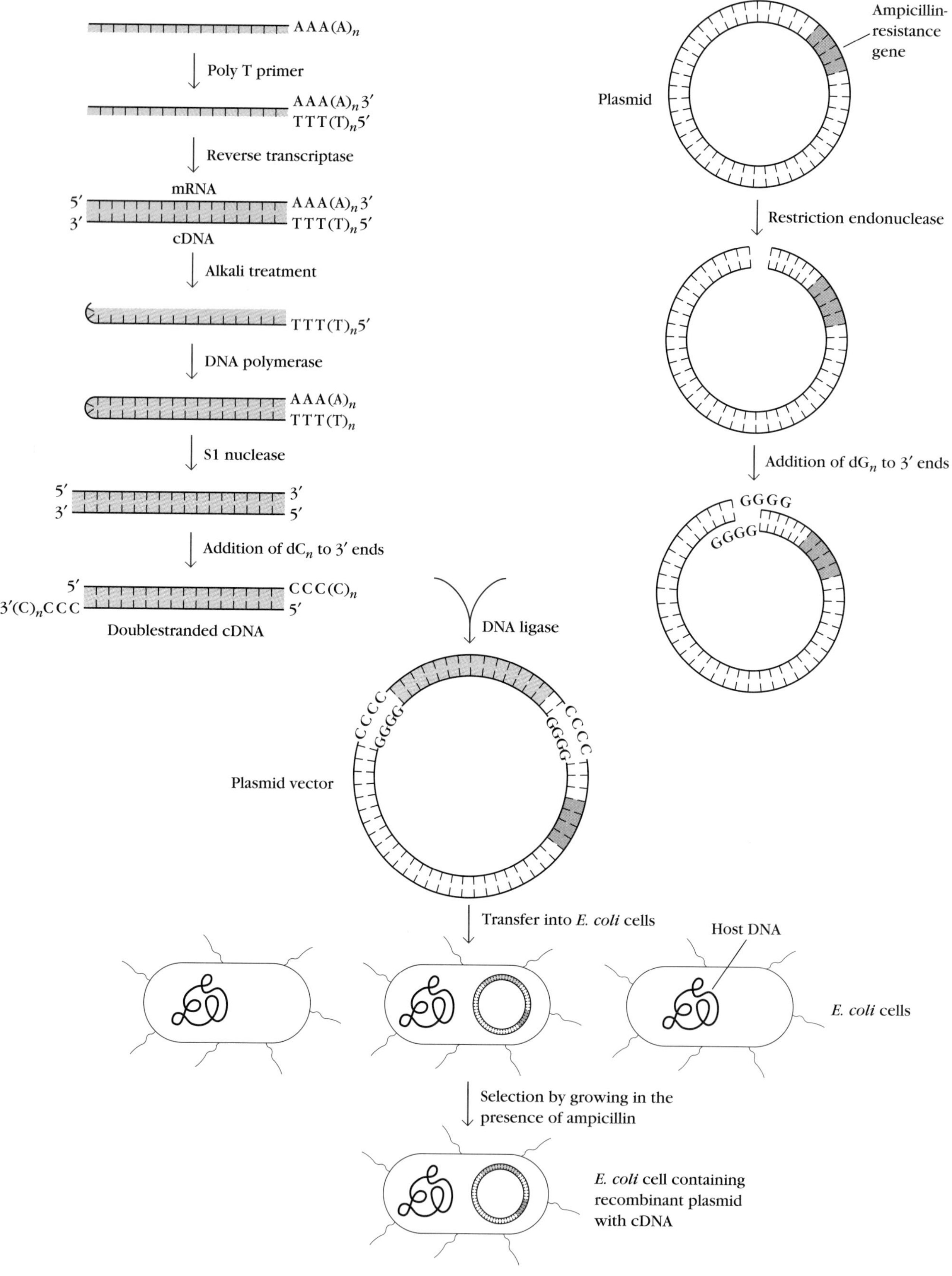

FIGURE 2-5 cDNA cloning using a plasmid vector. *(Left)* Formation of double-stranded cDNA is outlined. *(Right)* Plasmid DNA containing an ampicillin-resistance gene is cut with a restriction endonuclease that produces blunt ends. Following addition of a poly-C tail to the 3′ ends of the cDNA and of a poly-G tail to the 3′ ends of the cut plasmid, the two DNAs are mixed, annealed, and joined by DNA ligase, forming the plasmid vector. The vector is transferred into *E. coli* cells, which are grown in the presence of ampicillin to select cells containing the vector.

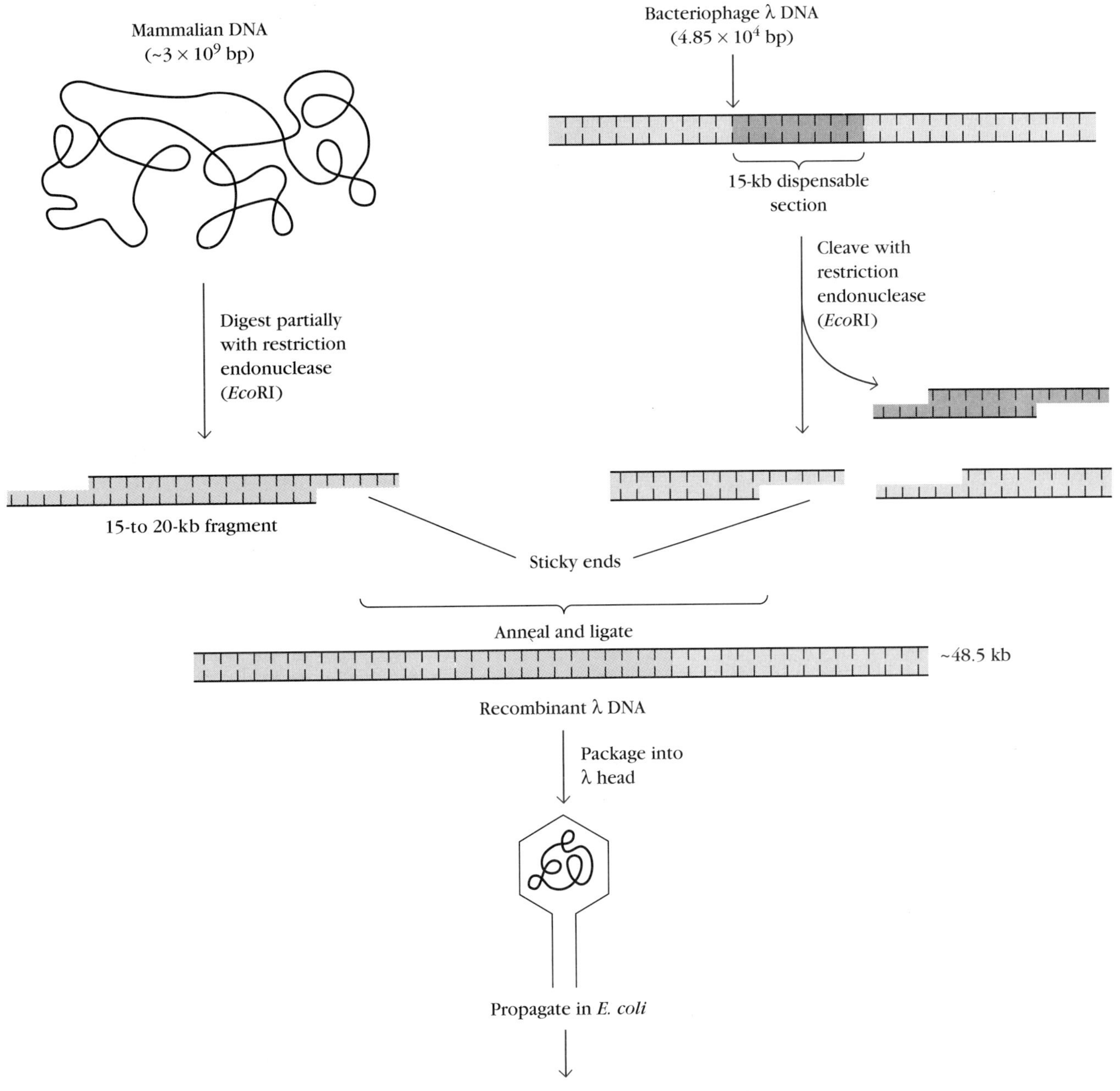

FIGURE 2-6 Genomic DNA cloning using bacteriophage λ as the vector. Genomic DNA is partially digested with *Eco*RI, producing fragments with sticky ends. The central 15-kb region of the λ phage DNA is cut out with *Eco*RI and discarded. The sticky ends of the genomic and λ DNA fragments are then annealed and ligated. After the resulting recombinant λ DNA is packaged into a phage head, it can be propagated in *E. coli.*

cosmid vector. A recombinant cosmid vector, although not a fully functional bacteriophage, can infect *E. coli* and replicate as a plasmid, generating a *cosmid library.* Even larger DNA fragments, approaching a megabase in length, can be cloned in yeast artificial chromosomes, which are linear DNA segments that can replicate in yeast cells.

Selection of DNA Clones

Once a cDNA or genomic DNA library is prepared, it can be screened to identify a particular DNA fragment by a process called in situ hybridization. The cloned bacterial colonies, yeast colonies, or phage plaques containing the recombinant DNA are transferred onto nitrocellulose or nylon filters by replica plating (Figure 2-7). The filter is then treated with NaOH, which both lyses the bacteria and denatures the DNA, allowing single-stranded DNA (ssDNA) to bind to the filter. The filter with bound DNA then is incubated with a radioactive probe specific for the gene of interest. The probe will hybridize with the colonies or plaques on the filter that contain the sought-after gene, and they can be identified by autoradiography. The position of the positive colonies or plaques on the filter shows where the corresponding clones can be found on the original agar plate.

Various radioactive probes can be used to screen a library. In some cases radiolabeled mRNA or cDNA serves as the probe. When the protein encoded by the gene of interest has been purified, it is possible to work backward from the amino acid sequence, using the genetic code, to determine the probable nucleotide sequence of the corresponding gene. A known sequence of five or six amino acid residues is all that is needed to synthesize radiolabeled oligonucleotide probes with which to screen a cDNA or genomic library for a particular gene. To cope with the degeneracy of the genetic code, peptides incorporating amino acids encoded by a limited number of codon sequences are usually chosen. Oligonucleotides representing all possible codon sequences for the peptide are synthesized and used as probes to screen the DNA library.

Southern Blotting

As noted already, DNA fragments generated by restriction-endonuclease cleavage can be separated on the basis of length by agarose gel electrophoresis. An elegant technique developed by E. M. Southern can be used to identify any fragment band containing a given gene sequence (Figure 2-8). In this technique, called *Southern blotting,* DNA is cut with restriction enzymes and the fragments are separated according to size by electrophoresis on an agarose gel. Then the gel is soaked in NaOH to denature the dsDNA, and the resulting ssDNA fragments are transferred onto a nitrocellulose or nylon filter by capillary action. After transfer, the filter is incubated with an appropriate radiolabeled probe specific for the gene sequence of choice. The probe hybridizes with the ssDNA fragment of interest, and the position of the fragment band is determined by autoradiography. Southern blot analy-

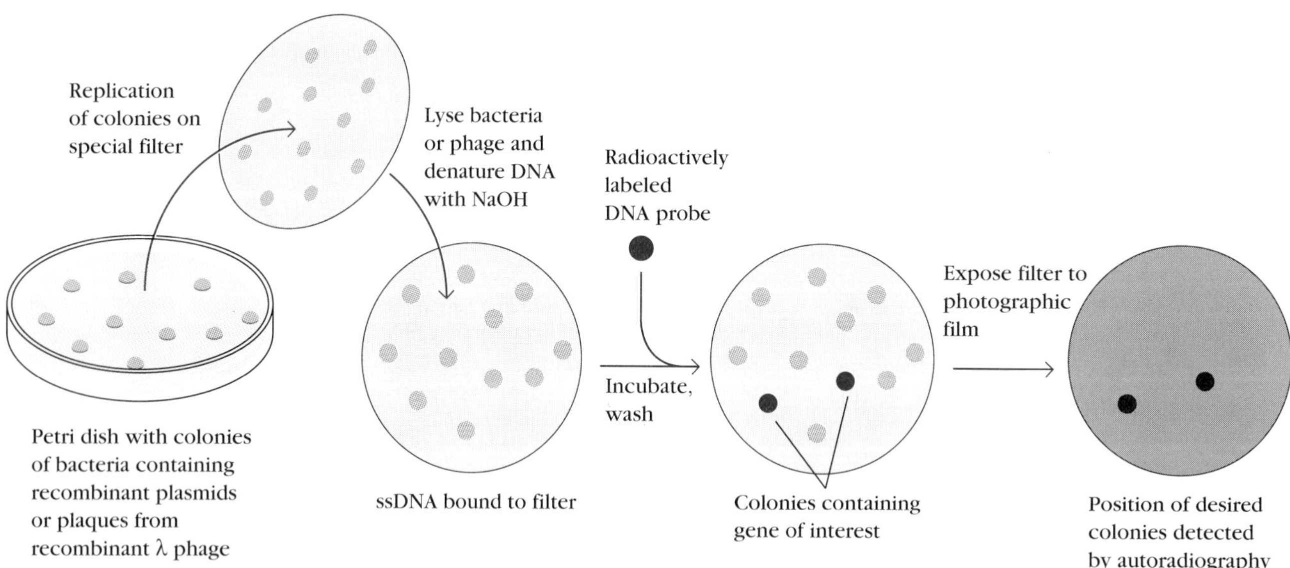

FIGURE 2-7 Selection of specific clones from a cDNA or genomic DNA library by in situ hybridization. A nitrocellulose or nylon filter is placed against the plate to pick up the bacterial colonies or phage plaques containing the cloned genes. The filter is then placed in a NaOH solution and heated, so that the denatured ssDNA becomes fixed to the filter. A radioactive probe specific for the gene of interest is incubated with the filter. The position of the colonies or plaques containing the desired gene is revealed by autoradiography.

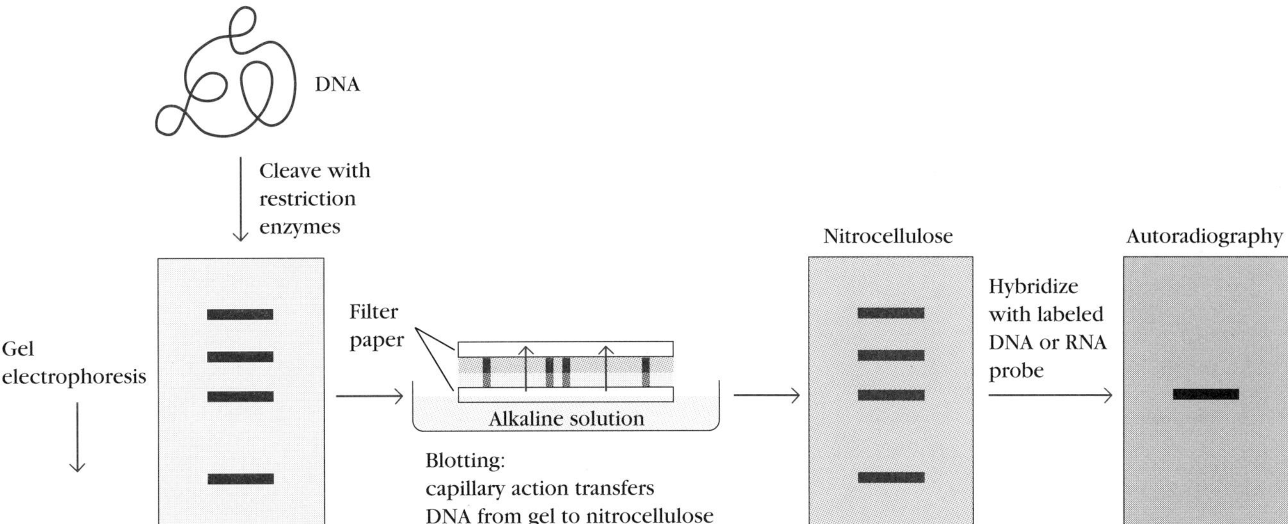

FIGURE 2-8 The Southern blot technique for detecting specific sequences in DNA fragments. The DNA fragments produced by restriction-enzyme cleavage are separated by size by agarose gel electrophoresis. The agarose gel is overlaid with a nitocellulose or nylon filter and a thick stack of paper towels. The gel is then placed in an alkaline salt solution, which denatures the DNA. As the paper towels soak up the moisture, the solution is drawn through the gel into the filter, transferring each ssDNA band to the filter. This process is called blotting. After heating, the filter is incubated with a radiolabeled probe specific for the sequence of interest; DNA fragments that hybridize with the probe are detected by autoradiography. [Adapted from James Darnell et al., 1990, *Molecular Cell Biology,* 2d ed., Scientific American Books.]

sis played a critical role in unraveling the mechanism by which diversity is generated for the immunoglobulin molecule and T-cell receptors.

Northern Blotting

Northern blotting (named for its similarity to Southern blotting) is used to detect the presence of specific mRNA molecules. In this procedure the mRNA is first denatured to ensure that it is in an unfolded, linear form. The mRNA molecules are then separated according to size by electrophoresis and transferred to a nitrocellulose filter to which the mRNAs will adhere. The filter is then incubated with a labeled DNA probe and subjected to autoradiography. Northern blot analysis is often used to determine how much of a specific mRNA is expressed in cells under different conditions. Increased levels of mRNA will bind more of the labeled DNA probe.

Polymerase Chain Reaction

The *polymerase chain reaction (PCR)* is a powerful technique for amplifying specific DNA sequences even when they are present at extremely low levels in a complex mixture (Figure 2-9). The procedure requires that the DNA sequences flanking the desired DNA sequence be known, so that short oligonucleotide primers can be synthesized. The DNA mixture is denatured into single strands by a brief heat treatment. The DNA is then cooled in the presence of an excess of the oligonucleotide primers, which hybridize with the complementary ssDNA. A temperature-resistant DNA polymerase (called Taq polymerase) is then added, together with the four deoxyribonucleoside triphosphates, and each strand is copied. The newly synthesized DNA duplex is separated by heating and the cycle is repeated. In each cycle there is a doubling of the DNA sequence; in only 25 cycles the desired DNA se-

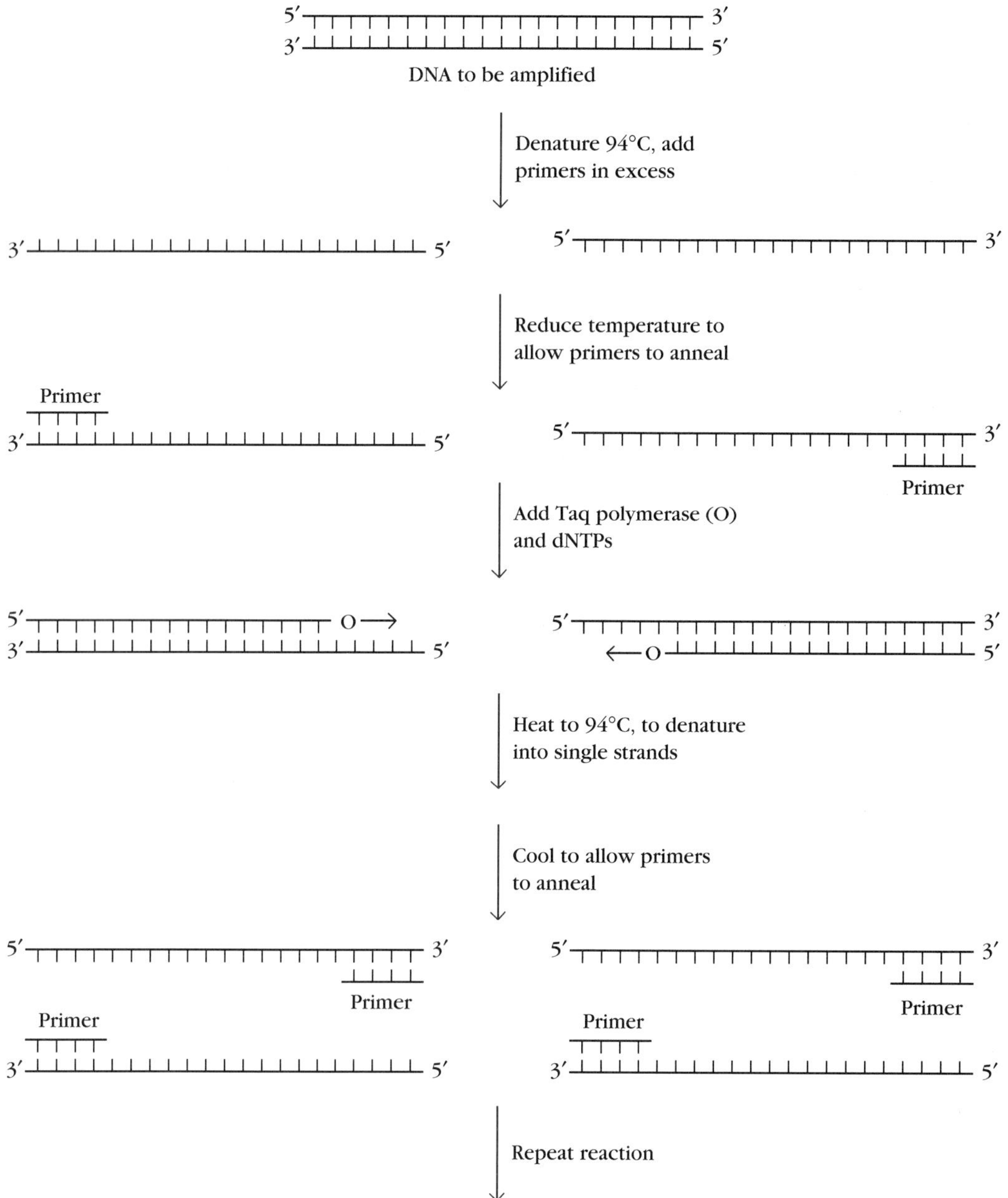

FIGURE 2-9 The polymerase chain reaction (PCR). DNA is denatured into single strands by a brief heat treatment and is then cooled in the presence of an excess of oligonucleotide primers complementary to the DNA sequences flanking the desired DNA segment. Taq polymerase, a heat-resistant DNA polymerase obtained from a thermophilic bacterium, is used to copy the DNA from the 3′ ends of the primers. Because all of the reaction components are heat stable, the heating and cooling cycle can be repeated many times, resulting in alternate DNA melting and synthesis, and rapid amplification of a given sequence. [Adapted from James Darnell et al., 1990, *Molecular Cell Biology,* 2d ed., Scientific American Books.]

quence can be amplified about a million-fold. The DNA amplified by PCR can be further characterized by Southern blotting, restriction-enzyme mapping, and direct DNA sequencing. The PCR has enabled immunologists to amplify genes encoding proteins that are important in the immune response, such as MHC molecules, the T-cell receptor, and immunoglobulins.

Analysis of DNA Regulatory Sequences

The transcriptional activity of genes is regulated by *promoter* and *enhancer* sequences. These sequences are *cis*-acting, meaning that they only regulate genes on the same DNA molecule. The promoter sequence lies upstream from the gene it regulates and includes a TATA box where the general transcription machinery, including RNA polymerase II, binds and begins transcription. The enhancer sequence confers a high rate of transcription on the promoter. Unlike the promoter, which always lies upstream from the gene it controls, the enhancer element can be located anywhere with respect to the gene (5′ of the promoter, 3′ of the gene, or even in an intron of the gene). The activity of enhancer and promoter sequences are controlled by *transcription factors,* which are *DNA-binding proteins.* These proteins bind to specific nucleotide sequences within promoters and enhancers and act either to enhance or suppress their activity. Enhancer and promoter sequences and their respective DNA-binding proteins have been identified by a variety of techniques including DNA footprinting, gel-shift analysis, and the CAT assay.

DNA Footprinting

Identification of the binding sites for DNA-binding proteins on enhancers and promoters can be achieved by a technique called *DNA footprinting* (Figure 2-10a).

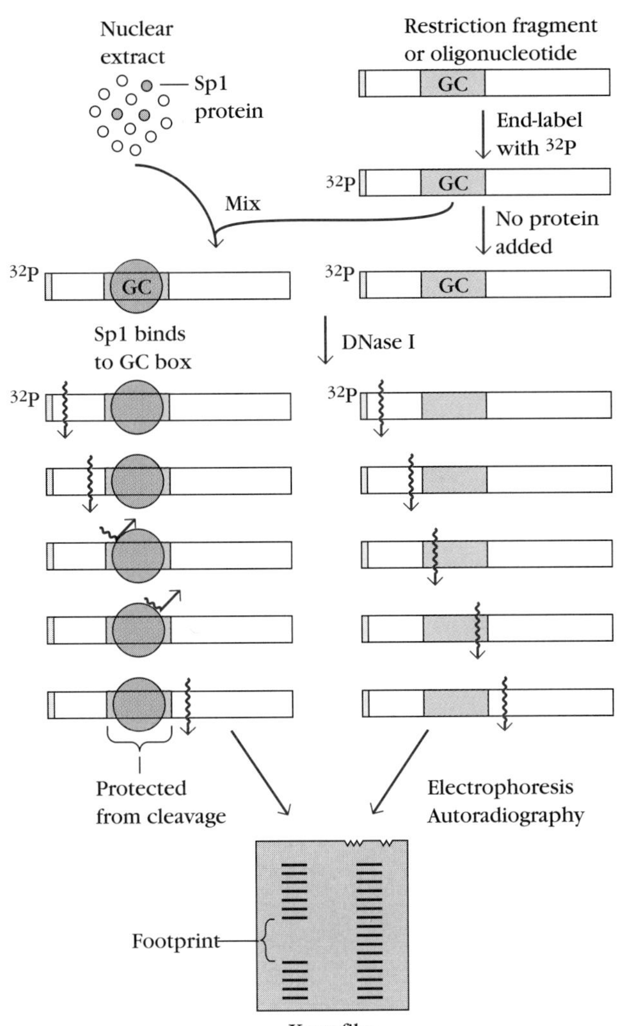

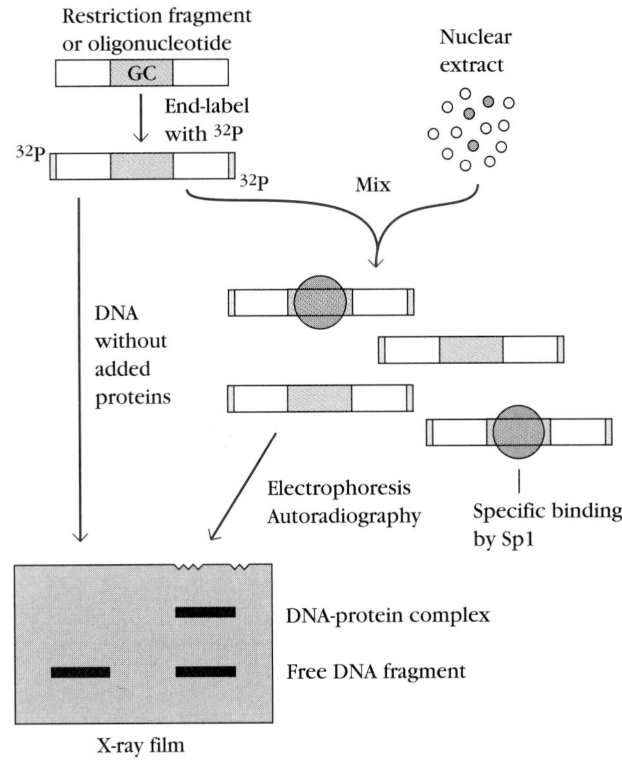

FIGURE 2-10 Identification of DNA sequences that bind protein by DNA-footprinting and gel-shift analysis. (a) In the footprinting technique, labeled DNA fragments containing a putative promoter or enhancer sequence are incubated in the presence and absence of a DNA-binding protein (e.g., Sp1 protein). After the samples are treated with DNase and the strands separated, the resulting fragments are electrophoresed; the gel then is subjected to autoradiography. A blank region (footprint) in the gel pattern indicates that protein has bound to the DNA. (b) In gel-shift analysis, a labeled DNA fragment is incubated with a cellular extract containing transcription factors. The electrophoretic mobility of the DNA-protein complex is slower than that of free DNA fragments. [Adapted from J. D. Watson et al., 1992, *Recombinant DNA: A Short Course,* 2nd ed., W. H. Freeman and Company.]

In this technique a cloned DNA fragment containing a putative enhancer or promoter sequence is first labeled at the 5′ end with ^{32}P. The labeled DNA is then divided into two fractions: One fraction is incubated with a nuclear extract containing a DNA-binding protein; the other DNA fraction is not incubated with the nuclear extract. Both DNA samples are then digested with a nuclease or a chemical that makes random cuts in the phosphodiester bonds of the DNA, and the strands are separated. The resulting DNA fragments are run on a gel to separate fragments of different sizes. In the absence of DNA-binding proteins, a complete ladder of bands is obtained on the electrophoretic gel. When a protein that binds to a site on the DNA fragment is present, it covers some of the nucleotides, protecting that stretch of the DNA from digestion. The electrophoretic pattern of such protected DNA will contain blank regions (or *footprints*). Each footprint represents the site within an enhancer or promoter that binds a particular DNA-binding protein.

Gel-Shift Analysis

Gel-shift analysis depends upon the reduction in electrophoretic mobility that occurs when a protein binds DNA, forming a DNA-protein complex. In this technique radioactively labeled cloned DNA containing an enhancer or a promoter sequence is incubated with a nuclear extract containing a DNA-binding protein (Figure 2-10b). The DNA-protein complex is then electrophoresed and its electrophoretic mobility is compared to that of DNA alone. A shift in the mobility indicates that a protein is bound to the DNA, retarding its migration on the electrophoretic gel.

CAT Assay

One way to assess promoter activity is to engineer and clone a construct containing a *reporter gene* and a promoter of interest. When this construct is transfected into eukaryotic cells, transcription will be initiated from the promoter. If the promoter is active, the reporter gene will be transcribed and its protein product can be measured. Generally reporter genes encode proteins that can be easily measured, such as the enzyme chloramphenicol acetyltransferase (CAT), which transfers the acetyl group from acetyl-CoA to the antibiotic chloramphenicol (Figure 2-11). The more active the promoter is, the more CAT will be produced within the transfected cell. By introducing mutations into promoter sequences and then assaying for promoter activity with the corresponding reporter gene, conserved sequence motifs have been identified within promoters that are necessary for promoter activity.

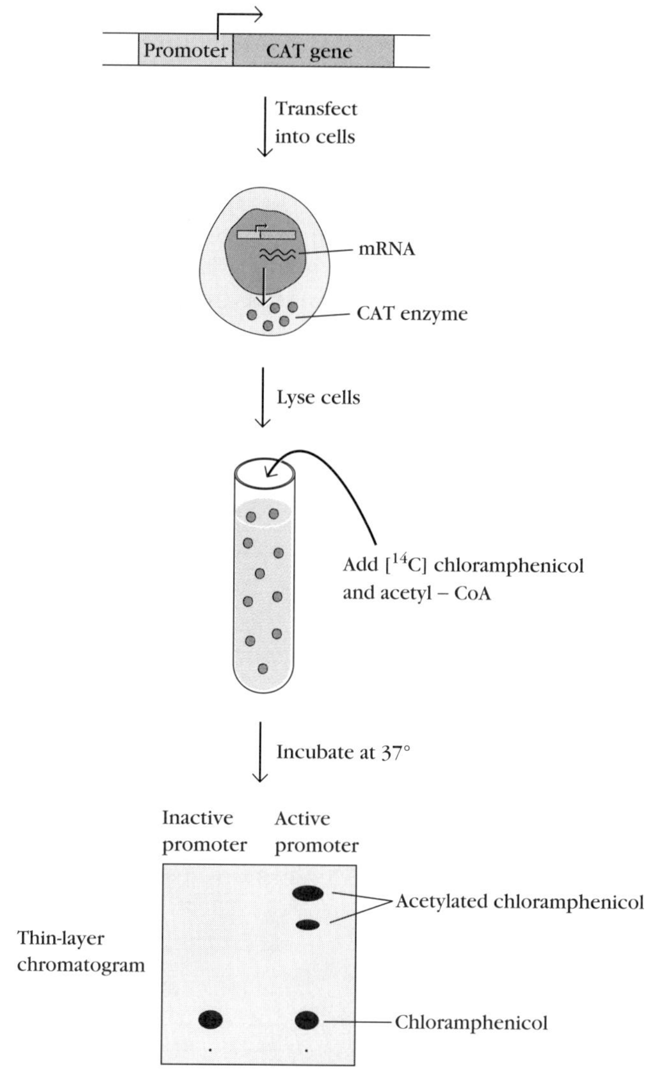

FIGURE 2-11 CAT assay for assessing functional activity of a promoter sequence. In this assay the promoter of interest is engineered with the gene encoding chloramphenicol acetyltransferase (CAT), and the construct is transfected into eukaryotic cells. If the promoter is active, the CAT gene will be transcribed and the CAT enzyme will be produced within the transfected cell. The presence of the enzyme can easily be detected by lysing the cell and incubating the cell lysate with [^{14}C]chloramphenicol and acetyl-CoA. The CAT enzyme will transfer the acetyl group from acetyl-CoA to the chloramphenicol forming acetylated chloramphenicol, which can be easily detected by thin-layer chromatography. [Adapted from J. D. Watson et al., 1992, *Recombinant DNA: A Short Course,* 2nd ed., W. H. Freeman and Company.

Gene Transfer into Mammalian Cells

A variety of genes involved in the immune response have been isolated and cloned by use of recombinant DNA techniques. The expression and regulation of these genes has been studied by introducing them into cultured cells and, more recently, into the germ line of animals.

Transfer of Cloned Genes into Cultured Cells

Diverse techniques have been developed for transfecting genes into cells. A common technique involves the use of a retrovirus in which a viral structural gene has been replaced with the cloned gene to be transfected. The altered retrovirus is then used as a vector for introducing the cloned gene into cultured cells. Because of the properties of retroviruses, the recombinant DNA integrates into the cellular genome with a high frequency. In an alternative method, the cloned gene of interest is complexed with calcium phosphate. The calcium phosphate–DNA complex is slowly precipitated onto the cells and the DNA is taken up by a small percentage of them. In another transfection method called *electroporation,* an electric current creates pores in cell membranes through which the cloned DNA is taken up. In both of these latter methods, the transfected DNA integrates, apparently at random sites, into the DNA of a small percentage of treated cells. Generally the cloned DNA being transfected is engineered to contain a selectable marker gene, such as one coding for resistance to neomycin. Following transfection the cells are cultured in the presence of neomycin. Because only the transfected cells are able to grow, the relatively small number of transfected cells in the total cell population can be identified and selected.

Transfection of cloned genes into cells has proved to be a highly effective technique in immunologic research. By transfecting genes involved with the immune response into cells lacking those genes, the product of a specific gene can be studied apart from interacting proteins encoded by other genes. For example, transfection of MHC genes into a mouse fibroblast cell line (L929 or simply L cells) has enabled immunologists to study the role of MHC molecules in antigen presentation to T cells. Transfection of the gene encoding the T-cell receptor has provided information about the antigen-MHC specificity of the T-cell receptor.

Transfer of Cloned Genes into Mouse Embryos

Development of techniques to introduce cloned foreign genes (called *transgenes*) into mouse embryos has permitted immunologists to study the effects of immune-system genes in vivo. If the introduced gene integrates stably into the germ-line cells, it will be transmitted to the offspring. Two techniques for producing transgenic mice are discussed in this section; one of these has been used to produce knock-out mice, which cannot express a particular gene product (Table 2-4).

Transgenic Mice

Transgenic mice are produced by injecting foreign cloned DNA into a fertilized egg (Figure 2-12). In the technically demanding process of producing transgenics, fertilized mouse eggs are held under suction at the end of a pipet and the transgene is micro-injected into one of the pronuclei with a fine needle. The transgene integrates into the chromosomal DNA of the pronucleus and is passed on to the daughter cells of

Table 2-4 Comparison of transgenic and knock-out mice

Characteristic	Transgenic mice	Knock-out mice
Cells receiving DNA	Zygote	Embryonic stem (ES) cells
DNA constructs used	Natural gene or cDNA	Mutated gene
Means of delivery	Microinjection into zygote and implantation into foster mother	Transfer of ES cells to blastocyst and implantation into foster mother
Outcome	Gain of a gene	Loss of a gene

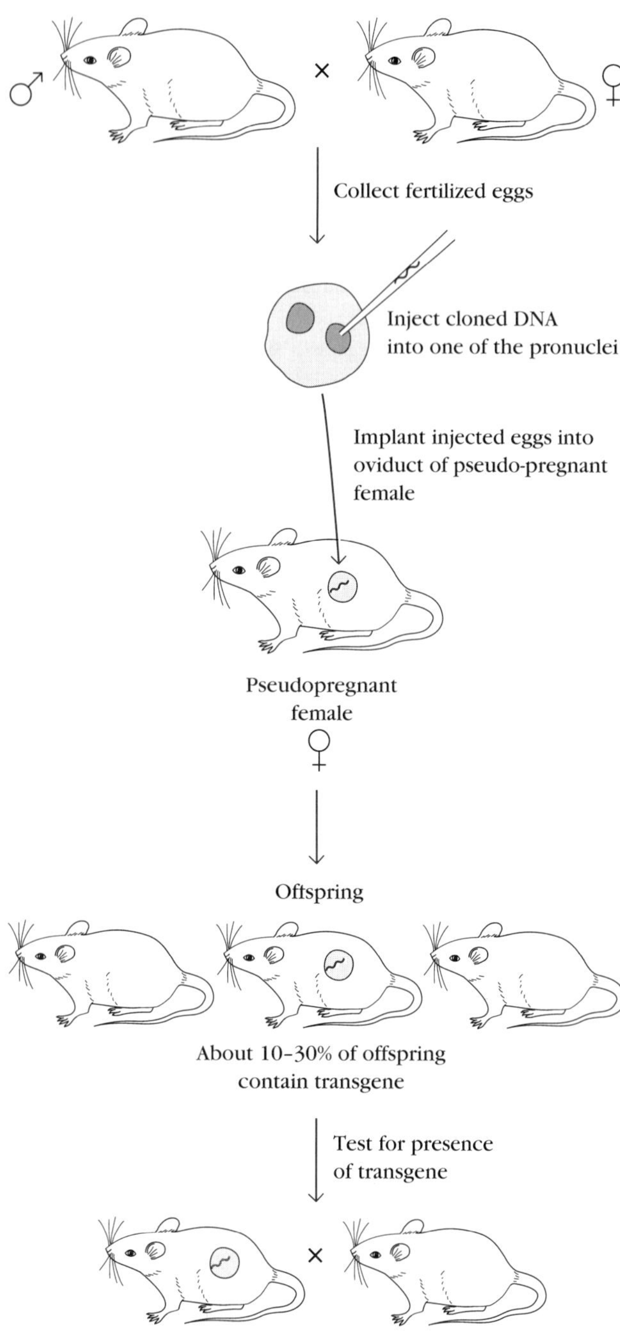

FIGURE 2-12 General procedure for producing transgenic mice. Fertilized eggs are collected from a pregnant female mouse. Cloned DNA (referred to as the transgene) is microinjected into one of the pronuclei of a fertilized egg. The eggs are then implanted into the oviduct of pseudo-pregnant foster mothers (obtained by mating a normal female with a sterile male). The transgene will be incorporated into the chromosomal DNA of about 10–30% of the offspring and will be expressed in all of their somatic cells. If a tissue-specific promoter is linked to a transgene, then tissue-specific expression of the transgene will result.

eggs that survive the process. The eggs are implanted in the oviduct of "pseudopregnant" females, and transgenic pups are born after 19 or 20 days of gestation. In general the efficiency of this procedure is low, with only one or two transgenic mice produced for every 100 fertilized eggs collected.

With transgenic mice immunologists have been able to study the expression of a given gene in a living animal. Although all the cells in a transgenic animal contain the transgene, differences in the expression of the transgene in different tissues has shed light on mechanisms of tissue-specific gene expression. By constructing a transgene with a particular promoter, one can control the expression of a given transgene. For example, the metallothionein promoter is activated by zinc. Transgenic mice carrying a transgene linked to a metallothionein promoter can therefore be induced to express the transgene at a particular time by addition of zinc to their water supply. Other promoters, such as the insulin promoter, are tissue-specific. By producing transgenics carrying a transgene linked to the insulin promoter, one can limit expression of the transgene to pancreatic cells.

Because a transgene is integrated into the chromosomal DNA within the one-celled mouse embryo, it will be integrated into both somatic cells and germline cells. The resulting transgenic mice thus can transmit the transgene to their offspring as a mendelian trait. In this way it has been possible to produce *lines* of transgenic mice in which every member of a particular line contains the same transgene. A variety of such transgenic lines are currently available and are widely used in immunologic research today. Included among these are lines carrying transgenes that encode immunoglobulin, T-cell receptor, class I and class II MHC molecules, various foreign antigens, and a number of cytokines. Several lines carrying oncogenes as transgenes also have been produced.

Gene-Targeted Knock-Out Mice

One of the limitations with transgenic mice is that the transgene is integrated randomly within the genome. To circumvent this limitation, researchers have developed a gene-targeting technique in which cloned DNA is introduced at specific DNA sequences in the chromosome by homologous recombination (Figure 2-13). In this technique, a desired gene is targeted to specific sites within the germ line of a mouse by introduction of cloned DNA into *embryonic stem cells (ES cells)*. These special cells, derived from the inner cell mass of a mouse blastocyst, are undifferentiated (pluripotent) cells that can differentiate in a variety of directions, generating distinct cellular lineages (e.g., germ cells, myocardium, blood vessels, myoblasts, nerve cells).

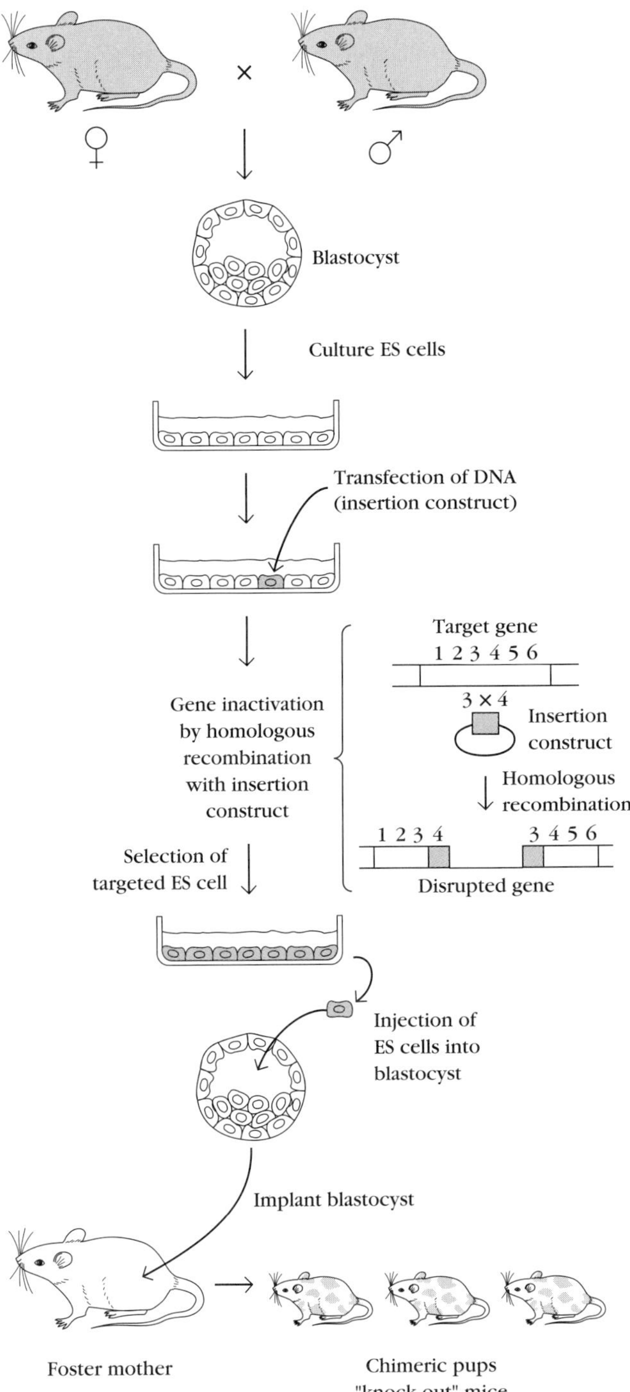

FIGURE 2-13 General procedure for producing knock-out mice. (a) Embryonic stem (ES) cells are obtained by culturing the inner cell mass of a mouse blastocyte on a feeder layer of fibroblasts or in the presence of leukemia inhibitory factor (LIF). Under these conditicns the ES cells grow but remain pluripotent. (b) A gene of interest is cloned and engineered in such a way that it is nonfunctional. This is often achieved by inserting the selection *neo* gene into one of the exons of the gene of interest. The engineered gene containing the desired mutation is then introduced into the ES cells by electroporation. As the transfected gene pairs with the homologous chromosomal DNA sequence, the mutation is introduced by recombination into the genome of the ES cell. After screening, the ES cells containing the mutant gene (purple) are injected into the blastocoel cavity of a preimplantation mouse embryo, and the blastocyst is surgically implanted into the uterus of a foster mother. The resulting pups are chimeric and contain cells from the host blastocyst and from the donor stem cells. [Adapted from M. R. Capecchi, 1989, *Science* **244**:1288.]

Cloned DNA containing a desired gene can be introduced into ES cells in culture by transfection, microinjection, or retroviral infection. The introduced DNA will pair with the chromosomal DNA in some ES cells and is then inserted by homologous recombination. If the introduced DNA includes a selection gene, then those ES cells containing the desired gene can be selected. After the altered ES cells are clonally expanded in cell culture, they are injected back into the blastocoelic cavity of a preimplantation mouse embryo; the blastocyst then is surgically implanted into a pseudopregnant female. The chimeric, transgenic offspring that develop are composed of cells derived from the genetically altered ES cells and cells derived from normal cells of the host blastocyst. When the germ-line cells are derived from the genetically altered ES cells, the genetic alteration can be passed on to the offspring. Often ES cells and recipient blastocysts are derived from mice having different coat colors, so that the chimeric offspring will have patches of both hair colors.

One of the advantages of the ES cell is the ease with which it can be genetically manipulated. For example, if mutant genes are introduced into ES cells, the transgenic mice carrying the mutant genes can be bred to produce mice homozygous for the mutation. These transgenic mice can then be used to assess the impact of a given mutation in a gene. In some cases the mutation so disrupts the desired gene that no functional gene product is expressed. Such transgenic mice, called *knock-out mice,* have been extremely helpful to immunologists trying to understand how the removal of a particular gene product affects the immune system. A variety of knock-out mice are being used in immunologic research, including mice lacking particular cytokines or MHC molecules.

Summary

1. Inbred strains allow immunologists to work routinely with syngeneic, or genetically identical, mice. With these strains, aspects of the immune response can be studied uncomplicated by unknown variables that could be introduced by genetic differences between animals.

2. In adoptive-transfer experiments, lymphocytes are transferred from one mouse to a syngeneic recipient mouse that has been exposed to a sublethal (or potentially lethal) dose of x-rays. The irradiation inactivates the immune cells of the recipient, so that one can study the response of only the transferred cells.

3. With in vitro cell-culture systems, populations of lymphocytes can be studied under more-defined conditions than are possible with in vivo animal systems. Such systems include primary cultures of lymphoid cells, cloned lymphoid cell lines, and hybrid lymphoid cell lines. Unlike primary cultures, cell lines are immortal and homogeneous. With cell lines, the intracellular events and cell products associated with individual subpopulations of lymphocytes can be investigated. Such studies are difficult, if not impossible, with the heterogeneous populations typical of primary cultures.

4. The ability to identify, clone, and sequence immune-system genes, using recombinant DNA techniques, has revolutionized the study of all aspects of the immune response. Both cDNA, which is prepared by transcribing mRNA with reverse transcriptase, and genomic DNA can be cloned. Generally, cDNA is cloned using a plasmid vector; the recombinant DNA containing the gene to be cloned is propagated in *E. coli* cells. Genomic DNA can be cloned with bacteriophage λ as the vector or with cosmid vectors, both of which are propagated in *E. coli.* Larger genomic DNA fragments can be cloned within yeast artificial chromosomes, which can replicate in yeast cells.

5. Transcription of genes is regulated by promoter and enhancer sequences; the activity of these sequences is controlled by DNA-binding proteins. Footprinting and gel-shift analysis can be used to identify DNA-binding proteins and their binding sites within the promoter or enhancer sequence. Promoter activity can be assessed by the CAT assay.

6. Cloned genes can be transfected (transferred) into cultured cells by several methods. Commonly, immune-system genes are transfected into cells that do not express the gene of interest. Cloned genes also can be incorporated into the germ-line cells of mouse embryos, yielding transgenic mice, which can transmit the incorporated transgene to their offspring. With transgenic mice, expression of a given gene can be studied in a living animal.

References

BARINAGA, M. 1989. Making transgenic mice: is it really that easy? *Science* **245**:590.

BELL, J. 1989. The polymerase chain reaction. *Immunol. Today* **10**:351.

BERGER, S. L., and A. R. KIMMEL (eds.). 1987. Guide to molecular cloning techniques. *Methods Enzymol.* **152**:(entire volume).

BURKE, D. T., G. F. CARLE, and M. V. OLSO. 1987. Cloning of large segments of exogenous DNA into yeast by means of artificial chromosome vectors. *Science* **236**:806.

CAMPER, S. A. 1987. Research applications of transgenic mice. *Biotechniques* **5**:638.

CAPECCHI, M. R. 1989. Altering the genome by homologous recombination. *Science* **244**:1288.

DENIS, K. A., and O. N. WITTE. 1989. Long-term lymphoid cultures in the study of B cell differentiation. In *Immunoglobulin Genes.* Academic Press, p. 45.

DEPAMPHILIS, M. L., S. A. HERMAN, E. MARTINEZ-SALAS et al. 1988. Microinjecting DNA into mouse ova to study DNA replication and gene expression and to produce transgenic animals. *Biotechniques* **6**(7):622.

KAVATHAS, P., and L. A. HERZENBERG. 1986. Transfection for lymphocyte cell surface antigens. In *Handbook of Experimental Immunology.* Vol. 3: Genetics and Molecular Approaches to Immunology. D. M. Weir (ed.). Blackwell Scientific Publications, p. 91.1.

KOLLER, B. H., and O. SMITHIES. 1992. Altering genes in animals by gene targeting. *Annu. Rev. Immunol.* **10**:705.

MCCUNE, J. M., et al. 1988. The SCID-Hu mouse; murine model for analysis of human hematolymphoid differentiation and function. *Science* **241**:1632.

MORRISON, S., and V. T. OI. 1986. Lymphoid cell gene transfer. In *Handbook of Experimental Immunology.* Vol. 3: Genetics and Molecular Approaches to Immunology. D. M. Weir (ed.). Blackwell Scientific Publications, p. 92.1.

OLD, R. W., and S. B. PRIMROSE. 1985. *Principles of Gene Manipulation: An Introduction to Genetic Engineering.* Blackwell Scientific Publications.

SAIKI, R. K., D. H. GELFAND, S. STOFFEL et al. 1988. Primer-directed enzymatic amplification of DNA with a thermostable DNA polymerase. *Science* **239**:487.

SCHLESSINGER, D. 1990. Yeast artificial chromosomes: tools for mapping and analysis of complex genomes. *Trends Genet.* **6**(8):254.

WATSON, J., M. GILMAN, J. WITKOWSKI, and M. ZOLLER. 1992. *Recombinant DNA: A Short Course,* 2nd ed. W. H. Freeman and Company.

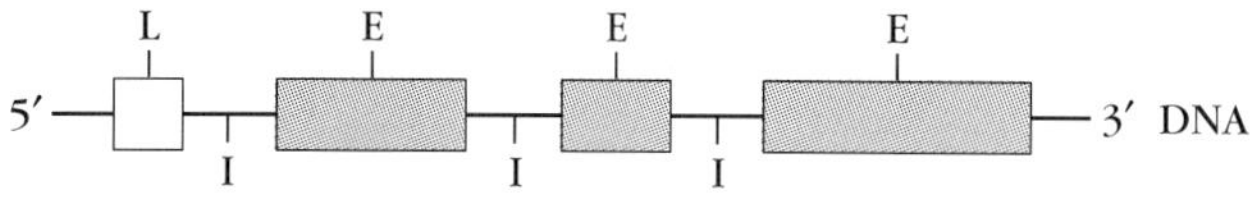

Study Questions

1. Explain why the following statements are false.
   a. The amino acid sequence of a protein can be determined from the nucleotide sequence of a genomic clone encoding the protein.
   b. Transgenic mice can be prepared by microinjection of DNA into a somatic-cell nucleus.
   c. Primary lymphoid cultures can be propagated indefinitely and are useful in studies on specific subpopulations of lymphocytes.

2. The gene diagrammed above, right contains one leader (L), three exons (E), and three introns (I). Illustrate the primary transcript, mRNA, and the protein product that could be generated from such a gene.

L E E E
5′ 3′ DNA
I I I

3. Why is it necessary to include a selectable marker gene in transfection experiments?

4. What would be the result if a transgene were injected into one cell of a four-cell mouse zygote rather than into a fertilized mouse egg before it divides?

5. A circular plasmid was cleaved with *Eco*RI, producing a 5.4-kb band on a gel. A 5.4-kb band was also observed when the plasmid was cleaved with *Hin*dIII. Cleaving the plasmid with both enzymes simultaneously resulted in a single band 2.7 kb in size. Draw a possible restriction map of this plasmid.

6. Explain briefly how you might go about cloning a gene for interleukin 2. Assume that you have available a monoclonal antibody to IL-2.

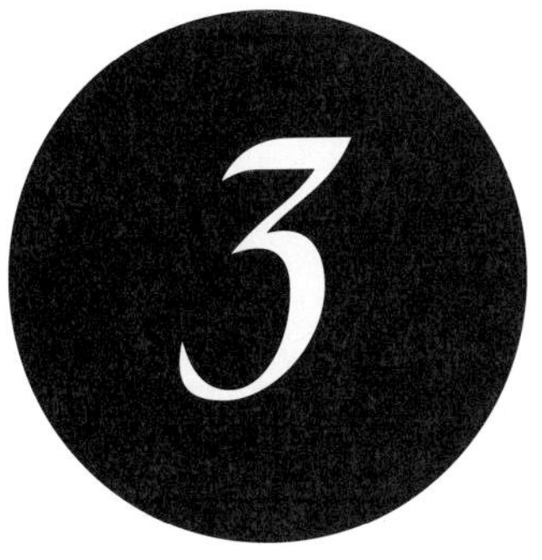

CELLS AND ORGANS OF THE IMMUNE SYSTEM

The immune system consists of many structurally and functionally diverse organs and tissues that are widely dispersed throughout the body. These organs can be classified on the basis of functional differences as *primary* and *secondary* lymphoid organs. The primary organs provide appropriate microenvironments for lymphocyte maturation. The secondary organs trap antigen from defined tissues or vascular spaces and provide sites where mature lymphocytes can interact effectively with that antigen. The blood vasculature and lymphatic systems interconnect these organs, uniting them into a functional whole.

Carried within the blood and lymph and populating the various lymphoid organs are the cells that participate in the immune response. The central cell of the immune system is the lymphocyte, which accounts for roughly 25% of the white blood cells in the blood and 99% of the cells in the lymph. There are approximately 10^{12} lymphocytes in humans, the equivalent in cellular mass to that of the brain or liver! These lymphocytes continuously recirculate between the blood and lymph and the various lymphoid organs, thereby providing a high degree of cellular integration to the immune system as a whole.

Cells of the Immune System

A variety of white blood cells, or *leukocytes,* participate in the development of an immune response (Table 3-1). Of these cells, only the lymphocytes possess the attributes of diversity, specificity, memory, and self/nonself recognition, the hallmarks of an immune response. All the other cells play accessory roles, serving to activate lymphocytes, to increase the effectiveness of antigen clearance by phagocytosis, or to secrete various immune effector molecules.

Hematopoiesis

In humans, *hematopoiesis,* the formation and development of red and white blood cells from stem cells, begins in the yolk sac in the first weeks of embryonic development. Here yolk-sac stem cells differentiate into primitive erythroid cells containing embryonic hemoglobin. In the third month of gestation, the stem cells migrate from the yolk sac to the fetal liver and then to the spleen; these two organs have major roles in hematopoiesis from the third to the seventh months of gestation. As gestation continues, the bone marrow becomes the major hematopoietic organ; by birth hematopoiesis has ceased within the liver and spleen.

It is remarkable that every functionally specialized, mature blood cell is derived from a common *stem cell.* In contrast to a unipotent cell, which differentiates into a single cell type, a hematopoietic stem cell is *pluripotent,* able to differentiate along a number of pathways and thereby generate erythrocytes, granulocytes, monocytes, mast cells, lymphocytes, and megakaryocytes. These stem cells are few in number, occurring with a frequency of one stem cell per 10^4 bone marrow cells.

The study of stem cells has been hampered by their low frequency and the inability of researchers to maintain them in tissue culture. As a result, little is known about the regulation of their proliferation and differentiation. By virtue of their capacity for self-renewal, stem cells are maintained at homeostatic levels throughout adult life; however, when there is an increased demand for hematopoiesis, stem cells display an enormous proliferative capacity. This can be demonstrated in mice whose hematopoietic systems have been completely destroyed by a lethal dose (950 rads) of x-rays. Such irradiated mice will die within 10 days unless they are infused with normal bone marrow cells from a syngeneic, or genetically identical, mouse. Although a normal mouse has 3×10^8 marrow cells, infusion of only 10^4–10^5 donor bone marrow cells (i.e., 0.01–0.1% of the normal level) is sufficient to completely restore the hematopoietic system, demonstrating the enormous proliferative and differentiative capacity of the few stem cells in the donor bone marrow.

Table 3-1 Normal adult blood-cell counts

Cell type	Cells/mm^3	%
Red blood cells	5.0×10^6	
Platelets	2.5×10^5	
Leukocytes	7.3×10^3	
Neutrophil		50–70
Lymphocyte		20–40
Monocyte		1–6
Eosinophil		1–3
Basophil		<1

Early in hematopoiesis, a pluripotent stem cell differentiates along one of two pathways, giving rise to either a *lymphoid stem cell* or a *myeloid stem cell* (Figure 3-1). Subsequent differentiation of lymphoid and myeloid stem cells generates committed *progenitor cells* for each type of mature blood cell. Progenitor cells have lost the capacity for self-renewal and are committed to a given cell lineage. The lymphoid stem cell generates T and B progenitor lymphocytes. The myeloid stem cell generates progenitor cells for erythrocytes, neutrophils, eosinophils, basophils, monocytes, mast cells, and platelets. Progenitor commitment depends on the acquisition of responsiveness to particular growth factors. When the appropriate growth factors are present, these progenitor cells proliferate and differentiate, giving rise to the corresponding type of mature red or white blood cells. The types and amounts of growth factors present in the microenvironment in which a particular stem cell resides controls its differentiation.

In adult bone marrow, the hematopoietic cells grow and mature on a meshwork of stromal cells, which are nonhematopoietic cells that support the growth and differentiation of the hematopoietic cells. Stromal cells include fat cells, endothelial cells, fibroblasts, and macrophages. Stromal cells influence hematopoietic stem-cell differentiation by providing a hematopoietic-inducing microenvironment consisting of a cellular matrix and either membrane-bound or diffusible growth factors. As hematopoietic stem cells differentiate in this microenvironment, their membranes acquire deformability, allowing the mature cells to pass through the sinusoidal wall into the sinuses of the bone marrow, from whence they enter the circulation.

Spleen Colony-Forming Assay

The earliest evidence proving that the various cell lineages in the bone marrow originate from pluripotent hematopoietic stem cells came from a classic

FIGURE 3-1 Regulation of hematopoiesis by cytokines that stimulate the proliferation and/or differentiation of various hematopoietic cells. In the absence of infection, bone-marrow stromal cells are the major source of hematopoietic cytokines. In the presence of infection, cytokines produced by activated macrophages and T_H cells induce additional hematopoietic activity, resulting in the rapid expansion of the WBC population that is necessary for fighting infection. IL = interleukin; CSF = colony-stimulating factor; EPO = erythropoietin.

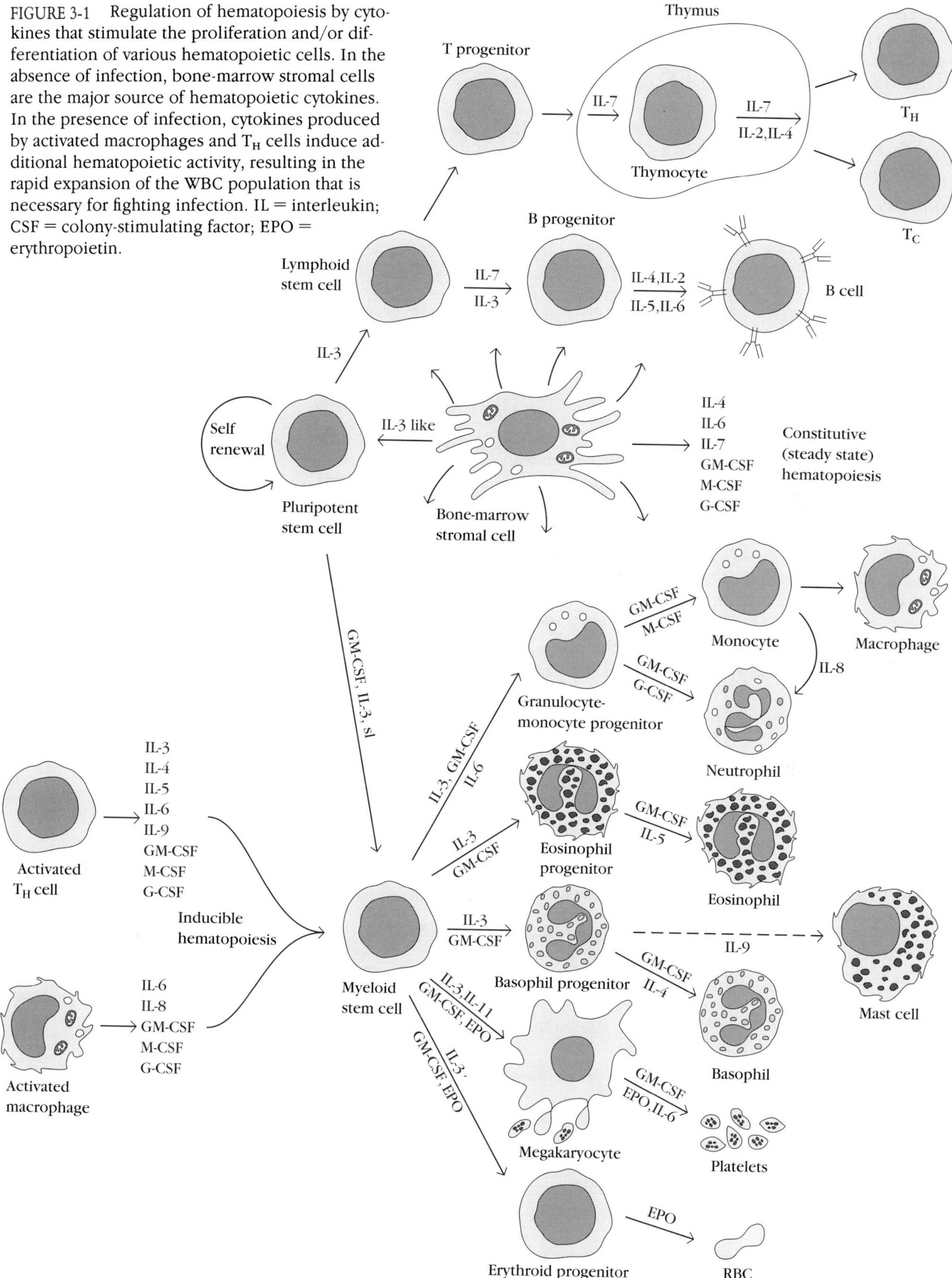

experiment of J. E. Till and E. A. McCulloch in 1961. Their examination of mice lethally irradiated with x-rays revealed extensive cellular loss specifically in the hematopoietic organs; especially noticeable were decreases in the cellular mass of the spleen except for the network of reticular connective cells. When Till and McCulloch injected low numbers of syngeneic bone marrow cells into these irradiated mice, some of these cells were carried to the spleen, where they formed visible nodules on the surface of the spleen, called *colony-forming units-spleen (CFU-S)*. The nodules resulted from clonal expansion of either a single pluripotent stem cell or progenitor cell present in the transplant. Dissection of these nodules revealed that some contained mixtures of differentiated cells: erythrocytes, granulocytes, monocytes, and megakaryocytes.

The actual proof that these differentiated cells were clonal progeny of a single stem cell was obtained in a modified experiment with marked bone marrow cells. Low-level x-irradiation (700 rads) induces random, nonlethal chromosomal damage in some cells; such chromosomal alteration can serve as a marker because all clonal progeny will express the same chromosomal alteration, which is visible by karyotype analysis. Till and McCulloch repeated their experiment, this time injecting low numbers of marked 700-rad x-irradiated bone marrow into the lethally irradiated mice. Examination of the resulting nodules revealed that all the cell types exhibited the identical chromosomal alteration, proving that all the cells were descendants of the same stem cell. Although lymphocytes were not present in the splenic nodules, they were found scattered throughout the spleen and also carried the same chromosomal alteration exhibited by the nodular colonies, proving that they also were derived from a common pluripotent stem cell.

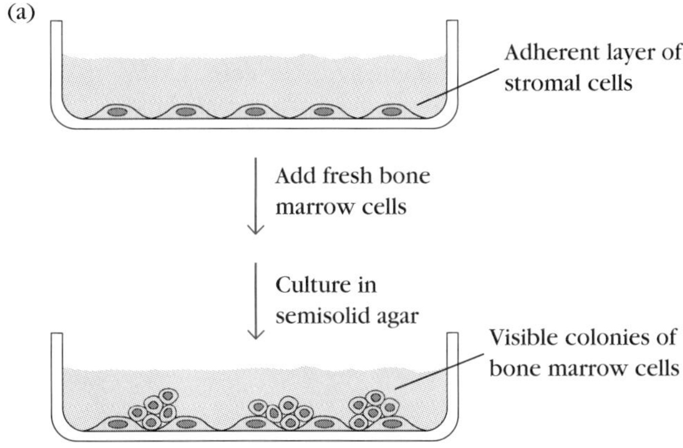

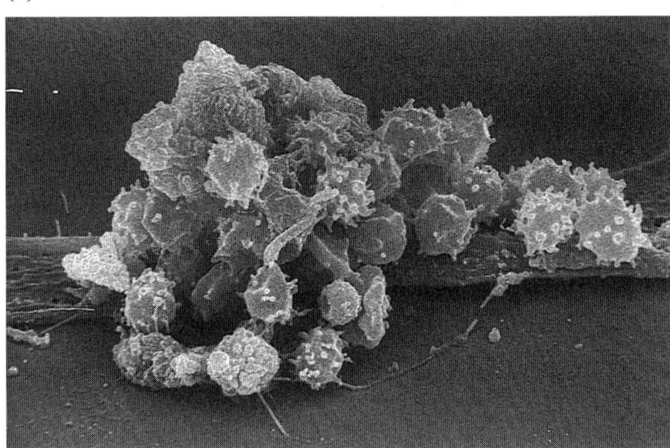

FIGURE 3-2 (a) Experimental scheme for culturing hematopoietic cells. Adherent bone-marrow stromal cells form a matrix on which the hematopoietic cells proliferate. Cells can be transferred to semisolid agar for colony growth, and the colonies analyzed for differentiated cell types. (b) Scanning electron micrograph of cells in long-term culture of human bone marrow. [Photograph from M. J. Cline and D. W. Golde, 1979, *Nature* **277**:180.]

Hematopoietic Growth Factors

Development of cell-culture systems that can support the growth and differentiation of lymphoid and myeloid stem cells led to identification of numerous hematopoietic growth factors. In these in vitro systems, bone-marrow stromal cells are cultured to form a layer of adherent cells; freshly isolated bone-marrow hematopoietic cells placed on this layer will grow and produce large visible colonies (Figure 3-2). If the cells are cultured on semisolid agar, the clonal progeny will be immobilized and can be analyzed for cell types. Colonies containing stem cells can be replated, producing mixed colonies containing a number of differentiated cell types; progenitor cells, which cannot be replated, produce lineage-restricted colonies.

Various growth factors have been shown to be required for the survival, proliferation, differentiation, and maturation of hematopoietic cells in culture. These growth factors, or *cytokines,* originally were detected in serum or in conditioned medium from in vitro cell cultures; they subsequently were defined on the basis of their ability to stimulate the formation of hematopoietic cell colonies in bone marrow cultures. Among the cytokines detected by this method was a family of acidic glycoproteins, the *colony-stimulating factors (CSFs),* named for their ability to induce the formation of distinct hematopoietic cell lineages. Four distinct colony-stimulating factors have been identified: multilineage colony-stimulating factor (multi-CSF), also known as interleukin 3 (IL-3); granulocyte-macrophage colony-stimulating factor (GM-CSF); macrophage colony-stimulating factor (M-CSF); and granulocyte colony-stimulating factor (G-CSF). Another important hematopoietic cytokine detected by this method is a glycoprotein called *erythropoietin*

TABLE 3-2 EFFECT OF CYTOKINES ON HEMATOPOIETIC CELLS

	Cytokines										
Target cells acted on in bone marrow	Multi-CSF (IL-3)	GM-CSF	G-CSF	M-CSF (CSF-1)	IL-4	IL-5	IL-6	IL-7	IL-8	IL-9	EPO
Pluripotent stem cell	+	+	−	−	−	−	−	−	−	−	−
Myeloid stem cell	+	+	−	−	−	−	+	−	−	−	−
Granulocyte-monocyte progenitor	+	+	+	+	−	−	−	−	−	−	−
Monocyte progenitor	+	+	−	+	−	−	−	−	−	−	−
Neutrophil progenitor	+	+	+	−	−	−	−	−	+	−	−
Eosinophil progenitor	+	+	−	−	−	+	−	−	−	−	−
Basophil progenitor	−	+	−	−	+	−	−	−	−	−	−
Mast cell	+	+	−	−	+	−	−	−	−	+	−
Megakaryocyte	+	+	−	−	−	−	−	−	−	−	+/−
Erythroid progenitor	+/−	+/−	−	−	−	−	−	−	−	−	+
Lymphoid stem cell											
B progenitor	−	−	−	−	+	−	−	+	−	−	−
T progenitor (thymus)	−	−	−	−	−	−	−	+	−	−	−

KEY: (+) = indicates cytokine acts on the indicated target cell to stimulate its proliferation and differentiation; (−) = no effect of the cytokine on the indicated cell. See Figure 3-1 for the position of the various target cells in the overall pathway of hematopoiesis.

(EPO); produced by the kidney, this cytokine induces terminal erythrocyte development and regulates red blood cell production. Other cytokines involved in hematopoiesis include interleukin 4 (IL-4), interleukin 5 (IL-5), interleukin 6 (IL-6), interleukin 7 (IL-7), interleukin 8 (IL-8), and interleukin 9 (IL-9). Many of these cytokines are secreted by bone-marrow stromal cells, activated T helper (T_H) cells, and activated macrophages.

Hematopoietic growth factors exert their biological activity at concentrations as low as 10^{-12} *M*, and biochemical purification of these cytokines initially was hampered by their low physiologic concentrations. A major breakthrough came when the genes encoding hematopoietic growth factors were cloned. By transfecting these cloned genes into cultured cells, researchers have obtained sufficient quantities of the various hematopoietic growth to determine their target cells and biological effects (Table 3-2).

The colony-stimulating factors act in a stepwise manner, inducing proper maturation of the hematopoietic cells. Multi-CSF (IL-3) acts early in differentiation, possibly even at the level of the pluripotent stem cell, to induce formation of all the nonlymphoid blood cells, including erythrocytes, monocytes, granulocytes (neutrophils, eosinophils, and basophils), and megakaryocytes. GM-CSF acts at a slightly later stage, but it also induces formation of all the nonlymphoid blood cells. M-CSF and G-CSF act still later to promote the formation of monocytes and neutrophils, respectively. The commitment of a progenitor cell to a given differentiation pathway has been shown to be associated with the expression on the cell of membrane receptors that are specific for particular cytokines. The macrophage progenitor cell, for example, bears specific receptors for M-CSF; the binding of M-CSF to these receptors stimulates cellular proliferation and differentiation in a concentration-dependent manner.

Regulation of Hematopoiesis

Hematopoiesis is a continuous process that generally maintains a steady state in which the production of mature blood cells equals their loss (principally as the cells age). The average erythrocyte has a life span of 120 days before it is phagocytosed and digested by macrophages in the spleen. The various white blood cells have life spans ranging from days for neutrophils to as long as 20–30 years for some T lymphocytes. To maintain steady-state levels, the average human must produce an estimated 3.7×10^{11} cells per day.

Hematopoiesis is regulated by complex mechanisms that affect all of the individual cell types. These regulatory mechanisms provide steady-state levels of the various red and white blood cells and yet have enough built-in flexibility so that production of blood cells can increase rapidly by ten- to twentyfold in response to hemorrhage or infection. Steady-state regulation of hematopoiesis is accomplished by the controlled production of cytokines by bone-marrow stromal cells. These cells have been shown to produce GM-CSF, M-CSF, G-CSF, IL-4, IL-6, and IL-7. Although multi-CSF (IL-3) is the earliest-acting cytokine, it has not been detected in stromal cells, but only in activated T_H cells. It is thought that some other, as yet unidentified, cytokine must be produced by bone-marrow stromal cells to maintain steady-state levels of the pluripotent stem cells.

In response to infections, localized influxes of white blood cells generate an inflammatory reaction that can limit the infection. The hematopoietic system is capable of rapid expansion and maturation of specific cell lineages to provide the necessary cells for such a localized inflammatory response. This inducible hematopoietic activity is regulated by activated T_H cells and activated macrophages, which secrete a number of cytokines that stimulate proliferation and differentiation of different white blood cells involved in the immune response. Among these cytokines are the colony-stimulating factors GM-CSF, G-CSF, and M-CSF, discussed previously, and the following interleukins: IL-3 (multi-CSF), IL-5, and IL-6, which stimulate early hematopoietic progenitor cells; IL-4, which stimulates the B progenitor and mast-cell progenitor; IL-8, which enhances neutrophil activity; and IL-9, which promotes mast-cell growth. The concerted actions of these factors induce localized hematopoietic activity to meet the needs of the immune system to fight infection (see Figure 3-1).

Production of different hematopoietic lineages can be regulated by changes in the local concentrations of cytokines or by differential expression of the receptors for the various cytokines in different lineages. Very little is known about how cytokine concentrations are regulated because the stromal-cell matrix in bone marrow, which creates unique microenvironments for the developing hematopoietic cells, has not been duplicated and studied in vitro. Likewise, although expression of cytokine receptors is known to vary among different hematopoietic lineages, the events determining this differential expression are not understood.

The effect of differential expression of cytokine receptors can be illustrated by the M-CSF receptor. Cells of the erythroid, lymphoid, eosinophilic, and megakaryocytic lineages lack M-CSF receptors, cells of the neutrophilic lineage express low levels of M-CSF receptors, and cells of the monocyte-macrophage lineage express high levels of M-CSF receptors. Since the level of receptor expression governs the responsiveness of a lineage to M-CSF concentrations, only cells of the monocyte-macrophage lineage respond to low concentrations of M-CSF; cells of the neutrophil lineage require much higher concentrations of M-CSF to induce a response, and the other hematopoietic lineages do not respond to M-CSF at all.

The binding of a CSF to its receptor causes some of the receptors to be internalized by the cell; internalization serves to down-modulate receptor expression by the cell. With fewer receptors on its membrane, the cell becomes progressively less responsive to the CSF, and proliferation of the lineage slows down. This down-modulation of CSF-receptor expression can even be induced by the binding of unrelated CSFs to their receptors. For example, when GM-CSF binds to its receptor, it induces the cell to down-modulate the expression of G-CSF and M-CSF receptors as well. This down-modulation of G-CSF and M-CSF receptors causes the lineages bearing these receptors to become less responsive to these CSFs.

Hematopoiesis can also be regulated by degradation of a CSF following its binding to a receptor. Experiments suggest that binding of M-CSF to its receptor results in degradation of the cytokine. As monocyte numbers increase, there is a corresponding increase in M-CSF receptors, leading to increased M-CSF degradation. The concentration of M-CSF would be expected to fall as cell numbers increase, thereby slowing further proliferation and differentiation of this lineage as long as the number of monocytes remains high.

PROGRAMMED CELL DEATH. In order for steady-state levels of the various hematopoietic cells to be maintained, cell division and differentiation in each of the lineages is balanced by a process called *programmed cell death*. Cells undergoing programmed cell death often exhibit distinctive morphologic changes, collectively referred to as *apoptosis* (Figure 3-3). These changes include a pronounced decrease in cell volume, modification of the cytoskeleton resulting in pronounced membrane blebbing, a condensation of the chromatin, and degradation of the DNA into oligonucleosomal fragments. Following these morphologic changes, an apoptotic cell sheds tiny membrane-bound apoptotic bodies containing intact organelles. Macrophages quickly phagocytose apoptotic bodies, ensuring that their intracellular contents, including

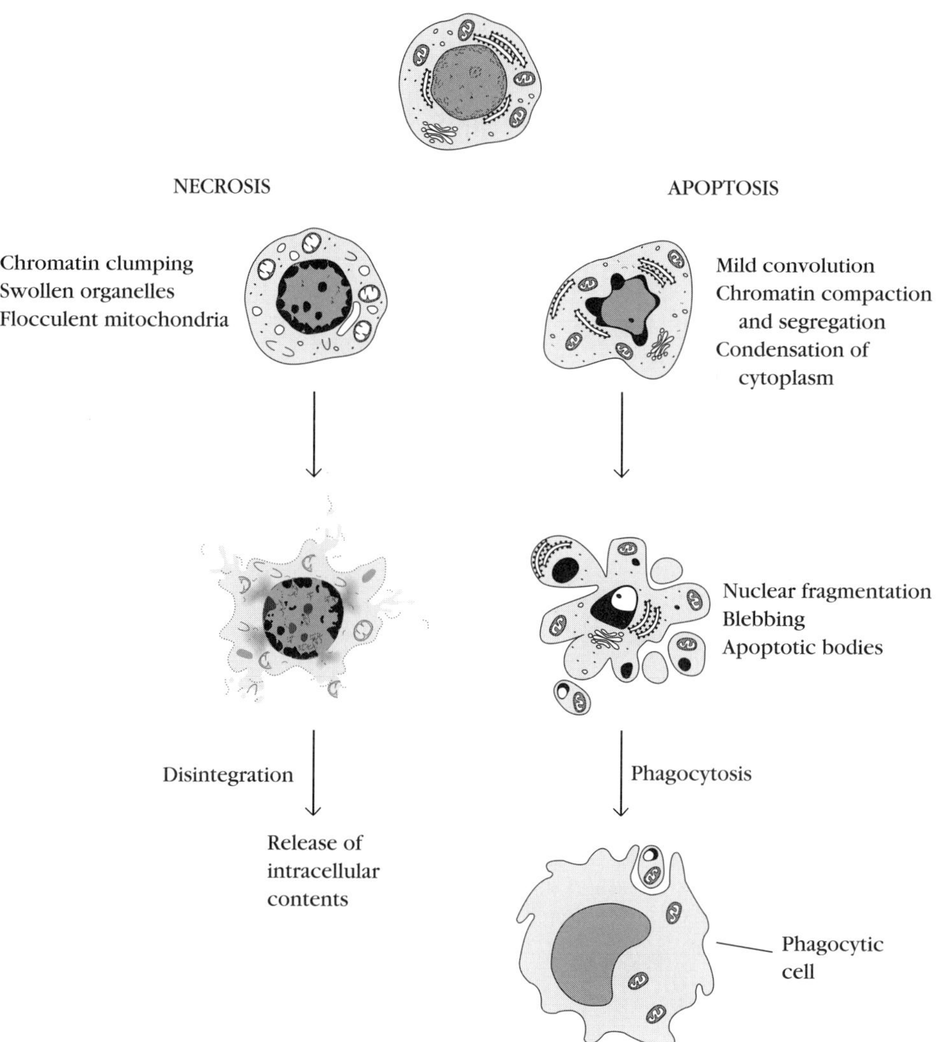

FIGURE 3-3 Comparison of morphologic changes that occur in apoptosis and necrosis. Apoptosis, which is associated with the programmed cell death of hematopoietic cells, does not induce a localized inflammatory response. In contrast, necrosis, the process leading to death of injured cells, results in release of the intracellular contents, which induce a localized inflammatory response.

proteolytic and other lytic enzymes, cationic proteins, and oxidizing molecules are not released into the surrounding tissue. In this way apoptosis occurs without inducing a localized inflammatory response. Apoptosis differs markedly from *necrosis,* the changes associated with cell death arising from injury. In necrosis the injured cell swells and bursts, releasing its intracellular contents, which are cytotoxic to other cells in the tissue; as a result, an inflammatory response develops.

Each of the cells produced by hematopoiesis has a characteristic life span and then dies by programmed cell death. In the adult human, for example, there are about 5×10^{10} neutrophils in the circulation. These cells have a life span of only 1 day and then die by programmed cell death. This death, coupled with constant neutrophil production, maintains steady-state levels of these cells. If programmed cell death fails to occur, a leukemic state may develop. Programmed cell death also plays a role in maintaining proper levels of hematopoietic progenitor cells. For example, when colony-stimulating factors are removed, progenitor cells undergo programmed cell death.

REGULATORY ABNORMALITIES AND LEUKEMIA. Abnormalities in the expression of hematopoietic cytokines or their receptors may result in some leukemias. Colony-stimulating factors are secreted by a limited number of cells, including activated T lymphocytes, macrophages, endothelial cells, and bone-marrow stromal cells. As mentioned above, each factor induces the proliferation and differentiation of only those hematopoietic stem cells that bear its receptor. Expression of the receptor for a growth factor appears to be linked to cellular differentiation following proliferation induced by earlier-acting growth factors. A defect in regulation of expression of either the growth factor or its receptor could lead to unregulated cellular proliferation. Failure to down-modulate receptor expression following GM-CSF activation may lead to a leukemic state. The binding of GM-CSF induces down-modulation of both G-CSF and M-CSF receptors on normal hematopoietic cells but not on leukemic cells (Figure 3-4a,b). This failure of GM-CSF to down-modulate the G-CSF or M-CSF receptors on leukemic cells may allow leukemic cells to respond to low levels of CSFs that would not induce the proliferation of normal down-modulated hematopoietic cells.

Inappropriate expression of a hematopoietic cytokine by a cell bearing a receptor for that cytokine could also lead to unregulated cancerous proliferation. Some findings suggest that this phenomenon occurs in some leukemias. For example, leukemic cells from some patients with acute myeloid leukemia have been shown to secrete GM-CSF, whereas normal myeloid cells do not secrete this growth factor (Figure 3-4c). Similarly, when normal myeloid cell lines bearing receptors for GM-CSF are transfected with cloned GM-CSF cDNA, they autostimulate their own growth in the absence of added GM-CSF (Figure 3-4d); if these transfected cells are injected into mice, the animals develop leukemias. Perhaps the strongest evidence that such abnormal autostimulation can lead to cancerous proliferation comes from the human adult T-cell leukemia associated with the HTLV-1 retrovirus, which infects human T cells and transforms them into leukemic cells. T cells infected with HTLV-1 begin to express the IL-2 receptor in the absence of previous antigen activation. Secretion of IL-2 by these same cells allows unregulated cellular proliferation resulting in leukemia. The molecular basis for this transformation is discussed in detail in Figure 25-4.

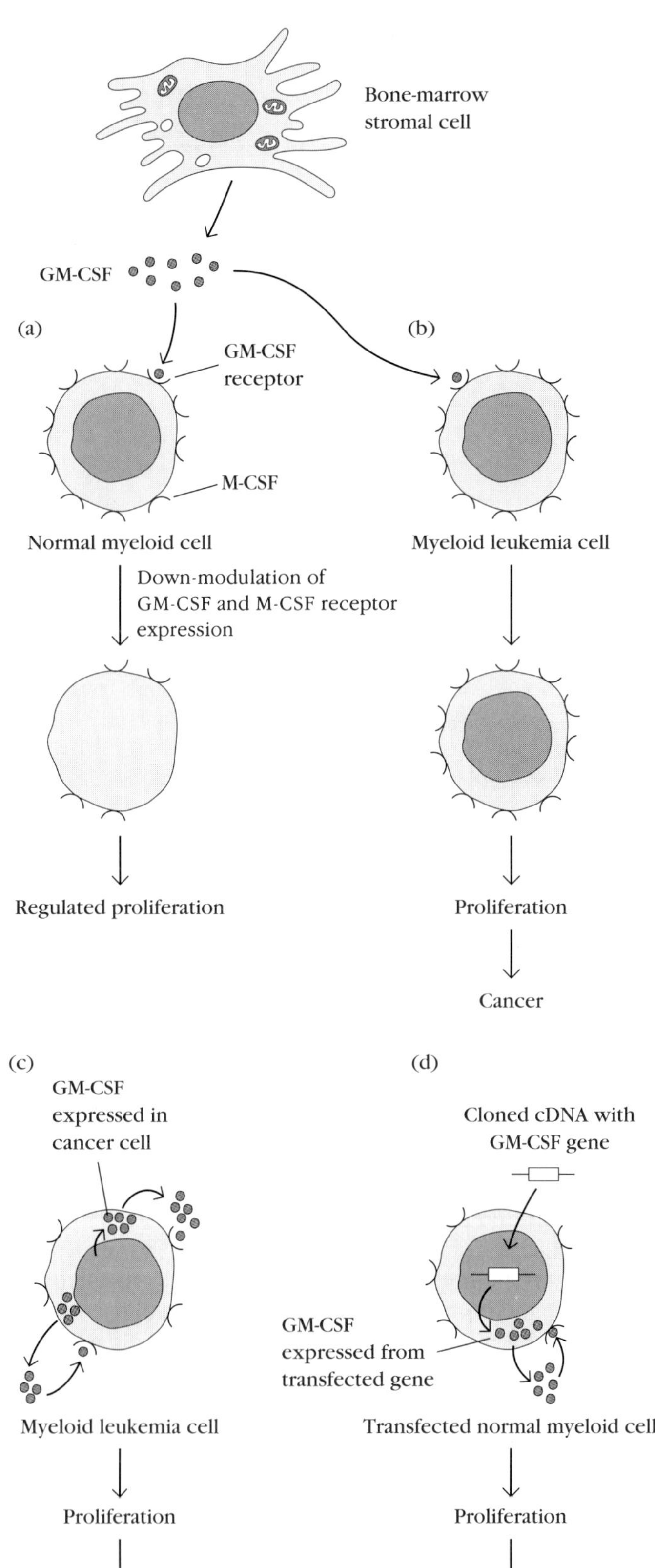

FIGURE 3-4 Possible role of regulatory abnormalities in hematopoiesis in generation of leukemia. (a) Down-modulation of expression of receptors for M-CSF and GM-CSF following GM-CSF activation of a normal myeloid stem cell results in regulated proliferation of monocyte and granulocyte lineages. (b) The absence of this down-modulation in myeloid leukemia cells might lead to leukemia. (c) Secretion of GM-CSF has been demonstrated in some myeloid leukemia cells. Such secretion, which does not occur with normal myeloid cells, might lead to autostimulation and unregulated proliferation. (d) Transfection of cDNA encoding GM-CSF has been shown to cause unregulated proliferation of the transfected cells. Injection of these transfected cells into mice results in leukemia.

Enrichment of Hematopoietic Stem Cells

I. L. Weissman and colleagues developed a novel way of enriching mouse pluripotent stem cells, which constitute only 0.05% of all bone marrow cells in mice. Their approach involved reacting bone marrow samples with fluorescent monoclonal antibodies specific for the differentiation antigens expressed on mature red and white blood cells. The labeled cells were then removed by flow cytometry with a fluorescence-activated cell sorter (Figure 3-5a). After each sorting, the remaining cells were assayed for their ability to restore hematopoiesis in a lethally x-irradiated mouse; this assay indicates the relative number of stem cells in a bone marrow sample. As long as the pluripotent stem cell was being progressively enriched, fewer and fewer cells were needed to restore hematopoiesis in this system. By removing those hematopoietic cells that express known differentiation antigens, these researchers were able to obtain a 50- to 200-fold enrichment of pluripotent stem cells. To further enrich the pluripotent stem cell, the remaining cells were incubated with various monoclonal antibodies raised against cells likely to represent early differentiation stages in hematopoiesis. One of these monoclonal antibodies recognized a differentiation antigen called stem-cell antigen 1 (Sca-1). With this monoclonal antibody, the remaining sample was so enriched in pluripotent stem cells that only 30–100 cells of the sample could restore hematopoiesis in a lethally x-irradiated mouse, whereas $1-3 \times 10^4$ nonenriched bone marrow cells were needed for restoration (Figure 3-5b).

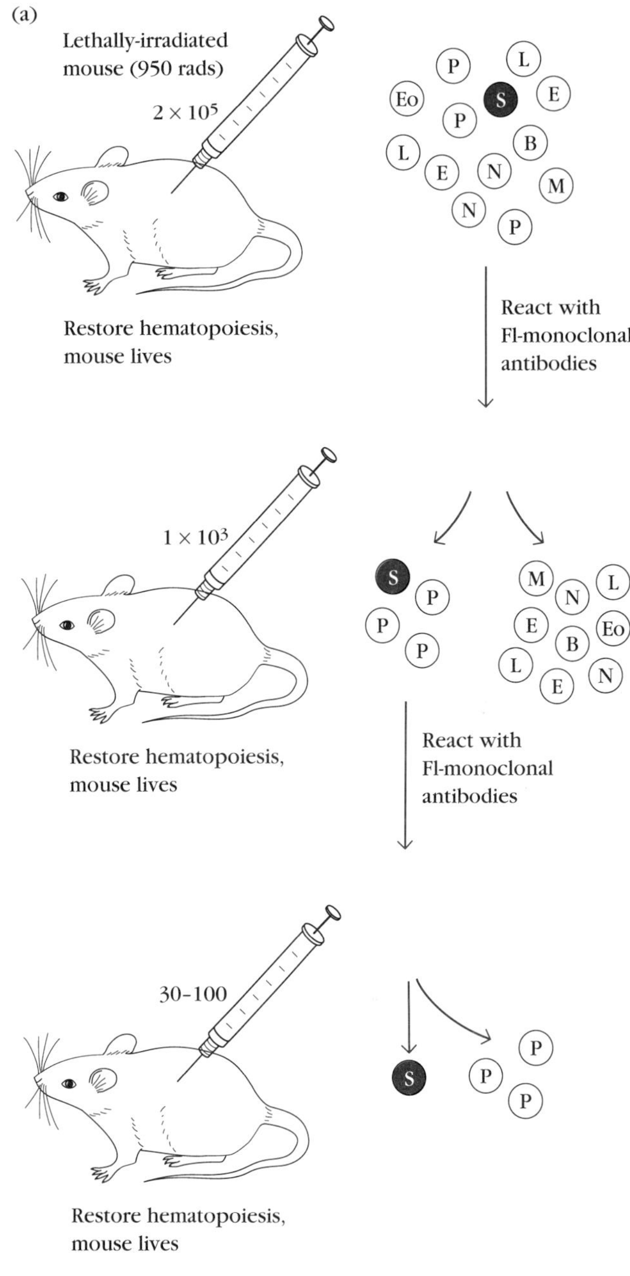

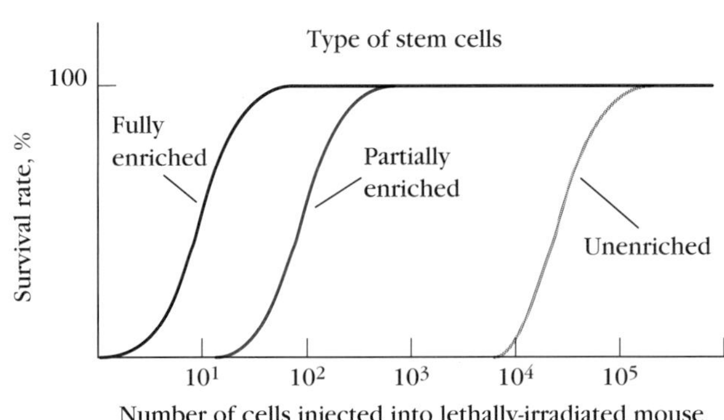

FIGURE 3-5 Enrichment of the pluripotent stem cell has been achieved with monoclonal antibodies specific for membrane molecules expressed on differentiated lineages but absent on undifferentiated lineages. (a) Removal of differentiated hematopoietic cells with monoclonal antibody: M = monocyte, N = neutrophil, L = lymphocyte, Eo = eosinophil, E = erythrocyte, B = basophil. The remaining cells were enriched in stem cells (S) and progenitor cells (P). (b) Assays of stem-cell preparations based on their ability to restore hematopoiesis in lethally irradiated mice. Only animals in which hematopoiesis occurs survive. Progressive enrichment of stem cells is indicated by the decrease in the number of injected cells needed to restore hematopoiesis. The fully enriched preparation was obtained by treating the partially enriched preparation with monoclonal antibody against Sca-1, an early differentiation antigen. A total enrichment of about 1000-fold is possible by this procedure.

Efforts are presently underway to identify and enrich the pluripotent stem cell in humans. One membrane molecule, called CD34, has been shown to be present on a small population (1–3%) of hematopoietic cells that can reconstitute the entire hematopoietic system, suggesting that the pluripotent stem cell is among the $CD34^+$ cell population. The next step is to further enrich the pluripotent stem cell from the $CD34^+$ population. One of the obstacles in identifying and characterizing the human pluripotent stem cell is the lack of an in vivo assay system comparable to that in mice. One experimental system that is being used to study the human pluripotent stem cell is *scid* mice implanted with fragments of human thymus and bone marrow (see Figure 2-1). Different subpopulations of $CD34^+$ human bone marrow cells are injected into these *scid*-human mice, and the development of various lineages of human cells in the bone marrow fragment subsequently is assessed. In the absence of human growth factors, only low numbers of granulocyte-macrophage progenitors develop. However, when human IL-3, GM-CSF, erythropoietin, and mast cell growth factor are administered along with $CD34^+$ cells, progenitor and mature cells of the myeloid, lymphoid, and erythroid lineages develop. This system has enabled researchers to study subpopulations of $CD34^+$ cells and to determine the effect of human growth factors on the differentiation of different hematopoietic lineages.

Clinical Uses of Pluripotent Stem Cells

TRANSPLANTATION OF BONE MARROW. Identification and enrichment of the pluripotent stem cell in humans will have a profound impact on the treatment of blood and immune-system diseases. Individuals with hematopoietic and immune-system dysfunctions caused by congenital disorders, cancer, chemotherapy, or radiation therapy require bone marrow transplants for survival. One problem with bone marrow transplantation is that marrow from an unrelated donor must be carefully matched for identity within the MHC (the probability of such a match is less than one in a million). Even with an MHC match, marrow from an unrelated donor fails to engraft about 10–20% of the time. In addition, the grafted bone marrow can cause graft-versus-host disease (GVHD) in which lymphocytes in the donor bone marrow begin to attack the recipient's cells. Transplantation of stem cells, rather than whole bone marrow, might increase acceptance of the foreign cells and decrease the incidence of GVHD. A recent advance in bone marrow transplantation is the availability of recombinant CSFs. Administration of recombinant GM-CSF or G-CSF along with the donor bone marrow dramatically increases stem-cell engraftment.

With new technologies for freezing human bone marrow in liquid nitrogen, individuals can donate their

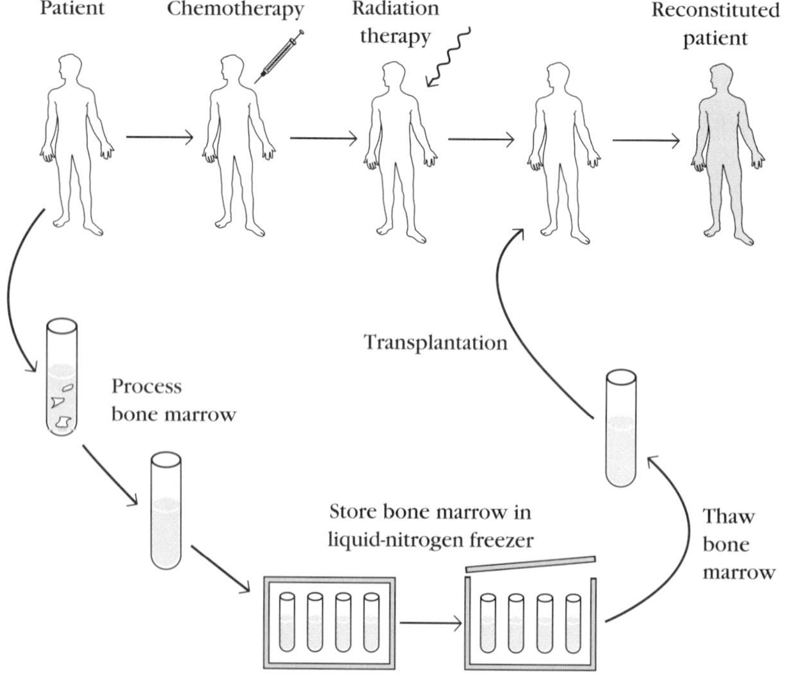

FIGURE 3-6 Autologous transplantation of bone marrow can be used to reconstitute the hematopoietic system of cancer patients whose blood cells have been injured by radiation and/or chemotherapy. Bone marrow is removed from the patient before treatment, stored, and reinfused at a later time. The amount of bone marrow that must be removed would be greatly reduced if a procedure for enriching pluripotent stem cells was available.

own bone marrow and receive it back at a later time. This procedure, known as *autologous transplantation,* has been used with cancer patients, permitting doctors to administer much higher doses of chemotherapy or radiation—doses that destroy the hematopoietic system. The frozen bone marrow is later reinfused into the patient where it reconstitutes the hematopoietic system (Figure 3-6). At the present time large volumes of bone marrow must be extracted and frozen to ensure that sufficient numbers of stem cells are present to reconstitute the hematopoietic system. If techniques for enriching the pluripotent stem cell are developed, autologous transplantation would be feasible with much smaller samples of bone marrow. In May 1992, CellPro Inc. reported successful enrichment of $CD34^+$ stem cells with a monoclonal antibody specific for CD34 (Figure 3-7). In the enrichment procedure used by CellPro, bone marrow is incubated with an anti-CD34 monoclonal antibody that is conjugated to biotin. The marrow cells are then passed through a column containing avidin-coated beads. Since avidin binds to biotin with high affinity, the antibody-coated $CD34^+$ stem cells are retained on the column, while the unlabeled cells pass through. After washing, the stem cells are eluted from the column by mechanical agitation. By using this procedure, CellPro scientists have isolated sufficient numbers of $CD34^+$ stem cells to perform autologous bone marrow transplantation. Clinical trials in patients with metastatic breast cancer and lymphoma are currently underway.

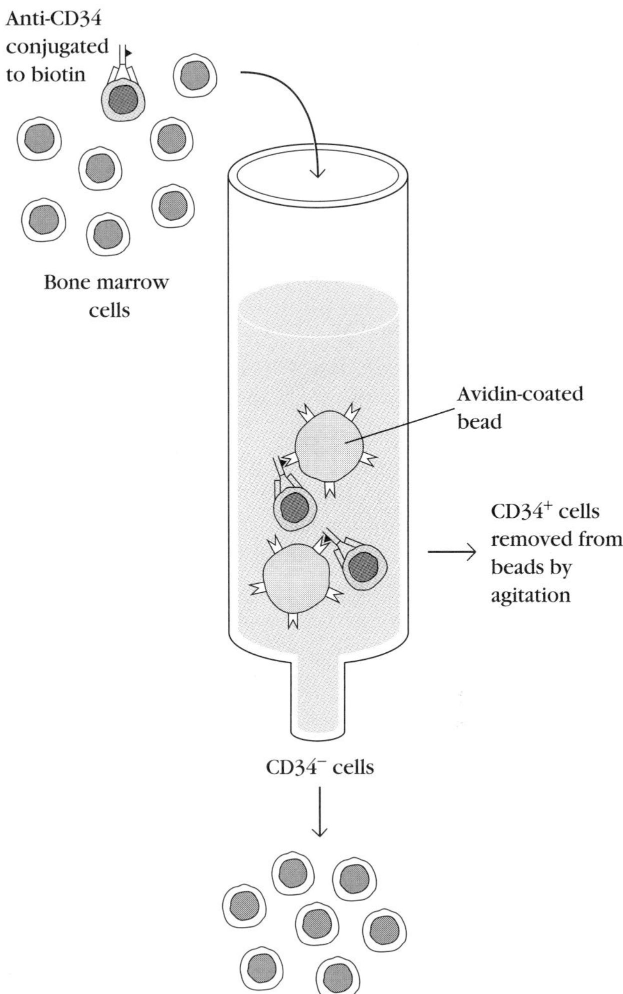

FIGURE 3-7 Enrichment of hematopoietic stem cells by affinity chromatography. CD34 is expressed on stem cells but not on other bone marrow cells. Cells that bind the anti-CD34 monoclonal antibody, which is conjugated to biotin, are retained on a column of avidin-coated beads, since avidin binds strongly to biotin. After the $CD34^-$ cells have passed through the column, the $CD34^+$ stem cells are removed by mechanical agitation.

GENE THERAPY WITH ENGINEERED STEM CELLS. Advances in genetic engineering may soon make gene therapy a realistic treatment for individuals with genetic disorders involving blood cells (e.g., sickle cell anemia, thalassemia, and severe combined immunodeficiency disease). In this approach, hematopoietic stem cells removed from an affected individual would be transfected with functional genes; the engineered stem cells then would be reinjected into the individual. Obviously, the ability to enrich stem cells would be helpful in this type of therapy. In a recent NIH study, $CD34^+$ cells were purified from pooled white blood cells from an individual with severe combined immunodeficiency disease (SCID) resulting from a defective gene encoding adenosine deaminase (ADA). The isolated cells were engineered with a good ADA gene. If some of the engineered $CD34^+$ cells are pluripotential stem cells, then all the white blood cells originating from the stem cells will be healthy. The advantage of using stem cells, rather than mature blood cells, in gene therapy is that they are self-renewing. In theory, patients only have to receive a single injection of engineered stem cells, whereas gene therapy with engineered mature lymphocytes or other blood cells requires periodic injections because these cells are not capable of self-renewal.

Lymphoid Cells

Lymphocytes are the white blood cells responsible for the immune response. Their characteristics account for the immune system's attributes of diversity, specificity, memory, and self/nonself recognition.

Lymphocytes, which constitute 20–40% of the body's white blood cells, circulate in the blood and lymph and are capable of migrating into the tissue spaces and lymphoid organs. The lymphocytes can be broadly subdivided on the basis of function and cell-membrane components into three populations: B cells, T cells, and null cells. All three cell types are small, motile, nonphagocytic cells, which cannot be distinguished morphologically. B and T lymphocytes that have not interacted with antigen—referred to as *virgin, naive,* or *unprimed*—are resting cells in the G_0 phase of the cell cycle. Known as *small lymphocytes,* these cells are only about 6 μm in diameter; their cytoplasm forms a barely discernible rim around the nucleus. Small lymphocytes have densely packed chromatin, few mitochondria, and a poorly developed endoplasmic reticulum and Golgi apparatus. These resting lymphocytes have a short life span (from a few days to a few weeks) and undergo programmed cell death. Interaction of unprimed B or T lymphocytes with antigen, in the presence of certain cytokines discussed later, rescues the cells from programmed cell death. Antigen-activated lymphocytes enter the cell cycle by progressing from G_0 into G_1 and subsequently into S, G_2, and M (Figure 3-8a). As they progress through the cell cycle, lymphocytes enlarge into 15-μm-diameter *blast cells,* called *lymphoblasts;* these cells have a higher cytoplasm : nucleus ratio and more organellar complexity than small lymphocytes.

The lymphoblasts proliferate and eventually differentiate into effector cells or into memory cells. Effector cells have short life spans, generally ranging from a few days to a few weeks. Plasma cells are the effector cell of the B-cell lineage. These cells have a characteristic cytoplasm developed for active secretion with abundant endoplasmic reticulum arranged in concentric layers and many Golgi vesicles (Figure 3-8b). The effector cells of the T-cell lineage include the T_H cell and the cytotoxic T lymphocyte (CTL). The memory cells are long-lived cells that reside in the G_0 phase of the cell cycle until activated by a secondary encounter with antigen.

Different lineages or maturational stages of lymphocytes can be distinguished by their expression of membrane molecules recognized by particular monoclonal antibodies. At first each membrane molecule identified by a particular monoclonal antibody was named by the individual researchers. This led to a plethora of designations for the same membrane molecule. In 1982 the First International Workshop on Human Leukocyte Differentiation Antigens was held to develop a uniform nomenclature for leukocyte membrane molecules. As a result of this workshop, all of the monoclonal antibodies that react with a particular membrane molecule were grouped together as a *cluster of differentiation (CD).* New monoclonal antibodies that recognize leukocyte membrane molecules are analyzed to determine if they fall within a given CD designation or are given a new CD designation if they identify a new membrane molecule. Although the CD nomenclature was originally developed for human leukocyte membrane molecules, the homologous membrane molecules found in other species, such as mice, are commonly referred to by the same CD designations. Table 3-3 lists some common CD molecules found on human lymphocytes.

The general characteristics and functions of B and T lymphocytes were discussed in Chapter 1 and are reviewed briefly in the following sections. These central cells of the immune system are examined in more detail in later chapters.

B Lymphocytes

The B lymphocyte derived its name from its site of maturation in the bursa of Fabricius in birds; the name turned out to be apt, for its major site of maturation in mammals is the bone marrow. Mature B cells can be distinguished from other lymphocytes by the presence of membrane-bound immunoglobulin (antibody) molecules, which serve as receptors for antigen. There are approximately 1.5×10^5 molecules of antibody on the membrane of a single B cell, with each molecule having an identical binding site for antigen. A number of other molecules are expressed on the membrane of the B cell (Figure 3-9a). A membrane molecule designated B220 (or CD45) is a marker of the B-cell lineage, first appearing during maturation on the precursor B cell and remaining throughout the life span of the B cell. Since the majority of B cells express class II MHC molecules, the cell is also classified as an antigen-presenting cell (APC). Mature B cells also express receptors for complement: CR1 (CD35), which binds to C3b, and CR2 (CD21), which binds to C3d. Receptors for the Fc portion of IgG, called FcγRII (CD32) are also expressed on the membrane of the B cell.

Appropriate interaction between antigen and the membrane-bound antibody on a naive B cell, together with T-cell and macrophage interactions, induces clonal selection of the B cell. In this process, the B cell divides repeatedly and differentiates, over a 4- to 5-day period generating a population of plasma cells and memory cells (see Figure 1-11). Plasma cells, which lack membrane-bound antibody, actively secrete one of the five classes of antibody. All clonal progeny from a given B cell secrete antibody molecules with the same antigen-binding specificity. Production of the memory cell is somewhat controversial. Some theories suggest that unequal division of an activated B cell generates both plasma and memory cells. Other

(a)

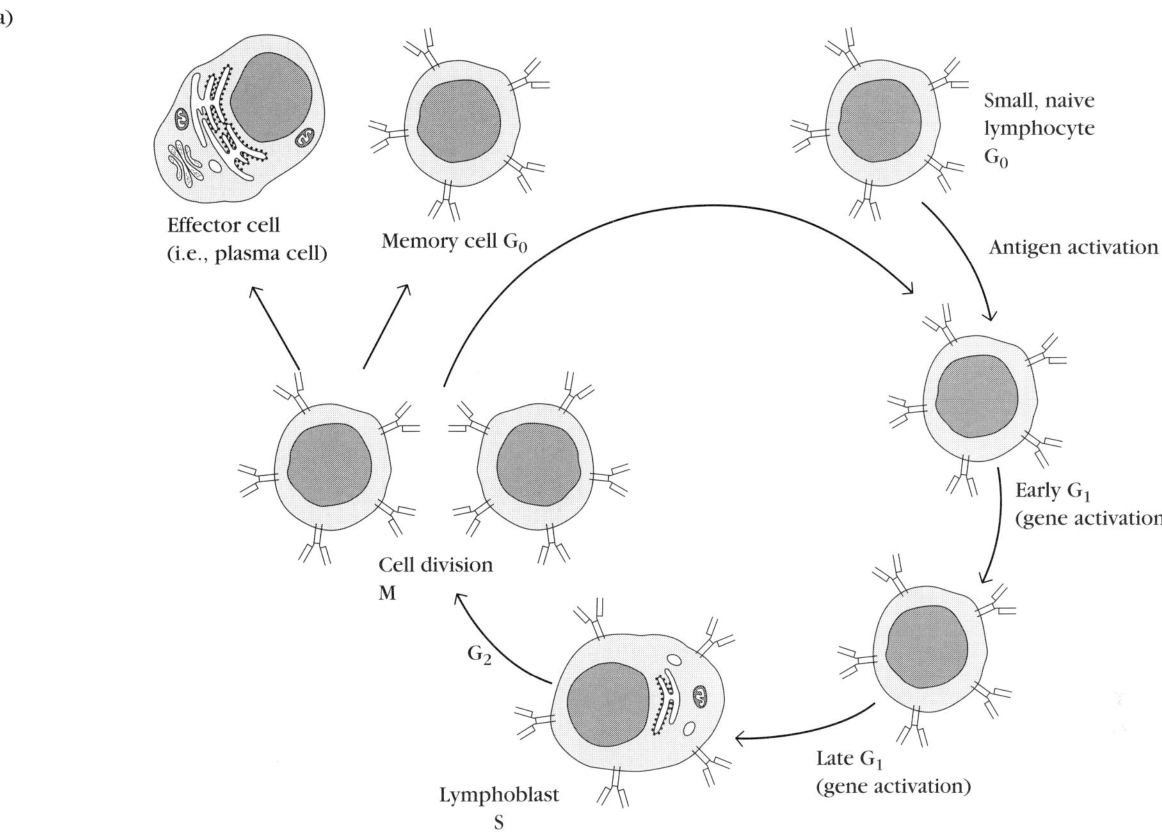

(b)

Small lymphocyte (T or B)
6 μm diameter

Blast cell (T or B)
15 μm diameter

Plasma cell (B)
15 μm diameter

FIGURE 3-8 Fate of antigen-activated small lymphocytes. (a) A small resting (unprimed) lymphocyte resides in the G_0 phase of the cell cycle. At this stage, B and T lymphocytes cannot be distinguished morphologically. Following antigen activation, a B or T cell enters the cell cycle and enlarges into a lymphoblast, which undergoes several rounds of cell division and eventually generates effector cells and memory cells. (b) Electron micrographs of a small lymphocyte *(left)* showing condensed chromatin indicative of a resting cell, an enlarged lymphoblast *(center)* showing decondensed chromatin, and a plasma cell *(right)* showing abundant endoplasmic reticulum arranged in concentric circles. The three cells are shown at different magnifications. [Part (b) courtesy of Dr. Joseph R. Goodman, Dept. of Pediatrics, University of California at San Francisco.]

TABLE 3-3 COMMON CD ANTIGENS USED TO DISTINGUISH FUNCTIONAL LYMPHOCYTE SUBPOPULATIONS

		B cell	T cell		NK cell
CD designation*	Function		T_H	T_C	
CD2	Adhesion molecule; signal transduction	−	+	+	+
CD3	Signal transduction element of T-cell receptor	−	+	+	−
CD4	Adhesion molecule that binds to class II MHC molecules; signal transduction	−	+ (usually)	− (usually)	−
CD5	Unknown	+ (subset)	+	+	−
CD8	Adhesion molecule that binds to class I MHC molecules; signal transduction	−	− (usually)	+ (usually)	+ (variable)
CD11a/CD18 (LFA-1)	Adhesion molecule that binds to ICAM-1 and ICAM-2	+	+	+	+
CD16 (FcγRIII)	Low-affinity receptor for Fc region of IgG	−	−	−	+
CD21 (CR2)	Receptor for complement (C3d) and Epstein-Barr virus	+	−	−	−
CD28	Receptor for co-stimulatory B7 molecule on antigen-presenting cells	−	+	+	−
CD32 (FcγRII)	Receptor for Fc region of IgG	+	−	−	−
CD35 (CR1)	Receptor for complement (C3b)	+	−	−	−
CD40	Signal transduction	+	−	−	−
CD45	Signal transduction	+	−	−	−
CD45R	Signal transduction	−	+	+	−
CD54 (ICAM-1)	Adhesion molecule that binds to CD11a/CD18 (LFA-1)	+	+	+	+
CD56	Adhesion molecule	−	−	−	+

* Synonyms are shown in parentheses.

theories suggest that the memory B cell may be a separate lineage which clonally expands following primary antigen exposure. This is discussed in Chapter 14.

T Lymphocytes

T lymphocytes derive their name from their site of maturation in the thymus. Like B lymphocytes, these cells have membrane receptors for antigen. The T-cell receptor for antigen is structurally distinct from immunoglobulin but does have some structural features in common with the immunoglobulin molecule, most notably in the structure of its antigen-binding site. What distinguishes the T-cell receptor from membrane-bound antibody on B cells is that it recognizes antigen only when the antigen is associated with a self-molecule encoded by genes within the major histocompatibility complex (MHC). This points to a fundamental difference between humoral and cell-mediated branches of the immune system. Whereas the B cell is capable of binding soluble antigen, the T-cell system is restricted to binding antigen displayed on self-cells. This antigen may be displayed together with MHC molecules on the surface of antigen-presenting cells or on virus-infected cells, cancer cells, and grafts.

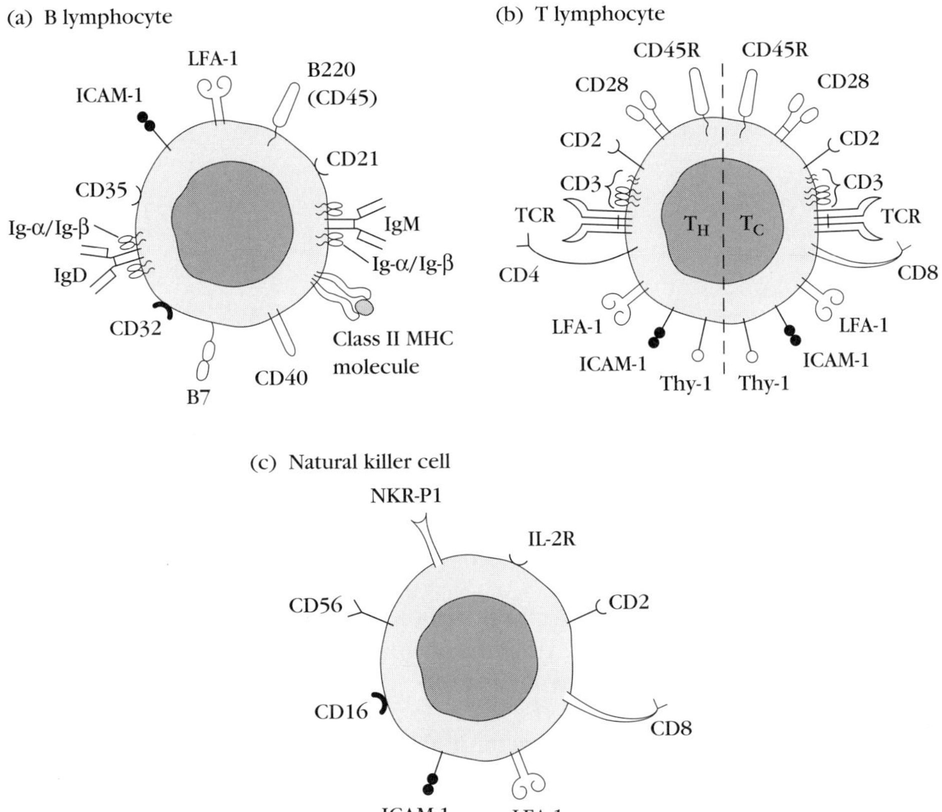

FIGURE 3-9 Schematic representation of some common membrane molecules present on mature lymphocytes and natural killer (NK) cells. Molecules involved in specific binding of antigen are shown in purple. CD16 (FcγRIII) on NK cells and CD32 (FcγRII) on B cells are receptors for the Fc region of IgG. CD21 and CD35 on B cells are receptors for complement components. Most T_H cells express CD4, whereas most T_C cells express CD8 (as do some NK cells).

The T-cell system has developed to eliminate these altered self-cells, which pose a threat to the normal functioning of the body.

Like B cells, T cells express distinctive membrane molecules (Figure 3-9b). The earliest marker of the T-cell lineage to appear is Thy-1, which is first expressed during T-cell maturation in the thymus and remains throughout the life span of the cell. All T-cell subpopulations express the T-cell receptor, but they can be distinguished by the presence of one or the other of two membrane molecules, CD4 and CD8. T cells that express CD4 recognize antigen associated with class II MHC molecules, whereas T cells expressing CD8 recognize antigen associated with class I MHC molecules. Thus the expression of CD4 versus CD8 corresponds to the MHC restriction of the T cell. In general, expression of CD4 and of CD8 also defines two major functional subpopulations of T lymphocytes. The $CD4^+$ T cells generally function as T helper (T_H) cells and are class II restricted; $CD8^+$ T cells generally function as T cytotoxic (T_C) cells and are class I restricted. T_H cells proliferate extensively following recognition of an antigen–class II MHC complex on an antigen-presenting cell. T_H cells secrete a variety of cytokines, sometimes called *lymphokines,* which play a central role in the activation of B cells, T_C cells, and a variety of other cells that participate in the immune response. The T_C cell is activated by interaction with an antigen–class I MHC complex on the surface of an altered self-cell (e.g., virus-infected cell) in the presence of appropriate cytokines (see Figure 1-14). This activation generates *cytotoxic T lymphocytes* (CTLs), which mediate killing of altered self-cells. By determining the number of $CD4^+$ and $CD8^+$ T cells, the ratio of T_H to T_C cells can be ascertained. This ratio is approximately 2:1 in normal human peripheral blood. This ratio may be significantly altered in immunodeficiency diseases, autoimmune diseases, and other disorders.

Another subpopulation of T lymphocytes—called *T suppressor (T_S)* cells—has been postulated. It is clear that some T cells mediate suppression of the humoral and the cell-mediated branches of the immune system, but no actual T_S cell has been isolated and cloned. For this reason, immunologists are still unsure whether T_S cells constitute a separate subpopulation or whether the observed suppression is simply the result of suppressive activities of the T_H and T_C subpopulations. The T_S cell is examined in more detail in Chapter 16.

The classification of $CD4^+$, class II-restricted cells as T_H cells and $CD8^+$, class I-restricted cells as T_C cells is not absolute. Instead, some functional T_H cells have been shown to express CD8 and recognize antigen associated with class I MHC, and some functional T_C cells are class II restricted and express CD4. Even the functional classification is not absolute. For example, many T_C cells have been shown to secrete a variety of cytokines and exert effects on other cells comparable to that exerted by T_H cells. The distinction between T_H and T_C cells, then, is not always clear; there can be ambiguous functional activities. However, because these ambiguities are the exception and not the rule, the general description of T helper cells as being $CD4^+$ and class II restricted and of T cytotoxic cells as being $CD8^+$ and class I restricted is adhered to, unless otherwise specified, throughout this text.

Null Cells

A small group of peripheral-blood lymphocytes, called null cells, fail to express the membrane molecules that distinguish T and B lymphocytes (Figure 3-9c). These cells also fail to display antigen-binding receptors of either the T- or B-cell lineage and therefore lack the attributes of immunologic specificity and memory. One functional population of null cells called *natural killer (NK)* cells are large, granulated lymphocytes; these cells constitute 5–10% of the peripheral-blood lymphocytes in humans.

The natural killer cell was first described in 1976, when it was shown that certain null cells display cytotoxic activity against a wide range of tumor cells in the absence of any previous immunization with the tumor. NK cells were subsequently shown to play an important role in host defense against tumor cells. NK cells can interact with tumor cells in two different ways. In some cases, an NK cell makes direct membrane contact with a tumor cell in a nonspecific, antibody-independent process. Some NK cells, however, express CD16, a membrane receptor for the carboxyl-terminal end of the antibody molecule. These NK cells can bind to antitumor antibodies bound to the surface of tumor cells and subsequently destroy the tumor; this specific process is called *antibody-dependent cell-mediated cytotoxicity*. The exact mechanism of tumor-cell killing by NK cells, the focus of much current experimental study, is discussed further in Chapter 15.

Several lines of evidence suggest that NK cells play an important role in host defense against tumors. For example, in humans, Chédiak-Higashi syndrome—an autosomal recessive disorder—is associated with an absence of NK cells and an increased incidence of lymphomas. Likewise, mice with an autosomal mutation called *biege* lack NK cells; these mutants are more susceptible than normal mice to tumor growth following injection with live tumor cells.

Mononuclear Cells

The mononuclear phagocytic system consists of circulating monocytes in the blood and macrophages in the tissues. During hematopoiesis in the bone marrow, granulocyte-monocyte progenitor cells differentiate into promonocytes, which leave the bone marrow and enter the blood, where they further differentiate into mature monocytes. Monocytes circulate in the bloodstream for about 8 h, during which time they enlarge; they then migrate into the tissues and differentiate into specific tissue macrophages.

Differentiation of a monocyte into a tissue macrophage involves a number of changes: The cell enlarges five- to tenfold; its intracellular organelles increase in both number and complexity; and it acquires increased phagocytic ability, produces higher levels of lytic enzymes, and begins to secrete a variety of soluble factors (Figure 3-10). Macrophages are dispersed throughout the body. Some take up residence in particular tissues becoming *fixed macrophages,* whereas others remain motile and are called *free,* or wandering, *macrophages.* Free macrophages move by amoeboid movement throughout the tissues. Fixed macrophages serve different functions in different tissues and are named to reflect their tissue location. In the liver they are called *Kupffer cells;* in the connective tissues, *histiocytes;* in the lung, *alveolar macrophages;* in the kidney, *mesangial cells,* and in the brain, *microglial cells.*

Macrophages are normally in a resting state, but in the course of an immune response, a variety of stimuli activate macrophages. Phagocytosis of particulate antigens serves as an initial activating stimulus. However, macrophage activity can be further enhanced by cytokines secreted by activated T_H cells, by mediators of the inflammatory response, and by bacterial cell-wall products. One of the most potent activators of macrophages is interferon gamma (IFN-γ) secreted by activated T_H cells. Compared with resting macrophages, activated macrophages have increased phagocytic activity, increased microbicidal activity, increased secretion of inflammatory mediators, and an increased ability to activate T cells. This increased activity enables these cells to more effectively eliminate potential pathogens. In addition, activated macrophages secrete various cytotoxic proteins that help them eliminate a broad range of pathogens, including virus-infected cells, tumor cells, and intracellular bacteria. Activated macrophages also express higher levels of class II MHC molecules, allowing them to function more effectively as antigen-presenting cells. Thus macrophages and T_H cells exhibit an interacting relationship during the immune response with each facilitating activation of the other.

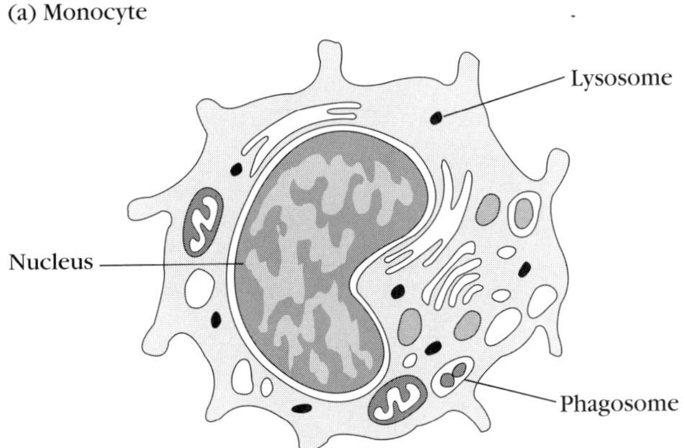

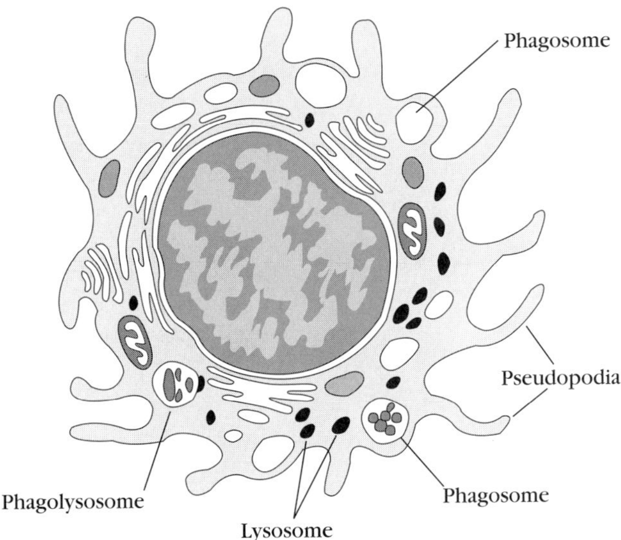

FIGURE 3-10 Drawings showing typical morphology of a monocyte and macrophage. Macrophages are five- to tenfold larger than monocytes and contain more organelles, especially lysosomes.

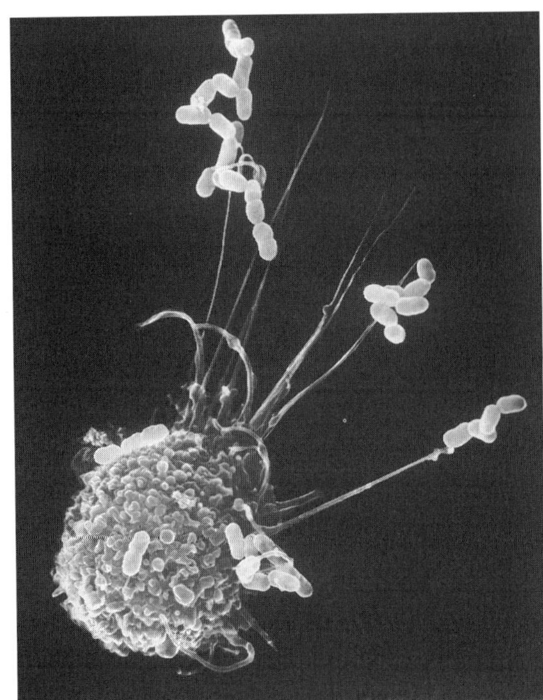

FIGURE 3-11 Scanning electron micrograph of a macrophage. Note the long pseudopodia extending toward and making contact with bacterial cells, an early step in phagocytosis. [Photograph by Lennart Nilsson; courtesy of Boehringer Ingelheim International GmbH.]

Phagocytosis

Macrophages are actively phagocytic cells capable of ingesting and digesting exogenous antigens such as whole microorganisms, insoluble particles, injured and dead host cells, cellular debris, and activated clotting factors. In the first step in phagocytosis, macrophages are attracted by and move toward a variety of substances generated in an immune response; this process is called *chemotaxis.* The next step in phagocytosis involves *adherence* of the antigen to the macrophage cell membrane. (Complex antigens, such as whole bacterial cells or viral particles, tend to adhere well and are readily phagocytosed; isolated proteins and encapsulated bacteria tend to adhere poorly and are less readily phagocytosed.) Adherence induces membrane protrusions, called *pseudopodia,* to extend around the attached material (Figure 3-11). The pseudopodia fuse enclosing the material within a membrane-bound structure called a *phagosome,* which then enters the endocytic processing pathway. In this pathway, a phagosome moves toward the cell interior, where it fuses with a *lysosome* to form a *phagolysosome.* Lysosomes contain hydrogen peroxide, oxygen free radicals, peroxidase, lysozyme, and various hydrolytic enzymes, which digest the ingested material. The digested contents of the phagolysosome are then eliminated in a process called *exocytosis* (Figure 3-12).

The phagocytic rate can be increased substantially in the presence of *opsonins,* which are molecules that bind to antigen and to macrophages. The macrophage membrane possesses receptors for certain classes of antibody and certain complement components. When an antigen (e.g., a bacterium) is coated with the appropriate antibody or complement component, it binds more readily to the macrophage membrane; as a result,

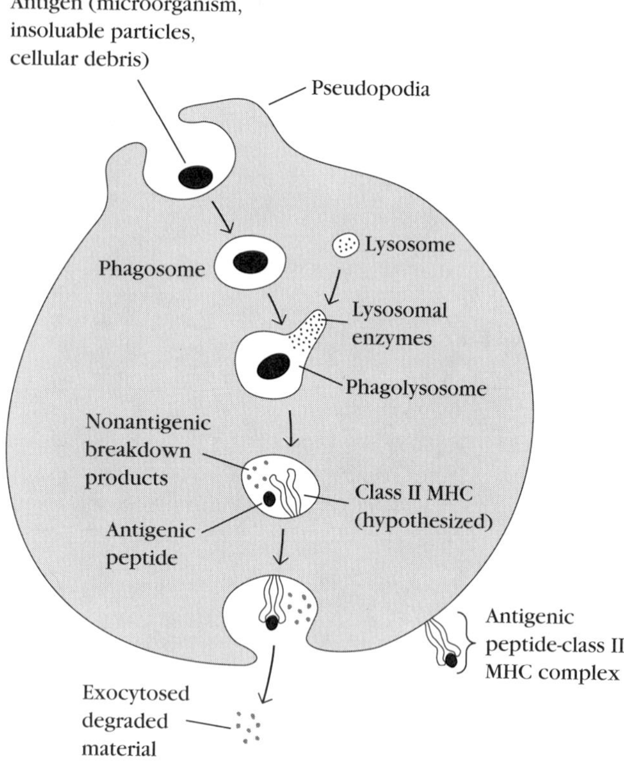

FIGURE 3-12 Phagocytosis and processing of exogenous antigen by macrophages. Following adherence of antigen to the macrophage membrane, long pseudopodia surround the attached material. Fusion of pseudopodia draws the material into the cell, forming a membrane-bound phagosome. Fusion of the phagosome with a lysosome produces a phagolysosome and results in release of the lysosomal contents. Most of the products from digestion of the ingested material are exocytosed. Some of the digested peptides are thought to interact with class II MHC molecules. The resulting antigenic peptide–class II MHC complexes then move to the cell surface where they are presented to T_H cells.

phagocytosis is enhanced. Thus antibody and complement function as opsonins; the entire process is called *opsonization*. In one study the rate of phagocytosis of an antigen was 4000-fold higher in the presence of specific antibody to the antigen than in its absence.

Antimicrobial and Cytotoxic Activities

A number of antimicrobial and cytotoxic substances produced by activated macrophages are responsible for the intracellular destruction of phagocytosed microorganisms (Table 3-4). In addition, these toxic substances can be released from macrophages to mediate potent antitumor activity. The toxic effects of these substances involve both oxygen-dependent and oxygen-independent mechanisms.

OXYGEN-DEPENDENT KILLING MECHANISMS. Activated phagocytes produce a number of *reactive oxygen intermediates* (ROIs) and *reactive nitrogen intermediates* (RNIs) that have potent antimicrobial activity. During phagocytosis a metabolic process known as the respiratory burst occurs in activated macrophages. This process results in the activation of a membrane-bound oxidase that catalyzes the reduction of oxygen to superoxide anion ($O_2^{\cdot -}$), a reactive oxygen intermediate that is extremely toxic to ingested microorganisms.

$$NAD(P)H + 2O_2 \rightarrow 2O_2^{\cdot -} + NAD(P) + H^+$$

The superoxide anion also generates other powerful oxidizing agents including hydroxyl radicals ($OH^{\cdot}$), singlet oxygen ($^1O_2$), and hydrogen peroxide (H_2O_2). As the lysosome fuses with the phagosome, myeloperoxidase together with a halide ion act on the hydrogen

TABLE 3-4 MEDIATORS OF ANTIMICROBIAL AND CYTOTOXIC ACTIVITY OF MACROPHAGES AND NEUTROPHILS

Oxygen-dependent killing	Oxygen-independent killing
Reactive oxygen intermediates	Defensins
$O_2^{\cdot -}$ (superoxide anion)	Tumor necrosis factor (macrophage only)
$OH^{\cdot}$ (hydroxyl radicals)	Lysozyme
$^1O_2$ (singlet oxygen)	Hydrolytic enzymes
H_2O_2 (hydrogen peroxide)	
HOCl (hypochlorous acid)	
NH_2Cl (monochloramine)	
Reactive nitrogen intermediates	
NO (nitric oxide)	
NO_2 (nitrogen dioxide)	
HNO_2 (nitrous acid)	

peroxide to produce longer-lived oxidants, including hypochlorite, which are toxic.

When macrophages are activated with bacterial cell-wall lipopolysaccharide (LPS) or muramyl dipeptide (MDP) together with a T-cell–derived cytokine (IFN-γ), they begin to express high levels of nitric oxide synthetase, which oxidizes L-arginine to yield citrulline and a reactive radical, nitric oxide (NO). Although NO itself has potent antimicrobial activity, it can combine with the superoxide anion ($O_2^{\cdot -}$) to yield even more potent antimicrobial substances. Recent evidence suggests that much of the antimicrobial activity of macrophages against bacterial, fungal, helminthic, and protozoal pathogens is due to NO and NO-derived substances.

OXYGEN-INDEPENDENT KILLING MECHANISMS. Activated macrophages contain lysozyme and hydrolytic enzymes whose degradative activities do not involve oxygen. A group of antimicrobial and cytotoxic peptides, commonly known as *defensins,* also are present in activated macrophages. These molecules are cysteine-rich cationic peptides of 29–35 amino acid residues. Each peptide contains six invariant cysteines, which form three intramolecular disulfide bonds. The disulfide bond between the amino-terminal and carboxy-terminal cysteine forms a circular molecule that is stabilized by the other two disulfide bonds into a folded triple-stranded β-sheet configuration. These circularized defensin peptides have been shown to form ion-permeable channels in bacterial and mammalian cell membranes. Defensins can kill a variety of bacteria including *Staphylococcus aureus, Streptococcus pneumoniae, Escherichia coli, Pseudomonas aeruginosa,* and *Hemophilus influenzae.*

RESISTANT PATHOGENS. Most phagocytosed microorganisms are killed as the contents of the lysosome are released into the phagosome. Some microorganisms, however, can survive and multiply within macrophages. These intracellular pathogens include *Listeria monocytogenes, Salmonella typhimurium, Neisseria gonorrhoea, Mycobacterium avium, Mycobacterium tuberculosis, Mycobacterium leprae, Brucella abortus,* and *Candida albicans.* Some of these pathogens prevent lysosome-phagosome fusion and proliferate within phagosomes; others have cell-wall components that render them resistant to the contents of lysosomes; and still others survive by escaping from phagosomes and proliferating within the cytoplasm of infected macrophages. These intracellular pathogens, which have developed a clever defense against the nonspecific phagocytic defense system, are shielded from a specific immunologic response. A unique cell-mediated immunologic defense mechanism, called delayed hypersensitivity, combats such pathogens; this mechanism is discussed Chapter 15.

Antigen Processing and Presentation

Not all of the antigen ingested by macrophages is degraded and eliminated by exocytosis. Experiments with radiolabeled antigens have demonstrated the presence of labeled antigen components on the macrophage membrane after most of the antigen has been digested and eliminated. As discussed in Chapter 1, phagocytosed antigen is degraded within the endocytic processing pathway into peptides that associate with class II MHC molecules; these peptide–class II MHC complexes then move to the macrophage membrane (see Figure 3-12). This presentation of antigen is a critical requirement for the activation of T_H cells, a central event in the development of both humoral and cell-mediated immune responses. The processing and presentation of antigen are examined in detail in Chapter 10.

Secretion of Factors

A number of important proteins central to development of immune responses are secreted by activated macrophages (Table 3-5). These include interleukin 1

TABLE 3-5 SOME FACTORS SECRETED BY ACTIVATED MACROPHAGES

Factor	Function
Interleukin 1 (IL-1)	Induces activation of T_H cells following interaction with antigen-MHC complexes; promotes inflammatory response and fever
Complement proteins	Promote elimination of pathogens and inflammatory response
Hydrolytic enzymes	Promote inflammatory response
Interferon alpha (IFN-α)	Activates cellular genes resulting in the production of proteins that confer an antiviral state on the cell
Tumor necrosis factor (TNF-α)	Kills tumor cells
Interleukin 6 (IL-6) GM-CSF G-CSF M-CSF	Promote inducible hematopoiesis

(IL-1), which acts on T_H cells and provides a costimulatory signal required for activation following antigen recognition. Interleukin 1 also acts on vascular endothelial cells, thus influencing the inflammatory response, and affects the thermoregulatory center in the hypothalamus, leading to the fever response.

Activated macrophages secrete a variety of other factors involved in the development of an inflammatory response. These include a group of serum proteins, called *complement,* that assist in the elimination of foreign pathogens and in the ensuing inflammatory reaction. The *hydrolytic enzymes* contained within their lysosomes can also be secreted by activated macrophages. The buildup of these enzymes within the tissues contributes to the inflammatory response and can, in some cases, lead to extensive tissue damage. Activated macrophages also secrete soluble factors, such as *tumor necrosis factor α (TNF-α),* that can kill a variety of cells. The secretion of these *cytotoxic factors* has been shown to contribute to tumor destruction by macrophages. Finally, as discussed earlier, activated macrophages secrete a number of cytokines that stimulate inducible hematopoiesis.

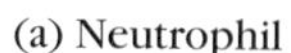

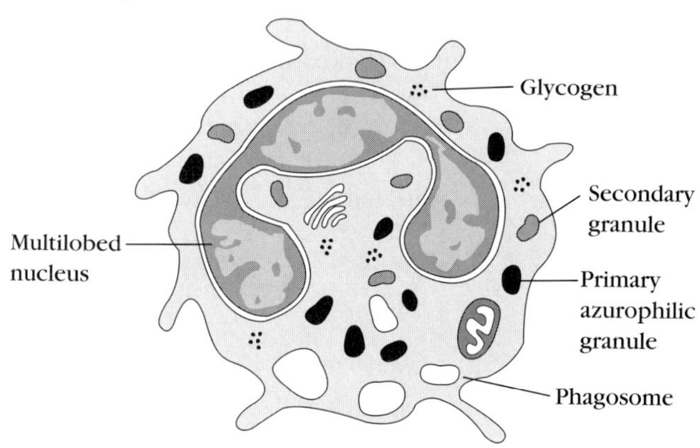

(b) Eosinophil

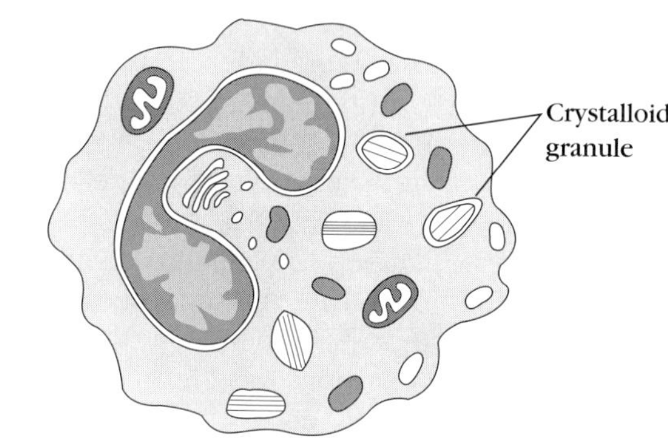

(c) Basophil

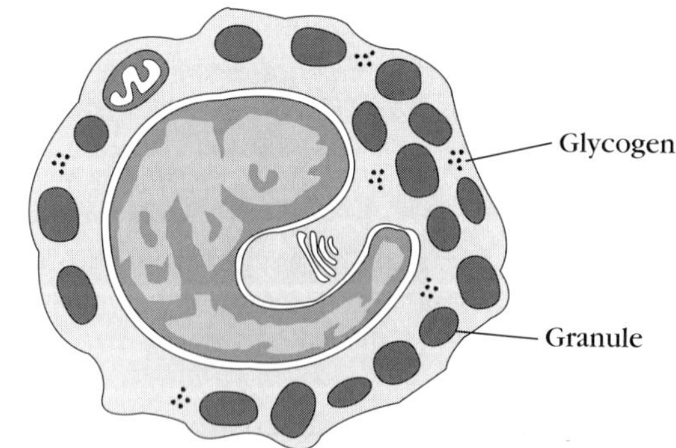

FIGURE 3-13 Drawings showing typical morphology of granulocytes. Note differences in the shape of the nucleus and in the number and shape of cytoplasmic granules.

Granulocytic Cells

The granulocytes are classified as *neutrophils, eosinophils,* or *basophils* on the basis of cellular morphology and cytoplasmic staining characteristics (Figure 3-13). The neutrophil, which has a granulated cytoplasm that stains with both acid and basic dyes, is often called a *polymorphonuclear leukocyte* for its multilobed nucleus. The eosinophil has a bilobed nucleus and a heavily granulated cytoplasm that stains with the acid dye eosin Y (hence its name). The basophil has a lobed nucleus and heavily granulated cytoplasm that stains with the basic dye methylene blue. Both neutrophils and eosinophils are phagocytic, whereas basophils are not. Neutrophils, which constitute 50–70% of the circulating white blood cells, are much more numerous than eosinophils (1–3%) or basophils (<1%).

Neutrophils

Neutrophils are produced in the bone marrow during hematopoiesis. They are released into the peripheral blood and circulate for 7–10 h before migrating into the tissues where they have a 3-day life span. In response to many types of infections the bone marrow releases increased numbers of neutrophils. The increased numbers of circulating neutrophils, called *leukocytosis,* is used medically to indicate the presence of an infection. Neutrophils generally are the first cell to arrive at a site of inflammation. Observation of neutrophil migration reveals that the cell first adheres to the vascular endothelium, then penetrates the gap between the endothelial cells lining the vessel wall, and finally penetrates the vascular basement membrane, moving out into the tissue spaces (this process is discussed in a later section). A number of substances generated in an inflammatory reaction serve as chemotactic factors that promote a buildup of neutrophils at an inflammatory site. Among these chemotactic factors are some of the complement components, components of the blood-clotting system, and products secreted by activated T_H cells.

Like macrophages, neutrophils are active phagocytic cells. The process of phagocytosis by neutrophils is similar to that described for macrophages, except that neutrophils contain lytic enzymes and bactericidal substances within primary and secondary granules. The larger, denser primary (or *azurophilic*) granules are a type of lysosome containing peroxidase, lysozyme, and various hydrolytic enzymes. The smaller, secondary granules contain collagenase, lactoferrin, and lysozyme. Both primary and secondary granules fuse with the phagosome, whose contents are then digested and eliminated much as they are in macrophages.

Neutrophils also employ both oxygen-dependent and oxygen-independent pathways to generate antimicrobial substances. Neutrophils are in fact much more able to kill ingested microorganisms than macrophages. Neutrophils exhibit a larger respiratory burst than macrophages and consequently are able to generate more reactive oxygen intermediates and reactive nitrogen intermediates (see Table 3-4). In addition, neutrophils express higher levels of defensins than macrophages.

Eosinophils

Eosinophils, like neutrophils, are motile, phagocytic cells that can migrate from the blood into the tissue spaces. Their phagocytic role is significantly less important than that of neutrophils, and it is thought that their major role is in defense against parasitic organisms. The secretion of the contents of eosinophilic granules results in damage to the parasite membrane.

Basophils

Basophils are not phagocytic and function by releasing pharmacologically active substances contained within their cytoplasmic granules. They have a major role in allergic responses during which they release the contents of their granules. Basophils are discussed in detail in Chapter 18 in the section on type I hypersensitive reactions.

Mast Cells

Mast-cell precursors, which are formed in the bone marrow during hematopoiesis, are released into the blood as undifferentiated precursor cells and do not differentiate until they leave the blood and enter the tissues. Mast cells can be found in a wide variety of tissues including the skin, connective tissues of various organs, and mucosal epithelial tissue of the respiratory, genitourinary, and digestive tracts. Like circulating basophils, these cells have large numbers of cytoplasmic granules containing histamine and other pharmacologically active substances. Mast cells, together with blood basophils, play an important role in the development of allergies and are discussed in more detail in Chapter 18.

Dendritic Cells

The dendritic cell acquired its name because it is covered with a maze of long membrane processes resembling dendrites of nerve cells. Dendritic cells have been very difficult to study because conventional procedures for isolating lymphocytes and accessory immune-system cells tend to damage the long dendritic processes, so that the cells fail to survive. Use of gentler dispersion techniques with enzymes has facilitated isolation of these cells for in vitro study.

In addition to their unusual dendritic shape, all types of dendritic cells share several structural and functional features. They express high levels of class II MHC molecules and function as important antigen-presenting cells for T-cell activation. After capturing antigen in the tissues, dendritic cells migrate to various lymphoid organs where they present the antigen to lymphocytes. Dendritic cells are found in nonlymphoid organs and tissues, in lymphoid organs, and in the blood and lymph (Table 3-6). The dendritic cells in each of these locations have morphologic and functional differences but may arise from a common progenitor cell and may represent various stages of a single lineage. Until the dendritic progenitor is

TABLE 3-6 DENDRITIC CELLS

Location	Cell type
Nonlymphoid organs	
Skin	Langerhans cells
Organs	Interstitial dendritic cells
Lymphoid organs	
T-cell areas	Interdigitating dendritic cells
B-cell areas	Follicular dendritic cells
Circulation	
Blood	Blood dendritic cells
Lymph	"Veiled" cells

identified, the relationship among the various dendritic cells remains unresolved.

The nonlymphoid dendritic cells include Langerhans cells of the epidermis and the interstitial dendritic cells that populate most organs (e.g., heart, lungs, liver, kidney, gastrointestinal tract). Nonlymphoid dendritic cells capture antigen and carry it to regional lymph nodes. As nonlymphoid dendritic cells enter the blood and lymph, they change morphologically and become "veiled" cells. In the blood these cells account for <0.1% of leukocytes. In organ transplants, resident populations of nonlymphoid dendritic cells may migrate from the transplanted organ to regional lymph nodes where they serve to activate recipient T cells against the foreign antigens of the transplanted organ. This process is discussed more fully in Chapter 24.

The lymphoid dendritic cells include interdigitating dendritic cells and follicular dendritic cells. Interdigitating dendritic cells are found in T-cell–rich regions of lymphoid organs including the spleen, lymph nodes, and thymus. T cells and interdigitating dendritic cells form large multicellular aggregates, which may enhance the likelihood of effective antigen-MHC presentation to T cells. Follicular dendritic cells were named for their exclusive location in organized structures of the lymph node called lymph follicles. Lymph follicles are rich in B cells, and follicular dendritic cells are thought to trap antigen, facilitating B-cell activation. Follicular dendritic cells express high levels of membrane receptors for antibody and complement. Circulating antibody-antigen complexes bound to these receptors have been shown to be retained on the dendritic-cell membrane for very long periods of time, ranging from weeks to months. An electron-dense layer of antigen-antibody complexes can be seen covering the dendritic processes of these cells in Figure 3-14. The presence of antigen-antibody complexes on the membrane of follicular dendritic cells is thought to play a role in the development of memory B cells within the follicle.

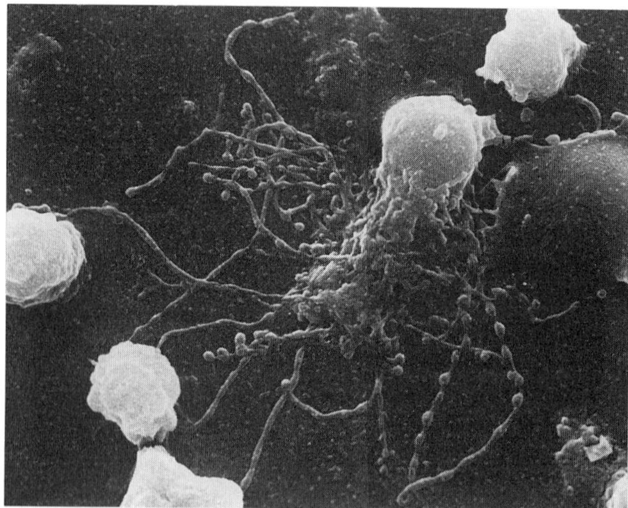

FIGURE 3-14 Scanning electron micrograph of follicular dendritic cells showing long "beaded" dendrites. The beads are coated with antigen-antibody complexes. The dendrites emanate from the cell body. [From A. K. Szakal et al., 1985, *J. Immunol.* **134**:1353. © 1985 American Association of Immunologists. Reprinted with permission.]

Organs of the Immune System

A number of morphologically and functionally diverse organs have various functions in the development of an immune response. These organs can be divided on the basis of function into the primary (or central) and secondary (or peripheral) lymphoid organs (Figure 3-15). Immature lymphocytes generated during hematopoiesis mature and become committed to a particular antigenic specificity within the primary lymphoid organs. Only after a lymphocyte has matured within a primary lymphoid organ is the cell immunocompetent (i.e., capable of mounting an immune response). In mammals, the primary lymphoid organs are the bone marrow, where B-cell maturation occurs, and the thymus, where T-cell maturation occurs.

A variety of peripheral lymphoid organs exist, each uniquely suited to trap antigen from defined tissues or vascular spaces and to provide sites where mature, immunocompetent lymphocytes can interact effectively with that antigen. The lymph nodes function to collect antigen from the intracellular tissue fluids, whereas the spleen filters blood-borne antigens. The respiratory and gastrointestinal tracts possess aggregations of mucosal-associated lymphoid tissue (MALT)—including Peyer's patches, tonsils, adenoids, and the appendix; these trap antigens entering through various mucous membrane surfaces.

Primary Lymphoid Organs

Thymus

T-cell progenitors formed during hematopoiesis enter the thymus gland as immature *thymocytes* and mature there to become antigen-committed, immunocompetent T cells. The thymus is a flat, bilobed organ situated above the heart. Each lobe is surrounded by a capsule and is divided into lobules, which are separated from each other by strands of connective tissue called *trabeculae.* Each lobule is organized into two

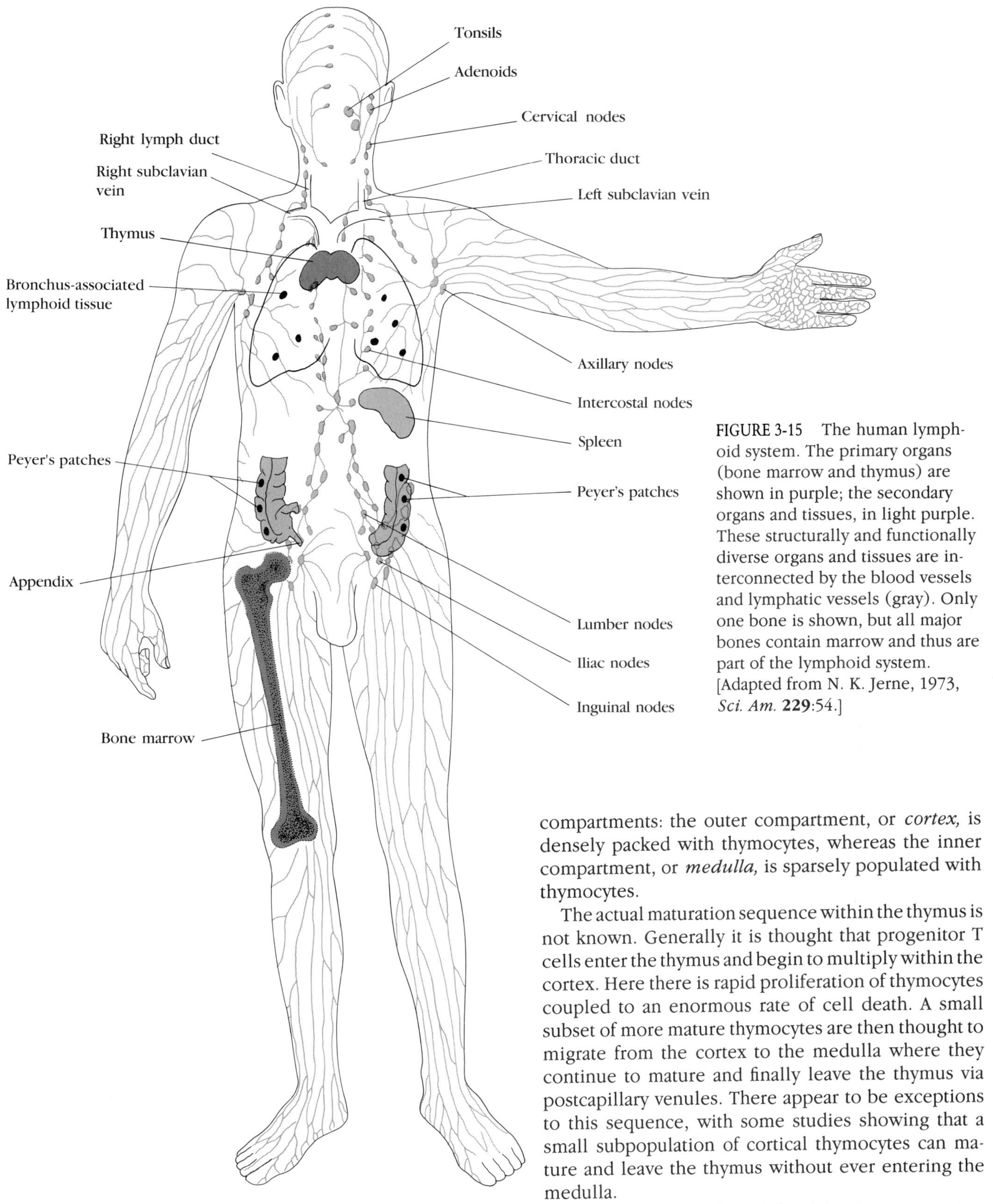

FIGURE 3-15 The human lymphoid system. The primary organs (bone marrow and thymus) are shown in purple; the secondary organs and tissues, in light purple. These structurally and functionally diverse organs and tissues are interconnected by the blood vessels and lymphatic vessels (gray). Only one bone is shown, but all major bones contain marrow and thus are part of the lymphoid system. [Adapted from N. K. Jerne, 1973, *Sci. Am.* **229**:54.]

compartments: the outer compartment, or *cortex,* is densely packed with thymocytes, whereas the inner compartment, or *medulla,* is sparsely populated with thymocytes.

The actual maturation sequence within the thymus is not known. Generally it is thought that progenitor T cells enter the thymus and begin to multiply within the cortex. Here there is rapid proliferation of thymocytes coupled to an enormous rate of cell death. A small subset of more mature thymocytes are then thought to migrate from the cortex to the medulla where they continue to mature and finally leave the thymus via postcapillary venules. There appear to be exceptions to this sequence, with some studies showing that a small subpopulation of cortical thymocytes can mature and leave the thymus without ever entering the medulla.

Both the cortex and medulla of the thymus are crisscrossed by a three-dimensional network of stromal cells composed of epithelial cells, interdigitating dendritic cells, and macrophages, which make up the framework of the organ and contribute to thymocyte maturation. Many of these stromal cells physically interact with the developing thymocytes (Figure 3-16). Some thymic epithelial cells in the outer cortex, called "nurse" cells, have long membrane processes that surround as many as 50 thymocytes, forming large multicellular complexes. Other cortical epithelial cells have long interconnecting cytoplasmic processes that form a network and have been shown to interact with numerous thymocytes as they traverse the cortex. Bone marrow–derived interdigitating cells are located at the junction of the cortex and medulla. These cells also have long processes that interact with developing thymocytes.

MATURATION AND SELECTION OF T CELLS. Thymic epithelial cells secrete several hormonal factors necessary for the differentiation and maturation of T lymphocytes. Four such hormonal factors have been characterized: α_1-thymosin, β_4-thymosin, thymopoietin, and thymulin. When bone marrow cells are cultured with these factors, T-cell lineage membrane molecules have been shown to appear, although the role of each of these factors in T-cell maturation remains unknown. Thymic stromal cells also secrete interleukin 7 (IL-7); this cytokine stimulates growth of thymocytes.

In the course of thymocyte maturation within the thymus, the antigenic diversity of the T-cell receptor is generated by a series of random gene rearrangements (see Chapter 11). After developing thymocytes begin to express antigen-binding receptors, they are subjected to a selection process, so that only T cells recognizing antigenic peptides in the context of self-MHC

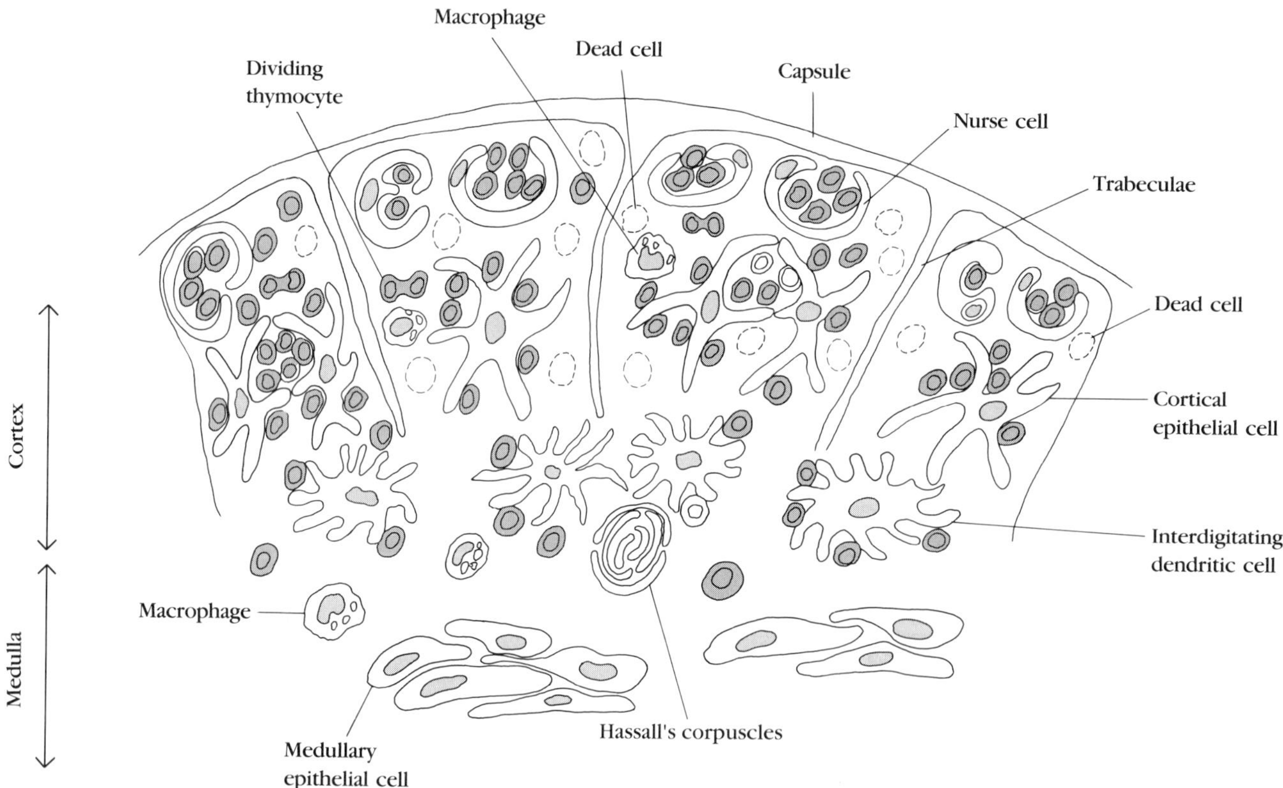

FIGURE 3-16 Diagrammatic cross section of a portion of the thymus, showing several lobules separated by connective tissue strands (trabeculae). Progenitor T cells produced in the bone marrow during hematopoiesis enter the thymus as immature thymocytes and mature into functional T-cell subpopulations. The outer cortex is densely populated and is thought to contain immature thymocytes (purple), which undergo rapid proliferation coupled with an enormous rate of cell death. The medulla is sparsely populated and is thought to contain more mature thymocytes. During their stay within the thymus, thymocytes interact with stromal cells (epithelial cells, interdigitating dendritic cells, and macrophages). These cells produce thymic hormones and express high levels of class I and class II MHC molecules. Several unique cells are also found in the thymus including the thymic "nurse" cell, an epithelial cell that engulfs up to 50 thymocytes with its long membrane processes and Hassall's corpuscles containing concentric layers of degenerating epithelial cells. [Adapted from W. van Ewijk, 1991, *Annu. Rev. Immunol.* **9**:591.]

molecules are released from the thymus. Thymic stromal cells, which express high levels of class I and class II MHC molecules, play a role in this selection process (see Chapter 12). The first step in this process is *positive selection* of those T cells bearing receptors that recognize self-MHC molecules. Any developing thymocytes that are unable to recognize self-MHC molecules are not selected and are thought to be eliminated by programmed cell death. In the second step, termed *negative selection,* potentially self-reactive thymocytes with a high-affinity receptor for self-antigen plus self-MHC (or self-MHC alone) are eliminated. By means of positive and negative selection in the thymus, only those cells are allowed to mature whose receptor recognizes an MHC molecule plus foreign antigen.

An estimated 95–99% of all thymocyte progeny undergo programmed cell death within the thymus without ever maturing. This high death rate probably results primarily from the elimination of thymocytes that cannot recognize foreign antigenic peptides displayed by self-MHC molecules and of thymocytes that recognize self-peptides displayed by self-MHC molecules. It is not known whether some sort of external signal, such as the presence or absence of a factor, initiates programmed cell death in those thymocytes that fail positive or negative selection. Some have suggested that the death of the majority of nonselected thymocytes may be induced by endogenous glucocorticoids. It has been known for some time that cortical thymocytes, especially in rodents, are extremely sensitive to glucocorticoids, whereas mature T cells are not. When mouse thymocytes are incubated with high physiologic levels of glucocorticoids, the cells begin to die within 1–2 h by apoptosis. The pronounced effect of glucocorticoids on the thymus can be seen in Figure 3-17. The role of apoptosis in thymic selection is discussed more fully in Chapter 12.

Relationship between Thymic Function and Immune Function. The first evidence implicating the thymus in immune function came from experiments involving neonatal thymectomy in which the thymus was surgically removed from newborn mice. These thymectomized mice showed a dramatic decrease in circulating lymphocytes of the T-cell lineage and an absence of cell-mediated immunity. A congenital birth defect in humans (DiGeorge syndrome) and in certain mice (nude mice) that involves failure of the thymus to develop provides further evidence. In both cases there is an absence of circulating T cells and of cell-mediated immunity and an increase in infectious disease.

The decline in immune functions that accompanies aging, leading to an increase in infections, autoimmunity, and cancer, probably results primarily from changes in the T-cell component of the immune system. The thymus reaches its maximal size at puberty and then atrophies, with a significant decrease in both cortical and medullary cells and an increase in the total fat content of the organ. Whereas the average weight of the thymus is 70 g in infants, its average weight is only 3 g in the elderly. This thymic involution, with the associated decrease in cortical size, medullary size, and hormonal production, precedes the decrease in immune function that is seen with aging. A number of

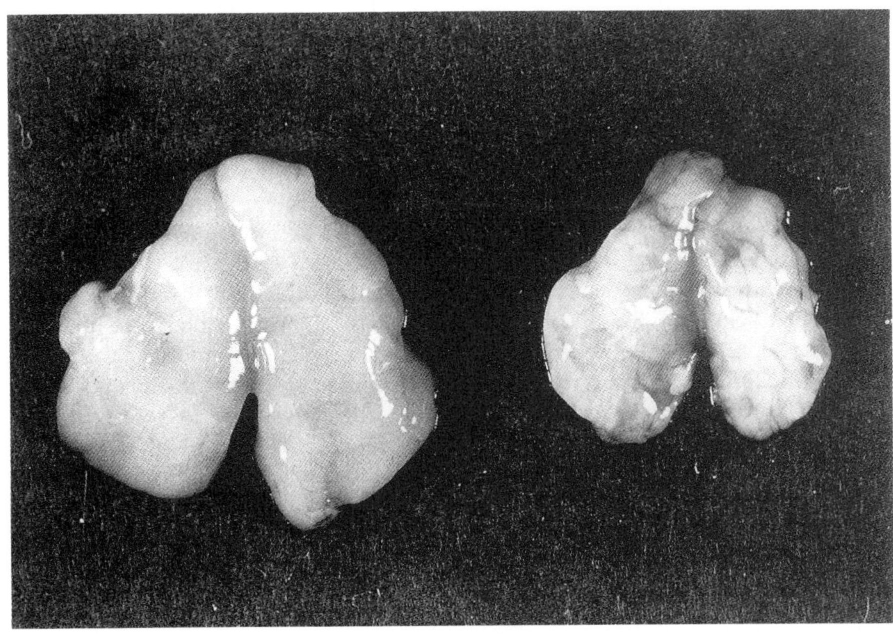

FIGURE 3-17 Effects of glucocorticosteroids on the rat thymus gland. A normal thymus *(left)* compared with the thymus of a rat 48 h following injection of a corticosteroid (5 mg/kg body weight). [From M. M. Compton and J. A. Cidlowski, 1992, *Trends in Endocrinology and Metabolism* **3**:17.]

experiments have been designed to look at the effect of age on the immune function of the thymus. In one experiment the thymus from a 1-day-old or 33-month-old mouse was grafted into thymectomized adult littermates. Mice receiving the newborn thymus graft showed a significantly larger improvement in immune function than mice receiving the 33-month-old thymus.

Bone Marrow

In birds a lymphoid organ called the bursa of Fabricius is the primary site of B-cell maturation. There is no bursa in mammals and no single counterpart to it as a primary lymphoid organ. Instead, regions of the bone marrow and possibly of other lymphoid tissues serve as the "bursal equivalent" where B-cell maturation occurs. Because B-cell development in mammals does not take place in a single anatomic structure, it is difficult to study B-cell development in mammals, and much remains unknown about this process.

Secondary Lymphoid Organs

As blood circulates under pressure, the fluid component of the blood *(plasma)* seeps through the thin wall of the capillaries into the surrounding tissue. Much of this fluid, called *interstitial fluid,* returns to the blood through the capillary membranes. The remainder of the interstitial fluid, now called *lymph,* flows from the connective tissue spaces into a network of tiny open lymphatic capillaries and then into a series of progressively larger collecting vessels called *lymphatic vessels* (Figure 3-18). The largest lymphatic vessel, the *thoracic duct,* empties into the left subclavian vein near the heart (see Figure 3-15). In this way the lymphatic system functions to capture fluid lost from the blood and return it to the blood, thus ensuring steady-state levels of fluid within the circulatory system. The heart does not pump the lymph through the lymphatic system; instead the flow of lymph is achieved as the lymph vessels are squeezed by movements of the body's muscles. A series of one-way valves along the lymphatic vessels ensure that lymph flows only in one direction.

When foreign antigen gains entrance into the tissues, it is picked up by the lymphatic system (which drains all the tissues of the body) and carried to various organized lymphoid tissues, which trap the foreign antigen. As lymph passes from the tissues to lymphatic vessels, it becomes progressively enriched in lymphocytes. Thus, the lymphatic system also serves as a means of transporting lymphocytes and antigen from the connective tissues to organized lymphoid tissues where the lymphocytes may interact with the trapped antigen.

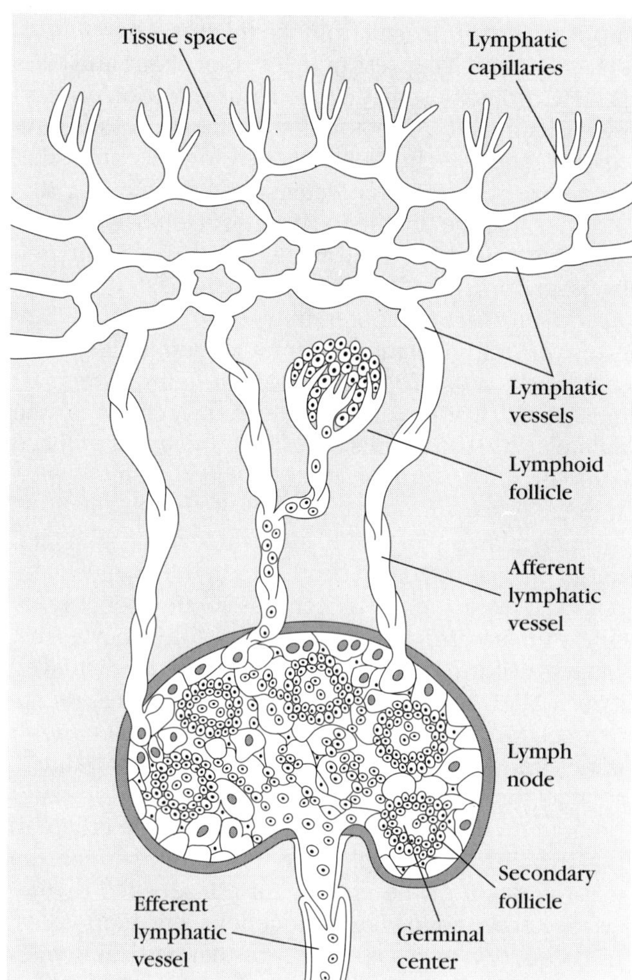

FIGURE 3-18 Lymphatic vessels. Small capillaries opening into the tissue spaces pick up interstitial tissue fluid and carry it into progressively larger lymphatic vessels, which carry the fluid, now called lymph, into regional lymph nodes. As lymph leaves the nodes, it is carried through larger efferent lymphatic vessels, which eventually drain into the circulatory system at the thoracic duct or right lymph duct (see Figure 3-15).

Various types of organized lymphoid tissues are located along the vessels of the lymphatic system. Some lymphoid tissue in the lung and lamina propria of the intestinal wall consists of diffuse collections of lymphocytes and macrophages. Other lymphoid tissue is organized into structures called *lymphoid follicles,* which consist of aggregates of various cells surrounded by a network of draining lymphatic capillaries. In the absence of antigen activation, a lymphoid follicle—called a *primary follicle*—comprises a network of follicular dendritic cells and small resting B cells. Following antigenic challenge, a primary follicle becomes a larger *secondary follicle*—a ring of concentrically packed B lymphocytes surrounding a center (the *germinal center*) in which large proliferating B lymphocytes, memory B cells, and plasma cells are interspersed with macrophages and follicular dendritic cells (Figure 3-19). The germinal center is a site of intense B-cell activation and contains large numbers of blast cells, called *centroblasts.* Interaction with antigen displayed on the membrane of follicular dendritic cells induces the B cells to proliferate and differentiate into plasma and memory cells. In the absence of antigen activation, the B cells appear to undergo programmed cell death within the germinal center. The germinal cell is discussed more fully in Chapter 14.

Lymphoid follicles are particularly abundant in the lamina propria of the intestines, in the upper airways and bronchi, and in the genital tract. Histologic sections have revealed more than 15,000 follicles along the intestines of a healthy child. Some lymphoid tissue is more highly organized. Peyer's patches in the small intestine, the tonsils, and the appendix all contain organized clusters of lymphoid follicles. Lymph nodes and the spleen have an even more complex organization; in addition to lymphoid follicles, these lymphoid organs possess distinct regions of T-cell and B-cell activity and are surrounded by a fibrous capsule.

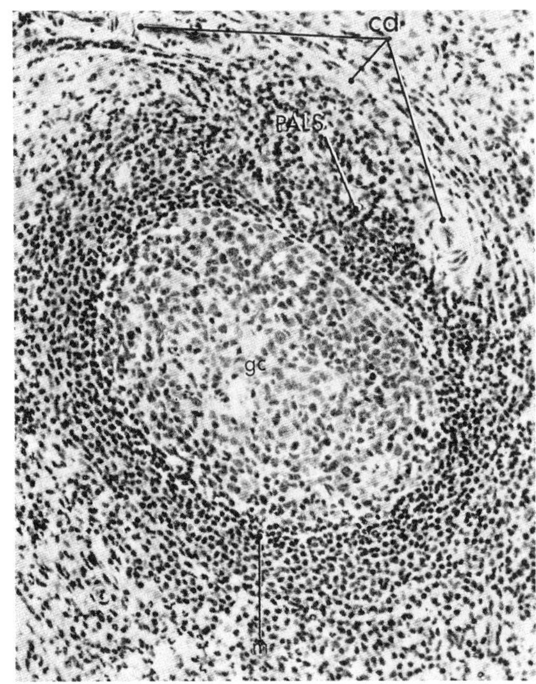

FIGURE 3-19 A secondary lymphoid follicle consisting of a large germinal center surrounded by a dense mantle of small lymphocytes. [From W. Bloom and D. W. Fawcett, 1975, *Textbook of Histology,* 10th ed., W. B. Saunders Co.]

Lymph Nodes

Lymph nodes are encapsulated bean-shaped structures containing a reticular network packed with lymphocytes, macrophages, and dendritic cells. Clustered at junctions of the lymphatic vessels, lymph nodes are the first organized lymphoid structure to encounter antigens that enter the tissue spaces. As lymph percolates through a node, any particulate antigen that is brought in with the lymph will be trapped by the cellular network of phagocytic cells and reticular dendritic cells. The overall architecture of a lymph node provides an ideal microenvironment for lymphocytes to effectively encounter and respond to trapped antigens.

Morphologically, a lymph node can be divided into three roughly concentric regions: the cortex, paracortex, and medulla each of which provides a distinct microenvironment (Figure 3-20). The outermost layer, the *cortex,* contains lymphocytes (mostly B cells) and macrophages arranged in primary follicles. Following antigenic challenge, the primary follicles enlarge into secondary follicles, each containing a germinal center. Intense B-cell activation and differentiation into plasma and memory B cells occurs in the germinal centers of lymph nodes. (In children with B-cell deficiencies, the cortex lacks primary follicles and germinal centers.) Beneath the cortex is the *paracortex,* which is populated with T lymphocytes and also contains dendritic cells thought to have migrated from tissues to the node. These dendritic cells express high levels of class II MHC molecules, which are necessary for antigen presentation to T_H cells. Lymph nodes taken from neonatally thymectomized mice show a severe depletion of cells in the paracortical region; the paracortex is therefore sometimes referred to as a thymus-dependent area in contrast to the cortex, which is a thymus-independent area. The innermost layer of a lymph node, the *medulla,* is more sparsely populated with lymphocytes, but many of these are plasma cells actively secreting antibody molecules.

As antigen is carried into a regional node by the lymph, it is trapped, processed, and presented together with class II MHC molecules by dendritic cells in the paracortex, resulting in T_H-cell activation. The initial activation of B cells is also thought to take place within the paracortex. Once activated, T_H and B cells migrate to the primary follicles of the cortex. Within a primary follicle, cellular interactions between follicular dendritic cells, B cells, and T_H cells take place, leading to development of a secondary follicle with a central germinal center. Follicular dendritic cells, which make up the cellular meshwork of the germinal center, trap antigen complexed with antibody and retain the antigen-antibody complexes on the membrane for long periods of time (see Figure 3-14). Antigen trapped on the membrane of these cells is thought to be particularly effective in activating B cells.

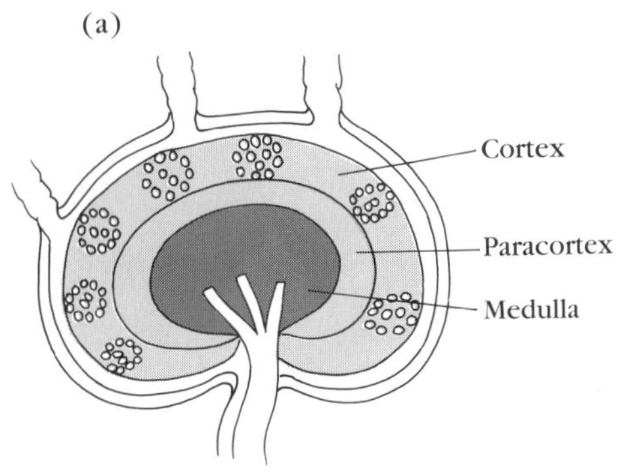

FIGURE 3-20 Structure of a lymph node. (a) The three layers of a lymph node provide distinct microenvironments. (b) The left side depicts the arrangement of reticulum and lymphocytes within the various regions of a lymph node. Macrophages and dendritic cells, which trap antigen, are present in the cortex and paracortex. T_H cells are concentrated in the paracortex; B cells are located primarily in the cortex within follicles and germinal centers. The medulla is populated largely by antibody-producing plasma cells. Lymphocytes circulating in the lymph are carried into the node via afferent lymphatics (purple arrows); they either enter the reticular matrix of the node or pass through it and leave via the efferent lymphatic vessel. The right side of (b) depicts the lymphatic artery and vein and the postcapillary venules. Lymphocytes in the circulation can pass into the node from the postcapillary venules by a process called extravasation *(inset).*

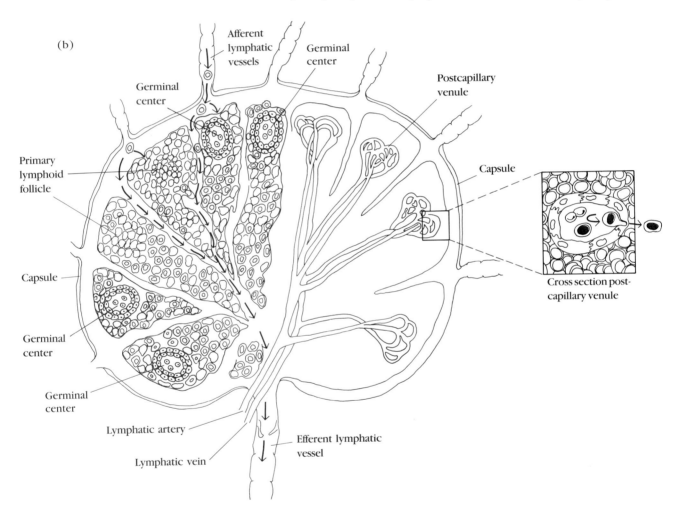

Follicular dendritic cells also produce growth factors that are essential for B-cell activation, as do T_H cells. The activated B cells in a node divide rapidly and either differentiate into plasma and memory B cells or die by programmed cell death. Plasma cells leave the germinal center and migrate to the medulla where they secrete large quantities of antibody.

Afferent lymphatic vessels pierce the capsule of a lymph node at numerous sites and empty lymph into the subcapsular sinus (see Figure 3-20). Lymph coming from the tissues percolates slowly inward through the cortex, paracortex, and medulla, allowing phagocytic cells and reticular dendritic cells to trap any bacteria or particulate material (e.g., antigen-antibody complexes) carried by the lymph. Following infection or introduction of other antigens into the body, the lymph leaving a node through its single efferent lymphatic vessel is enriched with antibodies newly secreted by medullary plasma cells and also has a 50-fold higher concentration of lymphocytes than the afferent lymph. The increase in lymphocytes is due in part to lymphocyte proliferation within the node in response to antigen, but most of the increase represents blood-borne lymphocytes that migrate into the node by passing between specialized endothelial cells lining the postcapillary venules of the node. Estimates are that 25% of the lymphocytes leaving a lymph node have migrated across this endothelial layer and entered the node from the circulation. Because antigenic stimulation within a node can increase this migration tenfold, the concentration of lymphocytes in nodes involved in an active immune response can increase greatly, resulting in visible swelling of the nodes. As discussed later in this chapter, factors released in lymph nodes during antigen stimulation are thought to facilitate this increased lymphocyte migration.

Spleen

The spleen is a large, ovoid secondary lymphoid organ situated high in the left abdominal cavity. Unlike lymph nodes, which are specialized to trap localized antigen from regional tissue spaces, the spleen is adapted to filtering blood and trapping blood-borne antigens, and thus can respond to systemic infections. The spleen is surrounded by a capsule that sends a number of projections (trabeculae) into the interior to form a compartmentalized structure. The compartments are of two types, the *red pulp* and *white pulp,* which are separated by a diffuse *marginal zone* (Figure 3-21). The splenic red pulp consists of a network of sinusoids populated with macrophages and numerous erythrocytes; it is the site where old and defective red blood cells are destroyed and removed. Many of the macrophages within the red pulp contain engulfed red blood cells or iron pigments from degraded hemoglobin. The splenic white pulp surrounds the arteries, forming a *periarteriolar lymphoid sheath (PALS)* populated mainly by T lymphocytes. The marginal zone, located peripheral to the PALS, is rich in B cells organized into primary lymphoid follicles. Upon antigenic challenge, these primary follicles develop into characteristic secondary follicles containing germinal centers (like those in the lymph nodes) where rapidly dividing B cells (centroblasts) and plasma cells are surrounded by dense clusters of concentrically arranged lymphocytes.

Unlike the lymph nodes, the spleen is not supplied by afferent lymphatics draining the tissue spaces. Instead, blood-borne antigens are carried into the spleen through the splenic artery, which empties into the marginal zone. As antigen enters the marginal zone, it is trapped by dendritic cells, which carry the antigen to the periarteriolar lymphoid sheath. Lymphocytes in

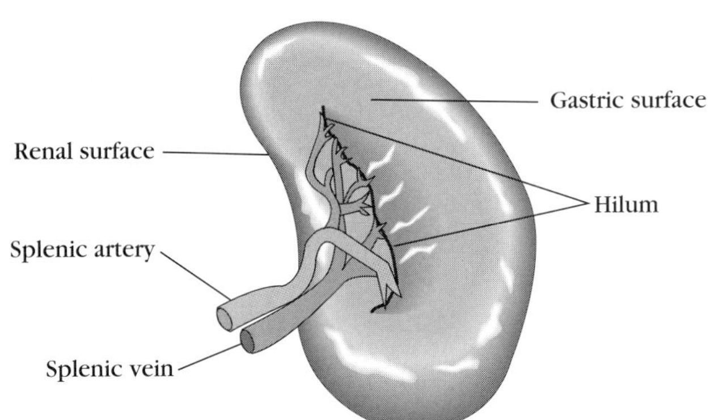

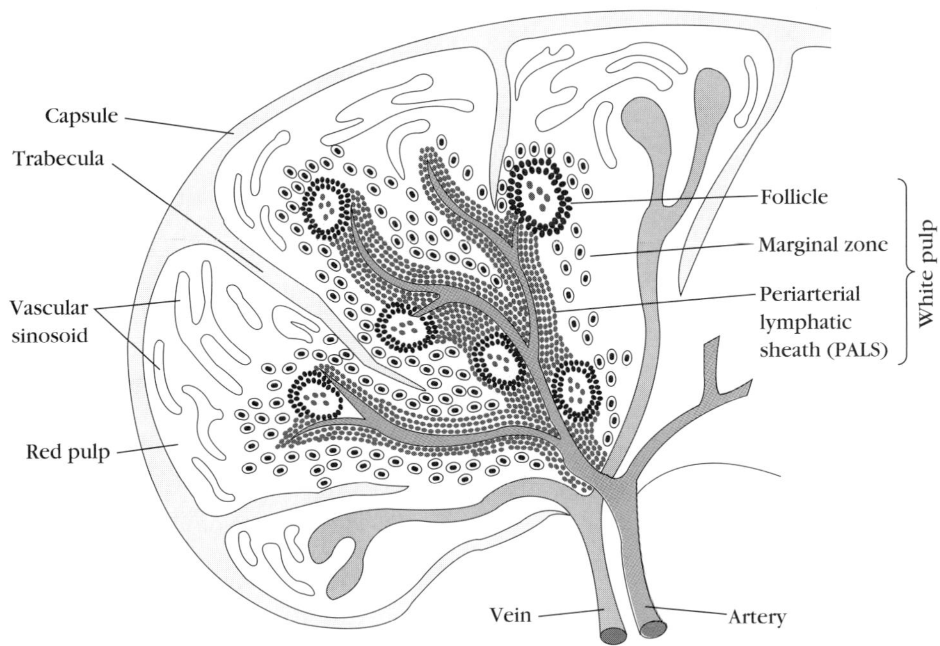

FIGURE 3-21 Structure of the spleen. (a) The spleen is specialized for trapping blood-borne antigens. (b) Diagrammatic cross section of the spleen. The arteriole blood supply pierces the capsule and divides into progressively smaller arterioles, ending in vascular sinusoids that drain back into the splenic vein. The erythrocyte-filled red pulp surrounds the sinusoids. The white pulp forms a sleeve around the arterioles (PALS), which contains numerous T cells. Closely associated with the PALS is the marginal zone, a B-cell–rich area containing lymphoid follicles that can develop into germinal centers.

the blood also enter the marginal zone in the sinuses and migrate to the periarteriolar lymphoid sheath. Experiments with radioactively labeled lymphocytes show that more recirculating lymphocytes daily pass through the spleen than through all the lymph nodes combined. The effects of splenectomy on the immune response depends on the age at which the spleen is removed. In children, splenectomy often leads to an increased incidence of bacterial sepsis caused primarily by *Streptococcus pneumoniae, Neisseria meningitidis,* and *Hemophilus influenzae.* Splenectomy in adults has less adverse effects, although it leads to some increase in blood-borne bacterial infections, or bacteremia.

Mucosal-Associated Lymphoid Tissue

The mucous membranes lining the digestive, respiratory, and urogenital system, which have a combined surface area of about 400 m², are the major sites of entry for most pathogens. The defense of these vulnerable membrane surfaces is provided by organized lymphoid tissues known collectively as *mucosal-associated lymphoid tissue (MALT).* Structurally these tissues range from loose clusters of lymphoid cells with little organization in the lamina propria of intestinal villi to organized structures such as the tonsils, appendix, and Peyer's patches (see Figure 3-15). The functional importance of MALT in the body's defense is attested to by its large population of antibody-producing plasma cells, whose number far exceeds that of plasma cells in the spleen, lymph nodes, and bone marrow combined.

The tonsils are found in three locations: lingual at the base of the tongue; palatine at the side of the back of the mouth; and nasopharyngeal (adenoids) in the roof of the nasopharynx. All three tonsil groups are nodular structures consisting of a meshwork of reticular cells and fibers interspersed with lymphocytes, macrophages, granulocytes, and mast cells. The B cells are organized into follicles and germinal centers; the latter are surrounded by regions showing T-cell activity. The tonsils play a role in defense against antigens entering through the nasal and oral epithelial routes.

Peyer's patches consist of 30–40 lymphoid nodules on the outer wall of the intestines. These structures also contain follicles from which germinal centers develop upon antigenic stimulation. The follicles, which are very close to the intestinal mucosal epithelium, are thought to be the sites where antigens penetrate the intestinal epithelium, thus facilitating accumulation of antigen within organized lymphoid structures.

The epithelial cells of mucous membranes play an important role in promoting the immune response by delivering small samples of foreign antigen from the lumina of the respiratory, digestive, and urogenital tracts to the underlying mucosal-associated lymphoid tissue. This antigen transport is carried out by specialized cells, called *M cells.* The structure of the M cell is striking: It contacts the lumen with broad membrane processes and contains a deep invagination, or pocket, in the basolateral plasma membrane; this pocket is filled with a cluster of B cells, T cells, and macro-

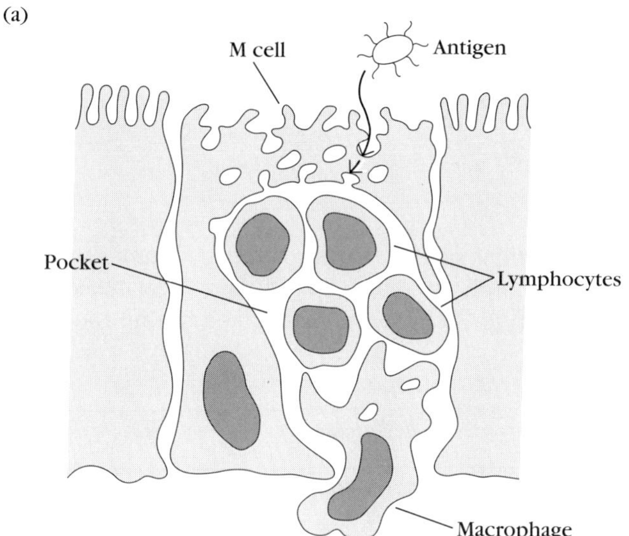

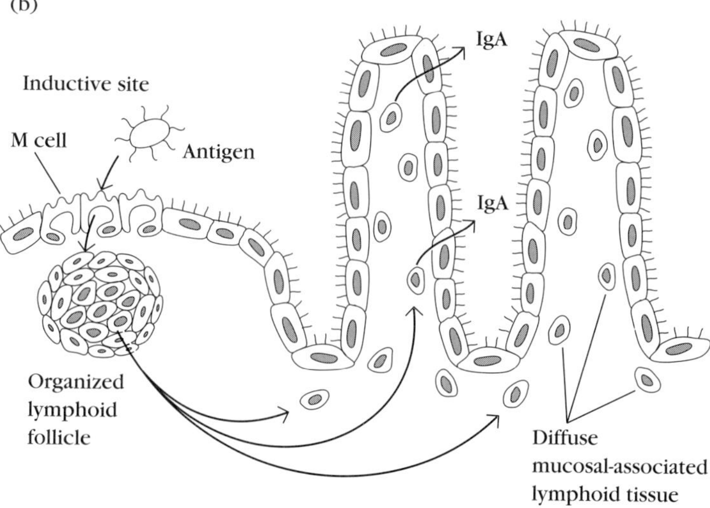

FIGURE 3-22 Structure of M cells and production of IgA at inductive sites. (a) M cells, located in mucous membranes, endocytose antigen present in the lumin of the digestive, respiratory, and urogenital tracts. The antigen is delivered to the cell's large basolateral pocket. (b) Diagram of mucous membrane showing secretion of IgA antibodies in response to antigen endocytosed by M cells at an inductive site. Activated B cells migrate from the lymphoid follicle to nearby mucosal-associated lymphoid tissue where they differentiate into IgA-producing plasma cells.

phages (Figure 3-22a). Luminal antigens are endocytosed into vesicles that are transported from the luminal membrane to the underlying pocket membrane. The vesicles then fuse with the pocket membrane, delivering the antigens to the clusters of lymphocytes contained within the pocket. M cells express class II MHC molecules, but it is not known whether antigen is processed within the endocytic vesicles and then presented with class II MHC to the T_H cells contained within the pocket.

M cells are located in so-called *inductive sites*—small regions of a mucous membrane that are underlain by organized lymphoid follicles (Figure 3-22b). Antigens transported across the mucous membrane by M cells activate B cells within these lymphoid follicles. The activated B cells leave the lymphoid follicle and migrate to diffuse mucosal-associated lymphoid tissue where they differentiate into plasma cells that secrete the IgA class of antibodies. These IgA antibodies are transported across the epithelial cells into the secretions of the lumen where they can interact with antigens present in the lumen (see Figure 5-14).

Leukocyte Recirculation

Lymphocytes are capable of a remarkable level of recirculation, continuously moving through the blood and lymph to the various lymphoid organs (Figure 3-23). James Gowans demonstrated the recirculation of lymphocytes in 1964 by isolating lymph from the thoracic duct of a rat, radiolabeling the lymphocytes, and then transfusing them into normal animals. By monitoring the location of the labeled cells at various time intervals, Gowans found that the lymphocytes spent 2–12 h in the blood before appearing in the lymph or lymphoid organs. As lymphocytes recirculate, they make contact with antigens presented on the surface of antigen-presenting cells in the peripheral lymphoid organs. This feature allows maximal numbers of antigenically committed lymphocytes to encounter and interact with antigen. Since only about one in 10^3–10^6 lymphocytes can recognize a particular antigen, it would appear that a large number of antigen-committed T or B cells must contact antigen on a given antigen-presenting cell within a relatively short period of time in order to generate a specific immune response. The odds of the small percentage of lymphocytes committed to a given antigen actually making contact with that antigen when it is present are greatly increased by the extensive recirculation of lymphocytes. Experiments have shown that when a particular antigen is injected, T cells specific for that antigen disappear from the circulation within 48 h, suggesting that all the specific T cells encounter the antigen in peripheral lymph organs and cease recirculating within that time period.

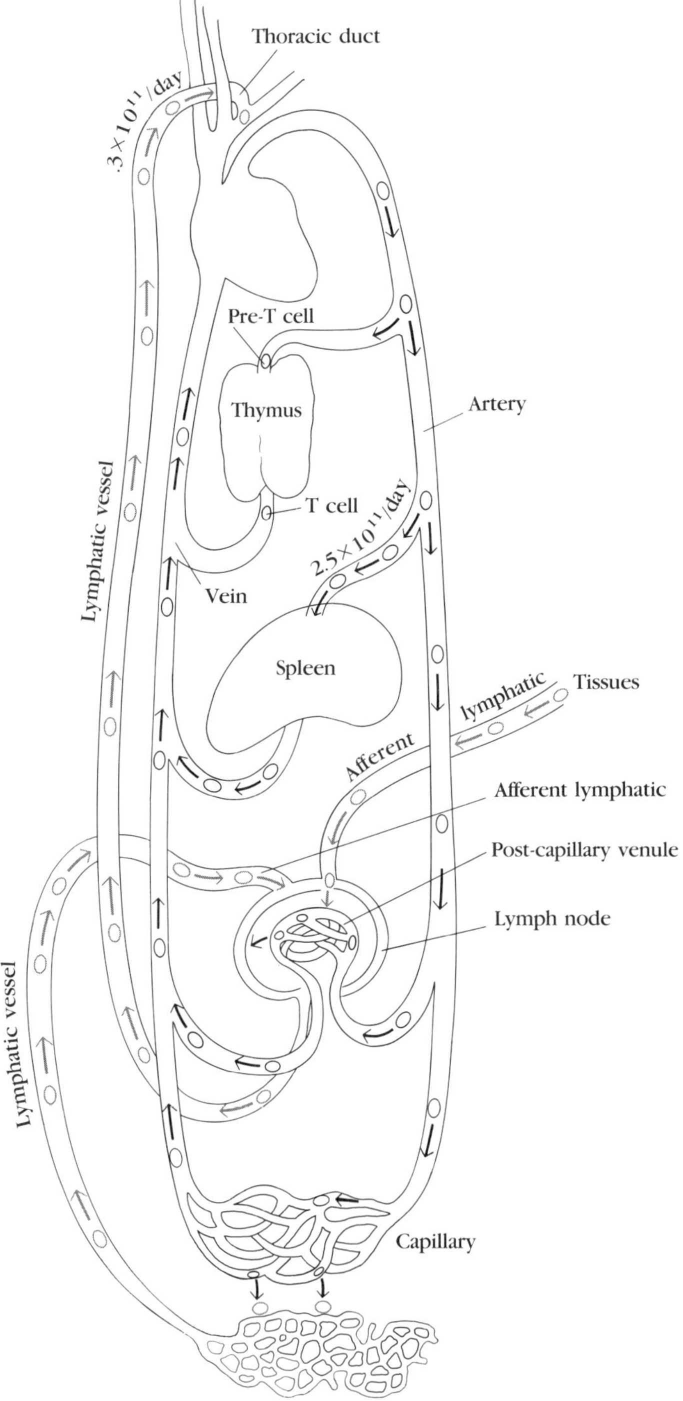

FIGURE 3-23 Diagram of lymphocyte recirculation through the blood (purple) and lymph vasculature (gray) to the major organs of the lymphatic system.

Cell-Adhesion Molecules

The vascular endothelium serves as an important "gatekeeper," regulating the movement of blood-borne molecules and leukocytes into the tissues. In order for circulating leukocytes to enter inflammatory tissue or peripheral lymphoid organs, the cells must adhere to and pass between the endothelial cells lining the walls of blood vessels, a process called *extravasation.* Endothelial cells express leukocyte-specific *cell-adhesion molecules (CAMs).* Some of these membrane proteins are expressed constitutively; others are only expressed in response to localized concentrations of cytokines produced during an inflammatory response. Recirculating lymphocytes, monocytes, and granulocytes bear receptors that bind to CAMs on the vascular endothelium, enabling these cells to extravasate into the tissues.

A number of endothelial CAMs and their corresponding leukocyte receptors have been cloned and characterized recently, providing new details about the extravasation process. Most of these CAMs and their ligands belong to three families of proteins: the immunoglobulin (Ig) superfamily, the integrin family, and the selectin family (Table 3-7 and Figure 3-24). Several endothelial cell-adhesion molecules, including ICAM-1, ICAM-2, and VCAM-1, have sequence homology with the immunoglobulins and thus are classified in the *immunoglobulin superfamily,* which is discussed in detail in Chapter 5.

The *integrin family* of adhesion molecules serve as receptors for ICAM-1, ICAM-2, and VCAM-1. The integrins are heterodimeric proteins (consisting of an α and a β chain) that facilitate leukocyte adherence to the vascular endothelium or other cell-to-cell interactions. Different integrins are expressed by different populations of leukocytes, allowing these cells to bind to different CAMs expressed along the vascular endothelium. The importance of integrin molecules in leukocyte extravasation is demonstrated by *leukocyte-adhesion deficiency (LAD),* an autosomal recessive disease characterized by recurrent bacterial infections and impaired healing of wounds. The deficiency stems from abnormal synthesis of the β chain of the integrin heterodimer present on all leukocytes. Leukocytes lacking integrin molecules cannot extravasate from the blood vessels to the tissues. As a result, an inflammatory response cannot develop in the tissues, and affected individuals have more frequent and more severe bacterial infections than normal individuals.

The *selectin family* of membrane glycoproteins have a characteristic extracellular structure consisting of three domains: a lectin domain, a domain having homology to epidermal growth factor, and a number of repeats related to complement-regulatory proteins. These molecules are sometimes referred to as *LEC-CAMs* in reference to their three domains. Molecules of the selectin family serve as adhesion molecules on vascular endothelial cells or as adhesion-molecule receptors on circulating leukocytes. Selectins bind to specific carbohydrate groups by means of their distal lectin domain.

In addition to their role in leukocyte adhesion to vascular endothelial cells, many adhesion molecules also serve to increase the strength of the functional interactions between cells of the immune system. Various adhesion molecules have been shown to contribute to the T_H-APC, T_H-B cell, and CTL-target cell interactions. These interactions are examined in later chapters.

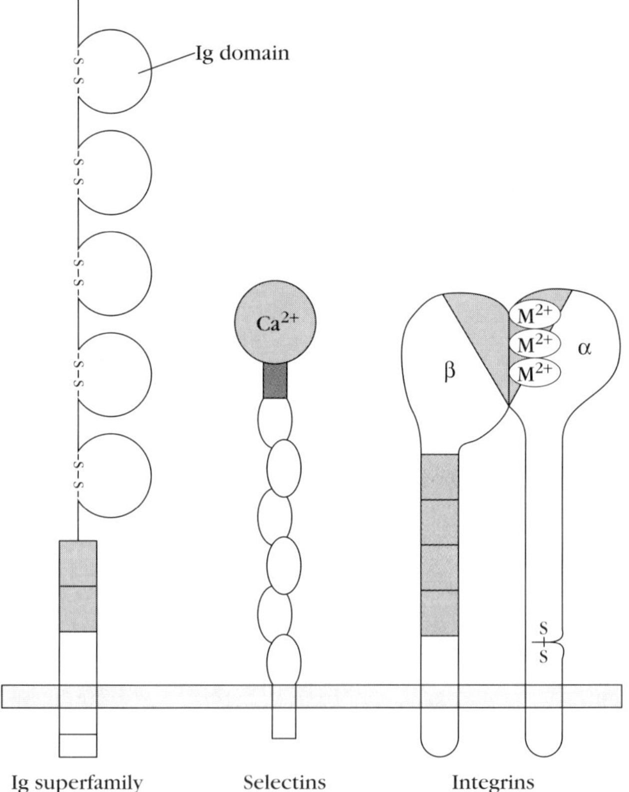

FIGURE 3-24 Major structural features of three families of cell-adhesion molecules (CAMs). (a) Adhesion molecules belonging to the immunoglobulin (Ig) superfamily contain Ig domains and fibronectin type III repeats (gray). (b) Selectin molecules contain a Ca^{2+}-dependent lectin domain (gray), a single domain with homology to epidermal growth factor (purple), and a series of repeats related to complement-binding proteins. (c) Integrins are heterodimers composed of an α and a β chain. The α chain contains three metal-binding sites (M^{2+}). The β chain contains four cysteine-rich repeats (purple). Both the α and β chains contribute to the ligand-binding site (gray). [Adapted from R. O. Hynes and A. D. Lander, 1992, *Cell* **68**:303.]

TABLE 3-7 SELECTED SURFACE MOLECULES INVOLVED IN LEUKOCYTE ADHESION TO ENDOTHELIAL CELLS

Adhesion molecule	Cellular distribution	Function	Ligands
Selectin family[*]			
L-selectin	Lymphocytes, neutrophils, monocytes	Homing receptor	Vascular addressin on HEVs of peripheral lymph nodes
		Adhesion receptor	Sialylated glycoprotein on activated vascular endothelium
E-selectin	Activated vascular endothelium	Cell-adhesion molecule	Sialylated glycoprotein on neutrophils, monocytes, and lymphocytes
P-selectin	Activated vascular endothelium	Cell-adhesion molecule	Sialylated glycoprotein on neutrophils
Integrin family			
VLA-4[†]	Lymphocytes, monocytes, neutrophils	Homing receptor	Vascular addressin on HEVs of Peyer's patches
		Adhesion receptor	VCAM-1 on activated vascular endothelium
LFA-1	Lymphocytes, neutrophils, monocytes	Adhesion receptor	ICAM-1 and ICAM-2 on HEVs and activated vascular endothelium
LPAM-1	Lymphocytes	Homing receptor	Unknown vascular addressins in Peyer's patches
Ig superfamily			
ICAM-1, ICAM-2	Activated vascular endothelium	Cell-adhesion molecule	LFA-1 (see above)
VCAM-1	Activated vascular endothelium	Cell-adhesion molecule	VLA-4 (see above)

[*] Synonyms are as follows: L-selectin—LECAM-1, MEL-14, and LAM-1; E-selectin—ELAM-1; and P-selectin—PADGEM, GMP-140, and CD62.
[†] VLA-4 is also known as LPAM-2.

Neutrophil Extravasation

As an inflammatory response develops, a variety of cytokines and other inflammatory mediators act upon the local blood vessels inducing increased expression of endothelial CAMs. The vascular endothelium is then said to be *activated,* or *inflamed.* Neutrophils are generally the first cell type to bind to activated endothelium and extravasate into the tissues. To accomplish this, neutrophils must recognize the inflamed endothelium and adhere strongly enough so that they are not swept away by the flowing blood. The bound neutrophils must then penetrate the endothelial layer and migrate into the underlying tissue (Figure 3-25a).

Activated endothelial cells express adhesion molecules of the selectin family, which interact with carbohydrate ligands on the neutrophil membrane, tethering the leukocyte briefly to the endothelial cell. The sheer force of the circulating blood detaches the neutrophil, but selectin molecules on another endothelial cell again tether the neutrophil; this process is repeated, so that the neutrophil tumbles end-over-end along the endothelium, a type of binding referred to as *rolling.* As the neutrophil rolls, it is activated by platelet-activating factor (PAF) expressed on the membrane of activated endothelial cells.

(a)

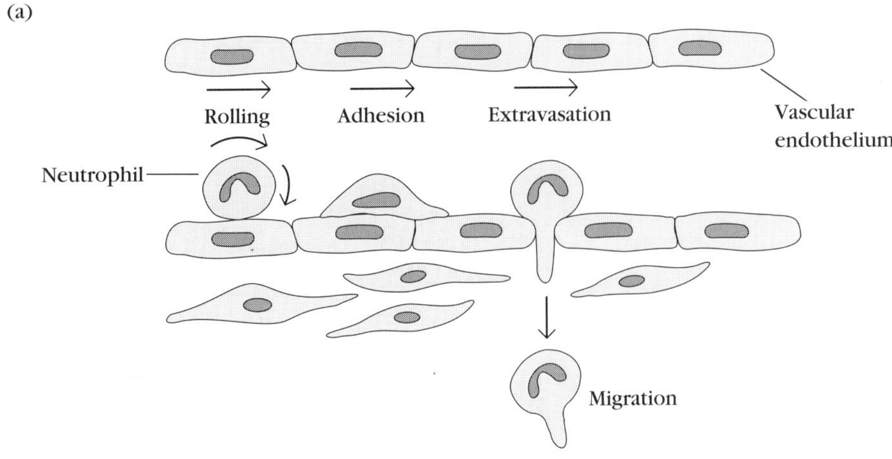

(b)

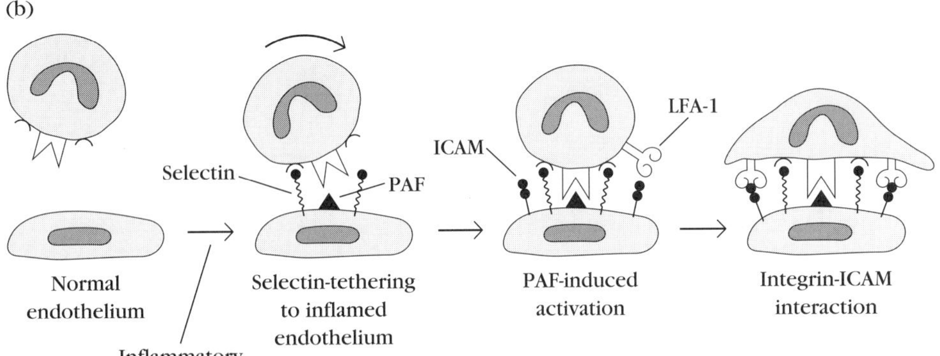

FIGURE 3-25 (a) General process of neutrophil adherence to and extravasation across activated (inflamed) vascular endothelium near an inflammatory site. (b) Interactions of cell-adhesion molecules that lead to adherence of neutrophils to vascular endothelium. PAF = platelet-activating factor. See text for details.

Platelet-activating factor increases the adhesiveness of neutrophils for endothelial cells by stimulating the expression of the integrin receptor LFA-1 on the neutrophil membrane (Figure 3-25b). Once LFA-1 is expressed by a neutrophil, it binds to ICAMs on an endothelial cell, thus strengthening adhesion of the neutrophil sufficiently to allow it to extravasate. As neutrophils arrive at the site of an infection, they begin to phagocytose particulate antigens and release a host of defensive antimicrobial agents to fight the infection. Since LFA-1 is only expressed by PFA-activated neutrophils, circulating neutrophils normally adhere only to regions of activated endothelium in the vicinity of an inflammatory response; this mechanism assures that neutrophils do not adhere to unactivated endothelium and thus do not extravasate into tissues unaffected by an inflammatory response. Circulating lymphocytes and monocytes also can bind to activated endothelium and extravasate into tissue where these cells participate in the inflammatory response.

Lymphocyte Extravasation

Various subsets of lymphocytes exhibit directed extravasation at inflammatory sites and secondary lymphoid organs. The recirculation of lymphocytes thus is carefully controlled to ensure that appropriate populations of B and T cells are recruited into different tissues. As with neutrophils, extravasation of lymphocytes involves a number of cell-adhesion molecules.

High-Endothelial Venules

Some regions of vascular endothelium found in postcapillary venules of various lymphoid organs are composed of specialized cells with a plump, cuboidal ("high") shape; such regions are called ***high-endothelial venules,*** or HEVs (Figure 3-26a,b). Each of the secondary lymphoid organs, with the exception of the spleen, contains HEVs. When frozen sections of lymph nodes, Peyer's patches, or tonsils are incubated with lymphocytes and washed to remove unbound cells, over 85% of the bound cells are found adhering to HEVs, even though HEVs account for only 1 – 2% of the total area of the frozen section (Figure 3-26c). The development of HEVs in lymphoid organs is influenced by cytokines produced in response to antigen capture. When animals are raised in a germfree environment, HEVs fail to develop. The need for antigenic activation of lymphocytes in maintaining HEVs can be demonstrated by surgically blocking the afferent lymphatic vasculature to a node, so that antigen entry to the node is blocked. Within a short period of time, the

HEVs show impaired function and eventually revert to a more flattened morphology.

High-endothelial venules express a variety of cell-adhesion molecules. Like other vascular endothelial cells, HEVs express CAMs of the immunoglobulin superfamily and selectin family. In addition, HEVs express some adhesion molecules that are distributed in a tissue-specific manner. These tissue-specific adhesion molecules have been called *vascular addressins* (VAs) because they serve to direct the extravasation of different populations of recirculating lymphocytes to particular lymphoid organs. The tissue-specific distribution of these addressin molecules can be demonstrated by differences in binding of monoclonal antibodies to HEVs. For example, some monoclonal antibodies bind only to vascular addressins in the HEVs of lymph nodes, whereas other monoclonal antibodies bind selectively to vascular addressins of Peyer's patches.

Homing of Lymphocytes

The differential migration of lymphocyte subsets into different tissues is called *trafficking,* or *homing.* In general naive (unprimed) T and B lymphocytes tend to home to various secondary lymphoid organs, such as the spleen, lymph nodes, or Peyer's patches. As discussed previously, the secondary lymphoid organs trap antigen and provide specialized microenvironments to support the clonal expansion and differentiation of antigen-activated lymphocytes into effector and memory cells. Recirculating naive lymphocytes have cell-surface receptors that recognize particular vascular addressins on the HEVs of different secondary lymphoid tissues (see Table 3-7). Because these receptors direct the circulation of various populations of lymphocytes

(a)

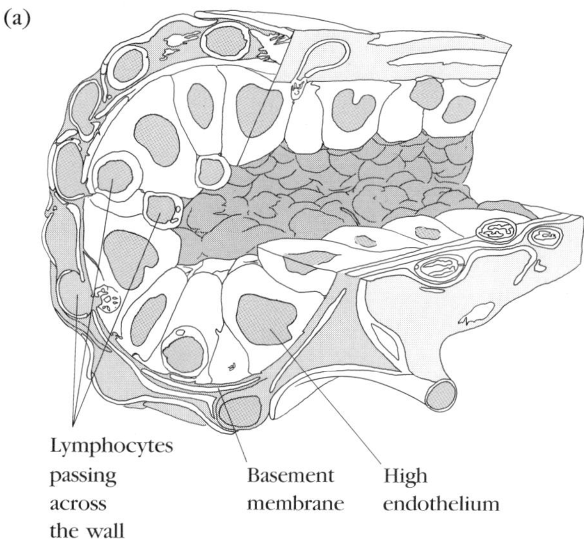

(b)

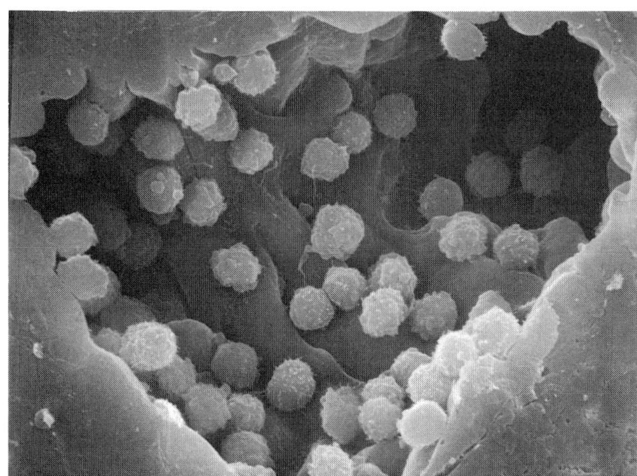

(c)

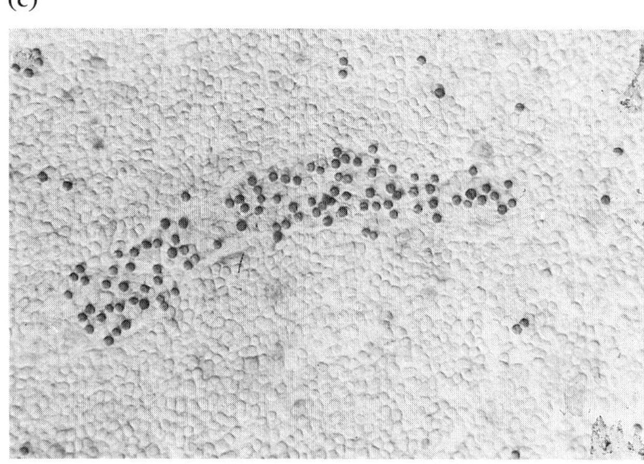

FIGURE 3-26 (a) Schematic diagram showing a cross section of a lymph node postcapillary venule with high endothelium. Lymphocytes are shown in various stages of attachment to the HEV and extravasation across the wall into the cortex of the node. (b) Scanning electron micrograph showing numerous lymphocytes bound to the surface of a high-endothelial venule. (c) Incubation of lymphocytes (darkly stained) with frozen sections of lymphoid tissue reveals that 85% of the lymphocytes are bound to HEVs (cross sections), which comprise only 1–2% of the total area of the tissue section. [Part (a) adapted from A. O. Anderson and N. D. Anderson, 1981, in *Cellular Functions in Immunity and Inflammation,* J. J. Oppenheim et al. (eds), Elsevier, North-Holland; part (b) from S. D. Rosen and L. M. Stoolman, 1987, *Vertebrate Lectins,* Van Nostrand Reinhold; part (c) from S. D. Rosen, 1989, *Curr. Opin. Cell Biol.* **1**:913.]

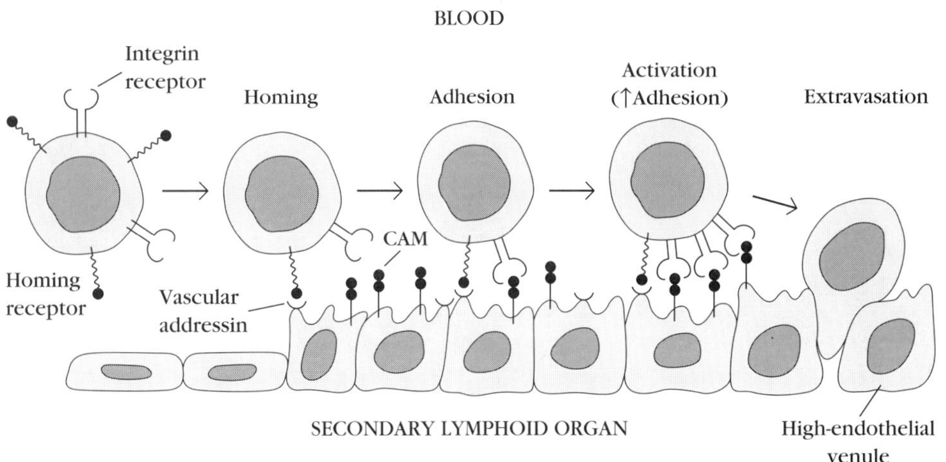

FIGURE 3-27 Interactions of cell-adhesion molecules involved in adhesion of lymphocytes to high-endothelial venules (HEVs). See text for details.

to particular lymphoid tissues, they have been called *homing receptors.* Different populations of lymphocytes express different homing receptors: B cells, for example, express VLA-4, a homing receptor for vascular addressins in MALT, whereas T cells express L-selectin, a homing receptor for addressins in peripheral lymph nodes. For this reason, B cells represent the majority of naive lymphocytes in Peyer's patches, whereas T lymphocytes predominate in lymph nodes.

Memory and effector lymphocytes display different homing properties. These cells are less likely to home to secondary lymphoid organs and instead home to sites of inflammation in the tissues (these sites are sometimes referred to as *tertiary lymphoid tissue*). Interestingly, memory lymphocytes exhibit selective homing to the type of tissue in which they first encountered antigen. Presumably this ensures that a particular memory cell will return to the tissue where it is most likely to re-encounter a subsequent antigenic threat.

Adhesion-Molecule Interactions

The adhesion of lymphocytes to HEVs or regions of inflamed endothelium and their subsequent extravasation is a multistep process involving a cascade of adhesion-molecule interactions (Figure 3-27). The first step usually involves the interaction of a homing receptor on a lymphocyte with a tissue-specific vascular addressin. Although this initial interaction is quite weak, the slow rate of blood flow in postcapillary venules, particularly in regions of HEVs, reduces the likelihood that the sheer force of the flowing blood will dislodge the tethered lymphocyte. In the second step, cellular adhesion is strengthened by binding of an integrin receptor on the lymphocyte with a CAM on the HEV. This latter interaction might involve binding of the integrin molecule VLA-4 to VCAM-1, or binding of the integrin LFA-1 to ICAM-1 or ICAM-2 (see Table 3-7; note that some molecules can function as both homing and adhesion receptors). This second interaction generates an activating signal that causes the lymphocyte to up-regulate its expression of integrin molecules. The increased expression of integrin molecules provides multiple adhesion receptors, strengthening the interaction between the lymphocyte and the HEV. The final step in the adhesion cascade is extravasation of the lymphocyte through the endothelium into the tissue. This step requires a reduction in the strength of adhesion between the lymphocyte and endothelium, so that the lymphocyte can extravasate through the endothelium.

Clinical Reduction of Extravasation

Although extravasation of leukocytes into the tissues is essential for the development of an effective inflammatory response, the response can sometimes be detrimental. Allergies, autoimmune diseases, microbial infections, transplants, and burns may be accompanied by a chronic inflammatory response. One way to reduce leukocyte extravasation, which is desirable in such cases, is to block the activity of various adhesion molecules with antibodies. In animal models, for example, antibodies to the integrin LFA-1 has been used to reduce neutrophil buildup in inflammatory tissue. Antibodies to ICAM-1 have also been used, with some success, in preventing the tissue necrosis associated with burns and in reducing the likelihood of kidney-graft rejection in animal models. The results with anti-ICAM-1 have been so encouraging that this antibody is now being tested in clinical trials on human kidney-transplant patients.

Summary

1. The cells that participate in the immune response are white blood cells, or leukocytes, all of which develop from a common pluripotent stem cell during hematopoiesis.

2. Various hematopoietic growth factors (cytokines) induce proliferation and differentiation of the different blood cells. This process is closely regulated to assure steady-state levels of each of the different types of blood cells. Cell division and differentiation of each of the lineages is balanced by programmed cell death by apoptosis.

3. The lymphocyte—the central cell of the immune system—is the only cell to possess the attributes of specificity, diversity, memory, and self/nonself recognition.

4. The monocyte, macrophage, and neutrophil are accessory immune-system cells whose primary function is to phagocytose and eliminate antigen. Phagocytosis is facilitated by opsonins such as antibody and complement, which increase the attachment of antigen to the membrane of the phagocyte.

5. In addition to phagocytosis, the macrophage plays an important role in T_H-cell activation by processing and presenting antigen in association with a class II MHC molecule and by secreting interleukin 1.

6. The primary lymphoid organs provide sites where lymphocytes mature and become antigenically committed. T lymphocytes mature within the thymus, and B lymphocytes mature within the bursa of Fabricius in birds and largely in the bone marrow in mammals.

7. The secondary lymphoid organs function to capture antigen and to provide sites where lymphocytes interact with that antigen and undergo clonal proliferation and differentiation into effector cells.

8. Lymphocytes undergo constant recirculation between the blood, lymph, lymphoid organs, and tissue spaces. Extravasation of lymphocytes and other leukocytes requires interaction between cell-adhesion molecules on the vascular endothelium and receptors for these CAMs on the circulating cells. Homing receptors on lymphocytes, which interact with tissue-specific adhesion molecules on high endothelial venules, direct recirculation of lymphocytes in a tissue-specific fashion.

References

BADWEY, J.A., and M. L. KARNOVSKY. 1986. Production of superoxide by phagocytic leukocytes: a paradigm for stimulus-response phenomena. *Curr. Topics Cell. Reg.* **28**:183.

BERG, E. L., L. GOLDSTEIN, M. A. JUTILA et al. 1989. Homing receptors and vascular addressins: cell adhesion molecules that direct lymphocyte traffic. *Immunol. Rev.* **108**:5.

DEXTER, T. M., and E. SPOONCER. 1987. Growth and differentiation in the hemopoietic system. *Ann. Rev. Cell Biol.* **3**:423.

DORSHKIND, K. 1990. Regulation of hematopoiesis by bone marrow stromal cells and their products. *Annu. Rev. Immunol.* **8**:111.

DUIJVESTIJN, A., and A. HAMANN. 1989. Mechanisms and regulation of lymphocyte migration. *Immunology Today* **10**:23.

DUSTIN, M. L., and T. A. SPRINGER. 1991. Role of lymphocyte adhesion receptors in transient interactions and cell locomotion. *Annu. Rev. Immunol.* **9**:27.

GALLATIN, M., T. P. ST. JOHN, M. SIEGELMAN et al. 1986. Lymphocyte homing receptors. *Cell* **44**:673.

GOLDE, D. W. 1991. The stem cell. *Sci. Am.* **255**(Dec.):86.

HYNES, R. O., and A. D. LANDER. 1992. Contact and adhesive specificities in the associations, migrations, and targeting of cells and axons. *Cell* **68**:303.

KAUSHANSKY, K. 1987. The molecular biology of the colony stimulating factors. *Blood Cells* **13**:3.

LAPIDOT, T., F. PFLUMIO, M. DOEDENS et al. 1992. Cytokine stimulation of multilineage hematopoiesis from immature human cells engrafted in SCID mice. *Science* **255**:1137.

LEHRER, R. I., A. K. LICHTENSTEIN, and T. GANZ. 1993. Defensins: antimicrobial and cytotoxic peptides of mammalian cells. *Annu. Rev. Immunol.* **11**:105.

MOORE, M. A. S. 1991. The clinical use of colony stimulating factors. *Annu. Rev. Immunol.* **9**:159.

NATHAN, C. F., and J. B. HIBBS. 1991. Role of nitric oxide synthesis in macrophage antimicrobial activity. *Curr. Opin. Immunol.* **3**:65.

NEUTRA, M. R., and J. P. KRAEHENBUHL. 1992. Transepithelial transport and mucosal defense I: the role of M cells. *Trends Cell Biol.* **2**:134.

OSBORN, L. 1990. Leukocyte adhesion to endothelium in inflammation. *Cell* **62**:3.

PICKER, L. J., and E. C. BUTCHER. 1992. Physiological and molecular mechanisms of lymphocyte homing. *Annu. Rev. Immunol.* **10**:561.

SHIMIZU, Y., W. NEWMAN, Y. TANAKA, and S. SHAW. 1992. Lymphocyte interactions with endothelial cells. *Immunol. Today* **13**:106.

SPANGRUDE, G. J., S. HEIMFELD, and I. WEISSMAN. 1988. Purification and characterization of mouse hematopoietic stem cells. *Science* **241**:58.

SPRINGER, T. A. 1990. Adhesion receptors of the immune system. *Nature* **346**:425.

STEINMAN, R. M. 1991. The dendritic cell system and its role in immunogenicity. *Annu. Rev. Immunol.* **9**:271.

TUSHINSKI, R. J., I. T. OLIVER, L. J. GUILBERT et al. 1982. Survival of mononuclear phagocytes depends on a lineage-specific growth factor that the differentiated cells selectively destroy. *Cell* **28**:71.

VAN EWIJK, W. 1991. T-cell differentiation is influenced by thymic microenvironments. *Annu. Rev. Immunol.* **9**:591.

WOODRUFF, J. J., L. M. CLARKE, and Y. H. CHIN. 1987. Specific cell-adhesion mechanisms determining migration pathways of recirculating lymphocytes. *Annu. Rev. Immunol.* **5**:201.

YEDNOCK, T. A., and S. D. ROSEN. 1989. Lymphocyte homing. *Adv. Immunol.* **44**:313.

Study Questions

1. For each of the following situations, indicate which type of lymphocytes would be expected to proliferate rapidly in lymph nodes and where in the nodes they would do so.
   a. Normal mouse immunized with a soluble protein antigen.
   b. Normal mouse with a viral infection.
   c. Neonatally thymectomized mouse immunized with a protein antigen.
   d. Neonatally thymectomized mouse immunized with the thymus-independent antigen bacterial lipopolysaccharide (LPS), which does not require the aid of T_H cells to activate B cells.

2. Do monocyte progenitor cells secrete M-CSF; do they express receptors for M-CSF? What would be the consequences to the cell if both M-CSF and the receptor for M-CSF were expressed?

3. List the primary lymphoid organs and summarize their functions in the immune response?

4. List the secondary lymphoid organs and summarize their functions in the immune response.

5. What cell types compose the stroma of the thymus? List two important functions of the thymic stromal cells.

6. Describe the processes of antigenic commitment and clonal selection. Indicate where these processes occur and how they contribute to the specificity and memory of the immune response.

7. Inflammatory mediators, including interferon gamma, interleukin 1, and tumor necrosis factor, cause induction of ICAMs on a wide variety of tissues. What effect might this induction have on the localization of immune cells?

8. In Weissman's method for enriching pluripotent stem cells, why is it necessary to use lethally irradiated mice?

9. What effect does thymectomy have on an adult mouse? On a neonatal mouse? Why should there be any difference?

10. How could you determine whether T cells and B cells tend to populate different areas of the secondary lymphoid organs?

11. In order to study the mechanism of lymphocyte homing, you are trying to find mice with homing defects. After an exhaustive search you identify two mice (designated A and B) whose lymphocytes fail to home to their own cervical lymph nodes, although they do home to other lymphoid tissue such as Peyer's patches. To determine the nature of these defects, you isolate lymphocytes from mouse A, mouse B, and a normal control mouse of the same strain, radiolabel these cells, and then inject samples of all three labeled cell preparations into all three mice. You then determine the presence (+) or absence (−) of the labeled lymphocytes in the cervical lymph nodes of each animal. The results, shown in the table below, indicate whether homing occurs.

Source of labeled lymphocytes	Presence (+) or absence (−) of labeled cells in cervical lymph node		
	Mouse A	Mouse B	Control mouse
Mouse A	−	+	+
Mouse B	−	−	−
Normal control mouse	−	+	+

   a. What kind of membrane defect might mouse A have?
   b. What kind of defect might mouse B have?
   c. Design an experiment to test your hypothesis.

ANTIGENS

Antigens are substances capable of inducing a specific immune response. The molecular properties of antigens and the way in which these properties ultimately contribute to immune activation are central to our understanding of the immune system. Some of the molecular features of antigens recognized by B or T cells are described in this chapter. The contribution made by the biological system to immunogenicity also is explored; ultimately the biological system determines whether a molecule that can bind to a B or T cell's antigen-binding receptor subsequently can induce an immune response. Fundamental differences in the way T and B lymphocytes recognize antigen determine which molecular features of an antigen are recognized by each branch of the immune system. These differences also are examined in this chapter and illustrated by typical viral and bacterial antigens.

Immunologic Properties of Antigens

Antigens can be defined on the basis of four immunologic properties: immunogenicity, antigenicity, allerogenicity, and tolerogenicity.

Immunogenicity is the ability to induce a humoral and/or cell-mediated immune response:

B cells + antigen → plasma cells + memory cells

T cells + antigen → T effector cells + memory cells

In this context, an antigen is more appropriately called an *immunogen. Antigenicity* is the ability to combine specifically with the final products of the above responses (i.e., antibodies and/or cell-surface receptors). Although all molecules possessing the property of immunogenicity also possess the property of antigenicity, the reverse is not true. Some small molecules, referred to as *haptens,* possess the property of antigenicity but are not capable, by themselves, of inducing a specific immune response. In other words, they lack immunogenicity.

Allerogenicity is the ability to induce various types of allergic responses. *Allergens* are immunogens that tend to activate specific types of humoral or cell-mediated responses having allergic manifestations. *Tolerogenicity* is the capacity to induce specific immunologic nonresponsiveness in either the humoral or the cell-mediated branch. Tolerogenicity and allerogenicity are discussed in Chapters 16 and 18, respectively.

TABLE 4-1 MOLECULAR WEIGHT OF SOME COMMON EXPERIMENTAL ANTIGENS USED IN IMMUNOLOGY

Antigen	Approx. molecular weight (Da)
Bovine gamma globulin (BGG)	150,000
Bovine serum albumin (BSA)	69,000
Flagellin (monomer)	40,000
Hen egg-white lysozyme (HEL)	15,000
Keyhole limpet hemocyanin (KLH)	>2,000,000
Ovalbumin (OVA)	44,000
Sperm whale myoglobin (SWM)	17,000
Tetanus toxoid (TT)	150,000

FACTORS THAT INFLUENCE IMMUNOGENICITY

In order to provide protection against infectious disease, the immune system must be able to recognize bacteria, bacterial products, fungi, parasites, and viruses as immunogens. Closer analysis has shown that the immune system actually recognizes particular macromolecules of an infectious agent, generally either proteins or polysaccharides. Proteins function as the most potent immunogens, with polysaccharides ranking second. In contrast, lipids and nucleic acids of an infectious agent generally do not serve as immunogens unless they are complexed to proteins or polysaccharides. Immunologists tend to use soluble proteins or polysaccharides as immunogens in most experimental studies of humoral immunity (Table 4-1). For cell mediated immunity, only proteins serve as immunogens. These proteins are not recognized directly; instead they must first be processed into small peptides and then presented in association with MHC molecules on the membrane of a cell before they can be recognized as immunogens.

Immunogenicity is not an intrinsic property of a macromolecule but rather is a condition dependent on a number of interrelated factors involved in the total biological system. For example, the common experimental antigen bovine serum albumin (BSA) is not immunogenic when reinjected into a cow, but it can serve as an excellent immunogen when injected into a rabbit. Generally, then, a macromolecule must be foreign to the animal exposed to it to exhibit immunogenicity. With a given foreign macromolecule, differences in the biological system can influence immunogenicity. This is illustrated most dramatically by comparisons of the immune response of different inbred strains of mice to peptide fragments of a complex protein such as sperm whale myoglobin. A peptide of sperm whale myoglobin that is immunogenic in one inbred strain may not be immunogenic in another inbred strain. The properties that most immunogens share in common and the contribution the biological system makes to the expression of immunogenicity are discussed in the next two sections.

Contribution of the Immunogen to Immunogenicity

Immunogenicity is determined, in part, by four properties of the immunogen: its foreignness, molecular weight, chemical composition and complexity, and ability to be degraded by macrophage enzymes.

Foreignness

In order to elicit an immune response, a molecule must be recognized as nonself by the biological system. The ability to recognize self-molecules is thought to arise during development by exposure of immature lymphocytes to self-components. Any molecule that is not exposed to immature lymphocytes during this critical period is later recognized as nonself, or foreign, by the immune system. When an antigen is introduced into an organism, the degree of its immunogenicity depends on the degree of its foreignness. Generally, the greater the phylogenetic distance between two species, the greater the genetic (and therefore the antigenic) disparity between them. For example, the antigen BSA would be expected to exhibit greater immunogenicity in a chicken than in a goat, which is more closely related to bovines. There are some exceptions to this rule: Some macromolecules (e.g., collagen and cytochrome *c*) were highly conserved throughout evolution and therefore display very little immunogenicity across diverse species lines. Conversely, some self-components (e.g., corneal tissue and sperm) are effectively sequestered from the immune system, so that if these tissues are injected even into the animal from which they originated, they will function as immunogens.

Molecular Size

There is a correlation between the size of a macromolecule and its immunogenicity. The best immunogens tend to have a molecular weight approaching 100,000 daltons (Da). Generally substances with a molecular weight less than 5000–10,000 Da are poor immunogens; however, in a few instances substances with a molecular weight less than 1000 Da have proved to be immunogenic.

Chemical Composition and Heterogeneity

Size and foreignness are not, by themselves, sufficient to make a molecule immunogenic; other properties are needed as well. For example, synthetic homopolymers (polymers composed of a single amino acid or sugar) tend to lack immunogenicity regardless of their size. Studies with copolymers composed of different amino acids has shed light on the contribution of chemical complexity to immunogenicity. Copolymers of sufficient size, containing two or more different amino acids, are immunogenic. The addition of aromatic amino acids, such as tyrosine or phenylalanine, has a profound effect on the immunogenicity of these synthetic polymers (for an example of copolymer structure, see Figure 4-4). For example, a synthetic copolymer of glutamic acid and lysine requires a minimum molecular weight of 30,000–40,000 Da for immunogenicity. The addition of tyrosine to the copolymer reduces the minimum size required for immunogenicity to between 10,000 and 20,000, and the addition of both tyrosine and phenylalanine reduces the minimum molecular weight for immunogenicity to 4000. All four levels of protein organization —primary, secondary, tertiary, and quaternary— contribute to the structural complexity of a protein and hence affect its immunogenicity (Figure 4-1).

Degradability

The development of both humoral and cell-mediated immune responses requires interaction of T_H cells with antigen that has been phagocytosed, processed, and presented in association with MHC molecules on the surface of macrophages or other antigen-presenting cells. Therefore, macromolecules that cannot be degraded and processed by antigen-presenting cells are poor immunogens. This can be illustrated by polymers of D-amino acids, which are stereoisomers of L-amino acids. Because the degradative enzymes within macrophages can only degrade proteins containing L-amino acids, polymers of D-amino acids cannot be processed by macrophages and thus are poor immunogens.

Large, insoluble macromolecules generally are more immunogenic than small, soluble ones because they are more readily phagocytosed and processed. Intermolecular chemical cross-linking, heat aggregation, and attachment to insoluble matrices have been routinely used to increase the insolubility of macromolecules, thereby facilitating their phagocytosis and increasing their immunogenicity.

Contribution of the Biological System to Immunogenicity

Even when the foreignness, size, complexity, and degradability of a macromolecule are sufficient to make it immunogenic, the development of an immune response will depend on certain properties of the biological system that the antigen encounters.

Genotype of the Recipient Animal

The genetic constitution of an immunized animal influences the type of immune response the animal manifests, as well as the degree of the response. For

–Lys–Ala–His–Gly–Lys–Lys–Val–Leu

(amino acid sequence of polypeptide chain)

PRIMARY STRUCTURE

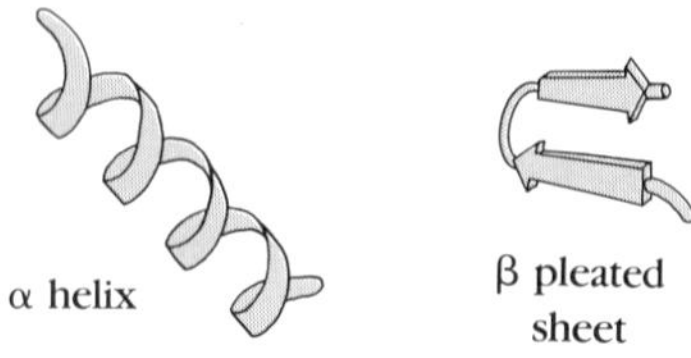

SECONDARY STRUCTURE

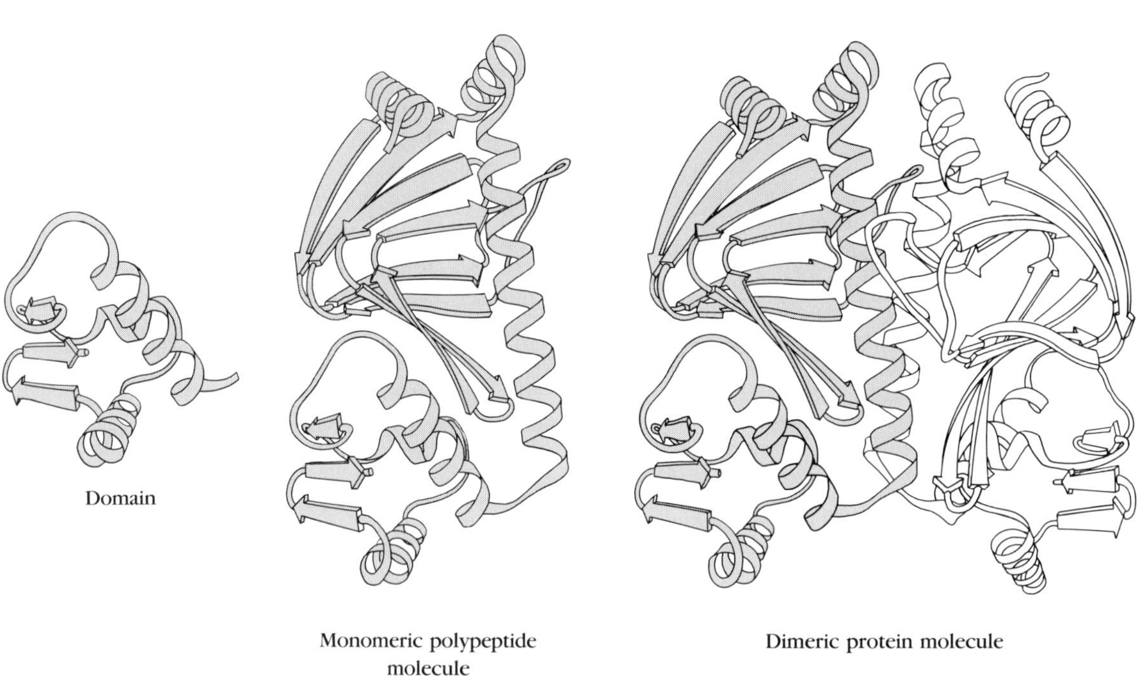

FIGURE 4-1 The four levels of protein organizational structure. The linear arrangement of amino acids constitute the primary structure. Folding of parts of a polypeptide chain into regular structures (e.g., α helices and β pleated sheets) generates the secondary structure. Tertiary structure refers to the folding of regions between secondary features to give the overall conformation of the molecule or portions of it (domains) with specific functional properties. Quaternary structure results from association of two or more polypeptide chains into a single polymeric protein molecule.

example, Hugh McDevitt showed that two different inbred strains of mice exhibited very different responses to a synthetic polypeptide immunogen. Following exposure to the immunogen, one strain produced high levels of serum antibody, whereas the other strain produced low levels. When the two strains were crossed, the F_1 generation showed an intermediate response to the immunogen. By backcross analysis, the F_1 gene controlling immune responsiveness was mapped to a subregion of the major histocompatibility complex (MHC). Numerous experiments with simple defined immunogens have demonstrated genetic control of immune responsiveness, largely confined to genes within the MHC (Table 4-2). These data indicate that the proteins encoded by the MHC, which function to present processed antigen to T cells, play a central role in determining the degree of immune responsiveness to an antigen.

The response of an animal to an antigen also is influenced by the genes encoding B-cell and T-cell receptors and by genes encoding various proteins involved in immune regulatory mechanisms. Genetic variability in all of these genes affects the immunogenicity of a given macromolecule in different animals. These genetic contributions to immunogenicity are discussed more fully in later chapters.

TABLE 4-2 EFFECT OF MHC HAPLOTYPE ON THE ANTIBODY RESPONSE TO THE SYNTHETIC COPOLYMERS (H,G)-A-L AND (T,G)-A-L IN MICE

MHC haplotype*	Representative mouse strains	Antibody response to (H,G)-A-L†	Antibody response to (T,G)-A-L‡
H-2^b	C57BL/6	Low	High
H-2^b	C3H.SW	Low	High
H-2^d	BALB/c	Intermediate	Intermediate
H-2^d	DBA/2	Intermediate	Intermediate
H-2^k	CBA	High	Low
H-2^k	C3H/HeJ	High	Low
H-2^s	B10.S	Low	Low
H-2^s	SJL	Low	Low

* The MHC haplotype is the entire set of closely linked MHC alleles inherited from the mother or the father. The haplotype is indicated by arbitrary superscripts. Since inbred strains are homozygous at each MHC loci (called H-2 in the mouse), a single superscript defines their haplotype.

† Copolymer consists of polylysine backbone with polyalanine side chains to which histidine and glutamic acid residues are attached at the end.

‡ Copolymer consists of polylysine backbone with polyalanine side chains to which tyrosine and glutamic acid residues are attached at the end (see Figure 4-4).

Immunogen Dosage and Route of Administration

For each experimental immunogen there will be some combination of optimal dosage and route of administration that will induce a peak immune response in a given animal. An insufficient dose will not stimulate an immune response either because it fails to activate enough lymphocytes or because it induces a nonresponsive state. Conversely, an excessively high dose also can fail to induce a response because it causes lymphocytes to enter a nonresponsive state. In mice the immune response to the purified pneumococcal capsular polysaccharide illustrates the importance of dose. A 0.5-mg dose of antigen fails to induce an immune response in mice, whereas a thousand-fold lower dose of the same antigen (5×10^{-4} mg) induces a humoral antibody response. This phenomenon of "immunologic unresponsiveness," or *tolerance,* is discussed in Chapter 16. A single dose of most experimental immunogens will not induce a strong response; rather, repeated administration over a period of weeks is required to stimulate a strong immune response. Such repeated administrations, or *boosters,* increase the clonal proliferation of antigen-specific T cells or B cells.

Experimental immunogens generally are administered parenterally—that is, by routes other than the digestive tract. Common administration routes are intravenous, intradermal, subcutaneous, intramuscular, and intraperitoneal. The route of antigen injection determines which immune organs and cell populations will be involved in the response. Antigen administered intravenously is carried first to the spleen, whereas antigen administered subcutaneously moves first to local lymph nodes. Differences in the lymphoid cells populating these organs generate differences in the quality of the subsequent immune response. For each new immunogen a dose-response curve must be established, with variations in dosage and route each contributing to peak responsiveness.

Adjuvants

Adjuvants (from Latin *adjuvare,* to help) are substances that, when mixed with an antigen and injected with it, serve to enhance the immunogenicity of that antigen. As seen in Figure 4-2, the antibody response to an influenza vaccine is much higher and longer-lasting when the vaccine is given with an adjuvant than when the vaccine is given alone. Adjuvants are often used to

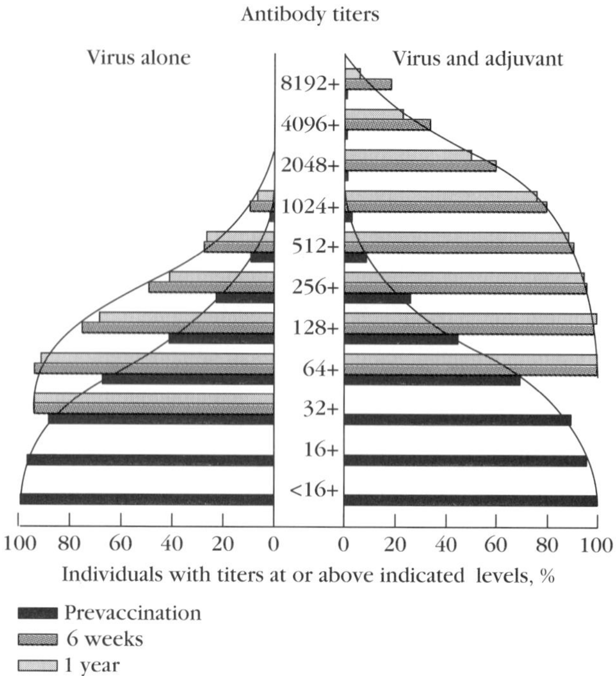

FIGURE 4-2 Effect of incomplete Freund's adjuvant on the immunogenicity of an influenza vaccine. Serum antibody titers to a major influenza antigen were measured before and at two times after immunization in 73 subjects immunized with the influenza vaccine alone and in 101 subjects immunized with the vaccine in adjuvant. The data are graphed as the percentage of individuals with serum antibody titers higher than that indicated by the central scale. The titer is the reciprocal of the last serum dilution to inhibit viral activity; thus, the greater the titer, the higher the antibody level. [Adapted from M. Zanetti et al., 1987, *Immunol. Today* **8**:23.]

boost the immune response when an antigen has low immunogenicity or when only small amounts of an antigen are available, limiting the immunizing dosage. For example, the antibody response in mice following immunization with BSA can be increased by fivefold or more if the BSA is administered with an adjuvant. Precisely how adjuvants augment the immune response is not entirely known, but several mechanisms appear to be involved (Table 4-3). As shown in the table, many adjuvants utilize more than one mechanism.

Some adjuvants have been shown to prolong the persistence of antigen in the immunized animals. For example, when an antigen is mixed with aluminum potassium sulfate (alum), the salt precipitates the antigen; injection of this alum precipitate results in a slower release of antigen from the injection site, so that the effective time of antigen exposure can be increased from a few days without adjuvant to several weeks with the adjuvant. The increased size of the antigen precipitate may also contribute to the adjuvant action of alum by increasing the likelihood of phagocytosis. Freund's water-in-oil adjuvants also function in this way. Freund's incomplete adjuvant contains antigen in aqueous solution, mineral oil, and an emulsifying agent such as mannide monooleate, which disperses the oil into small droplets surrounding the antigen; the antigen is then released very slowly from the site of injection. Freund's complete adjuvant, which contains heat-killed *Mycobacteria* in the water-in-oil emulsion, is more potent than the incomplete form because a muramyl dipeptide component of the mycobacterial cell wall activates macrophages, increasing production of interleukin 1 and thus augmenting the immune response by activating T_H cells.

TABLE 4-3 POSTULATED MODE OF ACTION OF SOME COMMONLY USED ADJUVANTS

	Postulated mode of action			
Adjuvant	Prolongs antigen persistence	Induces granuloma formation	Stimulates lymphocytes nonspecifically	Enhances co-stimulatory signal
Freund's incomplete adjuvant	+	+	−	+
Freund's complete adjuvant	+	++	−	+
Insoluble aluminum salts (alum)	+	+	−	?
Mycobacterium tuberculosis	−	+	−	?
Bordetella pertussis	−	−	+	?
Bacterial lipopolysaccharide (LPS)	−	−	+	+
Synthetic polynucleotides (poly IC/poly AU)	−	−	+	?

TABLE 4-4 COMPARISON OF ANTIGEN RECOGNITION BY T CELLS AND B CELLS

Characteristic	B cells	T cells
Interaction with antigen	Involves binary complex of membrane Ig and Ag	Involves ternary complex of T-cell receptor, Ag, and MHC molecule
Binding of soluble antigen	Yes	No
Involvement of MHC molecules	None required	Required to display processed antigen
Chemical nature of antigens	Protein, polysaccharide, lipid	Only protein
Epitope properties	Accessible, hydrophilic, mobile, often nonsequential (conformational) peptide	Internal, denatured, amphipathic, linear peptide that can bind to MHC molecule

Other adjuvants, such as synthetic polyribonucleotides and bacterial lipopolysaccharides, stimulate nonspecific lymphocyte proliferation and thus increase the likelihood of antigen-induced clonal selection of lymphocytes. Some adjuvants stimulate a local, chronic inflammatory response with an increase in phagocytic cells as well as lymphocytes. This cellular infiltration at the site of the adjuvant injection can often result in a dense, macrophage-rich mass of cells called a *granuloma.* Both alum and Freund's complete and incomplete adjuvants cause granuloma formation. The increased numbers of phagocytic cells at the site of the granuloma are thought to facilitate antigen processing and presentation and may also increase production of interleukin 1, thus stimulating activation of T_H cells.

An additional mechanism of adjuvant action has been revealed by more recent experiments. When a T_H cell recognizes antigen associated with a class II MHC molecule on the membrane of an antigen-presenting cell, the T_H cell needs a second signal, called a *co-stimulatory signal,* to become activated. One such co-stimulatory signal is generated by the interaction between two membrane molecules: B7, present on macrophages, and CD28, present on T_H cells. When antigen is injected with complete Freund's adjuvant, macrophages increase their expression of the B7 membrane molecule. Thus, the requisite co-stimulatory signal may be generated more easily in the presence of adjuvant than in its absence.

EPITOPES

As mentioned in Chapter 1, immune cells do not interact with, or recognize, an entire immunogen molecule; instead, lymphocytes recognize discrete sites on the macromolecule called *epitopes,* or *antigenic determinants.* Epitopes are the immunologically active regions of an immunogen that bind to specific membrane receptors for antigen on lymphocytes or to secreted antibodies. Interaction between lymphocytes and a complex antigen may involve several levels of antigen structure. In the case of protein antigens, the structure of an epitope may involve elements of the primary, secondary, tertiary, and even quaternary structure of the protein (see Figure 4-1). In the case of polysaccharide antigens, extensive side-chain branching via glycosidic bonds affects the overall three-dimensional conformation of individual epitopes.

T cells and B cells exhibit fundamental differences in antigen recognition (Table 4-4). B cells recognize soluble antigen when it binds to their membrane-bound antibody. Because B cells bind antigen that is free in solution, the epitopes they recognize tend to be highly accessible sites on the exposed surface of the immunogen. Such exposed epitopes generally contain hydrophilic amino acids and are often located at bends in the amino acid chain, imparting a greater degree of mobility to these residues. T cells, on the other hand, recognize processed peptides associated with MHC molecules on the surface of antigen-presenting cells and altered self-cells. T cells thus exhibit *MHC-restricted antigen recognition.* The CD4 subpopulation recognizes antigen in association with class II MHC molecules and generally functions as T helper cells, whereas the CD8 subpopulation recognizes antigen in association with class I MHC molecules and generally functions as T cytotoxic cells. The CD4 cell is therefore said to be class II restricted and the CD8 cell is said to be class I restricted. Subtle differences in the class I or class II MHC molecules expressed by different individuals influence their ability to recognize T-cell epitopes. Thus T-cell epitopes cannot be considered apart from their associated MHC molecules.

Determination of the conformation of an epitope is a time-consuming task requiring knowledge of its primary sequence and often of its three-dimensional structure, as well as information on the immune reactivity of each region of that structure. Some T-cell and B-cell epitopes have been identified by a technique called epitope mapping. In this technique, an immunogenic protein is fragmented with proteolytic enzymes into overlapping peptides, which are then tested for their ability to bind to an antibody elicited by the native protein or to induce T- or B-cell activation. This approach has been particularly useful in mapping T-cell epitopes since the T cell recognizes short linear peptides complexed with MHC molecules. This method is less effective for determining B-cell epitopes, which are often not contiguous amino acid sequences but instead are brought together in the tertiary folded configuration of the protein. These conformational B-cell epitopes cannot be identified by epitope mapping.

In a few cases B-cell epitopes have been identified by x-ray crystallographic analysis of Ag-Ab complexes. In this procedure beams of x-rays are passed through a crystal of an Ag-Ab complex. This analysis generates a three-dimensional space-filling model of every atom in the complex, allowing identification of the epitope and the contact residues of the antibody's antigen-binding site. Analysis of the x-ray diffraction patterns is extremely complex and takes years to complete. Consequently, only a few Ag-Ab complexes have been analyzed by this method. Needless to say, detailed understanding of epitope structure has not been attained for most immunogens.

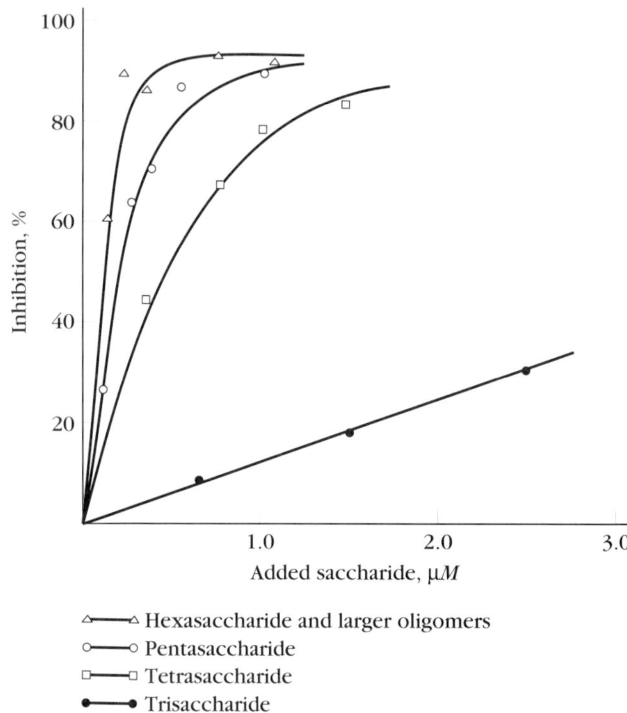

FIGURE 4-3 Ability of glucose oligomers of various sizes to inhibit the dextran-antidextran reaction. Rabbits were immunized with the glucose polymer dextran, and the antidextran antibodies produced were isolated and incubated with various short oligomers. Binding of the antidextran antibodies to dextran then was determined. Since the greatest inhibition would be expected with oligomers that bound most effectively to the dextran-binding site on the antibody molecules, these data can be used to estimate the size of the dextran epitope recognized by B cells. [Data from E. Kabat, 1974, *J. Am. Chem. Soc.* **76**:3709.]

Properties of B-Cell Epitopes

Several generalizations have emerged about properties of B-cell epitopes from studies with immunogens in which the conformation of the epitope recognized by B cells has been determined.

The size of a B-cell epitope is determined by the size of the antigen-binding site on the antibody molecules displayed by B cells. The binding of an antibody to an epitope involves weak noncovalent interactions, which operate only over short distances and therefore depend on complementarity between the antibody's binding site and the epitope to maximize these weak interactions. The size of the epitope recognized by a B cell thus is determined by the size, shape, and amino acid residues of the antibody's binding site.

In the 1950s, Elvin A. Kabat designed experiments to determine the size of the B-cell epitope on the glucose polymer dextran. In these experiments, he measured the ability of short glucose oligomers, varying in length from disaccharides to large oligosaccharides, to inhibit the binding of antidextran antibodies to dextran. Kabat reasoned that an oligomer constituting the entire epitope should be able to totally occupy the antibody's antigen-binding site and thus completely inhibit binding of the antibody to the epitope on the immunogen. As he increased the polymer size from trisaccharide to hexasaccharide, the oligomers showed increasing ability to inhibit the binding of antidextran antibodies to dextran (Figure 4-3). Since heptasaccharides and larger oligosaccharides showed the same inhibitory ability as the hexasaccharide, Kabat predicted that the hexasaccharide best approximated the size of the complete epitope and that additional sugar residues must lie outside the binding site on the antibody molecule. These early studies with small carbohydrate antigens suggested that the antibody's binding site was a cleft of sufficient size to bind six or seven amino acid or sugar residues.

As Ag-Ab complexes were analyzed with x-ray crystallography, a more detailed picture of epitope structure emerged. Smaller ligands such as carbohydrates, nucleic acids, peptides, and haptens were often found to bind to an antibody within a deep concave pocket. Crystallographic analysis of a small octapeptide hormone, called angiotensin II, revealed that the antibody made contact with the octapeptide within a deep and narrow groove of 725 Å^2. Within the groove, the peptide hormone was folded into a compact structure with two turns, which brought both amino and carboxyl termini close together. All eight amino acid residues of the octapeptide were shown to be involved in van der Waals contacts with 14 residues of the antibody groove.

X-ray crystallographic analysis of antibody complexed to globular protein antigens has yielded a very different picture of epitope structure. Analyses of monoclonal antibodies bound to hen egg-white lysozyme or neuraminidase (an envelope glycoprotein of influenza) have revealed that the antibody makes contact with the protein antigen across a large planar face. The interacting face between antibody and epitope has been observed as a somewhat flat to undulating surface in which protrusions on the epitope or antibody are matched by corresponding depressions on the respective antibody or epitope. These studies have revealed that 15–22 amino acids on the surface of the protein antigen make contact with a similar number of residues in the antibody's binding site; the surface area of this large complementary interface is between 650–900 Å^2. For these globular protein antigens, then, the epitope is entirely dependent on the tertiary conformation of the native protein.

Thus a different picture emerges of epitopes in globular protein antigens and in small peptide antigens. An epitope on a globular protein antigen appears to be considerably larger, occupying a more extensive surface area that is dependent on the tertiary structure of the protein; in contrast a smaller ligand, such as angiotensin II, folds into a compact structure that interacts with the antibody within a deep and narrow cleft. In Chapter 5 the nature of the interaction of the epitope with the antigen-binding site of the antibody is examined in more detail.

B-cell epitopes in native proteins generally are hydrophilic amino acids on the protein surface that are topographically accessible to membrane-bound or free antibody. A B-cell epitope must be accessible in order to be able to bind to an antibody. Amino acid sequences that are hidden within the interior of a protein cannot function as B-cell epitopes unless the protein is first denatured. Michael Sela demonstrated the importance of this topographical accessibility in experiments with synthetic branched copolymers in which the accessible amino acids attached to the backbone polypeptide chain were varied. One copolymer, (T,G)-A-L, consisted of a poly-L-lysine backbone with poly D,L-alanine side chains whose N-termini are capped with variable amounts of glutamic acid and/or tyrosine (Figure 4-4). Antibody to (T,G)-A-L reacted largely with the accessible tyrosine and glutamic acid residues at the end of each side chain. Furthermore,

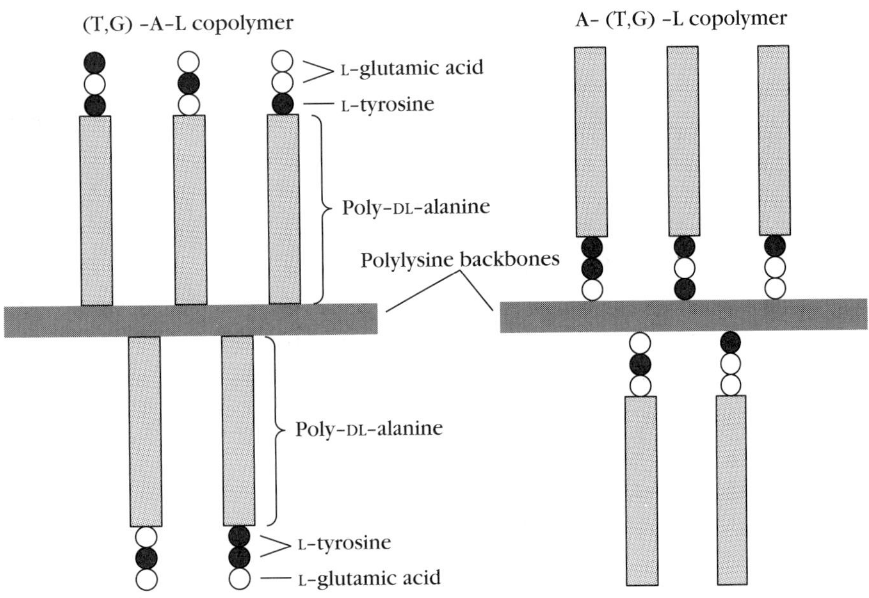

FIGURE 4-4 Antibodies elicited by immunization with the (T,G)-A-L copolymer react largely with the exposed tyrosine and glutamic acid residues. Anti-(T,G)-A-L antibodies do not react with the A-(T,G)-L copolymer in which the tyrosine and glutamic acid residues are buried. [Adapted from M. Sela, 1969, *Science* **166**:1365.]

the related synthetic copolymer A-(T,G)-L, in which poly D,L-alanine residues are in the accessible terminal positions and the glutamic acid and tyrosine residues are in a less accessible position, cannot react with the antibody to (T,G)-A-L.

The entire surface of globular protein antigens is thought to be potentially antigenic. In general, regions that tend to protrude on the surface of the protein are often recognized as epitopes. Because the residues are accessible, they are often hydrophilic. Of the crystallized Ag-Ab complexes analyzed to date, the interface between antibody and antigen possesses numerous complementary protrusions and depressions. Contact is made between 15–22 amino acids and has been shown to involve between 75–120 hydrogen bonds as well as ionic and hydrophobic interactions.

B-cell epitopes can contain sequential or nonsequential amino acids. Epitopes may be composed of *sequential* contiguous residues along the polypeptide chain or *nonsequential* residues from segments of the chain brought together by the folded conformation of the protein. Most antibodies elicited by globular protein antigens bind to the protein only when it is in its native conformation. Because denaturation of such antigens usually results in loss of the topographical structure of their epitopes, antibodies to the native protein fail to bind to the denatured protein.

Sperm whale myoglobin is an example of a protein antigen that contains several sequential epitopes. The three-dimensional structure of this protein has been determined by x-ray crystallography. The molecule has an abundance of α-helical regions and five distinct sequential epitopes, each containing six to eight

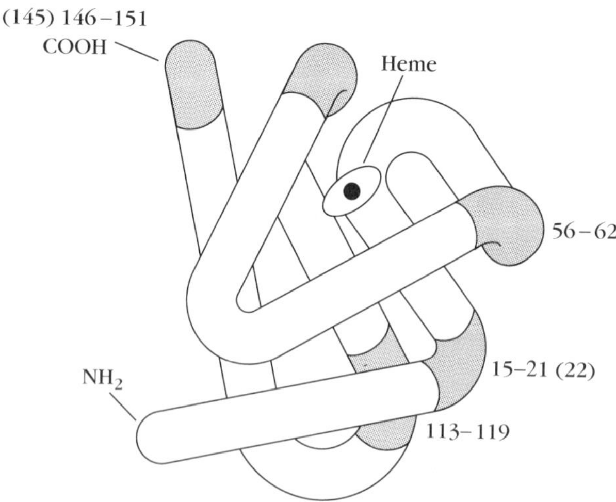

FIGURE 4-5 Diagram of sperm whale myoglobin showing locations of five sequential B-cell epitopes (light purple). [Adapted from M. Z. Atassi and A. L. Kazim, 1978, *Adv. Exp. Med. Biol.* **98**:9.]

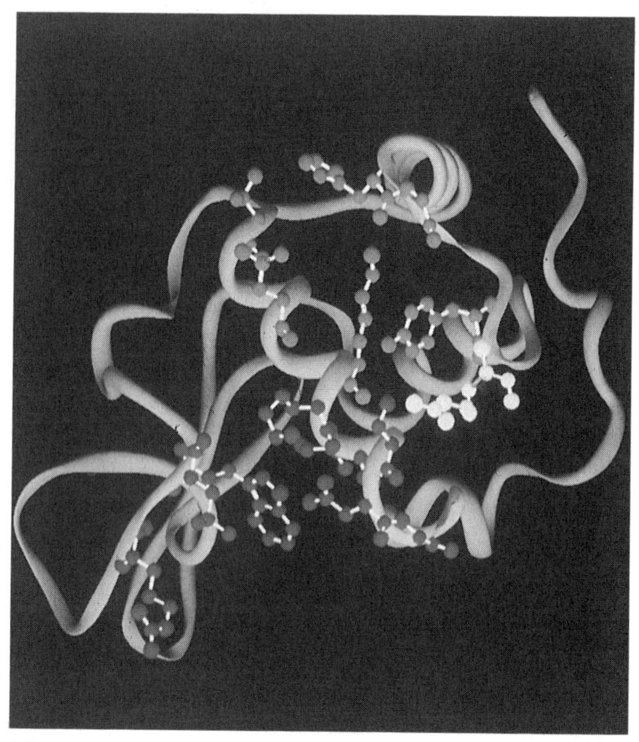

(a)

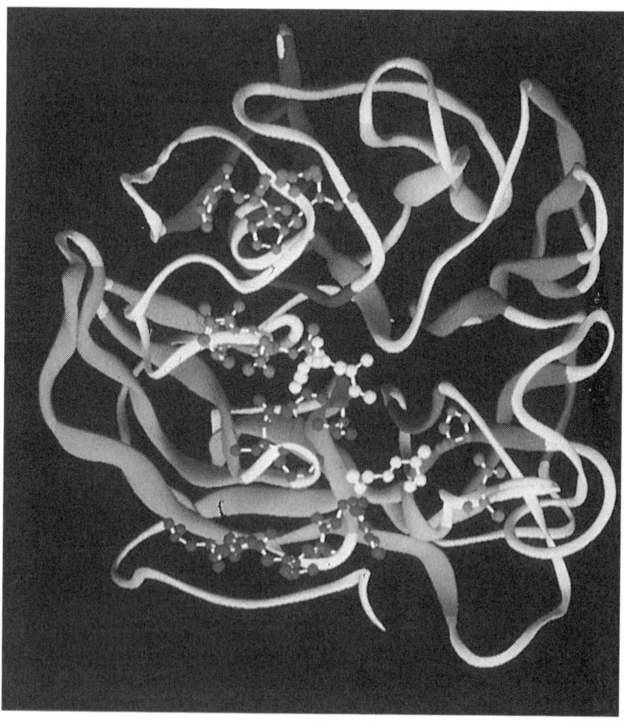

(b)

FIGURE 4-6 Ribbon diagrams of hen egg-white lysozyme (a) and influenza-virus neuraminidase (b) showing the location of one nonsequential epitope (conformational determinant) in each protein. The amino acids that have been shown to contact monoclonal antibody are indicated with shaded balls. [Adapted from W. G. Laver et al. 1990, *Cell* **61**:554.]

amino acids. Each of these epitopes is on the surface of the molecule at bends between the α-helical regions (Figure 4-5). Recently several additional nonsequential epitopes, or *conformational determinants,* also have been characterized for sperm whale myoglobin. The residues constituting these epitopes are far apart in terms of the primary amino acid sequence but close together in the tertiary structure of the molecule. Such epitopes thus are dependent on the native protein conformation for their topographical structure. The epitopes of hen egg-white lysozyme (HEL) and neuraminidase are well-characterized conformational determinants. Figure 4-6 shows the amino acid residues that make up one epitope of HEL and one epitope of neuraminidase. In each case the epitope is composed of nonsequential amino acids, far apart in the primary amino acid sequence, that have been brought together by the tertiary folding of the protein.

Sequential and nonsequential epitopes generally behave differently when a protein is fragmented or reduced. For example, appropriate fragmentation of sperm whale myoglobin can yield five fragments, each retaining one sequential epitope, as demonstrated by the observation that antibody can bind to each fragment. On the other hand, fragmentation of a protein or reduction of its disulfide bonds often destroys any nonsequential epitopes that it contains. For example, HEL has four intrachain disulfide bonds, which determine the final protein conformation. Antibodies to HEL recognize eight different epitopes, most of which are conformational determinants dependent on the overall structure of the protein. If the intrachain disulfide bonds of HEL are reduced with mercaptoethanol, the conformational determinants are lost and antibody to native HEL will not bind to reduced HEL. The inhibition experiment described in Figure 4-7 also dem-

(a) Hen egg-white lysosome

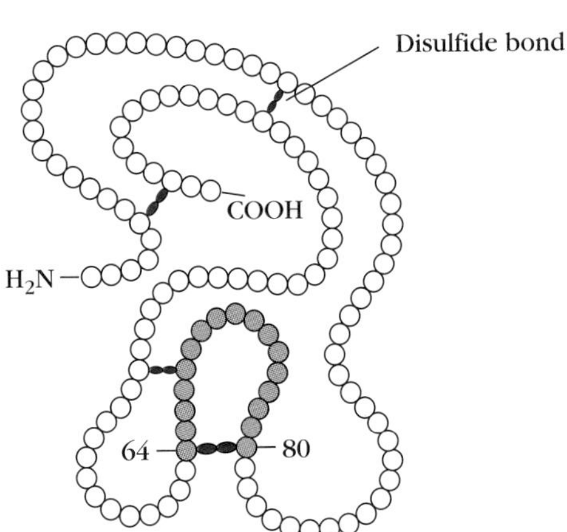

(b) Synthetic loop peptides

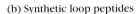

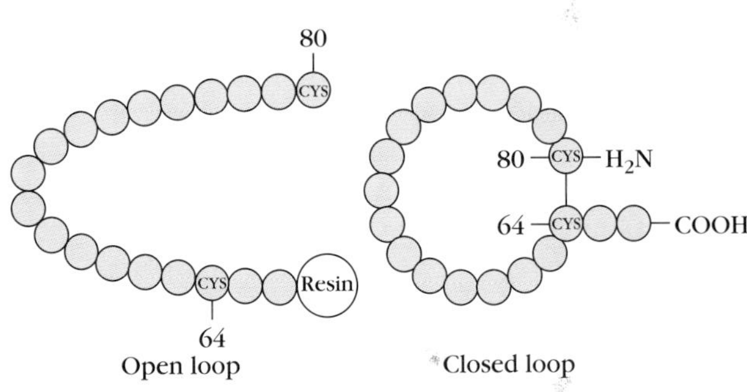

(c) Inhibition of reaction between HEL loop and anti-loop antiserum

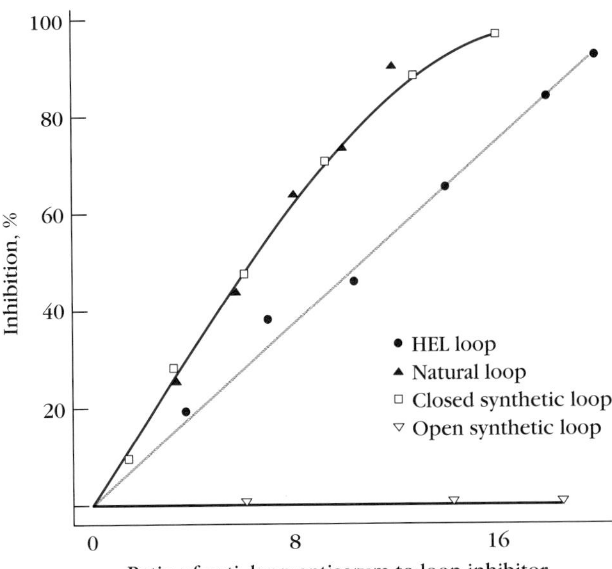

FIGURE 4-7 Experimental demonstration that binding of antibody to conformational determinants in hen egg-white lysozyme (HEL) depends on maintenance of the tertiary structure of the epitopes by intrachain disulfide bonds. (a) Diagram of HEL primary structure in which balls represent amino-acid residues. The loop (purple balls) formed by the disulfide bond between the cysteine residues at positions 64 and 80 constitutes one of the conformational determinants in HEL. (b) Synthetic open- and closed-loop peptides corresponding to the HEL loop epitope. (c) Inhibition of reaction between HEL loop epitope and anti-loop antiserum. Anti-loop antiserum was first incubated with HEL, the natural loop sequence, the synthetic closed-loop peptide, or the synthetic open-loop peptide; the ability of the antiserum to bind the natural loop sequence then was determined. The absence of any inhibition by the open-loop peptide indicates that it does not bind to the anti-loop antiserum. [Adapted from D. Benjamin et al., 1984, *Annu. Rev. Immunol.* **2**:67.]

TABLE 4-5 ANTIGEN RECOGNITION BY T AND B LYMPHOCYTES REVEALS QUALITATIVE DIFFERENCES

		Secondary immune response	
Primary immunization	Secondary immunization	Antibody production	Cell-mediated T_{DTH} response*
Native protein	Native protein	+	+
Native protein	Denatured protein	−	+

* T_{DTH} refers to a subset of $CD4^+$ T_H cells that mediate a type of cell-mediated response known as delayed-type hypersensitivity (see Chapter 15).

onstrates the importance of these disulfide bonds in determining the structure of HEL epitopes.

B-cell epitopes tend to be located in flexible regions of an immunogen and display site mobility. John A. Tainer and his colleagues analyzed the epitopes on a number of protein antigens (myohemerytherin, insulin, cytochrome *c*, myoglobin, and hemoglobin) by comparing the positions of the known B-cell epitopes with the atomic mobility of the same residues. Their analysis revealed that the major antigenic determinants in these proteins generally were located in the most mobile regions. These investigators propose that site mobility of epitopes maximizes complementarity with the antibody's binding site, giving rise to a higher-affinity interaction.

Complex proteins contain multiple overlapping B-cell epitopes. Until recently, it was dogma in immunology that a given globular protein had a small number of epitopes, each confined to a highly accessible region and determined by the overall conformation of the protein. However, it has been shown recently that most of the surface of a globular protein is potentially antigenic. This has been demonstrated by comparing the antigen-binding profiles of different monoclonal antibodies to various globular proteins. For example, when 64 different monoclonal antibodies to BSA were compared for their ability to bind to a panel of 10 different mammalian albumins, 25 different overlapping antigen-binding profiles emerged, suggesting that these 64 different antibodies recognized a minimum of 25 different epitopes on BSA. Similar findings have emerged for other globular proteins, such as myoglobin and HEL. The surface of a protein, then, must present a large number of potential antigenic sites. The subset of antigenic sites on a given protein that is selected by an individual animal is much smaller than the potential antigenic repertoire, and it varies from species to species and even among individual members of a given species. Within a given animal, certain epitopes are recognized as immunogenic, whereas others are not. Furthermore, some epitopes, referred to as *immunodominant,* induce a more pronounced immune response than other epitopes in a particular animal. It is thought that intrinsic topographical properties of the epitope as well as the animal's regulatory mechanisms influence the immunodominance of particular epitopes.

Properties of T-Cell Epitopes

Early studies by P. G. H. Gell and Baruj Benacerraf in 1959 suggested that there is a qualitative difference between the T-cell and the B-cell response to protein antigens. Gell and Benacerraf compared the humoral and cell-mediated responses to a series of native and denatured protein antigens (Table 4-5). They found that if primary immunization was with a native protein, then a secondary antibody response was elicited only with native protein, not with denatured protein. In contrast, the secondary cell-mediated response did not discriminate between native and denatured protein. In other words, a secondary T-cell–mediated response was induced by denatured protein even when the primary immunization had been with native protein. This observation puzzled immunologists until the 1980s, when it became clear that T cells do not recognize soluble native antigen but rather recognize antigen that has been processed and whose peptide fragments are presented in association with MHC molecules. For this reason, destruction of the conformation of a protein by denaturation does not affect its T-cell epitopes.

Because the T-cell receptor does not bind an epitope directly, experimental systems for studying T-cell epitopes must include antigen-presenting cells or target cells that can display the epitope together with an MHC molecule. In some systems, synthetic peptides are first allowed to interact with MHC molecules on antigen-presenting cells, and then T-cell proliferation is measured.

Oligomeric peptides function as T-cell epitopes. S. F. Schlossman synthesized polypeptide polymers containing oligomers of L-lysine residues separated by intervening sequences of D,L-lysine. He found that only oligomers with a minimum of seven contiguous L-lysines [(L-lysine)$_7$-D-lysine-L-lysine] were capable of stimulating T-cell proliferation. I. Berkower and J. Berzofsky tested the ability of peptides derived from sperm whale myoglobin (SWM), a complex protein antigen, to stimulate proliferation of a cloned $CD4^+$ T-cell line specific for SWM. The smallest peptide with stimulatory ability was an 11-aa peptide consisting of residues 136–146. However, most of the SWM peptides that were found to activate T cells contained on the order of 20 amino acids.

The antigen-binding cleft of an MHC molecule determines the nature and size of the peptide(s) that it can bind and consequently the maximal size of the T-cell epitope. Studies of the binding of peptides to class I MHC molecules have revealed that peptides of nine amino acid residues (nonamers) bind most strongly; peptides of 8–11 residues also bind but generally with lower affinity than nonamers. In the case of class II MHC molecules, peptides of 11–17 amino acid residues are preferentially bound.

Antigenic peptides recognized by T cells form trimolecular complexes with a T-cell receptor and a MHC molecule. Direct biochemical evidence for an interaction between defined T-cell peptide antigens and class I and class II MHC molecules has been obtained by several investigators. Crystallization of both class I and class II MHC molecules has revealed a small peptide, in the cleft of the molecule (see Color Plates 11 and 15). Antigens recognized by T cells must, therefore, possess two distinct interaction sites: one (the epitope) interacts with the T-cell receptor, and the other, called the *agretope,* interacts with a MHC molecule (Figure 4-8). Little is understood regarding the nature of the interaction between an agretope and a MHC molecule; the term agretope is not based on clear structural features but simply denotes the functional ability of an antigenic peptide to interact with a MHC molecule. Unlike B-cell epitopes, which can be viewed strictly in terms of their ability to interact with antibody, T-cell epitopes must be viewed in terms of a trimolecular complex involving a T-cell receptor, an antigenic peptide, and a MHC molecule.

The binding of a peptide to the cleft in a MHC molecule does not appear to have the kind of fine specificity exhibited in the interaction between an antibody and its epitope. Instead, a given MHC molecule can selectively bind a variety of different peptides. For example, the class II MHC molecule designated IA^d can bind peptides from ovalbumin (residues 323–339), hemagglutinin (residues 130–142), and lambda repressor (residues 12–26). This broad, but selective interaction suggests that the agretopes on these various peptides may share certain structural features, enabling them to bind to the same MHC molecule. More recent studies

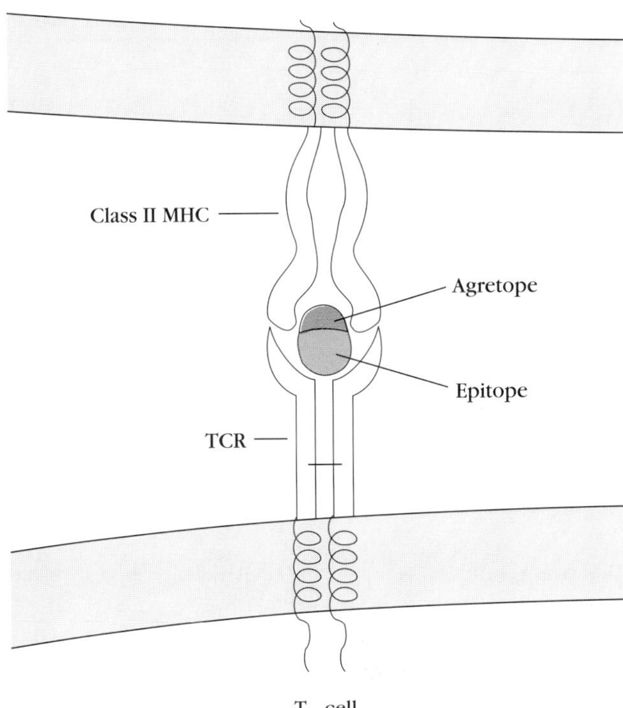

FIGURE 4-8 Schematic diagram of the ternary complex formed between a T-cell receptor (TCR), antigen, and MHC molecule. Antigens that are recognized by T cells have two distinct interaction sites: an agretope, which interacts with a class I or class II MHC molecule, and an epitope, which interacts with the T-cell receptor.

revealing common structural features, or motifs, among different peptides that bind to a single MHC molecule are discussed in Chapter 9.

Antigen processing is required to generate peptides that interact specifically with MHC molecules. As mentioned in Chapter 1, endogenous antigens and exogenous antigens appear to be processed by different intracellular pathways (see Figure 1-10). Endogenous antigens are processed into peptides within the cytoplasm, while exogenous antigens are processed within the endocytic pathway. Processing yields antigenic peptides that associate with class I or class II MHC molecules; the resulting peptide-MHC complexes are then presented on the cell surface where they can be recognized by T cells. The details of antigen processing and presentation are described in Chapter 10.

Antigens recognized by T cells often contain amphipathic peptides. J. Berzofsky and co-workers have suggested that the primary function of antigen processing may be to unfold an antigen and reveal internal regions

TABLE 4-6 POSITION OF KNOWN IMMUNODOMINANT T-CELL EPITOPES AND AMPHIPATHIC SEGMENTS IN VARIOUS PROTEIN ANTIGENS

Antigen	T-cell epitopes*	Amphipathic segments*	Amphipathic score†
Sperm whale myoglobin	69–78	64–78	14.2
	102–118	99–117	20.1
	132–145	128–145	15.3
Pigeon cytochrome *c*	93–104	92–103	4.3
Influenza hemagglutinin A/PR/8/34 Mt. S.	109–119	97–120	35.3
	130–140	—	—
	302–313	291–314	35.1
Pork insulin	(B)5–16	4–16	5.5
	(A)4–14	1–21	34.0
Chicken lysozyme	46–61	—	—
	74–86	72–86	8.9
	81–96	86–102	13.1
	109–119	—	—
Chicken ovalbumin	323–339	329–346	18.0
Hepatitis B virus pre S	120–132	121–135	8.7
Foot and mouth virus VP1	141–160	148–165	20.3
Beef cytochrome *c*	11–25	9–29	22.7
	66–80	58–78	23.6
Hepatitis B virus major surface antigen	38–52	36–49	7.3
	95–109	—	—
	140–154	—	—
λ Repressor protein CI	12–26	8–25	19.5
Rabies virus-spike glycoprotein precursor	32–44	29–46	20.2

* Positions of amino acid residues constituting epitopes and amphipathic segments are shown.

† Amphipathic score obtained from computer analysis of peptide segments within the proteins.

SOURCE: Adapted from H. Margalit et al., 1987, *J. Immunol.* **138**:2219.

that are amphipathic (i.e., possessing both hydrophobic and hydrophilic amino acid residues). The hydrophobic residues may act as agretopes, interacting with MHC molecules, and the hydrophilic residues may act as epitopes, interacting with T-cell receptors.

To determine whether there might be a correlation between amphipathic peptides and T-cell responsiveness, H. Margalit and her colleagues designed a computer program to analyze peptide sequences within proteins and assigned to each peptide segment an "amphipathic index" based on the amount of amphipathic α helices in it. Comparison of 23 known immunodominant T-cell peptides in various proteins with the amphipathic segments in the same proteins revealed that 18 of the T-cell peptides overlapped with highly amphipathic segments (Table 4-6). This correlation has been used to predict potential T-cell epitopes for synthetic peptide vaccines against a number of diseases, including malaria, influenza, and hepatitis (see Chapter 20). A somewhat similar approach has been used to demonstrate that the known T-cell epitopes in sperm whale myoglobin and hen egg-white lysozyme exhibit minimum protrusion; that is, they tend to be on the "inside" of the protein molecule (Figure 4-9).

Immunodominant T-cell epitopes are determined in part by the set of MHC molecules expressed by an individual. Various types of experiments have suggested that the MHC plays a significant role in determining which T-cell epitopes in a given antigen will be immunodominant in a given individual. For example, a correlation between the ability of a peptide to bind to a particular MHC molecule and the T-cell response to that peptide was shown in experiments of S. Buus, A. Sette, and H. M. Grey. They analyzed 14 synthetic peptides, representing overlapping sequences of the entire length of an immunogenic protein. Of these 14 peptides, three were shown to activate T_H cells, and each of these three peptides was also shown to bind to a class II MHC molecule expressed by the same strain of mice (Figure 4-10).

Another experimental approach for studying the role of the MHC in determining the immunodominance of T-cell epitopes involves transfection of class II MHC genes into a mouse fibroblast cell line called L cells. Since L cells are not antigen-presenting cells, they do not express their own class II MHC molecules. However, if a class II gene is transfected under the control of an active promoter, L cells will express the transfected class II gene product. Using this approach, N. Shastri transfected L cells with class II MHC genes that encoded either IA or IE. He then tested the ability of the transfected L cells to present various lysozyme peptides to different T_H clones known to be specific

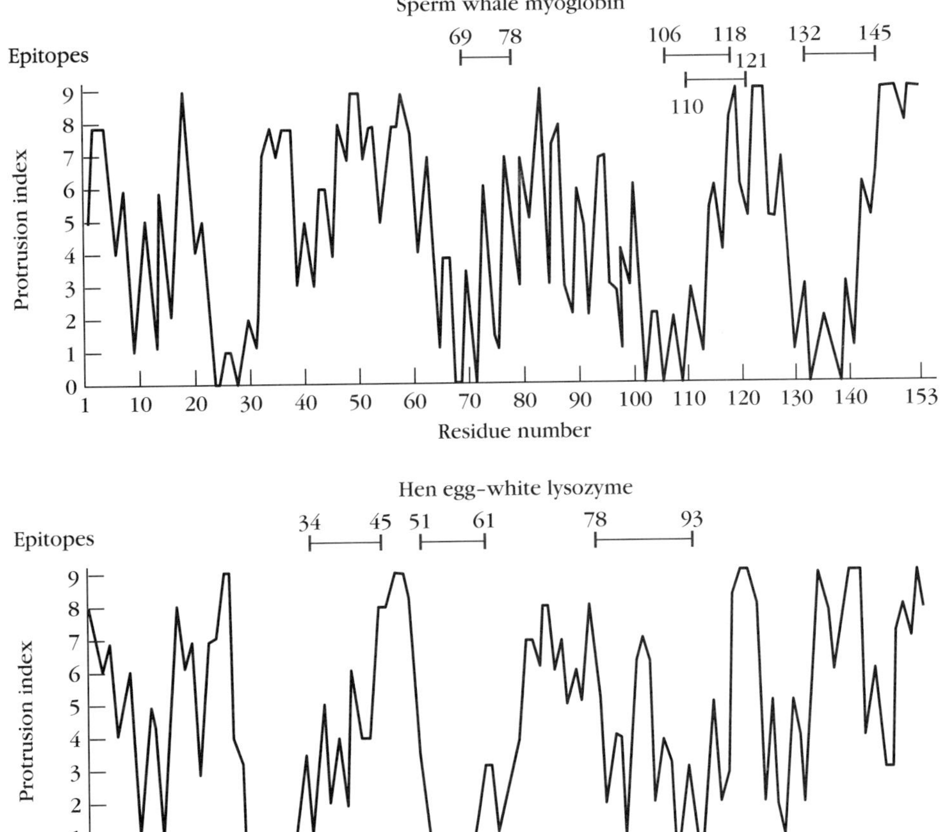

FIGURE 4-9 T_H cells tend to recognize internal peptides that are exposed during processing within antigen-presenting cells. The amino acids of two proteins (sperm whale myoglobin and hen egg-white lysozyme) have been plotted according to their protrusion in the tertiary conformation of the protein. The known T-cell epitopes for each protein are indicated by the purple bars. Notice that amino acid residues corresponding to the T-cell epitopes are residues with a minimum of protrusion. [From J. Rothbard et al., 1987, *Modern Trends in Human Leukemia,* vol. 7.]

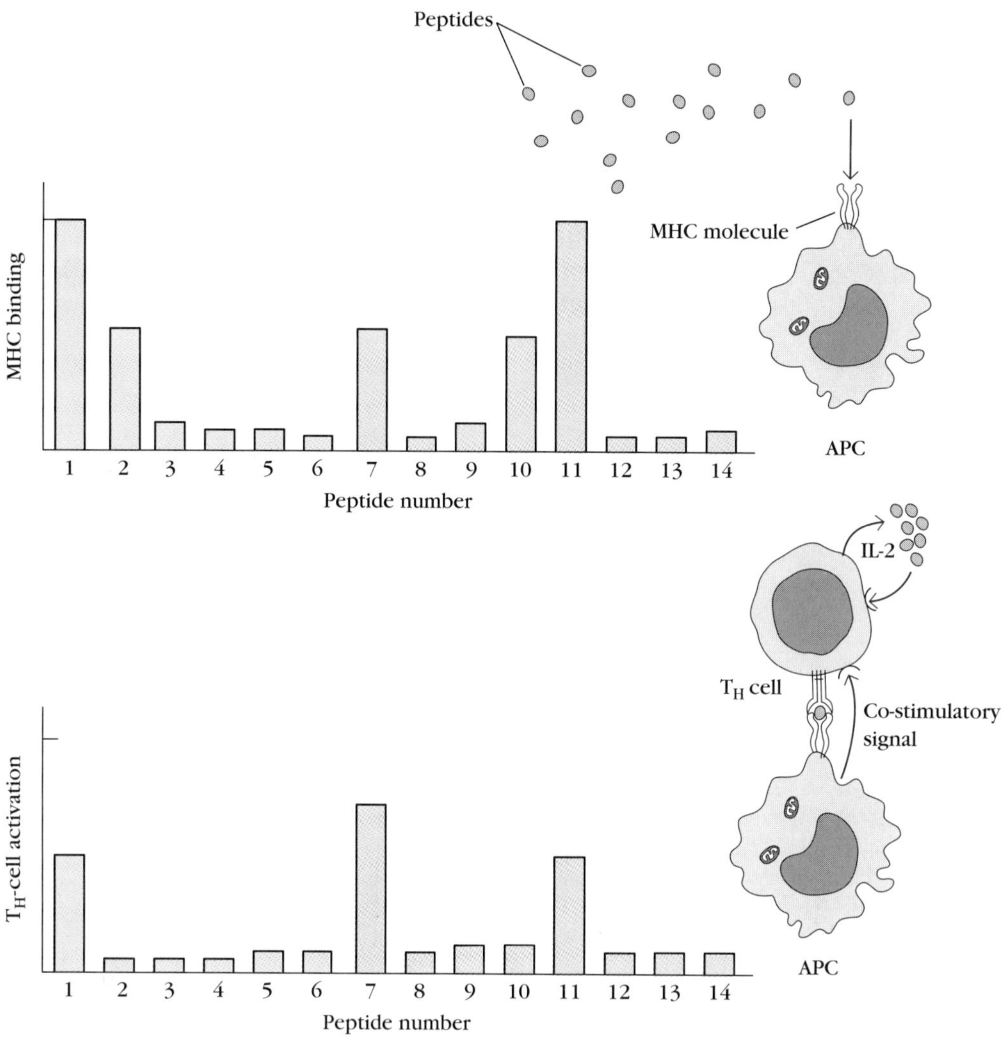

FIGURE 4-10 Correlation of MHC-binding ability and T-cell–activating ability of 14 synthetic peptides representing overlapping sequences of an immunogenic protein. Of the five peptides that bound to MHC molecules on mouse antigen-presenting cells *(top),* three also stimulated T-cell activation *(bottom).* These data suggest that binding to an MHC protein is necessary, but not sufficient, for a peptide to induce an immune response. [Adapted from H. M. Grey et al., 1989, *Sci. Am.* **261**(5):59.]

for lysozyme plus the IA or IE class II MHC molecule. He found that L cells transfected with the IA genes could present lysozyme peptide 74–86 but not peptide 85–96 to the IA-restricted clone; conversely, L cells transfected with the IE genes could present peptide 85–96 but not peptide 74–86 to the T_H-cell clone restricted for IE (Figure 4-11). In this system, then, one lysozyme T-cell epitope is immunodominant in the IA-restricted clone and another epitope is immunodominant in the IE-restricted clone, demonstrating that immunodominance is determined by the MHC molecules expressed.

Haptens and the Study of Antigenicity

The pioneering work of Karl Landsteiner in the 1920s and 1930s provided a simple, chemically defined system for studying the binding of an individual antibody to a unique epitope on a complex protein antigen. In Landsteiner's approach small organic compounds, called *haptens,* are chemically coupled to larger proteins, called *carriers* (Figure 4-12a). When the resulting *hapten-carrier conjugate* is used to immunize

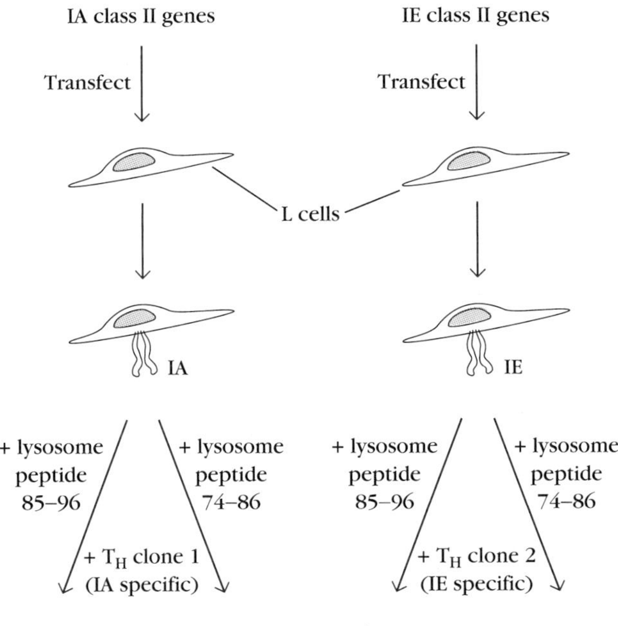

FIGURE 4-11 Experimental demonstration that MHC molecules exhibit differential interaction with antigenic peptides. In this experiment, the transfected L cells functioned as antigen-presenting cells to two T_H-cell clones, one specific for lysozyme plus class II IA MHC and the other specific for lysozyme plus class II IE MHC. The results indicate that each MHC molecule could present only one of the two lysozyme peptides.

animals, it functions as an immunogen, with antibodies being elicited both to the hapten determinant and to unaltered epitopes on the carrier protein; the hapten thus functions as an epitope. Since the chemical conjugation makes it possible for multiple molecules of a single hapten to be coupled to the carrier protein and to be accessible to the immune system, the hapten functions as the immunodominant determinant on a hapten-carrier conjugate. The beauty of the hapten-carrier system is that it provides immunologists with a chemically defined determinant that can be subtly modified by chemical means to determine the effect of various chemical structures on immune specificity.

In the system developed by Landsteiner, hapten alone does not stimulate clonal selection and the ensuing secretion of antibody. That happens only when a hapten is coupled to a protein carrier (Figure 4-12b). Although a hapten behaves as an antigen, in that it can react with antibody, its small size and minimal valency prevent it, by itself, from functioning as an immunogen. However, if multiple copies of a hapten are coupled to a large nonimmunogenic homopolymer, the molecule can sometimes behave as an immunogen; the homopolymer provides the requisite size, and the hapten provides the complexity and multivalency.

Landsteiner's studies with haptens demonstrated the fine specificity of the immune system. He immunized rabbits with a hapten-carrier conjugate and then tested the reactivity of the rabbit's immune sera to that

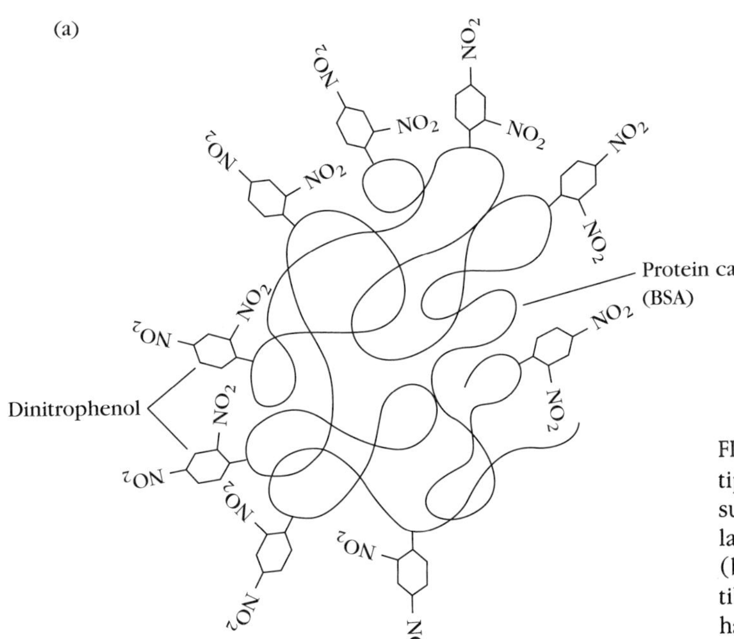

(b)

Injection with:	Antibodies formed:
Hapten (DNP)	None
Protein carrier (BSA)	Anti–BSA
Hapten–carrier conjugate (DNP–BSA)	Anti–DNP (major) Anti–BSA (minor)

FIGURE 4-12 (a) A hapten-carrier conjugate contains multiple copies of the hapten—a small organic compound such as dinitrophenol (DNP)—chemically linked to a large protein carrier such as bovine serum albumin (BSA). (b) Immunization with DNP alone elicits no anti-DNP antibodies, but immunization with DNP-BSA reveals that the hapten is the immunodominant epitope in a hapten-carrier conjugate.

hapten and to closely related haptens coupled to a different carrier protein. Thus he could measure, specifically, the reaction of the antihapten antibodies in the immune serum and not that of antibodies to the original carrier epitopes. Landsteiner tested whether an antihapten antibody could bind to other haptens having a slightly different chemical structure. If a reaction occurred, it was referred to as a *cross-reaction*. By observing which hapten modifications prevented or permitted cross-reactions, Landsteiner was able to gain insight into the specificity of the Ag-Ab interaction.

Landsteiner found that the overall configuration of a hapten plays a major role in determining whether it can react with a given antibody. He produced antisera to aminobenzene and its carboxyl derivatives (*o*-aminobenzoic acid, *m*-aminobenzoic acid, and *p*-aminobenzoic acid). Each antiserum was specific for the original immunizing hapten and did not react with any

TABLE 4-7 REACTIVITY OF ANTISERA WITH VARIOUS HAPTENS

	Reactivity with			
Antiserum against	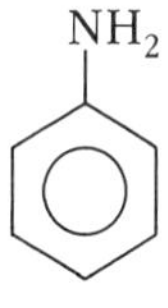 Aminobenzene (aniline) [NH_2]	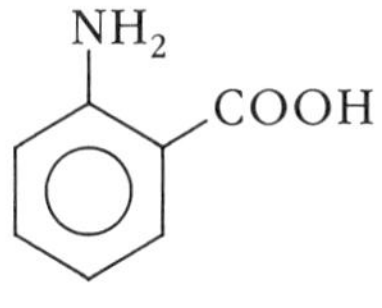 *o*-aminobenzoic acid [NH_2, COOH]	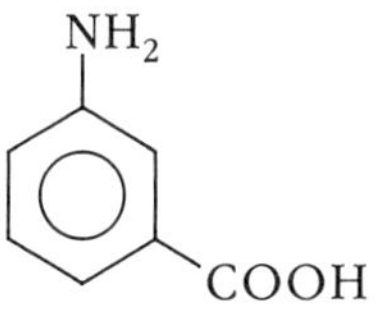 *m*-aminobenzoic acid [NH_2, COOH]	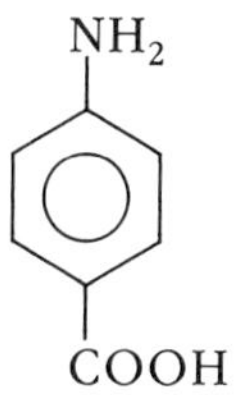 *p*-aminobenzoic acid [NH_2, COOH]
Aminobenzene	+++	0	0	0
o-aminobenzoic acid	0	+++	0	0
m-aminobenzoic acid	0	0	++++	0
p-aminobenzoic acid	0	0	0	+++±

	Reactivity with			
Antiserum against	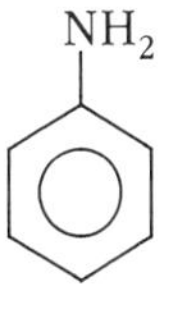 Aminobenzene (aniline) [NH_2]	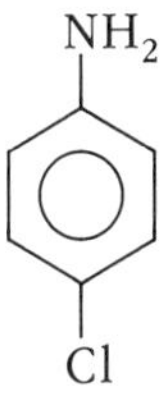 *p*-chloroaminobenzene [NH_2, Cl]	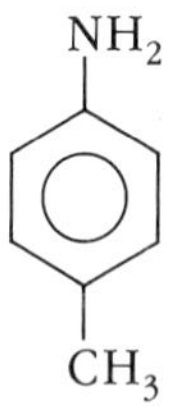 *p*-toluidine [NH_2, CH_3]	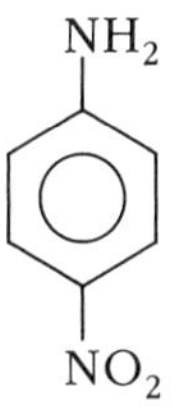 *p*-nitroaminobenzene [NH_2, NO_2]
Aminobenzene	+++	+	+±	+
p-chloroaminobenzene	+++	++	++	+±
p-toluidine	+±	++	++	+
p-nitroaminobenzene	+	++	+±	+

KEY: 0 indicates no reactivity; +++ and ++++ indicate strong reactivity; +±, and ++ indicate lesser degrees of reactivity.

SOURCE: Based on K. Landsteiner, 1962, *The Specificity of Serologic Reactions*, Dover Press. Modified by J. Klein, 1982, *Immunology: The Science of Self-Nonself Discrimination*, John Wiley Publishers.

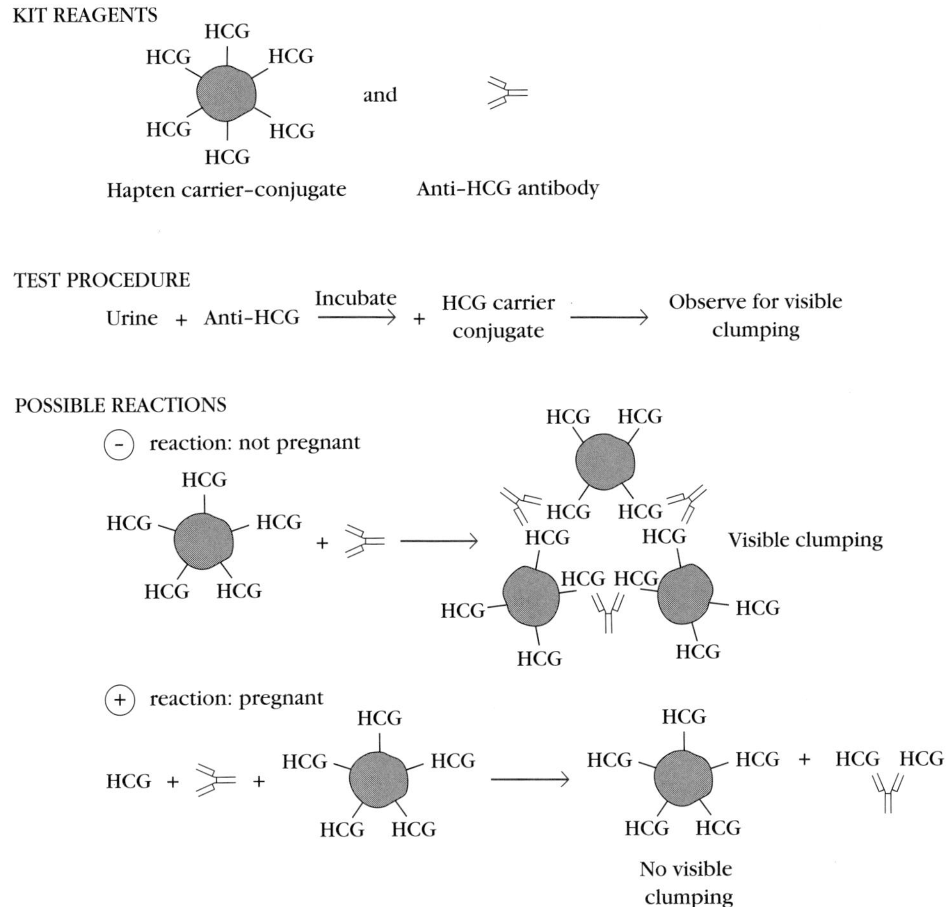

FIGURE 4-13 The home pregnancy test is a hapten-inhibition test that determines the presence or absence of human chorionic gonadotropin (HCG). If a woman is pregnant, her urine will contain HCG, which will bind to the anti-HCG antibodies in the test kit, thus inhibiting the subsequent binding of the antibody to the HCG-carrier conjugate. Because of this inhibition, no visible clumping occurs if HCG is present.

of the isomers. In contrast, if the overall configuration of the hapten was kept the same and the hapten was modified in the para position with various nonionic derivatives, then the antisera showed varying degrees of cross-reactivity (Table 4-7). In addition to demonstrating the specificity of the immune system, Landsteiner's work also demonstrated the enormous diversity of epitopes that the immune system is capable of recognizing.

Many biologically important substances, including drugs, peptide hormones, and steroid hormones can function as haptens. By conjugating these haptens to larger protein carriers, it is possible to produce hapten-specific antibody that can then be used to measure the presence of these substances in the body. The home pregnancy test kit, which determines the presence or absence of human chorionic gonadotropin (HCG) in a woman's urine, is a hapten-inhibition assay. If HCG (the hapten) is present in the urine, it inhibits the ability of the kit's anti-HCG antibodies to react with the kit's HCG-carrier conjugate. Since this reaction produces visible clumping, the absence of clumping indicates the presence of HCG, which is a sign of pregnancy (Figure 4-13).

Viral and Bacterial Antigens

The general properties of antigens discussed so far can be illustrated by a closer examination of viral and bacterial antigens. These antigens stimulate the immune response to viral and bacterial infection, thus triggering the body's most effective defense mechanism against infectious disease.

Viral Antigens

Animal viruses consist of nucleic acid (either DNA or RNA) surrounded by a protein coat, called a *capsid,* which is composed of protein subunits called *capsomers.* In simple viruses the capsomers are composed of a single protein; in more complex viruses several capsomer proteins may be present. A capsid with its enclosed nucleic acid is referred to as a *nucleocapsid;* a nucleocapsid may have helical or polyhedral symmetry. Some animal viruses are *naked,* but many have an additional lipoprotein *envelope,* which the virus acquires by modifying the host cell's plasma membrane as it leaves the cell in the process called *budding.* The complete viral particle is called a *virion* (Figure 4-14a). Protein—the principal constituent of animal viruses—is the only component of the capsid and a major component (sometimes in the form of glycoprotein) of the envelope. Proteins are also intimately associated with the viral nucleic acid as internal proteins of the nucleocapsid. Most of these proteins and glycoproteins can be recognized as immunogens by the immune system and will induce a humoral and/or a cell-mediated response.

B cells can recognize a variety of viral proteins and glycoproteins, including components of the envelope and interior components of the nucleocapsid, which may be released from infected host cells prior to complete viral assembly. The subunit structure of the capsid and repeating glycoprotein projections on many enveloped viruses provide the B cell with repeating epitopes. As discussed earlier, immunodominant B-cell epitopes tend to be residues that are accessible, hydrophilic, and mobile; thus surface sequences generated by the tertiary conformation of viral proteins function as the immunodominant B-cell epitopes. During the course of a viral infection, serum levels of antibody to envelope proteins, core proteins, and proteins associated with the viral genome all increase. These antibodies can facilitate virus clearance either by acting as opsonins to enhance phagocytosis or by activating the complement cascade leading to lysis of

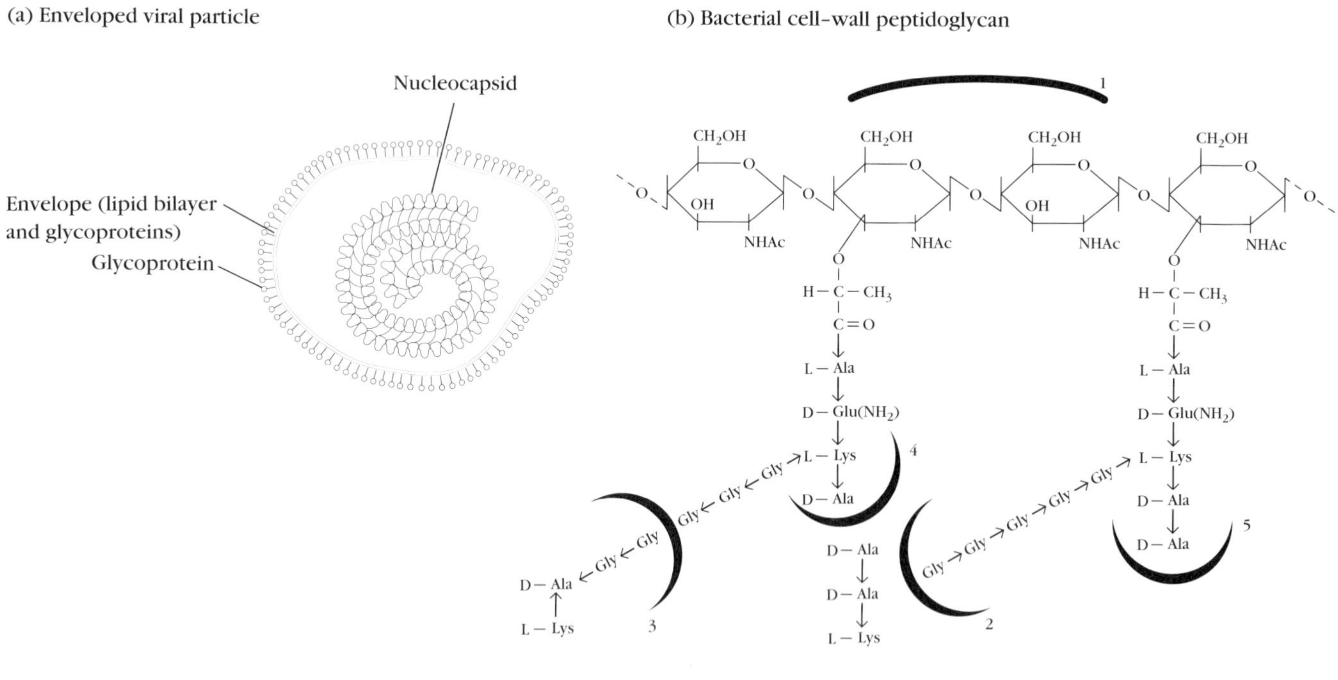

FIGURE 4-14 Viral and bacterial antigens. (a) Structure of an enveloped viral particle. The repeating envelope glycoproteins are B-cell epitopes, as are some internal core proteins; both can induce a humoral immune response. Internal proteins that are processed and presented on the membrane of virus-infected cells together with class I MHC molecules induce a cell-mediated response. (b) A portion of the primary structure of a bacterial cell-wall peptidoglycan showing five B-cell epitopes. [From B. Heymer, 1985, in *Immunology of the Bacterial Cell Envelope,* D. E. S. Stewart-Tull and M. Davis, eds., John Wiley and Sons.]

the enveloped viral particle. These antibodies often play a protective role by binding to viral envelope proteins or glycoproteins and preventing further infection of host cells. The presence of viral-specific antibodies is often used to determine whether an individual has been infected with a particular virus.

Although antibody is produced during a viral infection, in general a cell-mediated immune response is required for protective immunity to a virus. Both T_H and T_C cells can recognize viral proteins. T_H cells, which generally are class II MHC restricted, recognize viral proteins that have been internalized by antigen-presenting cells, either by phagocytosis in the case of macrophages or by receptor-mediated endocytosis in the case of the B cells. After processing in the endocytic pathway, antigenic peptides are displayed, together with a class II MHC molecule, on the membrane of these antigen-presenting cells. As mentioned already, the peptides recognized by T_H cells tend to be internal amino acid sequences that have amphipathic properties, enabling them to interact with both a class II MHC molecule and the T-cell receptor. Lymphokines produced by activated T_H cells then serve to activate either B cells or T_C cells.

As animal viruses replicate within the host cells, viral proteins are produced. These endogeneously produced antigens may be processed within the cytoplasm. The resulting peptides are then presented, together with a class I MHC molecule, on the membrane of the infected host cell, inducing a T_C-cell response. The epitopes recognized by T_C cells need not be major, exposed viral components such as the envelope glycoproteins; instead, they often are internal viral proteins produced within the infected host cell. For example, a major influenza antigen recognized by T_C cells is an internal protein called nucleoprotein, which is associated with the viral RNA genome. Activation of T_C cells in response to nucleoprotein peptides appears to play an important role in the elimination of influenza-infected host cells and in recovery from an influenza infection.

Some viruses are capable of substantial variation in the structure of their envelope glycoprotein components. Influenza virus, for example, constantly changes the amino acid sequence of its envelope glycoproteins. Either major amino acid variations *(antigenic shift)* or minor variations *(antigenic drift)* can give rise to new epitopes, allowing the virus to evade the immune system. This antigenic variation is the major cause of repeated influenza outbreaks. This process is discussed more fully in Chapter 20. Antigenic variation also is extensive in human immunodeficiency virus (HIV), the causative agent of AIDS. The frequent amino acid sequence changes in the proteins and glycoproteins of HIV not only enable the virus to evade the immune response but also pose a major obstacle to vaccine development (see Chapter 23).

Bacterial Antigens

Bacteria are single-cell prokaryotes, which lack a true membrane-bound nucleus. They are surrounded by a cell wall and in some cases enclosed in a capsule. Various structures (flagella, fimbriae, or pili) may protrude from the cell. Although a bacterium may secrete soluble products that can serve as immunogens, the major bacterial immunogens are epitopes on surface structures.

The cell wall of so-called *gram-positive* bacteria is composed largely of peptidoglycan, a network of polysaccharides cross-linked by short peptide chains. Intercalated within the gram-positive cell wall are various proteins, polysaccharides, and teichoic acids. Structural differences in these cell-wall components generate unique epitopes that can be recognized with antibody (Figure 4-14b). The gram-positive streptococci, for example, can be grouped on the basis of antigenic differences in their cell-wall carbohydrate.

Gram-negative bacteria have a thin peptidoglycan layer covered by an outer membrane containing phospholipid, protein, lipopolysaccharide, and lipoprotein. The lipopolysaccharide (LPS) is a major antigenic component of the gram-negative cell wall. The polysaccharide side chains of LPS consist of repeating linear trisaccharides or branched tetra- or pentasaccharides; a chain can include as many as 40 repeat units. The LPS of gram-negative cell walls thus presents the immune system with accessible and multivalent epitopes on the bacterial surface, which are referred to as *O antigens.* Differences in the O-antigen epitope structure of the polysaccharide side chains can induce specific antibodies, which can be used to classify gram-negative bacteria.

The bacterial capsule is a loose polysaccharide or polypeptide layer that lies outside the cell wall. The presence of a capsule is associated with virulence because it interferes with phagocytosis. Most capsules consist of repeating sequences of two or three sugars and have molecular weights as high as 140,000 Da. The accessibility of the capsule, as well as its repeating epitope structure, allows this bacterial component to generate a significant humoral antibody response. In the case of pneumococci, an estimated 4×10^6 antibody molecules can combine with the capsular epitopes expressed on a single bacterial cell. The binding

TABLE 4-8 CHARACTERISTICS OF THREE LECTIN MITOGENS

Characteristic	Concanavalin A (Con A)	Phytohemagglutinin (PHA)	Pokeweed mitogen (PWM)
Source	Jack beans	Kidney beans	Pokeweed
Molecular structure	Tetramer	Tetramer	Polymeric
Ligand	α-D-mannose and α-D-glucose	*N*-acetylgalactosamine	di-*N*-acetylchitobiose
Target cell(s)	T cells	T cells	T cells and B cells

of antibody to capsular epitopes provides another basis for typing bacteria. Differences in capsular polysaccharide sugars and their linkages define more than 80 pneumococcal types.

MITOGENS

Mitogens are agents that are able to induce cell division in a high percentage of T or B cells. Unlike immunogens, which activate only lymphocytes bearing specific receptors, mitogens activate many clones of T or B cells irrespective of their antigen specificity. Because of this ability, mitogens are known as *polyclonal activators.* A variety of diverse agents function as mitogens. A number of common mitogens are proteins (called *lectins*) that are derived from plants and bind sugars. Lectins recognize different glycoproteins on the surface of various cells, including lymphocytes. Lectin binding to the membrane glycoproteins often leads to agglutination, or clustering, of the cells, which is often followed by cellular activation. Some mitogens preferentially activate B cells, some preferentially activate T cells, and some activate both populations. Three common lectins with mitogenic activity are *concanavalin A (Con A), phytohemagglutinin (PHA),* and *pokeweed mitogen.* Each of these proteins binds to different carbohydrate residues in glycoproteins and are able to cross-link glycoproteins on the surface of cells (Table 4-8). Con A and PHA are T-cell mitogens; pokeweed mitogen is mitogenic for both T and B cells.

Not all mitogens are lectins. The lipopolysaccharide (LPS) component of the gram-negative bacterial cell wall functions as a B-cell mitogen. The mitogenic activity of LPS is due to its lipid moiety, which is thought to interact with the plasma membrane, resulting in a cellular activation signal through as-yet-unknown mechanisms.

An unusual group of substances, known as *superantigens,* are among the most potent T-cell mitogens known. Superantigens bind residues in the V_β domain of the T-cell receptor and residues in class II MHC molecules outside of the antigen-binding cleft (Figure 4-15). In this way a superantigen cross-links a T cell to a class II MHC molecule in an antigen-independent manner, resulting in the activation of a distinct set of V_β-expressing T cells. Included among the superantigens are the staphyloccocal enterotoxins (SEs) and toxic-shock syndrome toxin 1 (TSST1), which is produced by the gram-positive bacterium *Staphylococcal aureus.* These toxins appear to activate large numbers

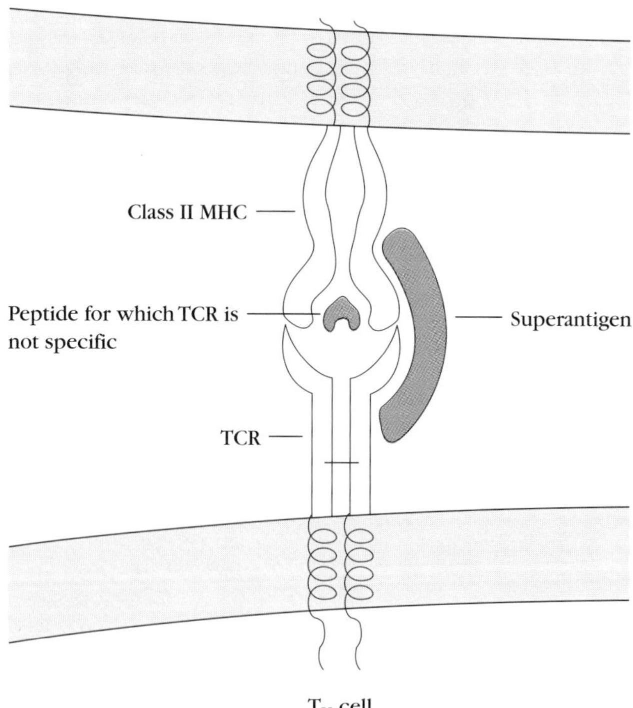

FIGURE 4-15 Schematic diagram of ternary complex formed between a T-cell receptor (TCR), superantigen, and MHC molecule. Superantigens bind to common sequences in class II MHC molecules and T-cell receptors that lie outside the normal antigen-binding sites (see Figure 4-8). T-cell activation by superantigens is not limited by the antigenic specificity of the T cell.

of T_H cells by cross-linking the T-cell receptors with any class II MHC molecule expressed on an antigen-presenting cell. Estimates are that one out of every five T cells can be activated by SEs, resulting in the release of abnormally high levels of cytokines. The high levels of cytokines released can lead to shock and death, seen most dramatically in tampon-related toxic shock syndrome caused by TSST1. These superantigens are discussed more fully in Chapters 13 and 21.

Summary

1. Immunogenicity is the ability of an antigen to induce an immune response within either the humoral or the cell-mediated branch of the immune system. Antigenicity is the ability of an antigen simply to interact specifically with free antibody and/or with antigen-binding receptors on lymphocytes. B cells and T cells recognize small sites called antigenic determinants, or epitopes, on a complex immunogen.

2. The foreignness, molecular size, chemical composition and complexity, and degradability of a substance influence its immunogenicity. In addition, several properties of the biological system that an antigen encounters affect its immunogenicity; these include the genotype of the recipient animal, the immunogen dosage and route of administration, and the presence or absence of adjuvants.

3. The size of B-cell epitopes—those epitopes recognized by membrane-bound antibody and free antibody—is determined by the size of an antibody's antigen-binding site. B-cell epitopes tend to be amino acid sequences within an antigen that are accessible, usually hydrophilic, and mobile. Sequential-B-cell epitopes consist of contiguous amino acid residues along the polypeptide chain, whereas nonsequential B-cell epitopes, also called conformational determinants, are formed from noncontiguous segments of the polypeptide chain that are brought into proximity by the three-dimensional folding of a protein.

4. T-cell epitopes—those epitopes recognized by T-cell receptors—tend to be slightly larger than B-cell epitopes and generally consist of internal amino acid sequences that are hydrophobic or more commonly amphipathic. T-cell epitopes are rendered accessible to the immune system by antigen processing, during which the protein is fragmented into small peptides that interact with class I MHC or class II MHC molecules; the resulting peptide-MHC complexes are then displayed on the surface of altered self-cells or antigen-presenting cells. The immunodominant T-cell epitopes are determined in part by the selective interactions of particular processed peptides with particular MHC molecules.

5. Haptens are small molecules that can bind to antibodies but cannot by themselves function as immunogens. The study of haptens has allowed immunologists to learn about the structural basis of antibody specificity.

References

BENJAMIN, D., J. BERZOFSKY, I. EAST et al. 1984. The antigenic structure of proteins: a reappraisal. *Annu. Rev. Immunol.* **2**:67.

BERZOFSKY, J. A., K. CEASE, J. CORNETTE et al. 1987 Protein antigenic structures recognized by T cells: potential applications to vaccine design. *Immunol. Rev.* **98**:9.

BERZOFSKY, J., S. BRETT, H. STREICHER, and H. TAKAHASHI. 1988. Antigen processing for presentation to T lymphocytes: function, mechanisms and implications for the T cell repertoire. *Immunol. Rev.* **106**:5.

BUUS, S., A. SETTE., and H. M. GREY. 1987. The interaction between protein-derived immunogenic peptides and IA. *Immunol. Rev.* **98**:115.

DEMOTZ, S., H. M. GREY, E. APPELLA, and A. SETTE. 1989. Characterization of a naturally processed MHC class II-restricted T cell determinant of hen egg lysozyme. *Nature* **342**:682.

GREY, H. M., A. SETTE, and S. BUUS. 1989. How T cells see antigen. *Sci. Am.* **261**(5):56.

HERMAN, A., J. W. KAPPLER, P. MARRACK, and A. M. PULLEN. 1991. Superantigens: mechanism of T-cell stimulation and role in immune responses. *Annu. Rev. Immunol.* **9**:745.

HUNT, D. F., R. A. HENDERSON, J. SHABANOWITZ et al. 1992. Characterization of peptides bound to the class I MHC molecule HLA-A2.1 by mass spectrometry. *Science* **255**:1261.

LAVER, W. G., G. M. AIR, R. G. WEBSTER, and S. J. SMITH-GILL. 1990. Epitopes on protein antigens: misconceptions and realities. *Cell* **61**:553.

MADDEN, D. R., J. G. GORGA, J. L. STROMINGER, and D. C. WILEY. 1992. The three-dimensional structure of HLA-B27 at 2.1 Å resolution suggests a general mechanism for tight peptide binding to MHC. *Cell* **70**:1035.

ROTHBARD, J. B., and M. L. GEFTER. 1991. Interactions between immunogenic peptides and MHC proteins. *Annu. Rev. Immunol.* **9**:527.

SILVER, M. L., H. C. GUO, J. L. STROMINGER, and D. C. WILEY. 1992. Atomic structure of a human MHC molecule presenting an influenza virus peptide. *Nature* **360**:367.

TAINER, J. A., E. GETZOFF, Y. PATERSON et al. 1985. The atomic mobility component of protein antigenicity. *Annu. Rev. Immunol.* **3**:501.

WERDELIN, O., S. MOURITSEN, B. PETERSEN et al. 1988. Facts on the fragmentation of antigens in presenting cells, on the association of antigen fragments with MHC molecules in cell-free systems and speculation on the cell biology of antigen processing. *Immunol. Rev.* **106**:181.

Study Questions

1. Indicate whether each of the following statements is true or false. If you think a statement is false, explain why.
   a. Most antigens induce a polyclonal response.
   b. A large protein antigen generally can combine with many different antibody molecules.
   c. A hapten can stimulate antibody formation but cannot combine with antibody molecules.
   d. MHC genes play a major role in determining the degree of immune responsiveness to an antigen.
   e. T-cell epitopes tend to be accessible amino acid residues that can interact with the T-cell receptor.
   f. B-cell epitopes are often nonsequential amino acids brought together by the tertiary conformation of a protein antigen.
   g. Both T_H and T_C cells recognize antigen that has been processed and presented with a MHC molecule.
   h. Each MHC molecule binds a unique peptide.
   i. Internal viral proteins of the nucleocapsid are not likely to be immunogenic because they are not accessible to the immune system.
   j. An influenza hemagglutinin peptide that induces potent proliferation of T_H cells in mice expressing the class II MHC molecule designated IA^k would also induce potent T_H-cell proliferation in mice expressing IA^d.

2. Two vaccines are described below. Would you expect either or both of them to activate T_C cells? Explain your answer.
   a. A UV-inactivated ("killed") viral preparation that has retained its antigenic properties but cannot replicate.
   b. An attenuated viral preparation that has low virulence but can still replicate within host cells.

3. You are trying to develop a synthetic peptide vaccine to induce cell-mediated immunity to malaria. As a first step, you screen peptides derived from the outer-coat protein of the microorganism that causes malaria for amphipathic properties. What is the rationale for this approach? What other factors must you take into consideration in developing a vaccine by this approach?

4. In the experiment outlined in Figure 4-11, why were MHC genes transfected into mouse L cells rather than into antigen-presenting cells such as macrophages?

5. What are the significant differences between T-cell and B-cell epitopes?

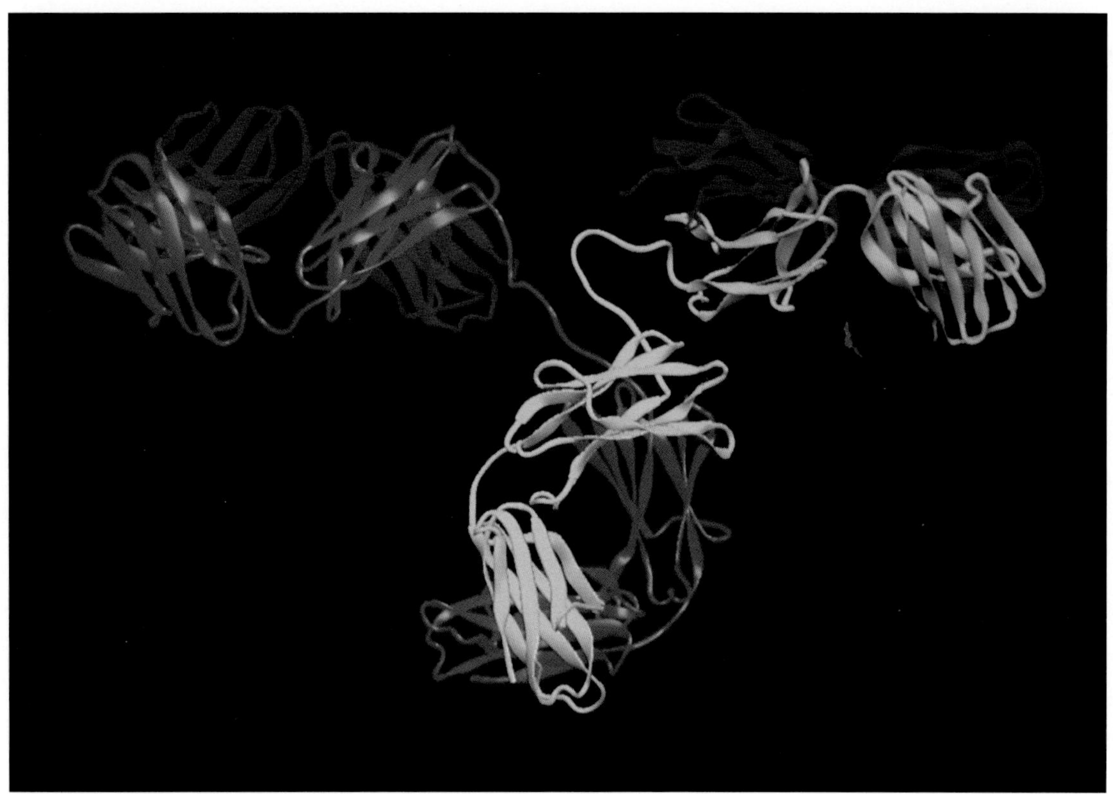

COLOR PLATE 1 Ribbon representation based on X-ray crystallography data of the structure of an intact monoclonal antibody to canine lymphoma depicting the heavy chains (yellow and blue) and light chains (red). The domain structure of the molecule is readily visible as is the extended conformation of the hinge region. [The laboratory of A. McPhearson provided this image based on the immunoglobulin structure determined by L. J. Harris. 1992. *Nature* **360**: 369.]

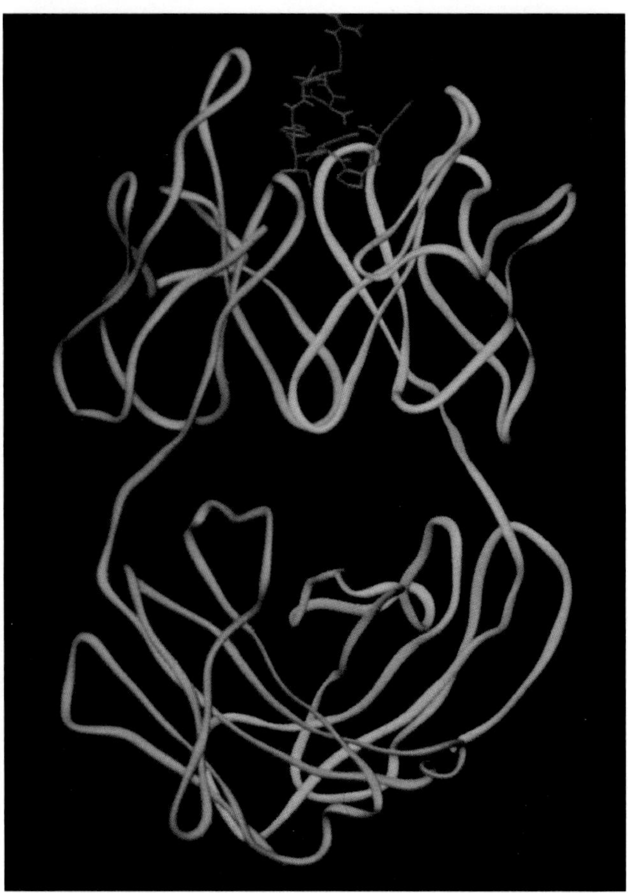

COLOR PLATE 2 Three-dimensional structure of an octapeptide hormone (angiotensin II) complexed to a monoclonal antibody Fab fragment. The angiotensin II peptide is shown in red, the heavy chain in blue, and the light chain in green. [From K. C. Garcia, P. M. Ronco, P. J. Verroust et al. 1992. *Science* **257**: 502.]

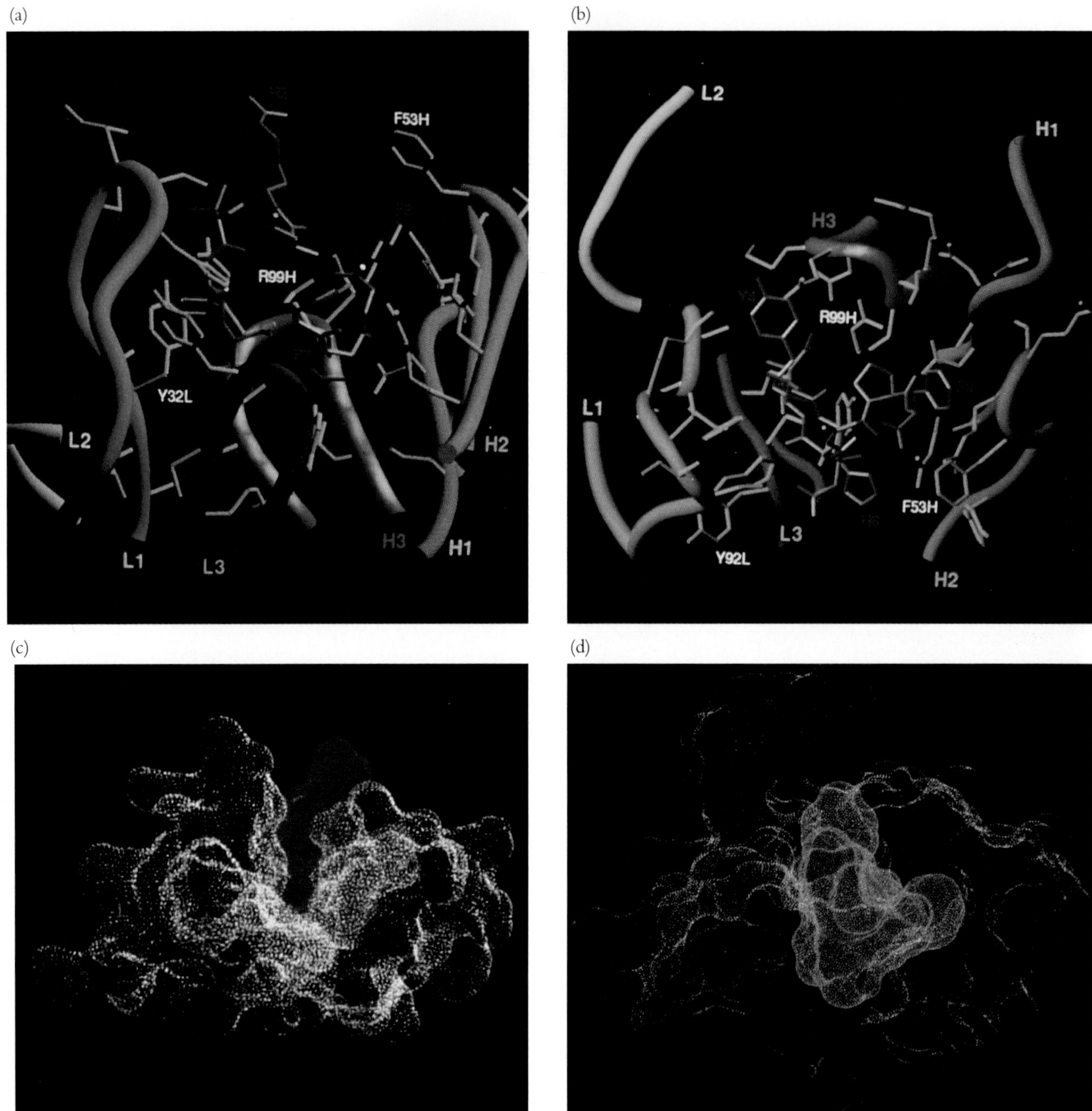

COLOR PLATE 3 (a) Side view and (b) front view of the three-dimensional structure of the combining site of an angiotensin II-Fab complex. The peptide is in red. The CDR main chains (different colors) are labeled L1, L2, L3, H1, H2, and H3. The side chains of the six CDRs within van der Vaals contact of the angiotensin peptide are shown in yellow. (c) Side view and (d) front view of the van der Vaals dot surface contact between the angiotensin II-Fab complex. [From K. C. Garcia, P. M. Ronco, P. J. Verroust et al. 1992. *Science* **257**: 502.]

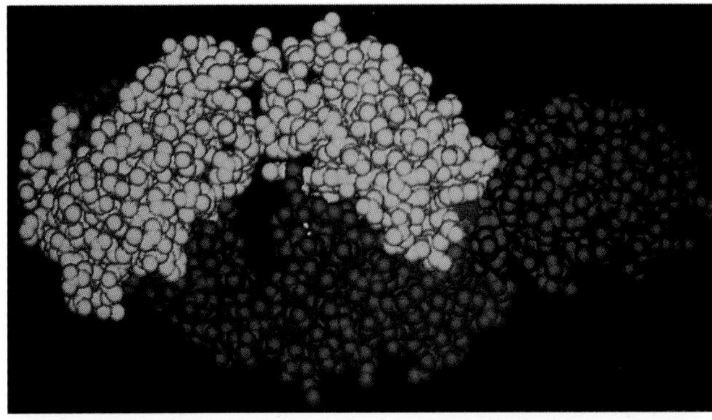

(b)

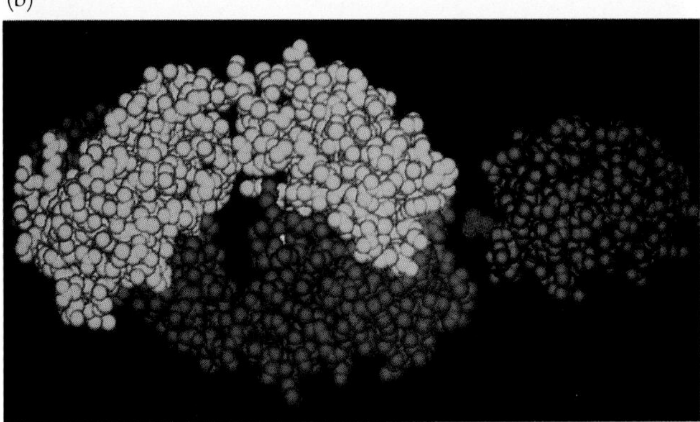

(c)

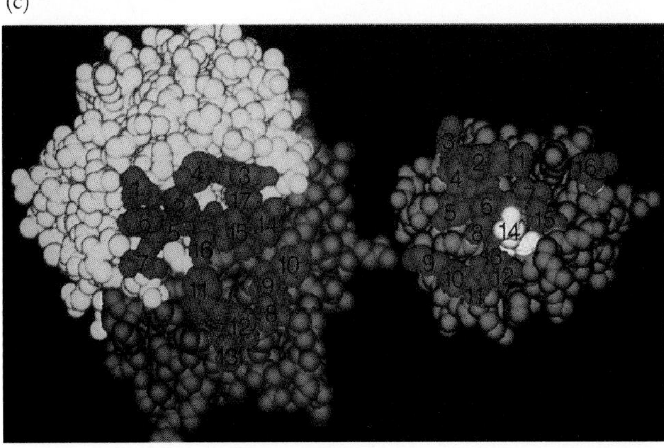

COLOR PLATE 4 (a) Interaction between hen egg lysozyme (HEL) and a Fab fragment of antibody to HEL determined by X-ray diffraction techniques depicting HEL (green), the Fab heavy chain (blue), and the light chain (yellow). Glutamine (red), an amino acid residue of lysozyme, fits into a pocket in the Fab fragment. (b) Representation of HEL and the Fab fragment when pulled apart showing complementary surface features. (c) View of the interacting surfaces of the Fab fragment and HEL obtained by rotating each of the molecules. The contacting residues are numbered and shown in red with the glutamine now in pink. [From A. G. Amit, R. A. Mariuza, S. E. V. Phillips, and R. J. Poljak, 1986. *Science* **233**: 747.]

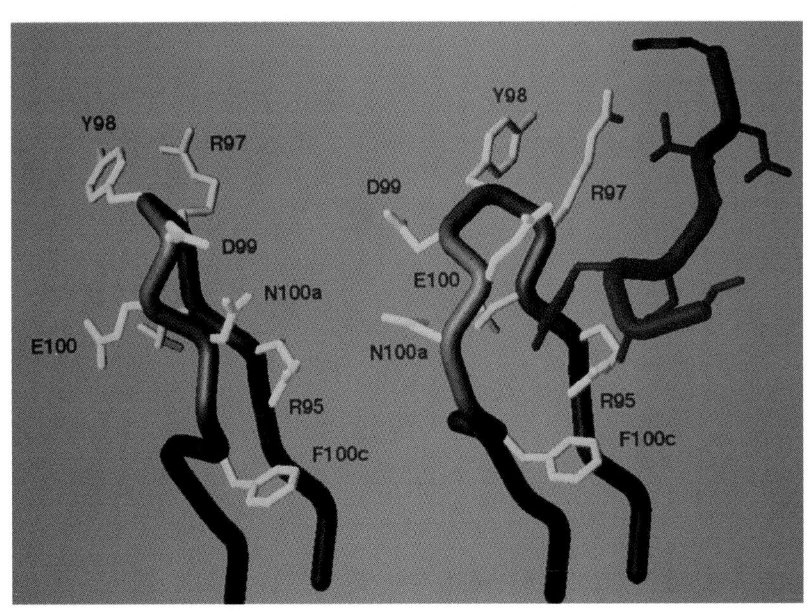

COLOR PLATE 5 Structural evidence of induced fit in the binding of an antigen to an antibody. Comparison of the heavy chain CDR3 loops of a bound and unbound Fab fragment reveals a major rearrangement in the heavy chain CDR3 loop following antigen binding. On the left, the heavy chain CDR3 loop is shown in blue with its side chains in yellow. On the right, the heavy chain CDR3 loop complexed to the hemagglutinin molecule is shown in green with its side chains in yellow. [From J. M. Rini, U. Schulze-Gahmen, I. A. Wilson. 1992. *Science* **255**: 959.]

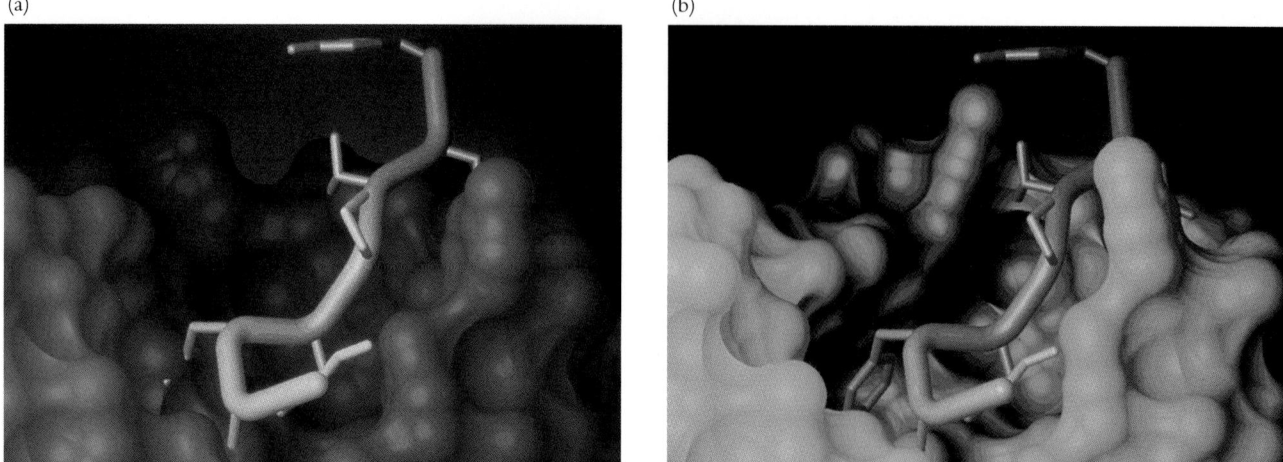

COLOR PLATE 6 The solvent-accessible surface of an unbound and bound peptide-Fab complex showing that peptide binding is accommodated by an alteration in the shape of the antibody binding pocket. The unbound Fab (a) contains an open, basin-shaped pocket whereas the bound Fab (b) has a prominant channel that interacts with the extended peptide and a pocket that interacts with the tyrosine residue. The peptide (pink) positioned over the Fab illustrates the difference in the shape of the free and bound combining sites. [From U. Schulze-Gahmen, J. M. Rini, M. Pique, and I. A. Wilson. 1992. *Science* **255**: 959.]

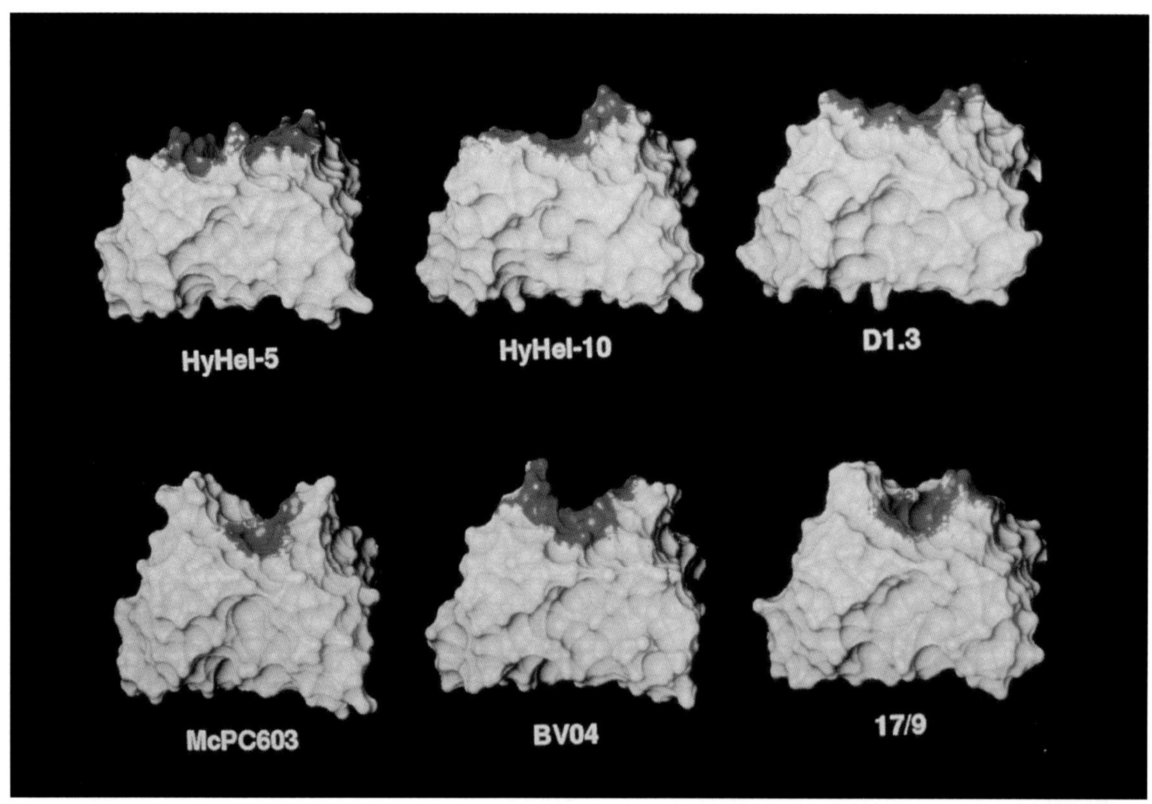

COLOR PLATE 7 The variable domains of six Fab fragments and their respective antigens: HyHel-5/lysozyme, HyHel-10/lysozyme, D1.3/lysozyme, McPC603/phosphocholine, BV04/single-stranded DNA, and 17/9, a peptide from influenza hemagglutinin are shown with their antigen-combining sites highlighted in dark gray. The binding sites for small molecules, such as phosphocholine (McPC603), appear as deep pockets; binding sites for large proteins, such as lysozyme, appear as flatter, more undulating surfaces. [From I. A. Wilson and R. L. Stanfield, 1993. *Current Opinion in Structural Biology* **3**: 113.]

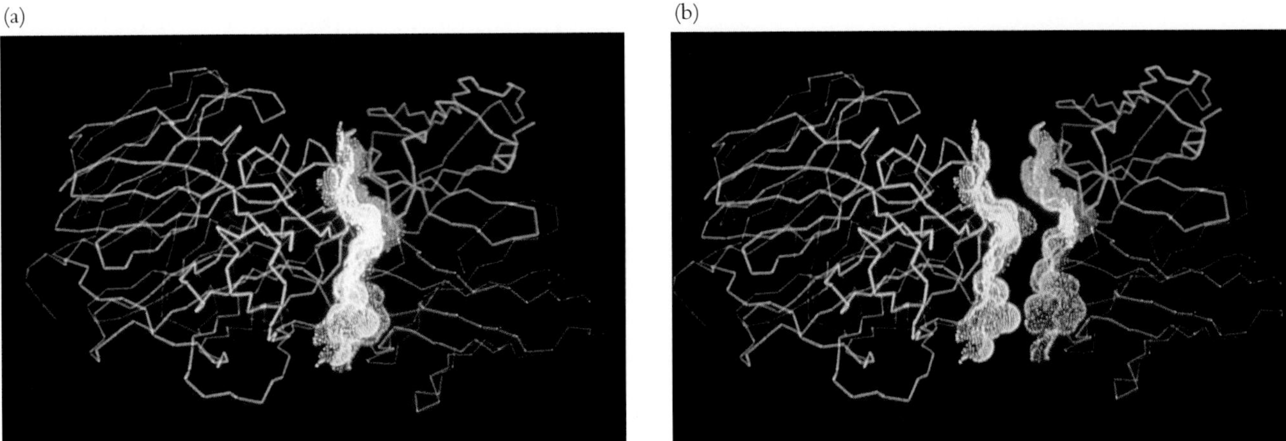

COLOR PLATE 8 Computer simulation of an antibody-antigen interaction based on X-ray crystallography data collected by P. M. Colman and W. R. Tulip. (a) Influenza virus antigen (yellow) interacting with antibody (variable heavy chain is red; variable light chain is blue). (b) The complementarity of the two molecules is revealed by separating the influenza virus antigen from the antibody by a distance of eight angstroms. [From G. J. V. H. Nossal. 1993. *Scientific American* **Sept**: 54.]

(a) (b)

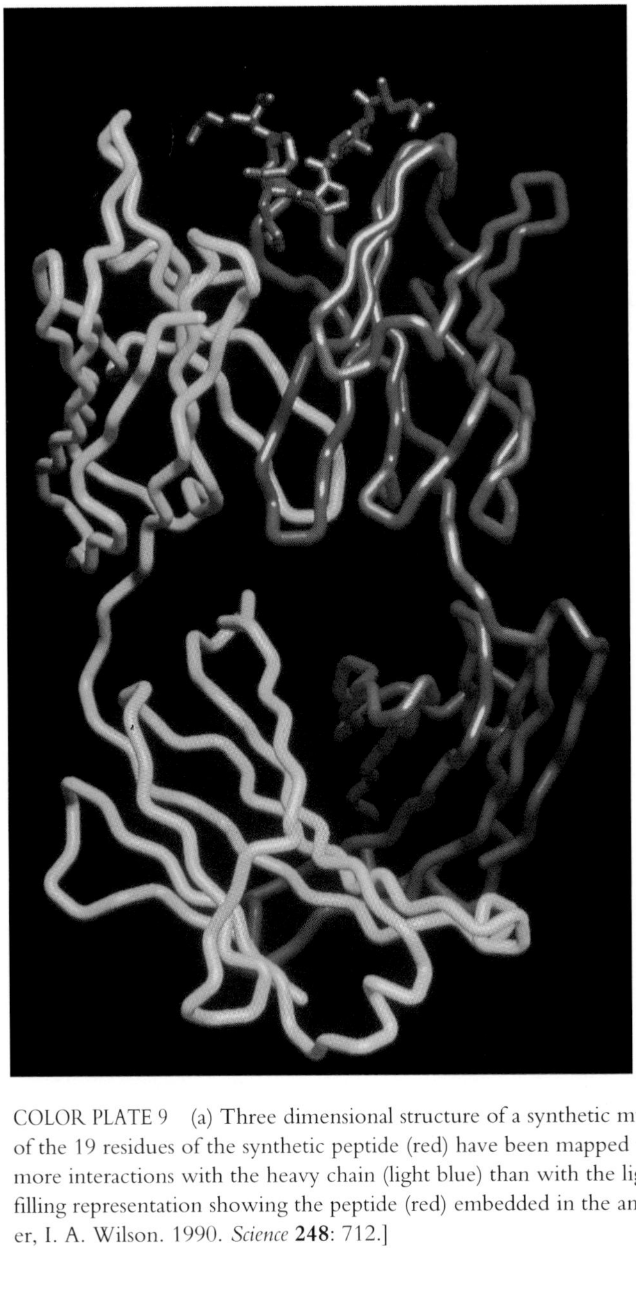

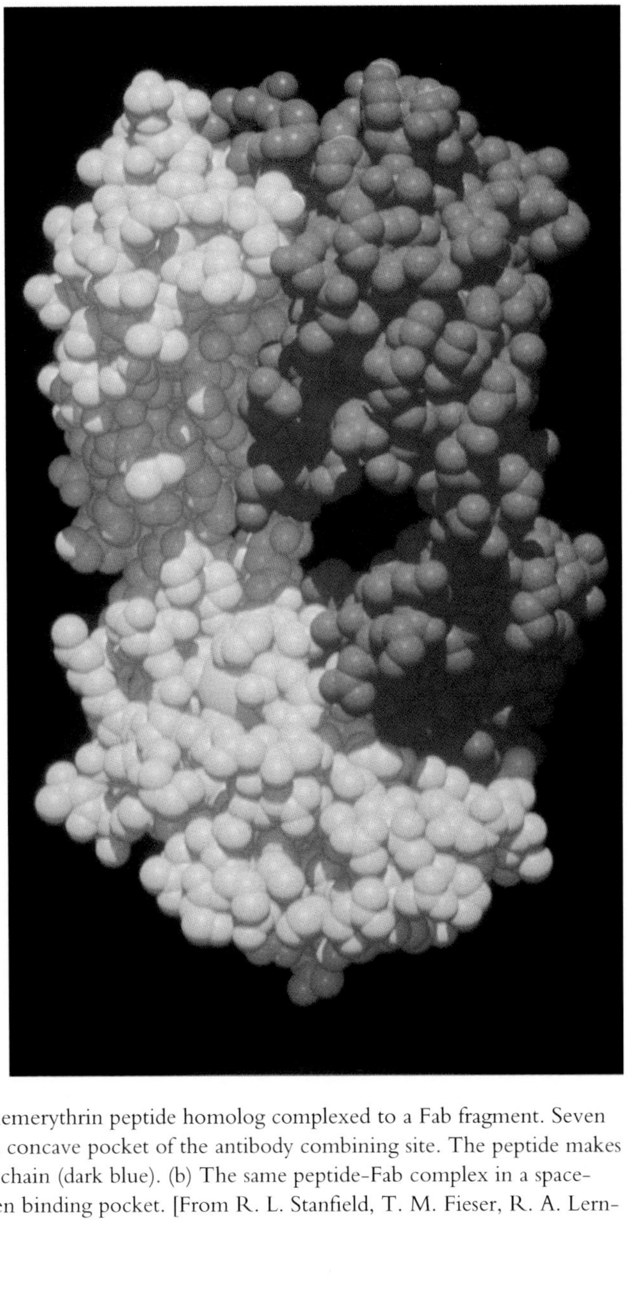

COLOR PLATE 9 (a) Three dimensional structure of a synthetic myohemerythrin peptide homolog complexed to a Fab fragment. Seven of the 19 residues of the synthetic peptide (red) have been mapped in a concave pocket of the antibody combining site. The peptide makes more interactions with the heavy chain (light blue) than with the light chain (dark blue). (b) The same peptide-Fab complex in a space-filling representation showing the peptide (red) embedded in the antigen binding pocket. [From R. L. Stanfield, T. M. Fieser, R. A. Lerner, I. A. Wilson. 1990. *Science* **248**: 712.]

(a)

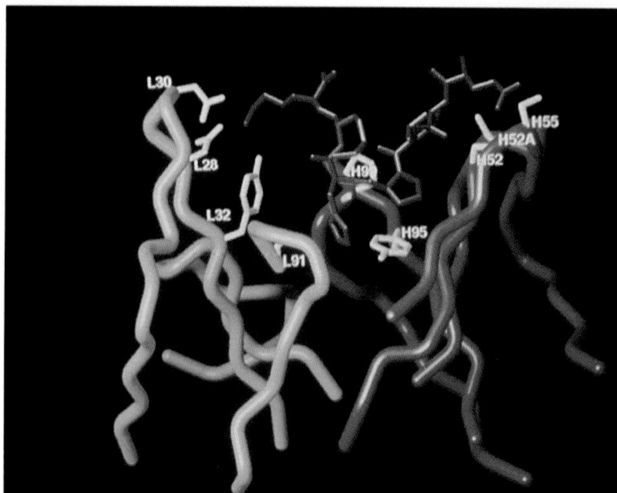

(b)

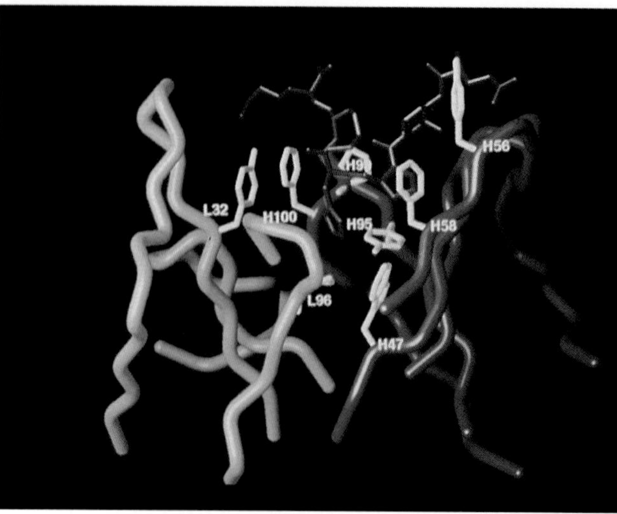

COLOR PLATE 10 (a) The antigen binding pocket of the myohemerythrin-Fab complex highlighting only the residues which form hydrogen bonds with the peptide antigen (red). The carbon-alpha backbones of the light chains (light blue) and heavy chains (dark blue) of the Fab fragment are shown; the side chains of the hydrogen bonding residues are highlighted in yellow. Side chains of hydrogen bonding residues are from CDR's L1, L3, H2, and H3. (b) Hydrophobic and aromatic residues of the Fab binding pocket fragment highlighting only the hydrophobic and aromatic Fab residues (shown in yellow). [From R. L. Stanfield, T. M. Fieser, R. A. Lerner, I. A. Wilson. 1990. *Science* **248**: 712.]

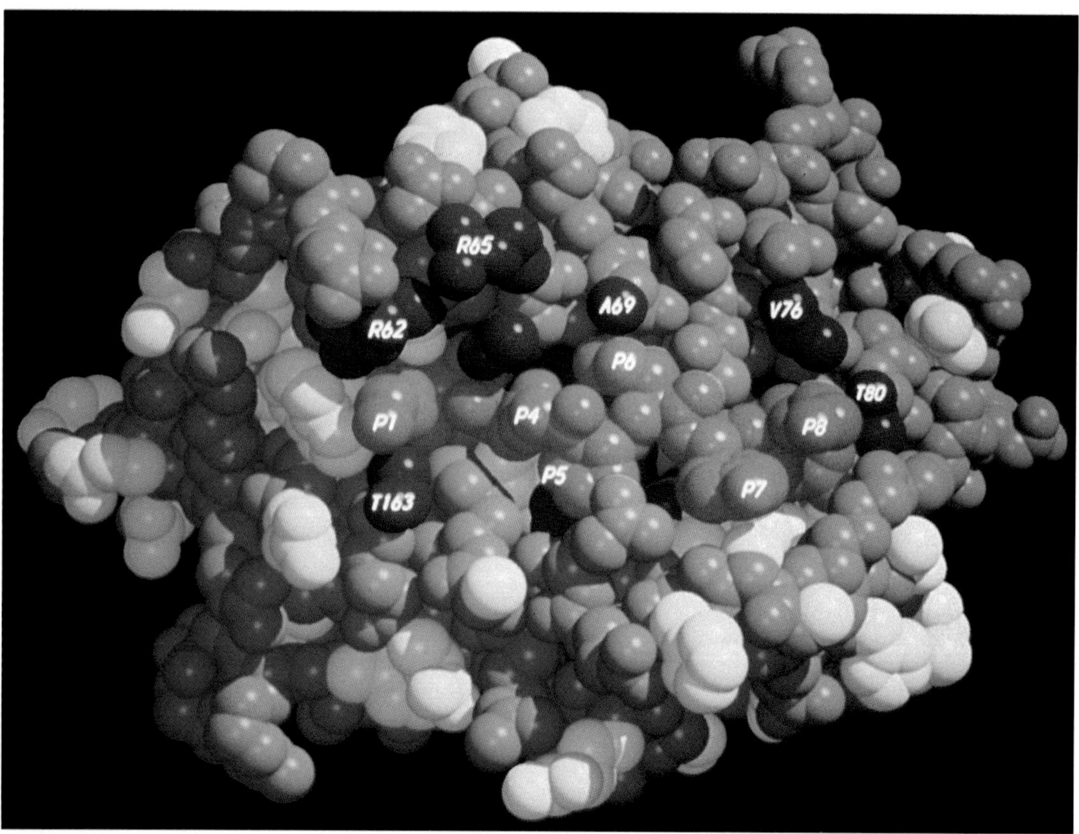

COLOR PLATE 11 Structure of a human class I MHC molecule bound to influenza nucleoprotein peptide 91-99 as determined by X-ray crystallography. The peptide is shown in orange. The MHC is depicted showing the conserved residues (blue), the polymorphic residues (red), and residues which are neither conserved nor polymorphic (light blue). Most (11/12) of the polymorphic residues are completely buried by the bound peptide and are not shown. Six polymorphic residues facing the solvent are shown; of these, four contact the bound peptide and all six can make contact with the T-cell receptor. [From M. L. Silver, H. C. Guo, J. L. Strominger, and D. C. Wiley. 1992. *Nature* **360**: 367.]

(a)

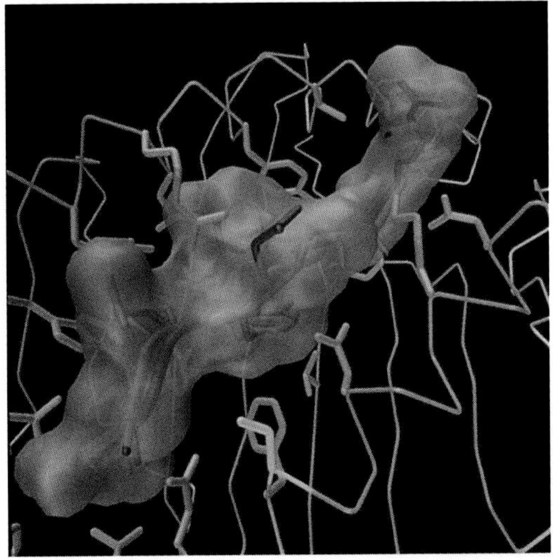

(b)

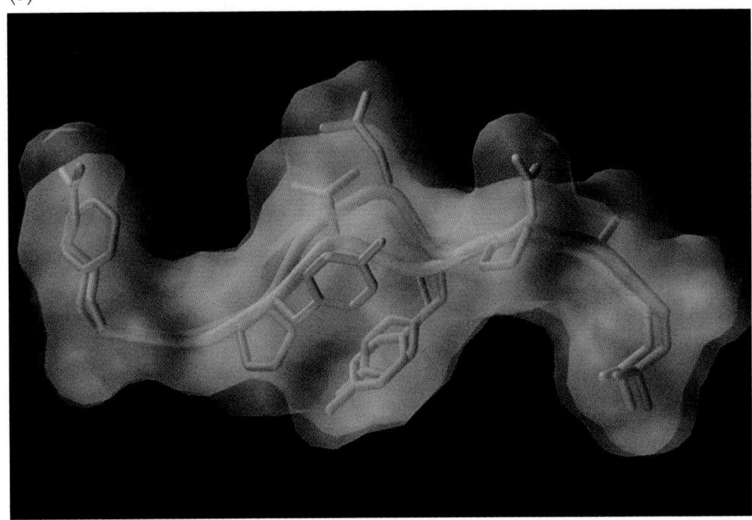

COLOR PLATE 12 (a) The antigen-binding groove of the class I K^b MHC molecule (magenta) complexed with two different viral nucleocapsid peptides: an octamer peptide of vesicular stomatitis virus (VSV-8), shown in yellow, and a nonamer peptide of Sendai virus (SEV-9), shown in blue. The tube representation of the peptides indicates that both peptides fit snugly into the groove by hydrogen bonds between the MHC and the backbone of each peptide. The peptide side chains contribute little to the binding energy. (b) Comparison of the conformation of the VSV-8 (yellow) and the SEV-9 (blue) peptides by the class I K^b MHC molecules. Both peptides adopt an extended conformation and the longer peptide is seen bulging in the middle in order to maintain the same 25 A amino to carboxyl termini distance as the octamer. [From D. H. Fremont, M. Pique, and I. A. Wilson, 1992. *Science* **257**: 891.]

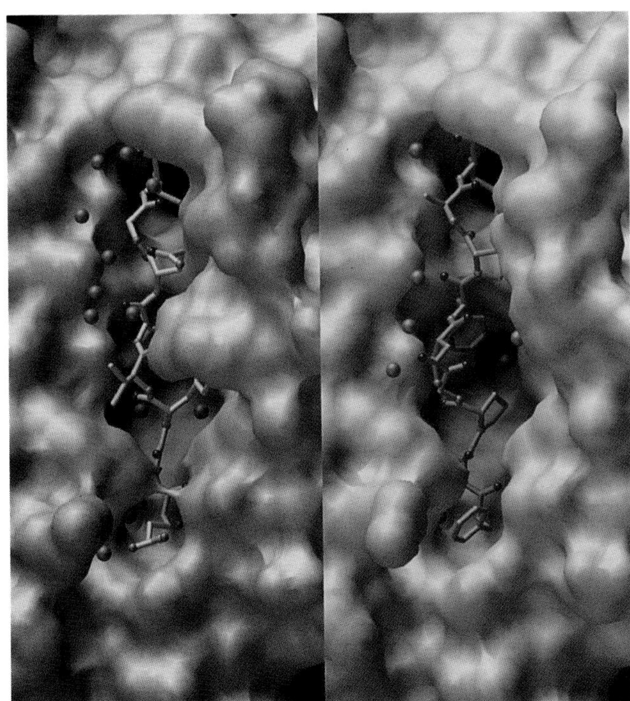

COLOR PLATE 13 Antigen peptides are deeply buried into the class I MHC binding groove. The solvent accessible area of a class I H-2K^b is shown, depicting the complex formed with vesicular stomatitis virus (VSV-8) peptide (left, in yellow) and Sendai virus nucleoprotein (SEV-9) (right, in blue). The amino termini of the peptides are shown at the bottom of the image and the H-2$K^b\alpha 1$ domains are on the left. Peptides oxygens and nitrogens are shown in red and blue, respectively. Water molecules (blue spheres) identified in the crystallographic experiment interact with the bound peptides. The majority of the surface of both peptides is inaccessible for direct T cell contact (VSV-8 is 83% buried; SEV-9 is 75% buried). Small, but potentially significant, conformational variation can be seen in the two H-2K^b surfaces, especially around the central region of the groove on the right side of the peptides ($\alpha 2$ helix) [From M. Matsumura, D. H. Fremont, P. A. Peterson, I. A. Wilson. 1992. *Science* **257**: 927.]

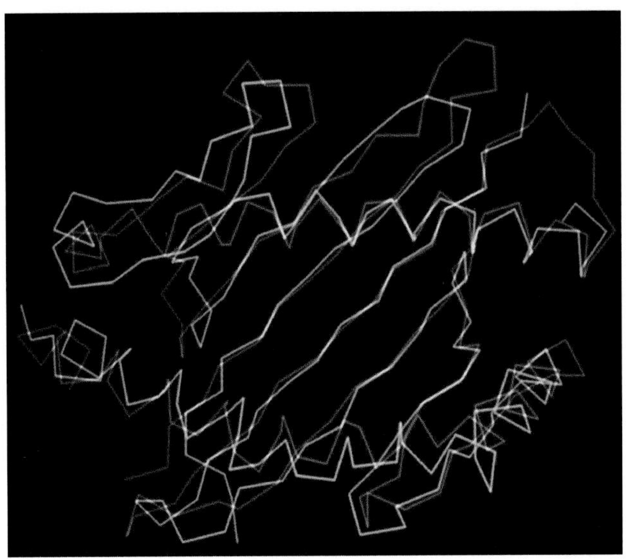

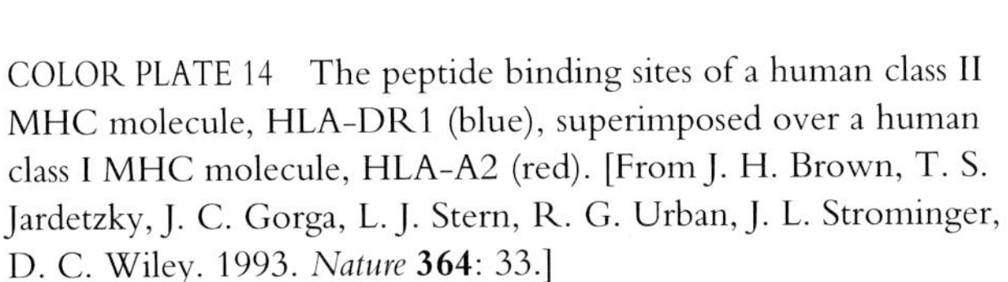

COLOR PLATE 14 The peptide binding sites of a human class II MHC molecule, HLA-DR1 (blue), superimposed over a human class I MHC molecule, HLA-A2 (red). [From J. H. Brown, T. S. Jardetzky, J. C. Gorga, L. J. Stern, R. G. Urban, J. L. Strominger, D. C. Wiley. 1993. *Nature* **364**: 33.]

(a)

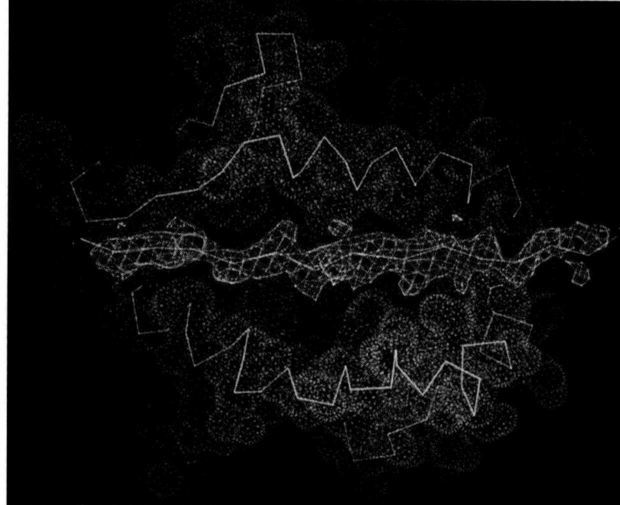

(b)

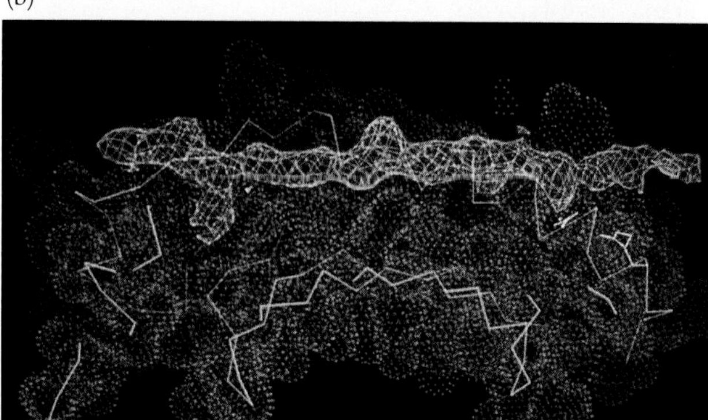

COLOR PLATE 15 X-ray crystallography of a peptide (red) bound to a human class II MHC molecule, DR1. The van der Waals surface of DR1 is shown in blue. (a) Top view showing the α1 domain on top and the β1 domain on bottom. (b) Side view showing the α1 domain helix behind the peptide and the β-sheet below. Here, the β1 domain helix was removed for clarity. [From J. H. Brown, T. S. Jardetzky, J. C. Gorga, L. J. Stern, R. G. Urban, J. L. Strominger, D. C. Wiley. 1993. *Nature* **364**: 33.]

(a)

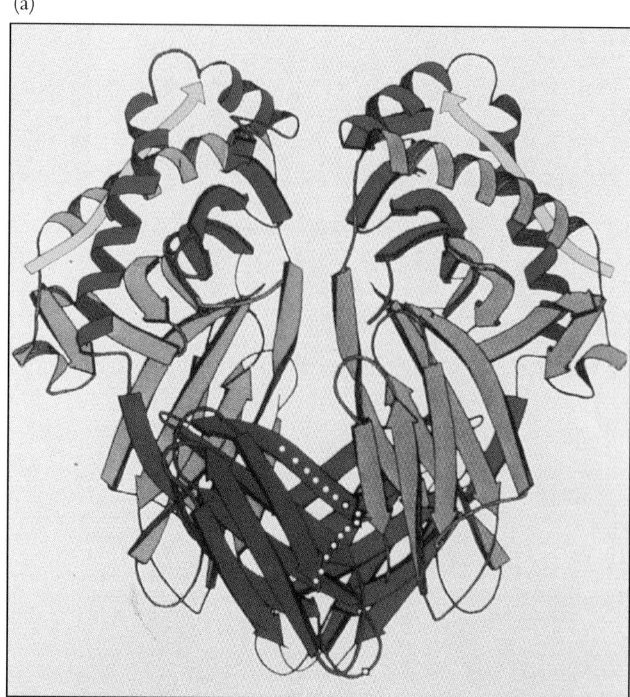

(b)

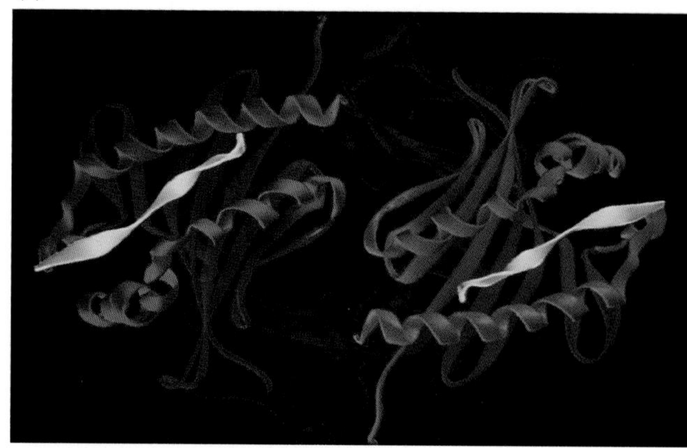

COLOR PLATE 16 (a) Ribbon representation and (b) top view of the antigen binding grooves of the class II DR1 molecule crystallized as a dimer of the αβ heterodimer. The crystallized dimer is shown with one DR1 molecule in red and the other DR1 molecule in blue. The peptides are shown in yellow. [From J. H. Brown, T. S. Jardetzky, J. C. Gorga, L. J. Stern, R. G. Urban, J. L. Strominger, D. C. Wiley. 1993. *Nature* **364**: 33.]

IMMUNOGLOBULINS: STRUCTURE AND FUNCTION

Immunoglobulins function as antibodies, the antigen-binding proteins that are present on the B-cell membrane and also are secreted by plasma cells. Secreted antibodies circulate in the blood and serve as the effectors of humoral immunity by searching out and neutralizing or eliminating antigens. Membrane-bound antibody confers antigenic specificity on B cells; antigen-specific proliferation of B-cell clones depends on interaction of membrane antibody and antigen. All immunoglobulins share certain structural features, bind to antigen, and participate in a limited number of effector functions. This chapter focuses on how the primary, secondary, and tertiary structure of immunoglobulins contribute to both their specificity and their effector functions.

Basic Structure of Immunoglobulins

It has been known since the turn of the century that antibodies—the effector molecules of humoral immunity—reside in the serum. Identification of the serum-protein fraction containing antibodies was accomplished in a classic experiment by A. Tiselius and E. A. Kabat in 1939. They immunized rabbits with a protein antigen, ovalbumin (the albumin of egg whites), and then divided the immunized rabbits' serum into two aliquots. The first serum aliquot was separated by electrophoresis into four fractions: albumin and the alpha (α), beta (β), and gamma (γ) globulins. The second serum aliquot was reacted with antigen, so that antibody bound to the ovalbumin was precipitated and could be removed; then the remaining serum proteins were electrophoresed. A comparison of the electrophoretic profiles of these two serum aliquots revealed that there was a significant drop in the γ-globulin peak in the aliquot that had been subjected to precipitation with antigen (Figure 5-1). Thus the γ-globulin fraction was identified as containing serum antibodies, which were called *immunoglobulins* to distinguish them from any other proteins that might be contained in the γ-globulin fraction.

In the 1950s and 1960s experiments by Rodney Porter and by Gerald Edelman elucidated the basic structure of the immunoglobulin (Ig) molecule. (These experiments were considered of such significance that the two investigators shared a Nobel prize in 1972.) Edelman's and Porter's experimental approaches were quite different. Porter cleaved the Ig molecule with enzymes to obtain fragments, whereas Edelman dissociated the molecule by reducing the interchain disulfide bonds. The results attained by these two approaches complemented each other and allowed the basic structure of the Ig molecule to be elucidated.

Using ultracentrifugation, both Porter and Edelman first separated the γ-globulin fraction of serum into a high-molecular-weight fraction with a sedimentation constant of 19S and a low-molecular-weight fraction with a sedimentation constant of 7S. They used the 7S fraction, containing a 150,000-MW γ-globulin designated as immunoglobulin G, or IgG, for their studies. Porter subjected IgG to brief digestion with the enzyme papain and separated the fragments. Although papain has general, nonspecific proteolytic activity and will eventually digest the entire IgG molecule, brief treatment cleaves only the most susceptible bonds. Papain digestion of IgG produced two identical fragments (each with a MW of 45,000) called *Fab* fragments because they retained their "antigen-binding" activity and one fragment (MW of 50,000) called the *Fc* fragments because it was found to crystallize during cold storage (Figure 5-2a). A similar experimental approach, but with the enzyme pepsin, was taken by Alfred Nisonoff. Brief pepsin digestion generated a single 100,000-MW fragment composed of two Fab-like fragments and designated $F(ab')_2$. Like the Fab fragments, the $F(ab')_2$ fragment was also able to visibly precipitate antigens. However, after pepsin digestion, the Fc fragment was not recovered because it had been digested into multiple fragments.

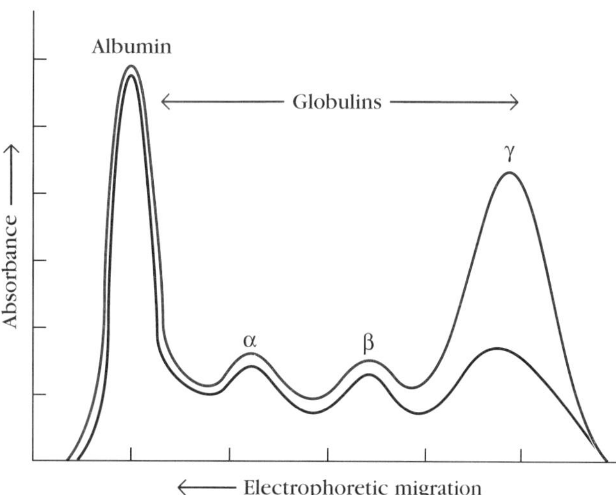

FIGURE 5-1 Experimental demonstration that antibodies are present in the γ-globulin fraction of serum proteins. After rabbits were immunized with ovalbumin (OVA), their antisera were pooled and electrophoresed, which separates the serum proteins based on electric charge. The purple line shows the electrophoretic pattern of untreated antiserum. The black line shows the pattern of antiserum that was incubated with OVA to remove anti-OVA antibody and then electrophoresed. [Adapted from A. Tiselius and E. A. Kabat, 1939, *J. Exp. Med.* **69**:119.]

The chain structure of IgG was first suggested by experiments of Edelman and his colleagues and later confirmed by Porter. Edelman reduced the disulfide bonds of IgG with mercaptoethanol and subjected the denatured protein to starch gel electrophoresis in 8 *M* urea, which reduces the intrachain as well as the interchain disulfide bonds and allows the molecule to unfold. Two electrophoretic bands were obtained, indicating that the IgG molecule contained more than one protein chain. Porter extended this study by doing a much milder mercaptoethanol reduction, so that only the interchain disulfide bonds were reduced. He then alkylated the exposed sulfhydryl groups with iodoacetamide to prevent random re-formation of the disulfide bonds and added an organic proprionic acid solvent to prevent aggregation. The sample was then chromatographed on a column that separates molecules on the basis of size (Figure 5-2b). This experiment revealed that the 150,000-MW IgG molecule was composed of two 50,000-MW polypeptide chains, designated as *heavy (H) chains,* and two 25,000-MW chains, designated as *light (L) chains.*

The remaining puzzle was to determine how the enzyme digestion products—Fab, $F(ab')_2$, and Fc—were related to the heavy-chain and light-chain reduction products. Porter answered this question by using antisera from goats that had been immunized with the Fab fragments and Fc fragments of rabbit IgG. He found that antibody to the Fab fragment could react with both the H and the L chains, whereas antibody to the Fc fragment reacted only with the H chain. These observations led to the conclusion that Fab consists of

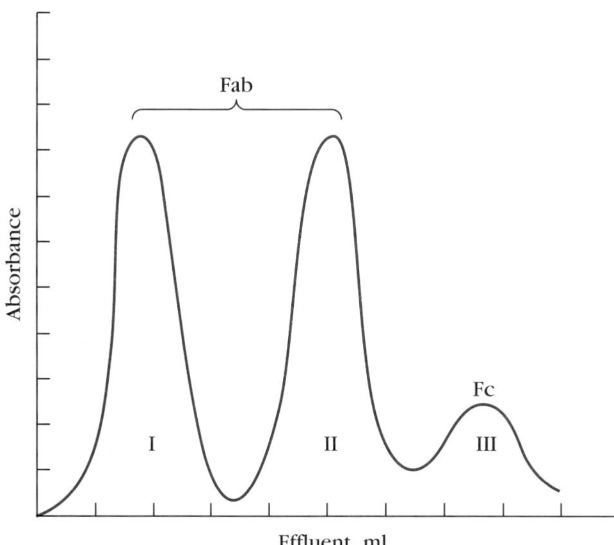

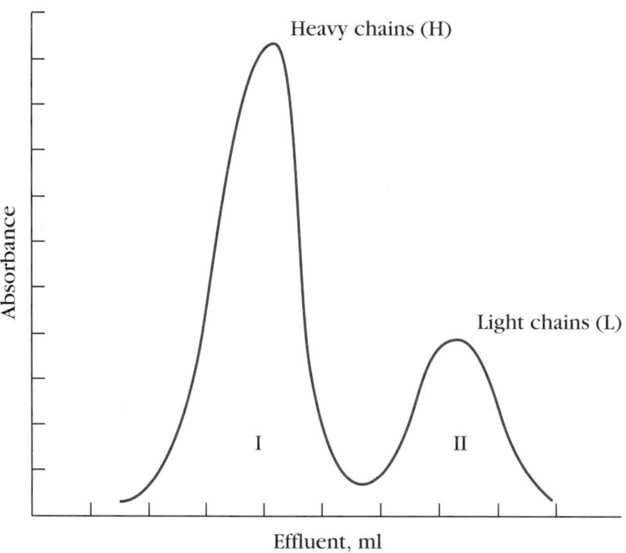

FIGURE 5-2 Separation of products resulting from enzymatic digestion or mild reduction of IgG. (a) Brief digestion of heterogeneous IgG with papain and separation of the digest on a carboxymethylcellulose column yields three peaks. Peaks I and II contain the 45,000-MW Fab fragments, and peak III contains the 50,000-MW Fc fragment. Digestion of homogeneous IgG yields a single Fab peak, which is the sum of peaks I and II. (b) Mild reduction of IgG and alkylation of the exposed sulfhydryl groups followed by gel filtration in proprionic acid yields two peaks. Peak I contains the 50,000-MW heavy chain, and peak II contains the 25,000-MW light chain. [Part (a) adapted from R. R. Porter, 1959, *Biochem. J.* **73**:119; part (b) adapted from J. B. Fleischman, 1962, *Arch. Biochem. Suppl.* **1**:1974.]

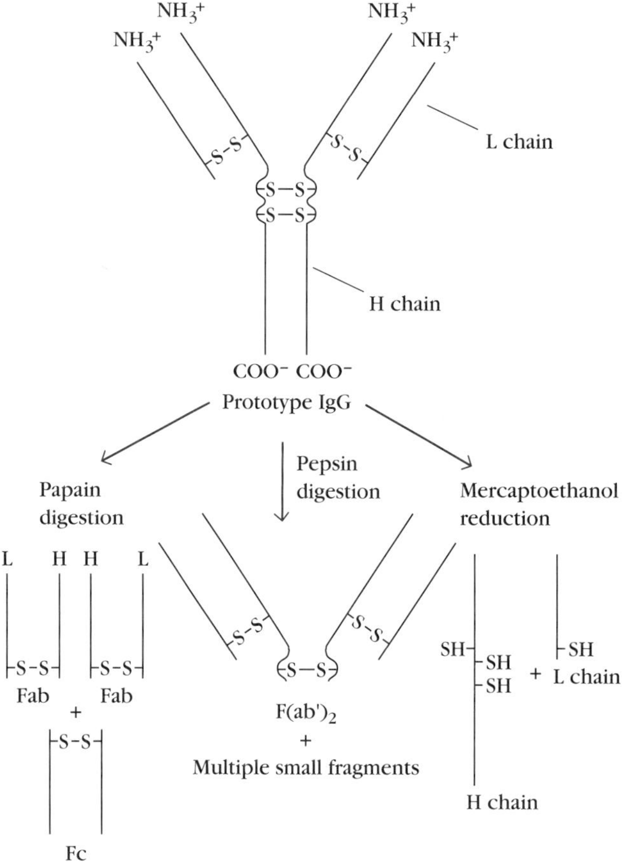

FIGURE 5-3 Prototype structure of IgG, proposed by Rodney Porter in 1962, showing chain structure and interchain disulfide bonds. The fragments produced by various treatments are also indicated.

portions of a heavy and a light chain and that Fc contains only heavy-chain components. Based on these results, Porter proposed a prototype structure for IgG, which has since been confirmed (Figure 5-3). According to this model, the IgG molecule consists of two identical H chains and two identical L chains, which are linked by disulfide bridges. The enzyme papain cleaves just above the interchain disulfide bonds linking the heavy chains, whereas the enzyme pepsin cleaves just below these disulfide bonds, so that the two proteolytic enzymes generate different digestion products. Mercaptoethanol reduction and alkylation allow separation of the individual heavy and light chains.

Immunoglobulin Sequencing Studies

Initial attempts to determine the amino acid sequence of the Ig heavy and light chains were unsuccessful because sufficient amounts of homogeneous protein were unavailable. Although the basic structure and chemical properties of different antibodies are similar, their antigen-binding specificities, and therefore their exact amino acid sequences, are very different. The γ-globulin fraction consists of a heterogeneous spectrum of antibodies that reflect all the different antigens that have induced an immune response in an animal. Even if immunization is done with a hapten-carrier conjugate, the antibodies formed just to the hapten alone are heterogeneous: They recognize different epitopes of the hapten and have different binding affinities. This heterogeneity of serum immunoglobulin rendered it unsuitable for sequencing studies.

Role of Multiple Myeloma

Sequencing analysis finally became feasible with the discovery of *multiple myeloma,* a cancer of antibody-producing plasma cells. In a normal individual, plasma cells are end-line cells that secrete specific antibody for a few days and then die. In multiple myeloma plasma cells are no longer end line but divide over and over in an unregulated way without requiring any activation by antigen to induce clonal proliferation. Although such a cancerous plasma cell, called a *myeloma cell,* has been transformed, its protein synthesizing machinery and secretory functions are not altered, and so the cell continues to secrete specific antibody. This antibody is indistinguishable from normal antibody molecules but is referred to as *myeloma protein* to denote its source. In a patient afflicted with multiple myeloma, myeloma protein can account for 95% of the serum immunoglobulins.

In general the antigenic specificity of the myeloma protein in an afflicted individual is unknown; it reflects a prior antigenic commitment of the cancerous plasma cell. A few myeloma proteins have been characterized, however, and shown to bind to known haptens or to known cell-surface determinants of common bacterial pathogens such as phosphorylcholine, a major cell-wall component of pneumococci. In such cases a plasma cell responsive to one of these common bacterial pathogens presumably has become a cancerous myeloma cell, secreting myeloma protein specific for a determinant on a normal pathogen. Most patients with multiple myeloma also secrete large amounts of excess light chains from their myeloma cells. These excess light chains were first discovered in the urine of myeloma patients and were named *Bence-Jones proteins* for their discoverer.

Multiple myeloma also occurs in other animals. In mice it can arise spontaneously, as it does in humans, or can be induced by injecting mineral oil into the peritoneal cavity. The clones of malignant plasma cells that develop are called *plasmacytomas* and are designated MOPCs, denoting the mineral-oil induction of plasmacytoma cells. A large number of mouse MOPC lines secreting different immunoglobulin classes are presently carried by the American type culture collection, a repository of cell lines commonly used in research.

Light-Chain Sequencing

When the amino acid sequences of several Bence-Jones proteins (light chains) were compared, a striking pattern emerged. The amino-terminal half of the chain, consisting of 100–110 amino acids, was found to vary among different Bence-Jones proteins. This region was called the *variable* (*V*) region. The carboxyl-terminal half of the molecule, called the *constant (C)* region, had two basic amino acid sequences, which were designated *kappa* (κ) and *lambda* (λ) (Figure 5-4a). In humans 60% of the light chains are kappa, and 40% are lambda, whereas in mice 95% of the light chains are kappa, and only 5% are lambda. A single antibody molecule expresses either κ light chains or λ light chains but never both.

A comparison of the amino acid sequences of λ light chains revealed minor differences on the basis of which λ light chains are classified into subtypes. In mice there are three subtypes ($\lambda1$, $\lambda2$, and $\lambda3$); in humans there are four subtypes. Single amino acid interchanges at two or three positions are responsible for the subtype differences.

Heavy-Chain Sequencing

For heavy-chain sequencing studies, myeloma proteins were reduced with mercaptoethanol and alkylated, and the heavy chains were separated by gel filtration in a denaturing solvent. When the amino acid sequences of several myeloma protein heavy chains were compared, a pattern similar to that observed with the light chains emerged. The amino-terminal 100–110 amino acids showed great sequence variation from one myeloma heavy chain to the next and was therefore called the variable (V) region. The remaining part of the protein revealed five basic amino acid sequence patterns (μ, γ, α, δ, and ϵ) corresponding to five different heavy-chain constant (C) regions (see Figure 5-4a). The length of the constant regions was approximately 330 amino acids for α, γ, and δ and 440 amino acids for μ and ϵ The heavy chains of a given antibody molecule determine the class of that antibody: IgM, IgG, IgA, IgD, or IgE. Each class can have either κ or λ light chains. A single antibody molecule has two identical heavy chains and two identical light chains (Table 5-1).

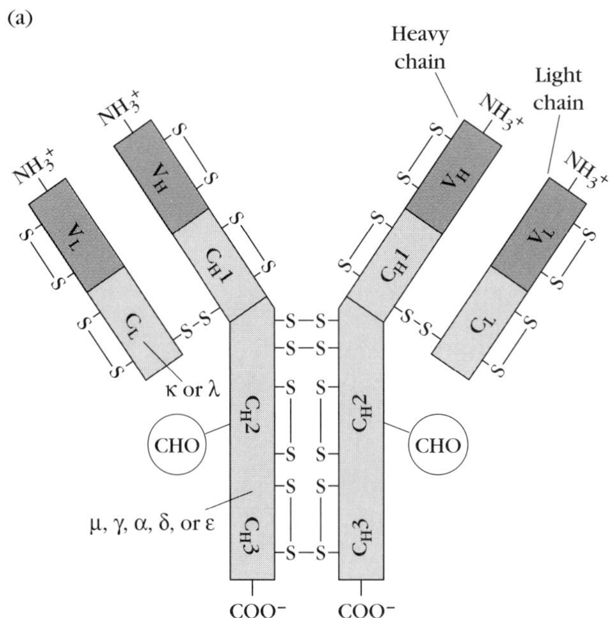

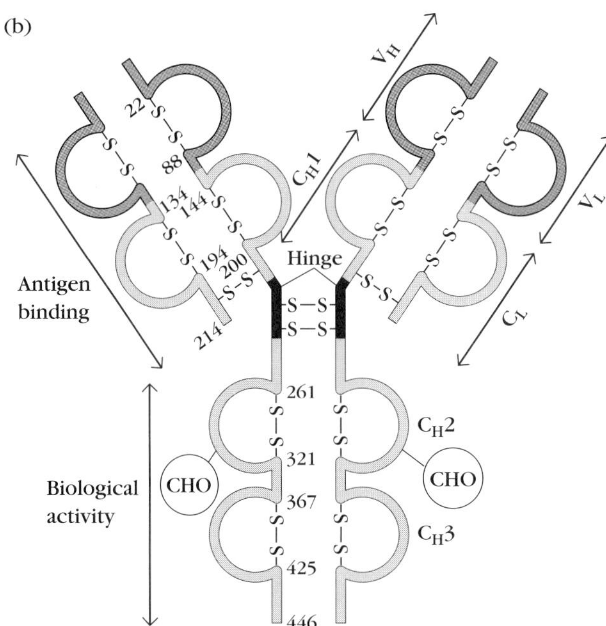

FIGURE 5-4 Primary and secondary structure of immunoglobulins derived from amino acid sequencing studies. (a) Each heavy and light chain in an immunoglobulin molecule contains an amino-terminal variable (V) region (purple) that consists of 100–110 amino acids and differs from one antibody to the next. The remainder of the molecule—the constant (C) region (gray)—exhibits limited variation that defines the κ or λ light chains and the μ, γ, α, δ or ϵ heavy chains. (b) Heavy and light chains are folded into domains, each containing about 110 amino acid residues and an intrachain disulfide bond that forms a 60-aa loop. Some heavy chains (γ, δ and α) also contain a proline-rich hinge region (black). The μ and ϵ heavy chains lack a hinge region but contain an additional domain in the central portion of the molecule.

TABLE 5-1 CHAIN COMPOSITION OF THE FIVE IMMUNOGLOBULIN CLASSES IN HUMANS

Class	Heavy chain	Light chain	Subclasses	Molecular formula
IgG	γ	κ or λ	$\gamma 1$, $\gamma 2$, $\gamma 3$, $\gamma 4$	$\gamma_2\kappa_2$ $\gamma_2\lambda_2$
IgA	α	κ or λ	$\alpha 1$, $\alpha 2$	$(\alpha_2\kappa_2)_n$ $(\alpha_2\lambda_2)_n$ $n = 1, 2, 3,$ or 4
IgM	μ	κ or λ	None	$(\mu_2\kappa_2)_n$ $(\mu_2\lambda_2)_n$ $n = 1$ or 5
IgD	δ	κ or λ	None	$\delta_2\kappa_2$ $\delta_2\lambda_2$
IgE	ϵ	κ or λ	None	$\varepsilon_2\kappa_2$ $\varepsilon_2\lambda_2$

Minor differences in the amino acid sequences of the α and of the γ heavy chains led to further classification of the heavy chains into subclasses. In humans there are two subclasses of α heavy chains ($\alpha 1$ and $\alpha 2$) and four subclasses of γ heavy chains ($\gamma 1$, $\gamma 2$, $\gamma 3$, and $\gamma 4$); in mice there are four subclasses of γ heavy chains ($\gamma 1$, $\gamma 2$a, $\gamma 2$b, and $\gamma 3$).

IMMUNOGLOBULIN FINE STRUCTURE

The structure of the immunoglobulin molecule is determined by its primary, secondary, tertiary, and quaternary protein structure. The primary amino acid sequence accounts for the variable and constant regions of the heavy and light chains. The secondary structure is formed as the extended polypeptide chain folds back and forth upon itself forming an antiparallel β pleated sheet (Figure 5-5a). The sheet is stabilized by an invariant intrachain disulfide bond and by hydrogen bonds that connect the peptide bonds in neighboring chains. The chains are then folded into a tertiary structure of compact globular domains, which are connected to neighboring domains by narrow, more exposed areas. Finally, the globular domains of adjacent heavy and light polypeptide chains interact in the quaternary structure, forming functional domains that enable the molecule to specifically bind antigen and, at the same time, perform a limited number of biological effector functions.

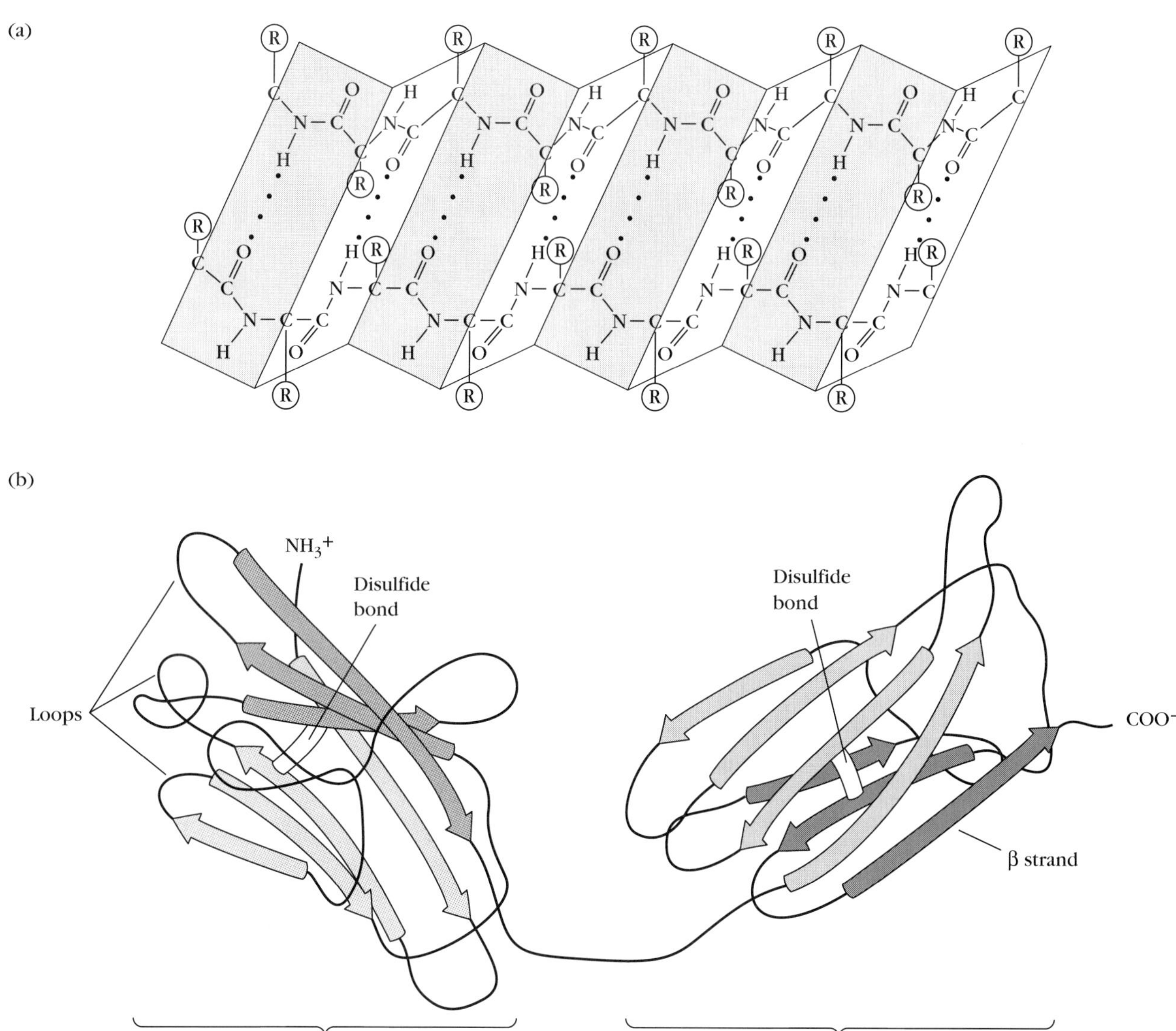

FIGURE 5-5 The immunoglobulin fold, the characteristic tertiary structure forming immunoglobulin domains, contains two antiparallel β pleated sheets. (a) Structural formula of a β pleated sheet containing two antiparallel β strands. The structure is held together by hydrogen bonds between peptide bonds in neighboring chains. The amino acid side groups (R) are arranged perpendicular to the plane of the sheet. (b) Diagram of immunoglobulin light chain depicting the immunoglobulin-fold structure of its variable and constant domains. The two β pleated sheets in each domain are held together by hydrophobic interactions and the conserved disulfide bond. Residues in the amino-terminal loop regions of the variable domains make up the antigen-binding site. Heavy-chain domains have the same characteristic structure. [Part (a) adapted from J. Darnell et al., 1990, *Molecular Cell Biology,* Scientific American Books, New York; part (b) adapted from M. Schiffer et al., 1973, *Biochemistry* **12**:4620.]

Immunoglobulin Domains

Careful analysis of the amino acid sequences of immunoglobulin heavy and light chains showed that both chains contain several homologous units of about 110 amino acid residues. Within each unit, termed a *domain,* an intrachain disulfide bond forms a loop of about 60 amino acids. Light chains contain one variable domain (V_L), and one constant domain (C_L); heavy chains contain one variable domain (V_H), and either three or four constant domains (C_H1, C_H2, C_H3, and C_H4), depending on the antibody class (Figure 5-4b).

X-ray crystallographic analysis revealed that immunoglobulin domains are folded into a characteristic compact structure known as the *immunoglobulin fold.*

This structure consists of a "sandwich" of two β pleated sheets, each containing three or four antiparallel β strands of amino acids, which are connected by loops of varying lengths (Figure 5-5b). The β strands are characterized by alternating hydrophobic and hydrophilic amino acids whose side chains are arranged perpendicular to the plane of the sheet—the hydrophobic amino acids are oriented toward the interior and the hydrophilic amino acids face outward. The two sheets are stabilized by the hydrophobic interactions between them and by the conserved disulfide bond. An analogy has been made to two pieces of bread, the butter between them, and a toothpick holding the slices together. The bread slices represent the two β pleated sheets; the butter represents the hydrophobic interactions between them; and the toothpick represents the intrachain disulfide bond.

Although variable and constant domains have a similar structure, there are subtle differences between them. The V domain is slightly longer than the C domain and contains an extra pair of β strands within the β-sheet structure, as well as an extra loop sequence connecting this pair of β strands. The basic structure of the immunoglobulin fold is uniquely suited to facilitate noncovalent interactions between domains across the faces of the β sheets (Figure 5-6). Interactions occur between identical domains (e.g., C_H2/C_H2, C_H3/C_H3, and C_H4/C_H4), and between nonidentical domains (e.g., V_H/V_L and C_H1/C_L). The structure of the immunoglobulin fold also allows for variable lengths

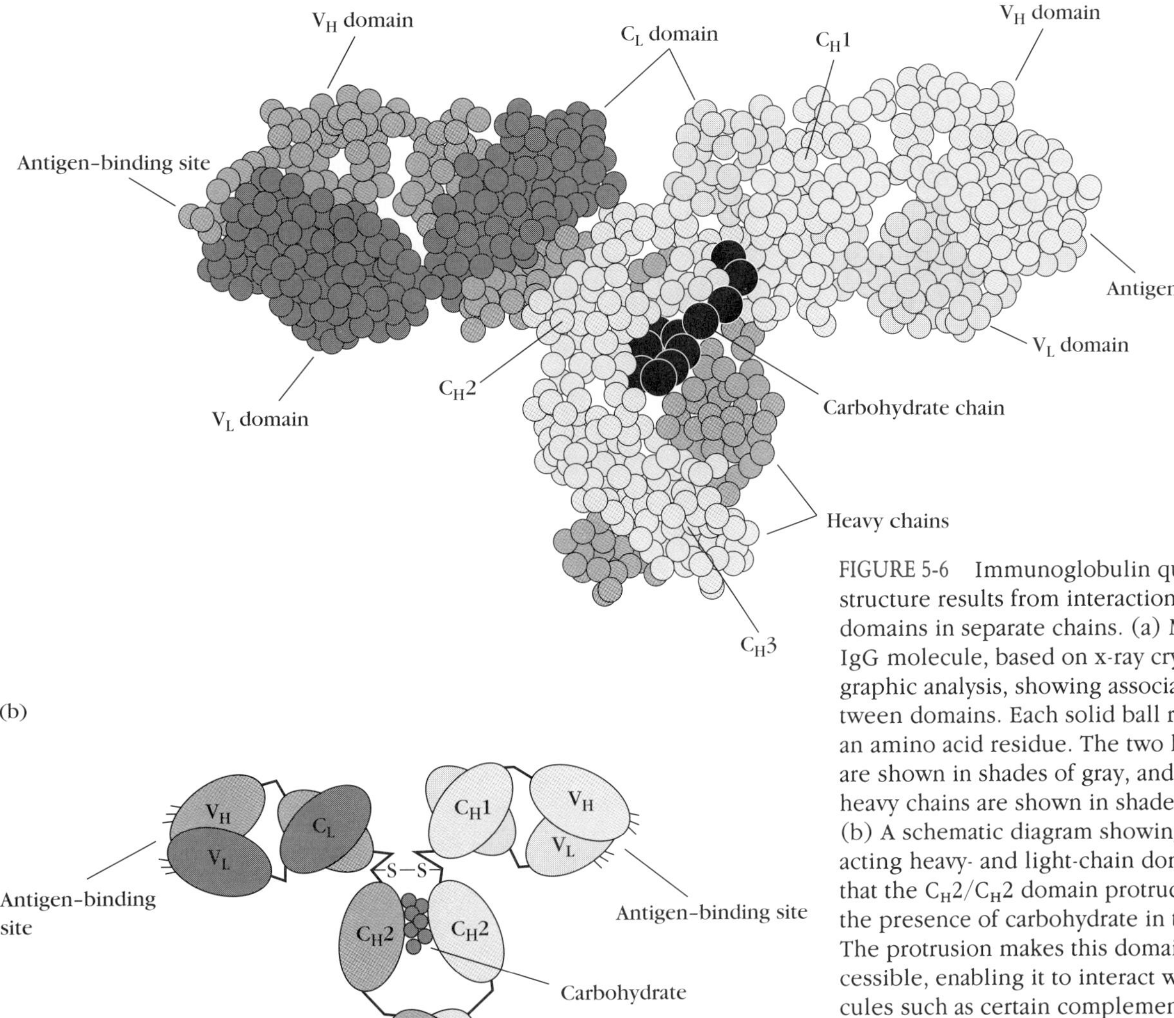

FIGURE 5-6 Immunoglobulin quaternary structure results from interactions between domains in separate chains. (a) Model of IgG molecule, based on x-ray crystallographic analysis, showing associations between domains. Each solid ball represents an amino acid residue. The two light chains are shown in shades of gray, and the two heavy chains are shown in shades of purple. (b) A schematic diagram showing the interacting heavy- and light-chain domains. Note that the C_H2/C_H2 domain protrudes due to the presence of carbohydrate in the interior. The protrusion makes this domain more accessible, enabling it to interact with molecules such as certain complement components. [Part (a) from E. W. Silverton et al., 1977, *Proc. Nat. Acad. Sci. USA* **74**:5140.]

(a)

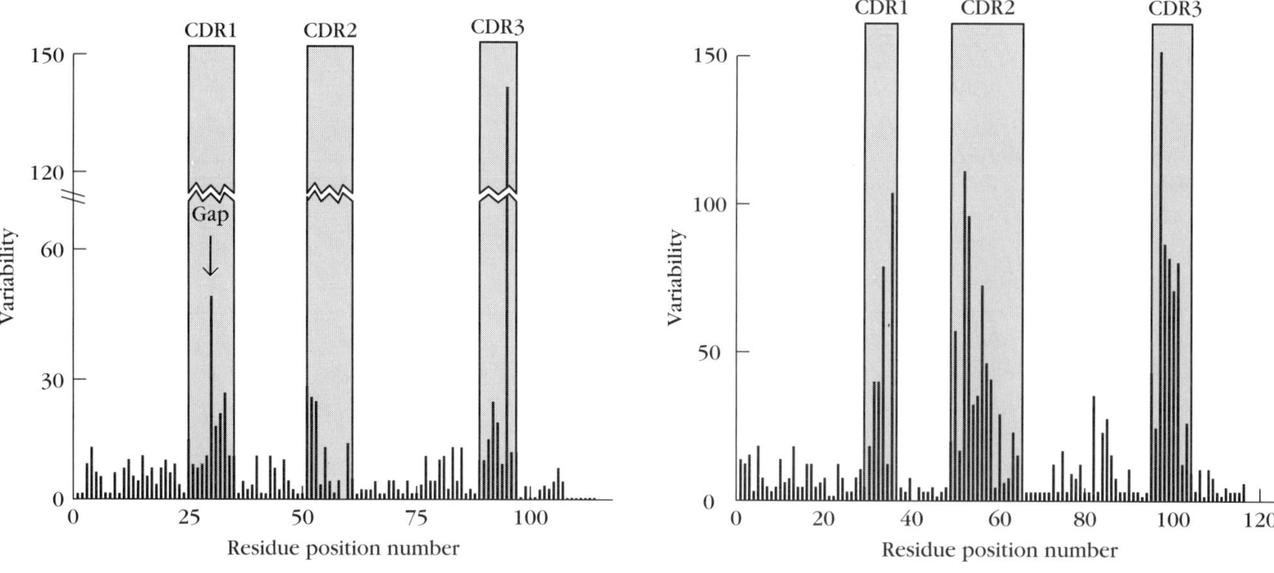

(b)

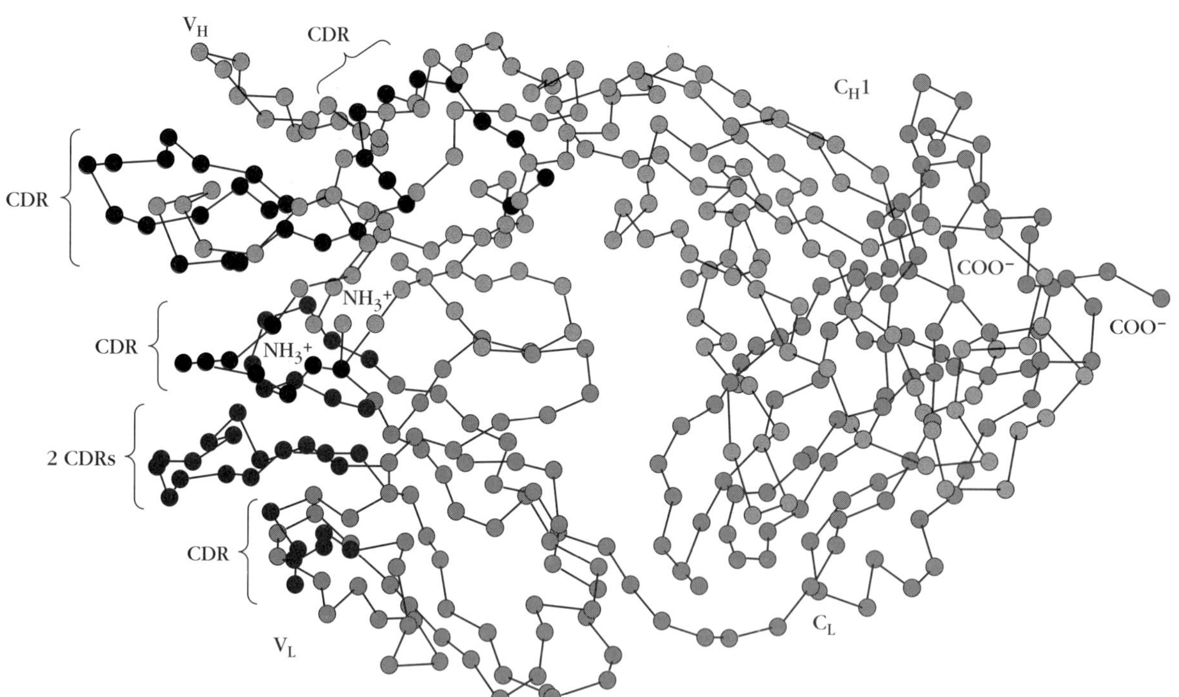

FIGURE 5-7 (a) Experimental demonstration of hypervariable regions in the V_L and V_H domains of human antibodies. Plots of amino acid variability at each position in antibodies with different specificities revealed three hypervariable regions, also called complementarity-determining regions (CDRs). (b) Model of a Fab fragment in which the α-carbon of each amino acid residue is represented by a ball. The residues making up the light-chain CDRs (black) and heavy-chain CDRs (purple) protrude from the molecule and thus are able to contact antigen. [Part (a) from E. A. Kabat et al., 1977, *Sequence of Immunoglobulin Chains,* U.S. Dept of Health, Education, and Welfare; part (b) from J. D. Capra and A. B. Edmundson, 1977, *The Antibody Combining Site,* © 1977, vol. 236R(1) Scientific American, Inc.]

and sequences of amino acids that form the loops connecting the β strands. As discussed later, the loop sequences of the V_H and V_L domains contain variable amino acids and constitute the antigen-binding site of the molecule.

Variable-Region Domains: Structure and Function

Detailed comparisons of the amino acid sequences of V_L and V_H domains revealed that the sequence variability is concentrated in several *hypervariable regions.* Three such hypervariable regions are present in each mouse and human heavy and light chain, constituting 15–20% of the variable domain (Figure 5-7a). The remaining 80–85% of the V_L and V_H domains exhibit far less variation; these stretches are referred to as the *framework regions (FRs).* The hypervariable regions form the antigen-binding site of the antibody molecule. Because the antigen-binding site is complementary to the structure of the epitope, the hypervariable regions are also called *complementarity-determining regions (CDRs).*

High-resolution x-ray crystallography has been used to determine the three-dimensional structure of the framework regions and complementarity-determining regions. The more conserved sequence of the framework regions generates the basic β pleated sheet structure of the V_H and V_L domains. The three heavy-chain and three light-chain CDRs are located on the loops that connect the β strands of the V_H and V_L domains (Figure 5-7b). The wide range of specificities exhibited by antibodies is a function of variations in the length and amino acid composition of the six CDR loops in each Fab fragment. The framework region thus acts as a scaffold supporting the six CDR loops. The framework regions of virtually all of the antibodies analyzed to date can be superimposed on one another; only the CDR loops show different orientations in different antibodies. This three-dimensional structure of the variable domain provides a rigid framework, which is necessary for overall antibody function; at the same time an enormous spectrum of antigen-binding specificities is achieved by the diversity within the six CDR loops.

The earliest evidence demonstrating the role of the hypervariable regions in binding antigen was obtained by L. Wofsy, H. Metzger, and S. J. Singer using an experimental technique called *affinity labeling.* This technique used a synthetic hapten as a labeling reagent that could bind specifically to an antibody forming a covalent bond with neighboring residues within the antibody's binding site. Identification of the amino acids covalently bound to the affinity label revealed that hypervariable amino acids within light- and heavy-chain CDRs constitute the antigen-binding site.

The three-dimensional structure of the antigen-binding site and the role of the CDRs in the binding of antigen have also been investigated by high resolution x-ray crystallography. To date, crystallographic analysis has been completed for about two dozen Fab fragments of monoclonal antibodies complexed either to large globular protein antigens or to a number of smaller antigens including carbohydrates, nucleic acids, peptides, and small haptens. In addition, complete x-ray pictures have recently been obtained for an intact antitumor monoclonal antibody (see Color Plate 1).

The results of these crystallographic studies have provided valuable insights into the structure of the V_H and V_L domains. For example, in binding to a large globular protein antigen (e.g., hen egg-white lysozyme or neuraminidase [an envelope glycoprotein of influenza]), the antibody contacts the protein antigen across a rather flat, undulating face. In the area of contact, protrusions or depressions on the antigen are matched by complementary depressions or protrusions on the respective antibody (see Color Plates 7 and 8). The surface area of this large complementary face is 650–900 Å^2; within this area some 15–22 amino acids on the protein antigen contact a similar number of residues in the antibody's binding site (see Color Plate 4). In antibodies that bind smaller antigens (e.g., the hapten phosphocholine or the octapeptide hormone angiotensin II), the antigen-binding site generally is smaller and appears more like a deep pocket in which the ligand is largely buried (see Color Plates 2 and 3; Table 5-2). For example, contact between phosphocholine (PC) and Fab fragment of anti-PC antibody occurs in a deep pocket of the antibody with a surface area of 161 Å^2, and the Fab to angiotensin II contacts the octapeptide within a deep, narrow groove with a surface area of 725 Å^2.

As the data in Table 5-3 indicate, a minimum of four of the six CDR loops in a Fab fragment make contact with the antigen's epitope. In the case of some antibodies, including that to angiotensin II, all six CDR loops in the Fab fragment contact the antigen (see Color Plate 3). In general, more residues in the three heavy-chain CDRs appear to contact antigen than in the light-chain CDRs. Thus, the V_H domain appears to contribute more to antigen binding than the V_L domain (see Table 5-3, right-hand columns). This dominant role of the heavy chain in antigen binding was demonstrated in a study in which a single heavy chain specific for a glycoprotein antigen of HIV was combined with various light chains of different antigenic specificity.

TABLE 5-2 CONTACT AREA BETWEEN FAB FRAGMENTS AND ANTIGENS*

Fab	Fab contact area (Å^2)	Antigen	Ag molecular weight (kDa)	Ag contact area (Å^2)	Ag buried contact area (Å^2)	% Antigen buried
Small antigens						
McPC603	161	Phosphocholine	169	169	137	81
DB3	286	Progesterone	314	277	246	89
Se155-4	297	Dodecasaccharide	1416	378	248	66
4-4-20	308	Fluoroscein	334	282	266	94
AN02	350	Dinitrophenyl spin-label	392	344	232	67
17/9	468	HA peptide	1055	742	436	59
BV04	515	d(pT)$_3$	932	687	454	66
B13/2	560	C-helix peptide	818	701	462	66
131	725	Angiotensin II	1046	ND	620	ND
Globular protein antigens						
D1.3	690	Lysozyme	14000	5564	680	12
HyHEL-10	721	Lysozyme	14000	5414	774	14
HyHEL-5	746	Lysozyme	14000	5436	750	14
NC41	916	Neuraminidase	50000	14638	899	6

KEY: Ag = antigen; HA = hemagglutinin; ND = not determined.

* Contact area determined by computer analysis of x-ray crystallographic data of Fab fragments bound to their respective antigens.

SOURCE: Adapted from I. A. Wilson and R. L. Stanfield, 1993, *Curr. Opin. Struc. Biol.* **3**:113.

All of the resulting hybrid antibodies exhibited affinity for the HIV glycoprotein antigen, indicating that the heavy chain alone was sufficient to confer specificity.

As more x-ray crystallographic analyses of Fab fragments were completed, it became clear that in some cases binding of antigen induces conformational changes in the antibody and/or antigen. Formation of the neuraminidase antigen–antibody complex is accompanied by a conformational change in side-chain orientation of both the epitope and the antigen-binding site of the antibody. This conformational change results in a closer fit between the epitope and the antibody's binding site. In some cases more significant conformational changes have been observed in the CDR loops upon antigen binding. For example, comparison of a Fab fragment before and after binding to a peptide antigen of influenza has revealed a visible conformational change in the heavy chain CDR3 loop following binding (Color Plates 5 and 6). Thus changes in the length and amino acid composition of the CDR loops, coupled with significant changes in the conformation of these loops upon antigen binding, enables a given antibody to more effectively assume a structure complementary to that of the epitope.

Constant-Region Domains: Structure and Function

The immunoglobulin constant-region domains are associated with various biological functions that are determined by the amino acid sequence of each domain.

C_H1 and C_L Domains

The C_H1 and C_L domains serve to extend the Fab arms of the antibody molecule, thereby facilitating interaction with antigen and increasing the maximum rotation of the Fab arms. These constant-region domains

TABLE 5-3 HYPERVARIABLE LOOPS USED IN ANTIGEN BINDING*

	Light chain			Heavy chain			Contribution to Ag binding (%)	
Fab fragment	CDR1	CDR2	CDR3	CDR1	CDR2	CDR3	V_L	V_H
B1312	+	−	+	+	+	+	22	78
17/9	+	−	+	−	+	+	26	74
DB3	+	−	+	+	+	+	35	65
4-4-20	+	−	+	+	+	+	40	60
Se155-4	+	−	+	+	+	+	40	60
HyHEL-5	+	+	+	+	+	+	41	59
131	+	−	+	+	+	+	41	57
BV04	+	+	+	+	+	+	43	57
HyHEL-10	+	+	+	+	+	+	43	57
D1.3	+	+	+	+	+	+	43	57
NC41	−	+	+	+	+	+	46	54
McPC603	−	−	+	+	+	+	47	53
AN02	+	+	+	−	−	+	61	39
Total	11	6	13	11	12	13		

* A + indicates that at least one residue in the CDR loop is involved in binding antigen; a − indicates that no residue in the CDR loop is involved in binding. The percentage contribution of the variable light-chain (V_L) and heavy-chain (V_H) domains to antigen binding was calculated from crystallographic data. See Table 5-2 for antigens bound by the listed Fab fragments.

SOURCE: Adapted from I. A. Wilson and R. L. Stanfield, 1993, *Curr. Opin. Struc. Biol.* **3**:113.

also help to hold the V_H and V_L domains together by virtue of the interchain disulfide bond between them (see Figure 5-4). More recent experiments have suggested that the C_H1 and C_L domains contribute to antibody diversity by allowing more random associations between V_H and V_L domains than would occur if this association were driven by the V_H/V_L interaction alone.

In one experiment, V_H and V_L domains from two antibodies having different known specifications (*a* and *b*) were prepared separately and then mixed. Each domain was shown to reassociate almost exclusively with its original partner to form V_La/V_Ha or V_Lb/V_Hb complexes (Figure 5-8a). In another experiment Fab fragments from antibody *a* and antibody *b* were mildly reduced and denatured to obtain V_HC_H1 and V_LC_L fragments from each antibody. When these longer fragments were mixed, random association occurred, yielding homogeneous complexes containing fragments from either antibody *a* or *b* and heterogeneous complexes containing one *a* and one *b* fragment (Figure 5-8b). As is discussed in Chapter 8, random rearrangements of the immunoglobulin genes generate unique V_H and V_L sequences for the heavy and light chains expressed by each B lymphocyte; association of the V_H and V_L sequences then generates a unique antigen-binding site. The results of these experiments suggest that the presence of C_H1 and C_L domains increases the number of stable V_H and V_L interactions that are possible, thus contributing to the overall diversity of antibody molecules that can be expressed by an animal.

Hinge Region

The γ, δ, and α heavy chains contain an extended peptide sequence between the C_H1 and C_H2 domains that has no homology with the other domains (see Figure 5-4b). This region, called the *hinge* region, is rich in prolines and is flexible, giving IgG, IgD, and IgA segmental flexibility. As a result, the two Fab arms can

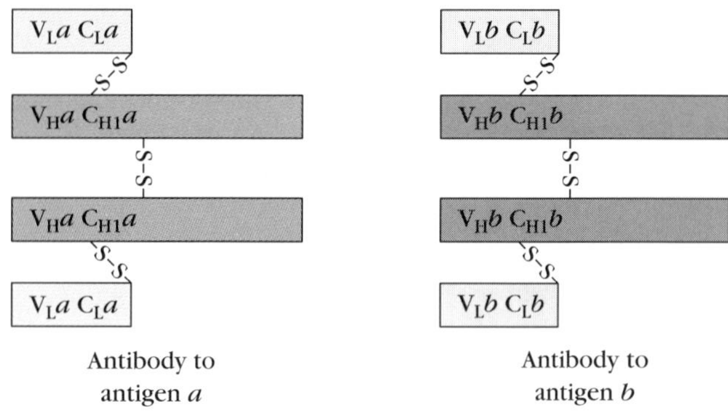

(a) $V_La + V_Lb + V_Ha + V_Hb \longrightarrow V_La/V_Ha + V_Lb/V_Hb$

Homogeneous complexes

(b) $V_La\ C_La + V_Lb\ C_Lb + V_Ha\ C_Ha + V_Hb\ C_Hb$

$V_La\ C_La/V_Ha\ C_Ha$ + $V_Lb\ C_Lb/V_Hb\ C_Hb$	$V_La\ C_La/V_Hb\ C_Hb$ + $V_Lb\ C_Lb/V_Ha\ C_Ha$
Homogeneous complexes	Heterogenous complexes

FIGURE 5-8 Experimental demonstration that C_H1 and C_L domains facilitate random association of heavy and light chains. Antibodies with two different specificities (*a* and *b*) were treated to obtain fragments corresponding to the V_L and V_H domains or longer fragments containing the V_HC_H1 and V_LC_L domains. Mixing of the V_H and V_L domains (a) or of the longer VC fragments (b) revealed that the presence of the C_H1 and C_L domains resulted in formation of heterogeneous complexes containing segments from both antibodies.

assume various angles relative to each other when antigen is bound. This flexibility of the hinge region can be visualized in electron micrographs of antigen-antibody complexes. For example, when a molecule containing two DNP groups reacts with anti-DNP antibody and the complex is captured on a grid, negatively stained, and observed with electron microscopy, large complexes (e.g., dimers, trimers, tetramers) are seen. The angle between the arms of the Y-shaped antibody molecules varies in the different complexes, reflecting the flexibility of the hinge region (Figure 5-9).

X-ray crystallographic analysis of an entire monoclonal antibody specific for canine lymphoma-cell membrane antigen has revealed that the hinge region serves as a sort of tether that allows the Fab components and the Fc to move (see Color Plate 1). In this way the Fab arms can move and twist to align the CDRs with epitopes displayed on the cell surface, and the Fc can move to maximize various effector functions such as complement activation or binding to Fc receptors.

Two prominent amino acids in the hinge region are proline and cysteine. The large number of proline residues in the hinge region confers an extended polypeptide conformation on it, making the hinge region particularly vulnerable to cleavage by proteolytic enzymes; it is this region that is cleaved with papain or pepsin (see Figure 5-3). The cysteine residues form interchain disulfide bonds that hold the two heavy chains together. The number of interchain disulfide bonds in the hinge region varies considerably among different classes of antibodies and between species. Although μ and ϵ chains lack a hinge region, they have an additional 110-aa domain (C_H2/C_H2) that has hingelike features.

Other Constant-Region Domains

In comparing the heavy-chain domains in the different immunoglobulin classes, the C_H2/C_H2 and C_H3/C_H3 domains of IgA, IgD, and IgG (containing α, δ, and γ heavy chains, respectively) correspond to the C_H3/C_H3 and C_H4/C_H4 domains in IgE and IgM (containing ϵ and μ heavy chains, respectively). As mentioned already, IgE and IgM lack the hinge region present in the other classes of immunoglobulin. In this region of the molecule, IgE and IgM have an additional immunoglobulin domain, designated C_H2/C_H2. The function of this domain in these classes has not yet been determined.

X-ray crystallographic analysis has revealed that the C_H2/C_H2 domain of IgA, IgD, and IgG (and the C_H3/C_H3 domain of IgE and IgM) are separated by oligosaccharide side chains; as a result these two globular domains are much more accessible than the other domains to the aqueous environment (see Figure 5-6b). This accessibility accounts for the important biological activity of these domains in the activation of complement components by the IgG and IgM classes of antibody molecules.

The carboxyl-terminal domain is designated C_H3/C_H3 in IgA, IgD, and IgG and C_H4/C_H4 in IgE and IgM. The amino acid sequence and the function of this domain in the secreted antibody of plasma cells differs from that in membrane-bound antibody on B cells (the latter is discussed in the next section). Secreted immunoglobulin (sIg) has a hydrophilic amino acid sequence of varying lengths at the carboxyl-terminal end. In secreted antibody the carboxyl-terminal domain together with the adjacent domain interact with Fc receptors on the surface of various cells. For example, IgG and IgM antibodies bind to Fc receptors on phagocytic cells, mediating opsonization. Some

(a)

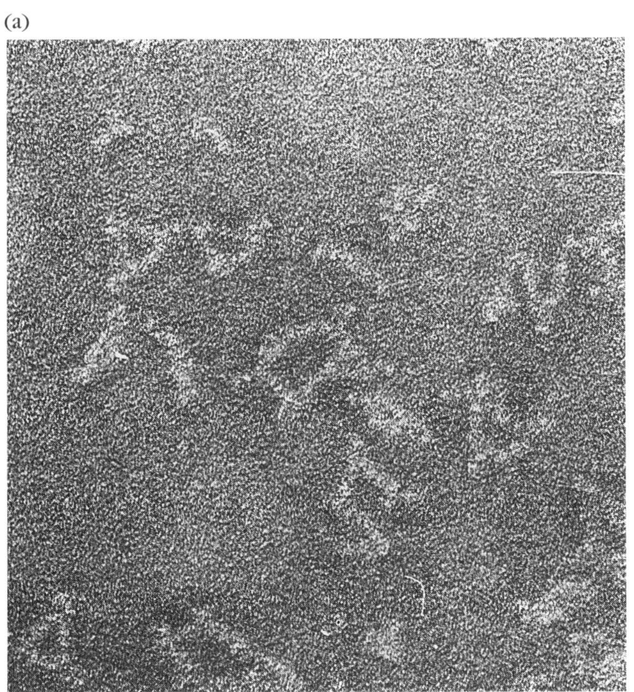

(b)

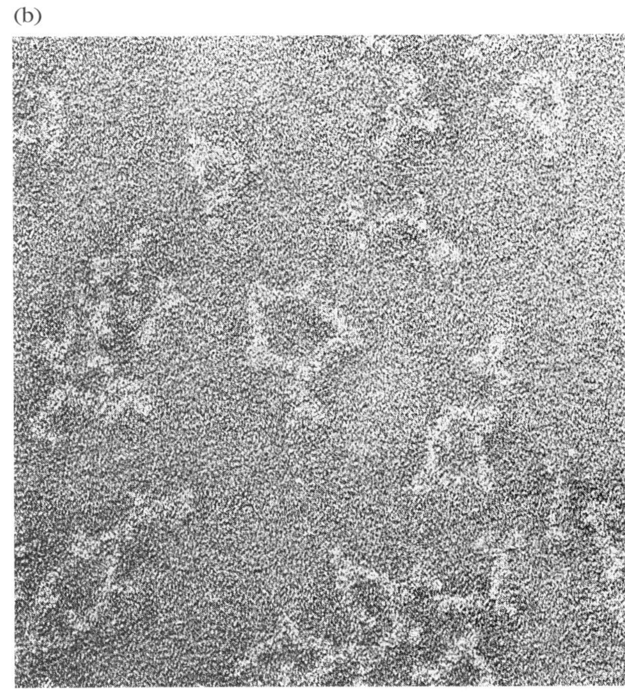

(c)

DNP ligand ●—●

O_2N—[benzene ring with NO_2]—N ∿∿∿∿ N—[benzene ring with NO_2]—NO_2

25Å

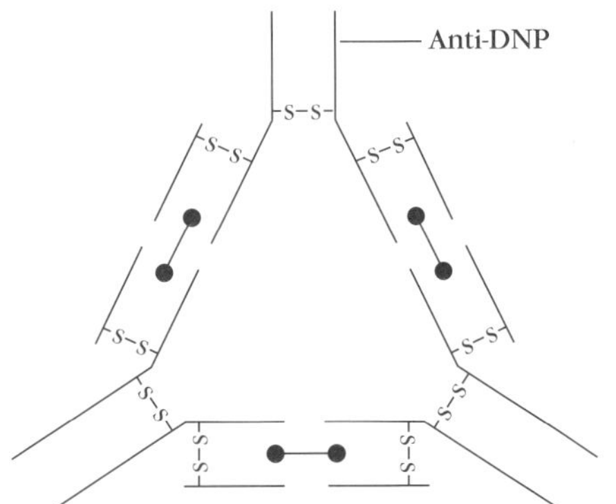

FIGURE 5-9 Reaction of a divalent DNP hapten with anti-DNP antibodies forms trimers (a) and tetramers (b), as well as other large antigen-antibody complexes. In these electron micrographs of negatively stained preparations, the antibody protein stands out as a light structure against the electron-dense background. Because of the flexibility of the hinge region, the angle between the arms of the antibody molecules varies. Schematic diagram of a trimer is shown in (c). [Photographs from R. C. Valentine and N. M. Green, 1967, *J. Mol. Biol.* **27**:615.]

subclasses of IgG bind to Fc receptors on placental cells and then are transferred across the placenta, allowing maternal IgG antibodies to protect the fetus. Binding of IgE to mast cells and basophils also is mediated by Fc receptors on these cells. As discussed in more detail later, formation of secretory IgA and IgM antibodies involves binding to Fc receptors on mucous membrane epithelial cells. The carboxyl-terminal domains of IgA and IgM also play a role in the polymerization of free IgA and IgM molecules. The presence of cysteine residues in this domain allows disulfide bonds to form between monomeric units, with the result that IgM is secreted by plasma cells as a pentamer and IgA is secreted as a dimer or trimer.

Immunoglobulin Receptor Complex

Not all immunoglobulin is expressed as secreted antibody. Instead, some immunoglobulin is produced in a form that enables it to be expressed on the membrane of B cells. The membrane-bound immunoglobulin expressed by a particular B cell determines the antigenic specificity of that cell.

Membrane Immunoglobulin

Membrane-bound immunoglobulin (mIg) differs from secreted immunoglobulin (sIg) in the carboxyl-terminal domain. The hydrophilic sequence present in sIg is replaced in mIg with three regions: an extracellular hydrophilic "spacer" sequence, a hydrophobic transmembrane sequence, and a short cytoplasmic sequence. The transmembrane sequence always contains 26 amino acid residues; the extracellular spacer sequence and cytoplasmic sequence vary in length among the immunoglobulin classes, called isotypes. Each of the five immunoglobulin isotypes and their subtypes can be expressed as membrane-bound antibody. B cells express different isotypes of mIg at different developmental stages. The immature B cell, called a pre-B cell, expresses only mIgM; mIgD appears later in maturation and is the predominant isotype on mature resting B cells. A memory B cell can express a variety of isotypes including combinations of mIgM, mIgG, mIgA, and mIgE. Even when different isotypes are expressed on a single cell, the antigenic specificity of all the membrane antibody molecules is the same, so that each antibody molecule binds to the same epitope. The genetic mechanism that allows a single B cell to express multiple isotypes all with the same antigenic specificity is discussed in Chapter 8.

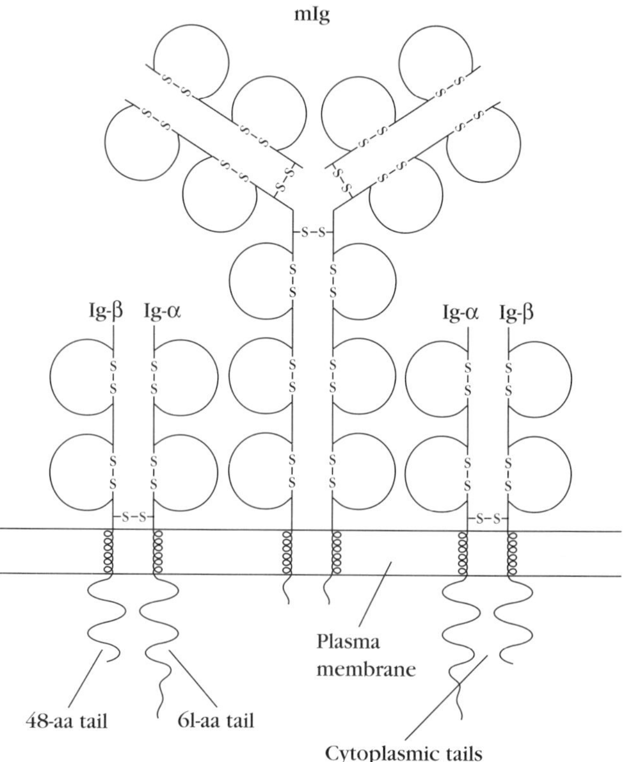

FIGURE 5-10 The B-cell antigen receptor (BCR) is composed of membrane-bound immunoglobulin (mIg) and a disulfide-linked heterodimer called Ig-α/Ig-β. The heterodimer contains the immunoglobulin-fold structure and cytoplasmic tails much longer than those in mIg. As depicted, each mIg molecule is thought to be associated with two heterodimer molecules. [Adapted from A. D. Keegan and W. E. Paul, 1992, *Immunol. Today* **13**:63 and M. Reth, 1992, *Annu. Rev. Immunol.* **10**:97.]

B-Cell Receptor Complex

Immunologists have long been puzzled about how mIg mediates an activating signal after contact with an antigen. The dilemma is that all isotypes of mIg have very short cytoplasmic tails: the mIgM and mIgD cytoplasmic tails contain only 3 amino acids; the mIgA tail, 14 amino acids; and the mIgG and mIgE tails, 28 amino acids. In each case, the cytoplasmic tail is too short to be able to associate with intracellular signaling molecules (e.g., tyrosine kinases and G proteins). Recent findings indicating that mIg does not constitute the entire B-cell antigen receptor appear to resolve this puzzle.

The B-cell receptor (BCR) recently has been shown to be a transmembrane protein complex composed of mIg and a disulfide-linked heterodimer called Ig-α/Ig-β. It is thought that two molecules of the heterodimer associate with one mIg molecule to form a single BCR (Figure 5-10). The Ig-α chain has a long cytoplasmic tail containing 61 amino acids; the tail of the Ig-β chain contains 48 amino acids. The tails in both Ig-α and Ig-β are long enough to interact with intracellular signaling molecules. In addition, both cytoplasmic tails in the heterodimer contain several tyrosine residues that can be phosphorylated by three members of the *src* family of tyrosine kinases: $p55^{blk}$, $p59^{fyn}$, and $p56^{lck}$. When mIg is cross-linked with an anti-Ig reagent, each of these protein kinases is activated. The kinases then act directly or indirectly to phosphorylate and activate a number of molecules involved in signal transduction in B cells. Discovery of the Ig-α/Ig-β heterodimer has substantially furthered understanding of B-cell activation, which is discussed in detail in Chapter 14.

Antigenic Determinants on Immunoglobulins

Since antibodies are glycoproteins, they can themselves function as potent immunogens to induce an antibody response. The antigenic determinants, or epitopes, on immunoglobulin molecules fall into three major categories: *isotypic, allotypic,* and *idiotypic* determinants, which are located in characteristic portions of the molecule (Figure 5-11).

Isotypic Determinants

Isotypes define constant-region determinants that distinguish each heavy-chain class and subclass and each light-chain type and subtype within a species. Each isotype is encoded by a separate constant-region gene, and all members of a species carry the same constant-region genes. Within a species, each normal individual will express all isotypes in their serum. Different species inherit different constant-region genes and therefore express different isotypes. Therefore, when an antibody from one species is injected into another species, the isotypic determinants will be recognized as foreign, inducing an antibody response to the isotypic determinants on the foreign antibody. Anti-isotype antibody is routinely used for research purposes to determine the class or subclass of serum antibody produced during an immune response or to characterize the class of membrane-bound antibody present on B cells.

Allotypic Determinants

Although all members of a species inherit the same set of isotype genes, multiple alleles exist for some of the genes. These alleles encode subtle amino acid differences, called allotypic determinants, that occur in some, but not all, members of a species. In humans, allotypes have been characterized for all four IgG subclasses, for one IgA subclass, and for the κ light chain. The γ chain allotypes are referred to as Gm markers. To date, 25 different Gm allotypes have been identified; they are designated by the class and subclass followed by the allele number, for example, G1m(1), G2m(23), G3m(11), G4m(4a). Of the two IgA subclasses, only the IgA2 subclass has allotypes, designated as A2m(1) and A2m(2). The κ light chain has three allotypes, designated κm(1), κm(2), and κm(3). Each of these allotypic determinants represents differences in one to four amino acids that are encoded by different alleles.

Antibody to allotypic determinants can be produced by injecting antibodies from one member of a species into another member of the same species who lacks the allotypic determinant. Antibody to allotypic determinants are sometimes produced by a mother during pregnancy in response to paternal allotypic determinants on the fetal immunoglobulins. Antibodies to allotypic determinants can also arise following a blood transfusion.

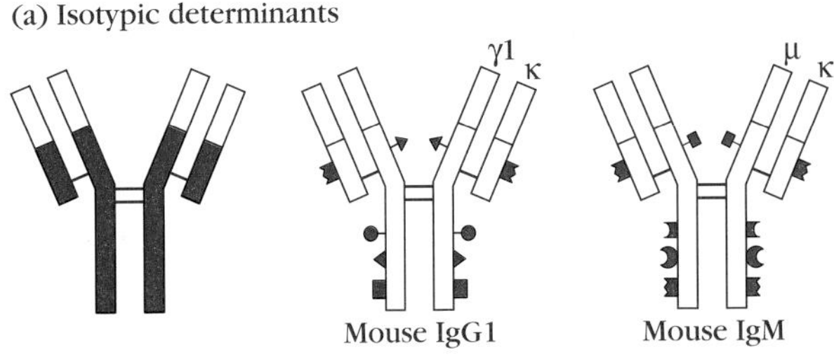

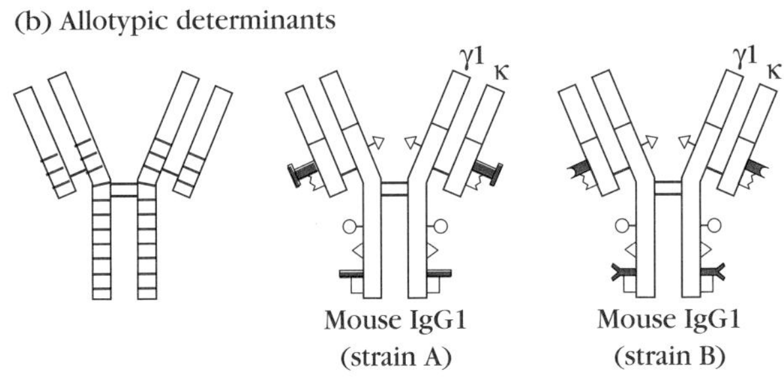

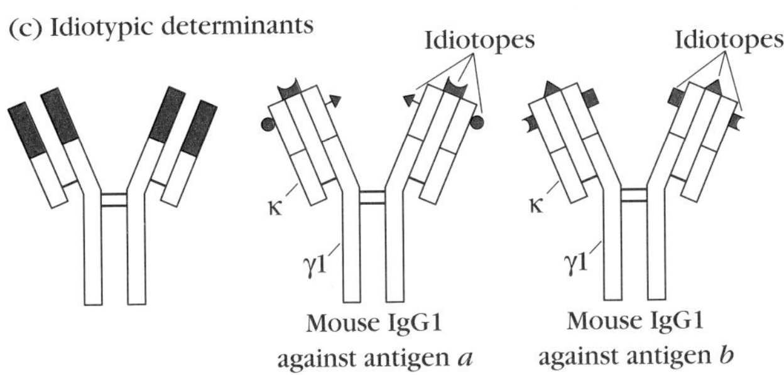

FIGURE 5-11 Antigenic determinants of immunoglobulins. (a) Isotypic determinants are constant-region determinants that distinguish each Ig class and subclass within a species. (b) Allotypic determinants are subtle amino acid differences encoded by different alleles. Allotypic differences can be detected by comparing the same antibody class among different inbred strains. (c) Idiotypic determinants are generated by the conformation of the amino acid sequences of the heavy- and light-chain variable region specific for each antigen. Each individual determinant is called an idiotope, and the sum of the individual idiotopes is the idiotype. For each type of determinant, the general location of determinants within the antibody molecule is shown *(left)* and two examples are illustrated (*center* and *right*).

Idiotypic Determinants

The unique amino acid sequence of the V_H and V_L domains of a given antibody can function not only as an antigen-binding site but also as an antigenic determinant. The idiotypic determinants are generated by the conformation of the heavy- and light-chain variable regions. Each individual antigenic determinant of the variable region is referred to as an *idiotope* (see Figure 5-11c). In some cases an idiotope may be the actual antigen-binding site, and in some cases an idiotope may comprise variable-region sequences outside of the antigen-binding site. Each antibody will present multiple idiotopes; the sum of the individual idiotopes is called the *idiotype* of the antibody.

Because the antibodies produced by individual B cells derived from the same clone have identical variable-region sequences, they all have the same idiotype. Some idiotypic determinants are shared by antibodies that are not clonally derived. These idiotypic determinants, called public idiotypic determinants, reflect the common usage of the same germ-line variable-region gene by different B cells from the same inbred strain. Anti-idiotype antibody is produced by minimizing isotypic or allotypic differences, so that the idiotypic difference can be recognized. Often a homogeneous antibody such as myeloma protein or monoclonal antibody is used. Injection of such an antibody into a syngeneic recipient will result in the formation of anti-idiotype antibody to the idiotypic determinants.

One of the earliest experiments demonstrating the presence of idiotypic determinants on antibodies was performed by J. Oudin and M. Michel at the Pasteur Institute in 1963. These researchers injected rabbit anti-*Salmonella* antibody into another rabbit of the same allotype. The rabbit produced antibody that bound to the immunizing antibody but did not bind with other rabbit antibodies from the same donor or with anti-*Salmonella* antibody from other rabbits. Anti-idiotype antibody is produced by animals during the course of an immune response and has been shown to play an important role in regulating the immune response; this phenomenon is discussed in Chapter 16.

Immunoglobulin Isotypes

The various immunoglobulin classes, or isotypes, have been mentioned briefly already. In this section, the structure and effector functions of each isotype are discussed in more detail. Each isotype is distinguished by unique amino acid sequences in the heavy-chain constant region that result in structural and functional differences among different isotypes. The structures of the five major isotypes are diagrammed in Figure 5-12. The molecular properties and biological activities of the immunoglobulin isotypes are listed in Table 5-4. The effector functions of each isotype results from interactions between its heavy-chain constant regions and other serum proteins or cell-membrane receptors.

Immunoglobulin G (IgG)

IgG, the most abundant isotype in serum, constitutes about 80% of the total serum immunoglobulin. The IgG molecule is a monomer consisting of two γ heavy chains and two κ or λ light chains. There are four IgG subclasses in humans, numbered in accordance with their decreasing average serum concentrations: IgG1 (9 mg/ml), IgG2 (3 mg/ml), IgG3 (1 mg/ml), and IgG4 (0.5 mg/ml). The four subclasses are encoded by different germ-line C_H genes whose DNA sequences are 90–95% homologous. The structural characteristics that distinguish these subclasses from one another are the size of the hinge region and the number and position of the interchain disulfide bonds between the heavy chains (Figure 5-13). The subtle amino acid differences between subclasses of IgG affect the biological activity of the molecule (see Table 5-4). IgG1, IgG3, and IgG4 readily cross the placenta and play an important role in protecting the developing fetus. Several IgG subclasses are activators of the complement system, although their effectiveness varies. The IgG3 subclass is the most effective complement activator, followed by IgG1; IgG2 is relatively inefficient at complement activation, and IgG4 is not able to activate the complement sequence at all. IgG also functions as an opsonin by binding to Fc receptors on phagocytic cells, but there are subclass differences in this function also. IgG1 and IgG3 bind with a high affinity to Fc receptors. IgG4 has an intermediate affinity, and IgG2 has an extremely low affinity.

Immunoglobulin M (IgM)

IgM accounts for 5–10% of the total serum immunoglobulin with an average serum concentration of 1.5 mg/ml. Monomeric IgM is expressed as membrane-bound antibody on B cells. IgM is secreted by plasma cells as a pentamer in which five monomer units are held together by disulfide bonds linking their carboxyl-terminal ($C_\mu4/C_\mu4$) domains and $C_\mu3/C_\mu3$

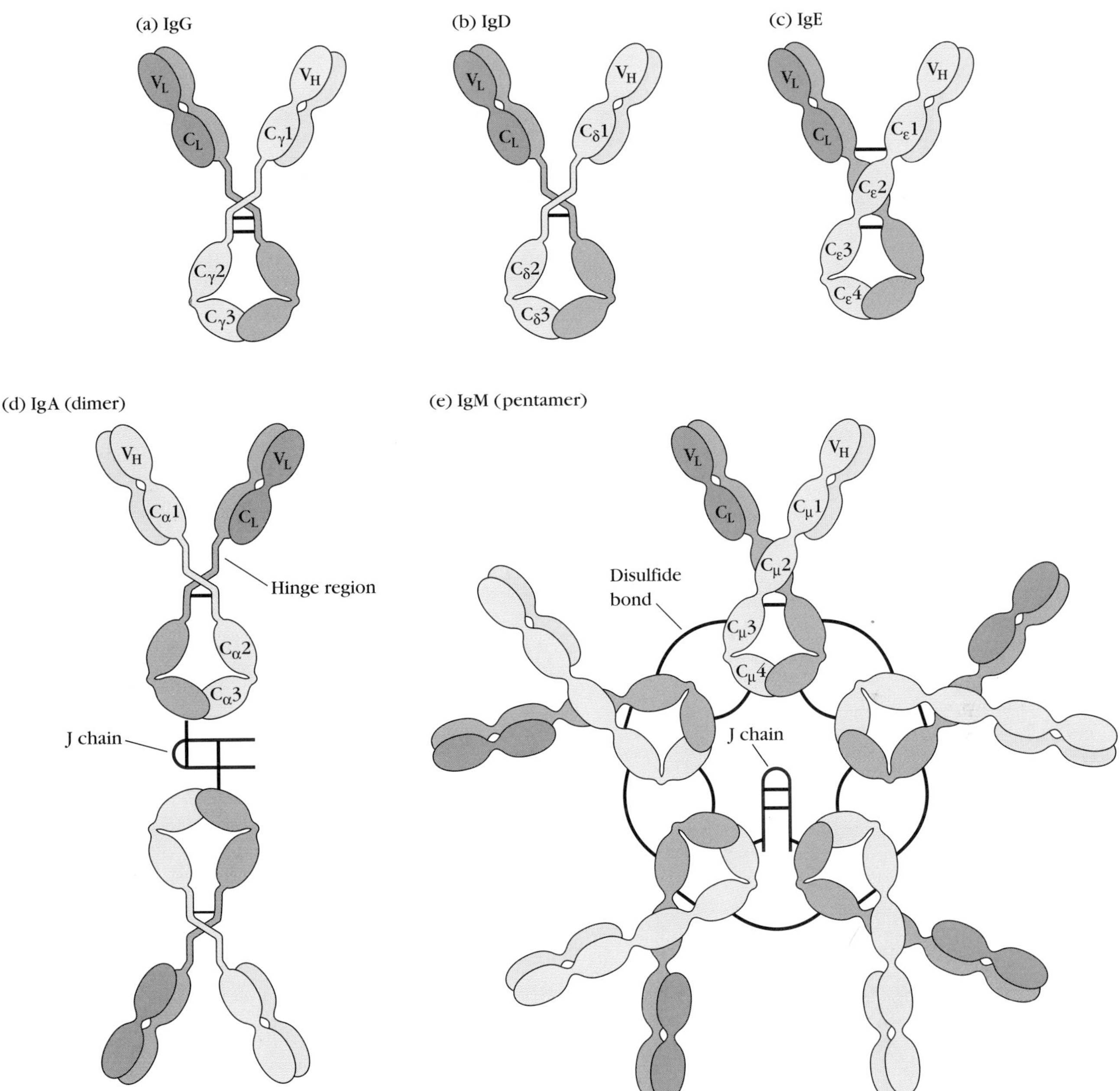

FIGURE 5-12 General structures of the five major isotypes of secreted antibody. Light chains are shaded gray and heavy chains are shaded purple; disulfide bonds are indicated by thick black lines. Note that the IgG, IgA, and IgD heavy chains contain four domains and a hinge region, whereas the IgM and IgE heavy chains contain five domains but no hinge region. The polymeric forms of IgM and IgA contain a polypeptide, known as the J chain (purple), that is linked by two disulfide bonds to the Fc region in two different monomers. Serum IgM is always a pentamer; most serum IgA exists as a monomer, although some dimers, trimers, and even tetramers sometimes are present. Not shown in these figures are intrachain disulfide bonds and disulfide bonds linking light and heavy chains (see Figure 5-4).

TABLE 5-4 PROPERTIES AND BIOLOGICAL ACTIVITIES* OF CLASSES AND SUBCLASSES OF SERUM IMMUNOGLOBULINS

Property/activity	IgG1	IgG2	IgG3	IgG4	IgA1	IgA2	IgM‡	IgE	IgD
Molecular weight†	150,000	150,000	150,000	150,000	150,000–600,000	150,000–600,000	900,000	190,000	150,000
Heavy-chain component	$\gamma 1$	$\gamma 2$	$\gamma 3$	$\gamma 4$	$\alpha 1$	$\alpha 2$	μ	ϵ	δ
Normal serum level (mg/ml)	9	3	1	0.5	3.0	0.5	1.5	0.0003	0.03
In vivo serum half-life (days)	23	23	8	23	6	6	5	2.5	3
Activates classical complement pathway	+	+/−	++	−	−	−	+++	−	−
Crosses placenta	+	+/−	+	+	−	−	−	−	−
Present on membrane of mature B cells	−	−	−	−	−	−	+	−	+
Binds to macrophage Fc receptors	++	+/−	++	+	−	−	+	−	−
Present in secretions	−	−	−	−	++	++	+	−	−
Induces mast-cell degranulation	−	−	−	−	−	−	−	+	−

* Activity levels indicated as follows ++ = high, + = moderate; +/− = minimal; and − = none.

† IgG, IgE, and IgD always exist as monomers, IgA can exist as a monomer, dimer, trimer, or tetramer. Membrane-bound IgM is a monomer, but secreted IgM in serum is a pentamer.

‡ IgM is the first isotype produced by the neonate and during a primary immune response.

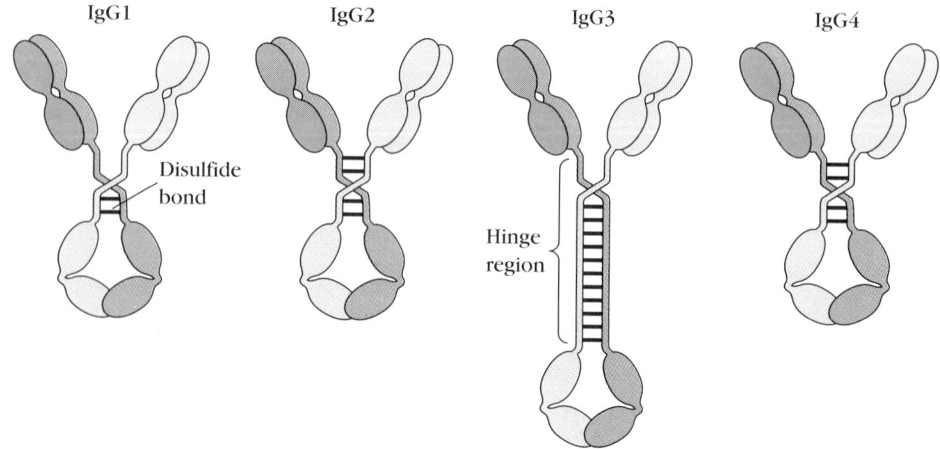

FIGURE 5-13 General structure of the four subclasses of human IgG, which differ in the number and arrangement of the interchain disulfide bonds (thick black lines) linking the heavy chains. The hinge region in IgG3 is four times as long as the hinge region in the other IgG subclasses and contains 11 interchain disulfide bonds.

domains (see Figure 5-12e). The five monomer subunits are arranged with their Fc regions in the center of the pentamer and the 10 antigen-binding sites on the periphery of the molecule. Each pentamer contains an additional Fc-linked polypeptide called the *J* (joining) *chain,* which is disulfide-bonded to the carboxyl-terminal cysteine residue of 2 of the 10 μ chains. The J chain appears to be required for polymerization of the monomers to form pentameric IgM; it is added just before secretion of the pentamer.

IgM is the first immunoglobulin class produced in a primary response to an antigen, and it is also the first immunoglobulin to be synthesized by the neonate. Because of its pentameric structure with 10 antigen-binding sites, serum IgM has a higher valency than the other isotypes. An IgM molecule can bind 10 small hapten molecules; however, because of steric hindrance, only 5 molecules of larger antigens can be bound simultaneously. The increased valency of pentameric IgM increases its capacity to bind such multidimensional antigens as viral particles and red blood cells (RBCs). For example, when RBCs are incubated with specific antibody, they clump together into large aggregates in a process called *agglutination.* It takes from 100 to 1000 times as many molecules of IgG as of IgM to achieve the same level of agglutination. A similar phenomenon occurs with viral particles—less IgM than IgG is required to neutralize viral infectivity. IgM is also more efficient than IgG at complement activation. Complement activation requires two Fc regions in close proximity, and the pentameric structure of a single molecule of IgM fullfills this requirement.

Because of its large size, IgM does not diffuse well and therefore is found in very low concentrations in the intercellular tissue fluids. The presence of the J chain allows IgM to bind to receptors on secretory cells, which transport it across epithelial linings to the external secretions that bathe mucosal surfaces. Although IgA is the major isotype found in these secretions, IgM also serves an important accessory role as a secretory immunoglobulin.

Immunoglobulin A (IgA)

Although IgA constitutes only 10–15% of the total immunoglobulin in serum, it is the predominant immunoglobulin class in external secretions such as breast milk, saliva, tears, and mucus of the bronchial, genitourinary, and digestive tracts. In serum, IgA exists primarily as a monomer, although polymeric forms such as dimers, trimers, and even tetramers are sometimes seen. The IgA of external secretions, called *secretory IgA,* consists of a dimer or tetramer, a J-chain polypeptide, and a polypeptide chain called *secretory component* (Figure 5-14a). The J-chain polypeptide is identical to that found in pentameric IgM and serves a similar function in facilitating the polymerization of both serum and secretory IgA. The secretory component is a 70,000-MW polypeptide produced by epithelial cells of mucous membranes. It consists of five immunoglobulin-like domains that bind to the Fc regions of the IgA dimer. This interaction is stabilized by a disulfide bond between the fifth domain of the secretory component and one of the α chains of the dimeric IgA. Surprisingly, daily production of secretory IgA is greater than that of any other immunoglobulin class. IgA-secreting plasma cells are concentrated along mucous membrane surfaces. Along the jejunum of the small intestines, for example, there are more than 2.5×10^{10} IgA-secreting plasma cells—a number that surpasses the total plasma cells of the bone marrow, lymph, and spleen combined! Each day humans secrete 5–15 g of secretory IgA into mucous secretions.

The plasma cells that secrete IgA home to subepithelial tissue, where that IgA binds tightly to a receptor for polymeric immunoglobulin molecules (Figure 5-14b). This *poly-Ig receptor* is expressed on the surface of most mucosal epithelia (e.g., the lining of the digestive, respiratory, and genital tracts) and on glandular epithelia in the mammary, salivary, and lacrimal glands. After polymeric IgA binds to the poly-Ig receptor, the receptor-IgA complex is transported across the epithelial barrier to the lumen. Transport of the poly-Ig receptor–IgA complex involves receptor-mediated endocytosis into coated pits and directed transport of the vesicle across the epithelial cell to the luminal membrane, where the vesicle fuses with the plasma membrane. The poly-Ig receptor is then cleaved enzymatically from the membrane and becomes the secretory component, which is bound to and released together with polymeric IgA into the mucous secretions. The secretory component masks sites susceptible to protease cleavage in the hinge region of secretory IgA, allowing the polymeric molecule to exist for a longer period of time in the protease-rich mucosal environment than would be possible otherwise. Pentameric IgM also is transported into mucous secretions by this mechanism, although it accounts for a much lower percentage of antibody in the mucous secretions than does IgA. It is thought that the poly-Ig receptor recognizes the J chain associated with both polymeric IgA and IgM antibodies.

Secretory IgA serves an important effector function at mucous membrane surfaces, which are the main entry sites for most pathogenic organisms. Because it is polymeric, secretory IgA can cross-link large antigens with multiple epitopes. Binding of secretory IgA to bacterial and viral surface antigens prevents attachment of the pathogens to the mucosal cells. Once

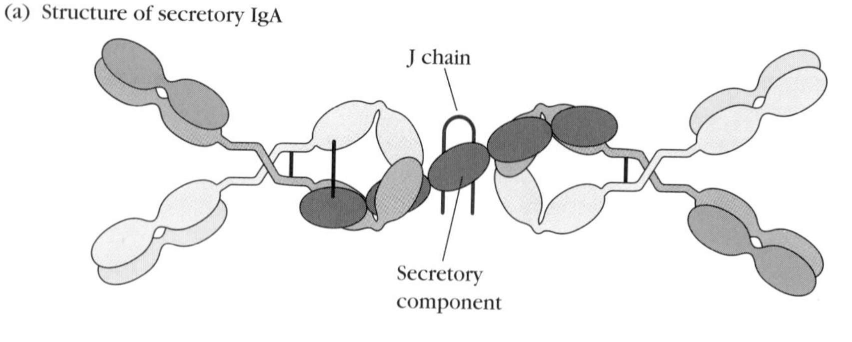

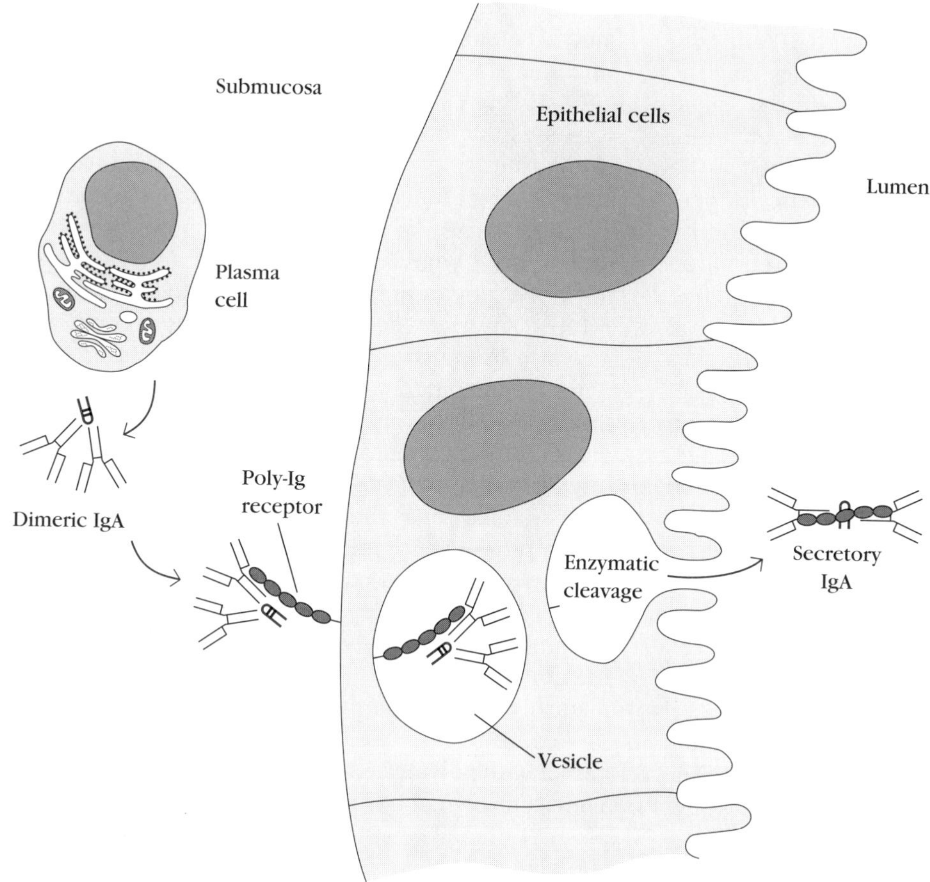

FIGURE 5-14 Structure and formation of secretory IgA. (a) Secretory IgA consists of at least two IgA molecules, which are covalently linked via a J chain and covalently associated with the secretory component. The secretory component contains five Ig-like domains and is linked to dimeric IgA by a disulfide bond (thick black line) between its fifth domain and one of the IgA heavy chains. (b) Secretory IgA is formed during transport through mucous membrane epithelial cells. Dimeric IgA binds to a poly-Ig receptor on the basolateral membrane of an epithelial cell and is internalized by receptor-mediated endocytosis. After transport of the receptor-IgA complex to the luminal surface, the poly-Ig receptor is enzymatically cleaved, releasing the secretory component bound to the dimeric IgA.

attachment is blocked, viral infection and bacterial colonization are inhibited. Complexes of secretory IgA and antigen are easily entrapped in mucous and then eliminated by the ciliated epithelial cells of the respiratory tract or by peristalsis of the gut. Secretory IgA has been shown to provide an important line of defense against bacteria such as *Salmonella, Vibrio cholerae, Neisseria gonorrhoea,* and viruses such as polio, influenza, and reovirus. Secretory IgA also is secreted in breast milk and plays an important role in protecting the newborn during the first months of life.

In order to enhance mucosal immunity, a purified antigen or attenuated virus vaccine must be administered orally or via another mucosal route and remain intact long enough to be taken up by M cells in mucosal epithelia. The polio vaccine, for example, is an attenuated virus that is administered orally on a sugar cube. After the attenuated polio virus binds to M cells along the mucous membranes of the digestive tract, the viral antigens are transported across the M cells into a basolateral pocket containing clusters of B cells, T cells, and macrophages (see Figure 3-22). Following B-cell activation, the B cells differentiate into plasma cells secreting dimeric IgA antibody. This dimeric antibody is then transported across the epithelia and released as secretory IgA into the lumen where it provides protection against a later challenge by a virulent polio virus. The inability to produce attenuated pathogens has hampered development of vaccines to induce secretory IgA production; this has been a major obstacle in developing a gonorrhea vaccine. One strategy currently being evaluated to get around this problem is to engineer an attenuated virus (e.g., the polio virus) with DNA encoding an antigen of choice (e.g., a surface antigen of the gonorrhea bacterium). The recombinant attenuated virus could then serve as a vehicle to express the antigen for sufficient time within the mucosal environment to induce IgA production.

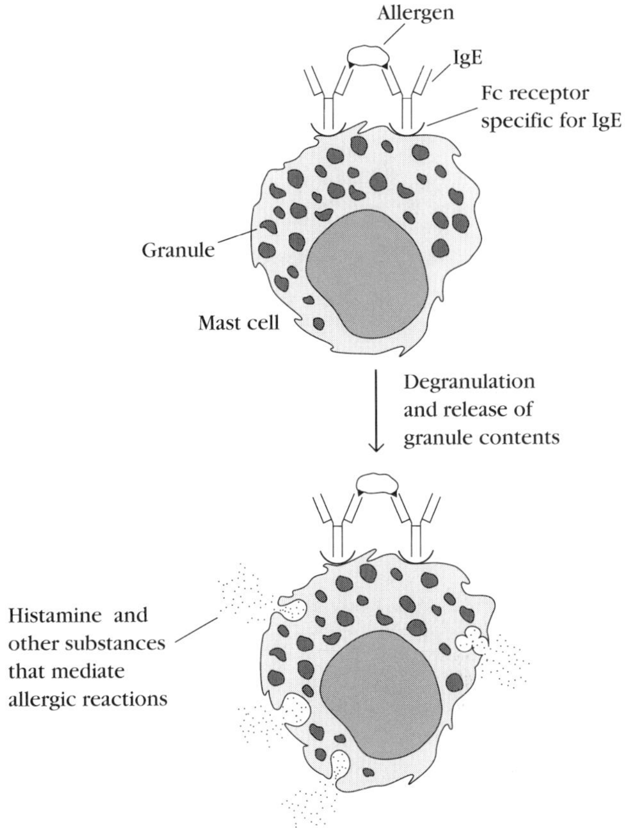

FIGURE 5-15 Allergen cross-linkage of receptor-bound IgE on mast cells induces degranulation, causing release of substances that mediate allergic manifestations.

Immunoglobulin E (IgE)

The potent biological activity of IgE allowed it to be identified in serum despite its extremely low average serum concentration (0.3 μg/ml). IgE antibodies mediate the immediate hypersensitivity reactions that are responsible for the symptoms of hay fever, asthma, hives, and anaphylactic shock. The presence of a serum component responsible for allergic reactions was first demonstrated in 1921 by K. Prausnitz and H. Kustner, who injected serum from an allergic person intradermally into a nonallergic individual. When the appropriate antigen was later injected at the site of injection, a wheal and flare (analogous to hives) developed there. This reaction, called the *P-K reaction,* was the basis for the earliest biological assay for IgE activity.

Actual identification of IgE was accomplished by K. and T. Ishizaka in 1966. They obtained serum from an allergic individual and immunized rabbits with it to prepare anti-isotype antiserum. The rabbit antiserum was then allowed to react with each class of human antibody known at that time (i.e., IgG, IgA, IgM, and IgD). In this way, each of the known anti-isotype antibodies was precipitated and removed from the rabbit anti-serum. What remained was an anti-isotype antibody specific for an unidentified class of antibody. This anti-isotype antibody turned out to completely block the P-K reaction. The new antibody was called IgE (in reference to the E antigen of ragweed pollen, which is a potent inducer of this class of antibody).

IgE binds to Fc receptors on the membranes of blood basophils and tissue mast cells. Cross-linkage of receptor-bound IgE molecules by antigen (allergen) induces degranulation of basophils and mast cells; as a result, a variety of pharmacologically active mediators present in the granules are released, giving rise to allergic manifestations (Figure 5-15). Localized mast-cell degranulation induced by IgE also may release mediators that facilitate a buildup of various cells necessary for antiparasitic defense (see Chapter 18).

Immunoglobulin D (IgD)

IgD was first discovered when a patient developed a multiple myeloma whose myeloma protein failed to react with anti-isotype antisera against the then-known isotypes: IgA, IgM, and IgG. When rabbits were immunized with this myeloma protein, the resulting antisera identified this same class of antibody at low levels in normal human serum. This new class, called IgD, has a serum concentration of 30 μg/ml and constitutes about 0.2% of the total immunoglobulin in serum. Its biological function is still not known. IgD, together with IgM, is the major membrane-bound immunoglobulin expressed by mature, B cells, and it is thought to function in the activation of a B cell by an antigen.

The Immunoglobulin Superfamily

The structures of the various immunoglobulin heavy and light chains described earlier share several features, suggesting that they have a common

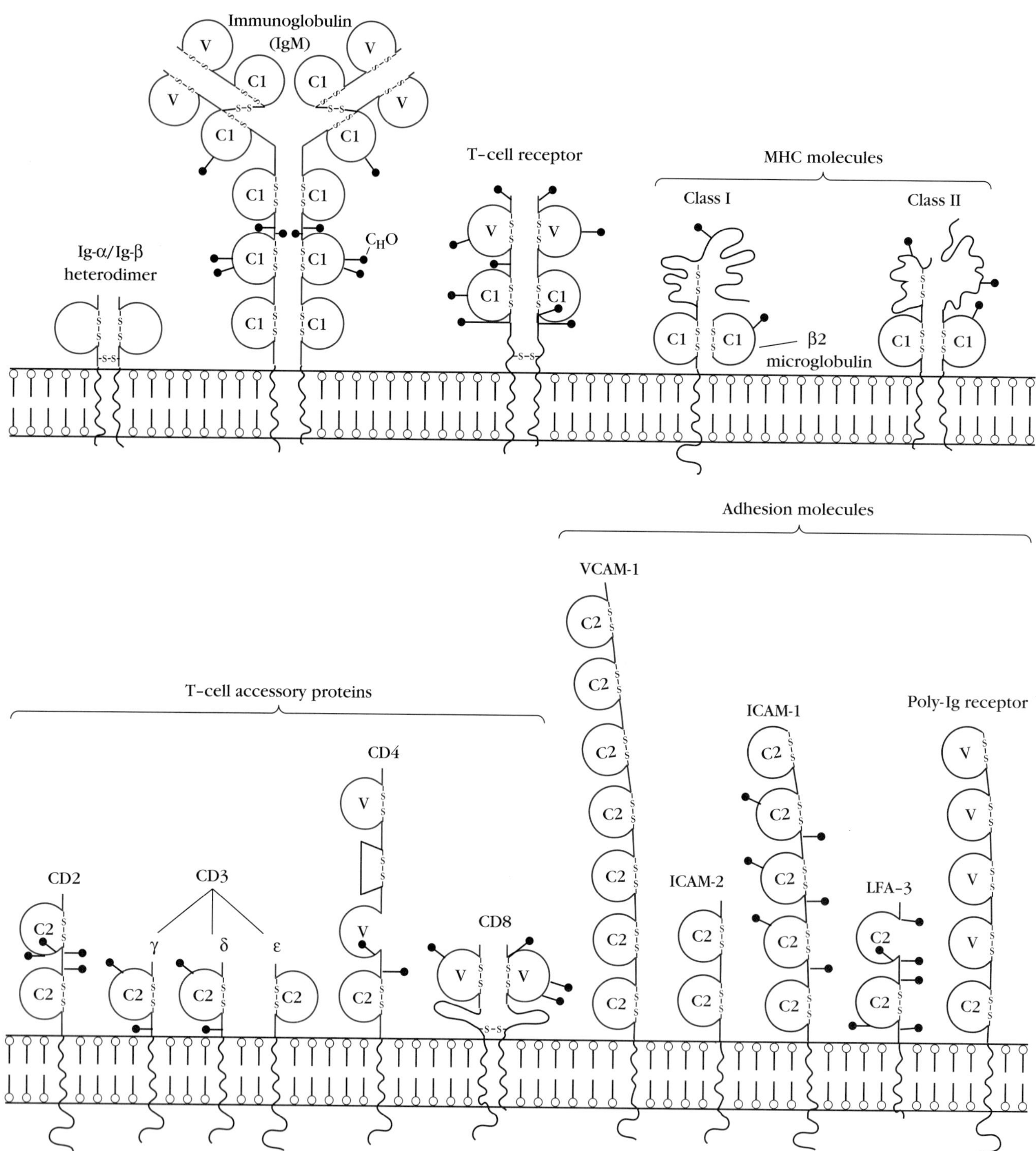

FIGURE 5-16 Some members of the immunoglobulin superfamily of structurally related glycoproteins, most of which are membrane bound. The loops shown in purple represent those portions of the molecule with the characteristic Ig-fold structure. In all cases the carboxyl-terminal end of the molecule is anchored in the membrane. Domains labeled C2 are shorter than the classical immunoglobulin constant-region domain (labeled C1) and exhibit equal homology with both variable- and constant-region domains.

evolutionary ancestry. In particular, all heavy- and light-chain classes have the immunoglobulin-fold domain structure (see Figures 5-4b and 5-5b). The presence of this characteristic structure in all immunoglobulin heavy and light chains suggests that the genes encoding them arose from a common primordial gene encoding a polypeptide of about 110 amino acids. Gene duplication and later divergence could then have generated the various heavy- and light-chain genes.

In the early 1970s β_2-microglobulin, a small invariant protein associated with class I MHC molecules, was sequenced. Surprisingly, its sequence showed homology to the immunoglobulin heavy- and light-chain constant-region domains, having a length of about 100 amino acids and a conserved intrachain disulfide bond spanning 60 amino acids. Later, x-ray crystallographic analysis revealed that β_2-microglobulin also has the β pleated-sheet structure characteristic of the immunoglobulin fold.

Since the discovery of an immunoglobulin-like domain in β_2-microglobulin, large numbers of membrane proteins have been shown to possess one or more regions homologous to an immunoglobulin domain. Each of these membrane proteins is classified as a member of the *immunoglobulin superfamily*. The term superfamily is used to denote proteins whose corresponding genes derived from a common primordial gene encoding the basic domain structure. These genes have evolved independently and do not share genetic linkage or function. Included in this group of proteins, in addition to the immunoglobulins themselves and β_2-microglobulin, are the following: the T-cell receptor; additional T-cell membrane proteins (e.g., CD2, CD4, CD8, CD28, and the γ, δ, and ϵ chains of CD3); class I and class II MHC molecules; the Ig-α/Ig-β heterodimer; various cell-adhesion molecules (e.g., VCAM-1, ICAM-1, ICAM-2, and LFA-3); the poly-Ig receptor; and platelet-derived growth factor (Figure 5-16). Numerous other proteins, some of them discussed in other chapters, belong to the immunoglobulin superfamily.

X-ray crystallographic analysis has not been accomplished for most members of the immunoglobulin superfamily. Nonetheless, the primary amino acid sequence of these proteins suggests that they all contain typical immunoglobulin-fold domains consisting of about 110 amino acids, arranged in antiparallel sheets of β pleated strands, usually with an invariant intrachain disulfide bond spanning 50–70 residues. Some proteins of the superfamily have V-like domains and some have C-like domains based on their homology to the immunoglobulin V or C domains. Other proteins have domains that fall between the classical V and C domains; that is, they are shorter than the classical immunoglobulin C domain and show equal homology to both V and C domains. These domains are designated C2 to distinguish them from the classical immunoglobulin C domains, which are called C1.

Since most members of the immunoglobulin superfamily cannot bind antigen, there must be some reason, apart from antigen binding, for so many membrane proteins to have a domain structure similar to the characteristic immunoglobulin fold. One possibility is that this structure may facilitate interactions between plasma-membrane proteins. As discussed earlier, interactions can occur between the faces of β sheets in homologous immunoglobulin domains (e.g., C_H2/C_H2 interaction) and those in nonhomologous domains (e.g., V_H/V_L and C_H1/C_L interactions). The observed associations between some members of the Ig superfamily may depend on similar interactions between nonhomologous Ig-fold domains. Among these associations are those between CD4 and a class II MHC molecule, or CD8 and a class I MHC molecule; between the T-cell receptor and an MHC molecule; between the poly-Ig receptor and polymeric IgA or IgM; and between the Ig-α/Ig-β heterodimer and membrane-bound immunoglobulin.

Summary

1. The basic structure of an antibody molecule consists of two identical light chains and two identical heavy chains, which are linked by disulfide bonds. Each heavy and light chain contains a variable sequence in the amino-terminal 110 amino acids and constant sequences in the remainder of the chain.

2. In any given antibody molecule, the constant region contains one of five basic heavy-chain sequences (μ, γ, δ, α, or ϵ) and one of two basic light-chain sequences (κ or λ). The heavy-chain constant-region sequences determine the five classes (isotypes) of antibody (IgM, IgG, IgD, IgA, and IgE) and the effector functions of the molecule.

3. The variable amino acid sequences are not randomly dispersed throughout the variable region but instead are clustered in several hypervariable regions, or complementarity-determining regions (CDRs). These regions form the antigen-binding site of the antibody molecule and determine its specificity.

4. The immunoglobulin molecule consists of a series of interacting domains, each of which is organized in a characteristic structure called the immunoglobulin fold. Immunoglobulin heavy and light chains are prototype members of a large group of proteins called the immunoglobulin superfamily. All members of this family contain the same basic immunoglobulin-fold domain structure. This basic structure may facilitate homologous and nonhomologous interactions between members of this family.

5. Immunoglobulins are expressed in two forms: secreted antibody produced by plasma cells and membrane-bound antibody present on the surface of B cells. Membrane-bound immunoglobulin associates with a recently discovered Igα/Igβ heterodimer to form the B-cell receptor. The antigenic specificity of a B cell is determined by the membrane-bound antibody that it expresses. The Igα/Igβ heterodimer of the B-cell receptor mediates the intracellular signals that lead to B-cell activation following interaction with antigen.

6. The five antibody isotypes differ in their ability to carry out various effector functions and in their average serum concentrations and their half-life. IgG, the most abundant isotype in serum, is particularly important in antigen clearance by various mechanisms; it also is the only isotype that can cross the placenta. Serum IgM exists as a pentamer; because of its high valency, IgM is more effective than other isotypes in viral neutralization, bacterial agglutination, and complement activation. IgA is the predominant isotype in external secretions including breast milk and mucus. In these secretions, secretory IgA exists as a dimer or tetramer linked by disulfide bonds to the J chain and secretory component. IgD and IgE are the two least abundant isotypes in serum. IgD (along with IgM) is the major isotype on mature B cells, and IgE mediates mast-cell degranulation.

References

ALZARI, P. M., M. B. LASCOMBE, and R. J. POLJAK. 1988. Three dimensional structure of antibodies. *Annu. Rev. Immunol.* **6**:555.

AMIT, A. G., R. A. MARIUZZA, S. E. PHILLIPS, and R. J. POLJAK. 1986. Three dimensional structure of an antigen-antibody complex at 2.8 Å resolution. *Science* **233**:747.

AREVALO, J. H., E. A. STURA, M. J. TAUSSIG, and I. A. WILSON. 1993. Three-dimensional structure of an anti-steroid Fab′ and progesterone-Fab′ complex. *J. Mol. Biol.* **231**:103.

DAVIS, D. R., E. A. PADLAN, and S. SHERIFF. 1991. Antibody-antigen complexes. *Annu. Rev. Biochem.* **59**:439.

GARCIA, K. C., P. M. RONCO, P. J. VERROUST et al. 1992. Three-dimensional structure of an angiotensin II-Fab complex at 3 Å: hormone recognition by an anti-idiotypic antibody. *Science* **257**:502.

GREENSPAN, N. S., and C. A. BONA. 1993. Idiotypes: structure and immunogenicity. *FASEB* **7**:437.

HARRIS, L. J., S. B. LARSON, K. W. HASEL et al. 1992. The three-dimensional structure of an intact monoclonal antibody for canine lymphoma. *Nature* **360**:369.

KOSHLAND, M. E. 1985. The coming of age of the J chain. *Annu. Rev. Immunol.* **3**:425.

KRAEHENBUHL, J. P., and M. R. NEUTRA. 1992. Transepithelial transport and mucosal defence II: secretion of IgA. *Trends in Cell Biol.* **2**:134.

RETH, M. 1992. Antigen receptors on B lymphocytes. *Annu. Rev. Immunol.* **10**: 97.

RETH, M., J. HOMBACH, J. WIENANDS et al. 1992. The B-cell antigen receptor complex. *Immunol. Today* **12**:196.

STANFIELD, R. L., T. M. FIESER, R. LERNER, and I. A. WILSON. 1990. Crystal structures of an antibody to a peptide and its complex with peptide antigen at 2.8 Å. *Science* **248**:712.

TULIP, W. R., J. N. VARGHESE, W. G. LAVER et al. 1992. Refined crystal structure of the influenza virus N9 neuraminidase-NC41 Fab complex. *J. Mol. Biol.* **227**:122.

UNDERDOWN, B. J., and J. M. SCHIFF. 1986. Immunoglobulin A: strategic defence initiative at the mucosal surface. *Annu. Rev. Immunol.* **4**:389.

WILLIAMS, A. F., and A. N. BARCLAY. 1988. The immunoglobulin superfamily—domains for cell surface recognition. *Annu. Rev. Immunol.* **6**:381.

WILSON, I. A., and R. L. STANFIELD. 1993. Antibody-antigen interactions. *Curr. Opin. Struc. Biol.* **3**: 113.

Study Questions

1. Indicate whether each of the following statements is true or false. If you think a statement is false, explain why.
   a. All myeloma protein molecules derived from a single myeloma clone have the same idiotype and allotype.
   b. A rabbit immunized with human IgG3 will produce antibody that reacts with all subclasses of IgG in humans.
   c. The presence of both IgM and IgD on a single B cell violates one of the tenets of clonal selection—the unispecificity of a given B cell.
   d. All immunoglobulin molecules on the surface of a given B cell have the same idiotype.
   e. All immunoglobulin molecules on the surface of a given B cell have the same isotype.
   f. The hypervariable regions make significant contact with the epitope.

g. All isotypes are normally found in each individual of a species.
h. The heavy-chain variable region (V_H) is twice as long as the light-chain variable region (V_L).
i. IgG functions more effectively than IgM in bacterial agglutination.

2. An energetic immunology student has isolated protein X, which he believes is a new isotype of human immunoglobulin.
   a. What structural features would protein X have to have in order to be classified as an immunoglobulin?
   b. You prepare rabbit antisera to whole human IgG, human κ chain, and human γ chain. Assuming protein X is, in fact, a new immunoglobulin isotype, to which of these antisera would it bind? Why?
   c. Devise an experimental procedure for preparing an antiserum that is specific for protein X.

3. IgG, which contains γ heavy chains, developed much more recently during evolution than IgM, which contains μ heavy chains. Describe two advantages and two disadvantages that IgG has in comparison with IgM?

4. Although the five immunoglobulin isotypes share many common structural features, the differences in their structures affect their biological activities.
   a. Draw a diagram of a typical IgG molecule that includes each immunoglobulin domain. Label the following on your diagram: H chains, L chains, interchain disulfide bonds, intrachain disulfide bonds, antigen-binding sites, Fab, Fc, and domains.
   b. How would you have to modify the diagram of IgG to depict an IgA molecule isolated from saliva.
   c. How would you have to modify the diagram of IgG to depict serum IgM.

5. Fill out the table abo‵ , right to indicate the properties of IgG molecules and their various parts. Use (+) if positive; (−) if negative, and (weak +) if slightly positive.

6. For each of the following immunization scenarios, state whether the anti-immunoglobulin antibodies would be formed to isotypic, allotypic, or idiotypic determinants:
   a. Anti-DNP antibodies produced in a BALB/c mouse are injected into a C57BL/6 mouse.
   b. Anti-BGG monoclonal antibody from a BALB/c mouse are injected into another BALB/c mouse.
   c. Anti-BGG antibodies produced in a BALB/c mouse are injected into a rabbit.
   d. Anti-DNP antibodies produced in a BALB/c mouse are injected into an outbred mouse.
   e. Anti-BGG antibodies produced in a BALB/c mouse are injected into the same mouse.

For use with question 5.

Property	Whole IgG	H chain	L chain	Fab	$F(ab')_2$	Fc
Binds antigen						
Bivalent antigen binding						
Bind to Fc receptors						
Fixes complement in presence of antigen						
Has V domains						
Has C domains						

7. In the table below, write YES or NO to indicate whether the rabbit antisera listed at the top reacts with the mouse antibody components listed at the left.

	Rabbit antisera to mouse antibody component				
	γ chain	κ chain	IgG Fab fragment	IgG Fc fragment	J chain
Mouse γ chain					
Mouse κ chain					
Mouse IgM whole					
Mouse IgG Fc fragment					

8. Where are the hypervariable regions located on an antibody molecule and what are their functions?

9. The characteristic structure of immunoglobulin domains, termed the immunoglobulin fold, also occurs in the numerous membrane proteins belonging to the immunoglobulin superfamily.
   a. Describe the typical features that define the immunoglobulin-fold domain structure.
   b. List three membrane proteins that belong to the immunoglobulin superfamily. How might the presence of the immunoglobulin-fold domain structure in these proteins facilitate their function?

10. A technician wanted to make a rabbit antiserum specific for mouse IgG. She injected a rabbit with purified mouse IgG and obtained an antiserum that reacted strongly with mouse IgG. To her dismay, however, the antiserum also reacted with each of the other mouse isotypes. Explain why she got this result. How could she make the rabbit antiserum specific for mouse IgG?

11. Match each immunoglobulin isotype (a–e) with the description(s) listed below (1–13) that are true about that isotype. Some of the descriptions may apply to more than one isotype; others may not apply to any isotype.

a. ______ IgA
b. ______ IgD
c. ______ IgE
d. ______ IgG
e. ______ IgM

1. Secreted form is a pentamer of the basic H_2L_2 unit
2. Binds to Fc receptors on mast cells
3. Multimeric forms have J chain
4. Present on the surface of mature, unprimed B cells
5. The most abundant immunoglobulin class in serum
6. Major antibody in secretions such as saliva, tears, and colostrum
7. Present on the surface of immature B cells
8. The first serum antibody made in a primary immune response
9. Plays an important role in immediate hypersensitivity
10. Plays an important role in protecting against pathogens that invade through the gut or respiratory mucosa
11. Multimeric forms present in secretions have secretory piece
12. Can fix complement by the classical pathway
13. Can participate in antibody-dependent cell-mediated cytotoxicity (ADCC)

12. Immunoglobulin molecules possess antigenic determinants that can induce formation of antibody. For each of the situations below, indicate whether the induced antibody would be specific for isotypic, allotypic, or idiotypic determinants on the immunogen.
   a. BALB/c mouse immunized with IgG from C57BL/6 mouse.
   b. C57BL/6 mouse immunized with IgG myeloma protein from C57BL/6 mouse.
   c. Rabbit immunized with IgG from C57BL/6 mouse.

ANTIGEN-ANTIBODY INTERACTIONS

The antigen-antibody interaction is a bimolecular association similar to an enzyme-substrate interaction but with the important distinction that it does not lead to an irreversible chemical alteration in either the antibody or antigen and therefore is reversible. The interaction between an antibody and an antigen involves various noncovalent interactions between the antigenic determinant, or epitope, of the antigen and the variable-region (V_H/V_L) domain of the antibody molecule, particularly the hypervariable regions, or complementarity-determining regions (CDRs). The exquisite specificity of antigen-antibody interactions has led to the development of a variety of immunologic assays. These assays can be used to detect the presence of either antibody or antigen and have played vital roles in diagnosing diseases, monitoring the level of the humoral immune response, and identifying molecules of biological or medical interest. These assays differ in their speed and their sensitivity; some are strictly qualitative, and others are quantitative. In this chapter, the nature of the antigen-antibody interaction is examined, and various immunologic assays that measure this interaction are described.

Strength of Antigen-Antibody Interactions

The noncovalent interactions that form the basis of antigen-antibody (Ag-Ab) binding include hydrogen bonds, ionic bonds, hydrophobic

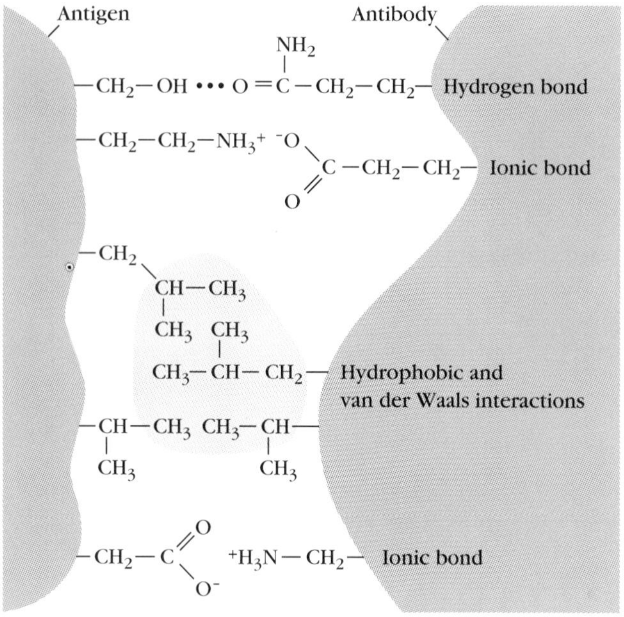

FIGURE 6-1 The interaction between an antibody and an antigen depends on four types of noncovalent forces: (1) ionic bonds between oppositely charged residues, (2) hydrogen bonds in which a hydrogen atom is shared between two electronegative atoms, (3) hydrophobic interactions in which water forces hydrophobic groups together to maximize hydrogen bonding of water molecules, and (4) van der Waals interactions between the outer electron clouds of two atoms. In an aqueous environment noncovalent interactions are extremely weak and depend upon close structural complementarity between antibody and antigen.

interactions, and van der Waals interactions (Figure 6-1). Because the strength of each of these interactions is weak (compared with that of a covalent bond), a large number of such interactions are required to form a strong Ag-Ab interaction. Furthermore, each of these noncovalent interactions operates over a very small distance, generally less than 1×10^{-7} mm (1 angstrom, Å); consequently, a strong Ag-Ab interaction depends on a very close fit between the antigen and antibody, which is reflected in the high degree of specificity characteristic of antigen-antibody interactions.

Antibody Affinity

The strength of the sum total of noncovalent interactions between a single antigen-binding site on an antibody and a single epitope is the *affinity* of the antibody for that epitope. Low-affinity antibodies bind antigen weakly and tend to dissociate readily, whereas high-affinity antibodies bind antigen more tightly and remain bound longer. The association between a binding site on an antibody (Ab) with a monovalent antigen (Ag) can be described by the equation

$$\text{Ag} + \text{Ab} \underset{k_{-1}}{\overset{k_1}{\rightleftharpoons}} \text{Ab} - \text{Ag}$$

where k_1 is the forward (association) rate constant and k_{-1} is the reverse (dissociation) rate constant. The ratio of k_1/k_{-1} is the association constant K, a measure of affinity. It can be calculated from the ratio of the concentration of bound Ag-Ab complex to the concentrations of unbound antigen and antibody, as follows:

$$K = \frac{k_1}{k_{-1}} = \frac{[\text{Ab} - \text{Ag}]}{[\text{Ab}][\text{Ag}]}$$

K values vary for different Ag-Ab complexes and depend upon both k_1, which is expressed in liters/mole/second (L/mol/s) and k_{-1}, which is expressed in 1/second. For small haptens, the forward rate constant can be extremely high; in some cases k_1 values can be as high as 4×10^8 L/mol/s, approaching the theoretical upper limit of diffusion-limited reactions (10^9 L/mol/s). For larger protein antigens, however, k_1 is smaller, with values in the range of 10^5 L/mol/s. The rate at which bound antigen leaves an antibody's binding site (i.e., the dissociation rate constant, k_{-1}) plays a major role in determining the antibody's affinity for an antigen. Table 6-1 illustrates the role of k_{-1} in determining the association constant K for several Ag-Ab interactions. For example, the k_1 for the DNP-L-lysine system is about one-fifth that for the fluorescein system, but its k_{-1} is 200 times greater; consequently, the K for the fluorescein system is about a thousandfold higher than K for the DNP-L-lysine system. Low-affinity Ag-Ab complexes have K values between 10^4 and 10^5 L/mol; high-affinity complexes can have K values as high as 10^{11} L/mol.

The association constant K can be determined by *equilibrium dialysis.* In this procedure a dialysis chamber containing two equal compartments separated by a semipermeable membrane is used. Antibody is placed in one chamber, and in the other chamber is placed a ligand that must be small enough to pass through the semipermeable membrane (Figure 6-2a). Suitable ligands include haptens as well as oligosaccharides and oligopeptides composing the epitope of complex polysaccharide or protein antigens. If a known amount of radioactively labeled ligand is used, the concentration of the antibody-bound ligand at equilibrium can be determined as follows: At equilibrium part of the labeled ligand will be bound to the

TABLE 6-1 FORWARD (k_1) AND REVERSE (k_{-1}) RATE CONSTANTS AND ASSOCIATION CONSTANT (K) OF THREE LIGAND-ANTIBODY INTERACTIONS

Antibody	Ligand	k_1 (L/mol/s)	k_{-1} (s^{-1})	K (L/mol)
Anti-DNP	ε-DNP-L-lysine	8×10^7	1	10^8
Anti-fluorescein	Fluorescein	4×10^8	5×10^{-3}	10^{11}
Anti-bovine serum albumin (BSA)	Dansyl-BSA	3×10^5	2×10^{-3}	1.7×10^8

SOURCE: Adapted from H. N. Eisen, 1990, *Immunology*, 3rd ed., Harper and Row Publishers.

antibody, and the unbound ligand will be equally distributed in both compartments. Thus the total concentration of ligand will be greater in the compartment containing antibody (Figure 6-2b). The difference in the ligand concentration in the two compartments represents the concentration of ligand bound to the antibody (i.e., the concentration of Ag-Ab complex). The higher the affinity of the antibody, the more ligand that is bound.

Since the total concentration of antibody in the equilibrium dialysis chamber is known, the equilibrium equation can be rewritten as

$$K = \frac{[\text{Ab} - \text{Ag}]}{[\text{Ab}][\text{Ag}]} = \frac{r}{(n - r)(c)}$$

where r = the ratio of the concentration of bound ligand to total antibody concentration, c = concentration

(a)

Control: No antibody present
(ligand equilibrates on both sides equally)

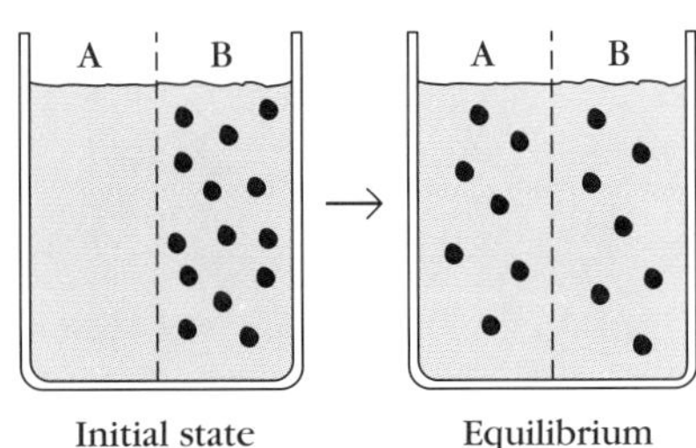

Experimental: Antibody in A
(at equilibrium more ligand in A due to Ab binding)

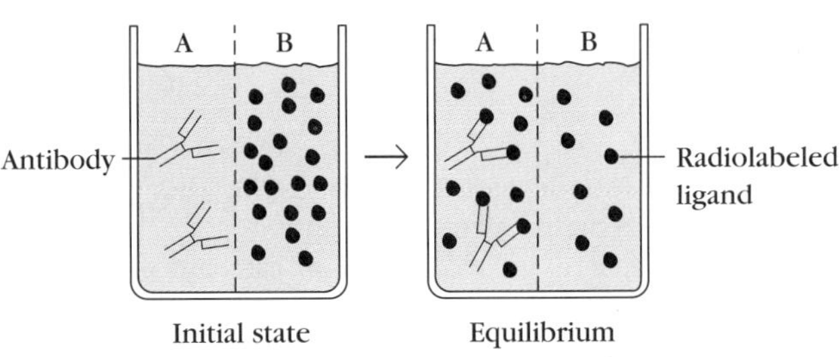

(b)

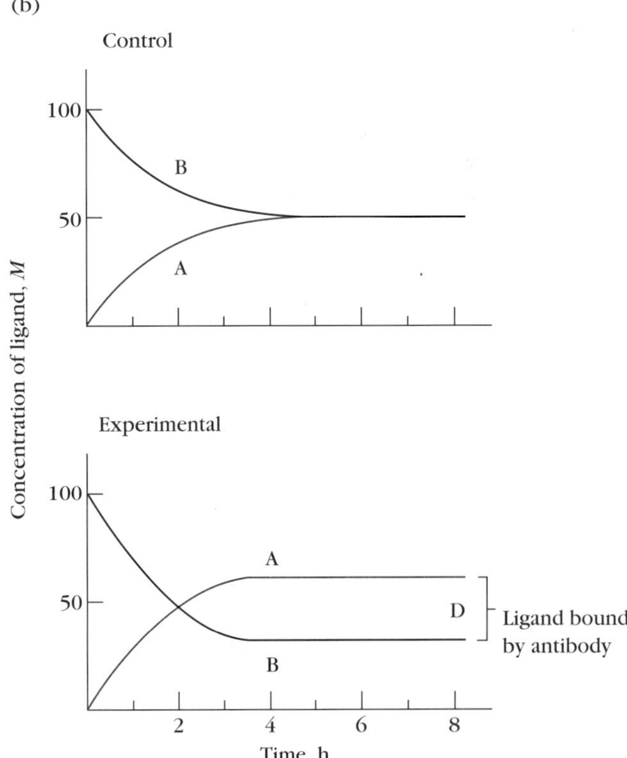

FIGURE 6-2 Determination of antibody affinity by equilibrium dialysis. (a) The dialysis chamber contains two compartments (A and B) separated by a semipermeable membrane. Antibody is added to one compartment and a radiolabeled ligand to another. At equilibrium the concentration of radioactivity in both compartments is measured. (b) Plot of concentration of ligand in each compartment with time. At equilibrium the difference in the concentration of radioactive ligand in the two compartments represents the amount of ligand bound to antibody.

of free ligand, and n = number of binding sites per antibody molecule. This expression can be rearranged to give the *Scatchard equation:*

$$\frac{r}{c} = Kn - Kr$$

Values for r and c can be obtained by repeating the equilibrium dialysis with the same concentration of antibody but with different concentrations of ligand. If K is a constant, that is, if all the antibodies within the dialysis chamber have the same affinity for the ligand, then a Scatchard plot of r/c versus r will yield a straight line with a slope of $-K$ (Figure 6-3a). As the concentration of unbound ligand c increases, r/c approaches 0, and r approaches n, the valency. For most antibody preparations, K is not a constant because antibodies (unless they are monoclonal) are heterogeneous and have a range of affinities. A Scatchard plot of heterogeneous antibody yields a curved line whose slope is constantly changing, reflecting the antibody heterogeneity (Figure 6-3b). With this type of Scatchard plot, it is possible to determine the average affinity constant K_0 by determining the value of K when half of the antigen-binding sites are filled:

$$K_0 = \frac{1}{(2-1)c} = \frac{1}{c}$$

Antibody Avidity

The affinity at one binding site does not always reflect the true strength of the antibody-antigen interaction. When complex antigens containing multiple, repeating antigenic determinants are mixed with antibodies containing multiple binding sites, the interaction of antibody with antigen at one site will increase the probability of reaction at a second site. The strength of such multiple interactions between a multivalent antibody and antigen is called the *avidity.* The avidity of an antibody is a better measure than the affinity of its binding capacity within biological systems (e.g., the reaction of an antibody with antigenic determinants on a virus or bacterial cell). High avidity can compensate

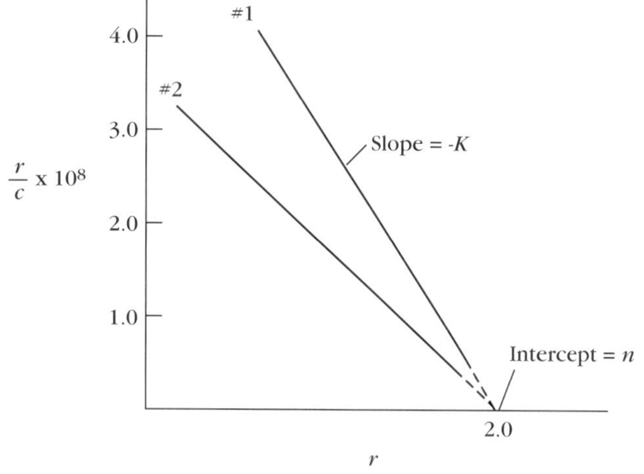

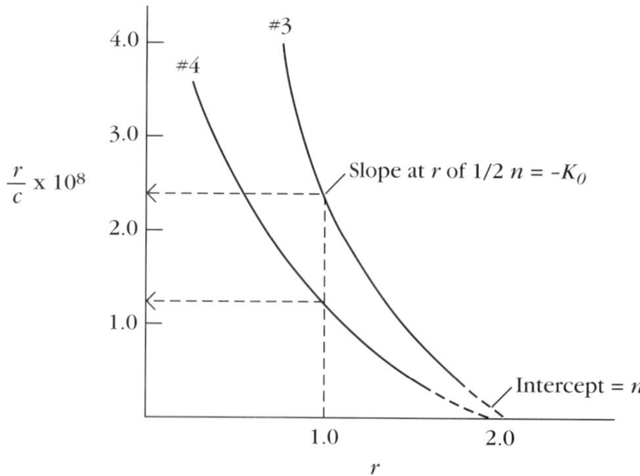

FIGURE 6-3 Scatchard plots are based on repeated equilibrium dialyses with a constant concentration of antibody and varying concentration of ligand. In these plots, r = moles bound ligand/mole antibody and c = free ligand. From a Scatchard plot, both the equilibrium constant (K) and the number of binding sites per antibody molecule (n), or its valency, can be obtained. (a) If all antibodies have the same affinity, then a Scatchard plot yields a straight line with a slope of $-K$. The Y intercept is the valence of the antibody, which is 2 for IgG. In this graph antibody #1 has a higher affinity than antibody #2. (b) If the antibodies have a range of affinities, a Scatchard plot yields a curved line, whose slope is constantly changing. The average affinity constant K_0 can be calculated by determining the value of K when one-half of the binding sites are occupied (i.e., when r = 1). In this graph antisera #3 has a higher affinity than antisera #4.

for low affinity. For example, secreted pentameric IgM often has a lower affinity than IgG, but the high avidity of IgM, resulting from its multivalence, enables it to bind antigen effectively.

Cross-Reactivity

Although Ag-Ab reactions are highly specific, in some cases antibody elicited by one antigen can cross-react with an unrelated antigen. Such cross-reactions occur if two different antigens share an identical epitope or if antibodies specific for one epitope also bind to an unrelated epitope possessing similar chemical properties. In the latter case the antibody's affinity for the cross-reacting epitope is usually less than that for the original epitope.

Cross-reactivity is often observed among polysaccharide antigens that contain similar oligosaccharide residues. The ABO blood-group antigens, for example, are glycoproteins expressed on red blood cells. Subtle differences in the terminal sugar residues distinguish the A and B blood-group antigens (see Figure 18-12). An individual lacking one or both of these antigens will have serum antibodies to the missing antigen(s). A type O individual thus has anti-A and anti-B antibodies; a type A individual has anti-B; and a type B individual has anti-A (Table 6-2). Cross-reactivity is the basis for the presence of these blood-group antibodies, which are induced in an individual not by exposure to red blood cell antigens but by exposure to cross-reacting microbial antigens present on common intestinal bacteria. These cross-reacting microbial antigens induce the formation of antibodies in individuals lacking these antigens. The blood-group antibodies, although elicited by microbial antigens, will cross-react with similar oligosaccharides on red blood cells.

A number of viruses and bacteria possess antigenic determinants identical to or similar to normal host-cell components. In some cases these microbial antigens have been shown to elicit antibody that cross-reacts with the host-cell components, resulting in a tissue-damaging autoimmune reaction. The bacterium *Streptococcus pyogenes,* for example, expresses cell-wall proteins called M antigens. Antibodies produced to streptococcal M antigens have been shown to cross-react with several myocardial and skeletal muscle proteins and have been implicated in heart and kidney damage following streptococcal infections. The role of other cross-reacting antigens in the development of autoimmune diseases is discussed in Chapter 19.

Table 6-2 ABO blood types

Blood type	Antigens on RBCs	Serum antibodies
A	A	Anti-B
B	B	Anti-A
AB	A and B	Neither
O	Neither	Anti-A and anti-B

Some vaccines also exhibit cross-reactivity. For instance, vaccinia virus, which causes cowpox, expresses cross-reacting epitopes with variola virus, the causative agent of smallpox. This cross-reactivity was the basis of Jenner's method of using vaccinia virus to induce immunity to smallpox, as mentioned in Chapter 1.

Precipitin Reactions

The interaction between an antibody and antigen in aqueous solution forms a lattice that eventually develops into a visible precipitate. While formation of the soluble Ag-Ab complex occurs within minutes, formation of the visible precipitate occurs more slowly and often takes a day or two to reach completion. The precipitate develops as neighboring antibody molecules within the lattic form ionic bonds with each other, causing the lattice to lose its charge and thus become insoluble.

Formation of an Ag-Ab lattice depends on the valency of both the antibody and antigen. The antibody must be bivalent; a precipitate will not form with monovalent Fab fragments. The antigen must either be bivalent or polyvalent; it must have at least two copies of the same epitope, or different epitopes that react with different antibodies present in polyclonal antisera. This requirement for bivalency or polyvalency of protein antigens can be illustrated by precipitin reactions involving myoglobulin. This protein antigen precipitates well with specific polyclonal antisera but fails to precipitate with a specific monoclonal antibody because it contains multiple, distinct epitopes but only a single copy of each epitope. Myoglobin thus can form a cross-linked lattice structure with polyclonal antisera but not with monoclonal antisera. Several common immunologic assays are based on precipitin reactions; the sensitivity of these assays varies considerably, as shown in Table 6-3.

TABLE 6-3 SENSITIVITY OF VARIOUS IMMUNOASSAYS

Assay	Sensitivity* (μg antibody N/ml)
Precipitin reaction in fluids	3–20
Precipitin reactions in gels	
Mancini radial immunodiffusion	0.2–1.0
Ouchterlony double immunodiffusion	3–20
Immunoelectrophoresis	3–20
Rocket electrophoresis	0.2
Agglutination reactions	
Direct	0.05
Passive agglutination	0.001–0.01
Agglutination inhibition	0.001–0.01
Radioimmunoassay	0.0001–0.001
Enzyme-linked immunosorbent assay (ELISA)	0.0001–0.001
Immunofluorescence	1.0

* The sensitivity depends upon the affinity of the antibody as well as the epitope density and distribution.

SOURCE: Adapted from N. R. Rose et al. (eds.), 1986, *Manual of Clinical Laboratory Immunology,* American Society for Microbiology, Washington, D.C.

Precipitin Reactions in Fluids

A quantitative precipitin reaction can be performed by placing a constant amount of antibody in a series of tubes and adding increasing amounts of antigen to the tubes. After the precipitate forms, each tube is centrifuged to pellet the precipitate, the supernatant is poured off, and the amount of precipitate is measured. Plotting the amount of precipitate against increasing antigen concentrations yields a precipitin curve. As Figure 6-4 shows, excess of either antibody or antigen interferes with maximal precipitation, which occurs in the so-called *equivalence zone,* when the ratio of antibody to antigen is optimal. As a large multimolecular lattice is formed at equivalence, the complex increases in size and precipitates out of solution. In the region of *antibody excess,* unreacted antibody is found in the supernatant along with small soluble complexes consisting of multiple molecules of antibody bound to a single molecule of antigen. In the region of *antigen excess,* unreacted antigen can be detected and small complexes are again observed, this time consisting of one or two molecules of antigen bound to a single molecule of antibody. Although the quantitative precipitin reaction is seldom used experimentally today, the principles of antigen excess, antibody excess, and equivalence apply to many Ag-Ab reactions.

The precipitin reaction can also be used as a rapid test for the presence of antibody or antigen. The inter-

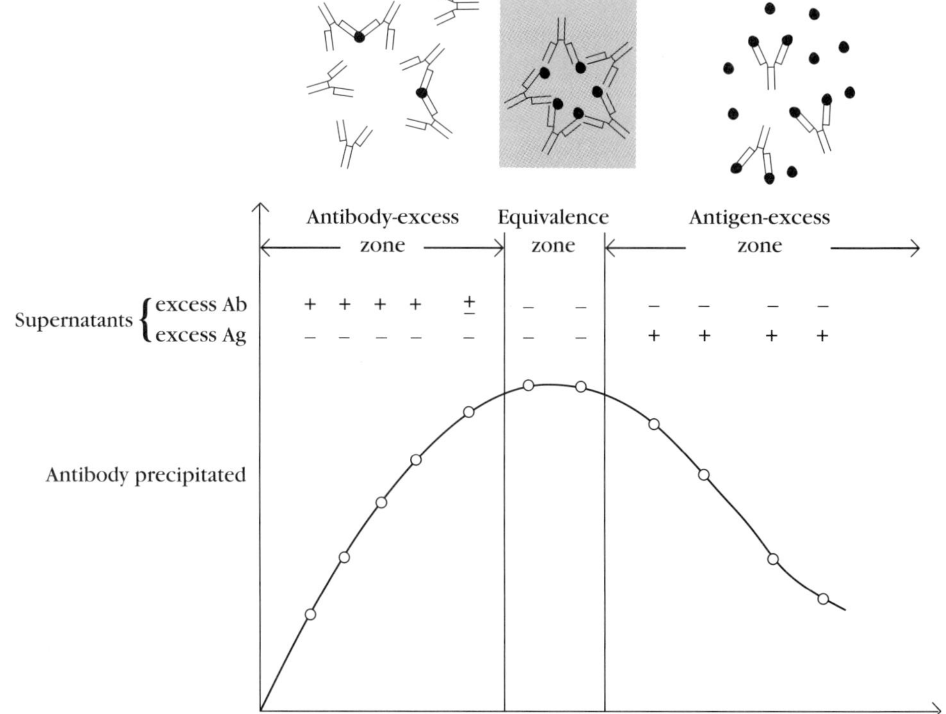

FIGURE 6-4 A precipitin curve for a system of one antibody and its antigen. This plot of the amount of antibody precipitated versus increasing antigen concentrations (at constant total antibody) reveals three zones: a zone of antibody excess in which precipitation is inhibited and excess antibody can be detected in the supernatant; an equivalence zone of maximal precipitation in which antibody and antigen form large insoluble complexes (purple) and neither antibody nor antigen can be detected in the supernatant; and a zone of antigen excess in which precipitation is inhibited and excess antigen can be detected in the supernatant.

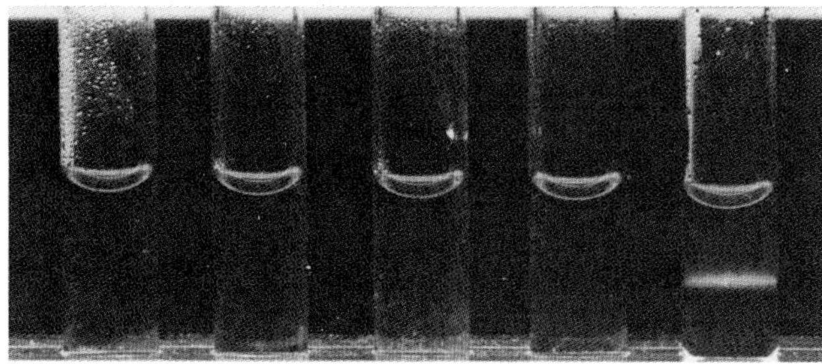

FIGURE 6-5 The interfacial, or ring, precipitin test is a rapid, qualitative method for determining the presence of antibody or antigen. The antiserum is placed in the bottom of a tube, and then the antigen solution is carefully layered on top. Formation of a visible line of precipitation in the tube at the extreme right indicates a positive reaction. The other four tubes are various controls (e.g., normal serum with antigen and antiserum with buffer). [From J. S. Garvey et al., 1977, *Methods in Immunology,* 3rd ed., W. A. Benjamin Inc., Advanced Book Program.]

facial, or ring, precipitin test is performed by adding antiserum to a small tube and layering antigen on top. If the antiserum contains antibodies specific for the test antigen, then the antibody and antigen diffuse toward each other and form a visible band of precipitation at the interface within a few minutes (Figure 6-5).

Precipitin Reactions in Gels

Immune precipitates can form not only in solution but also in an agar matrix. When antigen and antibody diffuse toward one another in agar or when antibody is incorporated into the agar and antigen diffuses into the antibody-containing matrix, a visible line of precipitation will form (Figure 6-6). As in a precipitin reaction in fluid, visible precipitation occurs in the region of equivalence, whereas no visible precipitate forms in regions of antibody or antigen excess. These *immunodiffusion* reactions can be used to determine relative concentrations of antibodies or antigens, to compare antigens, or to determine the relative purity of an antigen preparation. Two frequently used immunodiffusion techniques are the radial immunodiffusion (Mancini) method and the double-immunodiffusion (Ouchterlony) method; both are carried out in a semisolid medium like agar.

Radial Immunodiffusion (Mancini Method)

The relative concentrations of an antigen can be determined by a simple quantitative assay in which an antigen sample is placed in a well and allowed to diffuse

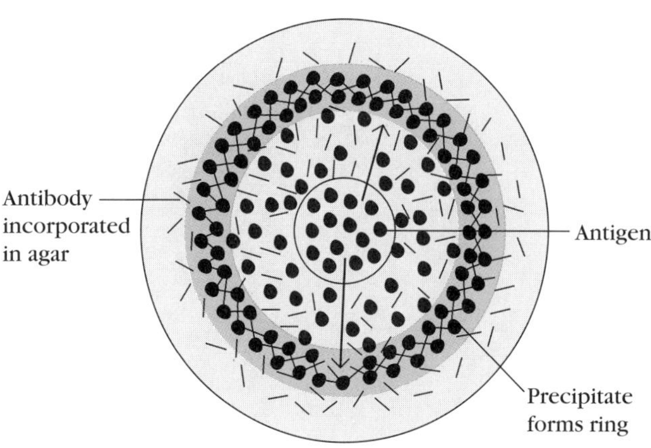

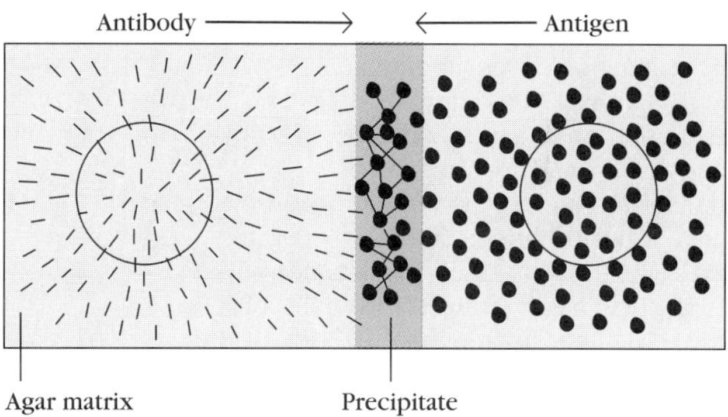

FIGURE 6-6 Diagrammatic representation of radial and double immunodiffusion in a gel. In both cases, large insoluble complexes form in the agar in the zone of equivalence, which are visible as a line of precipitation (purple). Only the antigen diffuses in radial immunodiffusion, whereas both the antibody and antigen diffuse in double immunodiffusion.

into agar containing a suitable dilution of an antiserum. As the antigen diffuses into the agar, the region of equivalence is established and a ring of precipitation forms around the well. The area of the precipitin ring is proportional to the concentration of antigen. By comparing the area of the precipitin ring with a standard curve (obtained by measuring the precipitin areas of known concentrations of the antigen), the concentration of the antigen sample can be determined. The Mancini technique is routinely used to quantitate serum levels of IgM, IgG, and IgA by incorporating class-specific anti-isotype antibody into the agar (Figure 6-7). The technique is also applied to determine concentrations of complement components in serum. This method cannot detect antigens present in

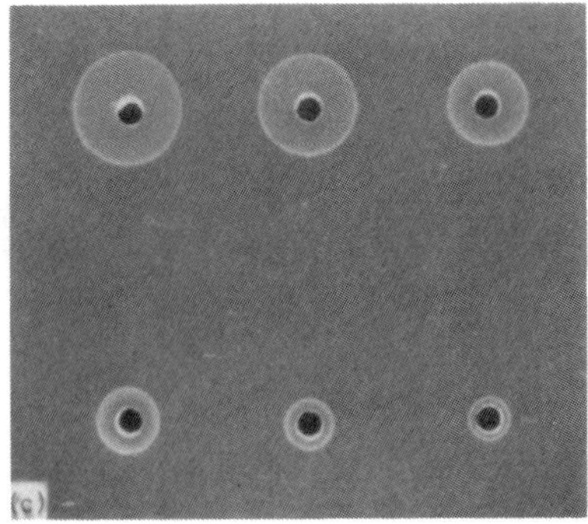

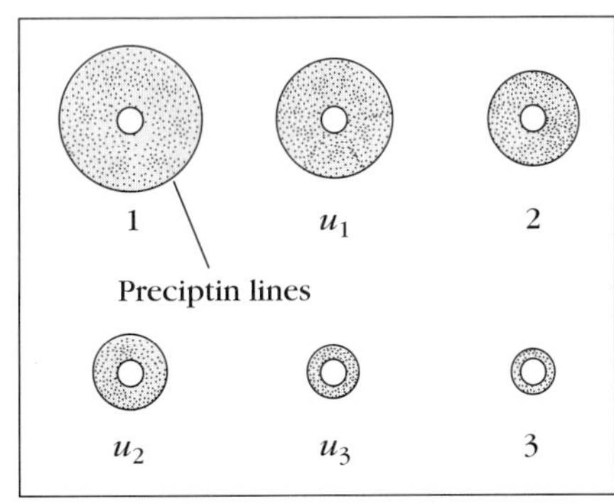

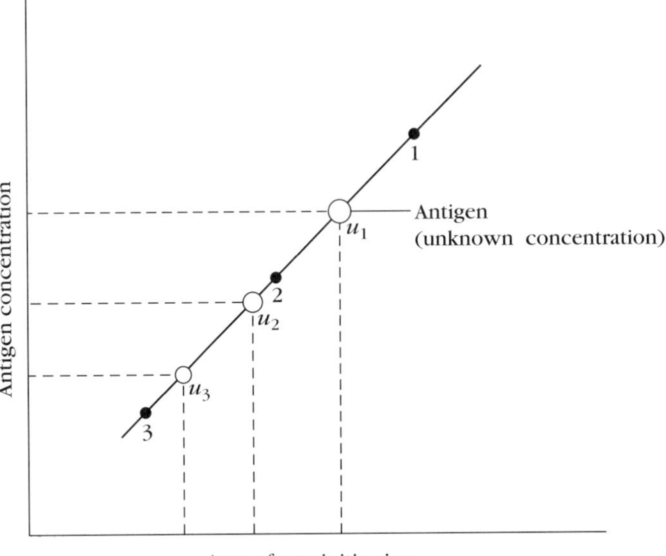

FIGURE 6-7 Determination of antigen concentration by radial immunodiffusion. The area of the ring of precipitation is proportional to the concentration of antigen. A standard curve can be obtained from the results with known concentrations of antigen (wells 1–3). From the standard curve, the antigen concentration can be determined in samples of unknown concentration (wells U_1, U_2, and U_3). [Photograph from D. M. Weir (ed.), 1986, *Handbook of Experimental Immunology,* Blackwell Scientific Publications.]

concentrations below 5–10 μg/ml; this moderate sensitivity is the major limitation of the radial immunodiffusion method.

Double Immunodiffusion (Ouchterlony Method)

In the Ouchterlony method both antigen and antibody diffuse radially from wells toward each other, thereby establishing a concentration gradient. As equivalence is reached, a visible line of precipitation forms. This simple technique is an effective qualitative tool for determining the relationship between antigens and the number of different Ag-Ab systems present. The pattern of the precipitin lines that form when two different antigen preparations are placed in adjacent wells indicate whether or not they share epitopes. For example, when two antigens share identical epitopes, the antiserum will form a single precipitin line with each antigen that will grow toward each other and fuse to form a pattern called ***identity*** (Figure 6-8a). If two antigens are unrelated, the antiserum will form independent precipitin lines that cross, a pattern that establishes ***nonidentity*** (Figure 6-8b). The lines cross because the unrelated antigen and antibody do not precipitate and therefore are free to diffuse past the precipitin line, forming the precipitin line of the unrelated antigen-antibody system. If two antigens share some epitopes but one or the other has a unique epitope, a pattern of ***partial identity*** is obtained (Figure 6-8c). Antibodies to the common epitope form a line of identity, but antibodies to the unique epitope(s) diffuse past the precipitin line to form a spur, which is a precipitin line formed with the unique epitope(s) of the more complex antigen.

One of the drawbacks of an Ouchterlony double-diffusion assay is that it takes 18–24 h before precipitin lines appear. This limitation can be overcome by using countercurrent electrophoresis. In this method

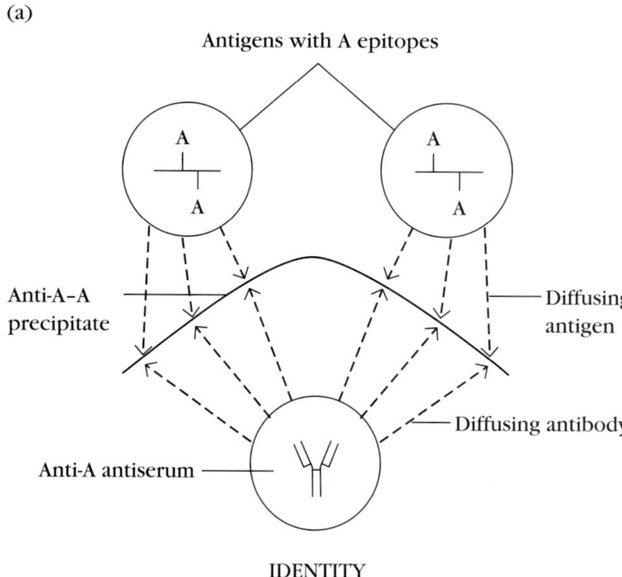

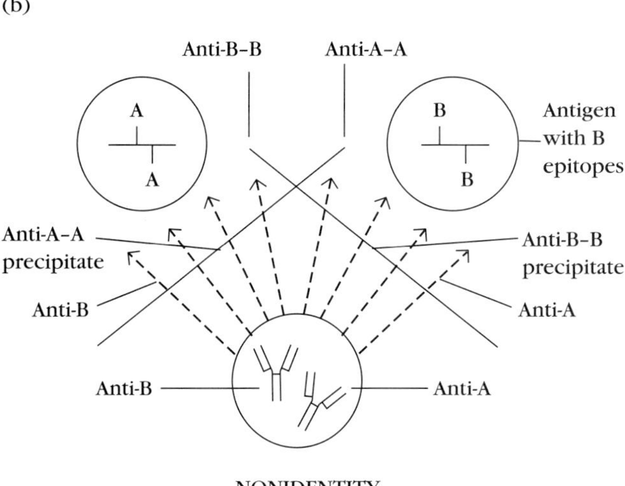

(c)

Anti-A–A precipitate spur

A B

B A

B

B

Anti A–AB/ Anti-B–AB precipitate

Anti-B–B precipitate

Anti-A

Anti-B

Anti-A

PARTIAL IDENTITY

FIGURE 6-8 Diagrams of possible precipitin patterns obtained in double immunodiffusion (Ouchterlony method) of antiserum with two different antigen preparations. The pattern of lines (purple) indicates whether the two antigens have identical epitopes (identity), partially identical epitopes (partial identity), or no epitopes in common (nonidentity).

positively charged antibody and negatively charged antigen are added to separate wells in a gel. An electric current is used to drive the immunodiffusion, forming a sharp precipitin line within minutes and with greater sensitivity than in Ouchterlony double diffusion.

Immunoelectrophoresis

Immunoelectrophoresis combines separation by electrophoresis with identification by double immunodiffusion (Figure 6-9a). An antigen mixture is first electrophoresed and separated by charge. Troughs are then cut into the agar gel parallel to the direction of the electric field, and antiserum is added to the troughs. The agar gel is then incubated in a humid chamber during which time antigen and antibody diffuse toward each other. The formation of precipitin bands with polyvalent or specific antiserum identifies individual antigen components. Immunoelectrophoresis is widely used in clinical laboratories to detect the presence or absence of proteins in the serum. The serum proteins are electrophoresed, and the individual serum components are identified with antisera specific for a given protein or immunoglobulin class (Figure 6-9b). Immunoelectrophoresis can determine whether a patient has an immunodeficiency disease. It can also show if a patient overproduces some serum protein, such as albumin, immunoglobulin, or transferrin. The immunoelectrophoretic pattern of serum from patients with multiple myeloma shows a heavy distorted arc caused by the large amount of myeloma protein, which is monoclonal and thereform uniformly charged.

Immunoelectrophoresis is a strictly qualitative technique that can detect antibody concentrations of 3–20 μg/ml. It is useful for detecting quantitative anomalies only when the departure from normal is striking, as in immunodeficiency and immunoproliferative disorders. A related technique, called rocket electrophoresis, permits quantitation of antigen levels as low as 0.2 μg/ml.

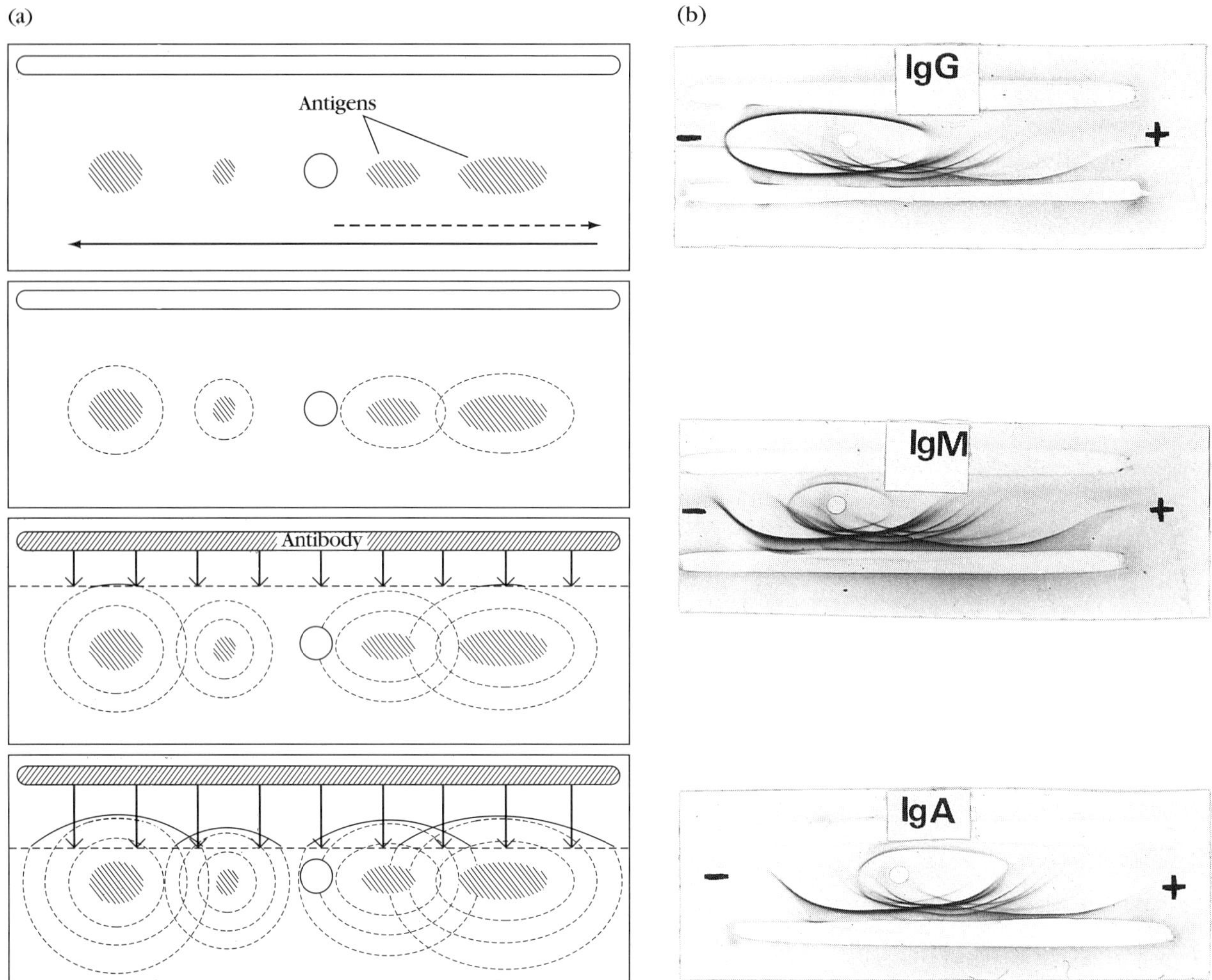

FIGURE 6-9 Immunoelectrophoresis of an antigen mixture. (a) An antigen preparation is first electrophoresed, which separates the component antigens on the basis of charge. Antiserum is then added to troughs on one or both sides of the separated antigens and allowed to diffuse; in time, lines of precipitation (purple) form where specific antibody and antigen interact. (b) Immunoelectrophoretic patterns of human serum. Goat antibody to whole human serum was placed in the bottom trough of each slide; goat antibody to human IgG, IgM, or IgA was placed in the top trough of each slide. After electrophoresis, the IgG, IgM, and IgA antibodies form a single line of precipitation with their respective antisera. The position of the human IgG, IgM, and IgA in the electrophoresed whole human serum sample can be determined by comparing the position of the single band at the top of each slide with the complex band pattern of the whole serum sample. [From J. S. Garvey et al., 1977, *Methods in Immunology,* 3rd ed., W. A. Benjamin Inc., Advanced Book Program.]

ROCKET ELECTROPHORESIS. In this technique negatively charged antigen is electrophoresed in a gel containing antibody. The precipitate formed between antigen and antibody has the shape of a rocket, the height of which is proportional to the concentration of antigen in the well (Figure 6-10). One limitation of rocket electrophoresis is the need for the antigen to be negatively charged for electrophoretic movement within the agar matrix. Some proteins, such as immunoglobulins, are not sufficiently charged to be quantitated by rocket electrophoresis; nor is it possible to quantitate several antigens in a mixture at the same time.

TWO-DIMENSIONAL IMMUNOELECTROPHORESIS. Several antigens in a complex mixture can be quantitated simultaneously with a modification of rocket electrophoresis called two-dimensional immunoelectrophoresis. In this technique antigen is first separated into components by electrophoresis. The gel is then laid over another agar gel containing antiserum, and electrophoresis is repeated at right angles to the first direction, forming precipitin peaks similar to those obtained with rocket electrophoresis. Measurement of the size of the peaks allows quantitation of a number of proteins in a complex antigen mixture (Figure 6-11).

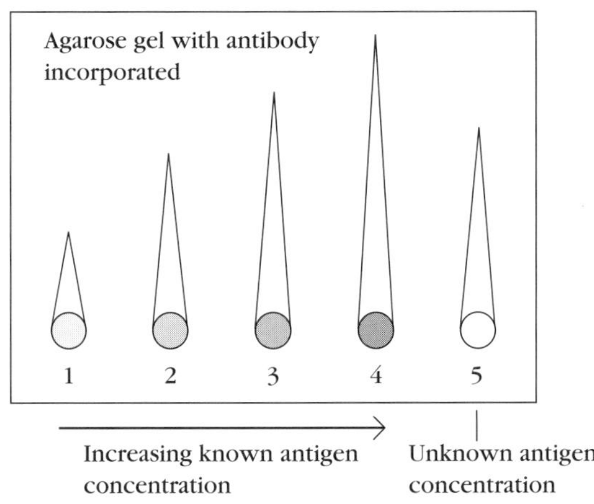

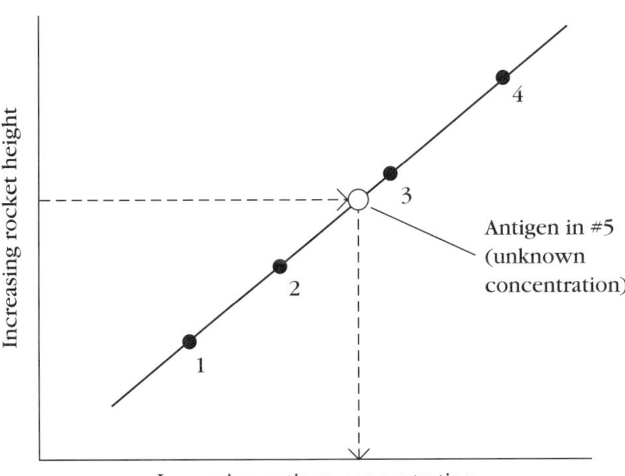

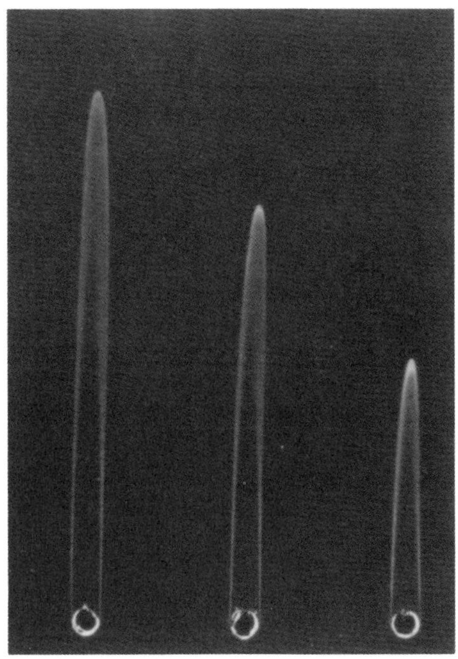

FIGURE 6-10 In rocket electrophoresis, antigen is electrophoresed in an agarose gel in which antibody has been incorporated. The height of the rocket-shaped line of precipitation (purple) that forms following electrophoresis for 2–3 h is proportional to the concentration of antigen. A sample of unknown antigen concentration (well 5) can be quantitated by reference to a standard curve. [Photograph from D. M. Weir (ed.), 1986, *Handbook of Experimental Immunology,* Blackwell Scientific Publications.]

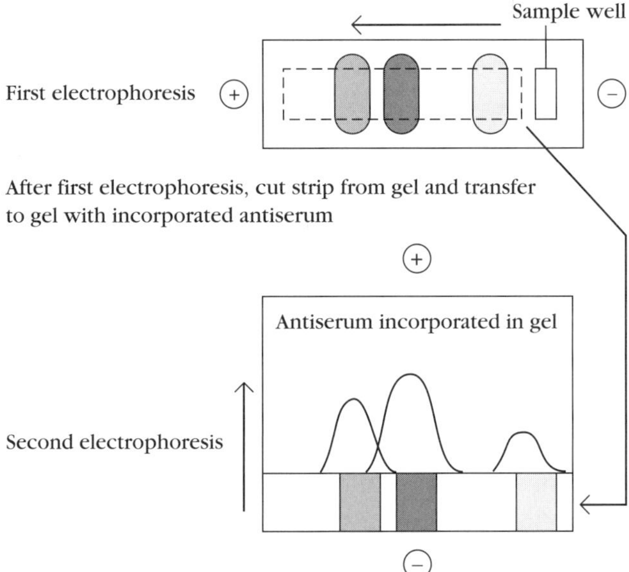

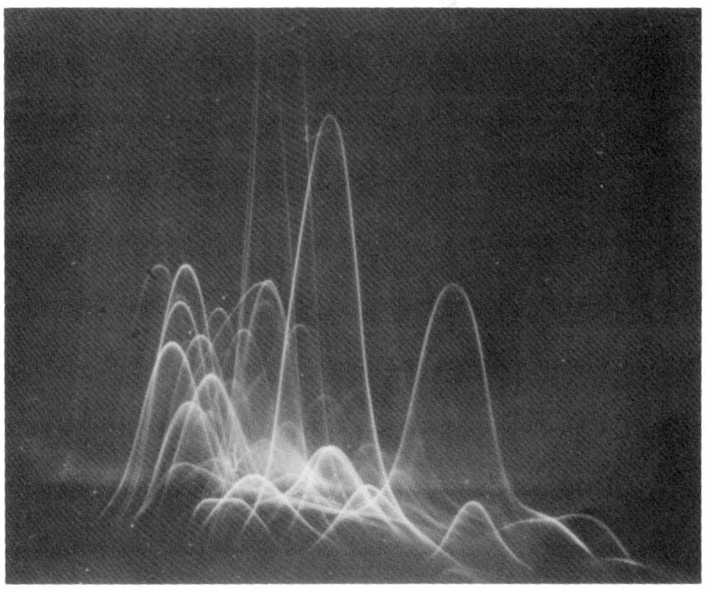

FIGURE 6-11 With two-dimensional immunoelectrophoresis, several antigens in a complex antigen mixture can be quantitated. The antigen sample is first electrophoresed; after the gel is laid over another gel containing antiserum, it is electrophoresed at right angles. The heights of the precipitin peaks (purple) in the second electrophoresis are proportional to the antigen concentrations, which can be determined by reference to standard curves. [Photograph from D. M. Weir (ed.), 1986, *Handbook of Experimental Immunology,* Blackwell Scientific Publications.]

Agglutination Reactions

The interaction between antibody and a particulate antigen results in visible clumping called *agglutination.* The agglutination reaction is similar in principal to the precipitation reaction. Just as antibody excess inhibits precipitation reactions, an excess of antibody inhibits agglutination reactions; this inhibition, called the *prozone effect,* can be caused by several mechanisms. First, high levels of antibody increase the likelihood that a single antibody molecule will bind to two or more epitopes on a single particulate antigen rather than cross-linking epitopes on two or more particulate antigens. The prozone effect can also occur at high concentrations of antibodies that bind to the antigen but do not induce agglutination; these antibodies, called *incomplete antibodies,* are often of the IgG class. At high concentrations of IgG, incomplete antibodies may occupy all of the antigenic sites, thus blocking access by IgM, which is a good agglutinator. The lack of agglutinating activity of an incomplete antibody may be due to restricted flexibility in the hinge region, making it difficult for the antibody to assume the required angle for optimal cross-linking of epitopes on two or more particulate antigens. Alternatively, the density of epitope distribution or the location of some epitopes in deep pockets of a particulate antigen may make it difficult for antibodies, specific for these epitopes, to agglutinate certain particulate antigens.

Hemagglutination

Agglutination reactions are routinely performed to type red blood cells (RBCs). In typing for the ABO antigens, RBCs are mixed on a slide with antisera to the A and B blood-group antigens. If the antigen is present on the cells, they agglutinate, forming a visible clump on the slide (see Table 6-2). Determination of which antigens are present on donor and recipient RBCs is the basis for matching blood types for transfusions.

At neutral pH, red blood cells are surrounded by a negative ion cloud that makes the cells repel one another; this repulsive force is called the zeta potential. Because of its size and pentameric nature, IgM can overcome the zeta potential and cross-link red blood cells, leading to agglutination. The smaller size and bivalency of IgG makes it less able to overcome the zeta potential. For this reason, IgM is more effective than IgG in agglutinating red blood cells. Antibodies to some RBC antigens (e.g., the Rh antigen) are of the IgG class exclusively. In order to agglutinate Rh^+ red blood cells with anti-Rh antibody, the zeta potential must be reduced. This is commonly done by placing the red blood cells in serum albumin, which has a high net negative charge that reduces the effect of the negative ion cloud surrounding the red cells, thus allowing anti-Rh antibody to agglutinate Rh^+ cells.

Bacterial Agglutination

A bacterial infection often elicits the production of serum antibodies specific for surface antigens of the bacterial cells. The presence of such antibodies can be detected by bacterial agglutination reactions. Serum from a patient thought to be infected with a given bacterium is serially diluted in a series of tubes to which the bacteria is added. The last tube showing visible agglutination will reflect the serum antibody titer of the patient. The *agglutination titer* is defined as the reciprocal of the last serum dilution that elicits a positive agglutination reaction. For example, if serial twofold dilutions of serum are prepared and if the dilution of 1/640 shows agglutination but the dilution of 1/1280 does not, then the agglutination titer of the patient's serum is 640. For some bacteria high-titer serum can be diluted up to 1/50,000 and still show agglutination.

The agglutination titer of an antiserum can be used to diagnose a bacterial infection. Patients with typhoid fever, for example, show a significant rise in the agglutination titer to *Salmonella typhi.* Agglutination reactions also provide a way to type bacteria. For instance, different species of the bacterium *Salmonella* can be distinguished by agglutination reactions with a panel of typing antisera.

Passive Agglutination

The sensitivity and simplicity of agglutination reactions can be extended to soluble antigens by the technique of *passive agglutination.* In this technique, a soluble antigen is mixed with red blood cells that have been treated with tannic acid or chromium chloride, both of which promote adsorption of the antigen to the surface of the cells. Serum containing antibody is serially diluted into microtiter plate wells, and the antigen-coated red blood cells are added to each well; agglutination is assessed by the size of the characteristic spread pattern of agglutinated red blood cells on the bottom of the well (Figure 6-12).

Passive hemagglutination is far more sensitive than precipitin reactions and can detect antibody concen-

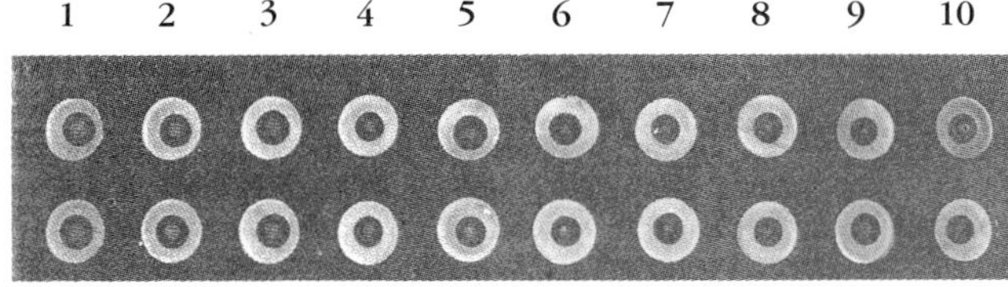

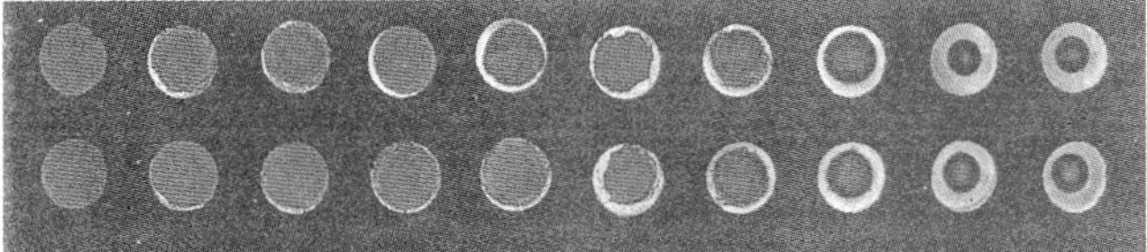

FIGURE 6-12 Passive hemagglutination test to detect antibodies against BSA-conjugated sheep red blood cells (SRBCs). *(Top)* The control wells contain only SRBCs, which settle into a solid "button." *(Bottom)* The experimental wells (in duplicate) contain a constant number of BSA-conjugated SRBCs plus serial dilutions of anti-BSA serum. The spread pattern in the experimental series indicates positive hemagglutination through tube 7, with a slightly positive reaction persisting at the next dilution in tube 8. [From J. S. Garvey et al., 1977, *Methods in Immunology,* 3rd ed., W. A. Benjamin Inc., Advanced Book Program.]

trations as low as 0.001 μg/ml. The sensitivities of precipitation and hemagglutination can be compared by testing an antiserum to hen ovalbumin in a tube-precipitation reaction and in passive hemagglutination with ovalbumin-coated red blood cells. Dilution of the antiserum by 1:5 results in loss of precipitation ability, whereas the antiserum still functions in passive agglutination out to a dilution of 1:10,000. Antigen can also be coupled to particles of latex or the mineral colloid bentonite.

Agglutination Inhibition

A modification of the agglutination assay, called agglutination inhibition, is a highly sensitive assay to detect small quantities of an antigen. One type of pregnancy test uses latex particles coated with human chorionic gonadotropin (HCG) and antibody to HCG (see Figure 4-13). The addition of urine from a pregnant woman, which contains HCG, inhibits agglutination of the latex particles, and so the absence of agglutination indicates pregnancy. Agglutination inhibition can also be used to determine if an individual is using certain types of illegal drugs such as cocaine or heroin. A urine or blood sample containing the suspected drug is first incubated with antibody specific for the drug. Then red blood cells or other particles coated with the drug are added. If the red blood cells are not agglutinated by the antibody, then it suggests that the individual may have been using the illicit drug. One problem with these tests is that some legal drugs have chemical structures similar to those of illicit drugs, and these legal drugs may crossreact with the antibody giving a false positive reaction. For this reason a positive reaction must be confirmed by a nonimmunologic method.

Agglutination inhibition is also widely used in clinical laboratories to determine if an individual has been exposed to certain types of viruses that cause agglutination of red blood cells. If an individual's serum contains specific antiviral antibodies, then the antibodies will bind to the virus and interfere with hemagglutination by the virus. This technique is commonly used in premarital testing to determine the immune status of women to rubella virus. The reciprocal of the last serum dilution to show inhibition of rubella hemagglutination is the titer of the serum. A titer greater than 10 (1:10 dilution) indicates that a woman is immune to rubella, whereas a titer of less than 10 is indicative of a lack of immunity and the need for immunization with the rubella vaccine.

Radioimmunoassay

Radioimmunoassay (RIA) is a highly sensitive technique that can detect antigen or antibody at concentrations less than 0.001 μg/ml. The technique was first developed by two endocrinologists, S. A. Berson and Rosalyn Yalow, in 1960 to determine levels of insulin–anti-insulin complexes in diabetics. Although their original attempts to publish a report of this research met with some resistance from immunologists, the technique soon proved its own value for quantitating hormones, serum proteins, drugs, and vitamins. In 1977, some years after Berson's death, the significance of the technique was acknowledged by the award of a Nobel prize to Yalow.

The principle of RIA involves competitive binding of radiolabeled antigen and unlabeled antigen to a high-affinity antibody. The antigen is generally labeled with a gamma-emitting isotope such as ^{125}I. The labeled antigen is mixed with antibody at a concentration that just saturates the antigen-binding sites of the antibody molecule, and then increasing amounts of unlabeled antigen of unknown concentration are added. The antibody does not distinguish labeled from unlabeled antigen, and so the two kinds of antigen compete for available binding sites on the antibody. With increasing concentrations of unlabeled antigen, more labeled antigen will be displaced from the binding sites. By measuring the amount of labeled antigen free in solution, it is possible to determine the concentration of unlabeled antigen.

Several methods have been developed for separating the bound antigen from the free antigen in RIA. One method involves precipitating the Ag-Ab complex with a secondary anti-isotype antiserum. For example, if the Ag-Ab complex contains rabbit IgG antibody, then goat anti-rabbit IgG can precipitate the complex. Another method makes use of the fact that protein A of *Staphylococcus aureus* has high affinity for IgG. If the complex contains an IgG antibody, the complex can be precipitated by mixing with formalin-killed *S. aureus.* After removal of the complex by either of these methods, the amount of free labeled antigen remaining in the supernatant can be quantitated in a gamma counter. A standard curve is then plotted of the percentage of bound labeled antigen versus known concentrations of unlabeled antigen. Once a standard curve had been plotted, unknown concentrations of the unlabeled antigen can be determined from the standard curve.

Various solid-phase RIAs have been developed that make it easier to separate the Ag-Ab complex from the unbound antigen. In some cases the antibody is covalently cross-linked to Sepharose beads. The amount of radiolabeled antigen bound to the beads can be quantitated after the beads have been centrifuged and washed. Alternatively, the antibody can be immobilized on polystyrene or polyvinylchloride and the amount of free labeled antigen in the supernatant can be determined in a gamma counter. In another approach, the antibody is immobilized on the walls of microtiter wells. This procedure is well suited for determining the concentration of a particular antigen in large numbers of samples. For example, a microtiter RIA has been widely used to screen for the presence of the hepatitis B virus (Figure 6-13). RIA screening of donor blood has sharply reduced the incidence of hepatitis B infections in recipients of blood transfusions.

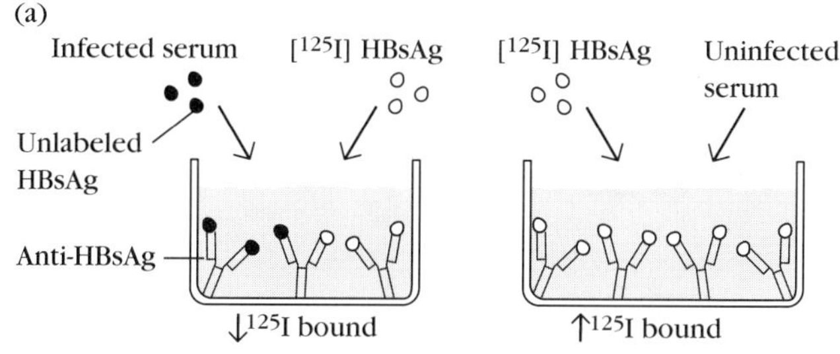

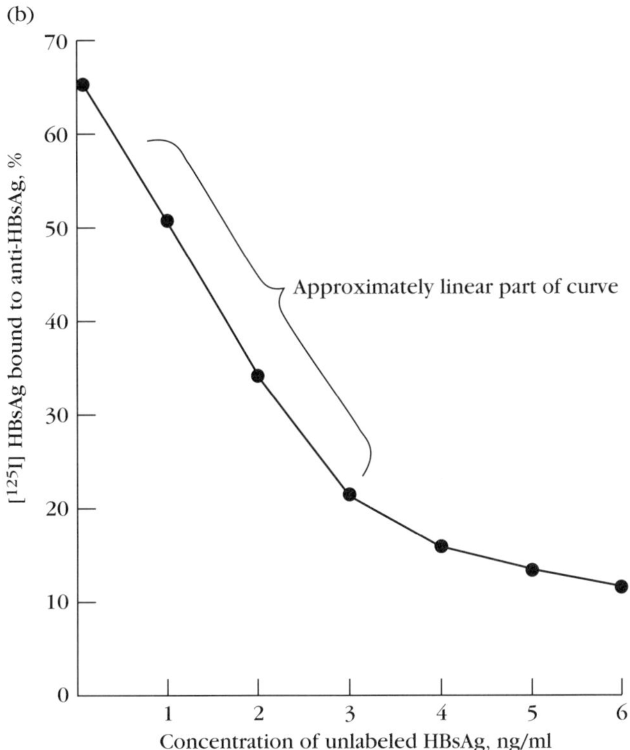

FIGURE 6-13 A solid-phase radioimmunoassay (RIA) to detect hepatitis B virus in blood samples. (a) Microtiter wells are coated with a constant amount of antibody specific for HBsAg, the surface antigen on hepatitis B virions. A serum sample and [^{125}I]HBsAg are then added. After incubation, the supernatant is removed and the amount of radioactivity bound to the antibody is determined. If the sample is infected, the amount of label bound will be less than in controls with uninfected serum. (b) A standard curve is obtained by adding increasing concentrations of unlabeled HBsAg to a fixed quantity of [^{125}I]HBsAg and specific antibody. From the plot of the percentage of labeled antigen bound versus the concentration of unlabeled antigen, the concentration of HBsAg in unknown serum samples can be determined from the linear portion of the curve.

Enzyme-Linked Immunosorbent Assay

Enzyme-linked immunosorbent assay, commonly known as *ELISA* (or *EIA*), is similar in principle to RIA but depends on an enzyme rather than a radioactive label. An enzyme conjugated to an antibody reacts with a colorless substrate to generate a colored reaction product. A number of enzymes have been employed for ELISA, including alkaline phosphatase, horseradish peroxidase, and *p*-nitrophenyl phosphatase. When mixed with suitable substrate, each of these enzymes generates a colored reaction product. These assays approach the sensitivity of RIAs and have the advantage of being safer and less costly. A number of variations of ELISA have been developed, allowing detection and quantitation of either antigen or antibody. Each type of ELISA can be used qualitatively to detect the presence of antibody or antigen. Alternatively, a standard curve based on known concentrations of antibody or antigen is prepared from which the unknown concentration of a sample can be determined.

An *indirect ELISA* is used to detect or quantitate *antibody* (Figure 6-14a). Serum or some other sample

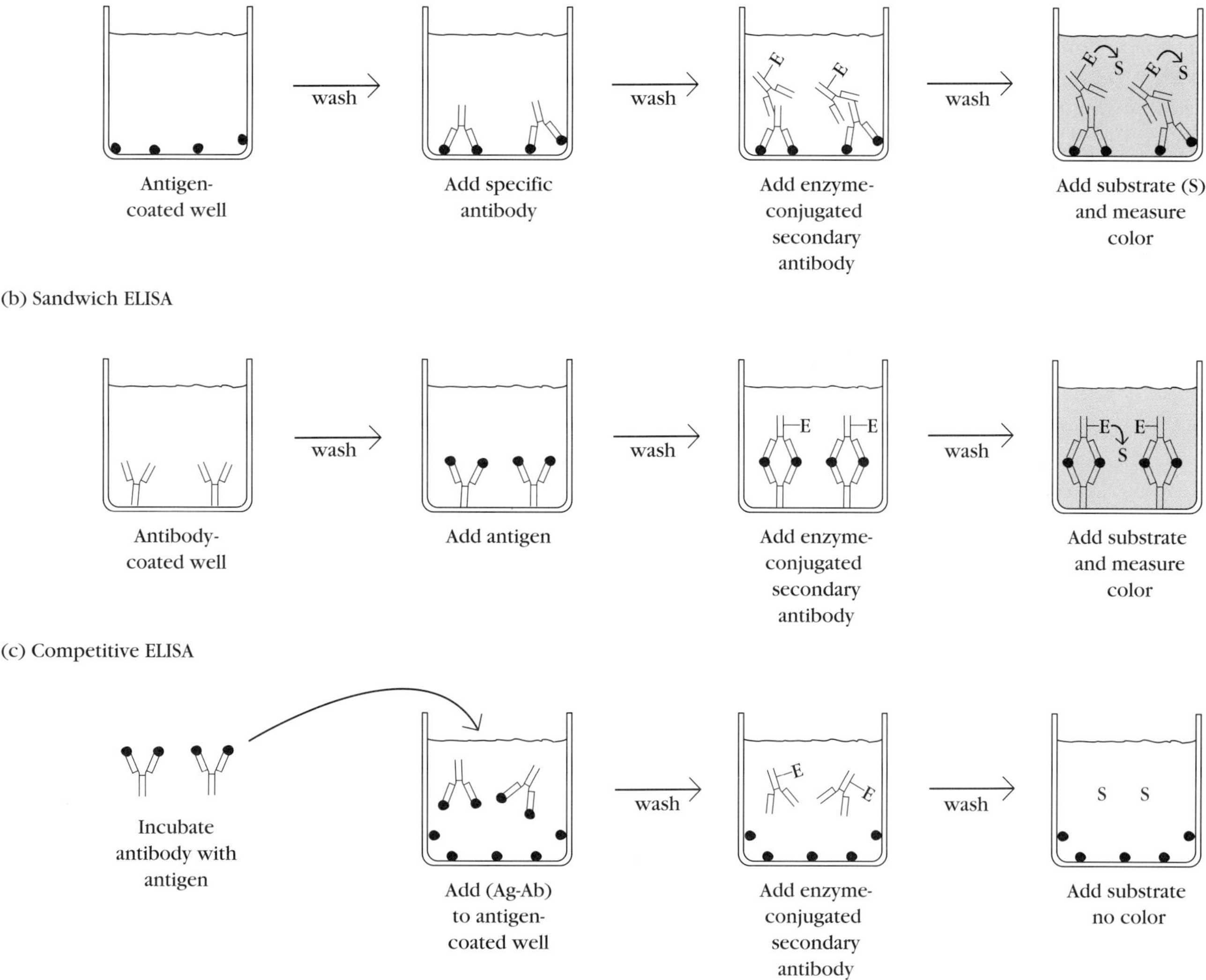

FIGURE 6-14 Variations in the enzyme-linked immunosorbent assay (ELISA) technique allow determination of antibody or antigen. Each assay can be used qualitatively or quantitatively by comparison with standard curves prepared with known concentrations of antibody or antigen. Antibody can be determined with an indirect ELISA (a), whereas antigen can be determined with a sandwich ELISA (b) or competitive ELISA (c). In the competitive ELISA, which is an inhibition-type assay, the concentration of antigen is inversely proportional to the color produced.

containing primary antibody (Ab_1) is added to an antigen-coated microtiter well and allowed to react with the bound antigen. After any free Ab_1 is washed away, the presence of antibody bound to the antigen is detected by adding an enzyme-conjugated secondary anti-isotype antibody (Ab_2), which binds to the primary antibody. Any free Ab_2 then is washed away, and a substrate for the enzyme is added. The colored reaction product that forms is measured by specialized spectrophotometric plate readers, which can measure the absorbance of a 96-well plate in less than a minute (see Figure 7-6).

An indirect ELISA has been the method of choice to detect the presence of serum antibodies against human immunodeficiency virus (HIV), the causative agent of AIDS. In this assay recombinant envelope and core proteins of HIV are adsorbed as solid-phase antigens to microtiter wells. Individuals infected with HIV will produce serum antibodies to epitopes on these viral proteins. Generally, serum antibodies to HIV can be detected by indirect ELISA within 6 weeks of infection (see Figure 23-20).

The technique of *sandwich ELISA* allows detection or quantitation of *antigen* (Figure 6-14b). In this case the antibody is immobilized on a microtiter well. A sample containing antigen is added and allowed to react with the bound antibody. After the well is washed, a second enzyme-linked antibody specific for a different epitope on the antigen is added and allowed to react with the bound antigen. After any free second antibody is removed by washing, substrate is added and the colored reaction product is measured.

Antigen can also be quantitated by another variation called *competitive ELISA* (Figure 6-14c). In this technique antibody is first incubated in solution with a sample containing antigen. The antigen-antibody mixture is then added to an antigen-coated microtiter well. The more antigen present in the sample, the less free antibody will be available to bind to the antigen-coated well. Addition of an enzyme-conjugated secondary antibody (Ab_2) specific for the isotype of the primary antibody can be used to quantitate the amount of primary antibody bound to the well as in an indirect ELISA. In the competitive assay, however, the higher the concentration of antigen in the original sample, the lower the absorbance.

Western Blotting

Identification of a specific protein in a complex mixture of proteins, or antibody to a given protein, can be accomplished by a technique known as Western blotting, named for its similarity to Southern blotting, which detects DNA fragments, and Northern blotting, which detects mRNAs. In Western blotting protein is electrophoretically separated on a polyacrylamide slab

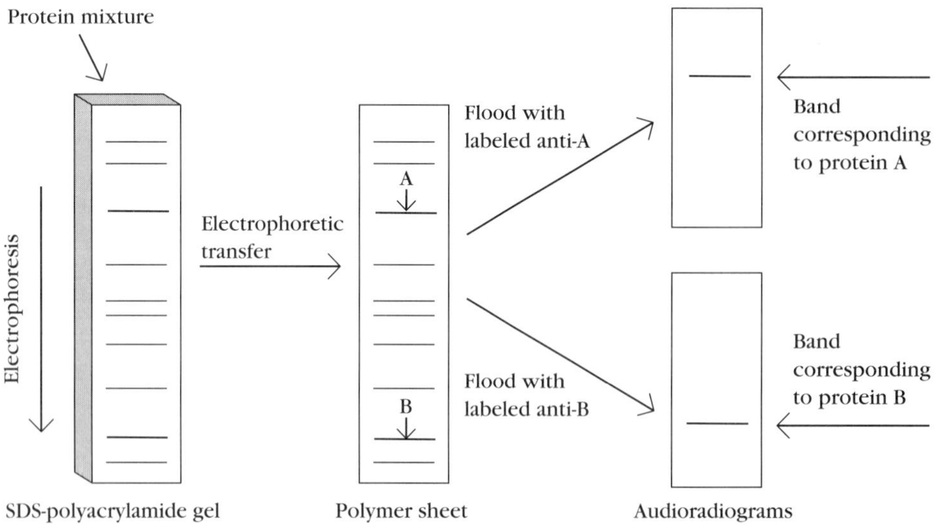

FIGURE 6-15 In Western blotting a protein mixture is separated by electrophoresis, and the protein bands are transferred by electrophoresis onto a nitrocellulose or other polymer sheet. After the sheet is flooded with radiolabeled specific antibodies, the various protein bands can be visualized by autoradiography.

gel in the presence of SDS. The protein bands are transferred to a nitrocellulose membrane by electrophoresis and the individual protein bands are identified by flooding the nitrocellulose membrane with radiolabeled polyclonal or monoclonal antibody. The Ag-Ab complexes that form are visualized by autoradiography (Figure 6-15). If labeled specific antibody is not available, Ag-Ab complexes can be detected by adding a secondary anti-isotype antibody that is either radiolabeled or enzyme-labeled; in this case the band is visualized by autoradiography or substrate addition. Western blotting can identify either a given protein antigen or specific antibody. For example, Western blotting has been used to identify the envelope and core proteins of HIV and the antibodies to these components in the serum of HIV-infected individuals.

Immunofluorescence

Binding of antibodies to cells or tissue sections can be visualized by tagging the antibody molecules with a fluorescent dye, or *fluorochrome.* The most commonly used fluorescent dyes are fluorescein and rhodamine. Both dyes can be conjugated to the Fc region of an antibody molecule without affecting the specificity of the antibody. Each of these dyes absorbs light at one wavelength and emits light at a longer wavelength. Fluorescein absorbs blue light (490 nm) and emits an intense yellow-green fluorescence (517 nm); rhodamine absorbs in the yellow-green range (515 nm) and emits a deep red fluorescence (546 nm). The fluorescence emitted light is generally viewed with a fluorescence microscope, which is equipped with a UV light source and excitation filters. By conjugating fluorescein to one antibody and rhodamine to another antibody, one can visualize two cell-membrane antigens simultaneously on the same cell.

Fluorescent-antibody staining of cell-membrane molecules or tissue sections can be direct or indirect (Figure 6-16). In direct staining the specific antibody (called the primary antibody) is directly conjugated with fluorescein; in indirect staining the primary antibody is unlabeled and is detected with an additional fluorochrome-labeled reagent. A number of reagents have been developed for indirect staining. The most common is a fluorochrome-labeled anti-isotype reagent such as fluorescein-labeled goat anti-mouse immunoglobulin. Another reagent is fluorochrome-labeled protein A from *Staphylococcus aureus;* this protein binds with high affinity to the Fc region of IgG antibody molecules. A third approach begins with a biotin-conjugated anti-isotype as the second antibody and then adds fluorochrome-conjugated avidin, a protein that binds to the biotin with extremely high

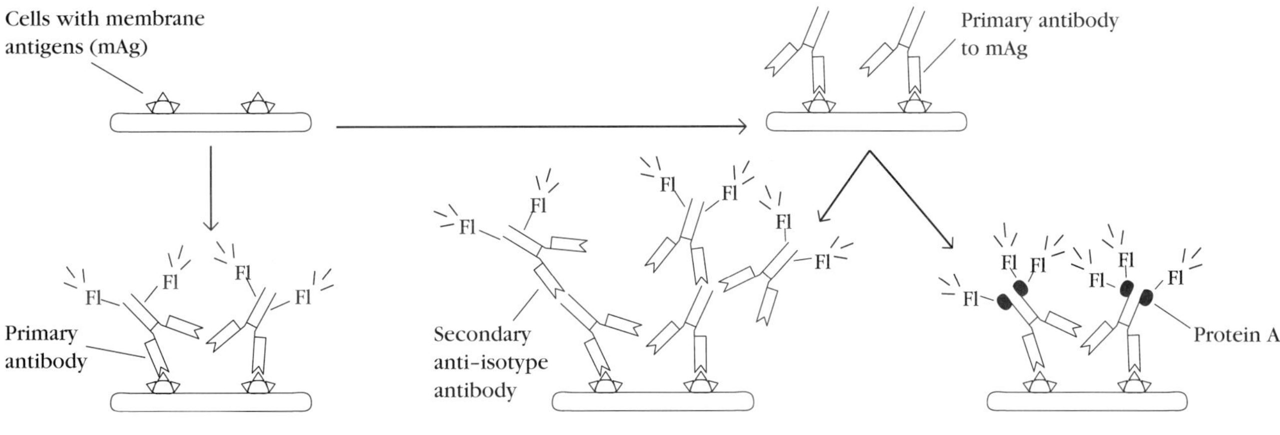

FIGURE 6-16 Direct and indirect immunofluorescence staining of membrane antigen (mAg). Cells are affixed to a microscope slide. In the direct method (a), cells are stained with anti-mAg antibody that is labeled with a fluorochrome (Fl). In the indirect methods (b and c), cells are first incubated with unlabeled anti-mAg antibody and then stained with a fluorochrome-labeled secondary reagent that binds to the primary antibody. Observation under a fluorescence microscope indicates whether the cells have been stained.

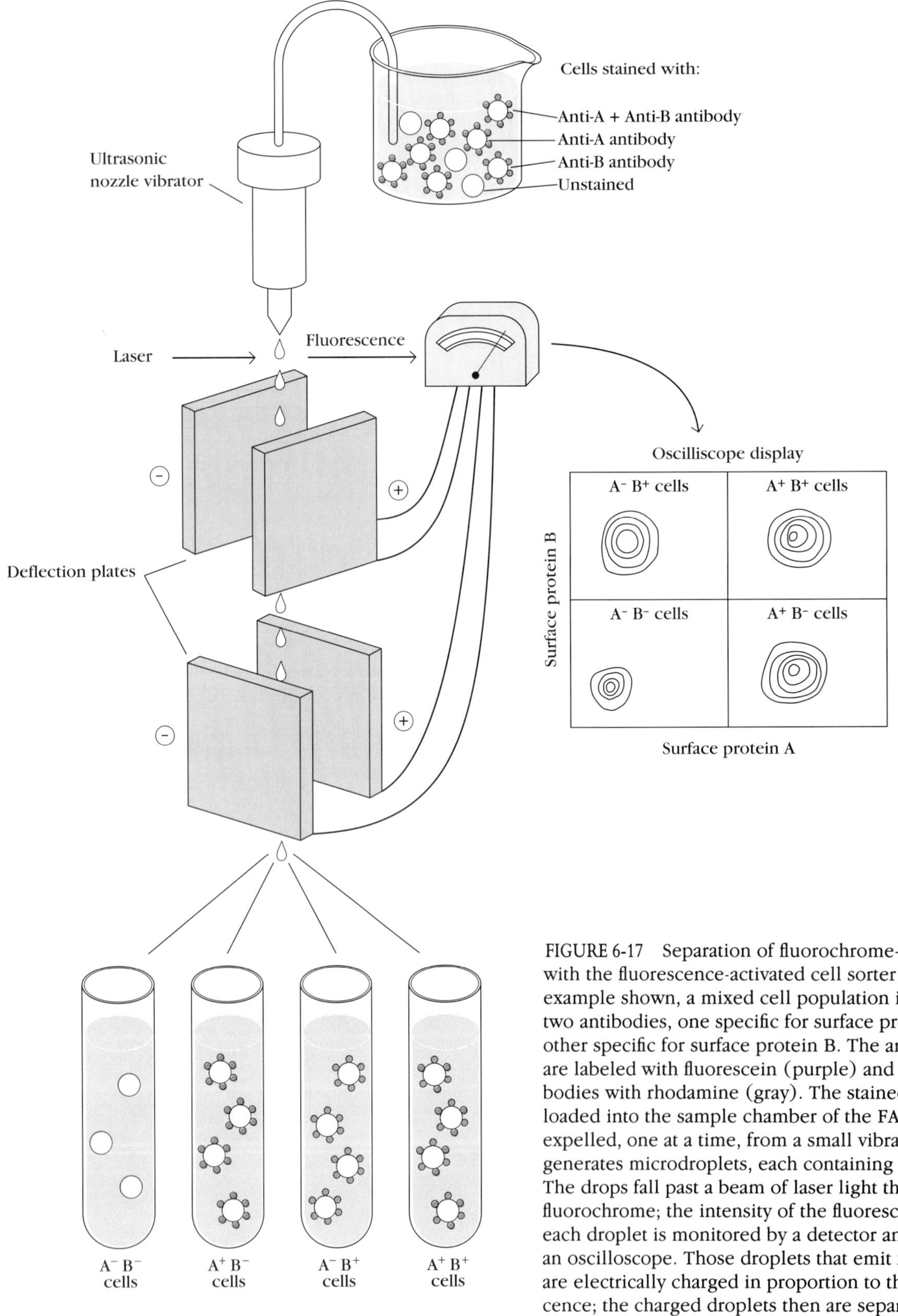

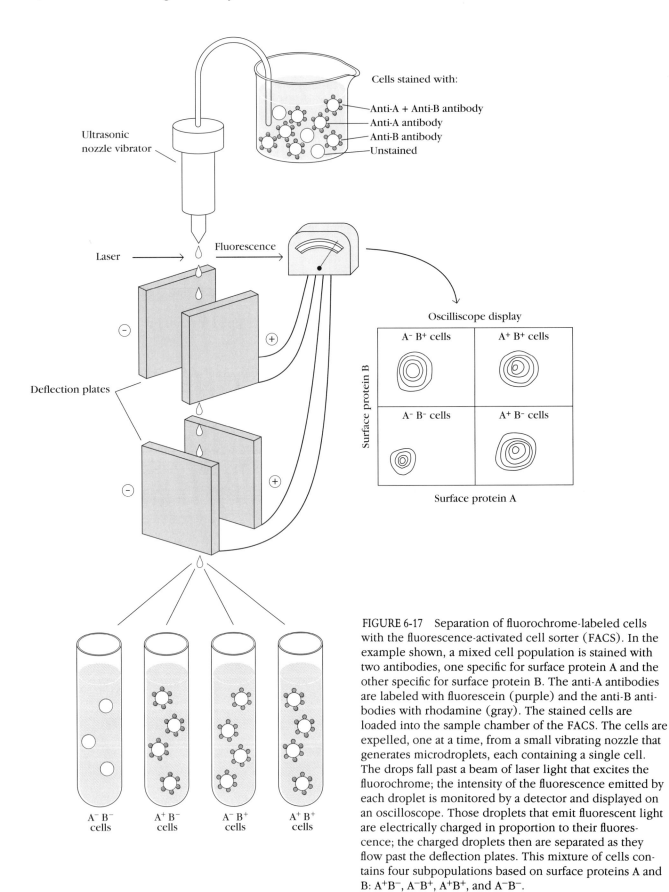

FIGURE 6-17 Separation of fluorochrome-labeled cells with the fluorescence-activated cell sorter (FACS). In the example shown, a mixed cell population is stained with two antibodies, one specific for surface protein A and the other specific for surface protein B. The anti-A antibodies are labeled with fluorescein (purple) and the anti-B antibodies with rhodamine (gray). The stained cells are loaded into the sample chamber of the FACS. The cells are expelled, one at a time, from a small vibrating nozzle that generates microdroplets, each containing a single cell. The drops fall past a beam of laser light that excites the fluorochrome; the intensity of the fluorescence emitted by each droplet is monitored by a detector and displayed on an oscilloscope. Those droplets that emit fluorescent light are electrically charged in proportion to their fluorescence; the charged droplets then are separated as they flow past the deflection plates. This mixture of cells contains four subpopulations based on surface proteins A and B: A^+B^-, A^-B^+, A^+B^+, and A^-B^-.

affinity. There are two advantages to indirect labeling. One is that the primary antibody does not need to be conjugated with label. Because the supply of primary antibody is often a limiting factor, it is advantageous to avoid loss of antibody in the course of labeling. The second advantage of indirect labeling is that sensitivity is increased because multiple fluorochrome reagents will bind to each primary antibody.

Immunofluorescence has a wide variety of applications. Fluorescent antibodies have been applied to identify a number of subpopulations of lymphocytes, notably the CD4 and CD8 T-cell subpopulations. Fluorescent antibodies can also be used to identify bacterial species, detect Ag-Ab complexes in autoimmune disease, detect complement components in tissues, and localize hormones and other cellular products stained in situ.

Subpopulations of lymphocytes labeled with fluorochrome-conjugated antibody can be analyzed and sorted on the basis of the intensity of fluorescent-antibody staining. Labeled cells can be separated in a specialized flow cytometer called a fluorescence-activated cell sorter (FACS), as illustrated in Figure 6-17. The FACS permits separation of fluorescein-stained and rhodamine-stained subpopulations and of high-, medium-, and low-staining cells. Recent advances in flow cytometry make it possible to analyze three fluorochromes on a single stained sample.

Immunoelectron Microscopy

The fine specificity of antibodies has made them powerful tools to identify intracellular tissue components by electron microscopy. In order to visualize the antibody, an electron-dense label is either conjugated directly to the Fc portion of the antibody molecule or an indirect labeling technique is employed in which the electron-dense label is conjugated to an anti-immunoglobulin reagent. A number of electron-dense labels have been employed including ferritin and colloidal gold. As the electron-dense label absorbs electrons, it can be visualized with the electron microscope as small black dots. In the case of immunogold labeling, different antibodies can be conjugated with different sizes of gold particles, allowing identification of several intracellular antigens within a cell by the size of the electron-dense gold particle attached to the antibody. These techniques have played an important role in demonstrating that class I and class II MHC molecules may be sequestered along different intracellular processing routes.

Summary

1. The Ag-Ab interaction depends on noncovalent interactions including hydrogen bonds, ionic bonds, hydrophobic interactions, and van der Waals interactions. The strength of this interaction depends on the number of these weak noncovalent interactions between antigen and antibody. The affinity of an antibody for an antigen refers to the strength of the noncovalent interactions between the antibody and antigen at a single binding site; the avidity reflects the overall strength of the interactions between a multivalent antibody and multivalent antigen at multiple sites.

2. The interaction of a soluble antigen and antibody forms an Ag-Ab complex that has a lattice structure and precipitates out of solution. Precipitin reactions can be performed in liquids or gels. They serve as simple methods for comparing antibodies or antigens; some versions can quantitate antibodies or antigens. Electrophoresis can be combined with precipitation in gels in a technique called immunoelectrophoresis. A variety of immunoelectrophoretic techniques have been developed, including countercurrent electrophoresis, rocket electrophoresis, and two-dimensional electrophoresis.

3. Agglutination reactions occur between antibody and a particulate antigen. In some cases the antigen is a membrane protein on a bacterial cell or red blood cell. In other cases the antigen may be attached to a latex particle or adsorbed on the surface of a red blood cell. Agglutination reactions are more sensitive than precipitin reactions and can often detect 100- or 1000-fold lower levels of antigen or antibody than can be detected with a precipitin reaction.

4. Radioimmunoassay utilizes radioactively labeled antigen or antibody and is therefore a highly sensitive technique. Liquid-phase RIA is based on the principle of competition between labeled and unlabeled antigen for a limited amount of antibody. In solid-phase RIA, antigen (or antibody) is immobilized on a solid matrix. The main advantage of this technique over liquid-phase RIA is its simplicity of performance and the ease with which bound Ag-Ab complex can be separated from unreacted antigen. Both types of RIA can be used to quantitate antibody or antigen.

5. The enzyme-linked immunosorbent assay (ELISA) involves principles similar to those of RIA but depends on an enzyme-substrate reaction that generates a colored reaction product rather than utilizing a radiolabel.

6. In Western blotting, antigen is separated by electrophoresis; then the antigen bands are electrophoretically transferred onto nitrocellulose and identified with labeled antibody.

7. Fluorescent-antibody staining can visualize antigen on cells. Various direct and indirect staining techniques have been developed. The fluorescence-activated cell sorter analyzes and sorts cells labeled with fluorescent antibody.

References

AXELSEN, N. H. 1983. *Handbook of Immunoprecipitation-in-Gel Techniques.* Blackwell Scientific Publications.

EDWARDS, R. 1985. *Immunoassay: An Introduction.* Heinemann Medical Books.

JOHNSTONE, A. (ed.). 1989. Immunological techniques. *Curr. Opin. Immunol.* **1**:927.

JOHNSTONE, A., and R. THORPE. 1987. *Immunochemistry in Practice,* 2d ed. Blackwell Scientific Publications.

POLAK, J. M., and S. VANNOORDEN. 1987. *An Introduction to Immunocytochemistry: Current Techniques and Problems.* Oxford Science Publishers.

WEIR, D. M. (ed.). 1986. *Handbook of Experimental Immunology,* 4th ed. Vols. I and II. Blackwell Scientific Publications.

Study Questions

1. Indicate whether each of the following statements is true or false. If you think a statement is false, explain why.
   a. Indirect immunofluorescence is a more sensitive technique than direct immunofluorescence.
   b. Most antigens induce a polyclonal response.
   c. A papain digest of anti-SRBC antibodies can agglutinate sheep red blood cells (SRBCs).
   d. A pepsin digest of anti-SRBC antibodies can agglutinate SRBCs.
   e. Indirect immunofluorescence can be performed using a Fab fragment as the initial nonlabeled antibody.
   f. For precipitation to occur, both antigen and antibody must be multivalent.
   g. The Ouchterlony technique is a quantitative precipitin technique.
   h. Precipitin tests are generally more sensitive than agglutination tests.

2. Briefly outline the ELISA test for HIV infection indicating which antigen and antibody are used.

3. You have obtained a preparation of purified albumin from normal bovine serum. To determine whether any other serum proteins remain in this preparation of BSA, you decide to use immunoelectrophoresis.
   a. What antigen would you use to prepare the antiserum needed to detect impurities in the BSA preparation?
   b. Assuming that the BSA preparation is pure, draw the immunoelectrophoretic pattern you would expect if the assay was performed with bovine serum in one well, the BSA sample in a second well, and the antiserum you prepared in (a) in the trough between the wells.

4. The labels from four bottles (A, B, C, and D) of hapten-carrier conjugates were accidentally removed. However, it was known that each bottle contained either hapten 1-carrier 1 (H1-C1), hapten 1-carrier 2 (H1-C2), hapten 2-carrier 1 (H2-C1), or hapten 2-carrier 2 (H2-C2). Ouchterlony assays with either anti-H1-C2 or anti-H2-C2 were performed. From the precipitin patterns shown below, determine which conjugate is in each bottle.

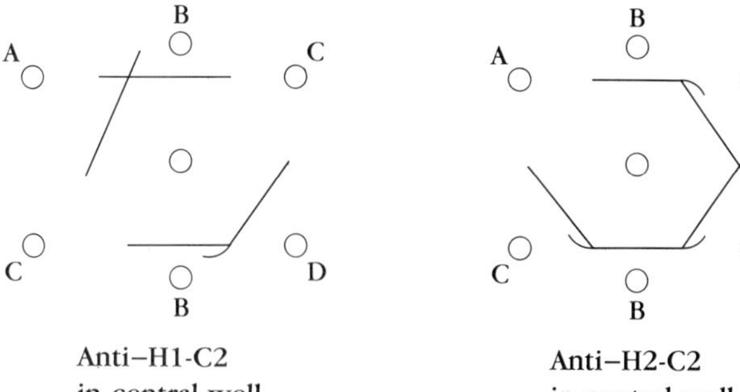

5. The concentration of a hapten can be determined by which of the following assays: (a) ELISA, (b) Ouchterlony method, (c) rocket electrophoresis, and (d) RIA.

6. You perform an Ouchterlony assay in which the central well contains goat antiserum against the

F(ab′)$_2$ fragment of pooled mouse IgG and the surrounding wells (1–6) contain six different test antigens. The resulting precipitin pattern is shown below.

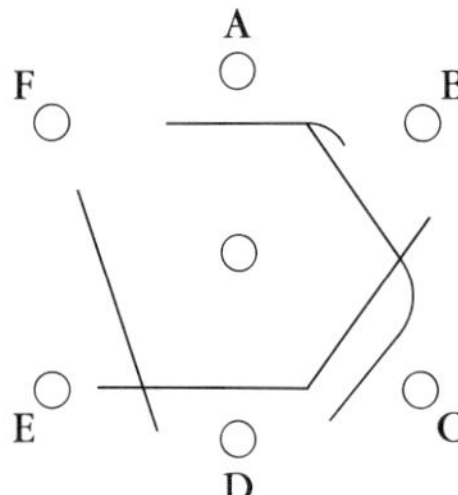

Based on this pattern, indicate which well contains each of the following test antigens:

a. ______ Fab fragment from an IgG myeloma protein ($\gamma_2\kappa_2$)
b. ______ Kappa (κ) light chains
c. ______ Gamma (γ) heavy chains
d. ______ Lambda (λ) light chains
e. ______ Fc fragment from IgG myeloma protein ($\gamma_2\lambda_2$)
f. ______ A mixture of γ heavy chains and κ light chains

7. You have a myeloma protein X whose isotype is unknown and several other myeloma proteins of known isotype (e.g., IgG, IgM, and IgA).
   a. How could you produce anti-isotype antibodies that could be used to determine the isotype of myeloma protein X?
   b. How could you use this anti-isotype antibody to measure the level of myeloma protein X in normal serum?

8. For each antigen or antibody listed below, indicate an appropriate assay method and the necessary test reagents. Keep in mind the sensitivity of the assay and the expected concentration of each protein.
   a. IgG in serum
   b. Insulin in serum
   c. IgE in serum
   d. Complement component C3 on glomerular basement membrane
   e. Anti-A antibodies to blood-group antigen A in serum
   f. Horsemeat contamination of hamburger
   g. Syphilis spirochete in a smear from a chancre

9. You want to develop a sensitive immunoassay for a hormone that occurs in the blood at concentrations around 10^{-7} *M*. You are offered a choice of three different antisera whose affinities for the hormone have been determined by equilibrium dialysis. The results are shown in the following Scatchard plots.

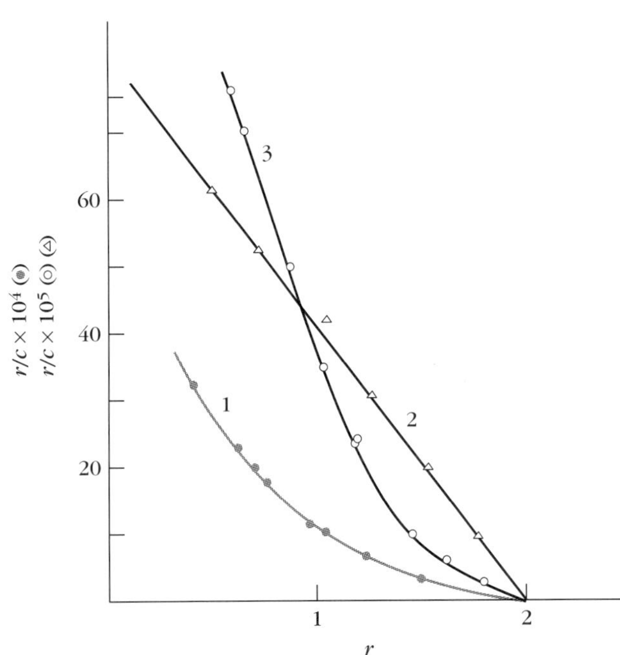

   a. What is the value of K_0 for each antiserum?
   b. What is the valence of each of the antibodies?
   c. Which of the antisera might be a monoclonal antibody?
   d. Which of the antisera would you use for your assay? Why?

10. In preparing a demonstration for her immunology class, an instructor purified IgG antibodies to sheep blood cells (SRBCs) and digested some of the antibodies into Fab, Fc, and F(ab′)$_2$ fragments. She placed each preparation in a separate tube, labeled the tubes with a water-soluble marker, and left them in an ice bucket. When the instructor returned for her class period, she discovered that the labels had smeared and were unreadable. Determined to salvage the demonstration, she relabeled the tubes 1, 2, 3, and 4 and proceeded. Based on the test results described below, indicate which preparation was contained in each tube and explain why you so identified the contents.

a. The preparation in tube 1 agglutinated SRBCs but did not lyse them in the presence of complement.

b. The preparation in tube 2 did not agglutinate SRBCs or lyse them in the presence of complement. However, when this preparation was added to SRBCs before the addition of whole anti-SRBC, it prevented agglutination of the cells by the whole anti-SRBC antiserum.

c. The preparation in tube 3 agglutinated SRBCs and also lysed the cells in the presence of complement.

d. The preparation in tube 4 did not agglutinate or lyse SRBCs and did not inhibit agglutination of SRBCs by whole anti-SRBC antiserum.

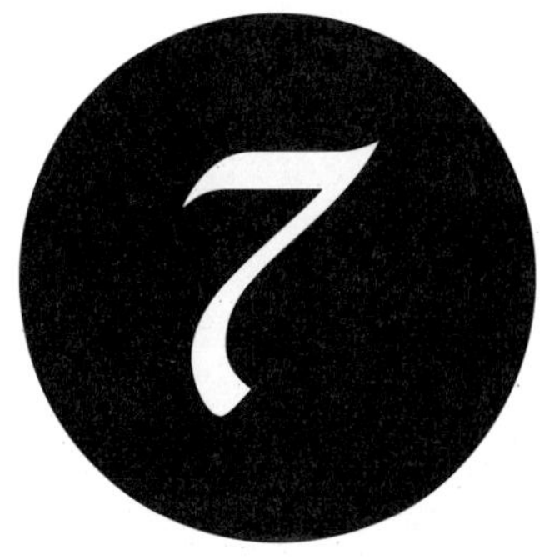

HYBRIDOMAS AND MONOCLONAL ANTIBODY

The serum antibodies produced in response to an antigen, even a purified one, are heterogeneous because the multiple epitopes on the antigen induce proliferation and differentiation of a variety of B-cell clones. Such a polyclonal antibody response facilitates the localization, phagocytosis, and complement-mediated lysis of antigen; it thus has clear advantages for the organism in vivo. Unfortunately, the antibody heterogeneity that increases immune protection in vivo often reduces the efficacy of an antiserum for various in vitro uses. Conventional heterogeneous antisera vary from animal to animal and contain undesirable nonspecific or cross-reacting antibodies. Removal of antibodies with unwanted specificities from a polyclonal antibody preparation is a time-consuming task involving repeated adsorption techniques. These methods often result in the loss of much of the desired antibody and seldom are very effective in reducing the heterogeneity of an antiserum.

An alternative, simpler approach is to generate pure (monospecific) clones of plasma cells in vitro from which monoclonal antibody with a single antigenic specificity can be obtained (Figure 7-1). For many years this approach was not technically feasible because plasma cells have a short life span and cannot be maintained in tissue culture. In 1975, Georges Kohler and Cesar Milstein devised a solution to this technical problem,

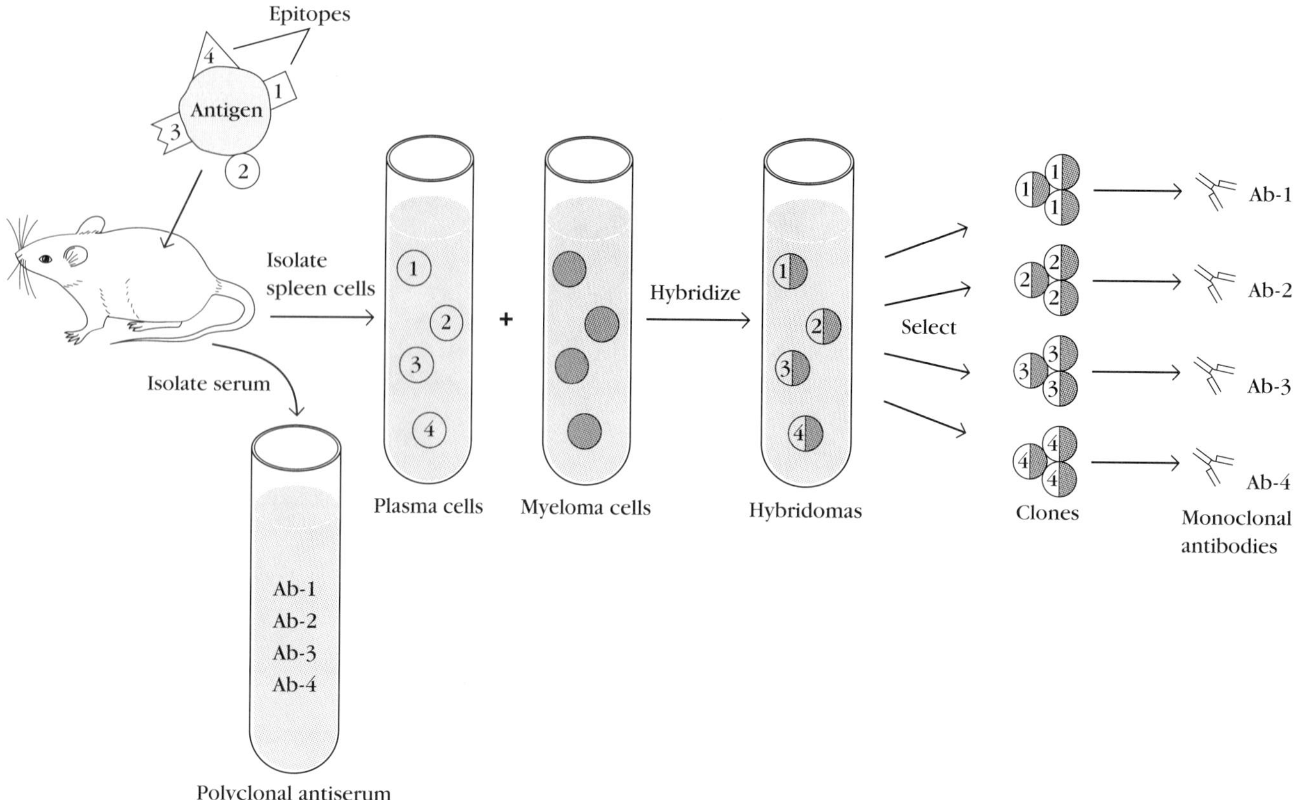

FIGURE 7-1 The conventional polyclonal antiserum produced in response to a complex antigen contains a mixture of antibodies, each specific for one of the four epitopes shown on the antigen. In contrast, a monoclonal antibody, which is derived from a single plasma cell, is specific for one epitope on a complex antigen. One method for obtaining monoclonal antibody is illustrated.

which was described briefly in Chapter 2. By fusing a normal B cell (plasma cell) with a myeloma cell (a cancerous plasma cell), they were able to generate a hybrid cell, called a hybridoma, that possessed the immortal-growth properties of the myeloma cell but secreted the antibody product of the B cell (see Figure 2-2). The resulting clones of hybridoma cells, which secrete large quantities of monoclonal antibody, can be cultured indefinitely. This basic procedure for producing monoclonal antibody is explained in detail in this chapter; several more recent methods for obtaining monoclonal antibody by genetic engineering techniques also are described.

The development of techniques for producing monoclonal antibody gave immunologists (and molecular biologists in general) a powerful and versatile research tool. The significance of the work by Kohler and Milstein was acknowledged when each was awarded a Nobel prize in 1984, along with the eminent theorist Niels Jerne. During the 1980s, monoclonal antibody technology moved out of the research laboratory and now forms the basis for a growing variety of commercial applications, some of which are described in this chapter.

Formation and Selection of Hybrid Cells

Since the early 1970s it has been possible to fuse one somatic cell with another to form a hybrid cell called a *heterokaryon.* Fusion can be achieved by incubating a suspension of two cell types with an inactivated enveloped virus called Sendai virus or with polyethylene glycol, both of which promote the fusion of plasma membranes. In this way the plasma membranes, cytoplasm, and nuclei of two separate cells are brought together into a single hybrid cell.

In the early 1970s L. D. Frye and M. Edidin used heterokaryons to study the fluidity of membrane proteins. In a classic experiment they fused a mouse fibroblast with a human fibroblast, generating a mouse-human heterokaryon, which was then exposed to

(a)

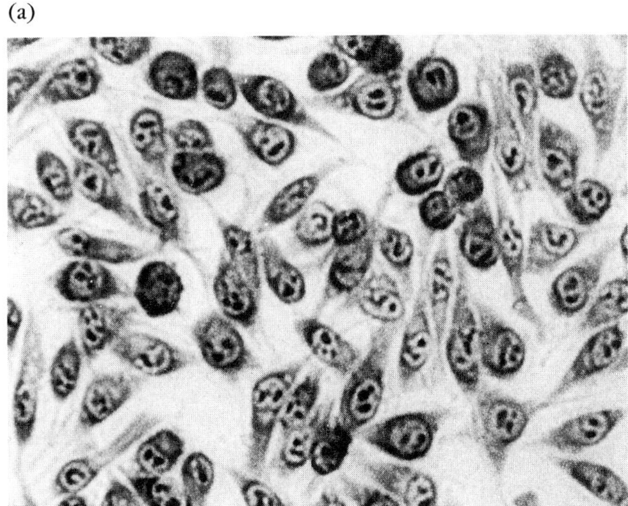

(b)

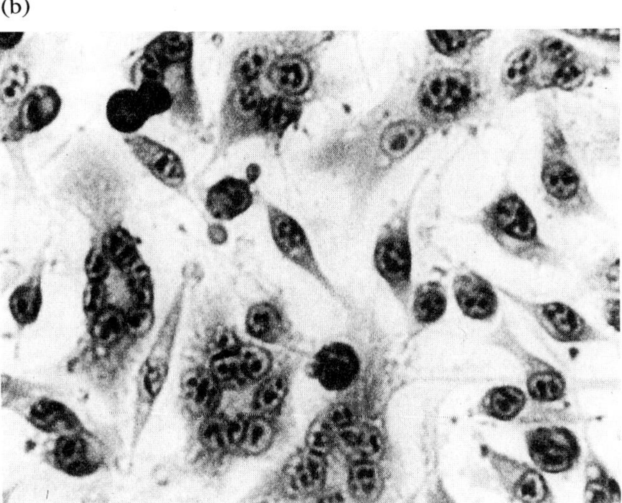

FIGURE 7-2 Heterokaryon formation. (a) Unfused cultured mouse cells. (b) Mouse cells fused by treatment with polyethylene glycol. There are two to five nuclei per heterokaryon. [From R. L. Davidson and P. S. Gerald, 1976, *Som. Cell Genet.* **2**:165.]

fluorescein- and rhodamine-tagged antibodies specific for the MHC molecules on human and mouse cells, respectively. Immediately after fusion the distribution of labeled antibody revealed that the mouse and human MHC molecules were confined to separate halves of the heterokaryon's plasma membrane. Within a short period of time, however, the fluorescein- and rhodamine-tagged antibodies were seen to diffuse and mix randomly over the surface of the heterokaryon, demonstrating the random diffusion of the mouse and human MHC molecules within the phospholipid bilayer of the heterokaryon's plasma membrane. This experiment was instrumental in the development of the fluid-mosaic model of the cell membrane by J. Singer and G. Nicholson in 1972.

A heterokaryon initially is multinucleated, having two to five separate nuclei (Figure 7-2). In the course of cell division the nuclear membranes disintegrate, and a single large nucleus is formed containing the chromosomes of both parent cells. At this stage the hybrid cell is unstable, and as it continues to divide, it loses a variable number of chromosomes from one or both parent cells until the fused cell stabilizes. Sometimes this random chromosome loss results in loss of a chromosome that is necessary for cell survival, and these hybrids die off. When mouse and human cells are fused, the hybrids eventually lose all of their human chromosomes. The reason for this disparate chromosome loss is not known but presumably is related to the phylogenetic distance between the two species. With selective culture conditions it is possible to select for mouse-human hybrid cells containing one or at most a few human chromosomes. These hybrids have been useful for mapping genes to particular human chromosomes by associating a particular gene function with a particular chromosome.

After fusion the hybrid cells must be separated from unfused parent cells (e.g., A cells and B cells). When Sendai virus or polyethylene glycol is the fusion agent, only a small percentage of the cells actually fuse, and some of the fused cells are homogeneous A-A or B-B cells rather than the desired A-B hybrid. In order to select for the hybrid cells, a selective medium called HAT is employed. HAT selection depends on the fact that mammalian cells can synthesize nucleotides by two different pathways—the de novo and the salvage pathways:

De novo pathway

Phosphoribosyl pyrophosphate + Uridylate

(blocked by aminopterin)

Nucleotides ⟶ DNA

Salvage pathway

(Catalyzed by HGPRT and TK enzymes)

Hypoxanthine + Thymidine

The de novo pathway, in which a methyl or formyl group is transferred from an activated form of tetrahydrofolate, is blocked by *aminopterin,* a folic acid analog (Figure 7-3). When the de novo pathway is blocked, cells utilize the salvage pathway, which bypasses the aminopterin block by converting purines and pyrimidines directly into DNA. The enzymes catalyzing the salvage pathway include hypoxanthine-guanine phosphoribosyl transferase (HGPRT) and thymidine kinase (TK). A mutation in either of these two enzymes blocks the salvage pathway. HAT

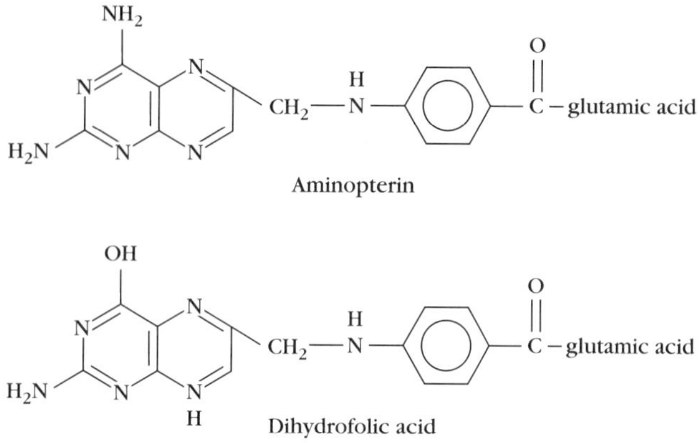

Aminopterin

Dihydrofolic acid

FIGURE 7-3 Aminopterin blocks DNA synthesis by the de novo pathway. It acts as an analog of dihydrofolic acid and binds with a high affinity to dihydrofolate reductase inhibiting purine synthesis.

medium contains aminopterin to block the de novo pathway and hypoxanthine and thymidine to allow growth via the salvage pathway. When two types of cells, each of which has a mutation in a different enzyme necessary for the salvage pathway, are fused, only the hybrid cells will contain the full complement of the necessary enzymes for growth on HAT medium via the salvage pathway. Culture in HAT medium thus allows only the hybrid cells to grow.

Production of Monoclonal Antibodies

The production of a given monoclonal antibody involves three basic steps: (1) generating B-cell hybridomas by fusing primed B cells and myeloma cells; (2) screening the resulting clones for those that secrete antibody with the desired specificity; and (3) propagating the desired hybridomas.

Generating B-Cell Hybridomas

In their innovative method for producing monoclonal antibodies, Kohler and Milstein applied the techniques of cell fusion and HAT selection of hybrid cells described in the previous section. Their general procedure is outlined in Figure 7-4. The use of myeloma cells that cannot grow in HAT medium (HGPRT$^-$ cells) assured that only hybridomas (hybrid myeloma-spleen cells) were selected. The unfused or fused spleen cells did not need to be selected because they were terminal cells of a differentiation series and were only capable of limited growth in vitro. After 7–10 days of culture in the HAT medium, most of the wells contained dead cells, but a few wells contained small clusters of viable cells, which could be visualized by using an inverted phase contrast microscope. Each cluster represented clonal expansion of a hybridoma (Figure 7-5). After HAT selection, single cells were transferred and cultured in separate wells in an effort to ensure the monoclonality of any secreted antibody. Wells containing single viable clusters were then screened for antibody production; antibody-positive clones were subcultured at low cell densities, again to ensure clonal purity in each microwell. The hybridoma clones obtained by this procedure were isolated, clonally expanded in culture, and shown by Kohler and Milstein to produce monoclonal antibodies, each specific for a single epitope on sheep red blood cells, the original antigen used in their experiments.

The first hybridomas obtained by Kohler and Milstein secreted not only antibody from the splenic B cell but also unwanted antibody from the myeloma cell as well as some hybrid antibody combining heavy or light chains from both original parent cells. To avoid this difficulty, an HGPRT$^-$, Ab$^-$ myeloma cell was chosen as the ideal fusion partner. This fusion partner has the immortal-growth properties of a cancer cell but does not secrete its own antibody gene product. Hybridomas generated with this fusion partner thus secrete only the antibody from the B-cell partner. These hybridomas can be propagated in tissue culture to give rise to large clones secreting homogeneous monoclonal antibody.

Screening for Monoclonal Antibody Specificity

Once pure clones of antibody-secreting hybridomas are obtained, they must be screened for the desired antibody specificity. Although some hybridomas will produce antibody specific for the antigen used for immunization, others will be specific for unwanted antigens. The supernatant of each hybridoma culture contains its secreted antibody and can be assayed for a particular antigen specificity in various ways.

Two of the most common screening techniques are ELISA and RIA, both of which are easily adapted to mass screening with 96-well microtiter plates. In both assays, antigen that reacts with the desired antibody is bound to the microtiter wells and washed to remove unbound antigen. Supernatant from each hybridoma well is added to separate wells. After incubation and more washing, an anti-isotype antibody directed against the isotypic determinants on the monoclonal antibody is added. In an ELISA this anti-isotype

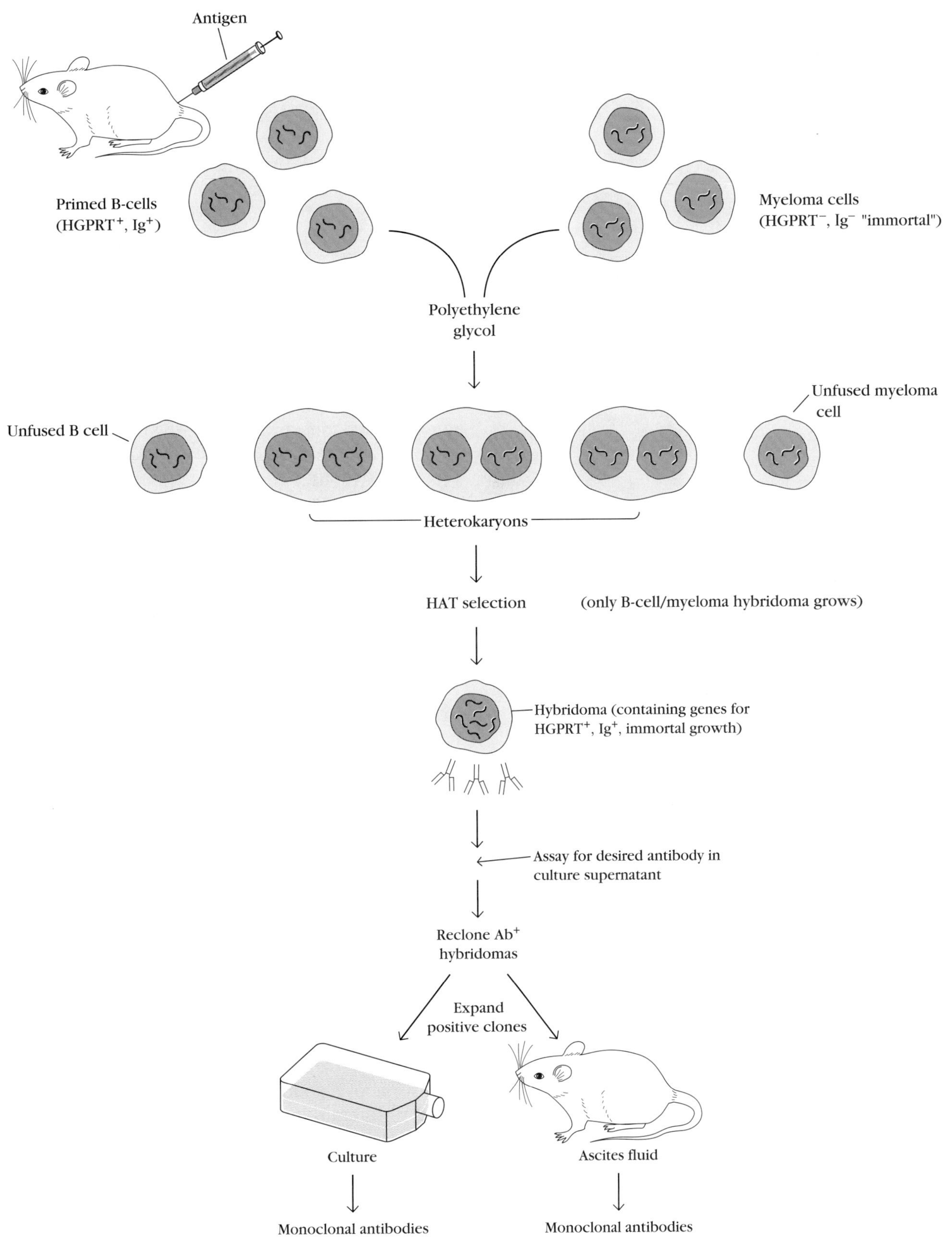

FIGURE 7-4 The procedure for producing monoclonal antibodies specific for a given antigen developed by G. Kohler and C. Milstein. Spleen cells from an antigen-primed mouse are fused with mouse myeloma cells ($HGPRT^-$ and Ig^-). The spleen cell provides the necessary enzymes for growth on HAT medium, while the myeloma cell provides immortal-growth properties. Unfused myeloma cells or myeloma/myeloma fusions fail to grow due to lack of HGPRT. Unfused spleen cells have limited growth and therefore do not need an enzyme deficiency for elimination with the HAT selection procedure.

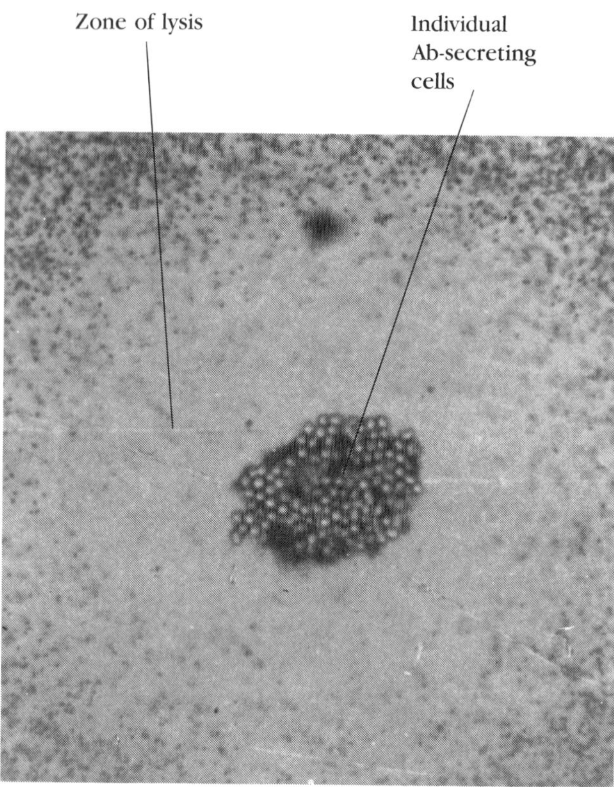

FIGURE 7-5 Viable hybridoma clone that appeared after culture for 7–10 days in HAT selection medium. The individual cells in the clone are visible. This particular clone secreted monoclonal antibody to sheep red blood cells (SRBCs). When SRBCs and complement were added, the anti-SRBC antibody diffusing out from the secreting cells caused complement-mediated lysis of the red blood cells, producing the visible clear zone. [From C. Milstein, 1980, *Sci. Am.* **243**:67.]

antibody is conjugated to an enzyme that produces a colored reaction product when the appropriate substrate is added (Figure 7-6). In an RIA the anti-isotype antibody is radiolabeled; bound label can be detected by counting the wells individually in a gamma counter, or the entire plate can be exposed to x-ray film.

If the desired monoclonal antibody is specific for a cell-membrane molecule, immunofluorescent techniques can be used for screening. In this case, target cells with the particular cell-membrane antigen are stained with the monoclonal antibody in microtiter wells and visualized by the addition of a fluorochrome-conjugated anti-isotype antibody (see Figure 6-17). Alternatively, a fluorescence-activated cell sorter can be modified to microsample labeled target cells taken from the microtiter wells.

Propagating Hybridomas Secreting Specific Monoclonal Antibodies

Once a hybridoma secreting a monoclonal antibody of the desired specificity has been identified, it should be recloned by limiting dilution to ensure that the culture is truly monoclonal. The cloned hybridoma can then be propagated in one of several ways to produce the desired monoclonal antibody. When a hybridoma is grown in tissue-culture flasks, the antibody is secreted into the medium at fairly low concentrations (10–100 μg/ml). A hybridoma also can be propagated in the peritoneal cavity of histocompatible mice, where it secretes the monoclonal antibody into the ascites fluid at much higher concentrations (1–25 mg/ml); the antibody can then be purified from the mouse ascites fluid by chromatography.

To meet the increased demand for monoclonal antibodies, biotechnology companies have been developing various techniques to increase yields. Damon Biotech Company encapsulates hybridomas in alginate gels, which allow nutrients to flow in and waste products and antibodies to flow out. In these capsules, hybridoma cells can achieve much higher densities than in tissue culture; as a result, 100-fold greater yields of antibody production have been attained by this method than with conventional tissue culture. A different approach has been taken by Celltech in England. In this company's method, hybridomas are grown in 1000-liter fermenters, which yield 100 grams of monoclonal antibody in a 2-week period. Further scale-ups to 10,000-liter fermenters are being developed.

Producing Human Monoclonal Antibody

The homogeneity and specificity of monoclonal antibodies make them particularly suitable for in vivo administration in humans for diagnostic or therapeutic purposes. However, a major obstacle to the clinical use of monoclonal antibodies in humans is that they are usually mouse antibodies and therefore are recognized as foreign, inducing an anti-isotype response. For human clinical intervention the use of human monoclonal antibodies is preferable, thus avoiding any anti-isotype response.

The production of human monoclonal antibody, however, has been hampered by a number of technical difficulties. First and foremost is the difficulty of obtaining antigen-primed B cells in humans (equivalent to the mouse spleen cells shown in Figure 7-4). Human hybridomas must be prepared from human peripheral blood, which contains few activated B cells

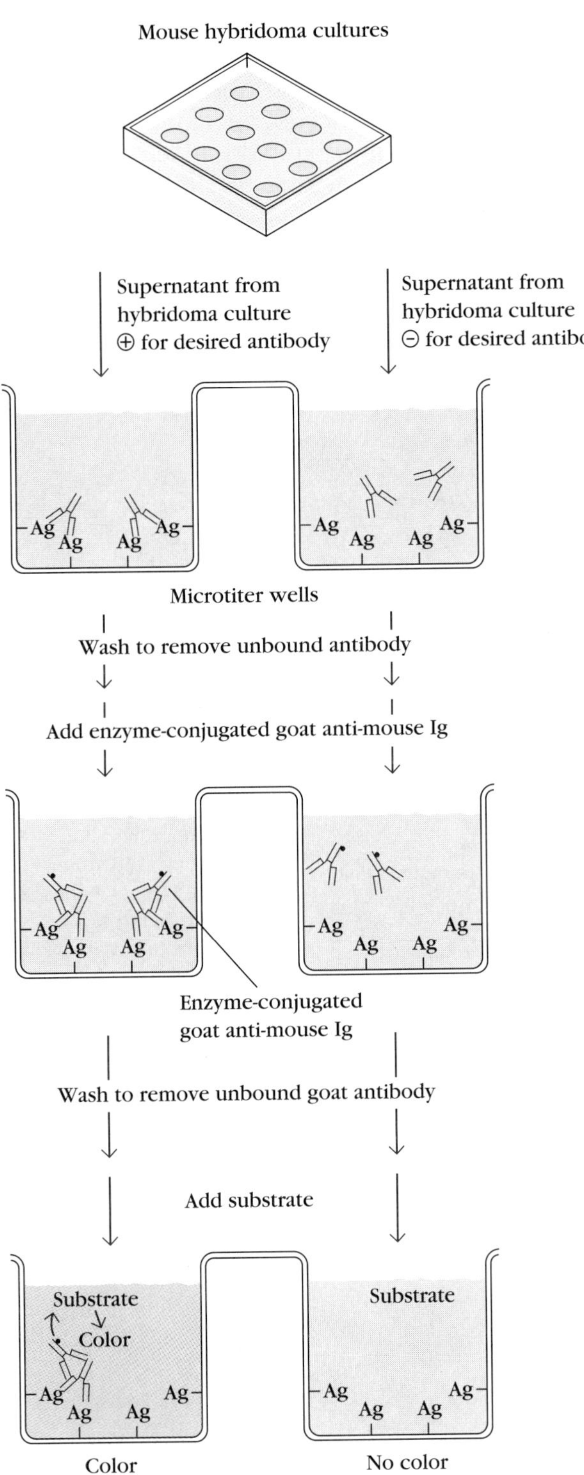

FIGURE 7-6 ELISA screening of mouse hybridomas for those secreting monoclonal antibody of desired specificity. Microtiter wells are coated with the desired antigen, and supernatant from each hybridoma culture is added to a well. After incubation to allow antibody to bind, the unbound antibody is washed away. An enzyme-conjugated goat anti-mouse antibody is then added. This anti-isotype antibody will bind to the mouse monoclonal antibody. After any unbound goat antibody is washed away, a substrate for the conjugated enzyme is added. If the original supernatant contains antibody specific for the antigen, a colored reaction product will be formed on addition of substrate *(left)*. The absence of color *(right)* indicates that the tested hybridoma does not secrete the desired antibody.

engaged in an immune response. It is possible to obtain B cells primed in response to the antigens in accepted vaccines, but one simply cannot immunize a human volunteer with the range of antigens that can be given to mice or other animals. Immunization in the human system must therefore be done using an in vitro cell-culture system. Because the in vitro system cannot mimic the normal microenvironment of lymphoid tissue, the B cells usually produce only low-affinity IgM antibody. Recently, this limitation was overcome by using an allogeneic system in which lymphocytes from two different individuals were cultured together. When antigen was added to the culture, the allogeneic cells in the culture had stimulated intense T-cell activity, providing sufficient helper activity to enable the B cells to produce higher-affinity antibody of the IgG class.

One way to avoid the need for in vitro priming of human B cells is to incorporate genes encoding human antibody within mice. *Scid*-human mice, for example, contain human B and T cells (see Figure 2-1). Following immunization of these mice, activated human B cells can be isolated and used to produce human monoclonal antibodies. Using another approach, GenPharm International has turned off the heavy- and light-chain genes within mice and then introduced yeast artificial chromosomes engineered with large DNA sequences containing human heavy- and light-chain genes. These mice are then able to produce human antibody.

Another major difficulty in producing human monoclonal antibodies has been finding a suitable fusion partner for the B cell—one that has the three important attributes: immortal growth, susceptibility to HAT selection, and inability to secrete its own antibody. The first human hybridomas were produced by fusing human peripheral-blood lymphocytes with human myeloma cells. Unlike mouse myeloma cells, these human myeloma cells did not display immortal growth in culture and instead exhibited a short life span in culture. So far, only a few human myeloma cell lines have been adapted to long-term culture, and these cells continue to secrete their own antibodies. In addition, the induction of mutations to allow for HAT selection increased the cells' instability. In an attempt to bypass these limitations of human fusion partners, some researchers have fused human B cells with mouse myeloma cells (Ab^-, $HGPRT^-$). These mouse-human hybrids have proved to be unstable, however, rapidly losing their human chromosomes and thus their antibody genes.

One way to circumvent these limitations of human myeloma cells is to avoid them altogether. Normal human B lymphocytes can be transformed with Epstein-Barr virus (EBV). When lymphocytes are cultured with antigen in the presence of EBV, some of the B cells acquire the immortal-growth properties of a transformed cell while continuing to secrete the desired antibody. Cloning of such primed, transformed cells has permitted production of human monoclonal antibody.

Uses for Monoclonal Antibodies

Monoclonal antibodies are the reagents of choice for a rapidly growing market of in vitro and in vivo diagnostic products and therapeutics. Total sales of monoclonal antibody products were about $1 billion in 1990. Initially, monoclonal antibodies were used primarily as in vitro diagnostic reagents. In vivo uses of monoclonal antibodies, in the area of in vivo diagnostic tests and immunotherapy, are predicted to expand greatly during the late 1990s. The Center for Exploitation of Science and Technology (CEST) estimates that the total market for therapeutic and imaging monoclonal antibodies will reach $1 billion in 1994, rising to $6 billion by the end of the century.

Purification of Proteins

Before the advent of monoclonal antibodies, the purification of minor protein components from a complex mixture of proteins often required numerous chromatographic steps and generally had low yields. However, monoclonal antibody can be made to even a minor protein (X) in a complex mixture, since any hybridoma clones that secrete antibody to proteins other than X are eliminated during the screening phase of monoclonal production. Once monoclonal antibody to a particular protein is available, it can be used to purify that protein.

This approach was used by D. S. Secher and D. C. Burke to obtain highly purified preparations of interferon, which previously had been purified from white blood cells to only a 1% purity level (i.e., 99% of the preparation was contaminating protein). In their work, Secher and Burke produced monoclonal antibody to interferon (IFN) using a partially purified preparation to immunize mice. They then attached the anti-IFN monoclonal antibody to beads, thus forming an *immunoadsorbent* column. When they passed a crude IFN preparation through this column, they achieved a

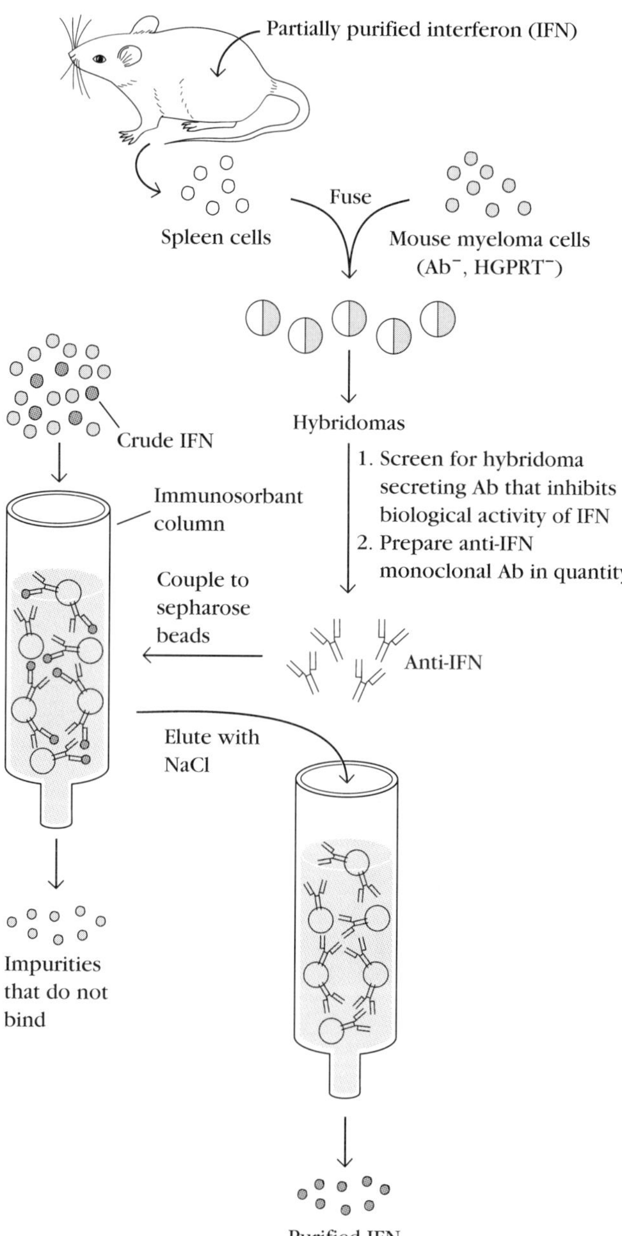

FIGURE 7-7 Purification of interferon (IFN) by use of an immunosorbent column. This technique can be used to purify any protein for which a monoclonal antibody is available.

5000-fold increase in interferon purity in a single passage (Figure 7-7). Large-scale production of interferon is now being performed by a number of biotechnology companies. Interferon is first produced in genetically engineered bacteria, and an anti-IFN immunoadsorbent column is then used to isolate the interferon from the bacterial products and other contaminants.

Identification and Isolation of Lymphocyte Subpopulations and Clones

Monoclonal antibodies can be used to identify and isolate various lymphocyte subpopulations that express characteristic patterns of membrane proteins. Since these proteins reflect the cells' state of differentiation, monoclonal antibodies specific for each of these membrane proteins can be applied to identify the various stages of lymphocyte differentiation. For example, as discussed in previous chapters, T helper cells express CD4 membrane protein and T cytotoxic cells express CD8 membrane protein in both humans and mice. If monoclonal antibodies to CD4 and CD8 are labeled with two different fluorochromes and incubated with a lymphocyte preparation, the T_H cells and T_C cells can then be separated in a fluorescence-activated cell sorter (Figure 7-8; see also Figure 6-17). Alternatively, a given subpopulation can be removed from a preparation by treating the preparation with monoclonal antibody and complement, causing lysis of the cells for which the monoclonal antibody is specific.

Monoclonal antibodies also can be made to cell-membrane proteins that are unique to certain lymphocyte clones. These antibodies, called *clonotypic* monoclonal antibodies, have been useful in the identification of proteins that are unique to a given cell lineage. For example, clonotypic monoclonal antibodies were instrumental in identification of the T-cell receptor, as is discussed in Chapter 11.

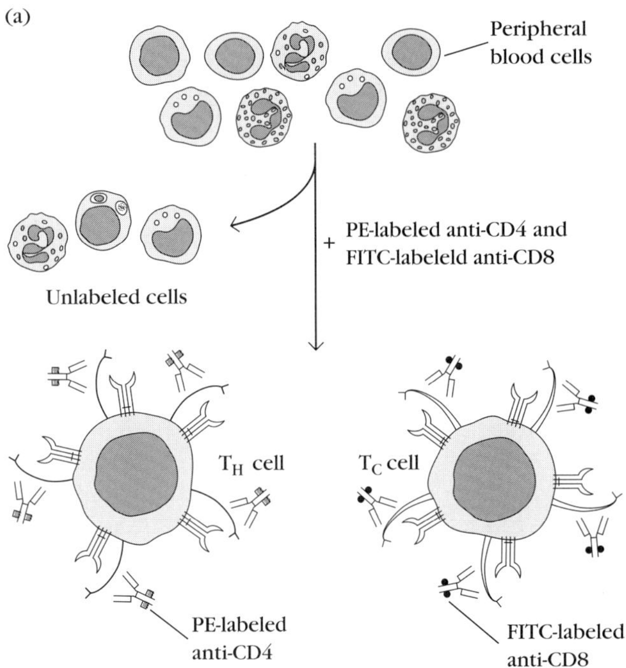

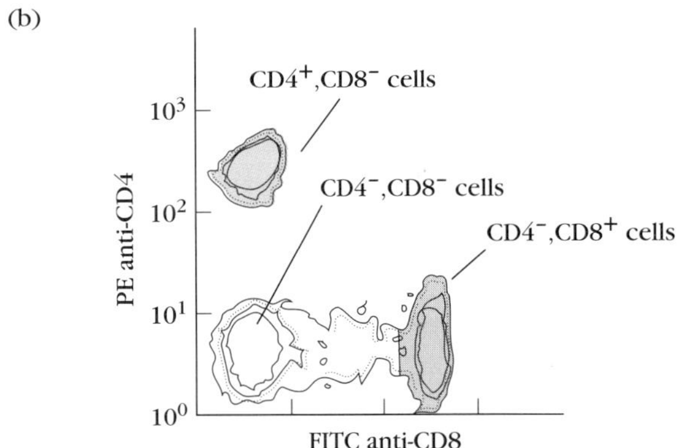

FIGURE 7-8 Separation of T_H cells and T_C cells from human peripheral-blood lymphocytes. (a) Monoclonal antibodies to CD4, which is generally present on T_H cells, and to CD8, which is generally present on T_C cells, are labeled with one of two fluorochromes: phycoerythrin (PE) or fluorescein isothiocyanate (FITC). When the labeled antibodies are incubated with peripheral lymphocytes, the T_H and T_C cells are labeled specifically. (b) Sorting in a FACS reveals three populations of cells, which can be separated.

Tumor Detection and Imaging

Monoclonal antibodies specific for certain tumor-associated membrane proteins can be produced; these proteins are present on tumor cells but are absent from normal cells (or present at much lower levels). Production of such monoclonal antibodies is a time-consuming task that involves screening of large numbers of hybridomas to identify clones secreting antibody specific for the tumor-associated antigens. The magnitude of this task is illustrated by the work of J. Minna, F. Cuttita, and S. Rosen, who immunized mice with human lung-cancer cells and fused the immunized spleen cells with mouse myeloma cells to generate hybridomas secreting monoclonal antibody to human lung-cancer cells. By screening 20,000 hybridoma clones, they were able to identify 80 clones that were specific for various lung-cancer cells and did not react against normal lung cells. One of these monoclonals displayed specificity for small-cell carcinoma of the lung, which accounts for 25% of human lung cancer in the United States. Monoclonal antibodies with such tumor specificity can be used either to detect the spread of tumors or to kill tumor cells.

Certain tumors shed tumor-specific antigen(s) into the blood, and the use of monoclonal antibodies for detection of such tumors has great potential. For example, in one study monoclonal antibody to a glycolipid antigen shed by colorectal tumors was able to detect this tumor-specific antigen in blood samples from 23 out of 33 patients with advanced colorectal cancer. A monoclonal antibody that detects a shed pancreatic tumor antigen also has been developed. This monoclonal antibody has considerable diagnostic value because the level of this pancreatic tumor antigen in the blood is indicative of the stage of tumor progression. The ability of monoclonal antibody to detect even low levels of this shed tumor antigen may allow early diagnosis of pancreatic cancer, which is not usually diagnosed until an advanced stage.

In another approach, radiolabeled monoclonal antibodies have been used to locate primary or metastatic tumors in patients. For example, monoclonal antibody to breast-cancer cells labeled with iodine-131 has been introduced into the blood to detect tumor spread to regional lymph nodes. This monoclonal imaging technique can detect breast-cancer metastases that would be undetected by other scanning techniques. Other researchers have labeled monoclonal antibody to breast-cancer cells with the metal gadolinium (Gd), which can be detected by magnetic resonance imaging (MRI) techniques. Following injection of Gd-labeled monoclonal antibody into the blood of breast-cancer patients, pinhead-sized metastases to regional lymph nodes have been visualized.

Although these approaches for detecting and localizing tumors have promise, there are a number of obstacles to widespread use of monoclonal antibodies in tumor detection and imaging. A major problem is that many tumors of a given type, such as breast cancer, do not share common tumor-specific membrane proteins. In one study five monoclonal antibodies to human breast tumors were reacted with breast-cancer biopsy tissue from 45 patients. Most of the biopsy samples reacted with only one of the five antibodies.

Tumor Killing

Monoclonal antibodies can also kill tumor cells, in some cases doing the job directly through complement-mediated lysis. Unconjugated monoclonal antibodies have been used with some success in treating human B-cell lymphomas and T-cell leukemias. In one remarkable study, Ronald Levy and his colleagues successfully treated a 64-year-old man with terminal B-cell lymphoma. At the time of treatment the lymphoma had metastasized to the liver, spleen, bone marrow, and peripheral blood. Because this cancer was of a B cell, the membrane-bound antibody on all the cancerous cells had the same idiotype. These researchers initially fused cancerous B-lymphoma cells from the patient with human myeloma cells to obtain a hybridoma secreting the B-lymphoma antibody. This monoclonal antibody bearing the identifying idiotype then served as an antigen to immunize mice, and the mouse spleen cells were fused with mouse myeloma cells. The resulting hybridomas were screened to find one that secreted monoclonal antibody specific for the B-lymphoma idiotype (Figure 7-9). When this mouse monoclonal antibody was injected into the patient, it bound specifically to the B-lymphoma cells because these cells expressed that particular idiotype. Since B-lymphoma cells are susceptible to complement-mediated lysis, the monoclonal antibody activated the complement system and lysed the lymphoma cells without harming other cells. After four injections with this anti-idiotype monoclonal antibody, the tumors began to shrink, and as of the last report this patient has been in complete remission.

Although a large number of tumor cells are resistant to complement-mediated lysis, tumor-specific monoclonal antibody can be conjugated to a lethal toxin or a radioisotope to form an *immunotoxin* capable of killing tumor cells. Several toxins lend themselves to this approach, including ricin, *Shigella* toxin, and diphtheria toxin, all of which inhibit protein synthesis and are so potent that a single molecule has been shown to kill a cell. Each of these toxins consists of two or more functionally distinct polypeptide components, one the toxin itself and the other a ligand that binds to receptors on cell surfaces; without the binding polypeptide the toxin cannot get into cells and therefore is harmless. An immunotoxin is prepared by replacing the binding polypeptide with a monoclonal antibody having specificity for a particular tumor cell (Figure 7-10a). In theory, the attached monoclonal antibody will target the toxin specifically to tumor cells, where it will cause cell death by inhibiting protein synthesis (Figure 7-10b). The high toxicity of the toxin is important, since very few molecules of an immunotoxin will actually make contact with the tumor mass. Several in vitro studies with toxin-conjugated monoclonal antibodies have demonstrated their ability to kill tumor cells without killing normal healthy cells.

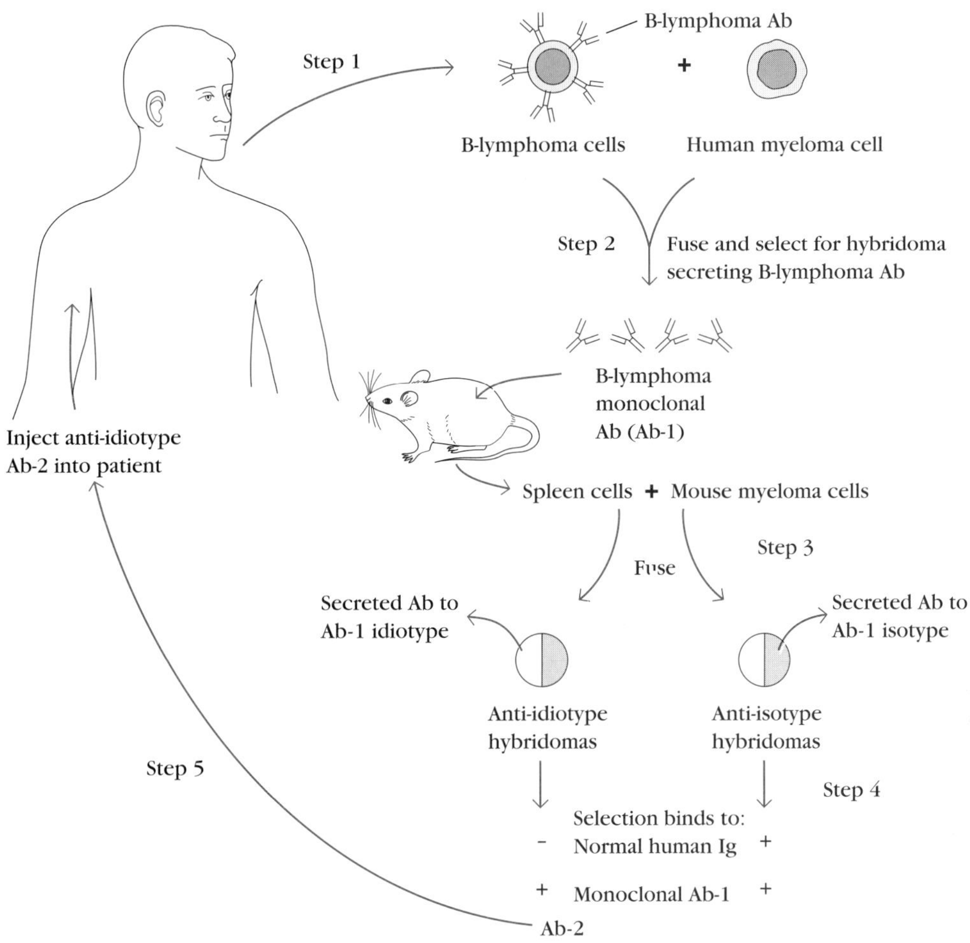

FIGURE 7-9 Treatment of a man with B-cell lymphoma with monoclonal antibody specific for idiotypic determinants on the B-lymphoma cells. Because all the lymphoma cells are derived from a single transformed B cell, they all express membrane-bound antibody (Ab-1) with the same idiotype (i.e., same antigenic specificity). In the procedure illustrated, monoclonal anti-idiotype antibody (Ab-2) against the B-lymphoma antibody was produced (steps 1–4). When this anti-idiotype antibody was injected into the patient (step 5), it bound to B-lymphoma cells, which then were susceptible to complement-mediated lysis.

A number of phase I or phase II clinical trials using immunotoxins have been completed and a number of other clinical trials are ongoing. Included among these trials are immunotoxins directed against cell-membrane antigens of melanoma, colorectal carcinoma, metastatic breast carcinoma, various lymphomas and leukemias, and graft-versus-host disease. In general the clinical responses reported in leukemia and lymphoma patients were quite good; in eight separate trials 12–75% of the patients exhibited partial or complete remission. In contrast, the responses in patients with larger tumor masses were disappointing. It is thought that the tumor mass may render most of the tumor cells inaccessible to the immunotoxin.

Diagnostic Reagents

More than 100 different monoclonal antibody diagnostic products are currently available. These include products for detecting pregnancy; diagnosing infectious protozoan, bacterial, and viral pathogens; monitoring therapeutic drug levels; detecting heart damage; matching histocompatibility antigens; detecting diabetes; and detecting tumor cells. Many of these test kits utilize strips of paper impregnated with an appropriate monoclonal antibody. Since the diagnostic products are relatively inexpensive to produce and are projected to have a growing market, many biotechnology companies have entered the field.

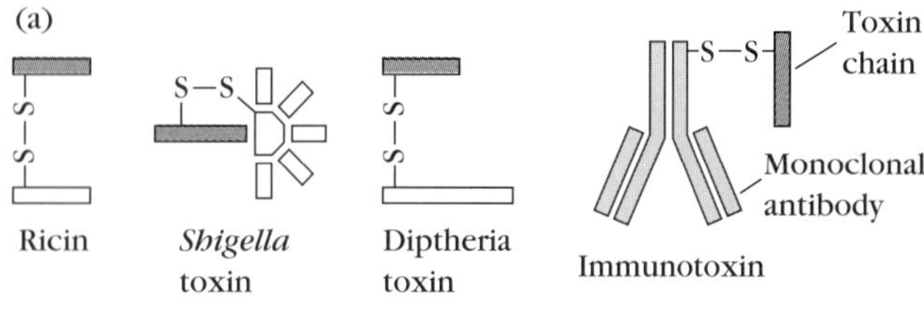

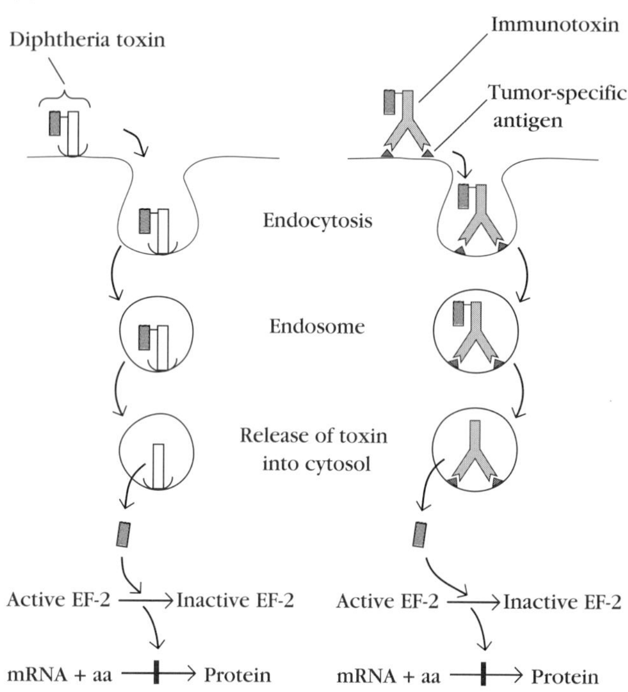

FIGURE 7-10 (a) Toxins used to prepare immunotoxins include ricin, *Shigella* toxin and diphtheria toxin. Each toxin contains an inhibitor chain (purple) and a binding component. To make an immunotoxin, the binding component of the toxin is replaced with a monoclonal antibody. (b) Diphtheria toxin binds to a cell-membrane receptor *(left)* and a diphtheria-immunotoxin binds to a tumor-associated antigen *(right)*. In either case the toxin is internalized in an endosome. The toxic chain is then released into the cytoplasm, where it inhibits protein synthesis by catalyzing the inactivation of elongation factor 2 (EF-2).

Engineered Monoclonal Antibodies

When mouse monoclonal antibodies are used as immunotoxins for tumor killing, they generally must be given in high concentrations to bind sufficient amounts of antibody to the tumor. However, these mouse monoclonal antibodies are recognized as foreign and evoke an antibody response. The induced human anti-mouse antibodies quickly reduce the effectiveness of the immunotoxin by clearing it from the bloodstream. In addition, circulating complexes of mouse and human antibodies can cause allergic reactions. In some cases the buildup of these complexes in organs such as the kidney can cause serious and even life-threatening reactions.

These undesirable reactions place limitations on the use of mouse monoclonal antibodies for tumor detection and killing in humans. Clearly, one way to overcome at least some of these complications is to use human monoclonal antibodies. However, as discussed previously, the development of human monoclonal antibodies has been hampered by considerable technical difficulties. Because of the problems in producing human monoclonal antibodies and the complications resulting from in vivo use of mouse monoclonal antibodies, researchers have begun engineering monoclonal antibody using recombinant DNA technology.

Chimeric Monoclonal Antibodies

One approach to engineering an antibody is to clone recombinant DNA containing the promoter, leader, and variable-region sequences from a mouse antibody gene and the constant-region exons from a human antibody gene (Figure 7-11). The antibody encoded by such a recombinant gene is a mouse-human chimera, commonly known as a ***humanized*** antibody. Its antigenic specificity, which is determined by the variable region, is derived from the mouse DNA; its isotype, which is determined by the constant region, is derived from the human DNA (Figure 7-12a). Because their constant regions are encoded by human genes, these chimeric antibodies have fewer mouse antigenic determinants and are far less immunogenic than mouse monoclonal antibodies when administered to humans. Another advantage of a chimeric antibody is that it retains the biological effector functions of the human antibody and is more likely to trigger complement activation or Fc receptor binding.

Because the mouse variable region in these humanized antibodies can also induce an antibody response in humans, chimeric antibodies containing only mouse CDRs have been developed. In this novel approach, the CDRs of a mouse antibody are grafted together with human framework regions to construct a variable region retaining the human β-strand framework with only the hypervariable loops of mouse origin (Figure 7-12b). These antibodies are less immunogenic in humans than humanized antibodies

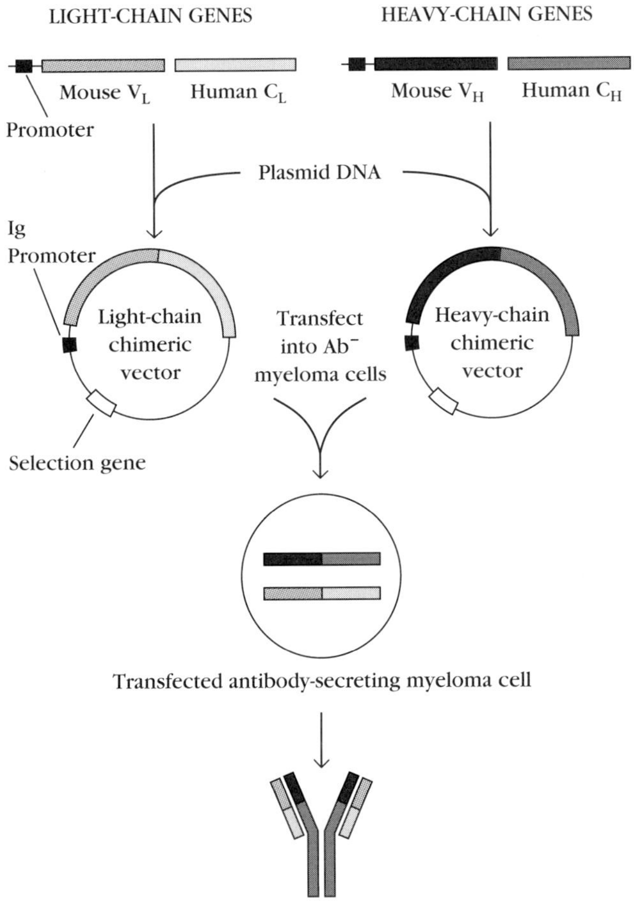

FIGURE 7-11 Production of chimeric mouse-human monoclonal antibodies. Chimeric mouse-human heavy- and light-chain λ expression vectors are produced. These vectors are transfected into Ab$^-$ myeloma cells. Culture in ampicillin medium selects for transfected myeloma cells, which secrete the chimeric antibody. [Adapted from M. Verhoeyen and L. Reichmann, 1988, *BioEssays* **8**:74.]

containing the entire mouse variable region. Since the hypervariable loops compose the antigen-binding site, sometimes CDR-grafted antibodies retain their ability to bind antigen. Often, however, CDR-grafted antibodies exhibit reduced binding affinity. In some cases, this can be corrected by introducing small mutations in the framework region that induce small changes in the three-dimensional configuration of the CDRs resulting in improved antibody affinity. CDR-grafted antibodies have been used in a number of clinical trials. In one study clinical remission was obtained in two patients with non-Hodgkin's lymphoma by giving them daily injections of CDR-grafted monoclonal antibody specific for a cell membrane antigen on the lymphoma cells. Table 7-1 lists some of the CDR-grafted monoclonal antibodies that are presently being assessed in clinical trials.

The chimera approach also can be used to engineer an antibody with a constant region possessing a given biological effector function. For example, the $\gamma 1$ constant region in humans is very effective at mediating complement lysis. By engineering antitumor antibodies with a $\gamma 1$ constant region, it is hoped that complement-mediated destruction of tumor cells can be enhanced. Another approach has been to replace the terminal constant-region domain with a toxin (Figure 7-12c). These antibodies serve as immunotoxins, and because they lack the terminal domain of the Fc, they are not able to bind to cells bearing Fc receptors.

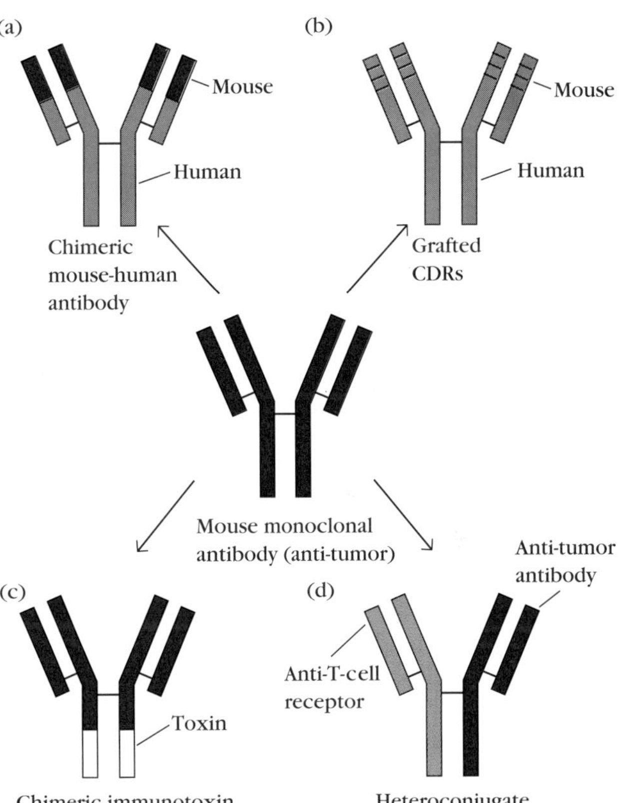

FIGURE 7-12 Recombinant DNA technology has allowed various monoclonal antibodies to be engineered. (a) Chimeric mouse-human monoclonal antibody containing the V_H and V_L domains of the mouse monoclonal antibody and the C_L and C_H domains of a human monoclonal antibody. (b) A chimeric monoclonal antibody containing only the CDRs of a mouse monoclonal antibody grafted within the framework regions of a human monoclonal antibody. (c) A chimeric monoclonal antibody in which the terminal Fc domain is replaced by a toxin. (d) A heteroconjugate in which one-half of the molecule is specific for a tumor antigen and the other half is specific for the CD3/T-cell receptor complex.

TABLE 7-1 THERAPEUTIC USES FOR CDR-GRAFTED ANTIBODIES

Target antigen	Clinical potential
CDw52 (surface molecule on leukocytes)	Lymphomas, systemic vasculitis, rheumatoid arthritis
CD3 (T-cell marker)	Organ transplantation
CD4 (T-cell marker)	Organ transplantation, rheumatoid arthritis, Crohn's disease
Receptor for interleukin 2	Leukemias and lymphomas, organ transplantation, graft-versus-host disease
Tumor necrosis factor α	Septic shock
Human immunodeficiency virus (HIV)	AIDS
Rous sarcoma virus (RSV)	Respiratory syncytial virus infection
Herpes simplex virus (HSV)	Neonatal, ocular, and genital herpes infection
Receptor for human epidermal growth factor (EGF)	Cancer
Placental alkaline phosphatase	Cancer
Carcinoembryonic antigen (CEA)	Cancer

SOURCE: Adapted from G. Winter and W. J. Harris, 1993, *Immunol. Today* **14**:243.

Monoclonal Antibody Heteroconjugates

Heteroconjugates are hybrids of two different antibody molecules (Figure 7-12d). Various heteroconjugates have been designed in which one half of the antibody has specificity for a tumor and the other half has specificity for a surface molecule on an immune effector cell, such as a NK cell, an activated macrophage, or a cytotoxic T lymphocyte (CTL). The heteroconjugate thus serves to cross-link the immune effector cell to the tumor. Some heteroconjugates have been designed to activate the immune effector cell when it is cross-linked to the tumor cell. For example, the T-cell receptor is always expressed as a complex with the associated membrane molecule CD3, which is involved in signal transduction. Heteroconjugates consisting of anti-CD3 and an antitumor monoclonal antibody have been shown to cross-link CTLs to tumor cells. Not only does the heteroconjugate cross-link the CTL to the tumor cell, but it also appears to activate the CTL so that it begins to mediate destruction of the tumor cell.

Monoclonal Antibodies Constructed from Immunoglobulin-Gene Libraries

Recently a new technology has been developed for generating monoclonal antibodies without hybrid-

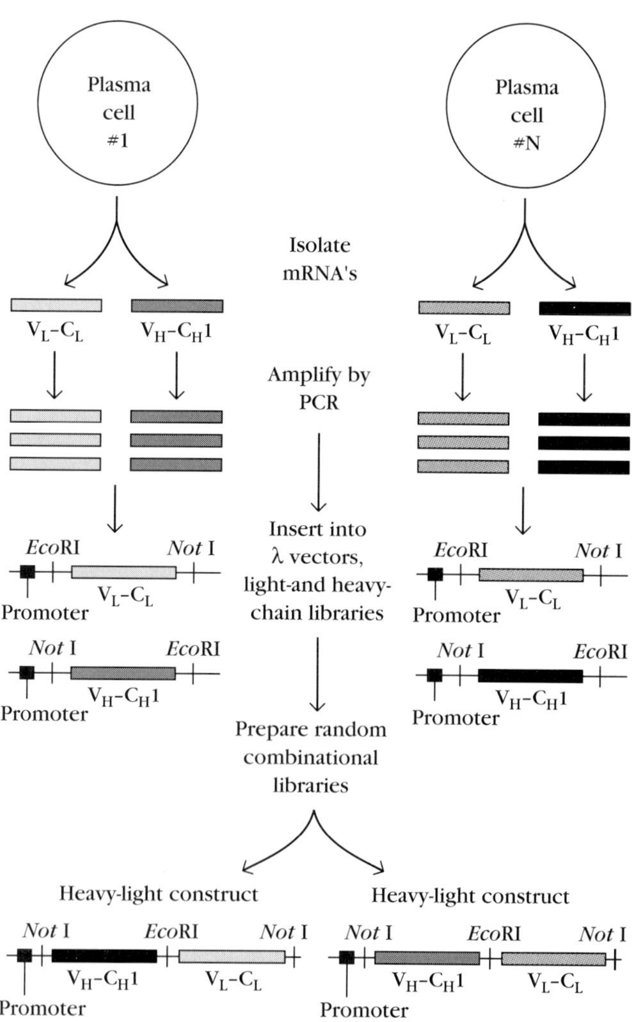

FIGURE 7-13 General procedure for producing gene libraries encoding Fab fragments. In this procedure isolated heavy- and light-chain genes are amplified by the polymerase chain reaction (PCR). Random combinations of heavy- and light-chain genes generate an enormous number of heavy-light constructs encoding Fab fragments. [Adapted from W. D. Huse et al., 1989, *Science* **246**:1275.]

omas or even immunization. In this approach, the polymerase chain reaction is used to amplify the DNA encoding antibody heavy-chain and light-chain Fab fragments from hybridoma cells or plasma cells (see Figure 2-9); separate heavy- and light-chain libraries then are constructed in bacteriophage λ. Each inserted gene contains an *Eco*RI restriction site, downstream of the heavy-chain genes and upstream of the light-chain genes. Cleavage with *Eco*RI and joining of the heavy- and light-chain genes yields numerous random heavy-light constructs (Figure 7-13). This procedure generates an enormous diversity of antibody combinations; clones containing these random combinations can be rapidly screened for those secreting antibody to a particular antigen. For example, in one study a million clones were screened in just 2 days, with over 100 being identified that produced antibody specific for the desired antigen. The technique has the potential of producing an enormous repertoire of antibody specificities without the limitations of antigen priming and hybridoma technology that currently complicate the production of monoclonal antibodies.

Catalytic Monoclonal Antibodies (Abzymes)

The binding of an antibody to its antigen is similar in many ways to the binding of an enzyme to its substrate. In both cases the binding involves weak, noncovalent interactions and exhibits high specificity and often high affinity. What distinguishes an antibody-antigen interaction from an enzyme-substrate interaction is that the antibody does not alter the antigen, whereas the enzyme catalyzes a chemical change in its substrate. The enzyme uses its binding energy to stabilize the transition state of the substrate, thus reducing the activation energy for chemical modification of the bound substrate.

Because of the similarities between antigen-antibody interactions and enzyme-substrate interactions, R. A. Lerner and his colleagues wondered whether some antibodies might behave like enzymes and catalyze chemical reactions. To investigate this possibility, they produced a hapten-carrier complex in which the hapten structurally resembled the transition state of an ester undergoing hydrolysis (Figure 7-14). Using this conjugate, they generated antihapten monoclonal antibodies. When these monoclonal antibodies were incubated with an ester substrate, some of them accelerated hydrolysis by about 1000-fold; that is, they acted like the enzyme that normally catalyzes the substrate's hydrolysis. The catalytic activity of these antibodies was highly specific; that is, they hydrolyzed only esters whose transition-state structure closely resembled that of the hapten in the immunizing conjugate.

Catalytic monoclonal antibodies have been generated that catalyze ester hydrolysis and carbonate

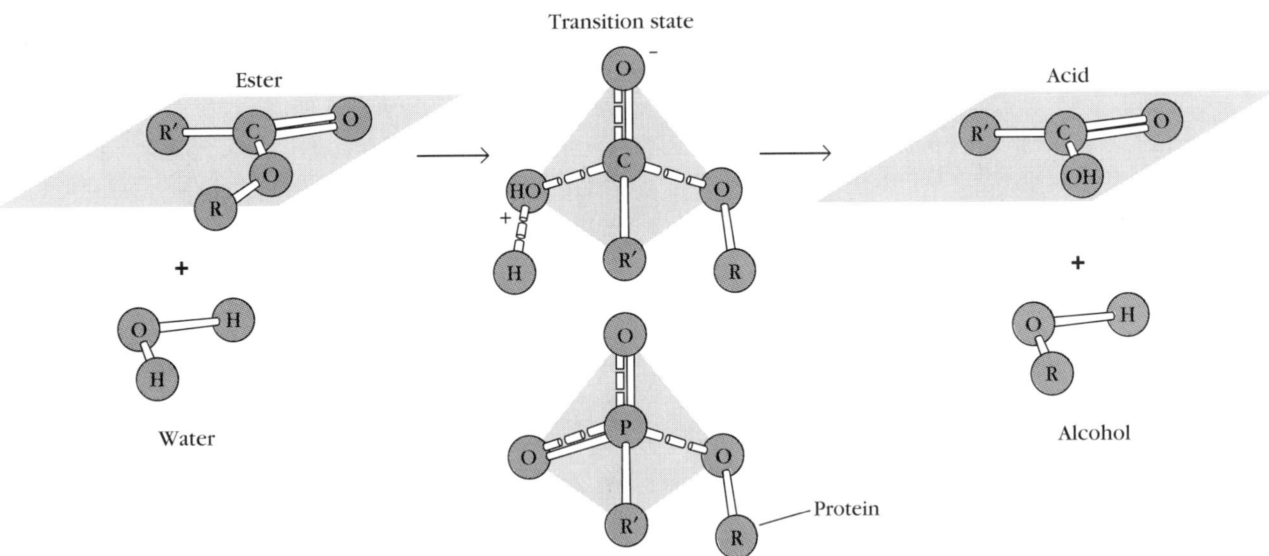

FIGURE 7-14 Because of its tetrahedral shape and partial negative charge, a phosphonate ester (PE) is an analog of the unstable transition state of an ester undergoing hydrolysis. Anti-PE monoclonal antibodies have been obtained by immunizing mice with a PE-carrier conjugate. Some of these anti-PE antibodies catalyze ester hydrolysis, presumably by binding to and stabilizing the transition state. [Adapted from R. A. Lerner and A. Tramontano, 1988, *Sci. Am.* **258**:58.]

hydrolysis. These antibodies have been called *abzymes* in reference to their dual role as antibody and enzyme.

The development of immunoglobulin-gene libraries was pioneered by Lerner to produce an enormous antibody repertoire without the requirement of antigen priming, so that large numbers of antibodies could be screened for their catalytic activity. As more and more abzymes are generated by this method, it may be possible to produce a battery of abzymes that cut peptide bonds at specific amino acid residues, much as restriction enzymes cut DNA at specific sites. Such enzymes would be invaluable tools in facilitating structural and functional analysis of proteins. Additionally, it may be possible to generate abzymes with the ability to dissolve blood clots or to cleave viral glycoproteins at specific sites, thus blocking viral infectivity. Abzymes are likely to represent a major technological advance that will impact on various branches of science in the coming years.

T-Cell Hybridomas

The hybridomas discussed so far are produced by fusion of primed B cells with cancerous plasma cells; these B-cell hybridomas secrete monoclonal antibody. T-cell hybridomas can be produced by fusing primed T cells with cancerous T cells (called thymoma cells) in a similar procedure. T-cell hybridomas do not secrete antibody, but rather possess other immunologic functions (e.g., secretion of cytokines and expression of T-cell receptors specific for a particular antigen-MHC molecule). Antigen-specific T helper and cytotoxic hybridomas have been cloned and have facilitated the identification of various T-cell–specific molecules. For example, an ovalbumin-specific, class II MHC-restricted T-cell hybridoma was used to identify the T-cell receptor for antigen (see Chapter 11). This particular T-cell hybridoma was produced by fusing a T_H cell specific for ovalbumin with a T-cell thymoma. The resulting hybridoma, which displayed the antigenic specificity and MHC restriction of the parent T_H cell, could be assayed for T_H function by its capacity to secrete interleukin 2 in response to ovalbumin on an appropriate antigen-presenting cell. Because T-cell hybridomas grow as tumors, large cell numbers can be attained within a short period of time; this property has facilitated the biochemical isolation and purification of various T-cell products, including several T-cell cytokines.

Summary

1. With the technique of cell fusion and HAT-medium selection, primed splenic lymphocytes can be fused with mouse myeloma cells ($HGPRT^-$, Ab^-). These hybrid cells, called B-cell hybridomas, continue to secrete the specific antibody of the primed B cell but possess the immortal-growth properties of the myeloma cell.

2. Unlike polyclonal antibodies, a monoclonal antibody is a homogeneous preparation specific for a single epitope on a complex antigen.

3. Monoclonal antibodies have been used to purify antigens, to detect cellular subpopulations, and to detect and kill specific tumor cells. In addition, monoclonal antibodies are presently used in over 100 diagnostic tests.

4. Recombinant DNA technology has been used to engineer chimeric monoclonal antibodies consisting of mouse variable regions and human constant regions. These chimeras do not elicit an anti-isotype response when injected into humans.

5. Monoclonal Fab fragments have been produced by random combination of heavy- and light-chain gene libraries constructed in bacteriophage λ. This procedure allows the production of monoclonal antibodies without antigen priming or hybridoma technology.

6. Several catalytic monoclonal antibodies, or abzymes, have been identified. Future screening of large numbers of monoclonal antibodies generated from immunoglobulin-gene libraries may identify other abzymes with useful catalytic functions.

7. T-cell hybridomas, produced by fusion of primed T cells with T-cell thymomas, have been useful in isolating and purifying various cytokines secreted by T cells.

References

DE YOUNG, G. 1986. Monoclonal antibodies: promises fulfilled. *High Technology* (Feb.):32.

HUSE, W. D., L. SASTRY, S. A. IVERSON et. al. 1989. Generation of a large combinatorial library of the immunoglobulin repertoire in phage lambda. *Science* **246**:1275.

JUNG, G., and H. J. MULLER EBERHARD. 1988. An in vitro model for tumor immunotherapy with antibody heteroconjugates. *Immunol. Today* **9**:257.

KOHLER, G., and C. MILSTEIN. 1975. Continuous cultures of fused cells secreting antibody of predefined specificity. *Nature* **256**:495.

LERNER, R. A., and S. J. BENKOVIC. 1988. Principles of antibody catalysis. *BioEssays* **9**:107.

LIU, A. Y., R. R. ROBINSON, K. E. HELLSTROM et al. 1987. Chimeric mouse-human IgG1 antibody that can mediate lysis of cancer cells. *Proc. Natl. Acad. Sci. USA* **84**:3439.

MARX, J. 1982. Monoclonal antibodies in cancer. *Science* **216**:283.

MILSTEIN, C 1980. Monoclonal antibodies. *Sci. Am.* **243**:66.

MORRISON, S. L., and V. T. OI. 1989. Genetically engineered antibody molecules. *Adv. Immunol.* **44**:65.

OLSNES, O., K. SANDVIG, O. W. PETERSEN, and B. VAN DEURS. 1989. Immunotoxin-entry into cells and mechanisms of action. *Immunol. Today* **10**:291.

REICHMAN, L., M. CLARK, H. WALDMANN, and G. WINTER. 1988. Reshaping human antibodies for therapy. *Nature* **332**:323.

VERHOEYEN, M., and L. RIECHMANN. 1988. Engineering of antibodies. *BioEssays* **8**:74.

VITETTA, E. S., P. E. THORPE, and J. W. UHR. 1993. Immunotoxins: magic bullets or misguided missiles? *Immunol. Today* **14**:252.

WINTER, G., and W. J. HARRIS. 1993. Humanized antibodies. *Immunol. Today* **14**:243.

WINTER, G., and C. MILSTEIN. 1991. Man made antibodies. *Nature* **349**:293.

Study Questions

1. Indicate whether each of the following statements is true or false. If you think a statement is false, explain why.
   a. An HGPRT$^+$ myeloma cell requires hypoxanthine for growth.
   b. When a heterokaryon initially is formed, it is multinucleated.
   c. Chromosome loss from heterokaryons occurs randomly.
   d. Hypoxanthine is added to HAT medium to prevent cell growth by the salvage pathway.
   e. An HGPRT$^+$ revertant myeloma cell would be a good fusion partner for production of B-cell hybridomas because it would not be able to grow in HAT medium.

2. The myeloma cells used in the production of B-cell hybridomas have three properties that make them suitable fusion partners. List these properties and explain why they are necessary for the production of hybridomas that secrete B-cell antibodies.

3. What would be the consequences if you omitted aminopterin from the HAT medium used to select hybridomas in the standard procedure for producing monoclonal antibodies.

4. In order to treat a patient with terminal B-cell lymphoma, Levy and his coworkers produced two hybridomas. One hybridoma was obtained by fusing B-lymphoma cells from the patient with human myeloma cells; the other was obtained by fusing primed mouse spleen cells with mouse myeloma cells.
   a. Why did the researchers produce these two hybridomas and what was the desired monoclonal antibody secreted by each?
   b. Outline a screening assay for identifying hybridomas that produce the desired monoclonal antibody. What kind of control should be included in the screening assay?

5. You immunize a mouse with human interleukin 2 (IL-2) and purify the antibodies against IL-2 from its serum. List three ways in which these antibodies differ from a monoclonal antibody specific for IL-2.

6. Polyclonal antibodies usually precipitate soluble protein antigens, whereas monoclonal antibodies to the same protein antigens often fail to do so. What might account for this difference?

7. Although monoclonal antibodies are by definition reactive with a single antigenic determinant, they sometimes react with more than one antigen. Explain this finding.

8. You have produced a monoclonal antibody that binds to a particular protein antigen, as determined by a solid-phase ELISA. Even though this antibody has a high affinity for the antigen, why might it fail to react in (a) an immunodiffusion assay, (b) a Western-blot assay, and (c) a tube precipitation assay.

9. You produced a monoclonal antibody A to HIV and suspect that it has been stolen by a colleague and is now being marketed by a biotechnology company as monoclonal B. You want to prove that the company's product is the same as the monoclonal antibody that you isolated.
   a. Describe two quick and inexpensive immunologic tests that you could perform to determine if monoclonal A and B might be identical.
   b. Assuming these initial tests suggest that the two antibodies are identical, what more expensive and time-consuming procedures could you use to

demonstrate unequivocally whether or not A and B are the same?

10. You fuse spleen cells having a normal genotype for immunoglobulin heavy chains (H) and light chains (L) with three myeloma-cell preparations differing in their immunoglobulin genotype as follows: (a) H^+, L^+; (b) H^-, L^+; and (c) H^-, L^-. For each hybridoma, predict how many unique antigen-binding sites theoretically could be produced and show the chain structure of the possible antibody molecules. For each possible antibody molecule indicate whether the chains would originate from the spleen (s) or from the myeloma (m) fusion partner (e.g., H_sL_s/H_mL_m).

11. An immunotoxin is prepared by conjugating a monoclonal antibody specific for a tumor antigen with diphtheria toxin. If the antibody part of the immunotoxin is degraded in vivo and the toxin is not, will normal cells be killed? Explain.

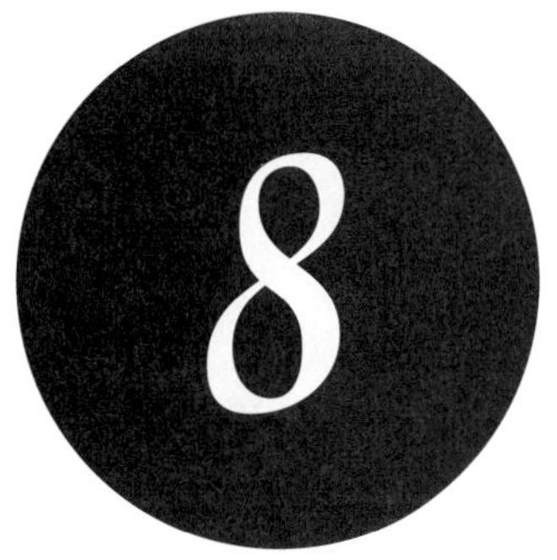

ORGANIZATION AND EXPRESSION OF IMMUNOGLOBULIN GENES

One of the most remarkable features of the vertebrate immune system is its ability to respond to an apparently limitless array of foreign antigens. As immunoglobulin sequence data accumulated, virtually every antibody molecule studied was found to contain a unique amino acid sequence in its variable region but only one of a limited number of invariant sequences in its constant region. The genetic basis of such tremendous variation coupled with constancy in a single protein molecule lies in the organization of the immunoglobulin genes. In germ-line DNA, multiple gene segments encode a single immunoglobulin heavy or light chain. These gene segments are carried in the germ cells but cannot be transcribed and translated into heavy and light chains until they are arranged into functional genes. During B-cell differentiation in the bone marrow, these gene segments are randomly shuffled by a dynamic genetic system capable of generating more than 10^8 specificities. This process is carefully regulated: B-cell differentiation from a progenitor B cell to a mature cell involves an ordered progression of immunoglobulin-gene rearrangements. By the end of this process a mature, immunocompetent B cell will contain a single, functional variable-region DNA sequence for its heavy chain, and a single, functional variable-region DNA sequence for its light chain, so that the individual B cell is antigenically committed to a

TABLE 8-1 SEQUENCE OF STAGES IN B-LYMPHOCYTE MATURATION AND DIFFERENTIATION

Cell stage	Site of maturation/ differentiation	Ig expressed	Isotype switching	Antigen required
Lymphoid stem cell	Bone marrow	None	No	No
Progenitor B cell	Bone marrow	None	No	No
Pre-B cell	Bone marrow	μ heavy chain	No	No
Immature B cell	Bone marrow	mIgM	No	No
Mature B cell	Periphery	mIgM + mIgD	No	No
Activated B cell	Periphery	Mostly mIg of various isotypes	Yes	Yes
Plasma cell	Periphery	Mostly secreted Ig of various isotypes	No	Yes
Memory cell	Periphery	mIg of various isotypes	Yes	Yes

specific epitope. After antigenic stimulation, further rearrangement of constant-region gene segments can generate changes in the isotype expressed, producing changes in the associated biological effector functions, without changing the specificity of the immunoglobulin molecule (Table 8-1).

This chapter describes the detailed organization of the immunoglobulin genes, the process of gene rearrangement, and the role of differential RNA processing of the primary transcript in the expression of immunoglobulin genes. The relationship of gene rearrangements to various stages in B-cell differentiation also is explored. Finally, the various mechanisms by which the dynamic immunoglobulin genetic system generates more than 10^8 different antibody specificities are discussed.

Genetic Model Compatible with Immunoglobulin Structure

The results of the immunoglobulin-sequencing studies discussed in Chapter 5 revealed a number of features of immunoglobulin structure that were difficult to reconcile with classic genetic models. Any viable model of the immunoglobulin genes has to account for (a) the vast diversity of antibody specificities, (b) the presence of a variable region at the amino-terminal end and of a constant region at the carboxyl-terminal end of heavy and light chains, and (c) the existence of isotypes with the same antigenic specificity, which result from the association of a given variable region with different heavy-chain constant regions.

Germ-Line and Somatic-Variation Models

It has been estimated that the mammalian immune system can generate more than 10^8 different antibody specificities, allowing an animal to respond to a vast number of potential antigens. Since antibodies are proteins and proteins are encoded by genes, it follows that this tremendous diversity in antibody structure must arise from a genetic system capable of generating tremendous diversity. For several decades immunologists sought to imagine a genetic mechanism that might generate such diversity. There emerged two very different sets of theories to explain the observed variability in antibody specificity at the gene level. The *germ-line* theories maintained that the genome contains a large repertoire of immunoglobulin genes sufficient to generate more than 10^8 different antibody specificities; thus no special genetic mechanisms were invoked to account for antibody diversity in these theories. In contrast, the *somatic-variation* theories maintained that the genome contains a relatively small number of immunoglobulin genes from which a large number of antibody specificities are generated in the somatic cells by mutational or recombinational mechanisms.

As the amino acid sequences of more and more immunoglobulins were determined, it became clear that there must be mechanisms not only for generating antibody diversity but also for maintaining constancy. In other words, whether diversity was generated by germ-line or somatic mechanisms, a paradox remained: How could stability be maintained in the constant (C) region while some kind of diversifying mechanism generated the variable (V) region?

Neither the germ-line nor somatic variation proponents could offer a reasonable explanation of this central feature of immunoglobulin structure. Germ-line proponents found it difficult to account for an evolutionary mechanism that could generate diversity in the variable part of each gene while preserving the constant region unchanged. Somatic-variation proponents found it difficult to conceive of a mechanism that could diversify the variable region of a single gene in the somatic cells without allowing a single alteration in the amino acid sequence encoded by the constant region.

The third structural feature of immunoglobulins requiring an explanation was first recognized when amino acid sequencing of the human myeloma protein called Til revealed that identical variable-region sequences were associated with both γ and μ heavy-chain constant regions. A similar phenomenon was observed in rabbits by C. Todd, who found that a particular allotypic marker in the heavy-chain variable region could be associated with α, γ, and μ heavy-chain constant regions. Considerable additional evidence has confirmed that a single variable-region sequence, defining a particular antigenic specificity, can be associated with multiple heavy-chain constant region sequences; in other words, different classes, or isotypes, of antibody (e.g., IgG, IgM) can be expressed having identical variable-region sequences.

Dryer and Bennett Two-Gene Model

In an attempt to develop a genetic model consistent with these findings about the structure of immunoglobulins, W. Dryer and J. Bennett suggested, in their classic theoretical paper of 1965, that two separate genes encode a single immunoglobulin heavy or light chain, one gene encoding the V region and one gene encoding the C region. They suggested that these two genes must somehow come together at the DNA level to form a continuous message that can be transcribed and translated to yield a single heavy or light protein chain. Moreover, they proposed that hundreds or thousands of V-region genes were carried in the germ line, whereas only single copies of C-region class and subclass genes need exist. The strength of this type of recombinational model (which combined elements of the germ-line and somatic-variation theories) was that it allowed for the great diversity of antibody specificities in the variable region while conserving invariant constant-region sequences to provide necessary biological effector functions. It suggested a way for a single V gene to join with various C-region genes and also for the association of innumerable V-region genes with a single C gene.

At first, support for the Dryer and Bennett hypothesis was indirect. The model could account for those immunoglobulins in which a single V region was combined with various C regions. By postulating a single constant-region gene for each immunoglobulin class and subclass, the model also could account for the conservation of necessary biological effector functions while allowing for evolutionary diversification of variable-region genes. Early studies of DNA hybridization kinetics using a radioactive constant-region DNA probe indicated that the probe hybridized with only one or two genes, confirming the model's prediction that only one or two copies of each constant-region class and subclass gene existed. Yet the evidence in support of the Dryer and Bennett model continued to be indirect, and there was stubborn resistance to their hypothesis in the scientific community. The suggestion that two genes coded a single polypeptide contradicted the existing one gene-one polypeptide principle and was without precedent in any system in cell or molecular biology.

As so often is the case in science, theoretical and intellectual understanding of immunoglobulin-gene organization progressed ahead of the available methodology. Although the Dryer and Bennett model provided a theoretical framework for reconciling the dilemma between immunoglobulin-sequence data and gene organization, actual validation of their hypothesis had to wait for several major technological advances in the field of molecular biology. These advances, described in Chapter 2, included mRNA isolation and purification, restriction-endonuclease cleavage of DNA, nucleic acid hybridization by Southern or Northern blotting, DNA cloning, DNA sequencing, and gene transfer by transfection or transgenic techniques. In time, the Dryer and Bennett hypothesis was proved to be essentially correct. Indeed, far more complex genetic mechanisms have been shown to be involved than could ever have been imagined at the time that Dryer and Bennett published their paper.

Early Verification of the Dryer and Bennett Hypothesis

In 1976 S. Tonegawa and N. Hozumi provided the first direct evidence that separate genes encode the V and C regions and are rearranged in the course of B-cell differentiation. The significance of this work in the field of immunology resulted in the award of the Nobel prize to Tonegawa in 1987.

In their experiments, Tonegawa and Hozumi first cleaved DNA from embryonic cells and from adult myeloma cells into fragments with various restriction endonucleases. These fragments were then separated by size by means of agarose gel electrophoresis and analyzed for their ability to hybridize with a radiolabeled κ-chain mRNA probe. The results showed that two separate restriction fragments from the embryonic DNA hybridized with the mRNA, whereas only a single restriction fragment of the myeloma DNA hybridized with the probe (Figure 8-1a). The interpretation of these results by Tonegawa and Hozumi was that during differentiation of lymphocytes from the embryonic state to the fully differentiated plasma-cell stage (represented in their system by myeloma cells), the V and C genes undergo rearrangement. In the embryo the V and C genes are separated by a large distance containing a restriction-endonuclease site, but during differentiation the V and C genes are brought closer together and the intervening restriction site is eliminated (Figure 8-1b).

In subsequent experiments, other researchers took an approach similar to that of Tonegawa and Hozumi but used the newly developed technique of Southern blotting, thus eliminating the need to elute the separated restriction DNA fragments from the gel slices (see Figure 2-8). These Southern-blot analyses permitted comparisons of the arrangement of the light-chain and heavy-chain genes in non-B cells (e.g., embryonic cells and liver cells) and in myeloma cells, which represent fully differentiated B cells. In each analysis the corresponding radiolabeled mRNA was used as the probe. In all these experiments, the variable- and constant-region genes of the embryonic DNA were shown to be separated by a large distance containing a restriction-enzyme site and therefore the respective radiolabeled mRNA probes hybridized with two bands: one band containing the variable-region sequence and one band containing the constant region sequence. In the fully differentiated plasma-cell stage (represented by the myeloma cell), the variable- and constant-region genes had rearranged and were now together on a single restriction DNA fragment and

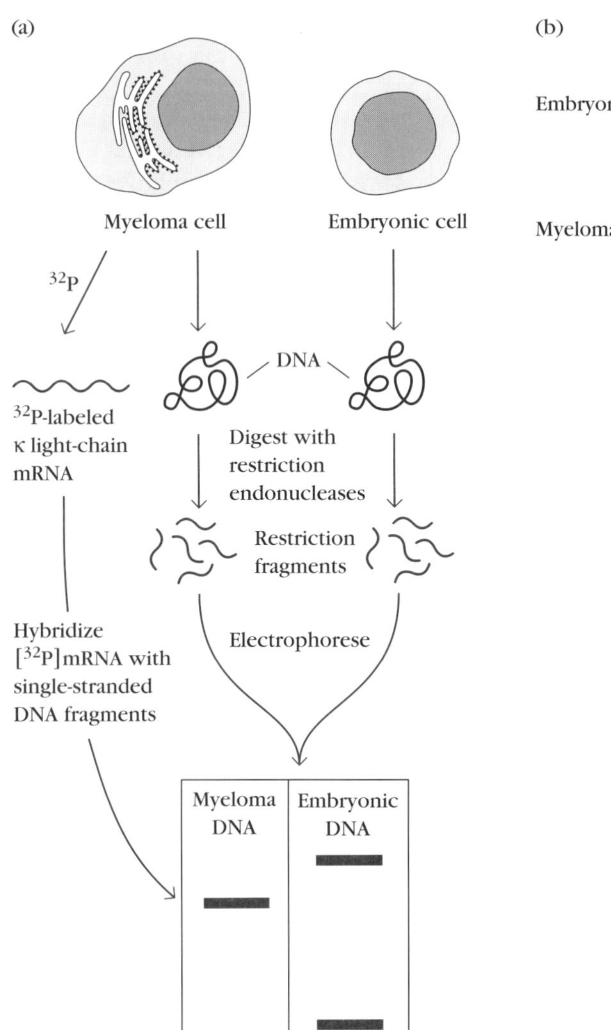

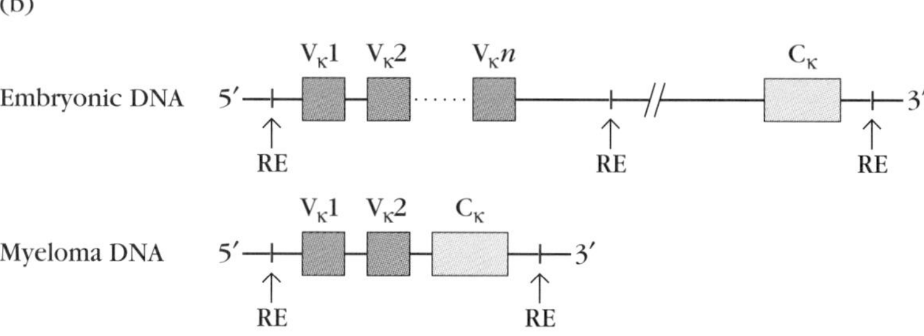

FIGURE 8-1 Experimental demonstration that genes encoding κ light chains are rearranged during B-cell development. (a) In this experiment, the myeloma cells are equivalent to differentiated plasma cells. The restriction-endonuclease digests of DNA from embryonic cells and myeloma cells were subjected to agarose gel electrophoresis. The gel was then cut into slices and the DNA fragments were eluted from the slice, denatured into single-stranded DNA, and incubated with ^{32}P-labeled mRNA encoding κ light chains. The mRNA probe hybridized with two bands from the germ-line embryonic DNA but with only a single band from the differentiated myeloma DNA. (b) Structure of embryonic and myeloma κ light-chain DNA compatible with the experimental results supports the Dryer and Bennett two-gene model. During development of B cells, κ exons ($V_κ$ and $C_κ$) are brought closer together and the restriction-endonuclease (RE) site between them is eliminated. [Adapted from N. Hozumi and S. Tonegawa, 1976, *Proc. Natl. Acad. Sci. USA* **73**:3628.]

therefore the radiolabeled mRNA probe hybridized with a single band. These results, analogous to those in Figure 8-1, demonstrated that the Dryer and Bennett two-gene model—one gene encoding the variable region and one gene encoding the constant region—applied to both heavy- and light-chain genes.

TABLE 8-2 CHROMOSOMAL LOCATIONS OF IMMUNOGLOBULIN GENES IN HUMAN AND MOUSE

	Chromosome	
Gene	Human	Mouse
λ Light chain	22	16
κ Light chain	2	6
Heavy chain	14	12

MULTIGENE ORGANIZATION OF IMMUNOGLOBULIN GENES

As cloning and sequencing of the light- and heavy-chain DNA was accomplished, even greater complexity was revealed than had been predicted by Dryer and Bennett. The κ and λ light chains and the heavy chains are encoded by separate multigene families situated on different chromosomes (Table 8-2). Each of these multigene families contains a series of coding sequences, called *gene segments.* The κ and λ light-chain families contain L, V, J, and C gene segments; the heavy-chain family contains L, V, D, J, and C gene segments. Functional immunoglobulin genes are generated during B-cell maturation by a process, to be described later, whereby the gene segments are rearranged and brought together. The rearranged VJ gene segments encode the variable region of the light chains; the rearranged VDJ gene segments encode the variable region of the heavy chain. The C gene segments encode the constant regions of the light or heavy chains. The L gene segment encodes a short *signal* or *leader* sequence that guides the heavy or light chain through the endoplasmic reticulum but is cleaved from the nascent polypeptide before assembly of the finished immunoglobulin molecule; thus amino acids corresponding to L gene segments do not appear in light and heavy chains.

λ-Chain Multigene Family

The first evidence that the light-chain variable region was actually encoded by two gene segments was provided when Tonegawa cloned the germ-line gene encoding the variable region of mouse λ light chain and determined its complete nucleotide sequence. When the nucleotide sequence was compared with the known amino acid sequence of the λ-chain variable region, an unusual discrepancy was observed. Although the first 97 amino acids of the λ-chain variable region corresponded to the nucleotide codon sequence, the remaining 13 carboxyl-terminal amino acids of the protein's variable region did not correspond to the sequential nucleotide sequence. It turned out that many base pairs away a separate, 39-bp gene segment, called J for joining, encoded the remaining 13 amino acids of the λ-chain variable region. Thus a functional λ variable-region gene contains two coding segments (or *exons*)—a 5′ V segment and a 3′ J segment—which are separated by a noncoding DNA sequence (or *intron*) in unrearranged germ-line DNA.

The λ multigene family in the mouse contains two V_λ gene segments, four J_λ gene segments, and four C_λ gene segments (Figure 8-2a). The $J_\lambda 4$ and $C_\lambda 4$ gene segments are defective genes, called pseudogenes, which are indicated with the psi symbol (ψ). The V_λ and J_λ gene segments encode the variable region of the λ light chain, and the three functional C_λ gene segments encode the constant regions of the three λ-chain subtypes (λ_1, λ_2, and λ_3). In humans there are an estimated 100 V_λ gene segments, 6 J_λ segments, and 6 C_λ segments.

κ-Chain Multigene Family

The κ-chain multigene family in the mouse contains approximately 300 V_κ gene segments, each with an adjacent leader sequence a short distance upstream (i.e., on the 5′ side). There are five J_κ gene segments (one of which is a nonfunctional pseudogene) and a single C_κ gene segment (Figure 8-2b). As in the λ multigene family, the V_κ and J_κ gene segments encode the variable region of the κ light chain, and the C_κ gene segment encodes the constant region. Since there is only one C_κ gene segment, there are no subclasses of κ light chains. Comparison of Figure 8-2a and b shows that the arrangement of the gene segments is quite different in the κ and λ gene families. The κ-chain multigene family in humans, which is similar to that in the mouse, contains approximately 100 V_κ gene segments, 5 J_κ segments, and a single C_κ segment.

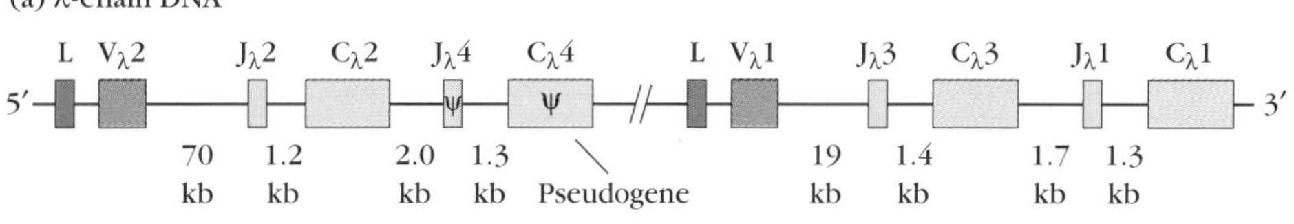

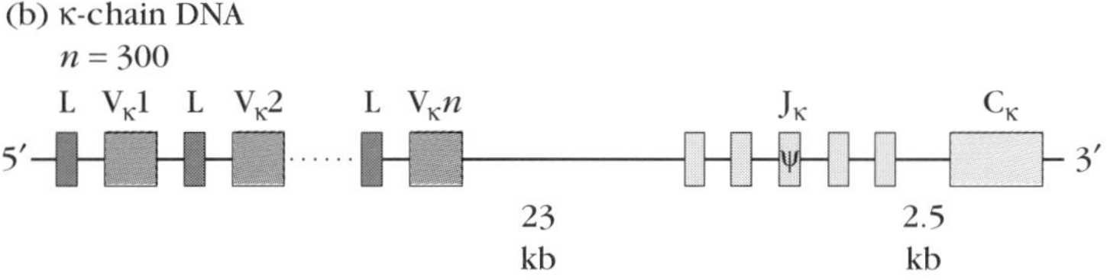

FIGURE 8-2 Germ-line organization of (a) λ light-chain, (b) κ light-chain, and (c) heavy-chain gene segments in the mouse. The λ and κ light chains are encoded by L, V, J, and C gene segments. The heavy chain is encoded by L, V, D, J, and C gene segments. The distances in kilobases (kb) separating the various gene segments in mouse germ-line DNA are shown below each diagram.

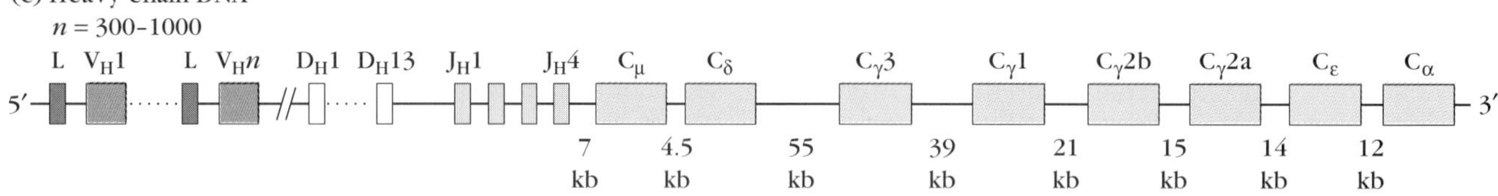

Heavy-Chain Multigene Family

The organization of the mouse immunoglobulin heavy-chain genes is similar to but more complex than that of the κ and λ light-chain genes (Figure 8-2c). An additional gene segment encodes part of the heavy-chain variable region. The existence of this gene segment was first proposed by Leroy Hood and his colleagues, who compared the heavy-chain variable-region amino acid sequence with the V_H and J_H nucleotide sequences. The V_H gene segment was found to encode amino acids 1 to 94 and the J_H gene segment was found to encode amino acids 98 to 113; however, neither of these gene segments carried the information to encode amino acids 95 to 97. When the nucleotide sequence was determined for rearranged myeloma DNA and compared with the germ-line DNA sequence, an additional nucleotide sequence was observed between the V_H and J_H gene segments. This nucleotide sequence corresponded to amino acids 95 to 97 of the heavy chain. Hood proposed that a third germ-line gene segment must join with the V_H and J_H gene segments to encode the entire variable region of the heavy chain. This gene segment, which encoded amino acids within the third complementarity-determining region (CDR3), was designated D, diversity, for its contribution to the generation of antibody diversity. Tonegawa and his colleagues located the D gene segments within mouse germ-line DNA with a cDNA D-region probe, which hybridized with a stretch of DNA lying between the V_H and J_H gene segments.

The heavy-chain multigene family on chromosome 12 in the mouse has an estimated 300–1000 V_H gene segments, located upstream from a cluster of about 13 D_H gene segments. As with the light-chain genes, each V_H gene segment has a leader sequence a short distance upstream from it. Downstream from the D_H gene segments are four J_H gene segments, followed by a series of C_H gene segments. Each C_H gene segment encodes the constant region of an immunoglobulin heavy-chain isotype. The C_H gene segments are organized into a series of coding exons and noncoding introns. Each exon encodes a separate domain of the heavy-chain constant region (see Figure 5-6b). A similar heavy-chain gene organization is found in humans with an estimated 75–250 V_H gene segments, 30 D_H segments, and 6 functional J_H segments followed by a series of C_H segments.

The conservation of important biological effector functions of the antibody molecule is maintained by the limited number of heavy-chain constant-region genes. In the mouse the C_H gene segments are arranged sequentially in the following order: C_μ–C_δ–$C_\gamma3$–$C_\gamma1$–$C_\gamma2b$–$C_\gamma2a$–C_ε–C_α. This sequential arrangement is no accident; it is generally related to the developmental appearance of the immunoglobulin classes in the course of an immune response. During B-cell differentiation there are notable changes in the classes of immunoglobulin expressed, while the specificity remains the same. The changes are accomplished by DNA rearrangements mediating class switching, which are discussed in a later section.

Variable-Region Gene Rearrangements

The previous sections have shown that the assembly of functional genes encoding immunoglobulin light and heavy chains involves recombinational events at the DNA level. Variable-region gene rearrangements occur in an ordered sequence during B-cell maturation in the bone marrow. The heavy-chain variable-region genes rearrange first, then the light-chain variable-region genes. At the end of this process, each B cell contains a single, functional variable-region DNA sequence for its heavy chain and a single, functional variable-region DNA sequence for its light chain. In other words, this process leads to generation of mature, immunocompetent B cells; each such cell is antigenically committed to a single epitope and expresses membrane-bound antibody on its surface. As is discussed in the next section, rearrangement of heavy-chain constant-region genes occurs later, generating changes in the immunoglobulin class expressed by a B cell without changing its antigenic specificity. Although variable-region gene rearrangements occur in an ordered sequence, they are random events that result in the random determination of B-cell specificity. The order, mechanism, and consequences of these rearrangements are described in this section.

V-J Rearrangements in Light-Chain DNA

Expression of both λ and κ light chains requires rearrangement of the variable-region V and J gene segments. In the case of the mouse λ light chain, DNA rearrangement can join the $V_{\lambda}1$ gene segment with either the $J_{\lambda}1$ or $J_{\lambda}3$ gene segments, or the $V_{\lambda}2$ gene segment can be joined with the $J_{\lambda}2$ gene segment. In the case of the mouse κ light chain, any one of the estimated 300 V_{κ} gene segments can be joined with any one of the four functional J_{κ} gene segments.

Rearranged κ and λ genes contain the following regions in order from the 5′ to 3′ end: a short leader (L) gene segment, a noncoding sequence (intron), a joined VJ gene segment, a second intron, and a C gene segment. Upstream from each leader gene segment is a promoter sequence. The rearranged light-chain sequence is transcribed by RNA polymerase from the L segment through the C segment, generating a light-chain primary RNA transcript (Figure 8-3). The introns in the primary transcript are removed by RNA-processing enzymes, and the resulting light-chain messenger RNA then exits from the nucleus. The light-chain mRNA binds to ribosomes and is translated into the

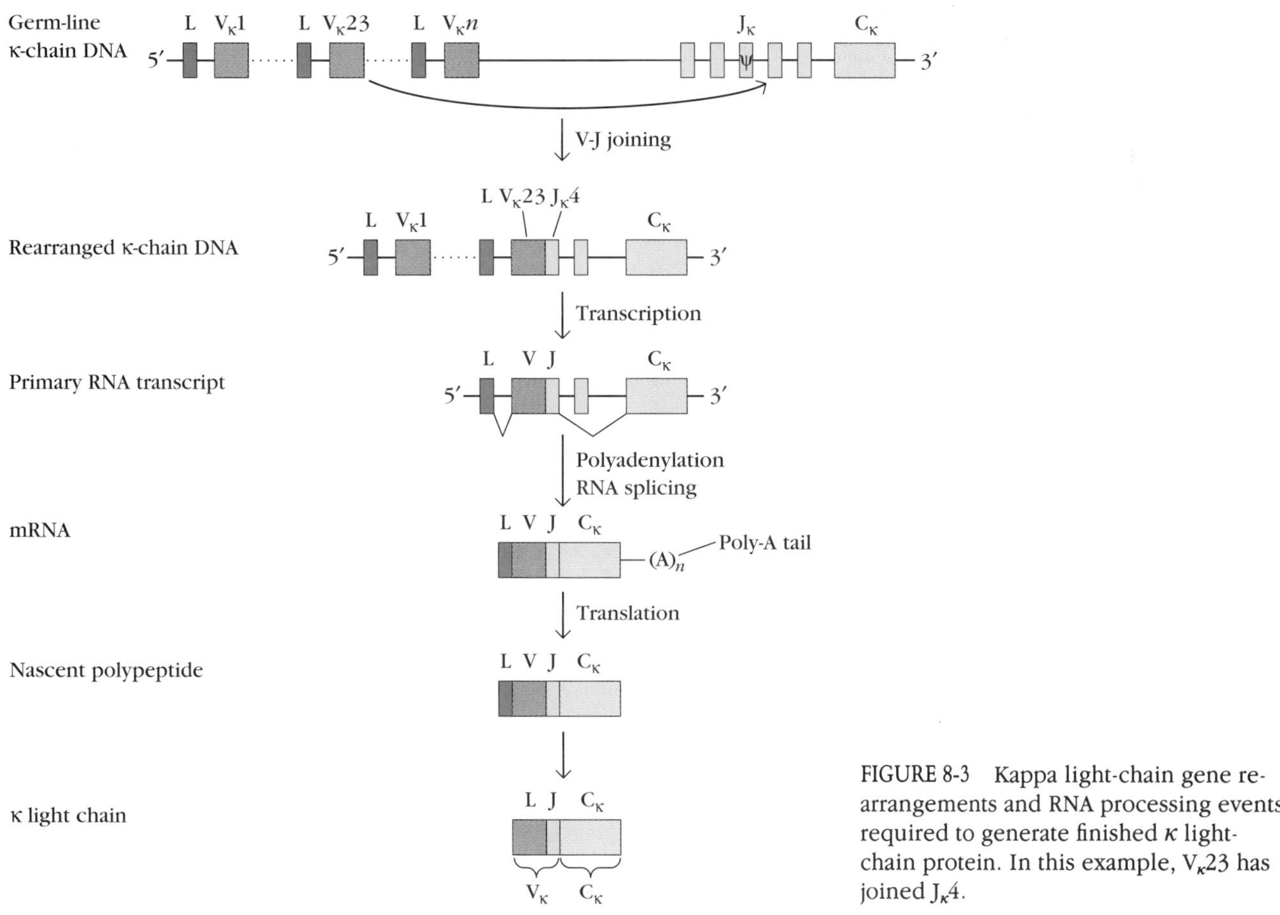

FIGURE 8-3 Kappa light-chain gene rearrangements and RNA processing events required to generate finished κ light-chain protein. In this example, $V_{\kappa}23$ has joined $J_{\kappa}4$.

light-chain protein. The leader sequence at the amino terminus pulls the growing polypeptide chain into the lumen of the rough endoplasmic reticulum and is then cleaved, so it is not present in the finished light-chain protein product.

V-D-J Rearrangements in Heavy-Chain DNA

Generation of a functional immunoglobulin heavy-chain gene requires two separate rearrangement events within the variable region. As illustrated in Figure 8-4, a D_H gene segment first joins to a J_H segment; the resulting D_HJ_H segment then moves next to and joins a V_H segment to generate a $V_HD_HJ_H$ unit that encodes the entire variable region. In heavy-chain DNA, variable-region rearrangement produces a rearranged gene consisting of the following sequences starting from the 5′ end: a short L segment, an intron, a joined VDJ segment, another intron, and a series of C gene segments. As with the light-chain genes, a promoter sequence is located a short distance upstream from each heavy-chain leader sequence.

Once heavy-chain gene rearrangement is accomplished, RNA polymerase can bind to the promoter sequence and transcribe the entire heavy-chain gene, including the introns. Initially, both C_μ and C_δ gene segments are transcribed. Differential polyadenylation and RNA splicing removes the introns and processes the primary transcript to generate mRNA, en-

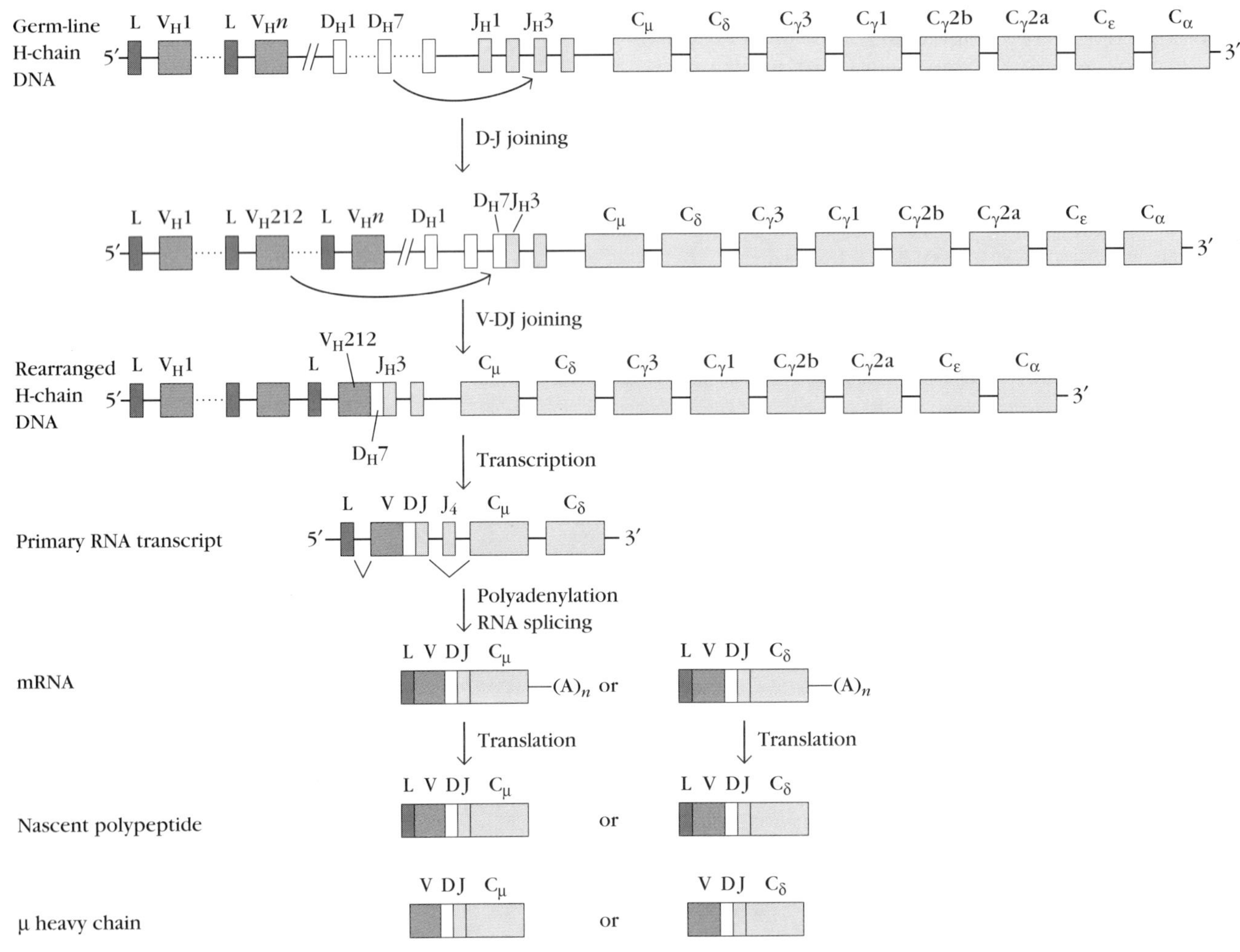

FIGURE 8-4 Heavy-chain gene rearrangements and RNA processing events required to generate finished μ heavy-chain protein. Two DNA rearrangements are necessary to generate a functional H-chain gene: a D_H to J_H rearrangement and a V_H to D_HJ_H rearrangement. In this illustration V_H212, D_H7, and J_H3 have been joined. Expression of functional heavy-chain genes, although generally similar to expression of light-chain genes, involves differential RNA processing, which generates several different products including μ and δ heavy chains.

coding either C_μ or C_δ. These two mRNAs then are translated, and the leader peptide of the resulting nascent polypeptide is cleaved, generating finished μ and δ chains. Since two different heavy-chain mRNAs are produced following heavy-chain variable-region gene rearrangement, a mature, immunocompetent B cell expresses both IgM and IgD with identical antigenic specificity on its surface.

Mechanism of Variable-Region DNA Rearrangements

Considerable research has been directed toward elucidating the mechanism by which variable-region gene rearrangements occur during maturation of B cells. The details of this process and the means by which it is regulated are discussed in this section.

Recombination Signal Sequences

Discovery of two closely related conserved sequences in variable-region germ-line DNA paved the way toward fuller understanding of the mechanism of gene rearrangements. DNA sequencing studies revealed the presence of unique DNA *recombination signal sequences* (RSSs) flanking each germ-line V, D, and J gene segment. One RSS is located 3′ to each V gene segment, 5′ to each J gene segment, and on both sides of each D gene segment. These sequences function as signals for the recombination process. Each RSS contains a conserved palindromic heptamer and a conserved AT-rich nonamer sequence separated by an intervening sequence of 12 or 23 base pairs (Figure 8-5a). Leroy Hood observed that the intervening 12- and 23-bp sequences correspond, respectively, to one and two turns of the DNA helix; for this reason the sequences are referred to as *one-turn signal sequences* and *two-turn signal sequences.* The V_κ signal sequence has a one-turn spacer, and the J_κ signal sequence has a two-turn spacer. In λ light-chain DNA this order is reversed; that is, the V_λ signal sequence has a two-turn spacer, and the J_λ signal sequence has a one-turn spacer. In heavy-chain DNA, a two-turn spacer occurs in the signal sequences of the V_H and J_H gene segments, and a one-turn spacer occurs in the signals on either side of the D_H gene segment (Figure 8-5b). Signal sequences having a one-turn spacer can only join with sequences having a two-turn spacer (the so-called *one-turn/two-turn joining rule*). This joining rule ensures that a V_L segment only joins to a J_L segment and not to another V_L segment; the rule likewise ensures that V_H, D_H, and J_H segments join in proper order and that segments of the same type do not join each other.

Joining of Gene Segments

Recent research has begun to unravel the mechanism of V-(D)-J recombination, which takes place at the junctions between RSSs and coding sequences. Recombination results in the formation of a *coding joint,*

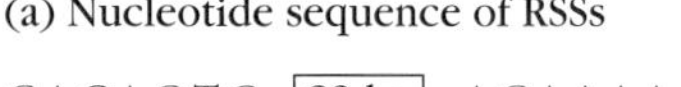

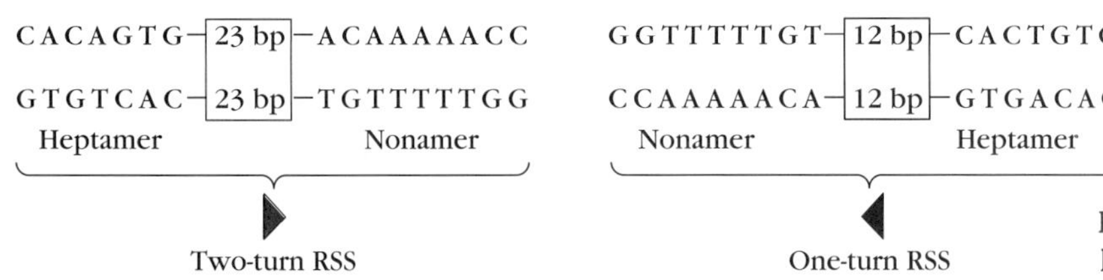

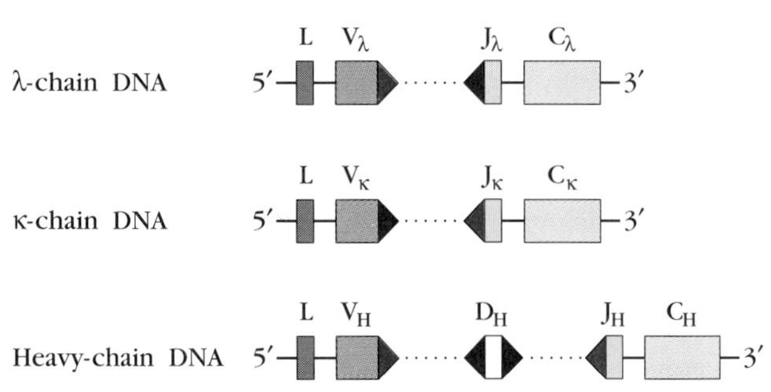

FIGURE 8-5 Two conserved sequences in light-chain and heavy-chain DNA function as recombination signal sequences (RSSs). (a) The signal sequences consist of conserved palindromic heptamer and conserved AT-rich nonamer sequences; these are separated by nonconserved spacers of 12 or 23 base pairs. (b) The two types of RSS—designated one-turn RSS and two-turn RSS—have characteristic locations within λ-chain, κ-chain, and heavy-chain germ-line DNA. During DNA rearrangement, gene segments having one-turn RSS can join only with segments having a two-turn RSS.

formed by joining of the coding sequences, and a *signal joint,* formed by joining of the RSSs (Figure 8-6). The relative transcriptional orientation of the gene segments to be joined determines the fate of the signal joint and intervening DNA. When the two gene segments are in the same transcriptional orientation, joining results in deletion of the signal joint and intervening DNA as a circular excision product (Figure 8-7). Less frequently, the two gene segments have opposite orientations. In this case joining occurs by inversion of the DNA resulting in the retention of both the coding joint and the signal joint (and intervening DNA) on the chromosome. In the human κ locus about half of the V_κ gene segments are inverted with respect to J_κ and joining is therefore by inversion.

According to the model diagrammed in Figure 8-6, gene-segment recombination is a multistep process involving the following sequence of events:

- Recognition of recombination signal sequences (RSSs) by recombinase enzymes
- Synapsis in which two signal sequences and the adjacent coding sequences (gene segments) are brought into proximity of each other
- Cleavage of the DNA by site-specific endonucleases at the juncture of the signal sequence and coding sequence
- Trimming of a few nucleotides from the coding sequence by a single-stranded endonuclease
- Optional addition of up to 15 nucleotides, called *N nucleotides,* at the cut ends of the V, D, and, J coding sequences of the heavy chain
- Repair and ligation to join the coding sequences and the signal sequences

One of the striking features of gene-segment recombination is the diversity of the coding joints that are formed between any two gene segments. This junctional diversity at the V-J and V-D-J coding joints is generated by a number of mechanisms: variation in trimming of the coding sequences, variation in N-nucleotide addition, and flexibility in joining the coding sequences. As discussed later, this variation contributes greatly to the diversity of the CDR3 region of the antigen-binding site.

Recombination-Activating Genes

Identification of the enzymes involved in recombination of V, D, and J gene segments began in the late 1980s and probably will receive research attention

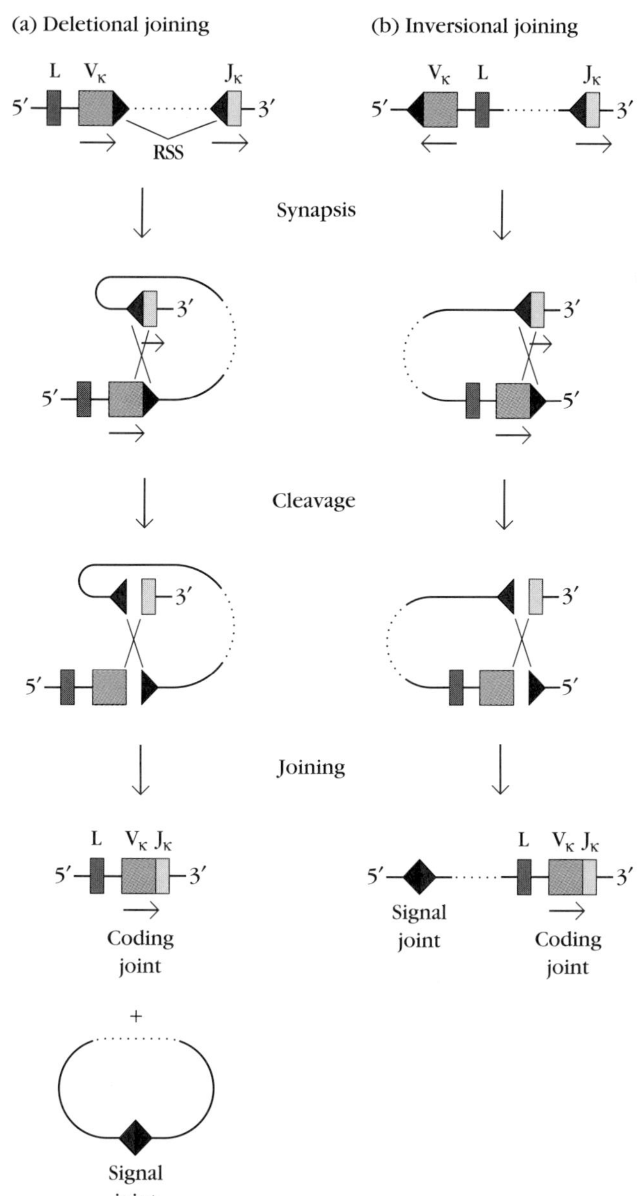

FIGURE 8-6 General process of recombination of immunoglobulin gene segments is illustrated with V_κ and J_κ. (a) Deletional joining occurs when the gene segments to be joined have the same transcriptional orientation (indicated by horizontal purple arrows). This process yields two products: (1) rearranged DNA containing the V_κ and J_κ gene segments plus the coding joint and (2) a circular excision product consisting of the recombination signal sequences (RSSs), signal joint, and intervening DNA. (b) Inversional joining occurs when the gene segments have opposite transcriptional orientations. In this case, the RSSs, signal joint, and intervening DNA are retained, and the orientation of one of the joined segments is inverted. In some cases, a few nucleotides may be deleted from or added to the cut ends of the coding sequences before they are rejoined. [Adapted from F. W. Alt, 1992, *Immunol. Today* **13**:306.]

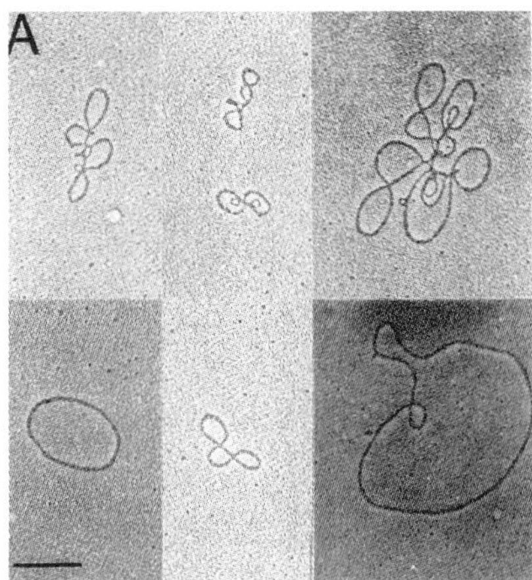

FIGURE 8-7 Circular DNA isolated from thymocytes in which the DNA encoding the chains of the T-cell receptor (TCR) undergoes rearrangement in a process analogous to that involving the immunoglobulin genes. Isolation of this circular excision product is direct evidence for the mechanism of deletional joining shown in Figure 8-6. [From K. Okazki et al., 1987, *Cell* **49**:477.]

throughout the 1990s. Two genes that act synergistically to mediate V-(D)-J joining are the recombination-activating genes designated *RAG-1* and *RAG-2,* which were first reported by David Schatz, Marjorie Oettinger, and David Baltimore in 1990. To identify these genes, the researchers first produced a retroviral construct that served as an assay system for recombination. This retroviral construct contained a promoter sequence, V_κ and J_κ gene segments with flanking signal sequences, and a gene that confers resistance to mycophenolic acid (Figure 8-8). The genes were arranged in such a way that the promoter was oriented in the opposite transcriptional orientation from that of the gene for mycophenolic acid resistance. If the V_κ and J_κ gene segments were rearranged by inversional joining, then the orientation of the gene for mycophenolic acid resistance would also be inverted, placing the gene in the correct 5′ to 3′ orientation to be transcribed from the promoter. A variety of cells were transfected with this construct; those cells that could rearrange the V_κ and J_κ gene segments acquired resistance to the mycophenolic acid, whereas those cells that could not rearrange the V_κ and J_κ gene segments were not resistant to mycophenolic acid. The results with this system demonstrated that only pre-B cells and pre-T cells were able to rearrange the V_κ and J_κ gene segments. (As is discussed in Chapter 11, the pre-T cell employs the same signal sequences in rearranging the genes for the T-cell receptor, which is why it also proved to be positive in this assay.) Mature B and T cells were unable to rearrange the retroviral construct, indicating that the recombinase activity is limited to an early stage in the maturation of both B and T cells.

Having established that the retroviral construct could be rearranged in pre-B cells, the research team then set out to isolate the recombination genes. First fibroblasts were transfected with the retroviral construct. Since fibroblasts do not express the recombination genes, the transfected cells could not rearrange the construct. Assuming that the recombination genes were located on a single locus, the researchers then transfected genomic DNA from pre-B cells into fibroblasts containing the retroviral construct. The presence of activated recombinase genes in the genomic DNA could be detected by the rearrangement of the

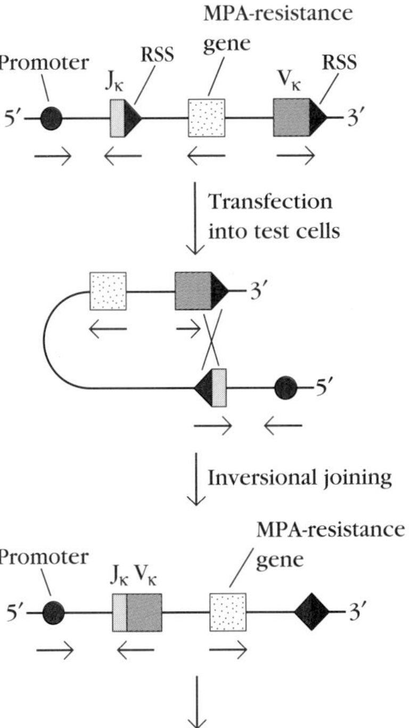

FIGURE 8-8 Assay system for demonstrating recombinase activity mediating immunoglobulin-gene recombination. If the test cells possess recombinase activity, then the transfected cells will be resistant to mycophenolic acid (MPA), as shown. If the test cells lack the enzymes for inversional joining, the MPA-resistance gene will not be expressed because its transcriptional orientation (horizontal purple arrows) is opposite to that of the promoter.

retroviral construct, which conferred resistance to mycophenolic acid upon the transfected fibroblasts. This experimental system led to identification of a gene that mediated recombination of the retroviral construct; it was named recombination-activating gene, or *RAG-1*. *RAG-1* mRNA was shown to be present in pre-B cells and pre-T cells, as well as cells of the central nervous system. The expression of *RAG-1* in the central nervous system is intriguing and suggests that similar recombination events may take place within the central nervous system.

It soon became apparent that *RAG-1* was not the whole story. When *RAG-1* cDNA was transfected into the fibroblasts, it was no more efficient at mediating recombination than the genomic DNA, although the purified cDNA would be expected to have a 100- to 1000-fold greater recombination efficiency than the genomic DNA. The puzzle was finally solved when the sequences of cDNA and genomic clones were compared. Although *RAG-1* contains two exons, most of the protein-coding region is in one exon of about 6.6 kb. The 18-kb genomic clone contained an additional 12-kb sequence of unknown function. To determine whether an additional gene was encoded in this 12-kb sequence of genomic DNA, the researchers transfected the fibroblasts with the *RAG-1* cDNA alone, with the genomic DNA alone, or with a mixture of both cDNA and genomic DNA. They found that co-transfection with both *RAG-1* cDNA and genomic DNA resulted in a 100-fold increase in the frequency of recombination compared with either DNA alone. These findings demonstrated the presence of a second closely linked gene, designated *RAG-2*. Co-transfection with both *RAG-1* and *RAG-2* increased recombination more than 1000-fold compared with genomic DNA in the fibroblast model system. Still to be determined is whether the RAG-1 and RAG-2 proteins play a direct role as part of the recombination machinery or whether they play a regulatory role leading to the expression of other, as yet unidentified enzymes, involved in recombination.

Several strains of mice with defects in various recombination genes have been developed and are proving valuable in unraveling the various steps in the recombination process. For example, knock-out mice with defects in either *RAG-1* or *RAG-2* are unable to initiate the recombination process because they cannot introduce double-strand DNA breaks between the recombination signal sequences (RSSs) and coding sequences in germ-line immunoglobulin DNA (see Figure 8-6). As a result of this defect, the V, D, and J gene segments remain unarranged. Since both B and T cells utilize the same recombination machinery, the *RAG-1*$^{-}$ and *RAG-2*$^{-}$ knock-out mice lack mature T and B cells and consequently exhibit a severe combined immunodeficiency.

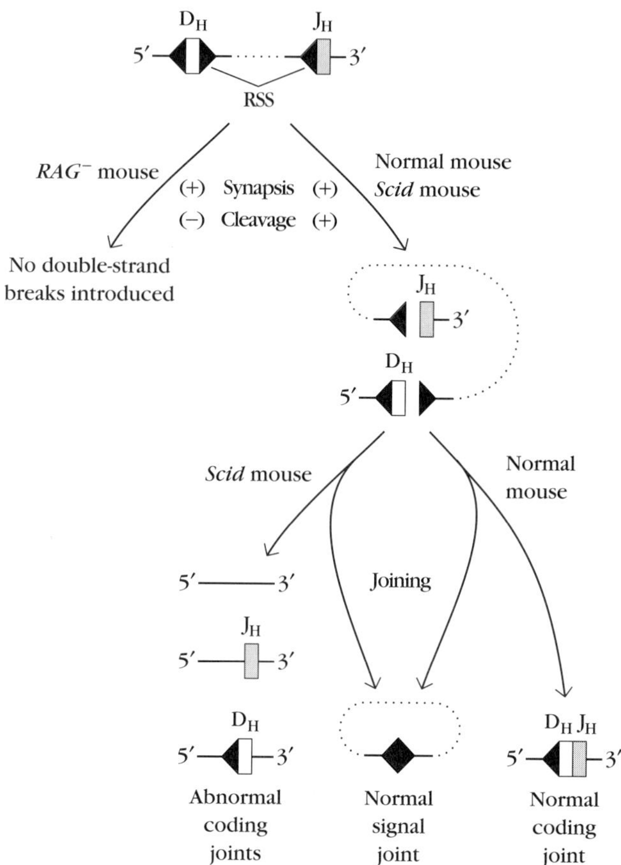

FIGURE 8-9 Recombination defects have been identified in *RAG*-deficient mice and *scid* mice. Mice lacking either *RAG-1* or *RAG-2* cannot even start the recombination process, whereas *scid* mice can, carrying out synapsis between D_H and J_H gene segments, introducing double-strand breaks to produce normal intermediates, and forming a normal signal joint. However, *scid* mice cannot properly join the coding sequences. Both types of defective mice lack mature B and T cells and thus exhibit a severe combined immunodeficiency. [Adapted from F. W. Alt, E. M. Oltz, F. Young et al., 1992, *Immunol. Today* **13**:306.]

Another recombination defect is found in CB-17 *scid* mice. These mice have an autosomal recessive mutation that impairs the V-(D)-J recombination process. *Scid* mice have a general absence of mature functional T and B cells and, like RAG^{-} mice, manifest a severe combined immunodeficiency (SCID). Unlike the *RAG* mutants, *scid* mice begin the recombination process normally: Synapsis occurs between the D and J gene segments; double-strand DNA breaks are properly introduced at the juncture of the recombination signal sequences and coding sequences; and the signal sequences are then rejoined. Joining of the coding sequences, however, occurs some distance from the D and J gene segments, resulting in deletion of one or both of the coding sequences (Figure 8-9).

Productive and Nonproductive Rearrangements

Although the double-strand DNA breaks that initiate V-(D)-J rearrangements are introduced precisely at the junctions of signal sequences and coding sequences, the subsequent joining of the coding sequences exhibits some flexibility. This flexibility in the joining process helps generate antibody diversity by contributing to the hypervariability of the antigen-binding site. (This phenomenon is covered in more detail in the section on generation of antibody diversity.)

Another consequence of joining flexibility is that gene segments may be joined out of phase, so that the triplet reading frame for translation is not preserved. In such a *nonproductive* rearrangement, the resulting VJ or VDJ unit will contain numerous stop codons, which interrupt translation (Figure 8-10). When gene segments are joined in phase, the reading frame is maintained. In such a *productive* rearrangement, the resulting VJ or VDJ unit can be translated in its entirety, yielding a complete variable-region polypeptide.

If one allele rearranges nonproductively, a B cell can then rearrange the other allele and may generate a productive rearrangement. If an in-phase rearranged heavy-chain and light-chain gene are not produced, the B cell dies by apoptosis. It is estimated that only one in three attempts at V_L-J_L, D_H-J_H, and V_H-D_HJ_H joining are productive. As a result, only about 8% of the pre-B cells in the bone marrow progress to maturity and leave the bone marrow as mature, immunocompetent B cells.

Allelic Exclusion

B cells, like all somatic cells, are diploid and contain both maternal and paternal chromosomes. Even though a B cell is diploid, it expresses the rearranged heavy-chain genes from only one chromosome and the rearranged light-chain genes from only one chromosome. This process, called *allelic exclusion,* ensures that functional B cells never contain more than one $V_HD_HJ_H$ and one V_LJ_L unit (Figure 8-11). This is, of

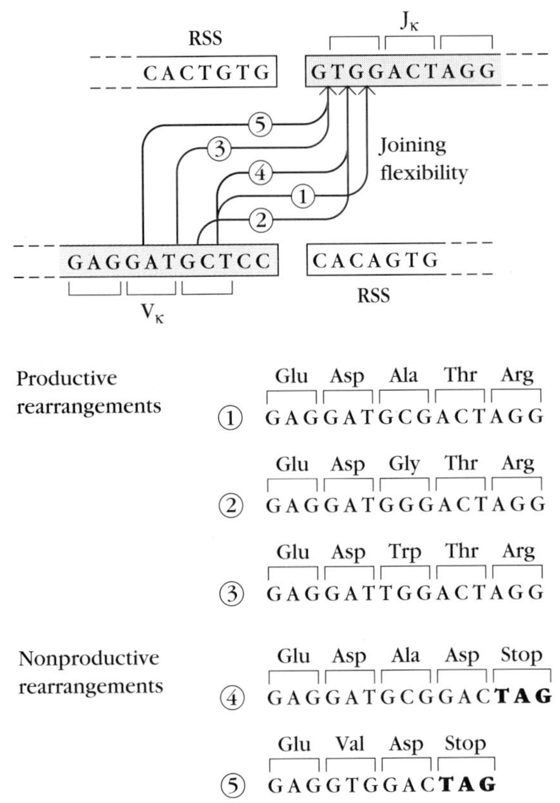

FIGURE 8-10 Junctional flexibility in the joining of immunoglobulin gene segments is illustrated with V_κ and J_κ. In-phase joining (purple arrows) generates a productive rearrangement, which can be translated into protein. Out-of-phase joining leads to a nonproductive rearrangement, which contains stop codons and is not translated into protein.

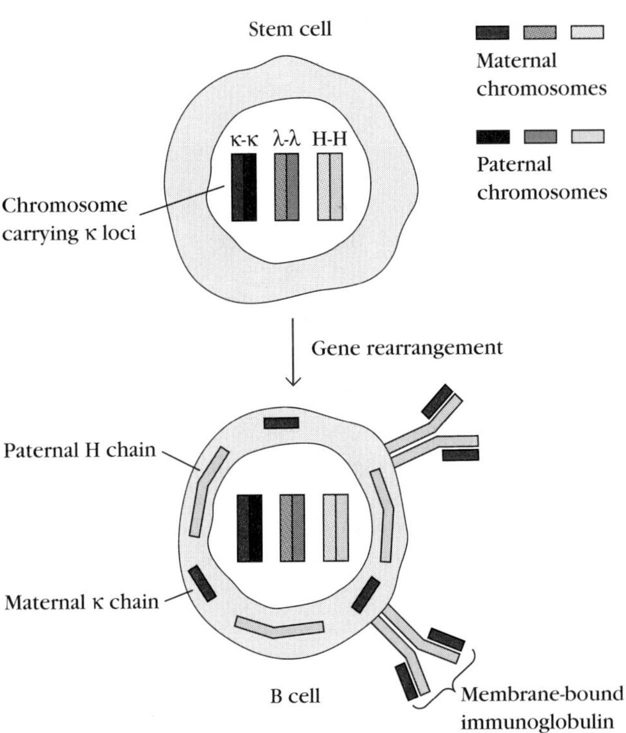

FIGURE 8-11 Because of allelic exclusion, the immunoglobulin heavy- and light-chain genes of only one parental chromosome are expressed per cell. This process ensures that a single B cell will be specific for a given epitope. The selection of which allele of each pair is rearranged to produce a functional gene is random. Only B cells and T cells exhibit allelic exclusion.

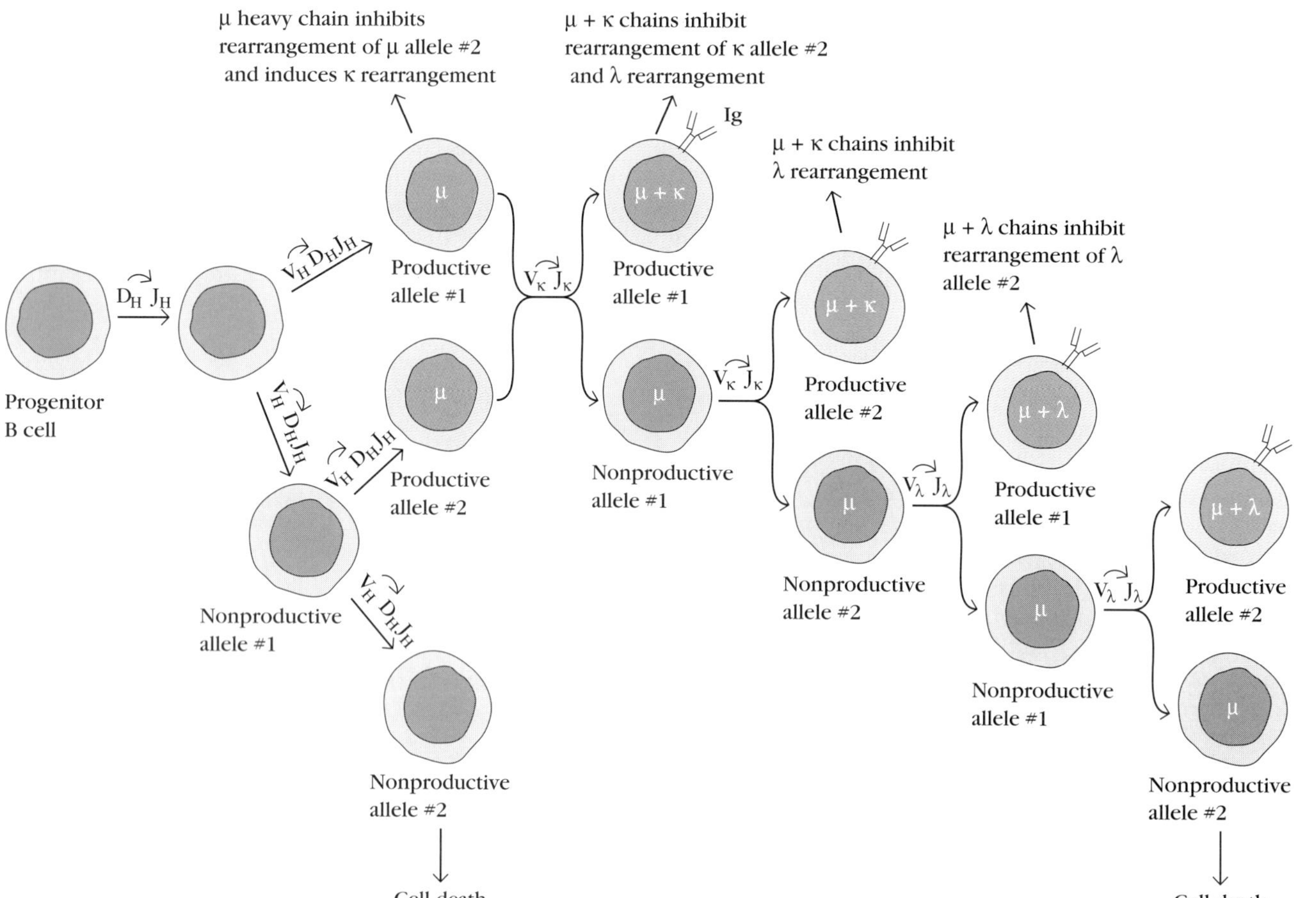

FIGURE 8-12 Model to account for allelic exclusion. Heavy-chain genes rearrange first, then κ light-chain genes, and finally λ light-chain genes. Once a productive heavy-chain gene rearrangement occurs, the μ protein product prevents rearrangement of the other heavy-chain allele and initiates light-chain gene rearrangement. Once a complete immunoglobulin is formed, further light-chain gene rearrangement ceases. If a nonproductive rearrangement occurs for one allele, then the cell attempts rearrangement of the other allele. [Adapted from G. D. Yancopoulos and F. W. Alt, 1986, *Annu. Rev. Immunol.* **4**:339.]

course, essential for the antigenic specificity of the B cell, because the expression of both alleles would render the B cell multispecific. The phenomenon of allelic exclusion suggests that once a productive V_H-D_H-J_H rearrangement and a productive V_L-J_L rearrangement have occurred, the recombination machinery is turned off, so that the heavy- and light-chain genes on the homologous chromosomes are not expressed.

G. D. Yancopoulos and F. W. Alt have proposed a model to account for allelic exclusion (Figure 8-12). They suggest that once a productive rearrangement is attained, its encoded protein is expressed and the presence of this protein acts as a signal to prevent further gene rearrangement. According to their model, the presence of μ heavy chains signals the maturing B cell to turn off rearrangement of the other heavy-chain allele and to turn on rearrangement of the κ light-chain genes. If a productive κ rearrangement occurs, κ light chains are produced and then pair with μ heavy chains to form a complete antibody molecule. The presence of this antibody then turns off further light-chain rearrangement. If κ rearrangement is nonproductive for both alleles, rearrangement of the λ-chain genes begins. If neither λ allele rearranges productively, the B cell presumably ceases to mature and soon dies by apoptosis.

Two studies with transgenic mice have supported the hypothesis that the protein products encoded by rearranged heavy- and light-chain genes regulate rearrangement of the remaining alleles. In one study, transgenic mice carrying a rearranged μ heavy-chain transgene were prepared (see Figure 2-12). The μ transgene product was expressed by a large percentage of the B cells, and rearrangement of the endogenous immunoglobulin heavy-chain genes was blocked. Similarly, cells from a transgenic mouse carrying a κ light-chain transgene did not rearrange the endogenous κ-chain genes when the κ transgene was expressed and was associated with a heavy chain to form complete immunoglobulin. These studies suggest that expression of the heavy- and light-chain proteins may indeed prevent gene rearrangement of the remaining alleles and thus account for allelic exclusion. Further discussion of allelic exclusion is presented later in the chapter.

Regulation of Immunoglobulin-Gene Transcription

Each V_H and V_L gene segment has a promoter located just upstream from the leader sequence (Figure 8-13). The promoter is a relatively short sequence of DNA extending about 200 bp upstream from the transcription initiation site. Like other promoters, the immunoglobulin promoters contain a highly conserved AT-rich sequence, called the TATA box, to which RNA polymerase II binds. After binding to the TATA box, the RNA polymerase starts transcribing the DNA from the initiation site, located about 25–35 bp downstream of the TATA box.

Effect of DNA Rearrangements on Transcription

The promoters associated with the immunoglobulin V gene segments bind RNA polymerase II very weakly. For this reason, the rate of transcription of V_H and V_L coding regions is almost negligible in unrearranged germ-line DNA. Following V-(D)-J rearrangement, however, the rate of transcription increases due to the effects of enhancer regions.

Enhancers are *cis*-acting DNA sequences that activate transcription from the promoter sequence. The mechanism by which enhancers activate transcription is still not known; it is thought that DNA-binding factors bound to the enhancer may alter chromatin structure in the vicinity, thereby facilitating the formation of a stable transcription-initiation complex at the promoter site. One heavy-chain enhancer is located within the intron between the last (3′) J gene segment and the first (5′) C gene segment (C_μ), which encodes the μ chain (see Figure 8-13). The location of this heavy-chain enhancer (ENH_{iH}) allows it to continue to function after class switching has occurred. Another heavy-chain enhancer ($ENH_{3'H}$) has been detected 3′ of the C_α gene segment. One κ light-chain enhancer (ENH_{ik}) is located between the J_κ segment and the C_κ segment, and another κ enhancer ($ENH_{3'k}$) is located 3′ of the C_κ segment. The λ light-chain enhancers are located 3′ of $C_\lambda4$ and 3′ of $C_\lambda1$.

In germ-line DNA, the variable-region promoters are about 250–300 kb away from the enhancers. Variable-region gene rearrangement brings a promoter within 2 kb of an enhancer, which is close enough for the enhancer to influence transcription. As a result, the rate of transcription of a rearranged V_LJ_L or $V_HD_HJ_H$ unit is as much as 10^4 times the rate of transcription of unrearranged V_L or V_H segments. The importance of the enhancer region in the transcription of immunoglobulin genes has been demonstrated experimentally. In one such study, B cells transfected with rearranged heavy-chain genes from which the enhancer had been deleted did not transcribe the genes.

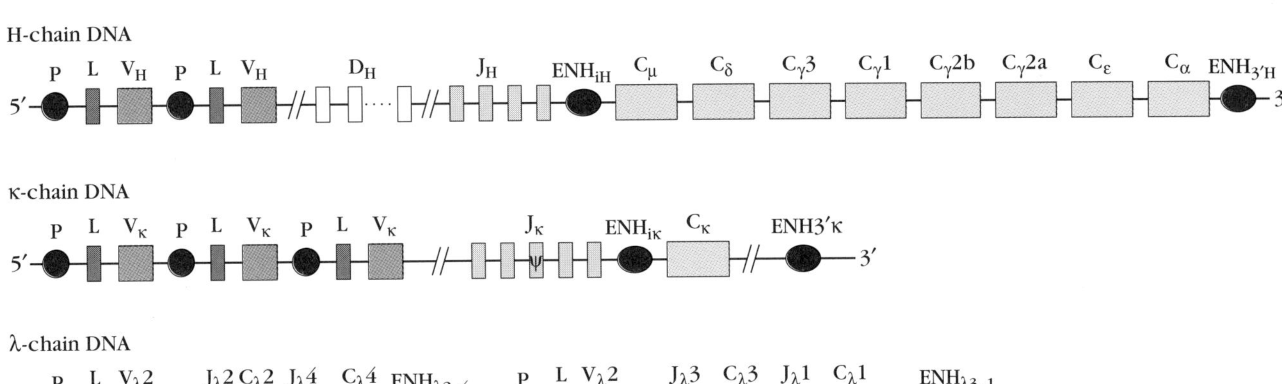

FIGURE 8-13 Location of the heavy-chain, κ light-chain, and λ light-chain promoter (P) and enhancer (ENH) sequences in mouse germ-line DNA. Variable-region DNA rearrangement moves an enhancer close enough to a promoter so that the enhancer can activate transcription from the promoter.

In contrast, B cells transfected with similar genes that contained the enhancer transcribed the transfected genes at a high rate.

Genes that regulate cellular proliferation or cell death, called *cellular oncogenes,* sometimes translocate to the immunoglobulin heavy- or light-chain loci. Here, under the influence of an immunoglobulin enhancer, the normally silent oncogene is activated, leading to increased expression of the oncogene product. Translocations of the c-*myc* and *bcl-2* oncogenes have each been associated with malignant B-cell lymphomas. The translocation of c-*myc* leads to constitutive expression of c-Myc and an aggressive B-cell lymphoma called Burkitt's lymphoma (see Figure 25-8). The translocation of *bcl-2* leads to suspension of apoptosis in programmed cell death in B cells, resulting in follicular B-cell lymphoma. This topic is covered in greater detail in Chapter 25.

Role of DNA-Binding Proteins

The activity of the immunoglobulin promoter and enhancer sequences are regulated by DNA-binding proteins. Some of these proteins are found in many cell types, whereas others are mostly restricted to cells of the lymphoid lineage. Evidence suggesting that lymphoid cells have lineage-restricted transcription factors was first demonstrated by experiments in which rearranged light-chain or heavy-chain DNA was introduced into the germ-line DNA of mouse embryos to yield transgenic mice carrying the rearranged genes in all their somatic cells. Even though all the cells in the transgenic mice contained the rearranged genes, these genes were expressed only in B cells and not in any other cells in the body. This finding suggests that B cells produce lineage-specific transcription factors that limit the transcription of the immunoglobulin genes to B-lineage cells.

The immunoglobulin heavy- and light-chain promoters contain a number of conserved sequences (or motifs) that are recognized by DNA-binding proteins (Figure 8-14a). The heavy-chain promoter includes a heptamer motif, an octamer motif (OCTA), a pyrimidine-rich motif (Py), two enhancer motifs (μE_3 and E), the TATA box, and a motif responsive to IL-5 plus antigen (VDSE). The light-chain promoter includes an octamer motif (OCTA), the TATA box, and a pentadecanucleotide motif. Different combinations of DNA-binding proteins bind to these motifs and act together to regulate gene transcription. Most of these conserved sequences and their associated DNA-bind-

(a) Ig promoters

Heavy-chain promoter

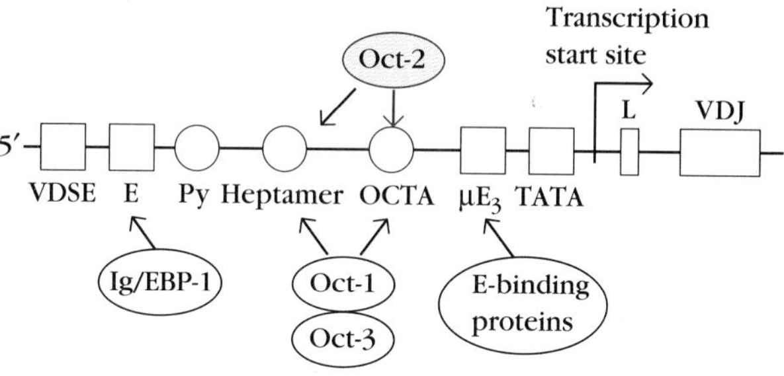

Light-chain promoter

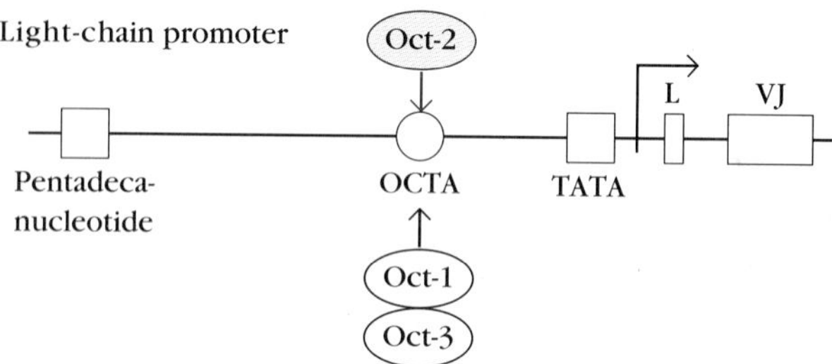

(b) Ig enhancers

Heavy-chain enhancer (ENH_{iH})

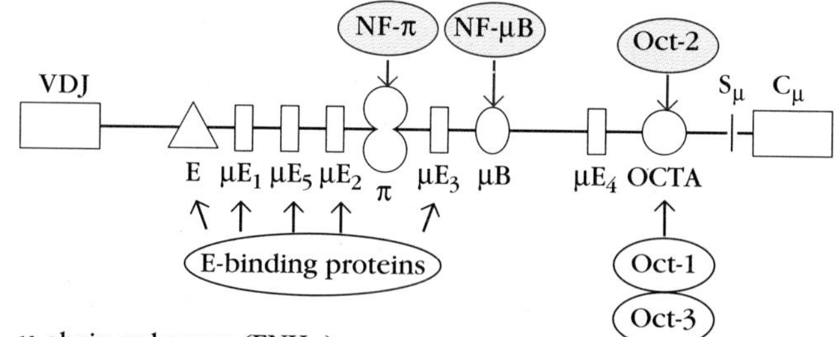

κ chain enhancer ($ENH_{i\kappa}$)

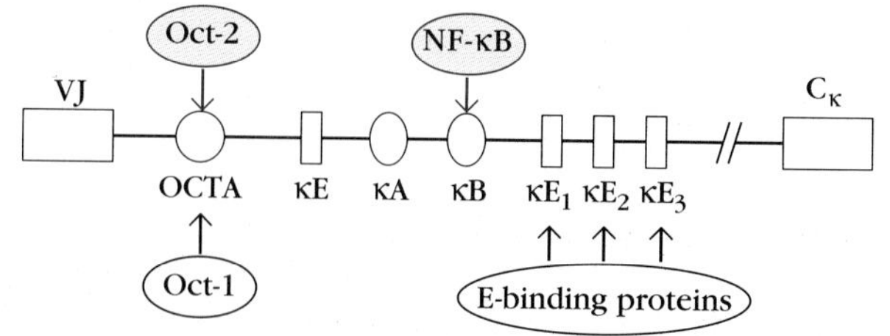

FIGURE 8-14 Location of conserved sequences (motifs) in the immunoglobulin (a) promoters and (b) enhancers in the mouse. Transcription factors that are B-lineage specific are shown in color above the promoter or enhancer sites to which they bind. Transcription factors that are present in many other cell types as well are shown below. Transcription of the immunoglobulin genes is regulated by these DNA-binding proteins.

ing proteins are found in a wide variety of cells. However, the OCTA motif and one of its associated DNA-binding proteins called Oct-2 is found only in B cells and a few other cell lineages.

Evidence that the OCTA sequence is regulated by B-lineage–specific DNA-binding factors came from engineering the OCTA sequence upstream of a TATA sequence on a β-globulin gene promoter. When the engineered β-globulin gene was transfected into B-cell lines and into fibroblast cells, the transfected B cells expressed 20-fold higher levels of the β-globulin gene than the transfected fibroblasts. The lineage-specific OCTA-binding protein, Oct-2, is expressed by B cells when D_H-J_H joining occurs. The positive regulatory role of Oct-2 on the immunoglobulin promoter can be demonstrated by transfecting the immunoglobulin gene and its promoter into a fibroblast cell line. The construct is inactive in these transfected cells unless the cell is also transfected with an Oct-2 expression vector.

The immunoglobulin enhancer regions are also regulated by lineage-specific factors (Figure 8-14b). The heavy-chain enhancer contains three sequences (π, μB, and OCTA) that are thought to bind lineage-specific transcription factors, as well as five E motifs (μE1–5) that bind factors that are not specific to B cells. The enhancer OCTA sequence is the same as the OCTA sequence in the immunoglobulin promoter; thus Oct-2 binds to both the heavy-chain promoter and enhancer. The κ light-chain enhancer also contains an OCTA sequence, various E motifs, and a lineage-specific sequence called κB that binds a protein called NF-κB. The κB motif also is present in the promoters of the genes encoding IL-2 and IFN-β and in the promoter sequence of the human immunodeficiency virus (HIV). Binding of NF-κB to the κB motif in each of these promoters results in enhanced transcription of the genes.

NF-κB is a heterodimer composed of two DNA-binding subunits (p50 and p65). In most of the wide variety of cells that express κB, this factor is retained in the cytoplasm in an inactive form complexed with inhibitor (I-κB). A variety of stimuli, including mitogens, various cytokines, and certain viruses, can induce release of NF-κB from I-κB. Once released, NF-κB enters the nucleus through nuclear pores and binds to the κB motif, thereby mediating gene activation (Figure 8-15). Unlike other cells, the mature B cell does not retain the inactive form of NF-κB in its cytoplasm. Instead, NF-κB is constitutively present in an active form in the nucleus of mature B cells. As discussed in Chapter 23, NF-κB also plays an important role in regulating transcription of the viral genome in HIV-infected T cells.

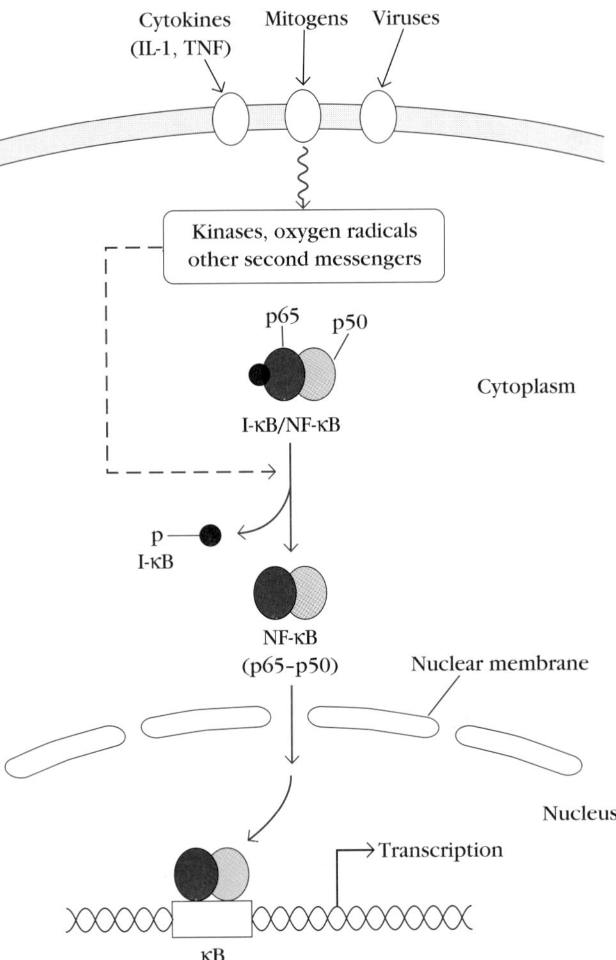

FIGURE 8-15 In most cells that express NF-κB, this heterodimeric transcription factor is present in the cytoplasm in an inactive form bound to an inhibitor (gray). Various stimuli can generate second messengers that induce release of NF-κB, which then enters the nucleus and binds to the κB enhancer sequence, stimulating transcription. In mature B cells, the active form of NF-κB is present constitutively. [Adapted from V. Blank et al., 1992, *Trends in Bio. Sci.* **17**:135.]

Generation of Antibody Diversity

As the organization of the immunoglobulin genes was deciphered, the sources of the vast diversity in the variable region began to come clear. The germ-line theory, mentioned earlier, argued that the entire variable-region repertoire is encoded in the germ line of the organism and is transmitted from parent to offspring via the germ cells (egg and sperm). The somatic-variation theory held that the germ line contains a limited number of variable genes, which are diversi-

TABLE 8-3 CUMULATIVE GENERATION OF MINIMUM ANTIBODY DIVERSITY IN THE MOUSE*

Mechanism of diversity	Heavy chain	Light chains κ	Light chains λ
	Estimated number of segments		
Multiple germ-line gene segments:			
V	300–1000	300	2
D	13	0	0
J	4	4	3
	Possible number of combinations†		
Combinatorial V-J and V-D-J joining	$300 \times 13 \times 4 = 1.6 \times 10^4$	$300 \times 4 = 1.2 \times 10^3$	$2 \times 3 = 6$
Junctional flexibility	+	+	+
N-region nucleotide addition	+	–	–
Somatic mutation	+	+	+
Combinatorial association of heavy and light chains	$>1.6 \times 10^4 \times (>1.2 \times 10^3 + >6) = \gg 1.9 \times 10^7$		

* Antibody diversity in humans is similar to that in the mouse.

† A + indicates mechanism makes a significant contribution to diversity but to an unknown extent. A – indicates mechanism does not operate.

fied in the somatic cells by mutational or recombinational events during development of the immune system. As the cloning and sequencing of the immunoglobulin genes was completed, both models were partially vindicated. The sources of antibody diversity in the mouse and the number of different specificities generated cumulatively by these mechanisms are summarized in Table 8-3. The total number of possible combinations is conservatively estimated to be $\approx 10^8$, the commonly quoted figure for the number of different antibody specificities that can be generated by the mammalian immune system.

Multiple Germ-Line V, D, and J Gene Segments

DNA hybridization studies have demonstrated that mouse germ-line DNA contains about 300 V_κ gene segments and 300—1000 V_H gene segments but only two V_λ gene segments. The existence of multiple J_L, D_H, and J_H segments expands the germ-line contribution to diversity. In the mouse, there appear to be 4 functional J_H, 4 functional J_κ, 3 functional J_λ, and an estimated 13 D_H gene segments. Although the numbers of germ-line genes are far fewer than predicted by early proponents of the germ-line model, multiple germ-line V, D, and J genes clearly do contribute to diversity of the antigen-binding sites in antibodies.

Combinatorial V-J and V-D-J Joining

The contribution of multiple germ-line gene segments to antibody diversity is magnified by the random rearrangement of these segments in somatic cells. The ability of any of the 300–1000 V_H gene segments to combine with any of the 13 D_H segments and any of the 4 J_H segments allows an enormous amount of diversity to be generated ($300 \times 13 \times 4 = 1.6 \times 10^4$ minimum possible combinations). Similarly, 300 V_κ gene segments randomly combining with 4 J_κ segments has the potential of generating 1.2×10^3 possible combinations. With only 2 V_λ and 3 J_λ gene segments, the combinatorial diversity of the λ light-chain DNA is much less.

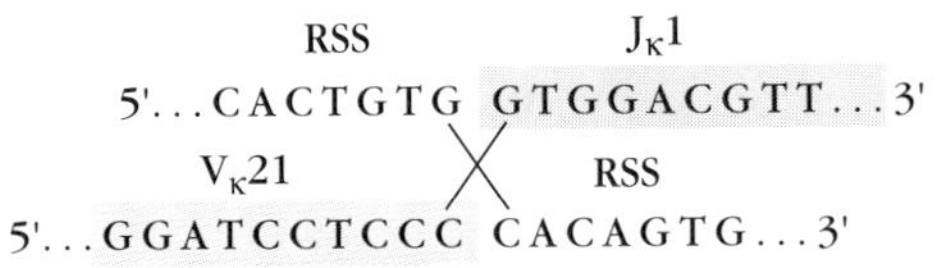

RSS $J_\kappa 1$
5'...CACTGTG GTGGACGTT...3'
$V_\kappa 21$ RSS
5'...GGATCCTCCC CACAGTG...3'

Pre-B cell lines	Coding joints ($V_\kappa 21\, J_\kappa 1$)	Signal joints (RSS/RSS)
Cell line #1	5'-GGATCC GGACGTT-3'	5'-CACTGTG CACAGTG-3'
Cell line #2	5'-GGATC TGGACGTT-3'	5'-CACTGTG CACAGTG-3'
Cell line #3	5'-GGATCCTC GTGGACGTT-3'	5'-CACTGTG CACAGTG-3'
Cell line #4	5'-GGATCCT TGGACGTT-3'	5'-CACTGTG CACAGTG-3'

FIGURE 8-16 Experimental evidence for junctional flexibility in immunoglobulin gene rearrangement. The nucleotide sequences flanking the coding joints between $V_\kappa 21$ and $J_\kappa 1$ and of the corresponding signal joints were determined in four pre-B cell lines. The sequence constancy in the signal joints contrasts with the sequence variability in the coding joints. Purple underline indicates nucleotides derived from $V_\kappa 21$ or its RSS; black underline indicates nucleotides derived from $J_\kappa 1$ or its RSS.

Junctional Flexibility

The enormous diversity generated by means of V, D, and J combinations is further augmented by a phenomenon known as *junctional flexibility*. As shown in Figure 8-6, the process of recombination involves both the joining of recombination signal sequences to form a signal joint and the joining of coding sequences to form a coding joint. Although the signal sequences are always joined precisely, joining of the coding sequences often is imprecise. In one study, for example, joining of the $V_\kappa 21$ and $J_\kappa 1$ coding sequences was analyzed in several pre-B cell lines. Sequence analysis of the signal and coding joints revealed precise joining of the signal sequences but flexible joining of the coding sequences (Figure 8-16).

As discussed earlier, this junctional flexibility leads to many nonproductive rearrangements, but it also generates several productive combinations encoding alternative amino acids at each coding joint (see Figure 8-10), thereby increasing antibody diversity. Coding joints have been shown to fall within the third hypervariable region (CDR3) in immunoglobulin heavy-chain and light-chain DNA (Table 8-4). Since the CDR3 hypervariable region makes up a significant portion of the antigen-binding site on the antibody molecule (see Color Plate 3), an amino acid change generated by junctional flexibility can have major impact in generating antibody diversity.

N-Region Nucleotide Addition

Variable-region coding joints have been shown to contain short amino acid sequences that are not encoded by the V, D, or J gene segments. These amino acids are encoded by N nucleotides that have been added during the joining process. N-region nucleotide addition, which occurs only during joining of heavy-chain V, D, and J gene segments, generates considerable heavy-

TABLE 8-4 SOURCES OF SEQUENCE VARIATION IN COMPLEMENTARITY-DETERMINING REGIONS OF IMMUNOGLOBULIN HEAVY- AND LIGHT-CHAIN GENES

Source of variation	CDR1	CDR2	CDR3
Sequence encoded by:	V segment	V segment	V_L-J_L junction V_H-D_H-J_H junctions
Junctional flexibility	−	−	+
N-nucleotide addition*	−	−	+
Somatic mutation	+	+	+

* N-nucleotide addition occurs only in heavy-chain DNA.

chain diversity. Up to 15 N nucleotides can be added to the D_H-J_H and V_H-D_HJ_H joints in a reaction thought to be catalyzed by terminal deoxynucleotidyl transferase (TdT). Evidence that TdT is responsible for N-nucleotide addition has come from transfection studies in fibroblasts. When fibroblasts were transfected with the RAG-1 and RAG-2 genes, V-D-J rearrangement occurred but no N nucleotides were present in the coding joints. However, when the fibroblasts were also transfected with the TdT gene, then V-D-J rearrangement was accompanied by addition of N nucleotides at the coding joints. Thus a complete heavy-chain variable region is encoded by a $V_HND_HNJ_H$ unit. The additional heavy-chain diversity generated by N-region nucleotide addition is quite large because N regions appear to consist of wholly random sequences. Since this diversity occurs at V-D-J coding joints, it is localized in the CDR3 of the heavy-chain genes.

Somatic Mutation

All the antibody diversity discussed so far stems from mechanisms that operate during formation of specific variable regions by gene rearrangement. The implicit assumption throughout this chapter has been that once a functional variable-region gene unit is formed, it is not altered. This assumption turns out to be false, and additional antibody diversity is generated in rearranged variable-region gene units by a process called *somatic mutation*. As a result of somatic mutation, individual nucleotides in VJ or VDJ units are replaced with alternative bases, thus potentially altering the specificity of the encoded immunoglobulins.

Comparisons of germ-line variable-region DNA sequences with the DNA sequences expressed by somatic cells has demonstrated somatic mutation in both light- and heavy-chain genes. In one such study, L. E. Hood and his colleagues investigated the antibody response in mice to the hapten phosphorycholine. This particular antigen-antibody system was chosen because a single V_H gene segment, T-15, was utilized by all the antibodies produced to phosphorylcholine. Hood cloned the T-15 germ-line DNA and sequenced it to determine the germ-line prototype sequence. He then sequenced the heavy-chain variable region in 19 phosphorylcholine-specific myeloma proteins and compared these with the germ-line V_H prototype sequence. Of the 19 expressed sequences, 10 were identical with the prototype sequence; the other 9 differed from the prototype by from one to eight amino acid substitutions. Of additional interest was the observation that all nine heavy-chain variable-region variants were present in the IgG or IgA myeloma proteins; none were present in IgM. This finding suggests a possible association of somatic mutation with class switching or, at least, that the additional cell divisions a cell undergoes in the process of class switching may increase the likelihood of somatic mutation occurring. Furthermore, the estimated rate of somatic mutation in B cells is quite high, being 10^{-3} mutations per base pair per cell division. This rate is 10^6 times higher than the spontaneous mutation rate in other genes, again suggesting that for some reason B cells are predisposed to somatic mutation.

The number of mutations generated by the process of somatic mutation has been shown to increase in the secondary and tertiary antibody responses to an antigen. Claudia Berek and Cesar Milstein were able to sequence the mRNA encoding antibodies produced in response to a primary, secondary, or tertiary immunization with a hapten-carrier conjugate. The hapten that they chose was 2-phenyl-5-oxazolone (phOx) coupled to a protein carrier. They chose this hapten because it had previously been shown to induce production of a majority of antibodies encoded by a single germ-line V_H and V_κ gene segment. Berek and Milstein immunized mice with the phOx-carrier conjugate and then used the mice spleen cells to prepare hybridomas secreting monoclonal antibodies specific for the phOx hapten. The mRNA sequence for the H chain and κ light chain of each hybridoma was then determined (Figure 8-17). They found that of 12 hybridomas obtained from mice seven days after a primary immunization, all used the V_H Ox-1 gene and all but one used the V_κ Ox-1 gene. Only a few hybridomas showed mutations from the germ-line sequence. By day 14 after primary immunization, analysis of eight hybridomas revealed that six continued to use the germ-line V_H Ox-1 gene and all continued to use the V_κ Ox-1 gene. Now, however, a majority of the hybridomas showed mutations from the germ-line sequence. Hybridomas analyzed from the secondary and tertiary responses showed a larger percentage utilizing germ-line V_H genes other than the V_H Ox-1 gene. In those hybridoma clones that utilized the V_H Ox-1 and V_κ Ox-1 gene segments, most of the mutations were clustered in the CDR1 and CDR2 hypervariable regions. As Figure 8-17 illustrates, the number of mutations progressively increased following primary, secondary, and tertiary immunizations. And even more interesting, the overall affinity of the antibodies also progressively increased from the primary to the secondary to the tertiary response. Although the process of somatic mutation is random, and can therefore generate antibodies of lower affinity as well as higher, the ability of an antigen to drive clonal expansion will selectively increase the proliferation of B cells that have higher-affinity membrane-bound antibody on their surface.

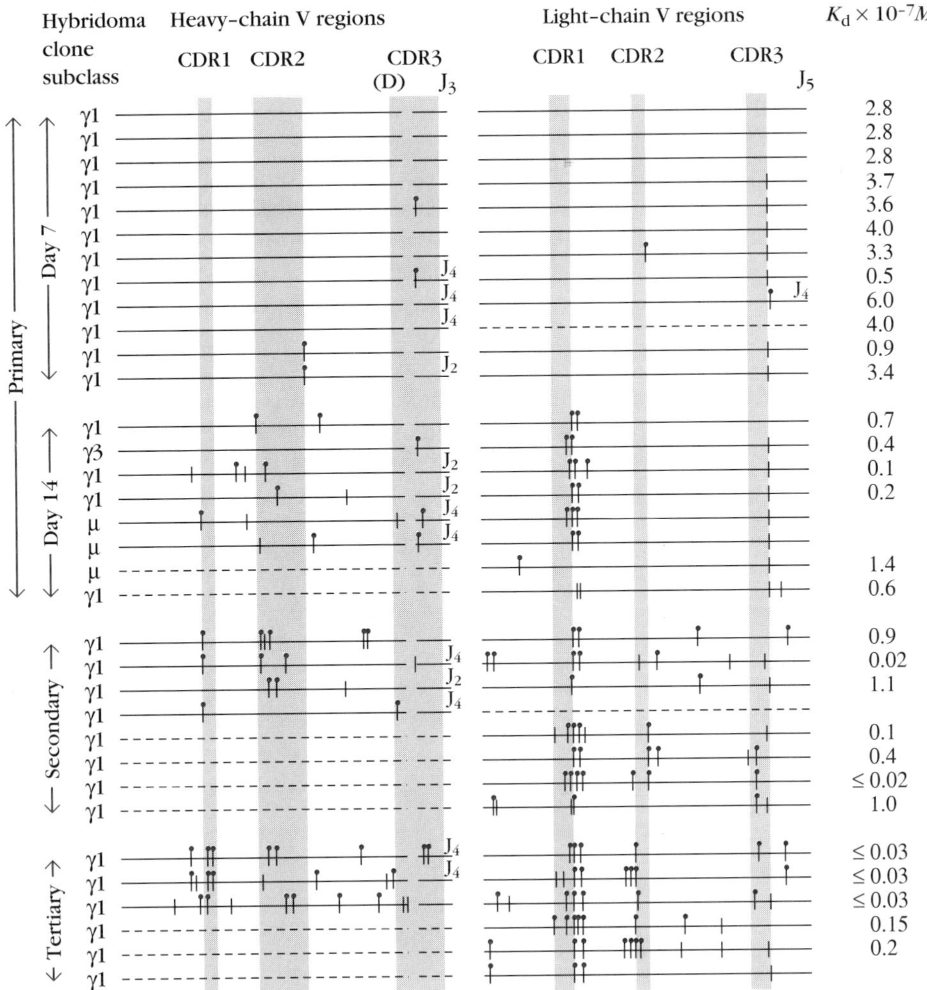

FIGURE 8-17 Experimental evidence for somatic mutation in variable regions of immunoglobulin genes. The diagram compares the mRNA sequences of the heavy and light chains from hybridomas specific for the phOx hapten. The horizontal solid lines represent the germ-line V_H and V_κ Ox-1 sequences; dashed lines represent sequences derived from other germ-line genes. Vertical lines show the position of mutations, and the purple circles indicate mutations that encode a different amino acid than the germ-line sequence. These data show that the frequency of mutation (1) increases in the course of the primary response and (2) is higher after secondary and tertiary immunizations than after primary immunization. Moreover, the dissociation constant (K_d) of the anti-phOx antibodies decreased in going from the primary to tertiary response, indicating an increase in the overall affinity of the antibody. Note also that most of the mutations are clustered within CDR1 and CDR2 of both the heavy and light chains. [Adapted from C. Berek and C. Milstein, 1987, *Immunol. Rev.* **96**:23.]

Association of Heavy and Light Chains

Estimates of the quantitative contribution of junctional flexibility, N-region nucleotide addition, and somatic mutation to the generation of antibody diversity are very imprecise; nonetheless these processes significantly increase the number of possible specificities that can be generated. The final source of antibody diversity is the combinatorial association of heavy and light chains. Because the specificity of an antibody's antigen-binding site is determined by the variable regions in both its heavy and light chains, combinational association of H and L chains also can generate diversity.

As shown in Table 8-3, a minimum of 1.6×10^4 heavy-chain genes and 1.2×10^3 κ light-chain genes can be generated in the mouse as a result of the variable-region gene rearrangements. Assuming that any one of the possible heavy-chain and light-chain genes can occur randomly in the same cell, then the minimum number of possible heavy- and light-chain combinations is 1.9×10^7. However, the actual number of possible antigenic specificities is considerably greater because of the unknown but significant number of nucleotide sequences introduced by junctional flexibility, N-region nucleotide addition, and somatic mutation. Some have estimated that total antibody diversity may be as high as 10^{11}.

Class Switching Among Constant-Region Genes

Following antigenic stimulation of a B-cell, the heavy-chain DNA can undergo a further rearrangement in which the $V_H D_H J_H$ unit can combine with any C_H gene segment. The exact mechanism of this process, called *class switching* is unclear, but evidence suggests that short DNA flanking sequences (termed *switch sites*) located 2–3 kb upstream from each C_H segment (except C_δ) are involved. These switch sites are rather large but are composed of multiple copies of short repeated sequences. One hypothesis is that a series of class-specific recombinase proteins bind to these switch sites and thereby facilitate DNA recombination. The choice of the particular immunoglobulin class to be expressed might then depend on the specificity of the recombinase protein expressed.

Various cytokines secreted by activated T_H cells have been shown to induce B cells to class-switch to a particular isotype. Interleukin 4 (IL-4), for example, induces class switching from C_μ to $C_\gamma 1$ or C_ϵ. K. Yoshida,

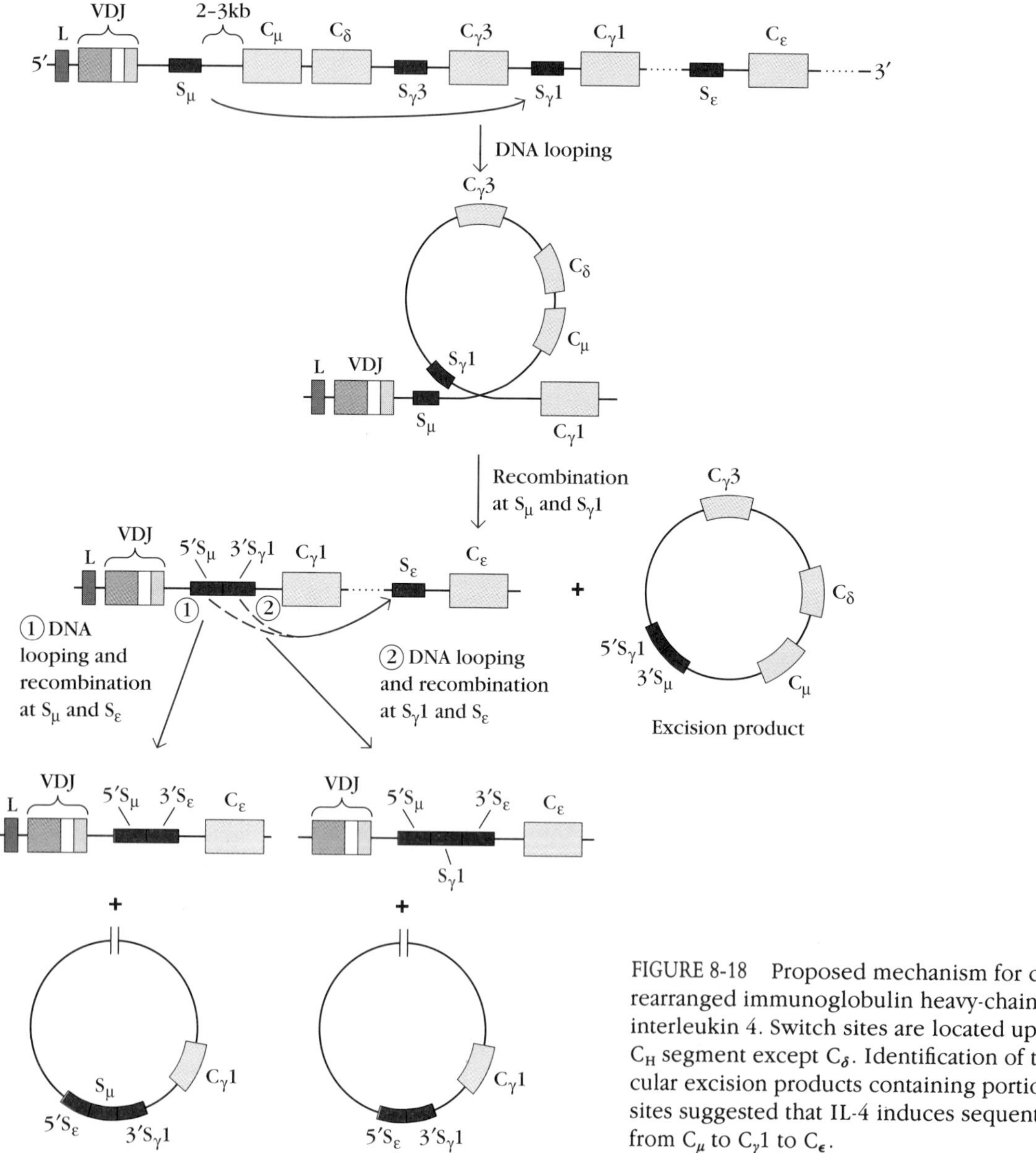

FIGURE 8-18 Proposed mechanism for class switching in rearranged immunoglobulin heavy-chain genes induced by interleukin 4. Switch sites are located upstream from each C_H segment except C_δ. Identification of the indicated circular excision products containing portions of the switch sites suggested that IL-4 induces sequential class switching from C_μ to $C_\gamma 1$ to C_ϵ.

H. Sakano, and colleagues have demonstrated that IL-4 induces class switching in a successive manner: first from C_μ to $C\gamma1$ and then from $C_\gamma1$ to C_ϵ (Figure 8-18). They were able to demonstrate this by identifying the circular excision products produced during class switching. The class switch from C_μ to $C_\gamma1$ was shown to generate a circular excision product containing C_μ together with the 5′ end of the $\gamma1$ switch site ($S_\gamma1$) and the 3′ end of the μ switch site (S_μ). The switch from $C_\gamma1$ to C_ϵ was shown to generate two circular excision products containing $C_\gamma1$ together with portions of the switch sites. The role of cytokines in immunoglobulin class switching is discussed more fully in Chapter 13.

Expression of Immunoglobulin Genes

As in the expression of other genes, post-transcriptional processing of immunoglobulin primary transcripts is required to produce functional mRNAs (see Figures 8-3 and 8-4). The first step in this RNA processing, which occurs while transcription is proceeding, is addition of a 7-methylguanosine residue to the 5′ end of the primary transcript. This forms the 5′ cap structure, which plays a role in translation of mRNA on the polyribosomes. Once transcription is completed, the primary RNA transcript is cleaved some 15–30 nucleotides downstream of a highly conserved AAUAAA sequence (called the *polyadenylation signal*). An enzyme called poly-A polymerase recognizes this signal sequence and adds sequential adenylate residues derived from ATP to the 3′ end of the primary transcript, forming a poly-A tail of about 250 residues.

Following capping and polyadenylation, the introns of a primary transcript are excised and their flanking exons are connected by a process called RNA splicing. Short, moderately conserved splice sequences, or splice sites, which are located at the intron-exon boundaries of a primary transcript, signal the positions at which splicing occurs. After heavy-chain and light-chain DNA rearrangement is completed, the DNA continues to contain intervening DNA sequences. These intervening sequences include noncoding introns and J gene segments not lost during V-D-J rearrangement. In addition the heavy-chain C gene segments are organized as a series of coding exons and noncoding introns. Each exon of the C_H gene segment corresponds to a domain or hinge region of the heavy polypeptide chain. Processing of the primary transcript in the nucleus removes each of these intervening sequences to yield the final mRNA product. The mRNA is then exported from the nucleus and goes to polyribosomes for translation into the complete H or L chain.

Differential RNA Processing of Primary Transcripts

The processing of an immunoglobulin primary transcript can also lead to production of different mRNAs. Such differential RNA processing of heavy-chain transcripts explains the production of secreted or membrane-bound forms of a particular immunoglobulin and the simultaneous expression of IgM and IgD.

Expression of Membrane-Bound or Secreted Immunoglobulin

As discussed in Chapter 5, a particular immunoglobulin can exist in a membrane-bound form or in a secreted form. The two forms differ in the amino acid sequence of the heavy-chain carboxyl-terminal domains (C_H3/C_H3 in IgA, IgD, and IgG and C_H4/C_H4 in IgE and IgM). The secreted form has a hydrophilic sequence of about 20 amino acids in the carboxyl-terminal domain; this is replaced in the membrane-bound form with a sequence of about 40 amino acids containing a hydrophilic segment, a hydrophobic transmembrane segment, and a short hydrophilic cytoplasmic segment at the carboxyl terminus (Figure 8-19a). For some time the existence of these two forms seemed inconsistent with the structure of germ-line heavy-chain DNA, which had been shown to contain a single C_H gene segment corresponding to each class and subclass (see Figure 8-2c).

The explanation of this apparent paradox came from DNA sequencing of the C_μ gene segment, which consists of four exons ($C_{\mu1}$, $C_{\mu2}$, $C_{\mu3}$, and $C_{\mu4}$) corresponding to the four domains of the IgM molecule. The $C_{\mu4}$ exon contains a nucleotide sequence at its 3′ end that encodes the hydrophilic sequence in the C_H4 domain of secreted IgM. Two additional exons called M1 and M2 are located just 1.8 kb downstream from the 3′ end of the $C_{\mu4}$ exon. The M1 exon encodes the transmembrane segment, and M2 encodes the cytoplasmic segment of the C_H4 domain in membrane-bound IgM. Later DNA sequencing revealed that all the C_H gene segments have two additional downstream M1 and M2 exons encoding the transmembrane and cytoplasmic segments.

The primary transcript produced by transcription of a rearranged μ heavy-chain gene contains two polyadenylation signal sequences, or poly-A sites. Site 1 is located at the 3′ end of the $C_{\mu4}$ exon and site 2 at the 3′ end of the M2 exon. If cleavage of the primary transcript and addition of the poly-A tail occurs at site 1, the M1 and M2 exons are lost. Excision of the introns and splicing of the remaining exons then produces mRNA encoding the secreted form of the μ heavy chain (Fig-

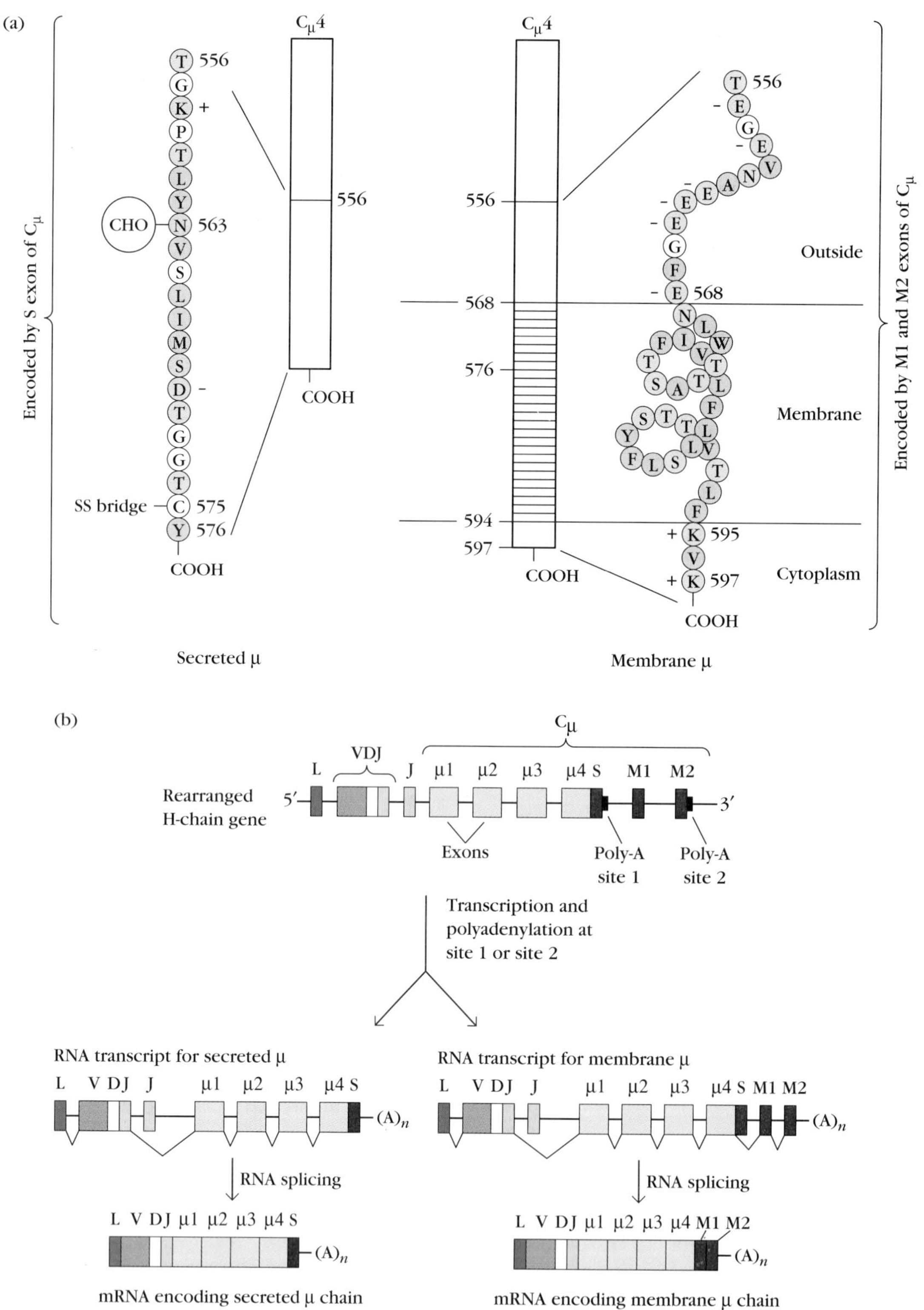

FIGURE 8-19 Expression of secreted and membrane forms of the μ heavy chain by alternative RNA processing. (a) Amino acid sequence of the carboxyl-terminal end of secreted and membrane μ heavy chains. Residues are indicated by the single-letter amino acid code. Hydrophilic residues are shaded purple, and hydrophobic residues are shaded gray. Charged amino acids are indicated with a + or −. The rest of the sequence is identical in both forms. (b) Structure of a rearranged heavy-chain gene showing the C_μ exons and poly-A sites. Polyadenylation of the primary transcript at either site 1 or site 2 produces two RNA transcripts. Subsequent splicing (indicated by V-shaped lines) generates mRNAs encoding secreted or membrane μ chains.

ure 8-19b). If cleavage and polyadenylation of the primary transcript occurs instead at site 2, then a different pattern of splicing occurs. The sequence of the $C_{\mu 4}$ exon contains a splice signal toward its 3′ end. Splicing enzymes, however, recognize this splice signal only if another splice signal lies downstream, as it does when the M1 and M2 exons are present. In this case, splicing removes the 3′ end of the $C_{\mu 4}$ exon that encodes the hydrophilic sequence of the secreted form and joins the remainder of the $C_{\mu 4}$ exon with the M1 and M2 exons, producing mRNA for the membrane form of the μ heavy chain.

Production of the secreted or membrane form of an immunoglobulin thus depends on differential processing of a common primary transcript. As noted previously, mature B cells produce only membrane-bound antibody, whereas differentiated plasma cells produce secreted antibodies. Presumably some mechanism exists in unprimed B cells and in plasma cells that directs RNA processing preferentially toward the production of mRNA encoding either the membrane form or secreted form of an immunoglobulin.

Simultaneous Expression of IgM and IgD

The phenomenon of differential RNA processing also explains the simultaneous expression of membrane-bound IgM and IgD by mature B cells. As mentioned already, transcription of rearranged heavy-chain genes in mature B cells produces primary transcripts containing both the C_μ and C_δ gene segments. One explanation for this is that the close proximity of C_μ and C_δ, which are only about 5 kb apart, and the lack of a switch site between them permits the entire VDJ$C_\mu C_\delta$ region to be transcribed into a long primary RNA transcript, about 15 kb long, which contains four poly-A sites (Figure 8-20a). Sites 1 and 2 are associated with C_μ, as

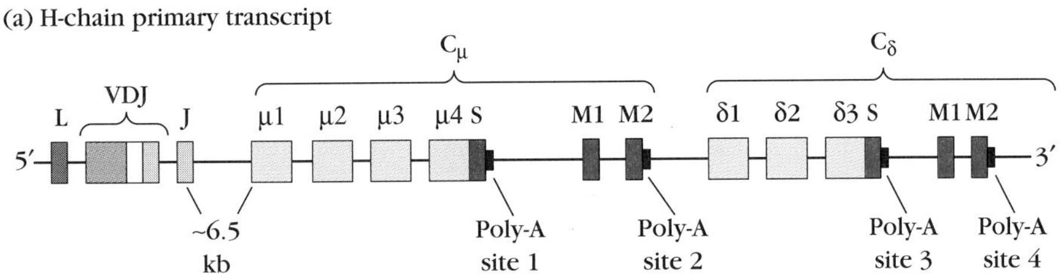

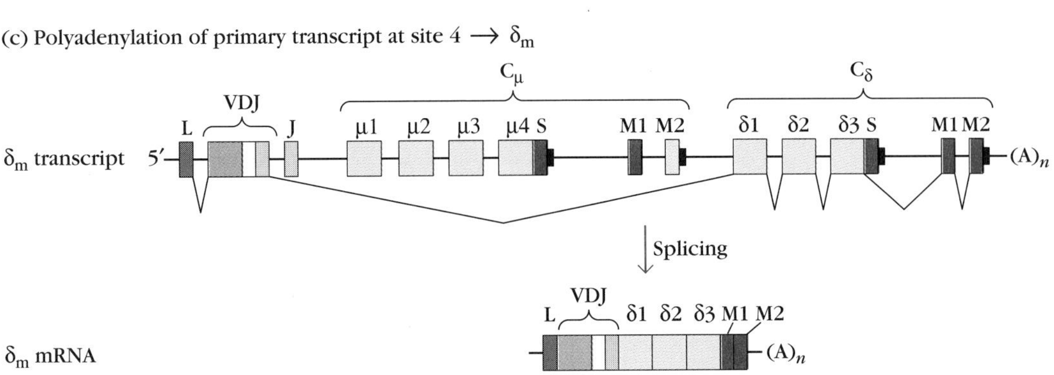

FIGURE 8-20 Expression of μ_m and δ_m heavy chains by alternative RNA processing. (a) Structure of rearranged heavy-chain gene showing C_μ and C_δ exons and poly-A sites. (b) Structure of μ_m transcript and μ_m mRNA resulting from polyadenylation at site 2 and splicing. (c) Structure of δ_m transcript and δ_m mRNA resulting from polyadenylation at site 4 and splicing. Both processing pathways can proceed in a given B cell.

described in the previous section; sites 3 and 4 are located at similar places in the C_δ gene segment. If the transcript is cleaved and polyadenylated at site 1 or 2 after the C_μ exons, then the mRNA will encode the membrane or secreted forms of the μ heavy chain (Figure 8-20b); if polyadenylation is instead further downstream at sites 3 or 4 after the C_δ exons, then RNA splicing will remove the intervening C_μ exons and produce mRNA for the membrane or secreted forms of the δ heavy chain (Figure 8-20c). Since the mature B cell expresses both IgM and IgD on its membrane, processing by both pathways must occur simultaneously.

Synthesis, Assembly, and Secretion of Immunoglobulins

Immunoglobulin heavy- and light-chain mRNAs are translated on separate polyribosomes of the rough endoplasmic reticulum (RER). Newly synthesized chains contain an amino-terminal leader sequence, which serves to guide the chains into the lumen of the RER where it is then cleaved off. The assembly of light (L) and heavy (H) chains into the disulfide-linked and glycosylated immunoglobulin molecule occurs as the chains pass through the cisternae of the RER into the Golgi apparatus and then into secretory vesicles, which fuse with the plasma membrane (Figure 8-21). The order of chain assembly varies among the immunoglobulin classes. In the case of IgM, the H and L chains assemble within the RER to form half-molecules, and then two half-molecules assemble to form the complete molecule. In the case of IgG, two H chains assemble, then an H_2L intermediate is assembled, and finally the complete H_2L_2 molecule is formed. Interchain disulfide bonds are formed, and the polypeptides are glycosylated as they move from the endoplasmic reticulum into the Golgi apparatus. If the molecule contains the transmembrane sequence of the membrane form, it becomes anchored in the membrane of a secretory vesicle and is inserted into the plasma membrane as the vesicle fuses with the plasma membrane. If the molecule contains the hydrophilic sequence of secreted immunoglobulins, it is

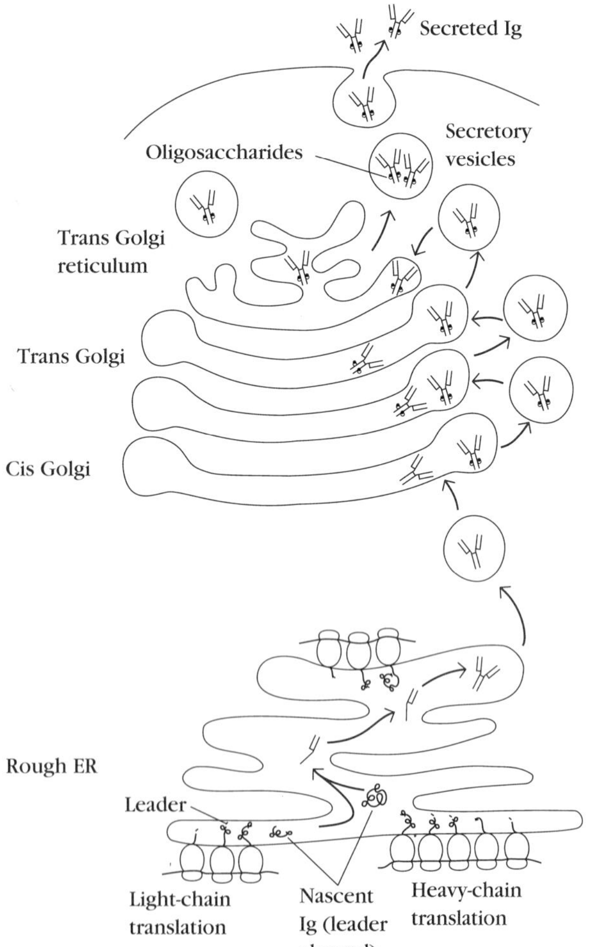

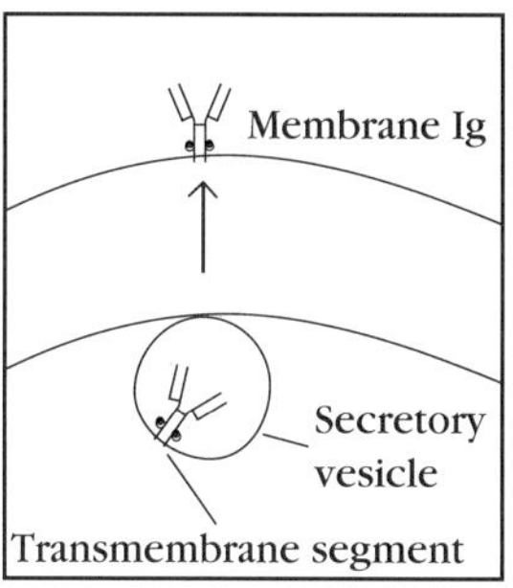

FIGURE 8-21 Synthesis, assembly, and secretion of the immunoglobulin molecule. The heavy and light chains are synthesized upon separate polyribosomes (polysomes). The assembly of the chains to form the disulfide-linked and glycosylated immunoglobulin molecule occurs as the chains pass through the cisternae of the rough endoplasmic reticulum (ER) into the Golgi apparatus and then into secretory vesicles. The main figure depicts assembly of a secreted antibody. The inset depicts a membrane-bound antibody, which contains the carboxyl-terminal transmembrane segment. This form becomes anchored in the membrane of secretory vesicles and then is inserted into the cell membrane when the vesicle fuses with the membrane.

transported as a free molecule in a secretory vesicle and is released from the cell when the vesicle fuses with the plasma membrane.

B-Cell Developmental Stages

The developmental process that results in generation of antibody-secreting B cells (plasma cells) can be divided into two phases: an *antigen-independent* phase, which occurs in the bone marrow, and an *antigen-dependent* phase, which occurs in the periphery. The development of mature B cells first occurs in the embryo and continues throughout life. Before birth, the yolk sac and fetal liver and bone marrow are the major sites of B-cell development; after birth, the bone marrow is the major site of B-cell development. Figure 8-22 outlines this developmental process and summarizes the properties of the intermediates.

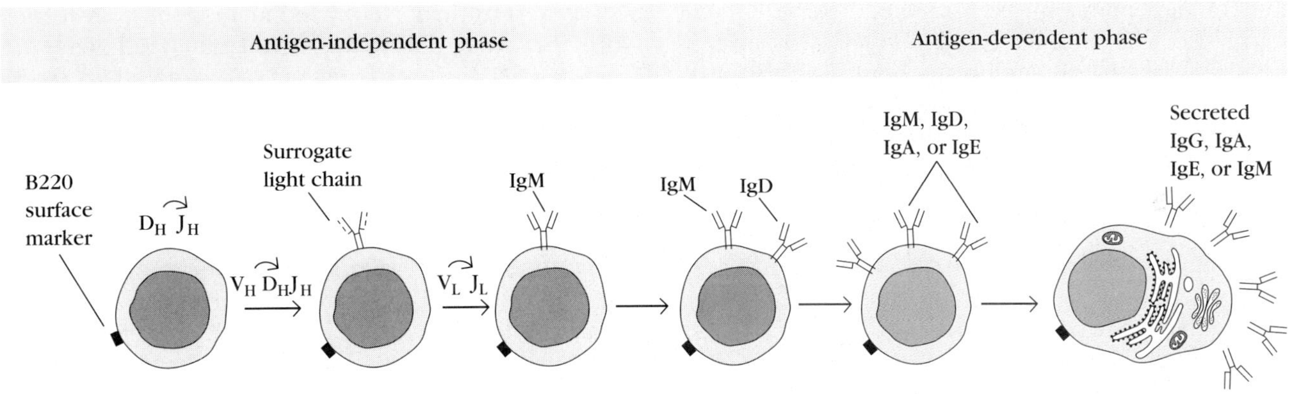

Antigen-independent phase

Antigen-dependent phase

B220 surface marker

$D_H J_H$

$V_H D_H J_H$

Surrogate light chain

$V_L J_L$

IgM

IgM IgD

IgM, IgD, IgA, or IgE

Secreted IgG, IgA, IgE, or IgM

	Pro-B cell	Pre-B cell	Immature B cell	Mature B cell	Activated B cell	Plasma cell
Heavy-chain genes	D_HJ_H	$V_HD_HJ_H$	$V_HD_HJ_H$	$V_HD_HJ_H$	$V_HD_HJ_H$	$V_HD_HJ_H$
Light-chain genes	Surrogate germ-line κ and λ	Surrogate germ-line κ and λ	V_LJ_L	V_LJ_L	V_LJ_L	V_LJ_L
RAG-1/ RAG-2	+	+	+	–	–	–
TdT	+	+	–	–	–	–
Membrane Ig:						
Heavy chain	–	μ	μ	μ + δ	μ + δ; or α, ε, or γ alone or + μ	–
Light chain	–	Surrogate light chain	κ or λ	κ or λ	κ or λ	–
Secreted Ig	–	–	–	–	Low levels	μ, γ, α, or ε
Class switching	–	–	–	–	+	–
Somatic mutation	–	–	–	–	+	–

FIGURE 8-22 Sequence of events in B-cell development and characteristics of the major intermediates. Changes in the RNA processing of heavy-chain transcripts following the pre-B cell stage lead to synthesis of both membrane-bound IgM and IgD by mature B cells and later to production of secreted Ig by plasma cells. See text for details. *RAG* = recombination-activating gene; TdT = terminal deoxyribonucleotidyl transferase.

The differentiation of hematopoietic precursor cells into mature immunocompetent B cells involves an orderly sequence of immunoglobulin gene rearrangements: first, D_H to J_H, then V_H to D_HJ_H, and finally V_L to J_L (see Figure 8-12). These sequential gene rearrangements, which occur in the absence of antigen, identify the different stages in B-cell maturation: *progenitor* B cell, *precursor* B cell, *immature* B cell, and *mature* B cell.

A mature B cell leaves the bone marrow expressing membrane-bound immunoglobulin (mIgM and mIgD) with a single antigenic specificity. These mature B cells circulate in the blood and lymph and are carried to the secondary lymphoid organs, most notably the spleen and lymph nodes (see Chapter 3). The antigen-dependent phase of B-cell development occurs in these sites. If a B cell interacts with the antigen for which its membrane-bound antibody is specific, the cell undergoes clonal expansion and differentiation, generating a population of antibody-secreting plasma cells and memory B cells.

Antigen-Independent Phase

B-cell development begins as lymphoid stem cells differentiate into the earliest distinctive B-lineage cell—the progenitor B cell (pro-B cell)—which expresses a lineage-specific cell-surface marker called B220. Pro-B cells proliferate within the bone marrow, filling the extravascular spaces between large sinusoids in the shaft of a bone. Proliferation and differentiation of pro-B cells into precursor B cells (pre-B cells) requires the microenvironment provided by the bone marrow stromal cells. If pro-B cells are removed from the bone marrow and cultured in vitro, they will not develop into more mature B-cell stages unless stromal cells are present. The stromal cells play two important roles: They interact directly with pro-B and pre-B cells, and they secrete various cytokines, notably IL-7, that support the developmental process.

At the earliest developmental stage pro-B cells require direct contact with stromal cells in the bone marrow. This interaction is mediated by several cell-adhesion molecules including CD44 on the pro-B cell and its ligand, hyaluronic acid, on the stromal cell. After contact is made with the stromal cell, a receptor on the pro-B cell, called c-Kit, interacts with a stromal-cell surface molecule known as stem-cell factor (SCF). This interaction activates c-Kit, which has tyrosine kinase activity, and the pro-B cell begins to divide and differentiate into a pre-B cell expressing a receptor for IL-7. Then IL-7 secreted by the stromal cells drives the maturation process, eventually inducing down-regulation of the adhesion molecules on the pre-B cells, so that the proliferating cells can detach from the stromal cells. At this stage pre-cells no longer require direct stromal-cell contact but continue to require IL-7 for growth and maturation.

Heavy-chain D_H-J_H gene rearrangement occurs in the pro-B cell stage followed by the V_H to D_HJ_H rearrangement in the pre-B cell stage. As would be expected, the recombination-activating genes *RAG-1* and *RAG-2,* which are required for both heavy-chain and light-chain gene rearrangements, are expressed during the pro-B and pre-B cell stages. In addition, the enzyme terminal deoxyribonucleotidyl transferase (TdT) is active during these early stages, allowing insertion of N nucleotides at the D_H-J_H and V_H-D_HJ_H coding joints.

Recent evidence has shown that the pre-B cell expresses the μ chain on its membrane associated with an unusual light-chain molecule called a *surrogate light chain.* The surrogate light chain consists of a V polypeptide sequence (called Vpre-B) and a C polypeptide sequence (called $\lambda 5$), which associate noncovalently to form a light chain-like structure. The genes encoding Vpre-B and $\lambda 5$ are located an unknown distance from the λ light-chain genes in mouse and human DNA. The surrogate light chain is first expressed on the membrane of the pro-B cell complexed with two other proteins (p130/p55) and without the μ heavy chain. Later the surrogate light chain appears with a truncated heavy-chain protein encoded by $D_HJ_HC\mu$, and finally it appears with a complete $V_HD_HJ_HC\mu$ chain in the pre-B cell stage. The complex consisting of the membrane-bound μ heavy chain and surrogate light chain is associated with the Ig-α/Ig-β heterodimer to form a pre-B cell receptor (Figure 8-23). Only pre-B cells that are able to express membrane-bound μ heavy chains in association with surrogate light chains are able to proceed along their differentiation pathway. If the heavy-chain rearrangement is nonproductive, the cell dies by apoptosis.

The function of the pre-B cell receptor has not yet been determined, but there is speculation that this receptor may recognize a ligand on the stromal-cell membrane, thereby generating a signal that prevents V_H to D_HJ_H rearrangement of the other heavy-chain allele (allelic exclusion) and inducing rearrangement of the κ light-chain locus. The critical role of the pre-B cell receptor was demonstrated with knock-out mice in which the $\lambda 5$ gene was disrupted. B-cell development in these mice was shown to be blocked at the pre-B cell stage. This finding suggests that a signal

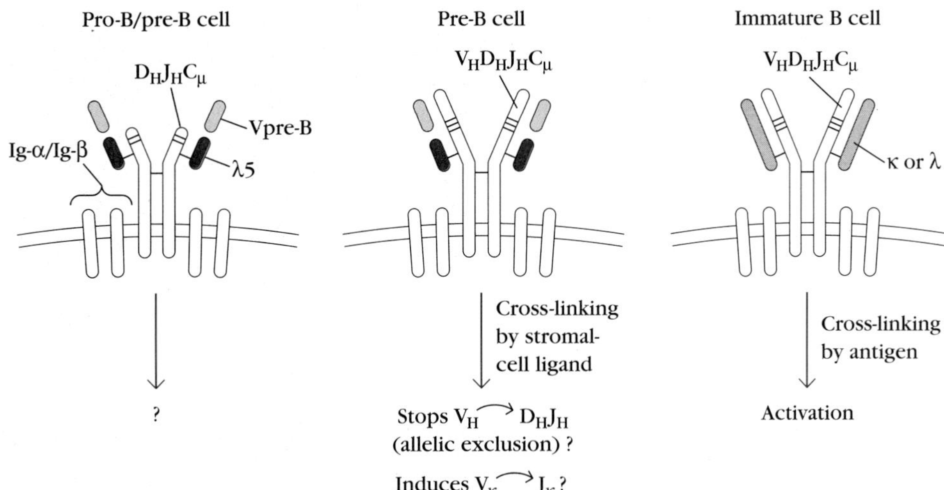

FIGURE 8-23 Schematic diagram of sequential expression of membrane immunoglobulin and surrogate light chain at different stages of B-cell differentiation in the bone marrow. The pre-B cell receptor contains a surrogate light chain consisting of a Vpre-B polypeptide and a λ5 polypeptide, which are noncovalently associated. The surrogate light chain is first expressed at the pro-B/pre-B cell stage with a truncated heavy-chain protein ($D_HJ_HC_\mu$). Later the surrogate light chain appears with a complete μ heavy chain. The immature B cell no longer expresses the surrogate light chain and instead expresses the κ or λ light chain together with the μ heavy chain.

generated through the pre-B cell receptor is necessary for maturation to proceed from the pre-B cell stage to the immature B-cell stage.

Continued development of a pre-B cell into an immature B cell requires a productive light-chain gene rearrangement. Only one light-chain isotype is expressed on the membrane of a B cell. As illustrated in Figure 8-12, this rearrangement begins with the κ gene segments; if it is productive, the cell stops light-chain rearrangement. If rearrangement of both κ alleles is nonproductive, the λ light-chain gene segments undergo rearrangement. Completion of the light-chain rearrangement commits the cell to a particular antigenic specificity determined by the cell's heavy-chain VDJ sequence and light-chain VJ sequence. As immature B cells are generated within the bone marrow, they are subject to a process of negative selection whereby those B cells with receptors specific for self-antigens are thought to be eliminated by apoptosis.

Further differentiation of immature B cells leads to the coexpression of IgD and IgM on the membrane, which characterizes mature B cells. This progression involves a change in RNA processing of the heavy-chain primary transcript to permit production of two mRNAs, one encoding the membrane form of the μ chain and the other encoding the membrane form of the δ chain (see Figure 8-20). The earliest mature cells in the bone marrow express low levels of IgD. These cells are exported from the bone marrow to peripheral lymphoid organs where the level of membrane IgD increases.

Antigen-Dependent Phase

Following export of mature B cells from the bone marrow, the subsequent steps in B-cell development and differentiation occur in the periphery and require antigen. In the absence of antigen activation, mature B cells in the periphery have a short life span, dying within a few days by apoptosis. Antigen-driven clonal selection of naive B cells leads to generation of plasma cells and memory B cells. As discussed in Chapter 14, memory B cells not only have a longer life span than naive B cells but also higher-affinity membrane-bound antibody, the result of a process known as *affinity maturation,* which involves somatic mutation in activated B cells.

Activated B cells can undergo class switching resulting in expression of isotypes other than IgM and IgD on the membrane. As a result, memory B cells often express membrane IgG, IgA, or IgE. Some memory B cells express a single isotype, whereas others express two isotypes (IgM + IgG, IgM + IgA, or IgM + IgE). It is not known how a memory B cell can express both

IgM and another isotype whose constant-region gene is 50 – 100 kb away. Possibly, the μ-chain mRNA is long lived, so that μ heavy chains continue to be expressed after class switching to another isotype occurs. Another possibility is that molecular mechanisms other than class switching are responsible for coexpression of IgM with IgG, IgA, or IgE. For example, some very long primary transcripts containing $V_HD_HJ_H$ and multiple C_H gene segments have been detected in memory B cells. Differential processing of such long transcripts might generate different isotypes within a given memory cell; this would be analogous to the coexpression of IgM and IgD in a mature B cell. At a later stage, class switching by the mechanism described earlier (see Figure 8-18) would lead to the irreversible deletion of intervening C_H segments, so that only a single isotype is expressed.

Plasma cells generally lack detectable membrane-bound immunoglobulin and instead synthesize high levels of secreted antibody. Differentiation of mature B cells into plasma cells must involve a change in RNA processing so that the secreted form of the heavy chain rather than the membrane form is synthesized. In addition, the rate of transcription of heavy- and light-chain genes increases significantly in plasma cells. Several authors have suggested that the increased transcription by plasma cells might be explained by their synthesis of higher levels of transcription factors that bind to immunoglobulin enhancers compared with less-differentiated B-lineage cells. Some mechanism also must coordinate the increase in transcription of heavy-chain and light-chain genes, even though these genes are on different chromosomes.

Summary

1. Immunoglobulin κ light chains, λ light chains, and heavy chains are encoded by three separate multigene families located on different chromosomes. In germ-line DNA, each multigene family contains numerous gene segments. The variable-region gene segments are designated V and J in light-chain DNA and V, D, and J in heavy-chain DNA. Multiple constant-region (C) gene segments also are present.

2. Functional light-chain and heavy-chain genes are generated by random rearrangement of the variable-region gene segments in germ-line DNA. Conserved DNA sequences, termed recombination signal sequences, flank each V, D, and J gene segment and direct the joining of segments. Each recombination signal contains a conserved heptamer sequence, a conserved nonamer sequence, and either a 12-bp (one-turn) or 23-bp (two-turn) spacer; the length, but not the nucleotide sequence, of these spacers is conserved. During rearrangement, gene segments flanked by a one-turn spacer join only to segments flanked by a two-turn spacer. This one-turn/two-turn joining rule assures proper V_L-J_L and V_H-D_H-J_H joining.

3. Immunoglobulin-gene rearrangements occur in sequential order, with heavy-chain rearrangements occurring first followed by light-chain rearrangements. These rearrangements are carefully regulated so that the immunoglobulin DNA of only one parental chromosome is rearranged to form a functional light-chain or heavy-chain gene. This allelic exclusion is necessary to assure that a mature B cell expresses immunoglobulin with a single antigenic specificity.

4. The various mechanisms contributing to antibody diversity can generate, at a minimum, about 10^8 possible combinations. Major sources of antibody diversity are the random joining of multiple V, J, and D germ-line gene segments and the random association of a given heavy-chain and light-chain in a particular cell. Other mechanisms that augment antibody diversity by a significant but unknown extent are junctional flexibility and N-region nucleotide addition, which produce variability in the nucleotide sequences at the coding joints between gene segments, as well as somatic mutation following antigenic stimulation.

5. Differential RNA processing of the immunoglobulin heavy-chain primary transcript generates either membrane-bound or secreted antibody. Differential processing is also responsible for expression of IgM alone by immature B cells and the coexpression of IgM and IgD by mature B cells.

6. After antigenic stimulation of mature B cells, additional rearrangement of their heavy-chain C gene segments can occur. Such class switching results in expression of different classes of antibody (IgG, IgA, and IgE) with the same antigenic specificity.

7. Differentiation of progenitor B cells into mature B cells has been correlated with variable-region gene rearrangements. This antigen-independent phase of B-cell differentiation occurs in the bone marrow. Dur-

ing the antigen-dependent phase of differentiation, antigenically primed B cells undergo class switching and changes in RNA processing. This phase leads to formation of B memory cells that express different membrane isotypes and plasma cells that secrete various isotypes.

References

AKIRA, S., K. OKAZAKI, and H. SAKANO. 1987. Two pairs of recombination signals are sufficient to cause immunoglobulin V-(D)-J joining. *Science* **238**:1134.

ALT, F. W., E. M. OLTZ, F. YOUNG et al. 1992. VDJ recombination. *Immunol. Today* **13**:306.

BEREK, C., and C. MILSTEIN. 1987. Mutation drift and repertoire shift in the maturation of the immune respose. *Immunol. Rev.* **96**:23.

BLANK, V., P. KOURILSKY, and A. ISRAEL. 1992. NF-κB and related proteins: Rel/dorsal homologies meet ankyrin-like repeats. *Trends Biochem. Sci.* **17**:135.

CALAME, K., and S. EATON. 1988. Transcriptional controlling elements in the immunoglobulin and T cell receptor loci. *Adv. Immunol.* **43**:235.

CHEN, J., and F. W. ALT. 1993. Gene rearrangement and B-cell development. *Curr. Opinion Immunol.* **5**:194.

CHUN, J. J. M., D. G. SCHATZ, M. A. OETTINGER et al. 1991. The recombination activating gene-1 (RAG-1) transcript is present in the murine central nervous system. *Cell* **64**:189.

HARRIMAN, W., H. VOLK, N. DEFRANOUX, and M. WABL. 1993. Immunoglobulin class switch recombination. *Annu. Rev. Immunol.* **11**:361.

HONJO, T., F. W. ALT, and T. H. RABBITS (eds.). 1989. *Immunoglobulin Genes.* Academic Press.

HOZUMI, N., and S. TONEGAWA. 1976. Evidence for somatic rearrangement of immunoglobulin genes coding for variable and constant regions. *Proc. Natl. Acad. Sci. USA* **73**:3628.

LASSOUED, K., C. A. NUNEZ, L. BILLIPS et al. 1993. Expression of surrogate light chain receptors is restricted to a late stage in pre-B cell differentiation. *Cell* **73**:73.

MELCHERS, F., H. KARASUYAMA, D. HAASNER et al. 1993. The surrogate light chain in B-cell development. *Immunol. Today* **14**:60.

OETTINGER, M. A. 1992. Activation of V(D)J recombination by RAG1 and RAG2. *Trends Genet.* **8**:413.

OETTINGER, M. A., D. G. SCHATZ, C. GORKA, and D. BALTIMORE. 1990. RAG-1 and RAG-2, adjacent genes that synergistically activate V(D)J recombination. *Science* **248**:1517.

PASCUAL, V., and J. D. CAPRA. 1991. Human immunoglobulin heavy-chain variable region genes: organization, polymorphism, and expression. *Adv. Immunol.* **49**:1.

RETH, M. 1992. Antigen receptors on B lymphocytes. *Annu. Rev. Immunol.* **10**:97.

ROLINK, A., and F. MELCHERS. 1993. B lymphopoiesis in the mouse. *Adv. Immunol.* **53**: 123.

ROTH, D. B., J. P. MENETSKI, P. NAKAJIMA et al. 1992. V(D)J recombination: broken DNA molecules with covalently sealed (hairpin) coding ends in scid mouse thymocytes. *Cell* **70**:983.

SCHATZ, D. G., M. A. OETTINGER, and M. S. SCHLISSEL. 1992. V(D)J recombination: molecular biology and regulation. *Annu. Rev. Immunol.* **10**:359.

SEN, R., and D. BALTIMORE. 1989. Factors regulating immunoglobulin gene transcription. In *Immunoglobulin Genes.* Academic Press.

STAUDT, L. M., and M. J. LENARDO. 1991. Immunoglobulin gene transcription. *Annu. Rev. Immunol.* **9**:373.

TONEGAWA, S. 1983. Somatic generation of antibody diversity. *Nature* **302**:575.

WALL, R., and M. KUEHL. 1983. Biosynthesis and regulation of immunoglobulin. *Annu. Rev. Immunol.* **1**:393.

YANCOPOULOS, G. D., and F. W. ALT. 1986. Regulation of the assembly and expression of variable region genes. *Annu. Rev. Immunol.* **4**:339.

Study Questions

1. Indicate whether each of the following statements is true or false. If you think a statement is false, explain why.

   a. V_λ gene segments sometimes join to C_κ gene segments.

   b. Immunoglobulin class switching usually is mediated by DNA rearrangements.

c. A separate exon encodes the transmembrane portion of each membrane immunoglobulin.
d. Although each B cell carries two alleles encoding the immunoglobulin heavy and light chains, only one allele is expressed.
e. Primary transcripts are processed into functional mRNA by removal of introns, capping, and addition of a poly-A tail.
f. The primary transcript is an RNA copy of the DNA and includes both introns and exons.

2. Draw a schematic diagram illustrating each of the following forms of immunoglobulin heavy-chain DNA, RNA, or protein in the mouse:
   a. The DNA arrangement in a liver cell.
   b. The DNA arrangement in a mature B cell.
   c. The primary RNA transcript in a mature B cell.
   d. The mRNA in a mature B cell.
   e. The protein product observed on the membrane of a mature B cell.
   f. The DNA arrangement in a plasma cell secreting IgE.

3. Explain why a V_H cannot join directly with a J_H in heavy-chain gene rearrangement?

4. Ignoring junctional flexibility, N-region neucleotide addition, and somatic mutation, how many different antibody molecules potentially could be generated from germ-line DNA containing 500 V_L and 4 J_L gene segments and 300 V_H, 15 D_H, and 4 J_H gene segments?

5. For each incomplete statement below (a–d), select the phrase(s) that correctly completes the statement. More than one choice may be correct.
   a. Recombination of immunoglobulin gene segments serves to
      (1) promote Ig diversification
      (2) assemble a complete Ig coding sequence
      (3) allow changes in coding information during B-cell maturation
      (4) increase the affinity of immunoglobulin for antibody
      (5) all of the above
   b. Somatic mutation of immunoglobulin genes accounts for
      (1) allelic exclusion
      (2) class switching from IgM to IgG
      (3) affinity maturation
      (4) all of the above
      (5) none of the above
   c. The frequency of somatic mutation in Ig genes is greatest during
      (1) differentiation of pre-B cells into mature B cells
      (2) differentiation of pre-T cells into mature T cells
      (3) generation of memory B cells
      (4) antibody secretion by plasma cells
      (5) none of the above
   d. Kappa and lambda light-chain genes
      (1) are located on the same chromosome
      (2) associate with only one type of heavy chain
      (3) can be expressed by the same B cell
      (4) all of the above
      (5) none of the above
   e. Generation of combinatorial diversity among immunoglobulins involves
      (1) mRNA splicing
      (2) DNA rearrangement
      (3) recombination signal sequences
      (4) one-turn/two-turn joining rule
      (5) switch sites

6. You have fluorescein (Fl)-labeled antibody to the μ heavy chain and a rhodamine (Rh)-labeled antibody to the δ heavy chain. Describe the fluorescent-antibody staining pattern of the following B-cell maturational stages assuming that you can visualize both membrane and cytoplasmic staining: (a) progenitor B cells; (b) pre-B cell; (c) immature B cell; (d) mature B cell; and (e) plasma cell.

7. What mechanisms generate the three hypervariable regions (complementarity-determining regions) of immunoglobulin heavy and light chains? Why is the third hypervariable region (CDR3) more variable than the other two (CDR1 and CDR2)?

8. You have been given a cloned myeloma cell line that secretes IgG with the molecular formula $\gamma_2\lambda_2$. Both the heavy and light chains in this cell line are encoded by genes derived from allele 1. Indicate the form(s) in which each of the genes listed below would occur in this cell line using the following symbols: G = germ-line form; R = productively rearranged form; NP = nonproductively rearranged form. State the reason for your choice in each case.
   a. Heavy-chain allele 1
   b. Heavy-chain allele 2
   c. κ-chain allele 1
   d. κ-chain allele 2
   e. λ-chain allele 1
   f. λ-chain allele 2

9. You have a B-cell lymphoma that has made nonproductive rearrangements for both heavy-chain alleles. What is the arrangement of its κ light-chain DNA? Why?

10. Indicate whether the class switches indicated below can occur (Yes) or cannot occur (No).
    a. IgM to IgD
    b. IgM to IgA
    c. IgE to IgG
    d. IgA to IgG
    e. IgM to IgG

11. Describe one advantage and one disadvantage of N-nucleotide addition during the rearrangement of immunoglobulin heavy-chain gene segments.

12. DNA was isolated from three sources: liver cells, pre-B lymphoma cells, and IgM-secreting myeloma cells. Each DNA sample was digested separately with *Bam*HI and *Eco*RI, and the digested samples were analyzed by Southern blotting. The *Bam*HI digests were treated with a radiolabeled $C_\mu 1$ probe (blot #1) and the *Eco*RI digests were treated with a radiolabeled C_κ probe (blot #2). Based on the restriction maps and Southern blots shown below, determine which DNA sample (designated A, B, or C) was isolated from the (a) liver cells, (b) pre-B lymphoma cells, and (c) IgM-secreting plasma cells.

13. X-ray crystallographic analyses of over two dozen antibody molecules bound to their respective antigens have revealed that in every case the CDR3 of both the heavy and light chains make contact with the epitope. Moreover, sequence analyses reveal that the variability of CDR3 is greater than that of either CDR1 or CDR2. What mechanisms account for the greater diversity in CDR3 than in the rest of the variable region?

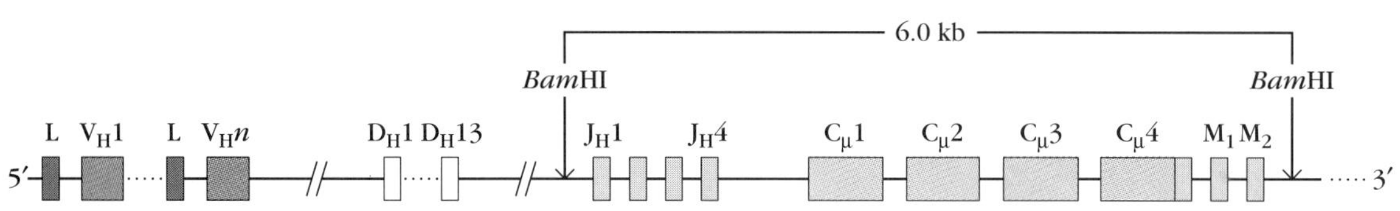

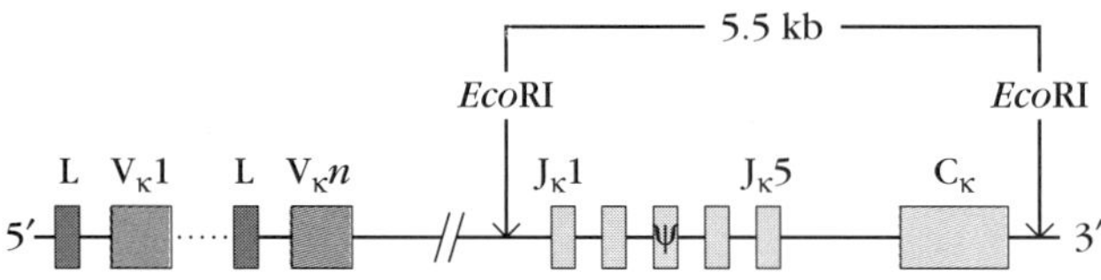

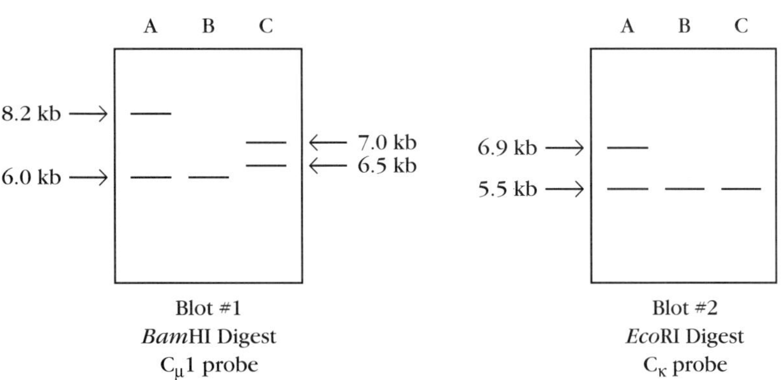

14. You wish to study the effect of the *RAG-1* gene on B-cell development in the bone marrow. You have available FITC-labeled anti-IgM monoclonal antibodies and rhodamine-labeled anti-IgD monoclonal antibodies. After treating bone marrow cells from normal mice and RAG-1^- mice with both antibodies, you subject each sample to FACS analysis. In the diagrams below, draw the FACS staining pattern you would expect with bone marrow cells from the (a) normal mice and (b) mice lacking the *RAG-1* gene. In both cases, label the cell population in each quadrant.

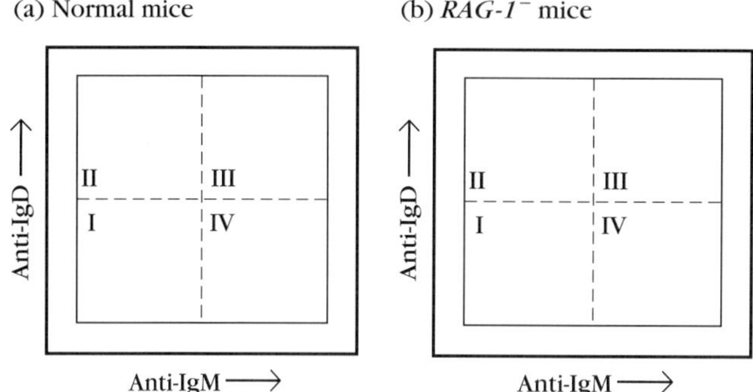

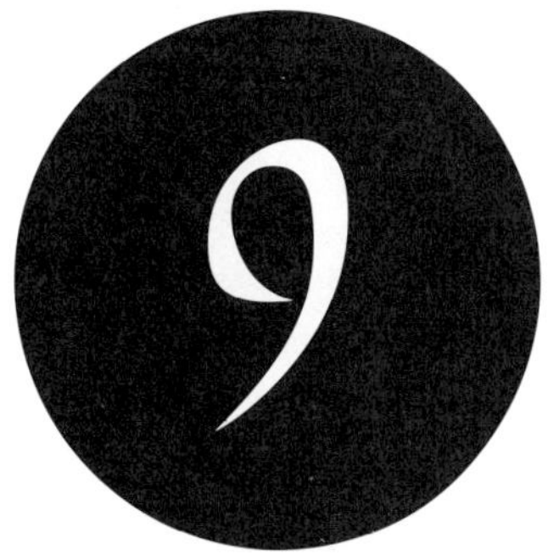

MAJOR HISTOCOMPATIBILITY COMPLEX

Every mammalian species studied to date possesses a tightly linked cluster of genes, the major histocompatibility complex (MHC), whose products are associated with intercellular recognition and with self/nonself discrimination. The MHC complex is a region of multiple loci that play major roles in determining whether transplanted tissue will be accepted as self (histocompatible) or rejected as foreign (histoincompatible).

The MHC plays a central role in the development of both humoral and cell-mediated immune responses. As discussed in previous chapters, T cells only recognize antigen when it is associated with an MHC molecule; thus MHC molecules play a critical role in antigen recognition by T cells. Because MHC molecules function as antigen-presenting structures, the particular set of MHC molecules expressed by an individual influences the repertoire of antigens to which that individual's T_H cells and T_C cells can respond. For this reason, the MHC partly determines the response of an individual to antigens of infectious organisms and the MHC has therefore been implicated in the susceptibility to disease and to the development of autoimmunity. This chapter examines the organization and inheritance of MHC genes, the structure of the MHC molecules, and the central function that these molecules play in producing an immune response.

General Organization and Inheritance of the MHC

The concept that the rejection of foreign tissue is the result of an immune response to cell-surface molecules (now called histocompatibility antigens) came from the work of R. A. Gorer and G. D. Snell in the mid-1930s. Gorer was using inbred strains of mice to identify blood-group antigens. In the course of these studies, he identified four groups of genes, designated I through IV, that encoded blood-cell antigens. Later work by Gorer and Snell established that the group II antigens were involved in the rejection of transplanted tumors and other tissue. Snell called these genes "histocompatibility genes"; their designation as histocompatibility-2 (H-2) genes was in reference to Gorer's group II blood-group antigens. The significant contribution of this early work of Snell was highlighted when he was awarded a Nobel prize in 1980.

Location and Function of MHC Regions

The major histocompatibility complex is a collection of genes arrayed within a long continuous stretch of DNA on chromosome 6 in humans and on chromosome 17 in mice. The MHC is referred to as the *HLA complex* in humans and as the *H-2 complex* in mice. Although the organization of genes is somewhat different in the human HLA and the mouse H-2 complex, certain features are common to both. In both cases the MHC genes are organized into regions encoding three classes of molecules: class I, class II, and class III. The class I genes encode glycoproteins expressed on the surface of nearly all nucleated cells, where they present peptide antigens of altered self-cells necessary for the activation of T_C cells. The class II genes encode glycoproteins expressed primarily on antigen-presenting cells (macrophages, dendritic cells, and B cells), where they present processed antigenic peptides to T_H cells. The class III genes encode somewhat different products some of which are also associated with the immune process. These include a number of soluble serum proteins (including components of the complement system), steroid 21-hydroxylase enzymes, and tumor necrosis factors.

Class I MHC molecules are encoded by the K and D regions in mice and by the A, B, and C regions in humans (Figure 9-1). Additional regions, designated Qa and Tla, also encode class I molecules in mice and are closely linked to the H-2 complex. Class II molecules are encoded by the I region in mice and by the D region in humans. The terminology is somewhat confusing, since the D region in mice encodes class I MHC molecules, whereas the D region in humans encodes class II MHC molecules! It is a relief that the class III molecules are encoded by regions with descriptive designations of S (for soluble protein) in the mouse and C4, C2, Bf (designating some of the individual complement proteins encoded here) in humans.

MHC Haplotypes

As discussed in more detail later, the loci constituting the MHC are highly *polymorphic;* that is, many alternate forms of the gene, or *alleles,* exist at each locus.

Mouse H-2 complex

Complex	H-2							Tla	
MHC class	I	II		III		I		I	I
Region	K	IA	IE	S		D		Qa	Tla
Gene products	H-2K	IA αβ	IE αβ*	Complement proteins	Tumor necrosis factor TNF-α TNF-β	H-2D	H-2L	Qa	Tla, Qa

Human HLA complex

Complex	HLA							
MHC class	II			III		I		
Region	DP	DQ	DR	C4, C2, BF		B	C	A
Gene products	DP αβ	DQ αβ	DR αβ	Complement proteins	Tumor necrosis factor TNF-α TNF-β	HLA-B	HLA-C	HLA-A

FIGURE 9-1 Simplified organization of the major histocompatibility complex (MHC) in the mouse and human. The MHC is referred to as the H-2 complex in mice and as the HLA complex in humans. In both species the MHC is organized into a number of regions encoding class I (purple), class II (light purple), and class III (gray) gene products. The class I and class II gene products shown in this figure are considered to be the classical MHC molecules. The *IEβ* gene is actually located in the IA region but for pedagogical reasons is shown in the IE region.

TABLE 9-1 H-2 HAPLOTYPES OF SOME MOUSE STRAINS

Prototype strain	Other strains with the same haplotype	Haplotype	H-2 alleles				
			K	IA	IE	S	D
CBA	AKR, C3H, B10.BR, C57BR	*k*	*k*	*k*	*k*	*k*	*k*
DBA/2	BALB/c, NZB, SEA, YBR	*d*	*d*	*d*	*d*	*d*	*d*
C57BL/10 (B10)	C57BL/6, C57L, C3H.SW, LP, 129	*b*	*b*	*b*	*b*	*b*	*b*
A	A/He, A/Sn, A/Wy, B10.A	*a*	*k*	*k*	*k*	*d*	*d*
A.SW	B10.S, SJL	*s*	*s*	*s*	*s*	*s*	*s*
A.TL		*t1*	*s*	*k*	*k*	*k*	*d*
DBA/1	STOLI, B10.Q, BDP	*q*	*q*	*q*	*q*	*q*	*q*

The MHC loci also are closely linked; for example, the recombination frequency within the H-2 complex is only 0.5%. For this reason, an individual inherits the alleles encoded by these closely linked loci as two sets, one from each parent. Each set of alleles is referred to as a *haplotype*. An individual inherits one haplotype from the mother and one haplotype from the father. In an outbred population the offspring are generally heterozygous at many loci and will express both maternal and paternal MHC alleles. The alleles are therefore codominantly expressed, that is both maternal and paternal gene products are expressed in the same cells. In inbred mice, however, each H-2 locus is homozygous because the maternal and paternal haplotypes are identical, and all offspring express identical haplotypes.

Certain inbred mice strains have been designated as prototype strains, and the haplotype expressed by these strains is designated by an arbitrary superscript (e.g., H-2^a, H-2^b, H-2^d, H-2^k). The arbitrary designation simply is a way of referring to the entire set of inherited alleles within a strain without having to refer to each allele individually (Table 9-1). If another inbred strain has inherited the same set of alleles as the prototype strain, its MHC haplotype is the same as the prototype strain, as illustrated in Figure 9-2a. For example, the

(a) Hypothetical allelic composition of mouse MHC haplotypes

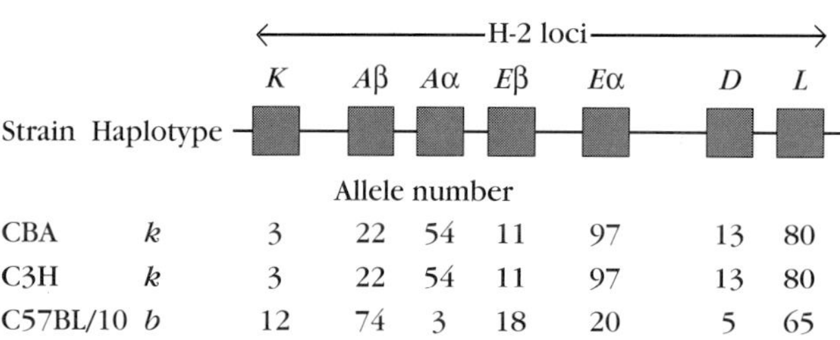

(b) Mating of inbred mouse strains with different MHC haplotypes

Homologous chromosomes with MHC loci

H-2^b parent H-2^k parent

b/b *k/k*

F$_1$ progeny (H-$2^{b/k}$)

b/k

(c) Mating of outbred mouse strains with different MHC haplotypes

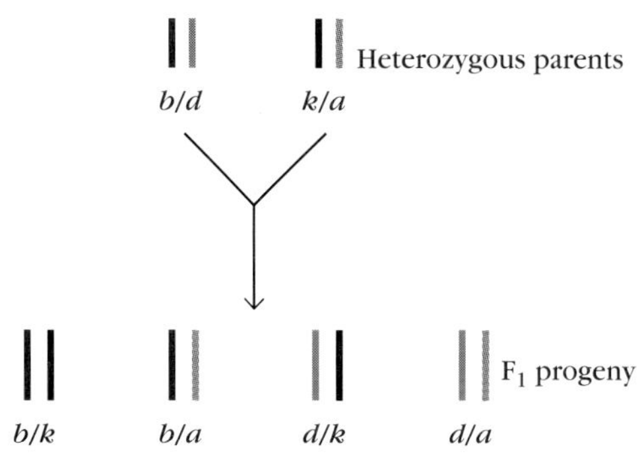

FIGURE 9-2 (a) Illustration of MHC haplotype designation. Strain CBA inherits a particular allele, indicated by a hypothetical number, at each MHC locus. The complete set of alleles is arbitrarily designated as the H-2^k haplotype. Any inbred strain (e.g., C3H) that has the same set of MHC alleles is designated as an H-2^k strain. Strains with a different set of MHC alleles (e.g., C57BL/10) are given a different haplotype designation. (b, c) Because the MHC loci are closely linked and inherited as a set, the MHC haplotype of F$_1$ progeny from mating of inbred and outbred strains can be predicted easily.

CBA, C3H and AKR strains all have the same MHC haplotype (H-2^k). The three strains differ, however, in genes outside the H-2 complex. If two inbred strains of mice having different MHC haplotypes are bred, the F_1 generation inherits haplotypes from both parental strains and therefore expresses both parental alleles at each MHC locus. For example, if strain C57BL/10 (H-2^b) is crossed with strain CBA (H-2^k), then the F_1 inherits both parental sets of alleles and is said to be H-$2^{b/k}$ (Figure 9-2b). Because such an F_1 expresses the MHC proteins of both parental strains on its cells, it is histocompatible with both strains and able to accept grafts from either parental strain.

As noted above, in an outbred population, each animal is generally heterozygous at each locus. Furthermore, both the maternal and paternal alleles at each MHC locus are expressed (this differs from expression of the immunoglobulin genes, which exhibit allelic exclusion, so that only one allele is expressed). The F_1 offspring of two heterozygous parents inherits one set of MHC alleles (i.e., one haplotype) from the father and one set from the mother (Figure 9-2c). Such an F_1 expresses only half of the paternal and half of the maternal class I MHC molecules on its nucleated cells. If this F_1 is grafted with tissue from either parent, it will recognize the foreign MHC molecules on the parental graft and reject the graft. Because the MHC loci are closely linked and are inherited as a haplotype, there is a one in four chance in outbred populations that siblings will inherit the same paternal and maternal haplotypes and therefore be histocompatible, assuming the father and mother have different haplotypes.

Congenic MHC Mouse Strains

Detailed analysis of the H-2 complex in mice was made possible by the development of congenic mouse strains. Two strains are *congenic* if they are genetically identical except at a single genetic locus or region. Any phenotypic differences that can be detected between congenic strains are related to the genetic region that distinguishes the strains. Congenic strains that are identical to each other except at the major histocompatibility complex can be produced by a series of crosses, backcrosses, and selections. Figure 9-3

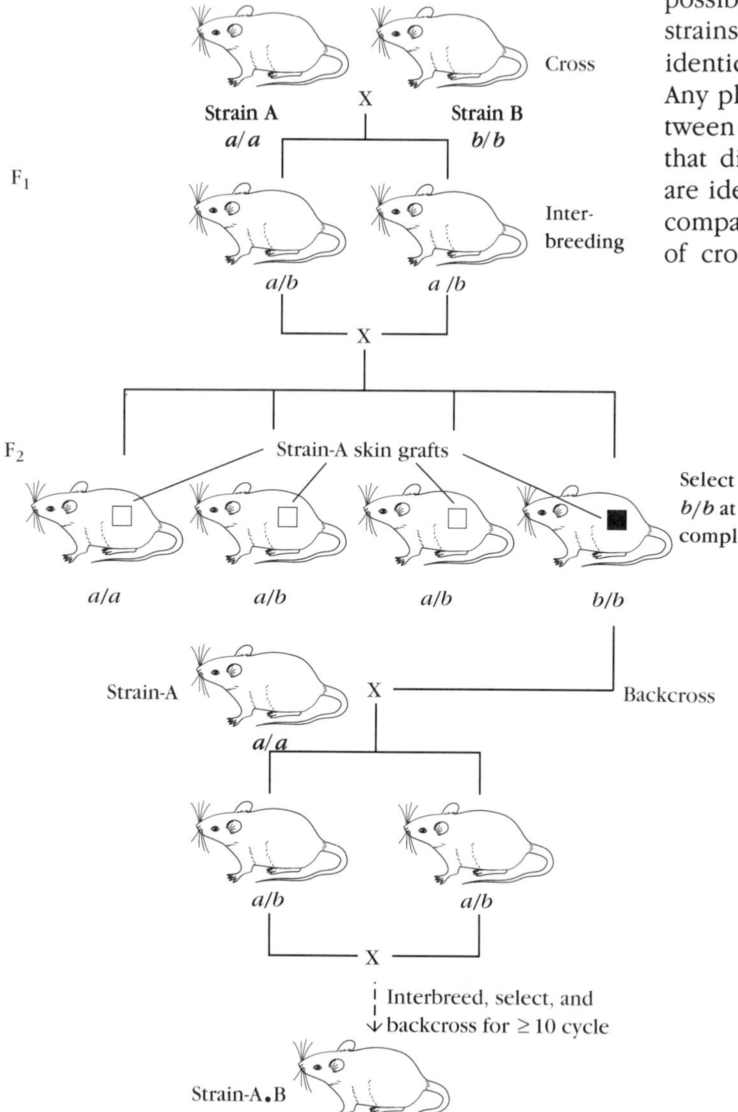

FIGURE 9-3 Production of congenic mouse strain A.B, which has the genetic background of parental strain A but the H-2 complex of strain B. Crossing inbred strain A (H-2^a) with strain B (H-2^b) generates F_1 progeny that are heterozygous (*a*/*b*) at all H-2 loci. The F_1 progeny are interbred to produce an F_2 generation, which includes *a*/*a*, *a*/*b*, and *b*/*b* individuals. The F_2 progeny homozygous for the B-strain H-2 complex are selected by their ability to reject a skin graft from strain A; any progeny that accept an A-strain graft are eliminated from future breeding. The selected *b*/*b* homozygous mice are then backcrossed to strain A; the resulting progeny are again interbred and their offspring are again selected for *b*/*b* homozygosity at the H-2 complex. This process of backcrossing to strain A, intercrossing, and selection for rejection of an A-strain graft is repeated for at least 12 generations. In this way A-strain homozygosity is restored at all loci except the H-2 locus, which is homozygous for the B strain.

outlines the steps by which the H-2 complex of homozygous strain B can be introduced into the background genes of homozygous strain A to generate a congenic strain, denoted A.B. The congenic strain will be genetically identical to strain A except for the MHC locus or loci contributed by strain B.

During production of congenic mouse strains, a crossover event sometimes occurs within the H-2 complex, yielding a recombinant strain that differs from the parental strains or the congenic strain at one or a few loci within the H-2 complex. Figure 9-4 illustrates several recombinant congenic strains that were obtained during production of a B10.A congenic strain. Such recombinant strains have been extremely useful in analyzing the MHC because they permit comparisons of functional differences between strains that differ in only a few genes within the MHC.

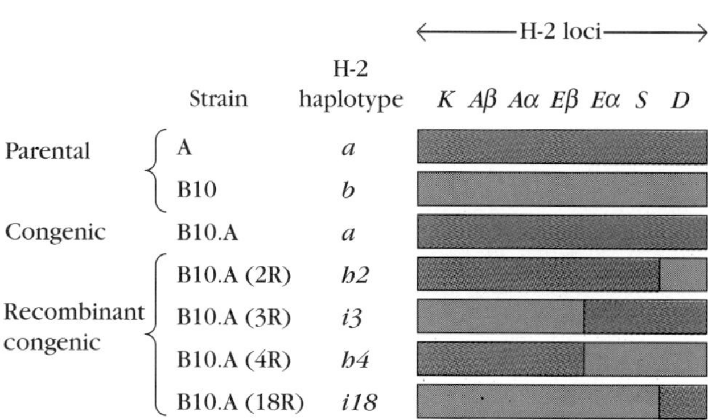

FIGURE 9-4 Examples of recombinant congenic mouse strains generated during production of the B10.A strain from parental strain B10 (H-2^b) and parental strain A (H-2^a). Crossover events within the H-2 complex produce recombinant strains, which have *a*-haplotype alleles (purple) at some H-2 loci and *b*-haplotype alleles (gray) at other loci.

Class I MHC Molecules and Genes

Class I MHC molecules contain a large α chain associated noncovalently with a much smaller β_2-microglobulin molecule (Figure 9-5). The α chain is encoded by genes within the A, B, and C regions of the human HLA complex and within the K and D/L regions of the mouse H-2 complex (see Figure 9-1). In the mouse, the genes in the Qa and Tla regions, which are downstream from the H-2 complex and closely linked to it, also encode class I MHC molecules. These genes, however, are less polymorphic than the classical class I

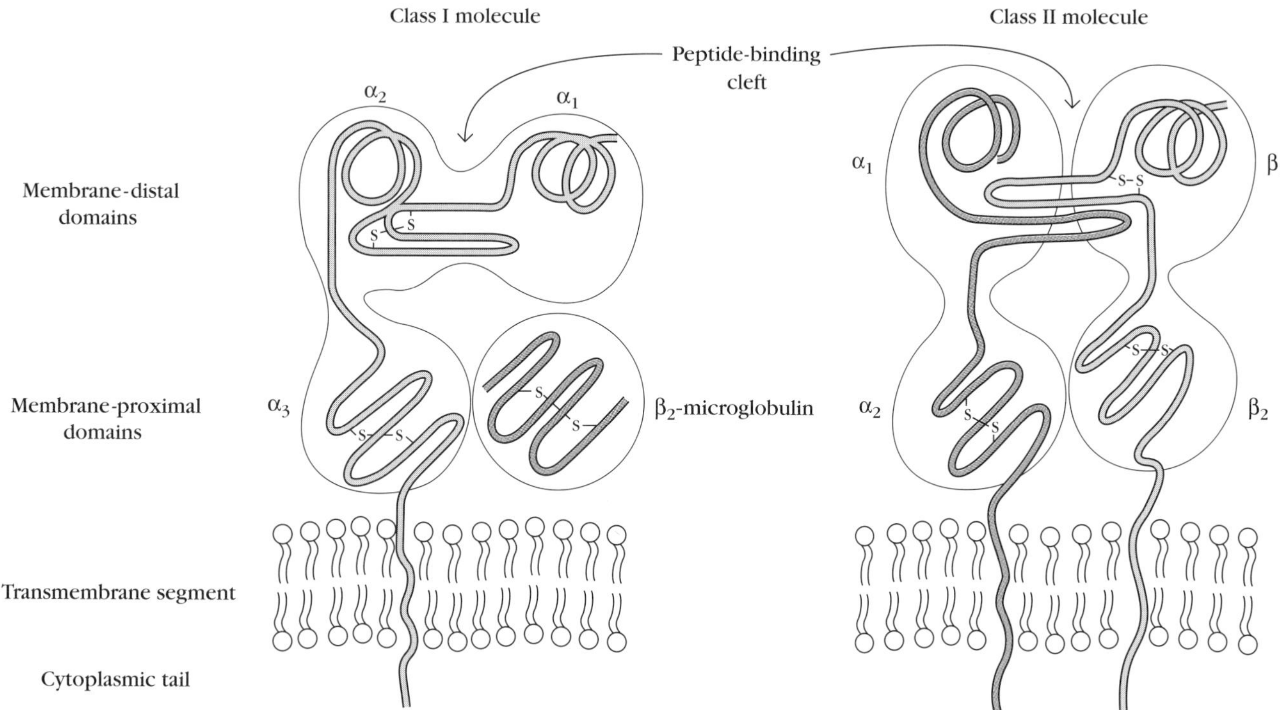

FIGURE 9-5 Schematic diagram of a class I and class II MHC molecule showing the external domains, transmembrane segment, and cytoplasmic tail. The peptide-binding cleft is formed by the membrane-distal domains in both class I and class II molecules. The membrane-proximal domains possess the basic immunoglobulin-fold structure; thus class I and class II MHC molecules are classified as members of the immunoglobulin superfamily.

MHC genes and show different patterns of expression. For example, the Tla gene products are expressed only in thymocytes, activated T cells, and some thymic leukemia cells, whereas class I MHC molecules are expressed in nearly all nucleated cells. In addition, a number of Qa gene products are expressed as secreted proteins, whereas class I MHC molecules are only expressed on membranes. Also, many of the genes in the Qa and Tla regions appear to be pseudogenes having no identified protein product. Class I MHC molecules function to present processed antigenic peptides produced in altered self-cells to $CD8^+$ T cells.

The isolation of class I MHC molecules is difficult because they are membrane bound and have a relatively low level of expression, accounting for at most only 1% of the membrane proteins. Their isolation from the membrane of lymphoid cell lines was ultimately achieved by two methods. In one method lymphoid cells are treated with Nonidet P-40 detergent, which extracts the class I molecule intact but renders it insoluble in aqueous solutions. In the other method cells are treated with the enzyme papain, which cleaves the exposed hydrophilic, soluble portion of the molecule from its hydrophobic, insoluble transmembrane tail.

Structure of Class I Molecules

As noted already, each class I MHC molecule consists of a heavy chain—the α chain—associated noncovalently with a light chain, which is β_2-microglobulin. The α chain is a polymorphic transmembrane glycoprotein of about 45 kilodaltons (kDa) encoded by class I MHC loci. The β_2-microglobulin is an invariant protein of about 12 kDa encoded by genes on a separate chromosome. Association of the α chain with β_2-microglobulin is required for expression of class I molecules on cell membranes. The α chain is anchored in the plasma membrane by its hydrophobic transmembrane segment and hydrophilic cytoplasmic tail.

Peptide mapping and amino acid sequencing have revealed that the α chain of class I MHC molecules is organized into three external domains each containing approximately 90 amino acids (α_1, α_2, and α_3), a transmembrane domain of about 40 amino acids, and a cytoplasmic anchor segment of 30 amino acids (Figure 9-6a). In size and organization β_2-microglobulin is similar to the α_3 external domain. Comparison of sequence data has shown that considerable homology exists between the α_3 domain, β_2-microglobulin, and the constant-region domains in immunoglobulins. The enzyme papain cleaves the α chain just 13 residues proximal to its transmembrane domain, releasing the extracellular portion of the molecule consisting of α_1, α_2, α_3, and β_2-microglobulin. Purification and crystallization of the extracellular portion revealed two pairs of interacting domains: a membrane-distal pair made up of the α_1 and α_2 domains and a membrane-proximal pair composed of the α_3 domain and β_2-microglobulin (Figure 9-6b).

The α_1 and α_2 domains interact to form a platform of eight antiparallel β strands spanned by two long α-helical regions. The structure forms a deep groove, or cleft, approximately 25 Å × 10 Å × 11 Å, with the long α helices as sides and the β strands of the β sheet as the bottom (Figure 9-6c). This groove is on the top surface of the molecule and is thought to be the peptide-binding site of the class I MHC molecule, having a sufficient size to bind a peptide of 8–20 amino acids. The great surprise in the x-ray crystallographic analysis of the class I molecule was the finding of a small peptide in the cleft that had cocrystallized with the molecule. It is speculated that this peptide may, in fact, be processed antigen bound to the α_1 and α_2 domains in this deep groove.

The α_3 domain and β_2-microglobulin are organized into two β pleated sheets each formed by antiparallel β strands of amino acids. As described in Chapter 5, this structure, known as the immunoglobulin fold, is characteristic of immunoglobulin domains. Because of this structural similarity, which is not surprising given the considerable sequence homology with the immunoglobulin constant regions, class I MHC molecules and β_2-microglobulin are classified as members of the immunoglobulin superfamily. The α_3 domain appears to be highly conserved among class I MHC molecules and contains a sequence that is recognized by the T-cell membrane molecule CD8. β_2-Microglobulin interacts extensively with the α_3 domain and also interacts with amino acids of the α_1 and α_2 domains. The interaction of β_2-microglobulin appears to be necessary for the proper conformation of class I MHC molecules. Peptide binding to the groove in the α_1/α_2 domain appears to enable the α_3 domain to interact with β_2-microglobulin, allowing the molecule to assume its proper conformation.

In the absence of β_2-microglobulin, the class I MHC α chain is not expressed on the cell membrane. This is illustrated by Daudi tumor cells, which are unable to synthesize β_2-microglobulin. These tumor cells possess class I MHC genes, which they can transcribe into mRNA. Although the mRNA is translated into protein, the cells do not express class I MHC α chains on the membrane. However, if Daudi cells are transfected with a functional gene encoding β_2-microglobulin, they will begin to express class I molecules on the membrane.

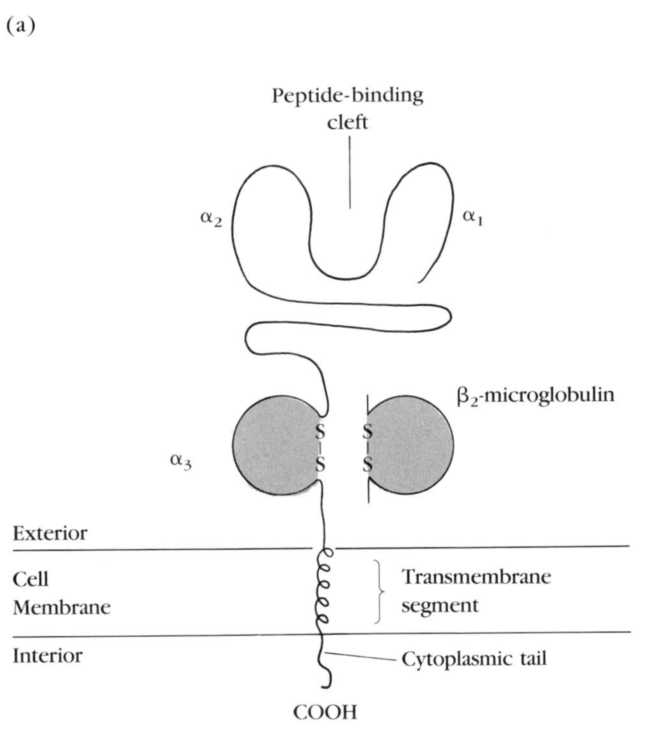

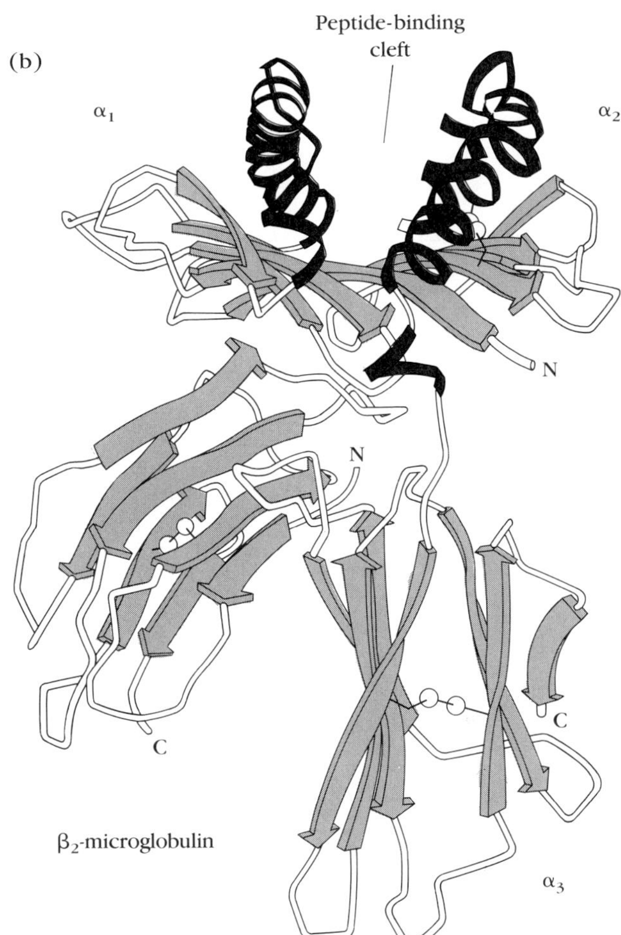

(c)

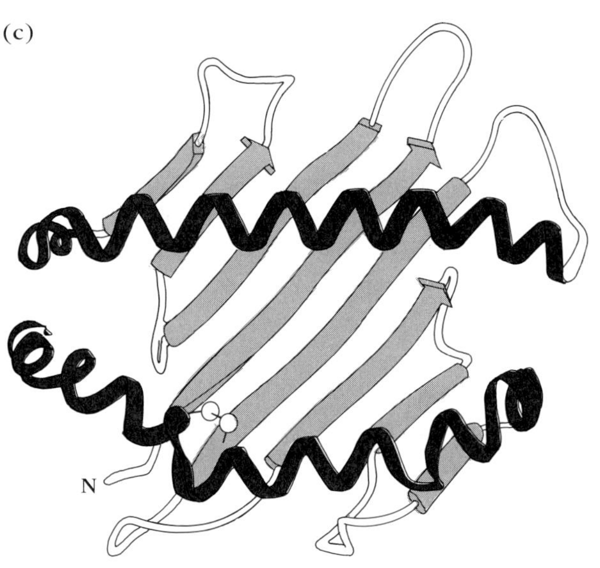

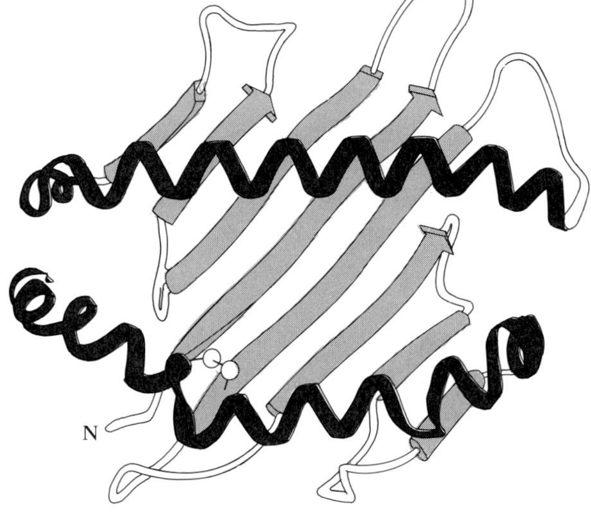

FIGURE 9-6 Structure of class I MHC molecules. (a) Schematic diagram showing various regions of a class I molecule. The α_3 domain and β_2-microglobulin have the immunoglobulin-fold structure (light purple). (b) Representation of the external domains of the human class I HLA-A2 molecule determined by x-ray crystallographic analysis. The β strands are depicted as thick arrows (light purple) and the α helices as spiral ribbons (dark purple). Disulfide bonds are shown as two interconnected spheres. (c) Representation of the α_1 and α_2 domains as viewed from top of a class I molecule showing the peptide-binding cleft consisting of a base of antiparallel β strands and sides of α helices.

Structure of Class I Genes

A number of class I MHC genes have been cloned and sequenced. Comparison of the amino acid sequence of the protein product with the DNA sequence has revealed that separate exons encode each domain (Figure 9-7a). The mouse *K, D, L, Qa,* and *Tla* genes and human *A, B,* and *C* genes all have a 5′ leader exon encoding a short signal peptide followed by five or six exons encoding the α chain of the class I molecule. The signal peptide serves to facilitate insertion of the α chain into the endoplasmic reticulum and is removed, after translation is completed, by proteolytic enzymes in the endoplasmic reticulum. The next three exons

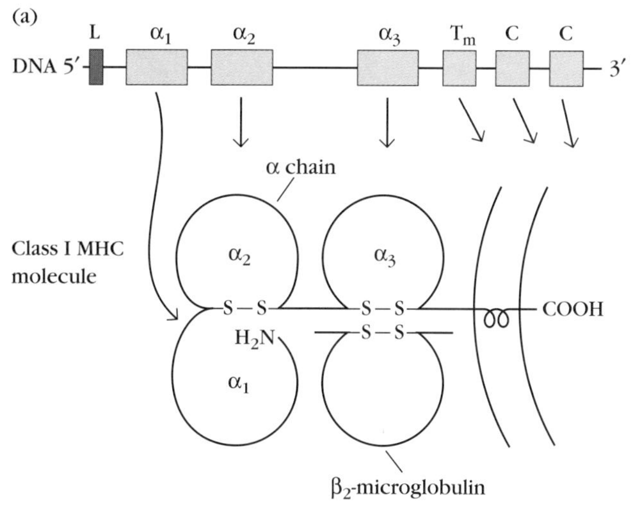

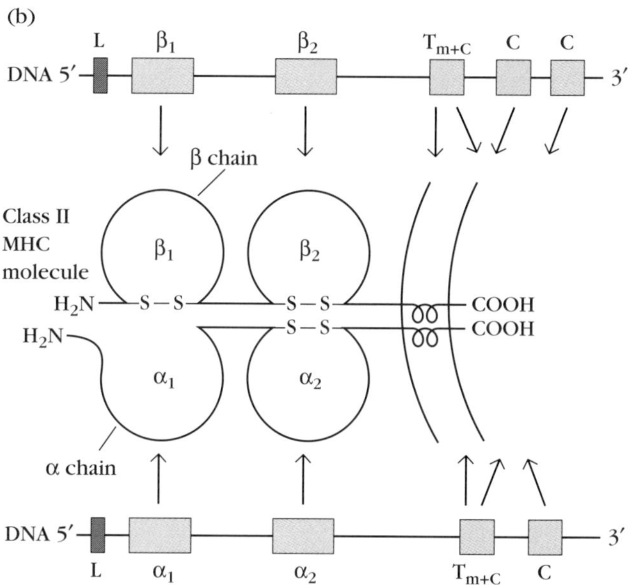

FIGURE 9-7 Schematic diagram of (a) class I and (b) class II MHC genes and molecules showing the correspondence between exons (purple) and the domains in the gene products. Each exon, with the exception of the leader (L) exon, encodes a separate domain of the MHC molecule. The gene encoding β_2-microglobulin is located on a different chromosome. T_m = transmembrane; C = cytoplasmic.

encode the extracellular α_1, α_2, and α_3 domains. The next downstream exon encodes the transmembrane region; finally a 3′-terminal exon or two exons encode the cytoplasmic domains.

Peptide Binding by Class I Molecules

Class I MHC molecules bind peptides and present these peptides to $CD8^+$ T cells (see Color Plates 11–13). In general these peptides are derived from endogenous proteins that have been degraded within the cytoplasm of the cell. Peptide binding by the cleft of a class I molecule does not exhibit the fine specificity characteristic of antigen binding by an antibody. Instead, a given MHC molecule can bind numerous different peptides, and some peptides can bind to several MHC molecules. Because of this broad specificity, the binding between a peptide and an MHC molecule is often referred to as "promiscuous."

Each type of class I MHC molecule (e.g., K, D, and L in mice or A, B, and C in humans) binds a unique set of peptides. A single nucleated cell expresses thousands of class I molecules, which collectively bind many different endogenous peptides. As discussed later, in a normal cell these are self-peptides derived from common intracellular proteins. H. G. Rammensee has estimated that a cell expresses about 200 copies of most intracellular proteins and about 1×10^5 copies of each class I MHC molecule, leading him to the conclusion that a single class I molecule is able to present at least 500 different peptides. In an altered self-cell (e.g., a virus-infected cell), some of these self-peptides are replaced with peptides derived from viral peptides. Each allelic form of a class I MHC molecule (e.g., H-$2K^k$ and H-$2K^d$) also binds a distinct set of peptides. This allelic variation and its influence on differences in immune responses among individuals are examined later in this chapter.

Identification of which peptides within a given antigen bind most effectively to various MHC molecules has important implications for vaccine development. Various approaches have been used to obtain information about the nature of the interaction between peptides and MHC molecules, a subject that is receiving considerable research attention. One approach is to digest antigens in vitro and then incubate the resulting peptides with cells expressing class I MHC molecules on their membrane. If the concentration of peptide is high enough, it can displace endogenously derived peptides from the MHC molecules on the cells. Studies of this type have shown which peptides from a complex protein are best able to be loaded onto a particular MHC molecule.

In another experimental approach, peptide–class I MHC complexes are isolated from cells, purified, and then denatured to release the bound peptide. In one such study, the bound peptides isolated from different class I molecules were found to have two unusual features: They generally were nonamers (nine residues), and they contained specific amino acids (or motifs) that appeared to be essential for binding of the peptide to a particular MHC molecule (Table 9-2).

The finding that the peptides most frequently isolated from class I MHC molecules are nonamers suggests that this peptide length is most compatible with the size of the peptide-binding cleft in class I molecules. Indeed, binding studies have shown that nonameric peptides bind to class I molecules with a 100- to 1000-fold higher affinity than do peptides that are either longer or shorter. The discovery of conserved motifs in peptides that bind to various MHC molecules may permit prediction of which peptides in a complex antigen will bind to a particular MHC molecule based on the presence or absence of these motifs.

Additional information about the interaction between peptides and class I MHC molecules has come from x-ray crystallographic analyses of peptide–class I MHC complexes. These studies have revealed certain common features in the way peptides bind to class I molecules. The peptide-binding cleft of class I MHC molecules is closed at both ends, thus limiting the size of peptide that can be accommodated (see Color Plate 11). Both ends of the peptide-binding cleft contain conserved amino acid residues that interact with the terminal amino acids of the peptide. As noted already, nonameric peptides are bound preferentially; the majority of contacts between class I MHC molecules and peptides involve the first two and last two amino acid residues of the peptide (i.e., residues 1, 2, 8, and 9). A bound peptide, which assumes an extended β structure, interacts with the MHC cleft at both ends but arches away from the floor of the cleft in the middle (Figure 9-8). Since the middle of the peptide does not make significant contact with the cleft of the MHC molecule, peptides that are slightly longer or shorter can be accommodated by slight differences in the number of residues that bulge away from the cleft. It is

(a)

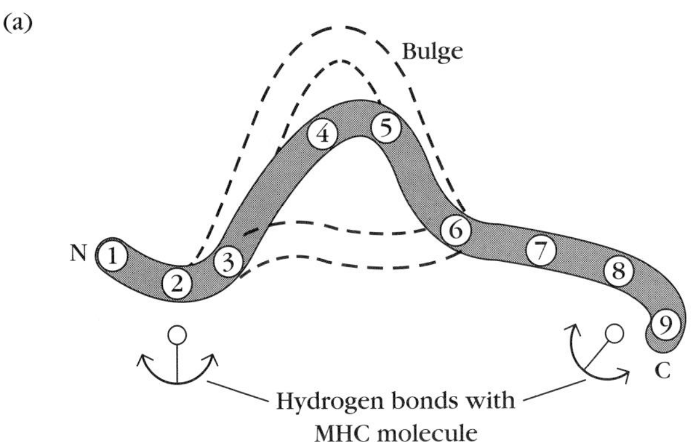

(b)

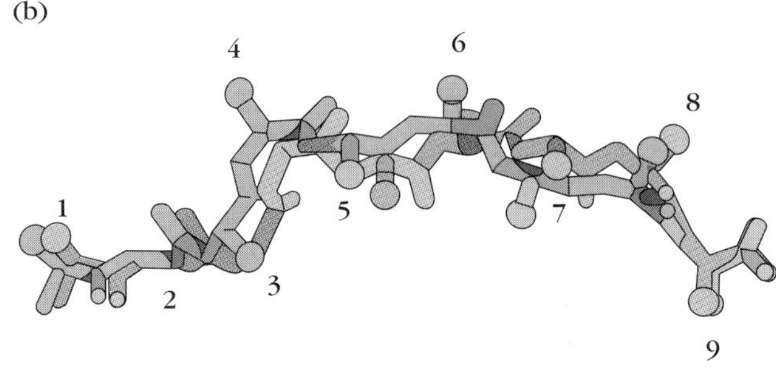

(c)

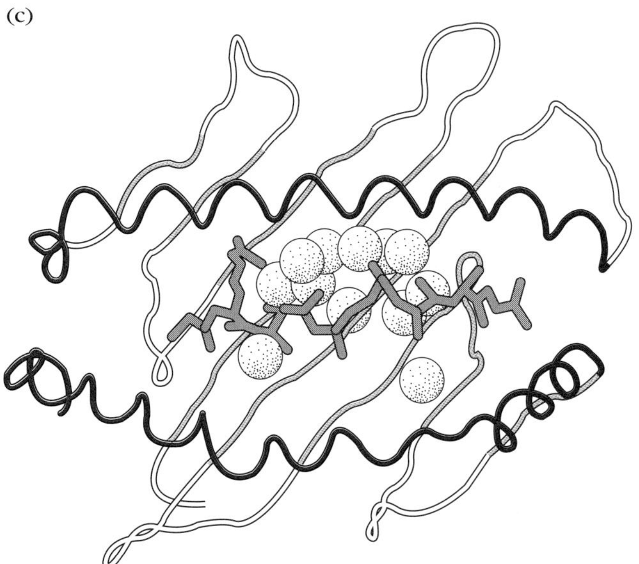

FIGURE 9-8 Interaction between peptides and binding cleft of class I MHC molecules. (a) Schematic diagram of conformational difference in bound peptides of different lengths. Longer peptides bulge in the middle, whereas shorter peptides are more extended. Contact with the MHC molecule is via hydrogen bonds involving residues 1/2 and 8/9. (b) Molecular models based on crystal structure of an influenza virus antigenic peptide (purple) and an endogenous peptide (gray) bound to a class I MHC molecule. Residues are identified by small numbers corresponding to those in part (a). (c) Representation of α_1 and α_2 domains of HLA-B27 and a bound antigenic peptide based on x-ray crystallographic analysis of the cocrystallized peptide-HLA molecule. The peptide (gray) arches up away from the β strands (light purple), which form the floor of the binding cleft, and interacts with twelve water molecules (white spheres). [Part (a) adapted from P. Parham, 1992, *Nature* **360**:300; part (b) adapted from M. L. Silver et al., 1992, *Nature* **360**:367; part (c) adapted from D. R. Madden et al., 1992, *Cell* **70**:1035.]

TABLE 9-2 OPTIMAL LENGTH AND BINDING MOTIF OF PEPTIDES EXTRACTED FROM CLASS I MHC MOLECULES ON MOUSE AND HUMAN CELLS

MHC restriction element	Peptide length	MHC-binding motif* Amino acid position 1	2	3	4	5	6	7	8	9
H-2K^b	8	—	—	—	—	Phe	—	—	Leu	
H-2K^d	9	—	Tyr	—	—	—	—	—	—	Ile
H-2D^b	9	—	—	—	—	Asn	—	—	—	Met
HLA-A2.1	9	—	Leu	—	—	—	—	—	—	Val
HLA-B27	9	—	Arg	—	—	—	—	—	—	—

* The position and identity of conserved amino acids in different peptides extracted from cells with a given MHC restriction element are shown.

SOURCE: Adapted from G. M. Bleek and S. G. Nathenson, 1992, *Trends Cell Biol.* **2**:202.

thought that the amino acids that arch away from the MHC molecule are more exposed and therefore can interact directly with the T-cell receptor.

The binding affinity of various peptides for MHC molecules has been determined by equilibrium dialysis (see Figure 6-2). In these experiments a labeled peptide was added to a solubilized class I or class II MHC molecule in a dialysis bag and the amount of labeled peptide bound to the MHC molecule at equilibrium was determined. Scatchard plots (see Figure 6-3) of the data revealed that the dissociation constant K_d of the peptide-MHC complex is approximately 10^{-6}; the rate of association is slow, but the rate of dissociation is even slower. What this means is that the peptide-MHC association is very stable under physiologic conditions; thus, most of the MHC molecules expressed on the membrane of a cell will be associated with a peptide.

CLASS II MHC MOLECULES AND GENES

Class II MHC molecules contain two different polypeptide chains, designated α and β. Both chains are encoded by genes within the D region of the human HLA complex and within the I region of the mouse H-2 complex (see Figure 9-1). The mouse I region is divided into two subregions—IA and IE, and the human D region is divided into at least three subregions—DP, DQ, and DR. Each of these subregions contains at least one α and one β gene, encoding the α and β chains of a class II MHC molecule. In addition both the mouse and the human class II regions contain some additional genes for which no protein product has been identified. The classical class II MHC molecules, which are expressed only by antigen-presenting cells, function to present processed antigenic peptides to $CD4^+$ T cells. The same methods described earlier for isolating class I MHC molecules have been used to isolate class II molecules.

Structure of Class II Molecules

Like class I MHC molecules, class II MHC molecules are membrane-bound glycoproteins that contain external domains, a transmembrane segment, and a cytoplasmic anchor segment. In mice there are two isotypic forms of class II molecules (IA and IE), and in humans there are three (DP, DQ, and DR). Amino acid sequencing comparisons of the mouse and human class II molecules suggests that there are structural and functional similarities between the IA and DQ molecules and between IE and DR; there does not appear to be a mouse equivalent for the human DP molecule. A class II MHC molecule contains a 33-kDa α chain and a 28-kDa β chain, which associate by noncovalent interactions (see Figures 9-5 and 9-9). An additional chain, called the invariant (Ii) chain, is transiently associated with the class II heterodimer during transport to the plasma membrane.

Each chain in a class II MHC molecule contains two external domains: α_1 and α_2 domains and β_1 and β_2

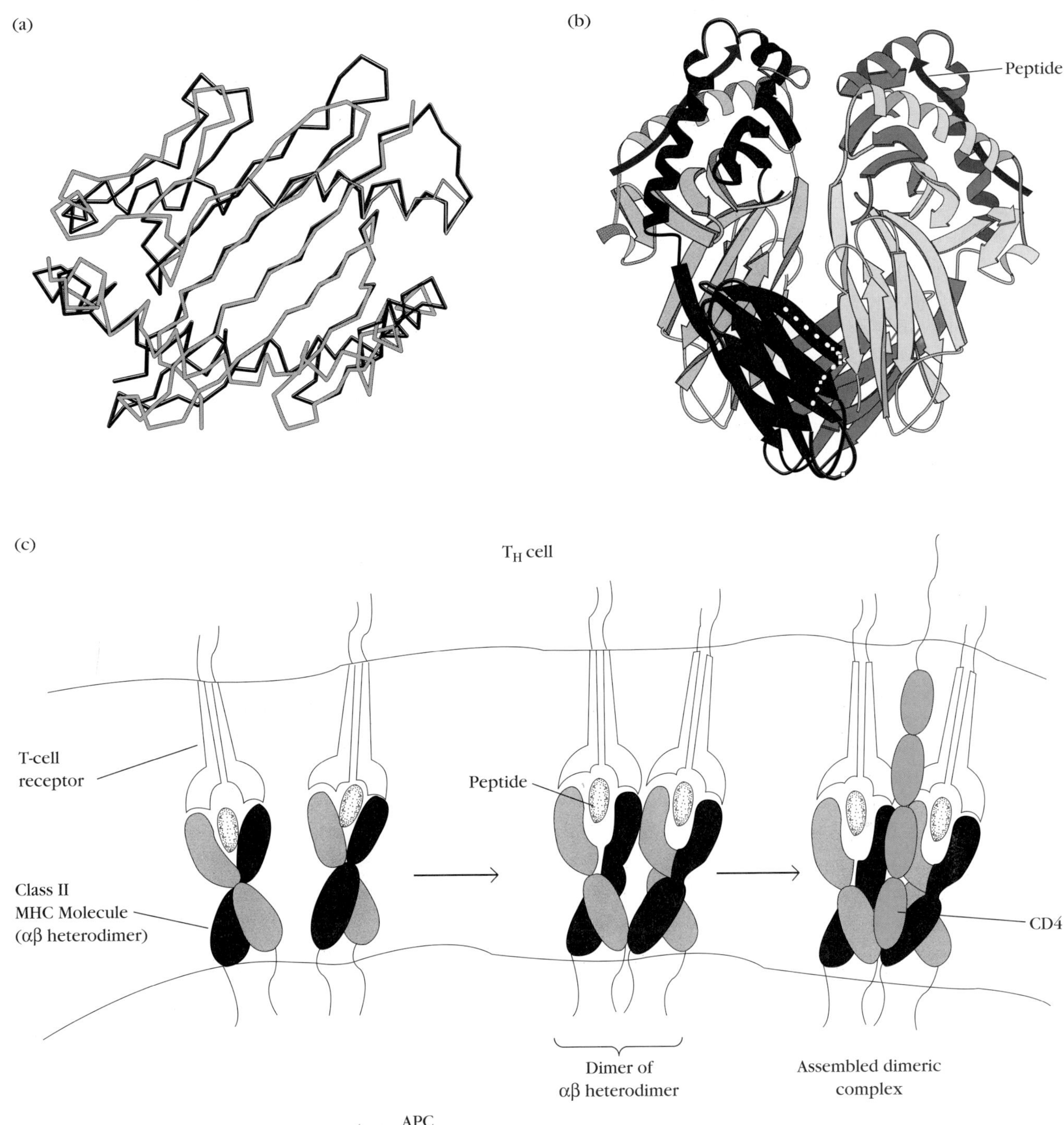

FIGURE 9-9 Structure of class II MHC molecules. (a) Models of membrane-distal domains of a class I MHC molecule (purple) and the class II HLA-DR1 molecule (gray) based on x-ray crystallographic analyses. Superimposition of the two molecules highlights the similarity in their structures. (b) Representation of crystallized HLA-DR1, which cocrystallized as a dimer of the *αβ* heterodimer (see Figure 9-5). One DR1 molecule is shaded purple, and the other is shaded gray. (c) Hypothetical model of in vivo assembly of class II MHC molecule, T-cell receptor, and CD4 to form a dimeric complex containing two molecules of each component. One CD4 is in the back and not shown; also not shown is CD3, which is associated with the T-cell receptor. [Adapted from J. H. Brown et al., 1993, *Nature* **364**:33.]

domains (see Figure 9-5). The membrane-proximal α_2 and β_2 domains, like the membrane-proximal α_3 domain of class I MHC molecules, bear sequence homology to the immunoglobulin-fold domain structure; for this reason, class II MHC molecules also are classified in the immunoglobulin superfamily. The membrane-distal domain of a class II molecule is composed of the α_1 and β_1 domains, which are thought to form an antigen-binding cleft for processed antigen.

Recently, the three-dimensional structure of a class II MHC molecule at 3.3 Å resolution was determined in the laboratories of D. C. Wiley and J. L. Strominger (see Color Plates 14–16). This accomplishment was no small feat, as it took nearly ten years to obtain sufficient quantities of pure human class II DR1 for crystallographic analysis. The overall three-dimensional structure of this class II molecule is similar to that of class I molecules. The antigen-binding cleft of HLA-DR1, like that in class I molecules, is composed of a floor of eight antiparallel β strands and sides of antiparallel α helices. The similarity is so great that the class II and class I antigen-binding clefts can be superimposed (Figure 9-9a).

The most striking difference between crystallized class I and class II molecules is that the latter occurs as a dimer of the $\alpha\beta$ heterodimer, a "dimer of dimers" (Figure 9-9b). The dimer is oriented so that the two peptide-binding clefts face in the opposite direction. Although it has not yet been determined whether this dimer form exists in vivo, Wiley and Strominger have speculated that it may facilitate the aggregation of two T-cell receptors (and the associated CD3 complex) and two CD4 molecules (Figure 9-9c). This aggregation may be necessary for signal transduction.

Structure of Class II Genes

Like class I MHC genes, the class II genes are organized into a series of exons and introns mirroring the domain structure of the α and β chains (Figure 9-7b). Both the α and the β genes encoding mouse and human class II MHC molecules have a leader exon, an α_1 or β_1 exon, an α_2 or β_2 exon, a transmembrane exon, and one or more cytoplasmic exons.

Peptide Binding by Class II Molecules

Class II MHC molecules bind peptides and present these peptides to $CD4^+$ T cells. In general these peptides are derived from exogenous proteins that have been degraded within the endocytic processing pathway. Like class I molecules, class II molecules can bind a variety of peptides.

In studies simiiar to those done with class I molecules, peptides have been isolated from class II MHC–peptide complexes. The isolated peptides generally contain 13–18 amino acid residues, and thus are slightly longer than the octameric and nonameric peptides that most commonly bind to class I molecules. The peptides that bind to class II molecules often have internal conserved "motifs," but unlike class I-binding peptides, they lack conserved motifs at the carboxyl-terminal end. Determination of the three-dimensional structure of the class II HLA-DR1 molecule has revealed that its peptide-binding cleft is open at both ends allowing a bound peptide to extend from both ends, much like a long hot dog in a bun (see Color Plate 15). This feature enables the class II molecule to bind longer peptides. Further clarification about the interaction between peptides and class II MHC molecules awaits the x-ray crystallographic analysis of more class II MHC-peptide complexes.

Polymorphism of Class I and Class II MHC Molecules

An enormous diversity is exhibited by the MHC molecules within a species. However, the source of the diversity of MHC molecules differs from that associated with antibodies and T-cell receptors. The diversity of antibodies and T-cell receptors is generated by a continual process of random gene rearrangements and thus it changes over time within an individual. In contrast, the diversity of MHC molecules results from *polymorphism,* that is, the presence of multiple alleles at a given genetic locus within a species. Thus, the MHC molecules expressed by an individual do not change over time, but they may differ significantly from those expressed by another individual of the same species.

The MHC, one of the most polymorphic genetic complexes known in higher vertebrates, possesses an extraordinarily large number of different alleles at each locus. These alleles differ in their DNA sequences from one individual to another, and consequently the gene products expressed by different individuals have unique structural differences. Analysis of human HLA class I molecules has so far revealed 23 *A* alleles, 49 *B* alleles, and 12 *C* alleles. In mice the polymorphism is equally staggering, with more than 55 alleles now identified at the *K* locus and 60 alleles identified at the *D* locus. The current estimate of actual polymorphism in both the human and mouse MHC, suggested by serologic and functional analysis, is on the order of 100 alleles for each locus.

This enormous polymorphism results in a tremendous diversity of MHC molecules within a species.

Given 100 different alleles for each class I and class II gene in the mouse H-2 complex, the theoretical diversity possible for the species is

$$100(K) \times 100(IA\alpha) \times 100(IA\beta) \times 100(IE\alpha) \times 100(IE\beta) \times 100(D) = 10^{12}!!$$

In humans the theoretical diversity is even larger, because humans have more class I and class II genes. However, because these genes are tightly linked and are inherited as a haplotype, the actual diversity within a species is less than the theoretical estimate. Still, this enormous polymorphism creates a major obstacle when it comes to matching MHC molecules for successful organ transplants.

A comparison of the amino acid sequences of several allelic MHC molecules encoded at a single locus reveals a sequence divergence of between 5 and 10%. This degree of variation is unusually high. Indeed, the sequence divergence among alleles of the MHC *within a species* is as great as the divergence observed for the genes encoding some enzymes (e.g., lactate dehydrogenase) *across species lines.* What is also unusual is that the sequence variation among MHC molecules is not randomly distributed along the entire polypeptide chain but instead is clustered in short stretches, largely within the membrane-distal α_1 and α_2 domains of class I molecules and α_1 and β_1 domains of class II molecules (Figure 9-10a).

The clustered distribution of the sequence variation in MHC molecules is thought to arise through *gene conversion,* a process whereby short donor DNA sequences base-pair with partially homologous DNA sequences in a recipient gene; excision repair or replication then inserts the donor sequence into the recipient DNA. By this process information is transferred unidirectionally from a donor DNA sequence to a partially

(a)

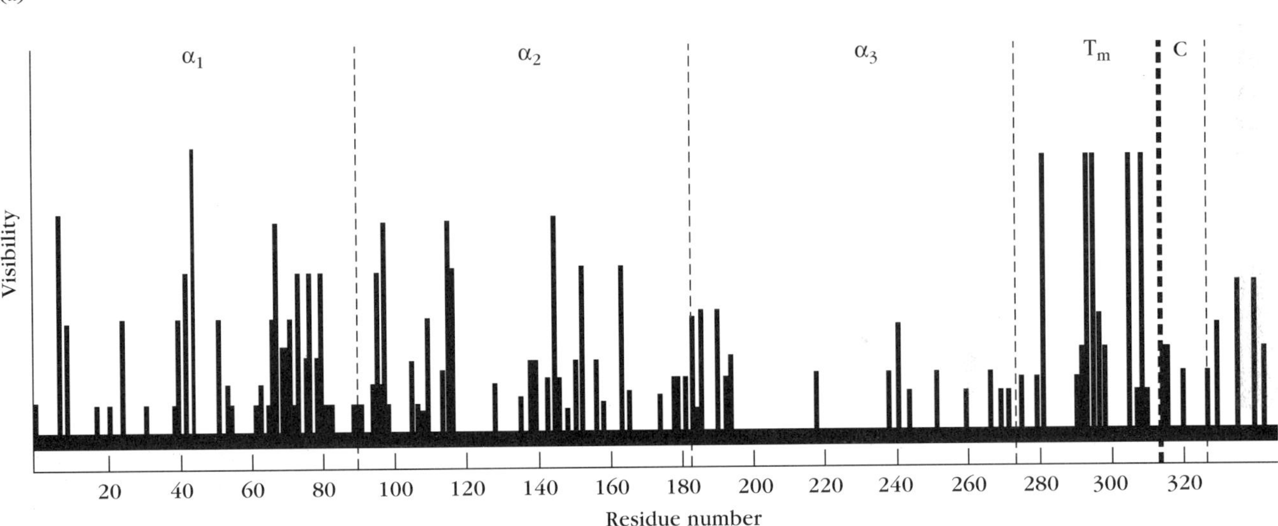

(b)

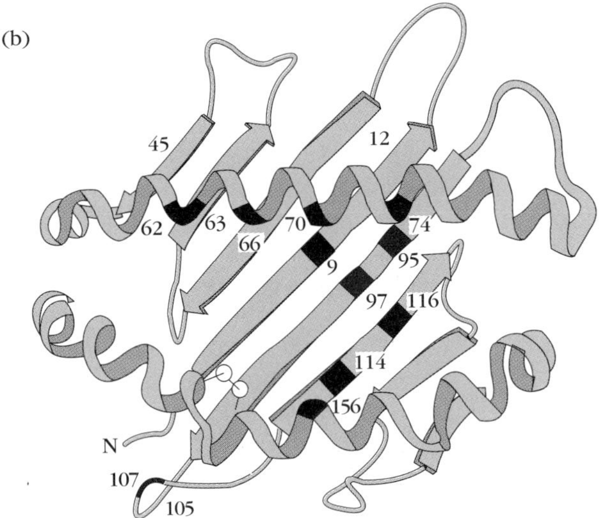

FIGURE 9-10 (a) Plots of variability in the amino acid sequence of allelic class I MHC molecules in humans versus residue position. In the external domains, most of the variable residues are in the membrane-distal α_1 and α_2 domains. (b) Location of polymorphic amino acid residues (black) in the α_1/α_2 domain of a human class I MHC molecule. [Part (a) adapted from R. Sodoyer et al., 1984, *EMBO J.* **3**:879; part (b) adapted from P. Parham, 1989, *Nature* **342**:617.]

homologous recipient DNA sequence. The molecular mechanism of gene conversion has not yet been defined, but conversion has been shown to occur in yeasts, trypanosomes, and human fetal globulin genes in addition to the class I and class II MHC genes. The large number of unexpressed pseudogenes in the MHC may serve as a pool of related gene sequences from which short, nearly homologous gene sequences can be transferred to functional class I or class II genes.

Some progress has been made in locating the polymorphic residues within the three-dimensional structure of the membrane-distal domains in class I and class II MHC molecules and in relating allelic differences to functional differences. For example, experiments described later show that different class II molecules preferentially bind various labeled peptides. In addition, studies with mutated and hybrid class II MHC molecules, as well as the recent x-ray crystallographic analysis of HLA-DR1, have located the peptide-binding site in the membrane-distal α_1/β_1 domain, the very region that displays localized polymorphism within class II MHC molecules. A number of researchers have suggested that such allelic differences in the class II molecules expressed by antigen-presenting cells may influence the cells' ability to recognize a particular peptide.

The polymorphic amino acids of class I MHC molecules also are clustered in the membrane-distal α_1/α_2 domain. Now that high-resolution x-ray crystallographic analyses of several class I molecules have been completed, the location of the polymorphic residues within the structure of the α_1/α_2 domain has been determined (Figure 9-10b). For example, of 17 amino acids previously shown to display significant polymorphism in the HLA-A2 molecule, 15 were shown by crystallographic analysis to be in the peptide-binding cleft of this molecule. The location of so many polymorphic amino acids within the binding site for processed antigen strongly suggests that allelic differences contribute to the observed differences in the ability of MHC molecules to interact with a given antigenic peptide.

Class III MHC Molecules

As noted earlier, several structurally and functionally diverse proteins are encoded within the third region of the MHC. These class III molecules include several complement components (C2, C4A, C4B, and factor B), two steroid 21-hydroxylase enzymes (21-OHA and 21-OHB), tumor necrosis factors α and β (TNF-α and TNF-β), and two heat-shock proteins.

Unlike class I and class II MHC molecules, the class III molecules are not membrane proteins and have no role in antigen presentation. It is not known why the class III genes are situated within the MHC complex. Some authors have speculated that the observed genetic association of certain MHC alleles with various diseases may in some cases reflect regulatory disorders of the class III region. For example, ankylosing spondylitis is strongly associated with an allele of the *B* locus of the HLA complex (the *HLA-B27* allele). This disease is characterized by destruction of cartilage, and it has been suggested that because of the close linkage of the *TNF-α* and *TNF-β* genes with the *HLA-B* locus, these cytokines may be involved in cartilage destruction. Systemic lupus erythematosus is another disease that is associated with certain alleles of the MHC. This disease is characterized by autoantibody production, deposition of immune complexes, and complement-mediated damage; it is possible that regulatory defects in the expression of class III complement components may contribute to the severity of this disease.

The heat-shock proteins are an unusual group of highly conserved proteins that are produced by cells in response to various stresses including heat shock (for which they were named), nutrient deprivation, oxygen radicals, and viral infection. Some heat-shock proteins are thought to bind incompletely or aberrantly folded proteins and may be involved in the intracellular trafficking of proteins necessary for proper antigen presentation. These proteins have been shown to associate with ribonucleoproteins in the nucleus during heat shock. Evidence suggesting that heat-shock proteins may be linked to certain autoimmune diseases is discussed in Chapter 19.

Mapping of the MHC

As noted already, the MHC is a large complex of genes located on chromosome 17 of mice and on chromosome 6 of humans. This complex is now known to contain nearly 100 genes; it spans some 2000 kb of mouse DNA and some 3500 kb of human DNA. Once congenic and recombinant congenic mouse strains became available, mapping of the position and function of the individual genes within the H-2 complex began. Initially, serologic and functional assays were used to assess the gene products encoded by the MHC genes. More recently, cloning of both mouse and human MHC genes has permitted restriction-enzyme mapping of the MHC. Detailed mapping of the MHC is progressing at a rapid pace, and additional genes are being identified within this complex each year.

Mapping Techniques

Serologic Mapping

When cells from one inbred strain are injected into a genetically different inbred strain, antibodies are elicited against the unique epitopes of the foreign MHC molecules. These antibodies can define different groups of MHC antigenic specificities. The epitopes that are unique to a given haplotype are *private specificities,* whereas epitopes shared by more than one haplotype are *public specificities.* Antisera specific for different public or private MHC antigenic specificities have been used to identify different MHC gene products and to determine whether or not they are encoded by separate loci. It was on the basis of early serologic results that the *K* and *D* loci of the mouse H-2 complex were first identified. Serologic studies eventually led to identification of the K, D, L, IA, and IE gene products and their mapping within the H-2 complex.

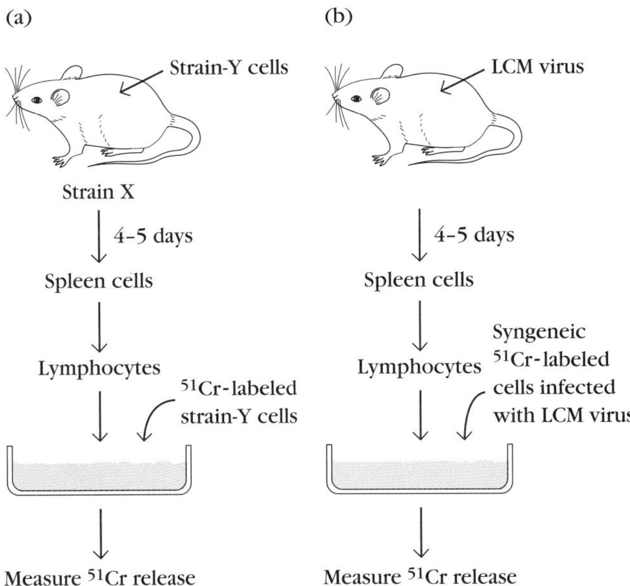

FIGURE 9-11 The in vitro cell-mediated lympholysis (CML) assay can measure the activity of cytotoxic T lymphocytes (CTLs) against allogeneic cells (a) or virus-infected cells (b). In both cases the release of ^{51}Cr into the supernatant indicates the presence of CTLs that can lyse the target cells.

Functional Mapping

A functional map of the mouse H-2 complex was developed by use of various assays based on the immunologic function of class I, II, and III MHC molecules. A few examples of these functional assays are described here; others are discussed in later chapters.

CLASS I FUNCTIONAL ASSAYS. When an animal is immunized with *allogeneic* cells (i.e., cells from a genetically distinct individual of the same species), it generates cytotoxic T lymphocytes (CTLs) specific for the MHC molecules on the allogeneic cells. The functional activity of the specific CTLs induced by the allogeneic cells can be assayed by *cell-mediated lympholysis* (CML). In the CML assay splenic lymphocytes from an immunized animal are incubated in vitro with the same allogeneic cells used for immunization except that the cells are labeled intracellularly with radioactive chromium-51 (^{51}Cr). As the immune CTLs attack the radiolabeled allogeneic cells, ^{51}Cr is released from the cells into the medium (Figure 9-11a). The amount of ^{51}Cr released into the culture medium is proportional to the level of cell-mediated cytotoxicity. CML assays performed with congenic recombinant mouse strains differing in various regions within the MHC have shown that a difference in either the K or the D region significantly affects CTL-mediated killing of allogeneic cells, indicating that this activity maps to the class I regions.

The CML assay also can be used to measure CTL-mediated killing of virus-infected cells. In this case, an animal is infected with a virus and the cytotoxic activity of its induced CTLs is assessed with syngeneic cells that have been infected with the same virus and intracellularly labeled with ^{51}Cr (Figure 9-11b). Such immune CTLs have been found to kill virally infected cells only if the class I MHC K or D regions of the target cells and the CTLs are identical, indicating that this activity maps to the class I region of the MHC.

CLASS II FUNCTIONAL ASSAYS. The earliest function associated with the class II MHC region—its ability to influence immune responsiveness to various antigens—was discovered quite unexpectedly by B. Benacerraf in 1963. He had been trying to produce homogeneous antibody by immunizing guinea pigs with simple synthetic immunogens containing a limited number of epitopes, such as DNP–poly-L-lysine (DNP-PLL). Much to his surprise, injection with DNP-PLL induced a good antibody response in some animals (designated as *responders*) but no antibody response in other animals (designated as *nonresponders*). Similar results were obtained with other simple synthetic polypeptides, such as a glutamic acid–alanine copolymer and a glutamic acid–tyrosine copolymer. The genetic control over responsiveness or nonresponsiveness was shown to be inherited in a simple mendelian fashion (Table 9-3). When responder guinea pigs were mated with nonresponder guinea pigs, all the F_1 offspring were responders;

TABLE 9-3 DEMONSTRATION OF MENDELIAN INHERITANCE OF IMMUNE RESPONSIVENESS TO SYNTHETIC PEPTIDE ANTIGENS IN GUINEA PIGS

	Immune response*				
Synthetic antigen	Strain 2	Strain 13	2×13 (F_1)	$F_1 \times 2$	$F_1 \times 13$
DNP–poly-L-Lys	+	−	+ (100%)	+ (100%)	+ (50%) − (50%)
Glu-Ala copolymer	+	−	+ (100%)	+ (100%)	+ (50%) − (50%)
Glu-Tyr copolymer	−	+	+ (100%)	+ (50%) − (50%)	+ (100%)

* Determined by production (+) or no production (−) of specific serum antibody following immunization with antigen. In crosses, the values in parentheses indicate the percentage of animals showing a + or − response.

backcrossing of the F_1 to the nonresponder parent yielded 50% nonresponders and 50% responders, suggesting that a single dominant genetic region controlled immune responsiveness.

Similar studies conducted by H. McDevitt with inbred mouse strains revealed that the MHC region controlled immune responsiveness to simple synthetic peptide antigens. The results of additional studies with congenic recombinant mouse strains showed this immune responsiveness mapped to a subregion between the class I K and D regions (Table 9-4). McDevitt designated this subregion as the Ir region, for immune responsiveness. This region is now known to comprise the IA and IE subregions encoding the class II MHC molecules and is referred to as the I region. Since these early studies with synthetic amino acid polymers, the immune response to a wide variety of antigens, both synthetic and naturally occurring, has been shown to be under the control of I-region genes in both IA and IE subregions. It was not until the late 1970s and early 1980s that the role of the I region in governing immune responsiveness began to be unraveled with the discovery of the central role of class II MHC molecules as antigen-presenting molecules for activation of T_H cells.

Class II MHC molecules also play a role in T-cell proliferation in response to antigens on allogeneic cells. For example, when lymphocytes from two different inbred strains are cultured together, the cells begin to proliferate in response to the antigenic differences on the allogeneic lymphocytes. The intensity of this *mixed lymphocyte reaction (MLR)* can be quantified by adding tritium-labeled thymidine to the culture medium. As the cells proliferate, the radioactive thymidine is incorporated into the DNA of the daughter cells. The extent of proliferation can be determined by

TABLE 9-4 EFFECT OF H-2 HAPLOTYPE ON IMMUNE RESPONSIVENESS OF MICE TO THE SYNTHETIC COPOLYMER ANTIGENS (H,G)-A-L AND (T,G)-A-L

	H-2 alleles						
Mouse strain	K	IA	IE	S	D	Response to (H,G)-A-L*	Response to (T,G)-A-L*
A	*k*	*k*	*k*	*d*	*d*	High	Low
A.TL	*s*	*k*	*k*	*k*	*d*	High	Low
B10.A (4R)	*k*	*k*	*b*	*b*	*b*	High	Low
B10	*b*	*b*	*b*	*b*	*b*	Low	High
B10.STA62	*w27*	*b*	*w27*	*w27*	*w27*	Low	High
A.SW	*s*	*s*	*s*	*s*	*s*	Low	Low

* Indicated by production of specific serum antibodies.

harvesting the cells, lysing them, and measuring the amount of radioactive thymidine incorporated into the DNA, which is directly proportional to the level of cell proliferation. When allogeneic lymphocytes are mixed together, both populations of lymphocytes proliferate. This type of reaction is called a *two-way MLR.* To measure the proliferative response of only one population of lymphocytes, a *one-way MLR* is performed; in this assay the proliferative response of one lymphocyte population is inhibited by treatment with x-rays to induce chromosomal damage or with mitomycin C to inhibit spindle formation. In the one-way MLR the untreated cells are referred to as *responders* and the treated cells, which can no longer proliferate, are called *stimulators* (Figure 9-12).

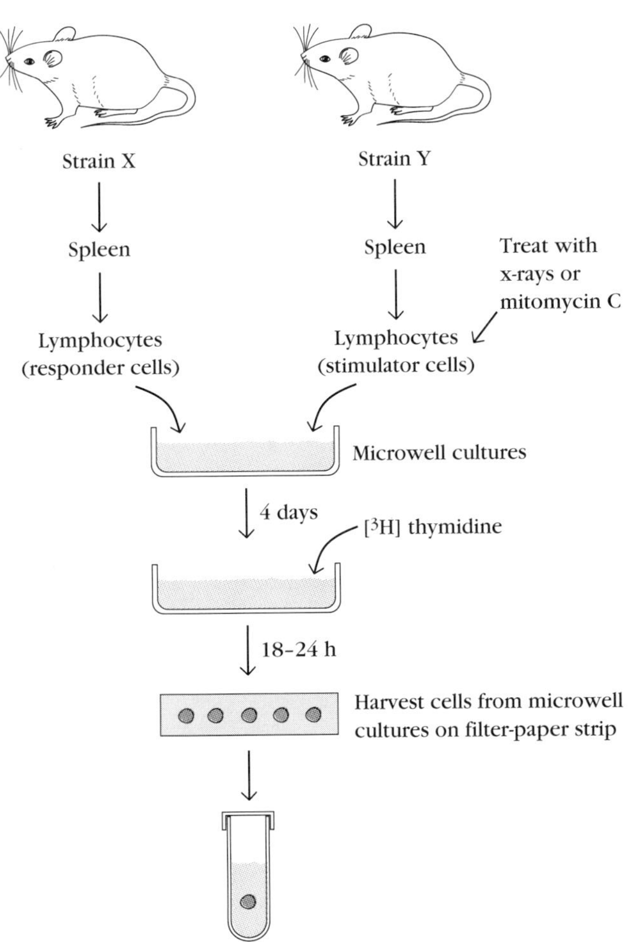

FIGURE 9-12 One-way mixed-lymphocyte reaction (MLR). This assay measures the proliferation of lymphocytes from one strain (responder cells) in response to allogeneic cells that have been x-irradiated or treated with mitomycin C to prevent proliferation (stimulator cells). The amount of [^{3}H]thymidine incorporated into the DNA is directly proportional to the level of proliferation.

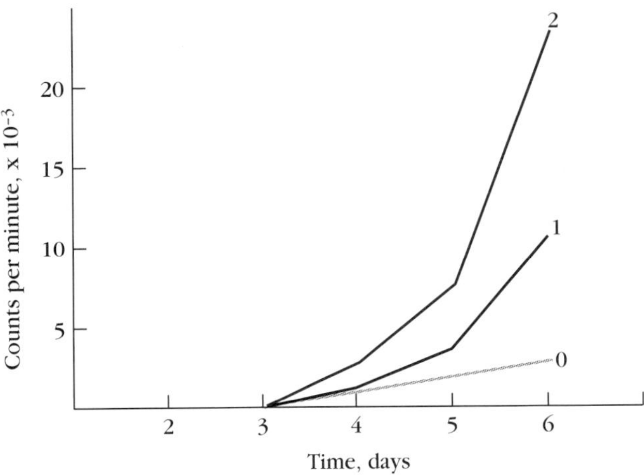

FIGURE 9-13 The amount of [^{3}H]thymidine uptake in a one-way MLR in which the stimulator and responder cells have no class II MHC differences (curve 0), have one class II MHC difference (curve 1), or have two class II MHC differences (curve 2). These results demonstrate that lymphocyte proliferation in response to allogeneic cells depends on differences in class II MHC molecules.

One-way MLRs with lymphocytes from different congenic recombinant mouse strains were used to determine which region of the MHC induced the strongest mixed-lymphocyte reaction. These experiments revealed that a difference between responder and stimulator cells in the class II MHC resulted in the most intense proliferative response (Figure 9-13). As is discussed later, the MLR measures proliferation of T_H cells; indeed, the critical role of class II MHC molecules in T_H-cell activation was first revealed by means of this assay.

Restriction-Enzyme Mapping

Molecular dissection of the MHC began in the early 1980s with the isolation of cDNA clones encoding class I, class II, or class III MHC molecules. In each case, mRNA encoding a particular MHC molecule was isolated and converted with reverse transcriptase into cDNA, which was then cloned (see Figure 2-5). Meanwhile, large fragments of chromosomal DNA from the BALB/c mouse strain were cloned in cosmid vectors (see Figure 2-6). These genomic DNA cosmid clones were then screened with a cDNA probe to identify the clones containing MHC genes.

The position of the individual MHC genes could then be determined by restriction-enzyme mapping. Each cosmid clone shown to hybridize with a cDNA probe was digested by several restriction endonucleases so that an ordered DNA map could be constructed (see Figure 2-4). The distal ends of the mapped region were subcloned, converted into single-stranded DNA,

DNA to be mapped (unknown gene sequence)

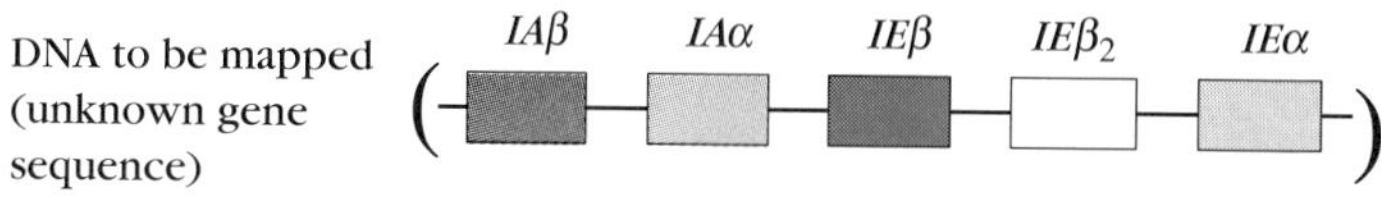

Step 1: Hybridize I-region cDNA probe with cosmid clones

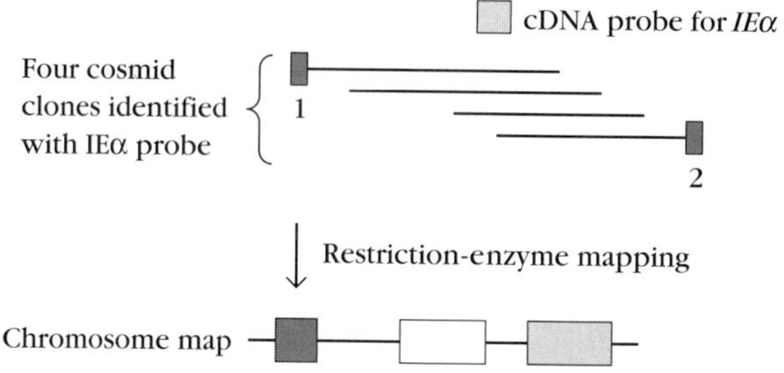

Step 2: Subclone 5′ and 3′ ends of cosmid clones to obtain new probes (1 and 2)

Step 3: Hybridize probes 1 and 2 with other cosmid clones

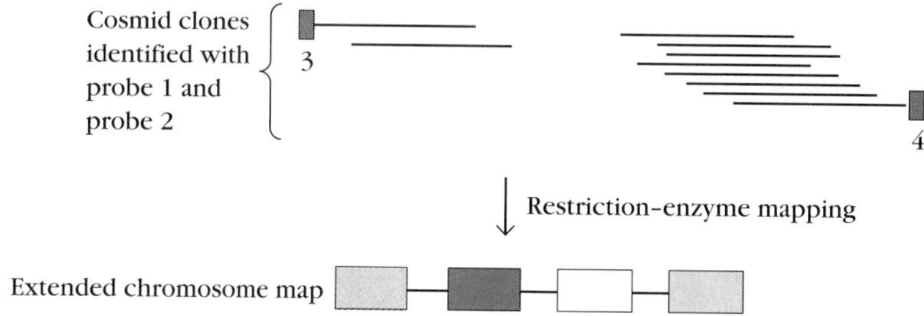

Step 4: Subclone 5′ and 3′ ends of cosmid clones to obtain new probes (3 and 4)

3 4

Step 5: Hybridize probes 3 and 4 with other cosmid clones

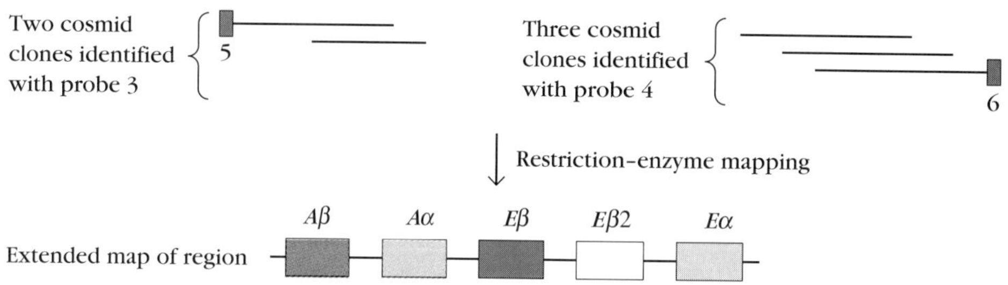

FIGURE 9-14 Mapping of I region of mouse H-2 complex by the technique of chromosome walking. Initially, an mRNA encoding an I-region gene product is converted into labeled cDNA with reverse transcriptase, and a series of large chromosomal fragments are cloned in cosmid vectors. The cDNA is used to probe the cosmid clones to identify those containing the I-region gene. Each identified clone is mapped by restriction-enzyme mapping and ordered relative to each other. The most distal 5′ and 3′ ends of the cosmid clones (numbered black boxes) are then subcloned and used as probes to identify still more cosmid clones. By repeating this process over and over, the map can be extended in both directions.

and used as probes to identify another set of overlapping cosmid clones. Each of these clones was again mapped by restriction-enzyme mapping and again the 5′ and 3′ ends were subcloned to serve as new probes that could recognize still more overlapping cosmid clones, thus extending the map in both the 5′ and 3′ directions (Figure 9-14). This technique, called *chromosome walking,* has made it possible to map large sequences of the mouse and human MHC complex.

Detailed Genomic Map of MHC Genes

Current understanding of the genomic organization of mouse and human MHC genes, based on reports through 1993, is diagrammed in Figure 9-15. Restriction-enzyme mapping has confirmed or corrected the earlier genomic maps derived from functional and serologic analyses. In addition to the "classical" MHC genes that had been recognized for some time (see

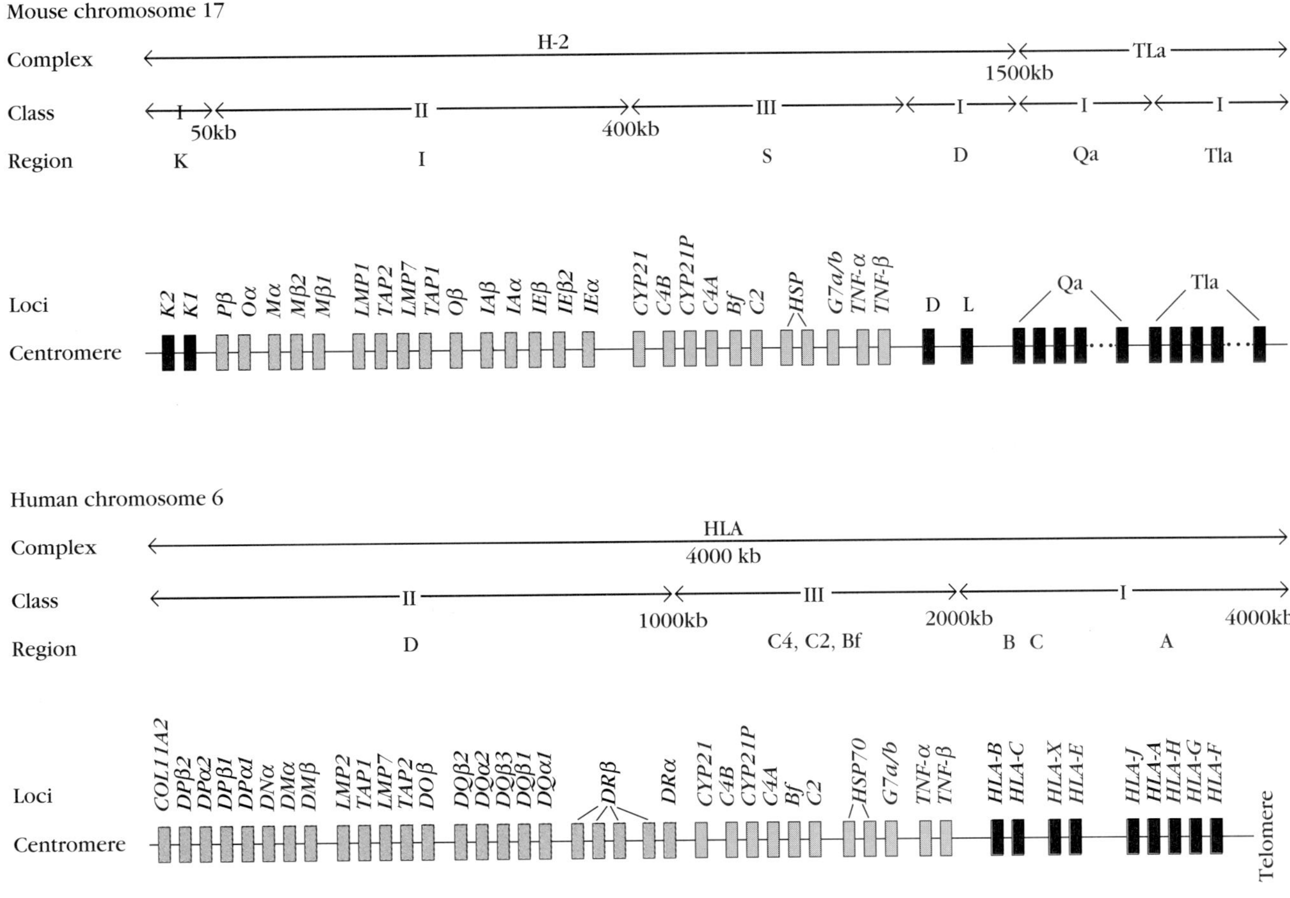

KEY

Gene	Encoded protein
C2, C4A, C4B, Bf	Complement components
COL11A2	Collagen
CYP21,CYP21P	Steroid 21-hydroxylases
G7a/b	Valyl-tRNA synthetase
HSP	Heat-shock protein
LMP1, LMP2, LMP7	Proteosome-like subunits
TAP1, TAP2	Peptide-transporter subunits
TNF-α, TNF-β	Tumor necrosis factors α and β

FIGURE 9-15 Detailed genomic map of the mouse and human MHC. Class I genes are shaded dark purple; class II genes, light purple; and class III genes, gray. In addition to the genes encoding the classical MHC molecules, molecular mapping has revealed numerous additional genes that encode nonclassical products. The functions of the proteins encoded by the nonclassical class I genes are largely unknown. In contrast, several of the nonclassical class II genes encode proteins with known functions. No pseudogenes are shown in this map. The mouse Hmt region is located downstream from Tla and is not shown.

Figure 9-1), molecular mapping has revealed a number of so-called "nonclassical" MHC genes that were not previously known. In a few cases, genes that had been identified by serologic or functional assays were not revealed by restriction-enzyme mapping. For example, early functional and serologic mapping identified a subregion called IJ in the mouse MHC, but cloning of the MHC showed that the I region does not include an IJ subregion, so other explanations must account for the functions attributed to the IJ subregion.

Map of Class I MHC

In humans the class I MHC region is about 1800 kb long and contains approximately 20 genes. In mice the class I MHC consists of two regions separated by the intervening class II and class III regions. Included within the class I region are the genes encoding the well-characterized classical class I MHC molecules designated HLA-A, HLA-B, and HLA-C in humans and H-2K, H-2D, and H-2L in mice. Many nonclassical class I genes, identified by molecular mapping, also are present in both the mouse and human MHC; the functions of these recently identified genes are only beginning to be unraveled.

In mice the nonclassical class I genes are located in three regions (Qa, Tla, and Hmt) downstream from the H-2 complex. In humans the nonclassical class I genes include the *HLA-E, HLA-F, HLA-G, HLA-H,* and *HLA-X* loci. A number of the nonclassical class I MHC genes are pseudogenes and do not encode a protein product, but others encode class I-like products of yet unknown function. In comparison with the classical class I genes, the nonclassical genes are less polymorphic and show more limited patterns of cellular expression.

The functions of the nonclassical class I MHC molecules remain largely unknown, although a few studies suggest that these molecules, like the classical class I MHC molecules, may present peptides to T cells. One intriguing finding is that the nonclassical class I molecule encoded by one *Hmt* locus is able to bind a self-peptide derived from a subunit of NADH dehydrogenase, an enzyme encoded by the mitochondrial genome. This particular self-peptide contains an amino-terminal formylated methionine. What is interesting about this finding is that peptides derived from prokaryotic organisms often have formylated amino-terminal methionine residues. One hypothesis is that this *Hmt*-encoded class I molecule may be uniquely suited to present peptides from prokaryotic organisms that are able to grow intracellularly within the cytoplasm of an infected cell. Such organisms include *Mycobacterium tuberculosis, Listeria monocytogenes, Brucella abortus,* and *Salmonella typhimurium.* Perhaps the limited polymorphism and unusual tissue distribution of nonclassical class I MHC molecules enables these molecules to present peptides from microorganisms that invade at specific tissue sites or infect specific types of cells.

Map of Class II MHC

The class II MHC region contains the genes encoding the α and β chains of the classical class II MHC molecules designated HLA-DR, HLA-DP, and HLA-DQ in humans and H-2IA and H-2IE in mice. Molecular mapping of the class II MHC has revealed additional β-chain genes in both mice and humans, as well as additional α-chain genes in humans (see Figure 9-15). In the human DR region, for example, there are three or four functional β-chain genes. All of the β-chain gene products can be expressed together with the α-chain gene product in a given cell, thereby increasing the number of antigen-presenting molecules on the cell. Although the human DR region contains just one α-chain gene, the DP and DQ regions each contain two functional α-chain genes.

Genes encoding nonclassical class II MHC molecules also have been identified in both humans and mice. In mice several class II genes ($O\alpha$, $O\beta$, $M\alpha$, and $M\beta$) encode nonclassical MHC molecules that exhibit limited polymorphism and a different pattern of expression than the classical IA and IE class II molecules. In the human class II region, nonclassical genes designated *DM, DN,* and *DO* have been identified. Some of these genes are pseudogenes, and others encode proteins of unknown function.

Mapping analysis of the class II MHC region also has revealed the presence, in both mice and humans, of two genes (*LMP2* and *LMP7*) that encode proteosome-like subunits and of two genes (*TAP1* and *TAP2*) that encode peptide-transporter subunits. As discussed in Chapter 10, proteosomes are thought to mediate cytoplasmic degradation of endogenous proteins into peptides, which then are transferred by peptide transporters into the lumen of the endoplasmic reticulum; here the peptides can interact with newly synthesized class I MHC molecules.

Map of Class III MHC

The class III region of the MHC in humans and mice contains a heterogeneous collection of more than 36 genes (see Figure 9-15). The class III region contains genes encoding several complement components, two steroid 21-hydroxylases, two heat-shock proteins, and two cytokines (TNF-α and TNF-β). The possible role of some of these class III MHC gene products in certain diseases was discussed previously. In addition, the genes encoding microsomal cytochrome P-450 and valyl-tRNA synthetase have been mapped to this region, as have many other genes encoding products whose functions are still unknown.

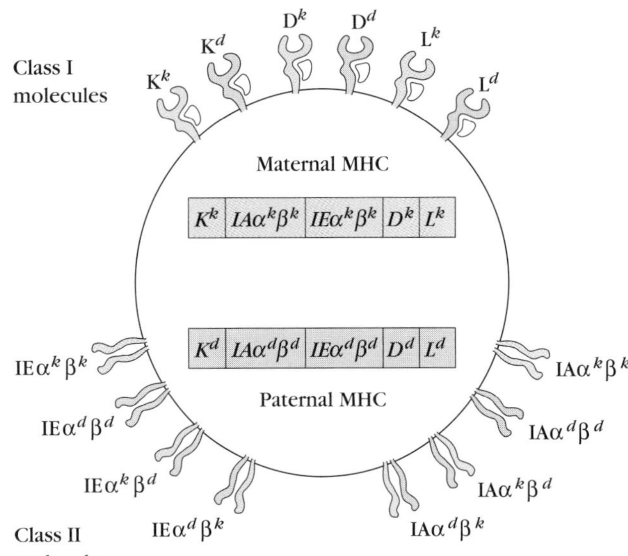

FIGURE 9-16 Diagram illustrating various MHC molecules expressed on antigen-presenting cells of a heterozygous H-$2^{k/d}$ mouse. Both the maternal (purple) and paternal (gray) MHC genes are expressed. Because the class II molecules are heterodimers, heterologous molecules containing one maternal-derived and one paternal-derived chain are produced. The β_2-microglobulin component of class I molecules is encoded by a gene on a separate chromosome and may be derived from either parent.

Expression of MHC Molecules

Cellular Expression

In general the classical class I MHC molecules are expressed on most somatic cells, but the level of class I MHC expression varies among different cell types. The highest levels of class I molecules are expressed by lymphocytes where they constitute approximately 1% of the total plasma-membrane proteins, or some 5×10^5 molecules per cell. In contrast, fibroblasts, muscle cells, liver hepatocytes, and neural cells express very low levels of class I MHC molecules. The low level of class I MHC molecules on liver transplants may reduce the likelihood of graft recognition by T cytotoxic lymphocytes of the recipient, thus contributing to the considerable success of such transplants. A few cell types (e.g., brain cells, sperm cells at certain stages of differentiation, and cells of the placenta) appear to lack class I MHC expression altogether.

As noted earlier, any particular MHC molecule can bind many different peptides. Since a single nucleated cell expresses many class I MHC molecules, each cell will display a large number of peptides in the peptide-binding clefts of its MHC molecules. If a cell is a normal healthy cell, its class I molecules will display self-peptides derived from common intracellular peptides. For example, self-peptides derived from cytochrome *c*, histones, and ribosomal protein have been eluted from class I MHC molecules on normal cells.

On the other hand, if a cell has been infected by a virus, then viral peptides, as well as self-peptides, will be displayed by its class I MHC molecules. A single virus-infected cell should be envisioned as having various class I molecules on its membrane, each displaying different sets of viral peptides. Because of individual allelic differences in the peptide-binding clefts of the classic class I MHC molecules, different individuals within a species will have the ability to bind different sets of viral peptides. Since the MHC alleles are codominantly expressed, a heterozygous individual expresses gene products encoded by both alleles at each MHC locus. An F_1 mouse, for example, expresses the *K*, *D*, and *L* from each parent (six different class I MHC molecules) on each of its nucleated cells (Figure 9-16). A similar situation occurs in humans; that is, a heterozygous individual expresses the *A*, *B*, and *C* alleles from each parent (six different class I MHC molecules) on the membrane of each nucleated cell.

Unlike class I MHC molecules, class II molecules are expressed only by antigen-presenting cells. These include macrophages, dendritic cells, B cells, thymic epithelial cells, and activated T cells in most species except the mouse. Among the various cell types that express class II MHC molecules, marked differences in expression have been observed. In some cases class II expression is related to the cell's differentiation stage. For example, class II molecules cannot be detected on pre-B cells but are expressed on the membrane of mature B cells. Some antigen-presenting cells, including B cells, dendritic cells, and Langerhans cells, constitutively express class II MHC molecules. In contrast, monocytes and macrophages that have not interacted with antigen express only low levels of class II molecules, but these cells increase their expression significantly after they have been activated.

Because each of the classical class II MHC molecules is composed of two different polypeptide chains, which are encoded by different loci, a heterozygous individual expresses not only the parental class II molecules but also heterologous hybrid molecules containing one parent's α chain and the other parent's β chain. For example, an H-2^k mouse expresses IA^k and IE^k class II molecules; similarly, an H-2^d mouse expresses IA^d and IE^d molecules. The F_1 progeny resulting from crosses of mice with these two haplotypes express four homologous parental class II molecules and four heterologous hybrid molecules as shown in Figure 9-16. Since the human MHC contains three classical class II genes (*DP*, *DQ*, and *DR*), a heterozygous individual expresses six homologous class II molecules and six heterologous molecules. The number of different class II molecules expressed by an individual is increased further by the presence of multiple β-chain genes in mice and humans, and in humans by multiple α-chain genes. The heterozygosity generated by these mechanisms presumably increases the number of different antigenic peptides that can be presented and thus is advantageous to the organism.

Regulation of MHC Expression

As the discussion in the previous section indicates, differential expression of the MHC genes occurs. Class II MHC genes are expressed only in a limited number of cell types, and the level of expression of both class I and class II genes varies among cell types. Research on the regulatory mechanisms that control this differential expression is still in the beginning stages.

Both class I and class II MHC genes are flanked by 5′ promoter sequences, which bind sequence-specific transcription factors. The promoter motifs and transcription factors that bind to these motifs are beginning to be identified. Transcriptional regulation of the MHC is mediated by both positive and negative elements. One way to analyze the effect of transcription factors on MHC expression is to fuse class II^+ and class II^- cells and see if the heterokaryon expresses the class II molecules or not. For example, when class II^+ B cells are fused with class II^- plasmacytomas, the resulting heterokaryon is always class II^-. This suggests that the plasmacytoma (representing a plasma cell) contains trans-acting factors that suppress class II MHC expression. On the other hand, when B cells (which express class II molecules constitutively) are fused with macrophages (which only express class II molecules after activation), the heterokaryon constitutively expresses class II MHC molecules, suggesting that positive transcription factors within the B cell promote class II MHC expression.

The expression of MHC molecules is also regulated by various cytokines. The interferons (alpha, beta, and gamma) and tumor necrosis factor have each been shown to increase expression of class I MHC molecules on cells. Interferon gamma (IFN-γ), for example, appears to induce the formation of a specific transcription factor that binds to the promoter sequence flanking the class I MHC genes. Binding of this transcription factor to the promoter sequence appears to up-regulate transcription of the class I genes. IFN-γ also has been shown to increase the level of class II MHC expression on a variety of non-antigen-presenting cells (e.g., skin keratinocytes, intestinal epithelial cells, vascular endothelium, placental cells, and pancreatic beta cells). Other cytokines influence MHC expression by limited cell types; for example, IL-4 appears to increase expression of class II molecules by resting B cells. Expression of class II molecules by B cells is down-regulated by IFN-γ; corticosteroids and prostaglandins also decrease expression of class II molecules.

As shown in Table 9-5, MHC expression also is influenced by a number of viruses including human cytomegalovirus (CMV), hepatitis B virus (HBV), and adenovirus 12 (Ad12). The mechanism by which these viruses cause decreased expression of class I MHC molecules is beginning to be unraveled. For example, during CMV infection a viral protein binds to β_2-microglobulin, preventing the transport of class I MHC α chains from the endoplasmic reticulum to the plasma membrane. Hepatitis B virus and adenovirus 12 appear to interfere with transcription of the class I MHC genes, presumably by blocking necessary transcription factors. Decreased expression of class I MHC molecules is likely to help viruses evade the immune response by reducing the likelihood that virus-infected cells would become targets for CTL-mediated destruction.

Probing MHC Structure and Function

Additional information about the structure and function of various MHC molecules has been obtained from studies with hybrid and mutated MHC genes and from transfection experiments.

TABLE 9-5 EFFECT OF SOME VIRUSES ON MHC EXPRESSION

Virus	Effect on expression*	
	Class I MHC	Class II MHC
Adenovirus (Ad12)	↓	
Cytomegalovirus (CMV)	↓	↓
Ectromelia virus	↓	
Hepatitis B virus (HBV)	↓	
Herpes simplex virus (HSV)	↓	
Human immunodeficiency virus (HIV)	↓	↑
Human papilloma virus 16 (HPV16)		↑
Measles virus	↑	↑
Moloney leukemia virus (MoMLV)	↑	
Rous sarcoma virus (RSV)	↓	↓
Simian immunodeficiency virus (SIV)		↑
Vaccinia virus	↓	
Vesicular stomatitis virus (VSV)	↓	
West Nile virus	↑	↑

* Increase (↑) and decrease (↓) in MHC expression are shown.

SOURCE: Adapted from D. J. Maudsley and J. D. Pound, 1991, *Immunol. Today* **12**:429.

Exon Shuffling and Site-Directed Mutagenesis

Hybrid class I and class II MHC genes can be constructed by shuffling of homologous exons using genetic engineering techniques. Since each exon encodes a separate protein domain, these hybrid genes can be used to produce MHC molecules containing domains from genetically distinct individuals. Figure 9-17 illustrates the production of MHC genes containing alleles from two different haplotypes. By means of such hybrid MHC genes, researchers have been able to assess the role of the membrane-distal α_1/α_2 and α_1/β_1 domains in class I and class II molecules, respectively, in antigen presentation and in antigen recognition by T cells. These experiments have revealed that both the

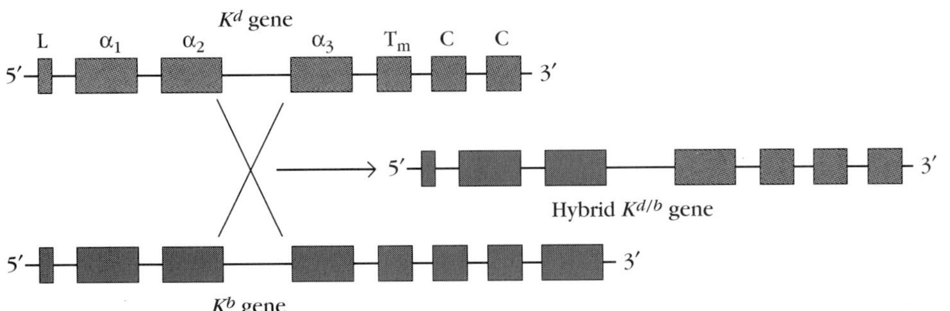

FIGURE 9-17 Hybrid class I and class II MHC genes can be constructed by exon shuffling. In this example, mouse class I *K* genes with the *b* (gray) or *d* (purple) haplotype were shuffled to produce a hybrid *K* gene containing some *b*-haplotype exons and some *d*-haplotype exons.

α_1 and the α_2 domains are required for class I MHC–restricted recognition by $CD8^+$ cells and that both the α_1 and the β_1 domain are required for class II MHC–restricted recognition by $CD4^+$ cells.

In another experimental approach, chemical or oligonucleotide-directed mutagenesis is used to induce single amino acid substitutions in the various external domains of class I and class II MHC molecules. The effect of these mutations on antigen presentation and activation of specific T-cell clones can then be studied. Experiments with mutated class I MHC molecules, for example, have confirmed the importance of both the α_1 and the α_2 domains in T_C-cell recognition, suggesting that the T-cell receptor interacts with residues in both domains. In some studies a single amino acid substitution in just one of the domains has been shown to inhibit antigen recognition by T_C cells.

Transfection of MHC Genes

Another way to study the function of a specific MHC gene is to transfect it into cells that do not express that particular MHC gene. In this way it is possible to study antigen presentation by a single MHC gene product, eliminating the complicating effect of other MHC gene products. For example, the L cell is not an antigen-presenting cell and therefore does not express any class II MHC molecules. For this reason, L cells transfected with a class II MHC gene express only the class II molecule encoded by the transfected gene. Transfection studies with genes encoding the class II IA and IE molecules have shown that these molecules differ in their ability to present particular peptides to T_H cells (see Figure 4-11).

In transfection experiments, a selection gene (e.g., thymidine kinase) is transfected in addition to the MHC gene. If the MHC gene is present in excess, most L cells that take up the selection gene also will take up the MHC gene. When the cells are cultured in the appropriate selection medium, only transfected cells will be able to grow. Transfection of MHC genes can be combined with exon shuffling or site-directed mutagenesis in a powerful experimental approach for studying the effect of various alterations in MHC molecules on T-cell activation.

MHC and Immune Responsiveness

As discussed earlier, immune responsiveness to exogenous antigens, as measured by the production of serum antibodies, is under the control of class II MHC genes. Two explanations have been proposed to account for the variability in immune responsiveness observed among different haplotypes (see Table 9-4). According to the ***determinant-selection*** model, different class II MHC molecules differ in their ability to bind processed antigen. The alternative ***holes-in-the-repertoire*** model suggests that T cells bearing receptors that recognize foreign antigens closely resembling self-antigens may be eliminated during thymic processing. Since the T-cell response to an antigen involves a trimolecular complex of the T cell's receptor, an antigenic peptide, and a MHC molecule (see Figure 4-8), both models may be correct. That is, the absence of a MHC molecule that can bind and present a given peptide *or* the absence of T-cell receptors that can recognize a given peptide–MHC molecule complex could result in the absence of immune responsiveness and so account for the observed relationship between MHC haplotype and immune responsiveness to exogenous antigens.

Determinant-Selection Model

The determinant-selection model assumes that the structure of a particular MHC molecule determines the strength of its association with any given antigen. Animals that respond, for example, to antigen A must express at least one class II MHC molecule whose structure facilitates interaction with antigen A, whereas animals that do not respond must express class II MHC molecules that do not interact effectively with antigen A. According to this model, the MHC polymorphism within a species will generate different patterns of responsiveness and nonresponsiveness to different antigens.

If this model is correct, then class II molecules from responder and nonresponder strains should show differential binding of antigen. Table 9-6 presents data on the binding of various radiolabeled peptides to class II IA and IE molecules with the H-2^d or H-2^k haplotype. Each of the listed peptides binds significantly to only one of the class II molecules. Furthermore, as predicted, the haplotype of the class II molecule showing the highest-affinity binding for a particular peptide generally is the same as the haplotype of responder strains for that peptide.

In other experiments the nonresponder status of some strains has been linked to the deletion of a class II MHC gene. For example, H-2^b and H-2^s haplotype mice have undergone deletion of the *IEα* gene and therefore do not express class II IE molecules. These

TABLE 9-6 DIFFERENTIAL BINDING OF PEPTIDES TO MOUSE CLASS II MHC MOLECULES AND CORRELATION WITH MHC RESTRICTION

Labeled peptide*	MHC restriction of responders†	Percentage of labeled peptide bound to‡			
		IA^d	IE^d	IA^k	IE^k
Ovalbumin (323–339)	IA^d	**11.8**	0.1	0.2	0.1
Influenza hemagglutinin (130–142)	IA^d	**18.9**	0.6	7.1	0.3
Hen egg-white lysozyme (46–61)	IA^k	0.0	0.0	**35.2**	0.5
Hen egg-white lysozyme (74–86)	IA^k	2.0	2.3	**2.9**	1.7
Hen egg-white lysozyme (81–96)	IE^k	0.4	0.2	0.7	**1.1**
Myoglobin (132–153)	IE^d	0.8	**6.3**	0.5	0.7
Pigeon cytochrome *c* (88–104)	IE^k	0.6	1.2	1.7	**8.7**
λ repressor (12–26)§	$IA^d + IE^k$	1.6	**8.9**	0.3	2.3

* Amino acid residues included in each peptide are indicated by the numbers in parentheses.

† Refers to class II molecule (IA or IE) and haplotype associated with a good response to the indicated peptides as determined by studies such as that shown in Table 9-4.

‡ Binding determined by equilibrium dialysis. Bold-faced values indicate binding was significantly greater ($p < 0.05$) than that of the other three class II molecules tested.

§ The λ repressor is an exception to the rule that high binding correlates with the MHC restriction of high-responder strains. In this case, the T_H cell specific for the λ peptide–IE^d complex has been deleted; this is an example of the hole-in-the-repertoire mechanism.

SOURCE: Adapted from S. Buus et al., 1987, *Science* **235**:1353.

strains are nonresponders to a synthetic Glu-Lys-Phe peptide and to pigeon cytochrome *c*. When an *IEα* gene is introduced into a fertilized egg in these nonresponding strains, the resulting transgenic mice express the class II IE molecule and are now able to respond to both the synthetic Glu-Lys-Phe peptide and to pigeon cytochrome *c*.

Holes-in-the-Repertoire Model

The influence of the MHC on immune responsiveness can also be caused by an absence of functional T cells capable of recognizing a given antigen–MHC molecule complex. A good example is documented in the peptide-binding data presented in Table 9-6. The λ repressor peptide (residues 12–26) binds best in vitro to IE^d, yet the MHC restriction for this peptide is known to be associated not with IE^d but instead with the IA^d and IE^k. The suggested explanation is that T cells recognizing this λ repressor peptide in association with IE^d may have been eliminated during thymic processing leaving a hole in the T-cell repertoire.

An absence of functional T cells capable of recognizing a given antigen–MHC complex has been observed in several experimental systems. For example, the synthetic peptide poly Glu-Tyr induces an immune response in DBA/2 mice but not in BALB/c mice, although both strains have the $H\text{-}2^d$ haplotype and the antigen-presenting cells of both strains are capable of presenting this peptide. T cells from the responder strain were shown to respond to poly Glu-Tyr on antigen-presenting cells from both responder and nonresponder strains, whereas T cells from the nonresponder strain did not respond to this peptide whether it was presented by responder or nonresponder antigen-presenting cells. These results suggest that the T cells specific for poly Glu-Tyr have been functionally inactivated or clonally deleted in the nonresponder strain. A number of elegant studies with transgenic mice designed to evaluate the role of self-tolerance in influencing the T-cell repertoire are described in later chapters.

MHC and Susceptibility to Infectious Diseases

As mentioned earlier, certain diseases have been shown to be associated with particular MHC alleles. Included among these diseases are a large number of autoimmune diseases, certain viral diseases, disorders of the complement system, certain neurologic disorders, and some types of allergies. In most MHC-associated diseases, however, a number of other genes, outside the MHC, as well as external environmental factors also appear to play a role; therefore, it has been difficult to unravel these associations. The relation of the MHC to autoimmune diseases is discussed in Chapter 19; the discussion here is limited to the relationship of the MHC to diseases caused by pathogenic organisms.

A number of hypotheses have been suggested to account for the role of the MHC in disease. Susceptibility to a given pathogen may reflect the role of particular MHC alleles in responsiveness or nonresponsiveness to the pathogen. Variations in antigen presentation by different MHC alleles may determine the effectiveness of the immune response to a given pathogen. If major epitopes on a given pathogen mimic certain self-MHC molecule, it is possible that an animal may lack functional T cells for that pathogen. Various MHC alleles may also provide binding sites for specific viruses, bacteria, or their products.

Some evidence suggests that a reduction in MHC polymorphism within a species may predispose that species to disease. Cheetahs, for example, have been shown to be far more susceptible to viral disease than other big cats. Because the present cheetah population arose from a limited breeding stock, the species suffers from a loss of MHC diversity. The increased susceptibility of cheetahs to various viral diseases may result from a reduction in the number of different MHC molecules available to the species as a whole and a corresponding limitation on the range of processed antigens with which these MHC molecules can interact. Thus the high level of MHC polymorphism that has been observed in various species may be advantageous by providing a broad range of antigen-presenting MHC molecules. Because of this extreme polymorphism, some individuals within a species probably will not be able to develop an immune response to any given pathogen and therefore will be susceptible to infection by it. On the other hand, and perhaps of more importance, MHC polymorphism ensures that at least some members of a species will be able to respond to any one of a very large number of potential pathogens. In this way, MHC diversity appears to protect a species from a wide range of infectious diseases.

In a few cases the presence or absence of certain MHC alleles has been associated with specific diseases. In chickens, for example, susceptibility to the virus causing Marek's disease has been linked to inheritance of certain MHC alleles. Chickens expressing the MHC *B19* allele are susceptible to the virus, whereas birds expressing the *B21* allele are not susceptible. An interesting link between the MHC and disease susceptibility in humans came from a study of Dutch immigrants to South America. In 1845 a group of Dutch immigrants consisting of 367 individuals from 50 families emigrated from Europe to South America. Within two weeks of their arrival an epidemic of typhoid fever killed 50% of the immigrants, and six years later an epidemic of yellow fever killed another 20% of the population. Thereafter the annual mortality rate was relatively low, and the survivors remained and intermarried. Recently the MHC polymorphism of the "selected" descendants of the survivors was analyzed and compared with that of a similar number of Dutch families living in the Netherlands. The descendants in South America exhibited significant relative decreases in some HLA alleles, such as *B7*, and significant increases in other alleles, such as *B13*, *Bw38*, and *Bw50*. It is hypothesized that these descendants may carry MHC alleles that enable them to respond more effectively to pathogens endemic to their South American environment.

Summary

1. The major histocompatibility complex (MHC) comprises tightly linked genes that encode proteins associated with intercellular recognition and antigen presentation to T lymphocytes. The MHC, called the H-2 complex in mice and the HLA complex in humans, is organized into three regions based on the type of molecules encoded. Class I molecules are encoded by the K and D regions in mice and the A, B, and C regions in humans. Class II molecules are encoded by the I region in mice and the D regions in humans. Class III molecules are encoded by the S region in mice and the C4, C2, Bf region in humans. Many alleles exist for each class I and class II MHC gene; the entire set of MHC alleles on a chromosome is referred to as its haplotype. A given animal may be homozygous or heterozygous for MHC haplotype.

2. Class I MHC molecules consist of a large glycoprotein α chain, encoded by the class I MHC genes, and a much smaller molecule of β_2-microglobulin, encoded by a gene outside of the MHC. The α chain contains three external domains (α_1, α_2, and α_3), a hydrophobic transmembrane segment, and a cytoplasmic tail. The latter two domains anchor the α chain to the plasma membrane, and the α_1 and α_2 domains interact to form a cleft that binds antigenic peptides. The class I MHC genes are organized as a series of exons and introns, with each exon encoding a separate domain of the α chain.

3. Class II MHC molecules are heterodimers composed of two noncovalently associated glycoproteins, the α and β chain, which are encoded by separate class II genes. Each chain contains two external domains, a transmembrane segment, and a cytoplasmic tail; each domain is encoded by a separate exon in the corresponding gene.

4. X-ray crystallographic analysis has been accomplished for several class I MHC molecules and one class II molecule. These analyses have revealed that the peptide-binding region in both class I and class II molecules is a deep cleft with a floor formed by eight antiparallel β strands and sides of two antiparallel α helices. The one class II molecule that has been crystallized did so as dimers of the $\alpha\beta$ heterodimer, suggesting that the molecule may be displayed on the membrane as a dimer.

5. Because portions of both class I and class II MHC molecules exhibit the immunoglobulin-fold structure, these molecules are considered members of the immunoglobulin superfamily. In addition to a similarity in structure, both class I and class II MHC molecules function to present antigen to T cells. Class I molecules, which are present on nearly all nucleated cells, present processed endogenous antigen to $CD8^+$ cells. Class II molecules, which are expressed on a limited number of antigen-presenting cells (macrophages, dendritic cells, B cells), present processed exogenous antigen to $CD4^+$ cells.

6. Class III MHC molecules include a diverse group of nonmembrane proteins that play no role in antigen presentation. Disturbances in the expression of some class III molecules (e.g., certain complement components, tumor necrosis factors, and heat-shock proteins) may be associated with certain autoimmune diseases.

7. Restriction-enzyme mapping of the MHC has supplemented earlier results obtained by serologic and functional analyses. The detailed genomic map of the MHC developed to date includes a number of "nonclassical" class I and class II genes. Some of these are pseudogenes, but others encode protein products whose functions are under study.

8. The interaction between MHC molecules and peptides has been studied with several different experimental approaches. Elution experiments and binding experiments have demonstrated that peptide length and the presence or absence of certain conserved motifs in peptides influence their ability to interact with class I and class II MHC molecules. Studies with hybrid and mutated genes have demonstrated that both membrane-distal domains in class I and class II MHC molecules are necessary for antigen presentation. Direct evidence of the interaction between a peptide and the cleft formed by the two membrane-distal domains in class I and class II molecules has been obtained from x-ray crystallographic analyses of peptide–MHC complexes.

9. Studies with congenic and recombinant congenic mouse strains and with L cells transfected with MHC genes have shown that MHC haplotype influences immune responsiveness and the ability to present antigen. The variation in amino acid sequences (i.e., the polymorphism) that gives rise to different haplotypes occurs primarily in the membrane-distal domains of class I and class II MHC molecules. The polymorphic residues in class I MHC molecules have been shown to be localized primarily in the peptide-binding cleft.

References

ACCOLLA, R. S., C. AUFFRAY, D. S. SINGER, and J. GUARDIOLA. 1991. The molecular biology of MHC genes. *Immunol. Today* **12**:97.

AJITKUMAR, P., S. S. GEIER, K. V. KESARI et al. 1988. Evidence that multiple residues on both the α-helices of the class I MHC molecules are simultaneously recognized by the T cell receptor. *Cell* **54**:47.

BENOIST, C., and D. MATHIS. 1990. Regulation of major histocompatibility complex class II genes: X, Y, and other letters of the alphabet. *Annu. Rev. Immunol.* **8**:681.

BJORKMAN, P. J., M. A. SAPER, B. SAMRAOUI et al. 1987. Structure of the human class I histocompatibility antigens. *Nature* **329**:506.

BJORKMAN, P. J., and P. PARHAM. 1990. Structure, function and diversity of class I major histocompatibility complex molecules. *Annu. Rev. Biochem.* **59**:253.

BROWN, J. H., T. S. JARDETSKY, J. C. GORGA et al. 1993. Three-dimensional structure of the human class II histocompatibility antigen HLA-DR1. *Nature* **364**:33.

GUO, H. C., T. S. JARDETZKY, T. P. J. GARRETT et al. 1992. Different length peptides bind to HLA-Aw68 similarly at their ends but bulge out in the middle. *Nature* **360**:364.

HEDRICK, S. M. 1992. Dawn of the hunt for nonclassical MHC function. *Cell* **70**:177.

KAPPES, D., and J. L. STROMINGER. 1988. Human class II major histocompatibility complex genes and proteins. *Annu. Rev. Biochem.* **57**:991.

KLEIN, J. 1986. *Natural History of the Major Histocompatibility Complex.* John Wiley and Sons.

KOLLER, B. H., D. E. GERAGHTY, R. DEMARS et al. 1989. Chromosomal organization of the human major histocompatibility complex class I gene family. *J. Exp. Med.* **169**:469.

LAWLOR, D. A., J. ZEMMOUR, P. D. ENNIS et al. 1990. Evolution of class I MHC genes and proteins: from natural selection to thymic selection. *Annu. Rev. Immunol.* **8**:23.

MADDEN, D. R., J. C. GORGA, J. L. STROMINGER, and D. C. WILEY. 1992. The three dimensional structure of HLA-B27 at 2.1 Å resolution suggests a general mechanism for tight peptide binding to MHC. *Cell* **70**:1035.

MATSUMURA, M., D. H. FREMONT, P. A. PETERSON, and I. A. WILSON. 1992. Emerging principles for the recognition of peptide antigens by MHC class I molecules. *Science* **257**:927.

PARHAM, P. 1992. Deconstructing the MHC. *Nature* **360**:300.

PETERS, P. J., J. J. NEEFJES, V. OORSCHOT, H. L. PLOEGH, and H. J. GEUZE. 1991. Segregation of MHC class II molecules from MHC class I molecules in the golgi complex for transport to lysosomal compartments. *Nature* **349**:669.

ROCHE, P. A., and P. CRESSWELL. 1990. Invariant chain association with HLA-DR molecules inhibits immunogenic peptide binding. *Nature* **345**:615.

SCHAEFFER, E. B., A. SETTE, D. J. JOHNSON et al. 1989. Relative contribution of determinant selection and holes in the repertoire to T cell responses. *Proc. Natl. Acad. Sci. USA* **86**:4649.

SILVER, M. L., H. C. GUO, J. L. STROMINGER, and D. C. WILEY. 1992. Atomic structure of a human MHC molecule presenting an influenza virus peptide. *Nature* **360**:367.

SPIES, T., M. BRESNAHAN, S. BAHRAM et al. 1990. A gene in the human major histocompatibility complex class II region controlling the class I antigen presentation pathway. *Nature* **348**:744.

TOWNSEND, A., C. OHLEN, J. BASTIN et al. 1989. Association of class I major histocompatibility heavy and light chains induced by viral peptides. *Nature* **340**:443.

TROWSDALE, J., J. RAGOUSSIS, and R. D. CAMPBELL. 1991. Map of the human MHC. *Immunol. Today* **12**:443.

Study Questions

1. Indicate whether each of the following statements is true or false. If you think a statement is false, explain why.
   a. A monoclonal antibody specific for β_2-microglobulin can be used to detect both class I MHC K and D molecules on the surface of cells.
   b. Antigen-presenting cells express both class I and class II MHC molecules on their membrane.

2. You wish to produce a syngeneic and a congenic mouse strain. Indicate whether each of the following characteristics applies to production of syngeneic (S), congenic (C), or both (S and C) mice.
   a. ____ Requires the greatest number of generations
   b. ____ Requires backcrosses
   c. ____ Yields mice that are genetically identical
   d. ____ Requires selection for homozygosity
   e. ____ Requires sibling crosses
   f. ____ Can be started with outbred mice
   g. ____ Yields progeny that are genetically identical to the parent except for a single genetic region

3. You have generated a congenic A.B strain mouse that has been selected for the MHC.
   a. Which strain provides the genetic background of this mouse?
   b. Which strain provides the haplotype of the MHC of this mouse?
   c. To produce this congenic strain, the F_1 progeny are always backcrossed to which strain?
   d. Why was backcrossing to the parent performed?
   e. Why was inbreeding performed?
   f. Why was selection necessary and what kind of selection was performed?

4. You cross a BALB/c(H-2^d) mouse with a CBA (H-2^k) mouse. What MHC molecules will the F_1 progeny express on its liver cells and on its macrophages?

5. To carry out studies on the structure and function of the class I MHC molecule K^b and the class II MHC molecule IA^b, you decide to transfect the genes encoding these proteins into a mouse fibroblast cell line (L cell) derived from the C3H strain (H-2^k). In the following table, indicate which of the listed MHC molecules will (+) or will not (−) be expressed on the membrane of the transfected L cells.

Transfected gene	MHC molecules expressed on the membrane of the transfected L cells					
	D^k	D^b	K^k	K^b	IA^k	IA^b
None						
K^b						
$IA\alpha^b$						
$IA\beta^b$						
$IA\alpha^b$ and $IA\beta^b$						

6. The SJL mouse strain, which has the H-2^s haplotype, has a deletion of the *IEα* locus.
   a. List the classical MHC molecules that are expressed on the membrane of macrophages from SJL mice.
   b. If the class II *IEα* and *IEβ* genes from a H-2^k strain are transfected into SJL macrophages, what additional classical MHC molecules would be expressed on the transfected macrophages.

7. Draw diagrams illustrating the general structure, including the domains, of class I MHC molecules, class II MHC molecules, and membrane-bound antibody on B cells. Label each chain and the domains within it, the antigen-binding regions, and regions that have the immunoglobulin-fold structure.

8. Where are most of the polymorphic amino acid residues located in MHC molecules? What is the significance of this location? How is MHC polymorphism thought to be generated?

9. As a student in an immunology laboratory class, you have been given spleen cells from a mouse immunized with the LCM virus. You determine the antigen-specific functional activity of these cells with two different assays. In assay 1, the spleen cells are incubated with macrophages that have been briefly exposed to the LCM virus; the production of interleukin 2 (IL-2) is a positive response. In assay 2, the spleen cells are incubated with LCM-infected target cells; lysis of the target cells represents a positive response in this assay. The results of the assays using macrophages and target cells of different haplotypes are presented in the accompanying table. Note that the experiment has been set up in a way to exclude alloreactive responses.
   a. The activity of which cell population is detected in each of the two assays?
   b. From the results of this experiment, which MHC molecules are required, in addition to the LCM virus, for specific reactivity of the spleen cells in each of the two assays?
   c. What additional experiments could you perform to unambiguously confirm the MHC molecules required for antigen-specific reactivity of the spleen cells?
   d. Which of the mouse strains listed in the table could have been the source of the immunized spleen cells tested in the functional assays? Give your reasons.

For use with Question 9.

Mouse strain used as source of macrophages and target cells	MHC haplotype of macrophages and virus-infected target cells				Response of spleen cells	
	K	*IA*	*IE*	*D*	IL-2 production in response to LCM-pulsed macrophages (assay 1)	Lysis of LCM-infected cells (assay 2)
C3H	*k*	*k*	*k*	*k*	+	−
BALB/c	*d*	*d*	*d*	*d*	−	+
BALB/c × B10.A(F_1)	*d/k*	*d/k*	*d/k*	*d/d*	+	+
A.TL	*s*	*k*	*k*	*d*	+	+
B10.A(3R)	*b*	*b*	*b*	*d*	−	+
B10.A(4R)	*k*	*k*	—	*b*	+	−

10. A T_C-cell clone recognizes a particular measles virus peptide when it is presented by H-2D^b. Another MHC molecule has an identical peptide-binding cleft as H-2D^b but differs from H-2D^b at several other amino acids in the α_1/α_2 domain. Predict whether the second MHC molecule could present this measles virus peptide to the T_C-cell clone. Briefly explain your answer.

11. How can you determine if two different inbred mouse strains have identical MHC haplotypes?

12. Red blood cells are not nucleated and do not express any MHC molecules. Why is this property fortuitous for blood transfusions?

ANTIGEN PROCESSING AND PRESENTATION

T-cell recognition of antigen requires that peptides derived from foreign antigen be displayed within the cleft of a MHC molecule on the membrane of a cell. The formation of these peptide-MHC complexes requires that a protein antigen be degraded into peptides by a sequence of events called *antigen processing.* The degraded peptides then associate with MHC molecules within the cell interior, and the peptide-MHC complexes are transported to the membrane where they are displayed *(antigen presentation).* As discussed briefly in Chapter 1, class I and class II MHC molecules associate with peptides that have been processed in different intracellular compartments. Class I MHC molecules bind peptides derived from endogenous antigens that have been processed within the cytoplasm of the cell (e.g., normal cellular proteins or viral and bacterial proteins produced within infected cells). Class II MHC molecules bind peptides derived from exogenous antigens that are internalized by phagocytosis or endocytosis and processed within the endocytic pathway. In this chapter the mechanism of antigen processing and the means by which processed antigen and MHC molecules are sequestered within different intracellular compartments for presentation are examined in more detail.

Self-MHC Restriction of T Cells

Both CD4$^+$ and CD8$^+$ T cells can only recognize antigen when it is presented on the membrane of a cell by a self-MHC molecule. This attribute, called *self-MHC restriction,* distinguishes recognition of antigen by T cells from that by B cells. Self-MHC restriction was first discovered in experiments in which T cells from one inbred strain were mixed with macrophages, B cells, or virus-infected cells from another inbred strain. In each experimental system a T-cell response to the antigen was obtained only if the T cells shared MHC alleles with the other cells in the mixture.

Beginning in the mid-1970s the now classic experiments of A. Rosenthal, E. Shevach, D. Katz, B. Benacerraf, D. Schreffler, R. Zinkernagel, and P. Doherty demonstrated self-MHC restriction in T-cell recognition. In their system Rosenthal and Shevach, for example, showed that antigen-specific proliferation of T_H cells only occurred in response to antigen presented by macrophages of the same MHC haplotype. In their experiment guinea pig macrophages from strain 2 were incubated with antigen. These "antigen-pulsed" macrophages then were mixed with T cells from the same strain (strain 2), a different strain (strain 13), or F_1 (2 × 13) animals, and the amount of T-cell proliferation in response to the antigen-pulsed macrophages was measured (Figure 10-1). The results showed that strain 2 macrophages only activated strain 2 and F_1 T cells but not strain 13 T cells. Similarly, strain 13 antigen-pulsed macrophages only activated strain 13 and F_1 T cells but not strain 2 T cells. When the studies were later expanded to inbred strains of mice, congenic and recombinant congenic strains that differed from each other only in selected regions of the H-2 complex were used as the source of macrophages and T cells. These experiments confirmed that the CD4$^+$ T_H cell is only activated by antigen-pulsed macrophages that share class II MHC alleles. Antigen recognition by the CD4$^+$ T_H cell is therefore class II MHC restricted.

The self-MHC restriction of CD8$^+$ T cells was first demonstrated by Zinkernagel and Doherty in 1974. In their experimental system mice first were immunized with lymphocytic choriomeningitis (LCM) virus; several days later their spleen cells, which included T_C cells specific for the virus, were isolated and incubated with LCM-infected target cells of the same or different haplotype (Figure 10-2). They found that the T_C cells only killed syngeneic virus-infected target cells. Later studies with congenic and recombinant congenic strains showed that the T_C cell and the virus-infected target cell must share class I molecules encoded by the K or D regions of the MHC. Thus antigen recognition by CD8$^+$ T_C cells is class I MHC restricted.

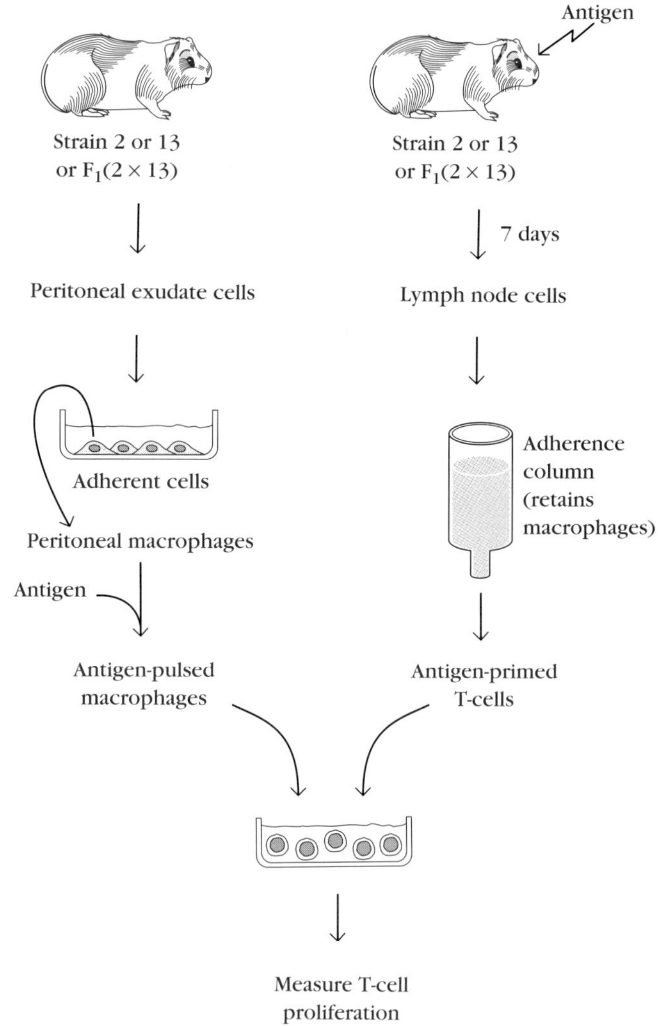

Antigen-primed T-cell	Antigen-pulsed macrophages: Strain 2	Strain 13	$F_1(2 \times 13)$
Strain 2	+	−	+
Strain 13	−	+	+
$F_1(2 \times 13)$	+	+	+

FIGURE 10-1 Experimental demonstration of self-MHC restriction of T_H cells. Peritoneal exudate cells from strain 2, strain 13, or F_1 (2 × 13) guinea pigs were incubated in plastic petri dishes allowing enrichment of macrophages, which are adherent cells. The peritoneal macrophages were then incubated with antigen, generating "antigen-pulsed macrophages." These antigen-pulsed macrophages were incubated in vitro with antigen-primed T cells from strain 2, strain 13, or F_1 (2 × 13) guinea pigs and the degree of T-cell proliferation was assessed. The results indicated that T_H cells could only proliferate in response to antigen presented by macrophages that shared MHC alleles. [Adapted from A. Rosenthal and E. Shevach, 1974, *J. Exp. Med.* **138**:1194).]

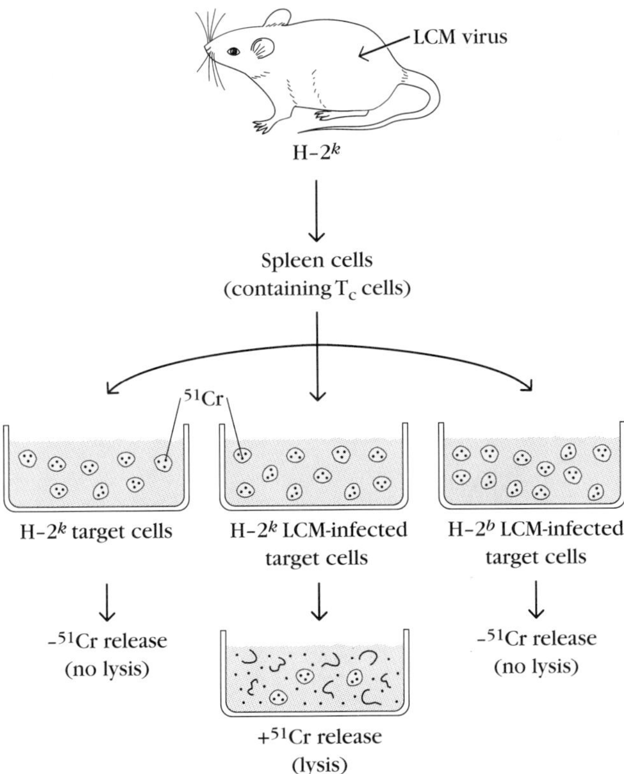

FIGURE 10-2 Classic experiment of Zinkernagel and Doherty demonstrating that antigen recognition by T_C cells exhibits MHC restriction. H-2^k mice were primed with the lymphocytic choriomeningitis (LCM) virus to induce cytotoxic T lymphocytes (CTLs) specific for the virus. Spleen cells from this LCM-primed mouse were then added to target cells of different H-2 haplotypes that were intracellularly labeled with ^{51}Cr (dots) and either infected or not with the LCM virus. CTL-mediated killing of the target cells, as measured by the release of ^{51}Cr into the culture supernatant, occurred only if the target cells were infected and had the same MHC haplotype as the CTLs.

Role of Antigen-Presenting Cells

Early Evidence for Antigen Processing and Presentation

As early as 1959 immunologists were confronted with data that suggested T cells and B cells recognized antigen by different mechanisms. These findings were difficult to reconcile with the then-current concepts about the function of immune cells. As mentioned in Chapter 4, P. G. H. Gell and B. Benacerraf discovered that when a primary antibody response and cell-mediated response were induced by a protein in its native conformation, then a secondary antibody response (mediated by B cells) could be induced only by native antigen, whereas a secondary cell-mediated response could be induced by either the native or denatured antigen (see Table 4-6). The dogma of the 1960s, which persisted until the 1980s, was that cells of the immune system recognize the entire protein in its native conformation. The experiment of Gell and Benacerraf was viewed as an interesting enigma, but its implications were completely overlooked until the early 1980s when several research groups began to obtain results that contradicted the prevailing dogma.

Among these results were those of K. Ziegler and E. R. Unanuae outlined in Figure 10-3. These researchers observed that T_H-cell activation by bacterial protein antigens was prevented by treating the antigen-presenting cells with paraformaldehyde prior to antigen exposure. However, if the antigen-presenting cells were allowed to ingest the antigen and then were fixed with paraformaldehyde 1–3 h later, T_H-cell activation still occurred. During that interval of 1–3 h, the antigen-presenting cells had processed the antigen and had displayed it on the membrane in a form able to activate T cells. R. P. Shimonkevitz showed that internalization and processing could be bypassed if antigen-presenting cells were exposed to peptide digests of an antigen instead of the native antigen (see Figure 10-3 *bottom*). In these experiments, antigen-presenting cells were treated with glutaraldehyde and then incubated with native ovalbumin or with ovalbumin that had been subjected to partial enzymatic digestion. The digested ovalbumin was able to interact with the glutaraldehyde-fixed antigen-presenting cells, thereby activating ovalbumin-specific T_H cells, whereas the native ovalbumin failed to do so. Taken together, these findings suggest that antigen processing is a metabolic process that digests proteins into peptides, which can then be displayed on the membrane of the antigen-presenting cell together with a class II MHC molecule.

At about the same time, A. Townsend and his colleagues began to identify the proteins of influenza virus that were recognized by T_C cells. Contrary to their expectations, they found that internal proteins of the virus, such as matrix and nucleocapsid proteins, were often recognized by T_C cells better than were the more exposed envelope proteins. Moreover, Townsend's work revealed that T_C cells recognized short linear peptide sequences of the influenza protein. In fact, when target cells were incubated in vitro with synthetic peptides corresponding to sequences of internal influenza proteins, the target cells could be recognized by T_C cells and subsequently lysed just as well as when the target cells had been infected with live influenza virus.

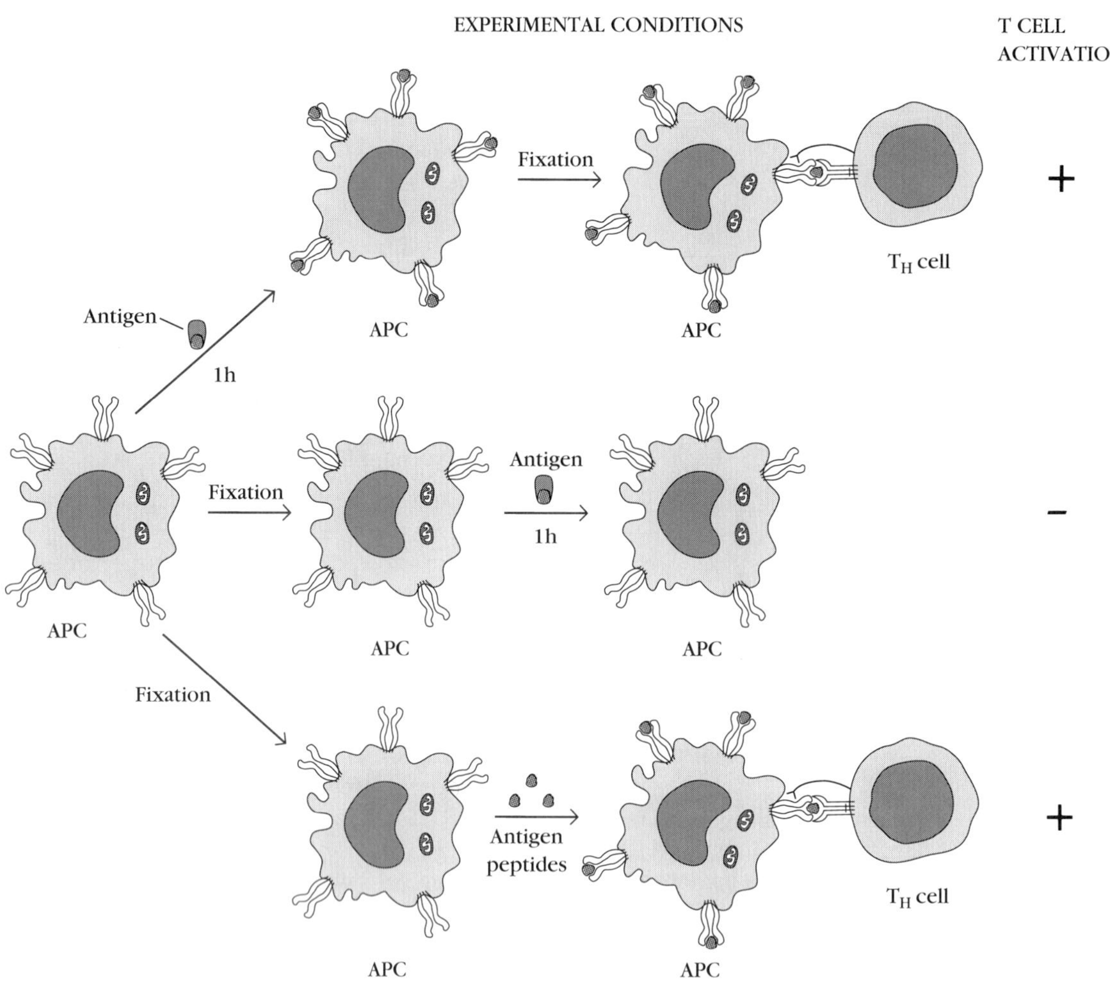

FIGURE 10-3 Experimental demonstration that antigen processing is necessary for T_H-cell activation. *(Middle)* When antigen-presenting cells (APCs) are fixed before exposure to antigen, they are unable to activate T_H cells. *(Top)* In contrast, APCs fixed at least 1 h after antigen exposure can activate T_H cells. *(Bottom)* When APCs are fixed before antigen exposure and incubated with peptide digests of the antigen (rather than native antigen), they also can activate T_H cells. T_H-cell activation is determined by measuring a specific T_H-cell response (e.g., cytokine secretion).

Cells That Function in Antigen Presentation

Cells that are able to present peptides to T cells are referred to as *antigen-presenting cells* (APCs). Since cells expressing either class I or class II MHC molecules can present peptides to T cells, technically they could be classified as antigen-presenting cells. However, by convention, those cells that display peptides associated with class I MHC molecules to $CD8^+$ T_C cells are referred to as *target cells;* only those cells that display peptides associated with class II MHC molecules to $CD4^+$ T_H cells are called antigen-presenting cells. This convention is followed throughout this text.

A variety of cells can function as antigen-presenting cells. The distinguishing feature of these cells is their ability to constitutively express class II MHC molecules (Table 10-1). These cells internalize exogenous antigen either by phagocytosis or by endocytosis, process the antigen within the endocytic pathway, and display the resulting antigenic peptides together with class II MHC molecules on their membrane. Among the cells that constitutively express class II MHC molecules and function as APCs are monocytes and macrophages, B cells, dendritic cells, Langerhans cells, thymic dendritic and epithelial cells, and venular endothelial cells (in humans).

Several other types of cells also can be induced to express class II MHC molecules during a sustained inflammatory response and thus can function as APCs for short periods of time (see Table 10-1). These include thyroid epithelial cells, glial cells, pancreatic

TABLE 10-1 CELLS THAT FUNCTION AS ANTIGEN-PRESENTING CELLS

Constitutive expression of class II MHC molecules
B cell
Dendritic cells
Langerhans cells
Macrophage/Monocyte
Thymic dendritic cell
Thymic epithelial cell
Vascular endothelial cell (human)
Inducible expression of class II MHC molecules*
Fibroblast (skin)
Glial cell (brain)
Pancreatic beta cell
Thyroid epithelial cell
Vascular endothelial cell(nonhuman)

* Occurs during inflammatory response.

beta cells, skin fibroblasts, and vascular endothelial cells.

Because nearly all nucleated cells express class I MHC molecules, virtually any nucleated cell is able to function as a target cell presenting endogenous antigens to T_C cells. Most often target cells are cells that have been infected by a virus or some other intracellular microorganism. However, target cells can also be altered self-cells such as cancer cells, aging body cells, or allogeneic cells from a graft.

ANTIGEN PROCESSING

Intracellular (endogenous) and extracellular (exogenous) antigens present different challenges to the immune system. Extracellular antigens are eliminated by secreted antibody, whereas intracellular antigens are most effectively eliminated by cytotoxic T lymphocytes (CTLs). To mediate these responses, the immune system uses two different antigen-presenting pathways: Exogenous antigens are processed in the *endocytic pathway* and presented on the membrane with class II MHC molecules, and endogenous antigens are processed in the *cytosolic pathway* and presented on the membrane with class I MHC molecules (Figure 10-4).

Endocytic Processing Pathway

Antigen-presenting cells can internalize antigen by phagocytosis, endocytosis, or both. Macrophages internalize antigen by both processes, whereas most other APCs are not phagocytic and therefore internalize exogenous antigen only by endocytosis (either receptor-mediated endocytosis or pinocytosis). B cells, for example, internalize antigen very effectively by receptor-mediated endocytosis using antigen-specific membrane antibody as the receptor. Once an

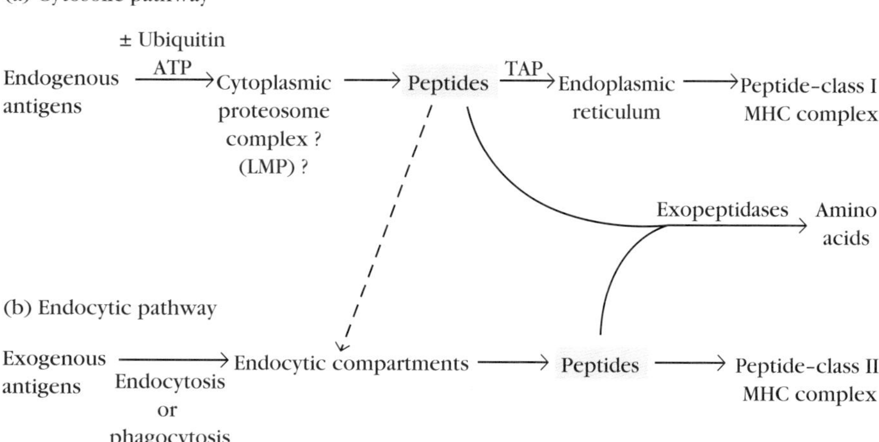

FIGURE 10-4 Overview of cytosolic and endocytic pathways for processing antigen. The resulting antigenic peptides associate with class I or class II MHC molecules, and the peptide-MHC complexes then are transported to the cell membrane. TAP = transporter of antigenic peptides.

antigen is internalized, it is degraded into peptides within compartments of the endocytic processing pathway. Internalized antigen takes 1–3 h to transverse the endocytic pathway and appear at the cell surface in the form of peptide–class II MHC complexes. The endocytic pathway appears to involve three increasingly acidic compartments: early endosomes (pH 6.0–6.5); late endosomes, or endolysosomes (pH 5.0–6.0); and lysosomes (pH 4.5–5.0). Internalized antigen moves from early to late endosomes and finally to lysosomes, encountering hydrolytic enzymes in each compartment (Figure 10-5). Lysosomes, for example, contain a unique collection of more than 40 acid-dependent hydrolases including proteases, nucleases, glycosidases, lipases, phospholipases, and phosphatases. Within the compartments of the endocytic pathway, antigen is degraded into oligopeptides of about 13–18 residues, which bind to class II MHC molecules. Because these enzymes are optimally active at acidic pHs, antigen processing can be inhibited by chemical agents, such as chloroquine, that increase the pH of the compartments or by protease inhibitors, such as leupeptin.

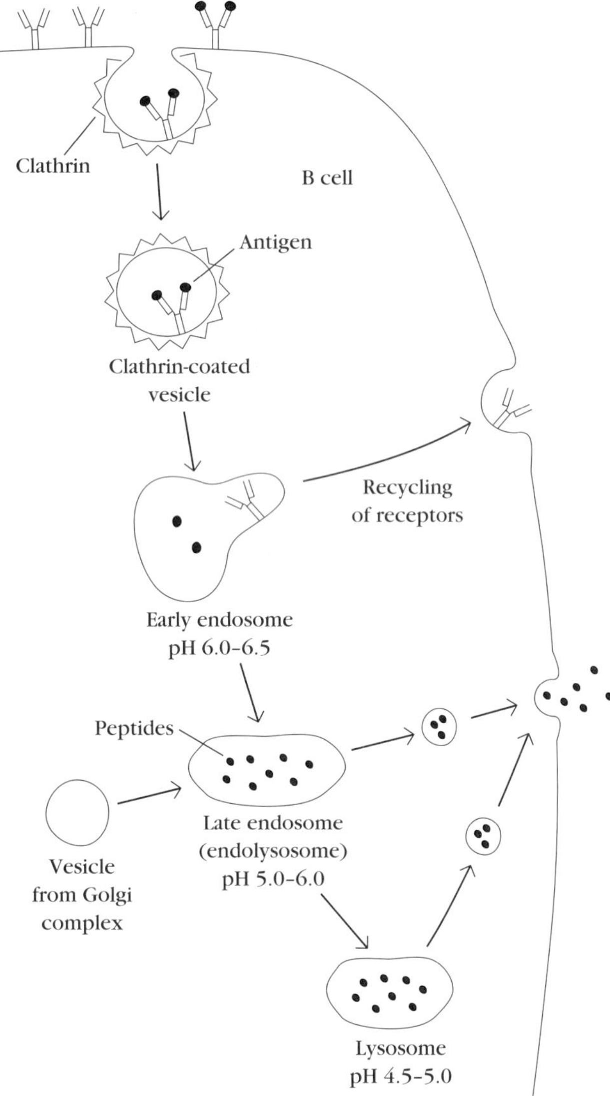

FIGURE 10-5 Endocytic processing pathway involves several acidic compartments in which exogenous antigen is degraded into peptides that ultimately associate with class II MHC molecules transported in vesicles from the Golgi complex. The figure shows a B cell, which internalizes antigen by receptor-mediated endocytosis with the membrane-bound antibody functioning as an antigen-specific receptor.

The mechanism by which internalized antigen moves from one endocytic compartment to the next has not been conclusively demonstrated. Some have suggested that early endosomes from the periphery move inward to become late endosomes and finally lysosomes. Others have suggested that small transport vesicles carry antigens from one compartment to the next, in a manner similar to the way in which small transport vesicles carry proteins from one compartment of the Golgi complex to the next. Eventually the endocytic compartments, or portions of them, return to the cell periphery where they fuse with the plasma membrane. In this way, the surface receptors may be recycled.

Cytosolic Processing Pathway

Endogenous antigens, such as those produced by a virus replicating within a cell, are degraded within the cytoplasm into peptides that can associate with class I MHC molecules. Soluble protein antigens that are experimentally delivered into the cytoplasm of a cell also have been shown to be degraded into peptides that can be presented by class I MHC molecules to T_C cells. (One way to deliver soluble protein antigens into the cytoplasm is to load them inside membrane liposomes; as these fuse with the plasma membrane, the antigen is released into the cytoplasm.) The pathway by which endogenous antigens are degraded, although not fully elucidated, may be similar to that involved in the turnover of normal intracellular proteins.

In eukaryotic cells protein levels are carefully regulated. Every protein is subject to continuous turnover and is degraded at a rate that is generally expressed in terms of its half-life. Some proteins (e.g., transcription factors, cyclins, and key metabolic enzymes) appear to have very short half-lives; denatured, misfolded, or otherwise abnormal proteins also are degraded rapidly. Intracellular proteins are degraded into short peptides by a cytosolic proteolytic system possessed by all cells. Those proteins that are targeted for prote-

(a)

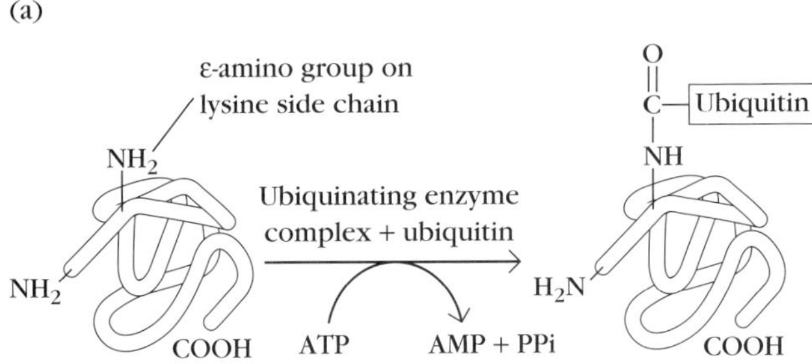

(b)

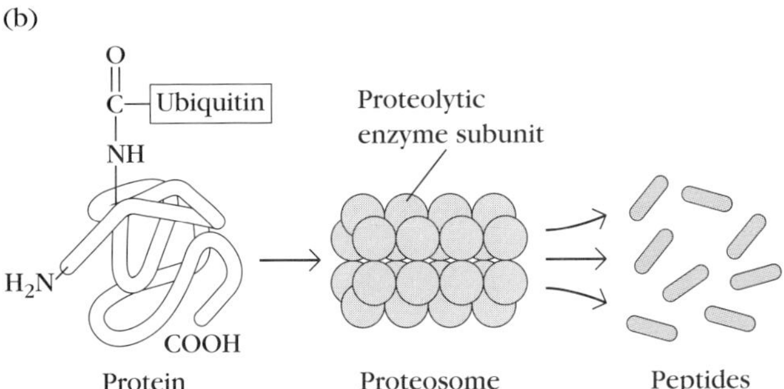

FIGURE 10-6 Cytosolic proteolytic system for degradation of intracellular proteins. (a) Proteins to be degraded often are covalently linked to a small protein called ubiquitin. In this reaction, which requires ATP, a ubiquinating enzyme complex links several ubiquitin molecules to a lysine ϵ-amino group near the amino terminus of the protein. (b) Degradation of ubiquitin-protein complexes occurs within the central channel of proteosomes, generating a variety of peptides. Proteosomes are large cylindrical particles whose subunits have proteolytic activity.

olysis often have a small protein, called *ubiquitin,* attached to them (Figure 10-6a). Such ubiquitin-protein conjugates can be degraded by *proteosomes,* which are large, cylindrical particles containing four rings of protein subunits with a central channel of 10–20 Å. A proteosome, described by John Monaco as a "big ball of degradative enzymes," can cleave three or four different types of peptide bonds in an ATP-dependent process (Figure 10-6b). Degradation of ubiquitin-protein complexes is thought to occur within the central hollow of a proteosome, thus avoiding proteolysis of other proteins within the cytoplasm.

Some researchers have suggested that the immune system may utilize this general pathway of protein degradation to produce small peptides for presentation with class I MHC molecules. Two proteosome-like subunits are now known to be encoded in the class II region of the MHC. These subunits are part of a large cytoplasmic proteolytic complex called the *low-molecular-mass polypeptide* (LMP). The LMP and the proteosome have a large number of subunits in common, and the two structures may be structurally and functionally related.

Antigen Presentation

Antigen presentation involves the association of antigenic peptides with class I or class II MHC molecules and movement of the peptide-MHC complexes to the cell membrane. Like other proteins, MHC molecules are synthesized on polysomes within the rough endoplasmic reticulum (RER), while antigenic peptides are generated in either the endocytic or cytosolic processing pathway. Class I MHC molecules appear to bind antigenic peptides within the RER, whereas class II molecules do not. In both cases, however, binding of peptide helps to stabilize the association between the MHC chains.

Assembly and Stabilization of MHC Molecules

Insight into the role of peptide in the assembly of class I MHC molecules within the RER came from studies of cell lines with defects in this process. Cells with mutations in peptide presentation by class I molecules were induced by treating the cells with a mutagen. After mutagenizing the cells, those cells that continued to express class I molecules on their membrane were selectively eliminated (via complement-mediated lysis) with anti-class I antibody. However, mutant cells that no longer expressed class I MHC molecules on the membrane survived. One such mutant cell line generated by this procedure is a mouse cell line called RMA-S. This particular cell line expresses about 5% of the normal levels of class I MHC molecules on its membrane. Although RMA-S cells continue to synthesize normal levels of class I α chains and β_2-microglobulin, both molecules remain intracellular instead of appearing on the membrane. A clue to the mutation in the RMA-S cell line was the discovery by A. Townsend and his colleagues that "feeding" these cells predigested peptides restored their level of membrane class I molecules to normal. They suggested that peptide might be required to stabilize the interaction between the class I α chain and β_2-microglobulin. This led them to speculate that the RMA-S cell line might have a defect in antigen processing or peptide transport. The ability to restore expression of class I MHC molecules on the membrane by feeding the cells predigested peptides would be compatible with either type of defect.

More recent studies have demonstrated that peptide does indeed stabilize the association between the class I α chain and β_2-microglobulin (Figure 10-7a). Moreover, peptides containing eight or nine residues are most efficient in this stabilization. As discussed in

(a)

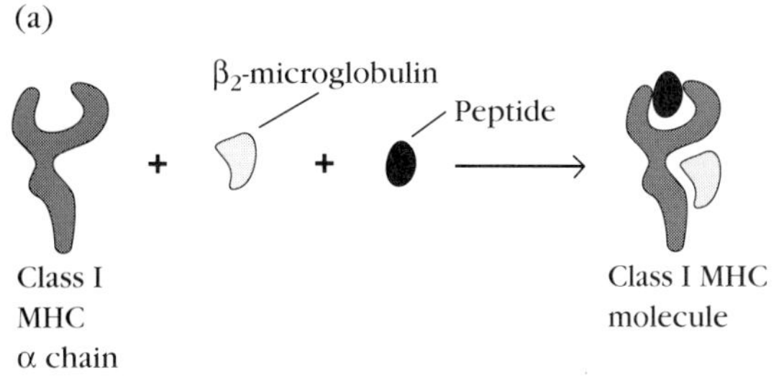

(b)

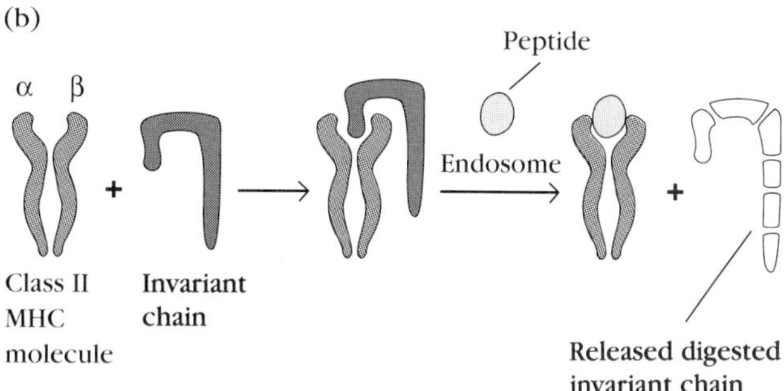

FIGURE 10-7 Assembly and stabilization of MHC molecules. (a) Binding of an antigenic peptide to a class I MHC α chain within the endoplasmic reticulum stabilizes the association of the α chain with β_2-microglobulin. (b) Within the endoplasmic reticulum, the noncovalently associated α and β chains of a class II MHC molecule bind an invariant chain. As long as the invariant chain occupies the peptide-binding cleft, the class II molecule cannot bind peptide.

Chapter 9, peptides of this length bind preferentially to the peptide-binding cleft of class I MHC molecules (see Table 9-2). In the absence of peptide, the assembly of class I MHC molecules in the RER is inhibited. Subsequent experiments with the RMA-S cell line showed that the defect in these cells is in the protein that transports peptides from the cytoplasm to the RER. In these experiments, RMA-S cells transfected with a functional transporter gene were able to express class I molecules on the membrane. The role of the transporter protein is examined in the next section.

Since antigen-presenting cells express both class I and class II MHC molecules, some mechanism must exist to prevent class II MHC molecules from binding to the same set of antigenic peptides as the class I molecules. Recent studies have shown that when a class II MHC molecule is synthesized within the RER, it associates with another protein called the *invariant (Ii) chain.* This protein interacts with the peptide-binding cleft of the class II molecule, preventing any endogenously derived peptides from binding to the cleft while the class II molecule is within the RER (Figure 10-7b). In addition to its role in preventing peptide binding to class II MHC molecules, the invariant chain also appears to be involved in the folding of the class II α and β chains, their exit from the RER, and the subsequent routing of class II molecules to the endocytic processing pathway.

As a class II molecule enters the endocytic pathway, the low pH and proteolysis cause release of the invariant chain. Within the acid environment of the endosome, the class II molecule assumes a more open conformation, called a floppy state, that is able to bind peptide. As with class I MHC molecules, peptide binding is required to maintain the structure and stability of class II MHC molecules. Once a peptide has bound, the peptide–class II complex is transported to the plasma membrane, where the neutral pH appears to enable the complex to assume a compact, stable form. Peptide is bound so strongly in this compact form that it is very difficult to replace a class II–bound peptide on the membrane with another peptide at physiologic conditions.

Segregation of MHC Molecules

Early evidence suggesting that class I and class II MHC molecules present antigenic peptides derived from different processing pathways was obtained from experiments with two clones of T_C cells specific for influenza virus. One clone was a typical $CD8^+$, class I–restricted T_C cell, but the other was an atypical $CD4^+$, class II–restricted T_C cell. As discussed in Chapter 3, the association between T-cell function and MHC restriction is not absolute. Indeed, an increasing number of reports have described cross-functional T-cell lines —that is, $CD4^+$, class II–restricted T_C clones and $CD8^+$, class I–restricted T_H clones.

L. A. Morrison and T. J. Braciale analyzed two T_C cell lines: one a typical T_C line that recognized influenza hemagglutinin (HA) associated with a class I MHC molecule and the other an atypical T_C line that recognized influenza HA associated with a class II MHC molecule. These researchers sought to determine whether antigen is processed along different pathways for association with class I or class II MHC molecules. In one set of experiments, target cells that expressed both class I and class II MHC molecules were incubated with infectious influenza virus or with UV-inactivated influenza virus. (The UV-inactivated virus retained its antigenic properties but was no longer capable of replicating within the target cells.) The target cells were then incubated with the class I–restricted or class II–restricted T_C cells and subsequent lysis of the target cells was determined. Their results, presented in Table 10-2, show that the class II–restricted T_C cells responded to target cells treated with infectious or noninfectious influenza virions, whereas the class I–restricted T_C cells responded to

TABLE 10-2 EFFECT OF ANTIGEN PRESENTATION ON ACTIVATION OF CLASS I AND CLASS II MHC-RESTRICTED T_C CELLS

	CTL activity†	
Treatment of target cells*	Class I restricted	Class II restricted
Infectious virus	+	+
UV-inactivated virus (noninfectious)	−	+
Infectious virus + emitine	−	+
Infectious virus + chloroquine	+	−
Hemagglutinin protein	−	+
Hemagglutinin gene	+	−
Synthetic hemagglutinin peptides	+	+

* Target cells, which expressed both class I and class II MHC molecules, were treated with the indicated preparations of influenza virus or other agents. Emetine inhibits viral protein synthesis, and chloroquine inhibits the endocytic processing pathway. The influenza hemagglutin (HA) gene was introduced into target cells as part of a recombinant vaccinia virus vector that contained the HA gene but no HA polypeptide.

† Determined by lysis (+) or no lysis (−) of the target cells.

SOURCE: Adapted from T. J. Braciale et al., 1987, *Immunol. Rev.* **98**:95.

target cells treated with infectious virions but not to target cells treated with noninfectious virions. Similarly, target cells that had been treated with infectious influenza virions in the presence of emitine, which inhibits viral protein synthesis, stimulated the class II–restricted T_C cells but not the class I–restricted T_C cells. Just the opposite results were obtained with target cells that had been treated with infectious virions in the presence of chloroquine, a drug that blocks the endocytic processing pathway.

These results support the distinction between exogenous and endogenous antigens and the preferential association of exogenous antigens with class II MHC molecules and of endogenous antigens with class I MHC molecules. In other words, the mode of antigen entry into cells and its subsequent processing within either the endocytic processing pathway (exogenous antigens) or cytosolic pathway (endogenous antigens) determines whether the resulting antigenic peptides associate with class I or class II MHC molecules. In the Morrison and Braciale experiments, association of viral antigen with class II MHC molecules did not require viral replication or protein synthesis. On the other hand, association of viral antigen with class I MHC molecules required replication of the influenza virus and viral protein synthesis within the target cells. These findings and other evidence suggest that routing of class I and class II MHC molecules to separate intracellular compartments dictates whether they interact with peptides derived from cytosolic degradation of endogenously synthesized proteins or with peptides derived from endocytic degradation of exogenous antigens.

Class I Endogenous Pathway

The current model of the pathway by which endogenous antigens are processed and presented is shown in Figure 10-8 *(left)*. As mentioned earlier, endogenous antigens are thought to be degraded within the cytoplasm by a proteosome-like complex called the LMP.

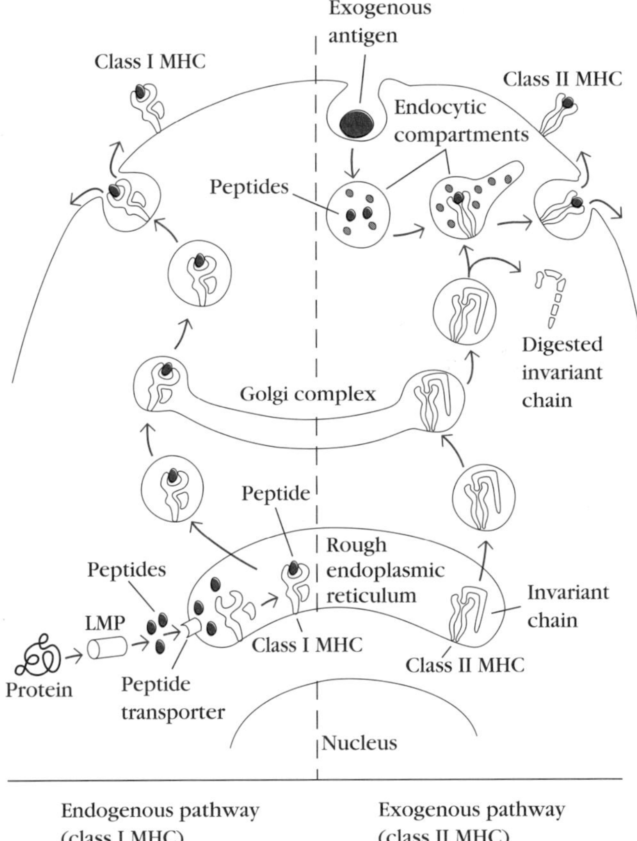

FIGURE 10-8 Model of separate antigen-presenting pathways for endogenous and exogenous antigens. The mode of antigen entry into cells and the site of antigen processing appear to determine whether antigenic peptides associate with class I MHC molecules in the rough endoplasmic reticulum or with class II molecules in endocytic compartments. Some elements of this model have not been experimentally demonstrated. See text for details.

The resulting cytosolic peptides appear to be transported by a heterodimeric protein designated TAP (transporter of antigenic peptides) across the membrane of the RER (Figure 10-9). Once in the RER, cytosolic peptides bind to newly synthesized class I α chains, inducing a conformational change that enables an α chain to associate with β_2-microglobulin.

The A and B chains of TAP are encoded by two genes (*TAP1* and *TAP2*) that map within the class II MHC region adjacent to two genes encoding two of the subunits of the LMP (see Figure 9-15). Both the transporter genes and the LMP genes are polymorphic; that is, different allelic forms of these genes exist within the population. Allelic differences in LMP-mediated proteolytic cleavage of protein antigens or in the transport of different peptides from the cytoplasm into the RER may contribute to the observed variation among individuals in their response to different endogenous antigens.

The functions of the LMP and peptide transporter presented here have by no means been conclusively demonstrated as yet. The finding that transfection of the genes encoding TAP restores membrane expression of class I MHC molecules in the mouse RMA-S cell line suggests a central role for the peptide transporter in antigen processing and presentation. However, the evidence is at best circumstantial. The suggested role of the LMP is even more controversial. A human mutant cell line, designated T2, which cannot express class I MHC molecules on the membrane, has been shown to have a large deletion in both the LMP and peptide-transporter genes. Membrane expression of class I molecules can be restored by transfecting T2 cells with the transporter genes, even though the transfected cells continue to lack LMP. This finding raises serious doubts about the postulated role of the LMP in protein processing; if the LMP is involved in processing, then cells appear to also possess alternative mechanisms for processing endogenous proteins.

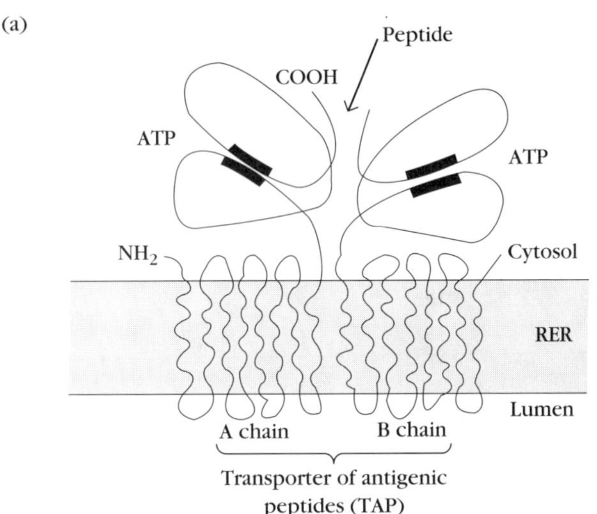

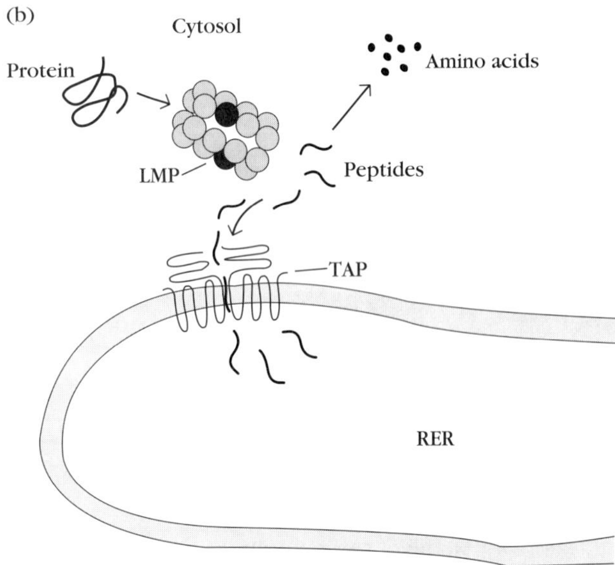

FIGURE 10-9 (a) Schematic diagram of the structure of TAP (transporter of antigenic peptides), which is anchored in the membrane of the rough endoplasmic reticulum (RER). The chains of the TAP heterodimer are encoded by *TAP1* and *TAP2.* (b) TAP is thought to transport peptides generated in the cytosolic processing pathway into the RER.

Class II Exogenous Pathway

As discussed previously, newly synthesized class II α and β chains associate with an invariant chain within the RER. This association precludes binding of class II MHC molecules with peptides derived from endogenous antigens or other intracellular proteins. Class II molecules, together with the associated invariant chains, are thought to be routed from the RER through the Golgi complex to the endocytic pathway (see Figure 10-8 *right*).

The role of the invariant chain in routing of class II molecules has been demonstrated in transfection experiments with cells that lack the genes encoding class II MHC molecules and the invariant chain. Immunofluorescent labeling of cells transfected only with class II MHC genes revealed that the class II molecules were localized within the Golgi complex. However, in cells transfected with both the class II MHC genes and invariant-chain gene, the class II molecules were localized in the cytoplasmic vesicular structures of the endocytic pathway. It is not known at what stage class II molecules and the associated invariant chain enter the endocytic pathway. Once inside an endocytic compartment, the invariant chain appears to be degraded by proteolytic enzymes, thus exposing the peptide-binding cleft of the class II molecules. As noted earlier, the low pH within endocytic compartments induces class II molecules to assume an open (floppy) conformation that facilitates binding of antigenic peptides.

Clinical Applications

The accumulating knowledge about different antigen-processing pathways has important implications for the design of new vaccines. If a class I–restricted cell-mediated response is desired, then a vaccine must be processed within the cytosolic pathway. This requirement is met by attenuated live vaccines capable of limited growth within the cytoplasm of infected cells and by several other types of vaccines developed in recent years. Vaccines intended to elicit a humoral antibody response, on the other hand, must possess epitopes that are recognizable by B cells (see Table 4-4). Once recognized by a B cell, the vaccine will be endocytosed and then processed within the endocytic pathway. An in-depth discussion of various approaches to designing vaccines is presented in Chapter 20.

Some evidence suggests that defects in antigen processing or presentation may contribute to certain autoimmune diseases. For example, D. Faustman and her colleagues found that expression of class I MHC molecules on cells from diabetic patients was significantly lower than that on cells from normal controls. Furthermore, nonobese diabetic (NOD) mice, which have a similar reduction in class I MHC expression, have been shown to have a genetic defect in the gene encoding the peptide-transport protein. Faustman has speculated that a defect in transporter function may be responsible for the reduction in class I MHC expression in both the NOD mouse and human diabetics. She has suggested that autoimmune diabetes may develop in individuals who are unable to present self-peptides together with class I MHC molecules to developing thymocytes during T-cell maturation in the thymus; as a result self-reactive T cells are not eliminated as they normally are. Faustman's theory is controversial, and so far no evidence for a defect in the peptide-transport protein in human diabetics has been reported. Indeed, some other mechanism may be responsible for the decreased expression of class I MHC molecules in NOD mice and human diabetics.

Summary

1. T-cell recognition of antigen requires that antigenic peptides be displayed within the cleft of a self-MHC molecule on the membrane of a cell. This requirement is called self-MHC restriction. In general, $CD4^+$ T_H cells are class II MHC restricted, whereas $CD8^+$ T_C cells are class I MHC restricted.

2. Peptide-MHC complexes are formed by degradation of a protein antigen by one of two different antigen-processing pathways. Those cells that process and present peptides associated with class II MHC molecules are called antigen-presenting cells (APCs); those that process and present peptides associated with class I MHC molecules are called target cells.

3. Endogenous antigens are thought to be degraded into peptides within the cytoplasm by a large proteolytic enzyme complex, called the LMP, which may be related to the proteosome. The resulting antigenic peptides are transported by TAP, a heterodimeric protein, across the membrane of the rough endoplasmic reticulum (RER), where they assemble with class I MHC molecules. Binding of peptide by a class I molecule stabilizes the association between the class I α chain and β_2-microglobulin. Peptide–class I complexes then are transported from the RER through the Golgi complex to the plasma membrane.

4. Exogenous antigens are degraded by various hydrolytic enzymes within the acidic endocytic compartments. Within the RER, class II MHC molecules are associated with the invariant chain, which blocks binding of peptides. Class II molecules with the associated invariant chain are routed to endocytic compartments, where the invariant chain is degraded by proteolytic enzymes. The class II molecules then assume a more open conformation that can bind antigenic peptides. The peptide–class II complexes are then transported to the plasma membrane.

References

ATTAYA, M., S. JAMESON, C. K. MARTINEZ et al. 1992. Ham-2 corrects the class I antigen-processing defect in RMA-S cells. *Nature* **355**:647.

BRODSKY, F. M. 1992. Antigen processing and presentation: close encounters in the endocytic pathway. *Trends in Cell Biol.* **2**:109.

DEMARS, R., and T. SPIES. 1992. New genes in the MHC that encode proteins for antigen processing. *Trends in Cell Biol.* **2**:81.

GERMAINE, R. N., and D. H. MARGULIES. 1993. The biochemistry and cell biology of antigen processing and presentation. *Annu. Rev. Immunol.* **11**:403.

GOLDGERG, A. L., and K. L. ROCK. 1992. Proteolysis, proteosomes and antigen presentation. *Nature* **357**:375.

KELLY, A., S. H. POWIS, L. A. KERR et al. 1992. Assembly and function of the two ABC transporter proteins encoded in the human major histocompatibility complex. *Nature* **355**:641.

MONACO, J. J. 1992. A molecular model of MHC class-I-restricted antigen processing. *Immunol. Today* **13**:173.

POWIS, S. J., E. V. DEVERSON, W. J. COADWELL et al. 1992. Effect of polymorphism of an MHC-linked transporter on the peptides assembled in a class I molecule. *Nature* **357**:211.

SADEGH-NASSERI, S., and R. N. GERMAIN. 1992. How MHC class II molecules work: peptide-dependent completion of protein folding. *Immunol. Today* **13**:43.

SPIES, T., V. CERUNDOLO, M. COLONNA et al. 1992. Presentation of viral antigen by MHC class I molecules is dependent on a putative peptide transporter heterodimer. *Nature* **355**:644.

TEYTON, L., and P. A. PETERSON. 1992. Invariant chain—a regulator of antigen presentation. *Trends in Cell Biol.* **2**:52.

TROWSDALE, J., I. HANSON, I. MOCKRIDGE et al. 1990. Sequences encoded in the class II region of the MHC related to the ABC superfamily of transporters. *Nature* **348**:741.

VAN BLEEK, G. M., and S. G. NATHENSON. 1992. Presentation of antigenic peptides by MHC class I molecules. *Trends in Cell Biol.* **2**:202.

Study Questions

1. Define the following terms:
   a. Self-MHC restriction
   b. Antigen processing
   c. Endogenous antigen
   d. Exogenous antigen

2. L. A. Morrison and T. J. Braciale conducted an experiment to determine whether antigens presented by class I or II MHC molecules are processed in different pathways. Their results are summarized in Table 10-2.
   a. Why were the class I–restricted T_C cells not able to respond to target cells infected with killed influenza virus?
   b. Why did chloroquine inhibit the response of the class II–restricted T_C cells?
   c. What effect does emitine exert?

3. Antigen-presenting cells have been shown to present lysozyme peptide 46–61 together with the class II IA^k molecule. When CD4$^+$ T_H cells are incubated with APCs and native lysozyme or the synthetic lysozyme peptide 46–61, T_H-cell activation occurs.
   a. If choloquine is added to the incubation mixture, presentation of the native protein is inhibited, but the peptide continues to induce T-cell activation. Explain why this occurs.
   b. If chloroquine addition is delayed for 3 h, presentation of the native protein is not inhibited. Explain why this occurs.

4. Predict whether T_H-cell proliferation or CTL-mediated cytolysis of target cells will occur with the following mixtures of cells. The CD4$^+$ T_H cells are from lysozyme-primed mice, and the CD8$^+$ CTLs are from influenza-infected mice. Use R to indicate a response and NR to indicate no response.
   a. ____ H-2^k T_H cells + lysozyme-pulsed H-2^k macrophages.
   b. ____ H-2^k T_H cells + lysozyme-pulsed H-2$^{b/k}$ macrophages.
   c. ____ H-2^k T_H cells + lysozyme-primed H-2^d macrophages.
   d. ____ H-2^k CTLs + influenza-infected H-2^k macrophages.
   e. ____ H-2^k CTLs + influenza-infected H-2^d macrophages.
   f. ____ H-2^d CTLs + influenza-infected H-2$^{d/k}$ macrophages.

T-CELL RECEPTOR

Although the antigen-specific nature of T-cell responses clearly implies that they possess an antigen-specific and clonally restricted receptor, the nature of the T-cell receptor for antigen was unknown as recently as the early 1980s. Relevant experimental results were contradictory and difficult to conceptualize within a single model because the T-cell receptor differs from the B-cell antigen-binding receptor in two important ways. First, the T cell does not secrete its receptor as the B cell does, so that any assessment of receptor structure and specificity had to rely on complex cellular assays. Second, the T-cell receptor (TCR) is specific not for antigen alone but for antigen in association with one of the molecules of the major histocompatibility complex. This property prevents purification of the T-cell receptor by antigen-binding techniques and adds complexity to any experimental system designed to investigate the receptor. In 1982, the authors of a workshop report, titled "T-Cell Receptors: Through a Glass Darkly," summarized the workshop by stating, "At present we approach the T-cell receptor as the blind men in the fable approached the elephant. Even with our eyes wide open, we do not know if one person's helper T cell is in any way related to another's, nor whether molecules isolated from different T cells are encoded by the same or independent genes."

Within two years of this workshop, new investigative tools—notably monoclonal antibodies and nucleic acid probes—were used to isolate T-cell receptors and their genes for the first time. Shortly thereafter, the T-cell receptor was identified as a heterodimer composed of either α and β or γ and δ chains. Surprisingly, the genomic organization and the mode of generation of diversity for each chain were found to be similar to that of the B-cell receptor's immunoglobulin chains. In addition, the T-cell receptor was found to be associated on the membrane with a signal transducing complex called CD3. A similar signal transducing complex was recently discovered for the B-cell receptor. Also discovered was the important difference that distinguishes the T-cell receptor from immunoglobulins—the restricted ability of the T-cell receptor to recognize antigen only as a complex with self-MHC molecules. The knowledge that emerged in the 1980s about the structure, specificity, and function of T-cell receptors has provided a framework for greater understanding of cell-mediated immunity and of the similarities and differences between B cells and T cells.

T-Cell Receptors

In the 1970s and early 1980s investigators learned much about T-cell function but were thwarted in their attempts to identify and isolate its antigen-binding receptor. Several properties, unique to the T-cell receptor, hampered its identification.

Functional Assays for the T-Cell Receptor

Because the T cell does not secrete its antigen-binding receptor, complex cellular assays are required to assess TCR structure, specificity, and function. The general practice is to challenge T cells with antigen and then measure various functions indicative of T-cell activation. For example, activation of T helper (T_H) cells can be assayed by proliferation of the T_H cells, by secretion of various cytokines, or by the ability of activated T_H cells to activate B cells and T cytotoxic (T_C) cells. Activation of T_C cells can be assayed by lysis of target cells or by secretion of cytokines such as interferon gamma (IFN-γ). The requirement for complex cellular assays to assess TCR structure or specificity made it difficult to tell whether an agent that specifically stimulated or blocked the T-cell's response did so directly by acting on the receptor or indirectly by acting on some other required component of the cellular function being assessed.

Early Studies of the T-Cell Receptor

Even before the T-cell receptor was isolated, researchers had demonstrated several properties related to its general structure and interaction with antigen. Early experiments to determine whether the T-cell receptor is similar in structure to immunoglobulins yielded somewhat conflicting results. Although T cells failed to stain with fluorescent anti-isotype antibodies directed against immunoglobulin heavy- and light-chain constant-region determinants, a low percentage of T cells did stain with fluorescent anti-idiotype antibodies. The latter finding suggested that the T-cell receptor has a variable region with some structural features in common with immunoglobulins. The debate concerning whether the T-cell receptor was partly encoded by immunoglobulin genes was settled in the early 1980s by M. Kronenberg, L. Hood, and their colleagues. These researchers demonstrated that T cells do not contain any functional rearranged immunoglobulin genes; thus the T-cell receptor is distinct from the immunoglobulins and is encoded by its own separate genes.

By the early 1970s, it was recognized that one could generate T_C cells specific for hapten-conjugated target cells. For example, mice primed with syngeneic target cells that had been chemically modified with the hapten TNP produced T_C cells that lysed the TNP target cells in vitro. Yet these same T_C cells failed to bind free TNP or a TNP-BSA conjugate. Why did the T_C cells not bind the soluble antigen? The answer came when it was shown that T cells recognize antigen only when it is associated with class I or class II MHC molecules.

Since the T-cell receptor does not bind soluble antigen, its specificity cannot be assessed by simple antigen-binding assays similar to those used to determine an antibody's specificity. Rather, complex cellular assays had to be devised to study TCR specificity. In a classic experiment described in Chapter 10, R. Zinkernagel and P. Doherty showed in 1974 that T_C cells can bind a viral antigen only when it is presented in the proper context of a class I self-MHC molecule (see Figure 10-2). Other experiments performed during this same time period by D. Katz and B. Benaceraff and by E. M. Shevach and A. Rosenthal demonstrated that T_H cells also exhibit MHC restriction, recognizing antigen only in the context of class II self-MHC molecules.

Two models were proposed to explain the MHC restriction of the T-cell receptor. The *dual-receptor model* envisioned a T cell as having two separate receptors, one for antigen and one for class I or class II MHC molecules. The *altered-self model* proposed that there is a single receptor capable of recognizing foreign antigen complexed to a self-MHC molecule.

Unlike the dual-receptor model, in which an antigen and MHC molecule are recognized separately, the altered-self model predicts that a single receptor recognizes an alteration in MHC molecules induced by their association with foreign antigens.

The debate between proponents of these two models was waged for a number of years, until an elegant experiment by J. Kappler and P. Marrack provided a means to test each model. Two preparations of T cells with specificities for different antigen–class II MHC complexes were used for the experiment: one preparation was a T-cell hybridoma specific for ovalbumin (OVA) in the context of class II MHC molecules with the H-2^k haplotype; the other preparation was a normal T cell reactive to keyhole limpet hemocyanin (KLH) in the context of an H-2^f class II MHC molecule. The experimenters fused these two cells to produce a T-cell hybridoma expressing the receptors of both fusion partners (Figure 11-1). If the dual-receptor model were correct, then the hybrid cells should express separate receptors for each antigen and separate receptors for each class II MHC molecule; therefore, the hybrid cells should respond to both antigens presented by either H-2^k or H-2^f antigen-presenting cells. In fact, Kappler and Marrack found that the hybrid cells continued to respond only to OVA presented by H-2^k cells and to KLH presented by H-2^f cells. In other words, the original specificity for antigen and MHC haplotype appeared to segregate together in the membrane of these hybrid cells. This finding provided early support for the altered-self model.

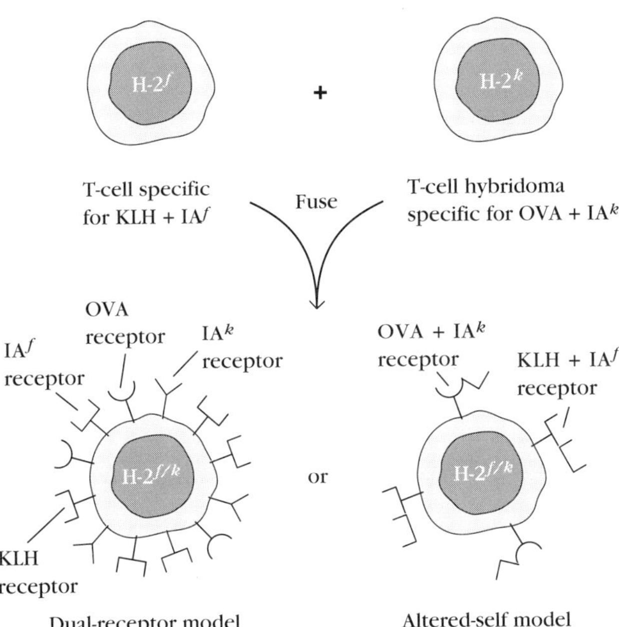

Response of fused cells				
		Expected response		
Antigen	MHC on APCs	Dual-receptor model	Altered-self model	Actual response
OVA	IA^k	+	+	+
OVA	IA^f	+	–	–
KLH	IA^k	+	–	–
KLH	IA^f	+	+	+

FIGURE 11-1 Fusion of T cells with two different specificities allowed the dual-receptor (DR) and altered-self (AS) models of T-cell antigen recognition to be tested. One fusion partner was specific for ovalbumin (OVA) + the class II MHC molecule IA^k on antigen-presenting cells (APCs), and the other was specific for keyhole limpet hemocyanin (KLH) + IA^f. Comparison of the expected responses of the fused cells, assuming the dual-receptor or altered-self model to be correct, with the actual responses supports the altered-self model. [Based on J. Kappler et al., 1981 *J. Exp. Med.* **153**:1198.]

Isolation of T-Cell Receptors with Monoclonal Antibodies

Identification and isolation of the T-cell receptor finally was accomplished by producing large numbers of monoclonal antibodies to various T-cell clones and then screening these monoclonal antibodies to find one that was clone specific, or *clonotypic*. This approach was based on the assumption that since the T-cell receptor is specific for both antigen and a MHC molecule, there should be significant structural differences in the receptor from clone to clone. Identification of the T-cell receptor using this approach was first accomplished by J. P. Allison in 1982, closely followed by E. Reinherz and S. Schlossman and by J. Kappler and P. Marrack.

The experimental approach of Kappler and Marrack illustrates how clonotypic monoclonal antibody can be used to identify and isolate the T-cell receptor. They had characterized a T_H-cell clone (hybridoma) that was specific for OVA and the H-2^d haplotype. This particular clone responded to OVA on an H-2^d antigen-presenting cell (APC) by secreting interleukin 2 (IL-2), which could be assayed in the culture supernatant. Kappler and Marrack set out to produce various monoclonal antibodies to membrane proteins of this antigen-specific T-cell clone, hoping to find a clonotypic monoclonal antibody that reacted only with the antigen-specific clone and not with other, related T-cell clones. After immunizing mice with the T-cell clone, they fused the spleen cells from the immunized mice with Ab^-, $HGPRT^-$ myeloma cells to make various hybridomas secreting monoclonal antibodies to epitopes on the T_H cells. They screened the wells for a monoclonal antibody that blocked IL-2 secretion by the immunizing T_H clone in response to OVA on H-2^d antigen-presenting cells. They reasoned that such a monoclonal antibody would be specific for the T-cell receptor if it was clonotypic and specifically inhibited the response of the immunizing clone to its antigen–class II molecule. Kappler and Marrack were, indeed, successful in identifying such a clonotypic monoclonal antibody, as the data in Table 11-1 show. Once having obtained a specific anti-TCR antibody, they used this antibody preparation to precipitate the T-cell receptor from a solubilized membrane extract of the original T_H clone. The clonotypic antibody precipitated a disulfide-linked glycoprotein that contained a 40-kDa α chain and a 43-kDa β chain.

By taking a similar approach, Allison isolated a similar $\alpha\beta$ heterodimer from the T-cell membrane. He carried the characterization of the T-cell receptor one step further by showing that some antisera bound to $\alpha\beta$ heterodimers from all T-cell clones, whereas other antisera was clone specific. This finding suggested that the TCR α and β chains, like the immunoglobulin heavy and light chains, each have a constant and variable amino acid sequence. Later, a second TCR heterodimer consisting of δ and γ chains was also identified. The great majority of T cells (more than 95%) express the $\alpha\beta$ heterodimer; the remaining 2–5% of T cells express the $\gamma\delta$ heterodimer.

TABLE 11-1 INHIBITION OF IL-2 SECRETION BY T_H CELLS SPECIFIC FOR OVALBUMIN (OVA) ON H-2^d APCs WITH CLONOTYPIC MONOCLONAL ANTIBODIES

Antigen	APC haplotype	Clonotypic antibody	IL-2 secretion by T cells (units/ml)
OVA	H-2^d	−	2000
OVA	H-2^d	+	5
—	H-2^d	−	5
OVA	H-2^k	−	5

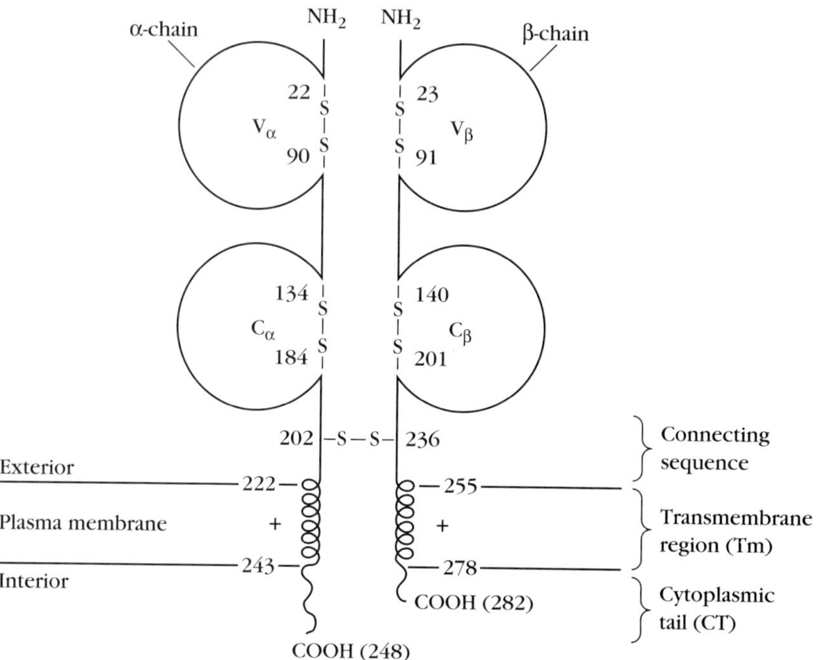

FIGURE 11-2 Schematic diagram of the $\alpha\beta$ T-cell receptor. Each chain is thought to contain two immunoglobulin-fold domains; each variable-region domain (V_α and V_β) contains three hypervariable regions equivalent to the CDRs in antibodies. The structure of the $\gamma\delta$ T-cell receptor is similar. Numbers indicate residue positions in the TCR molecule.

Structure of T-Cell Receptors

Amino acid sequencing analyses of the $\alpha\beta$ and $\gamma\delta$ TCR heterodimers revealed that their domain structure is strikingly similar to that of the immunoglobulins; thus, they are classified as members of the immunoglobulin superfamily (see Figure 5-16). Both chains of each TCR heterodimer exhibit marked variation in the amino-terminal amino acids but conservation in the carboxyl-terminal amino acids. However, the T-cell receptor has not yet been analyzed by x-ray crystallography, so its three-dimensional structure can only be inferred from its homology to immunoglobulin molecules. Each chain has two domains marked by an intrachain disulfide bond spanning 60–75 amino acids. These domains—one variable (V) domain and one constant (C) domain—are thought to have a structure similar to that of the immunoglobulin fold. Three complementarity-determining regions (CDRs), which appear to be equivalent to the CDRs in immunoglobulin light and heavy chains, have been identified in the V domain of each TCR chain.

In addition to the C domain, each TCR chain contains a short connecting sequence, which has a cysteine residue involved in disulfide linking of the two chains in the TCR heterodimer. Following the connecting region is a transmembrane region of 21 or 22 amino acids, anchoring each chain in the plasma membrane. Finally, each TCR chain contains a short cytoplasmic tail of 5–12 amino acids at the carboxyl-terminal end (Figure 11-2).

Organization and Rearrangement of TCR Genes

The genes encoding the $\alpha\beta$ and $\gamma\delta$ T-cell receptors are expressed only in cells of the T-cell lineage. The four TCR loci (α, β, γ, and δ) have a germ-line organization that is remarkably similar to the multigene organization of the immunoglobulin (Ig) genes. As with the Ig genes, separate V, D, and J gene segments rearrange during T-cell maturation to form functional genes encoding an $\alpha\beta$ or $\gamma\delta$ T-cell receptor.

Identifying and Cloning the TCR Genes

In order to identify and isolate the TCR genes, S. M. Hedrick and M. M. Davis sought to isolate mRNA encoding the α and β chains from a T_H-cell clone. This was no easy task. Because the T cell does not secrete its antigen-binding receptor, the receptor mRNA does not represent a sizable fraction of the mRNA, as it does, for example, in the plasma cell, where immunoglobulin is a major secreted cell product and mRNAs encoding the heavy and light chains are relatively easy to purify. The successful scheme of Hedrick and Davis for isolating TCR genes depended on a number of well-thought-out assumptions, which proved to be correct.

Hedrick and Davis reasoned that the mRNA encoding the T-cell receptor must, like the mRNAs encoding other integral membrane proteins, be bound to polyribosomes rather than to free cytoplasmic ribosomes. They therefore isolated the membrane-bound polyribosomal mRNA from a T_H-cell clone and used reverse transcriptase to synthesize ^{32}P-labeled cDNA probes (Figure 11-3). Because only 3% of lymphocyte mRNA is in the membrane-bound polyribosomal fraction, this step eliminated the 97% of the mRNA that did not encode any integral membrane protein.

Hedrick and Davis next used a technique called DNA subtractive hybridization to remove all the [^{32}P]cDNA that was not unique to T cells from their preparation. Their rationale for this step was that since T cells and B cells are derived from a common progenitor cell, they should express many genes in common. Earlier measurements by Davis had shown that 98% of the genes expressed in lymphocytes are common to B cells and T cells. Hedrick and Davis sought to enrich for the 2% of the expressed genes that are unique to T cells, which should include the genes encoding the T-cell receptor. Therefore, by hybridizing B-cell mRNA with their T_H-cell [^{32}P]cDNA, they were able to remove, or subtract, all the cDNA that was common to B cells and T cells. The unhybridized [^{32}P]cDNA remaining after this step presumably represented the expressed polyribosomal mRNA that was unique to the T_H-cell clone, including the mRNA encoding its T-cell receptor.

Cloning of the unhybridized [^{32}P]cDNA generated a library from which 10 different cDNA clones were identified on first analysis. To determine which of these T-cell–specific cDNA clones might represent the T-cell receptor, Hedrick and Davis used these clones as probes to look for genes on the genomic DNA that rearranged in mature T cells. This approach was based on the assumption that since the $\alpha\beta$ T-cell receptor appeared to have constant and variable regions, its genes should undergo DNA rearrangements like those observed in B cells. The two investigators isolated genomic DNA from T cells, B cells, liver cells, and macrophages, cleaved it with restriction endonucleases, and subjected each DNA sample to Southern-blot analysis (see Figure 2-8) using the 10 [^{32}P]cDNA probes to identify unique T-cell genomic DNA sequences. They looked for bands that showed DNA rearrangement in T cells but not in liver cells, B cells, or macrophages. One cDNA probe showed the same Southern-blot patterns for DNA isolated from liver cells, B cells, and macrophages but six different patterns for the DNA from six different mature T-cell lines (see Figure 11-3). These patterns presumably represented rearranged TCR genes. Such results would be expected if rearranged TCR genes occur only in mature T cells. The observation that all six T-cell lines showed different Southern-blot patterns is consistent with the differences in TCR specificity to be expected in each cell line.

The cDNA clone identified by the Southern-blot analyses shown in Figure 11-3 has all the hallmarks of a putative TCR gene: It represents a gene sequence that rearranges, is expressed as a membrane-bound protein, and is expressed only in T cells. This cDNA clone was found to encode the β chain of the T-cell receptor. Later, cDNA clones were identified encoding the α chain, the γ chain, and finally the δ chain.

TCR Multigene Families

Germ-line DNA contains four TCR multigene families each encoding one of the receptor chains. As in the case of Ig genes, functional TCR genes are produced by gene rearrangements involving V and J segments in the α-chain and γ-chain families and V, D, and J segments in the β-chain and δ-chain families. In the mouse the α-, β-, and γ-chain gene segments are located on chromosomes 14, 6, and 13, respectively. The δ-chain gene segments are located on chromosome 14 between the V_α and J_α segments. This location of the δ-chain gene family is significant: A productive rearrangement of the α-chain gene segments deletes C_δ, so that the $\alpha\beta$ TCR receptor cannot be coexpressed with the $\gamma\delta$ receptor in a given T cell.

Mouse germ-line DNA contains about 100 V_α and 50 J_α gene segments and a single C_α segment. The δ-chain gene family contains about 10 V gene segments, which are largely distinct from the V_α gene

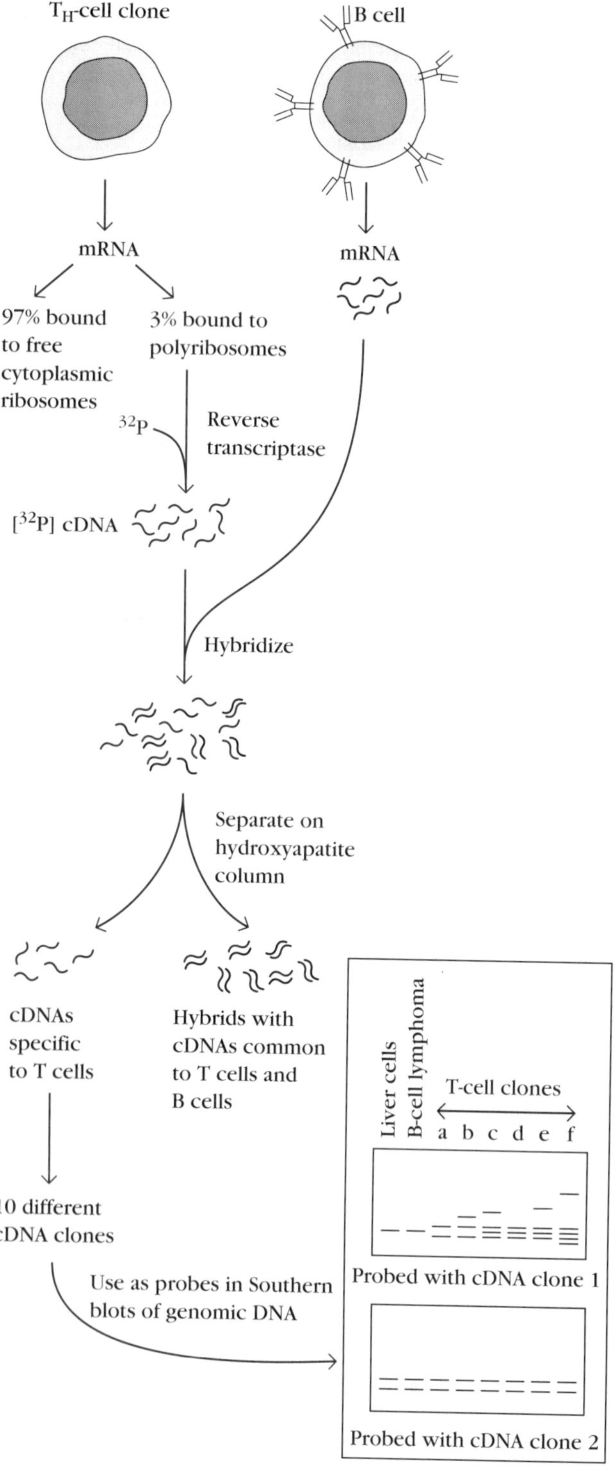

FIGURE 11-3 Production and identification of a cDNA clone encoding the T-cell receptor. The flow chart outlines the procedure used by S. Hedrick and M. Davis to obtain [32P]cDNA clones corresponding to T-cell–specific mRNAs. The technique of DNA subtractive hybridization enabled them to isolate [32P]cDNA unique to the T-cell. *(Inset)* The labeled cDNA clones were used as probes in Southern-blot analyses of genomic DNA from liver cells, B-lymphoma cells, and six different T_H-cell clones (a–f). Probing with cDNA clone 1 produced a distinct blot pattern for each T-cell clone, whereas probing with cDNA clone 2 did not. Assuming that the liver cells and B cells contained unrearranged germ-line DNA and that each of the T-cell clones contained different rearranged TCR genes, the results using cDNA clone 1 as the probe identified the T-cell receptor. The cDNA clone 2 identified another T-cell membrane molecule encoded by DNA that does not undergo rearrangement. [Based on S. Hedrick et al., 1984, *Nature* **308**:153.]

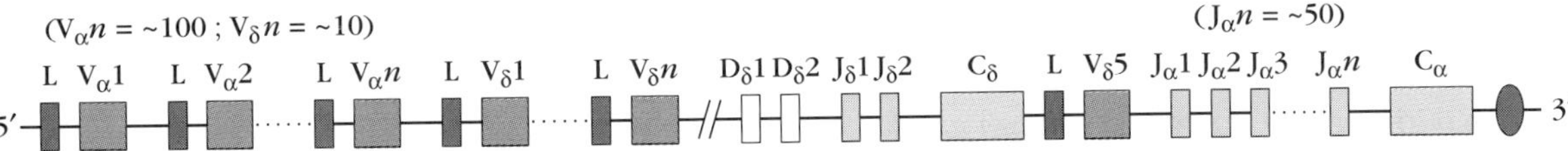

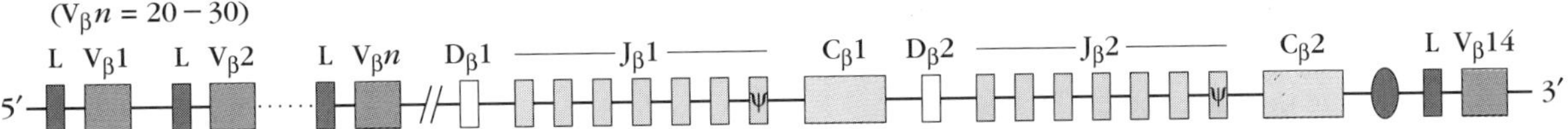

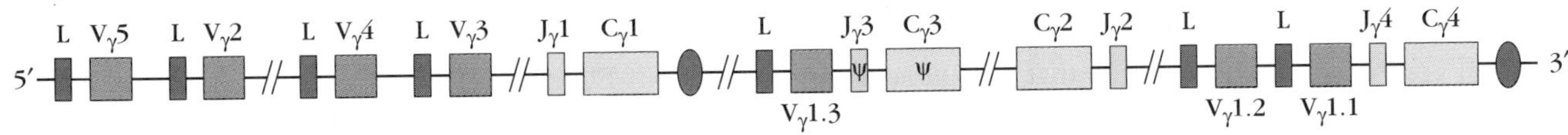

FIGURE 11-4 Germ-line organization of the mouse TCR α-, β-, γ-, and δ-chain gene segments. Each C gene segment is composed of a series of exons and introns, which are not shown. The organization of TCR gene segments in humans is similar, although the number of the various gene segments differs in some cases (see Table 11-2). [Adapted from D. Raulet, 1989, *Annu. Rev. Immunol.* **7**:175 and M. Davis, 1990, *Annu. Rev. Biochem.* **59**:475.]

segments, although some sharing of V segments has been observed in rearranged α- and δ-chain genes. Two D_δ and two J_δ gene segments and one C_δ segment also have been identified. The β-chain gene family has 20–30 V gene segments and two repeats of D, J, and C segments, each repeat consisting of one D_β, six J_β, and one C_β. The γ-chain gene family consists of seven V_γ segments and three different functional J_γ-C_γ repeats. The organization of the gene segments within each multigene family is shown in Figure 11-4. The organization of the TCR multigene families in humans is generally similar to that in mice, although the number of segments differs (Table 11-2).

Variable-Region Gene Rearrangements

The mechanisms by which TCR germ-line DNA is rearranged to form functional receptor genes appear to be similar to the mechanisms used in Ig-gene rearrangements. For example, conserved heptamer and nonamer recognition signal sequences (RSSs), containing either 12-bp (one-turn) or 23-bp (two-turn) spacer sequences, have been identified flanking each V, D, and J gene segment in TCR germ-line DNA. The recognition signals in T cells have similar heptamer and nonamer sequences as those in B cells (see Figure 8-5). All of the TCR-gene rearrangements follow the one-turn/two-turn joining rule observed for the Ig genes. A recombinase enzyme recognizes the heptamer and nonamer recognition signals and catalyzes V-J and V-D-J joining by the same deletional or inversional mechanisms that occur in the Ig genes (see Figure 8-6). Circular excision products thought to be generated by looping-out and deletion in TCR rearrangement have been shown to be present in thymocytes. Like the pre-B cell, the pre-T cell has also been shown to express the recombination-activating

TABLE 11-2 TCR MULTIGENE FAMILIES IN HUMANS

Gene	Chromosome location	No. of gene segments			
		V	D	J	C
α Chain	14	50		70	1
δ Chain*	14	3	3	3	1
β Chain†	7	57	2	13	2
γ Chain‡	7	14		5	2

* The δ-chain gene segments are located between the V_α and J_α segments.

† There are two repeats each containing 1 D_β, 6 or 7 J_β, and 1 C_β.

‡ There are two repeats each containing 2 or 3 J_γ and 1 C_γ.

SOURCE: Data from P. A. H. Moss et al., 1992, *Annu. Rev. Immunol.* **10**:71.

genes (*RAG-1* and *RAG-2*). These genes either encode a part of the recombination machinery or play a role in regulating expression of other as yet unidentified enzymes involved in recombination.

A number of experiments have suggested that T cells utilize the same recombinase enzyme system as B cells in V-(D)-J joining. In one experiment G. D. Yancopoulos transfected unrearranged TCR *β*-chain genes into B-lineage precursor cells having active recombinase activity. He found that the recombinase enzyme of the B cells could rearrange the transfected TCR *β*-chain genes. Studies with *scid* mice, which lack functional T and B cells, also have shed light on the mechanisms of V-D-J joining during Ig-gene and TCR-gene rearrangements. As discussed in Chapter 8, *scid* mice show abnormal gene rearrangements such that the D and/or J gene segment is deleted during D-J joining in both Ig and TCR DNA (see Figure 8-9). This finding lends support to the notion that the same recombinase enzyme may be involved in V-D-J rearrangements in B cells and in T cells and that a defect in this recombinase system may give rise to the immunodeficiency in *scid* mice.

As noted already, the Ig genes are not normally rearranged in T cells and the TCR genes are not rearranged in B cells, suggesting that mechanisms must exist for regulating the recombinase enzyme system in each cell lineage. Presumably, differences in chromatin configuration of the Ig genes and TCR genes within B- and T-cell lineages account for the preferential rearrangement of Ig genes in B cells and TCR genes in T cells.

Allelic Exclusion of TCR α and β Genes

As with the Ig genes, rearrangement of the TCR *β*-chain genes also exhibits allelic exclusion. Once a productive rearrangement occurs for one *β*-chain allele, the rearrangement of the other *β* allele is inhibited. Allelic exclusion appears to be less stringent for the TCR *α*-chain genes. For example, analyses of T-cell clones expressing a functional *αβ* T-cell receptor revealed a number of clones with productive rearrangements for both *α*-chain alleles. Furthermore, when an immature T-cell lymphoma expressing a particular *αβ* T-cell receptor was subcloned, several subclones were obtained that expressed the same *β*-chain allele but a different *α*-chain allele from the original parent clone.

Studies with transgenic mice also indicate that allelic exclusion is less stringent for TCR *α*-chain genes than for *β*-chain genes. Mice carrying a productively rearranged *αβ*-TCR transgene do not rearrange and express the endogenous *β*-chain genes. However, the endogenous *α*-chain genes sometimes are expressed at varying levels in place of the already rearranged *α*-chain transgene. Since allelic exclusion is not complete for the TCR *α* chain, more than one *α* chain occasionally is expressed on the membrane of a given T cell. The obvious question is how do the rare T cells that express two *αβ* T-cell receptors maintain a single antigen-binding specificity? One possibility, suggested by some researchers, is that when a T cell expresses two different *αβ* T-cell receptors, only one is self-MHC restricted.

Structure of Rearranged TCR Genes

The general structure of rearranged TCR genes is shown in Figure 11-5. The variable regions of T-cell receptors are, of course, encoded by rearranged VDJ and VJ sequences. In TCR genes, combinatorial joining of V gene segments appears to generate CDR1 and CDR2, whereas junctional flexibility and N-region nucleotide addition generate CDR3. Rearranged TCR genes also contain a short leader (L) sequence upstream of the joined VJ or VDJ sequences. The amino acids encoded by the leader sequence are cleaved as the nascent polypeptide enters the endoplasmic reticulum.

The constant region of each TCR chain is encoded by a C gene segment that has multiple exons corre-

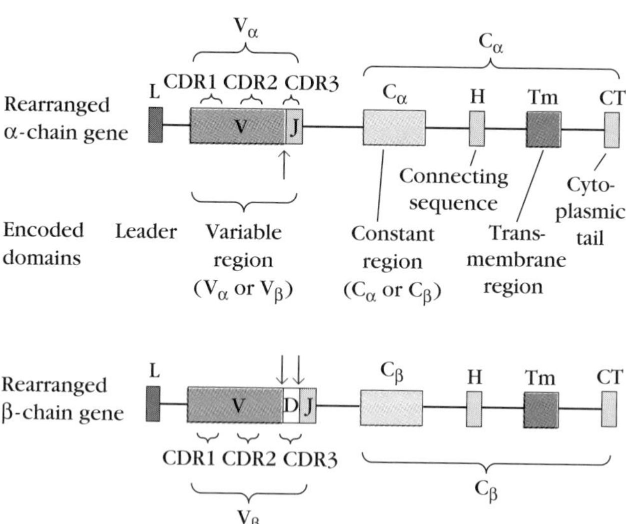

FIGURE 11-5 Schematic diagram of rearranged TCR genes showing the exons encoding the various domains of the *αβ* T-cell receptor and approximate position of the CDRs. Junctional diversity (purple arrows) generates CDR3 (see Figure 11-6). The leader sequence is cleaved from the nascent polypeptide chain and is not present in the finished protein. The structures of the rearranged *γ*- and *δ*-chain genes are similar although additional junctional diversity can occur in *δ*-chain genes.

sponding to the structural domains in the protein (see Figure 11-2). The first C-region exon encodes the majority of the C domain. Next is a short exon encoding the connecting sequence, followed by exons encoding the transmembrane region and cytoplasmic tail. As described in Chapter 8, differential RNA processing of the constant region in immunoglobulin heavy-chain primary transcripts produces either secreted or membrane-bound antibody. Since there is no secreted form of the T-cell receptor, such differential processing of TCR primary transcripts does not occur.

Generation of TCR Diversity

Although TCR germ-line DNA contains far fewer V gene segments than Ig germ-line DNA, a number of features contribute to generating many more antigenic specificities among T-cell receptors than antibodies. Table 11-3 and Figure 11-6 compare the generation of diversity among antibody molecules and TCR molecules.

Combinatorial joining of variable-region gene segments generates a large number of random gene combinations for all the TCR chains, as it does for the Ig heavy- and light-chain genes. For example, 100 V_α and 50 J_α gene segments can generate 5×10^3 possible VJ combinations for the TCR α chain. Similarly, 25 V_β, 2 D_β, and 12 J_β, gene segments can give 6×10^2 possible combinations. Although there are fewer TCR V_α and V_β gene segments than immunoglobulin V_H and V_κ segments, this difference is offset by the greater number of J segments in TCR germ-line DNA. Assuming that the antigen-binding specificity of a given T-cell receptor depends upon the variable region in both chains, random association of 5×10^3 V_α combinations with 6×10^2 V_β combinations can generate a minimum of 3×10^6 possible combinations for the $\alpha\beta$ T-cell receptor.

As illustrated in Figure 11-6b, the location of one-turn (12-bp) and two-turn (23-bp) recognition signal sequences in TCR β- and δ-chain DNA differs from that in Ig heavy-chain DNA. Because of the arrangement of the recognition signal sequences in TCR germ-line

TABLE 11-3 COMPARISON OF POSSIBLE DIVERSITY IN MOUSE IMMUNOGLOBULIN AND TCR GENES

Mechanism of diversity	Immunoglobulins		$\alpha\beta$ T-cell receptor		$\gamma\delta$ T-cell receptor	
	H chain	κ chain	α chain	β chain	γ chain	δ chain
	Estimated number of segments					
Multiple germ-line gene segments						
V	300	300	100	25	7	10
D	12	0	0	2	0	2
J	4	4	50	12	3	2
	Possible number of combinations*					
Combinatorial V-J and V-D-J joining	$300 \times 12 \times 4 = 1.4 \times 10^4$	$300 \times 4 = 1.2 \times 10^3$	$100 \times 50 = 5 \times 10^3$	$25 \times 2 \times 12 = 6 \times 10^2$	$7 \times 3 = 21$	$10 \times 2 \times 2 = 40$
Alternative joining of D gene segments	−	−	−	+ (some)	−	+ (often)
Junctional flexibility	+	+	+	+	+	+
N-region nucleotide addition†	+	−	+	+	+	+
Somatic mutation	+	+	−	−	−	−
Total estimated diversity‡	~10^{11}		~10^{15}		~10^{18}	

* A + indicates mechanism makes a significant contribution to diversity but to an unknown extent. A − indicates mechanism does not operate.

† See Figure 11-6d for theoretical number of combinations generated by N-region addition.

‡ Total estimated diversity includes contribution from combinatorial association of chains.

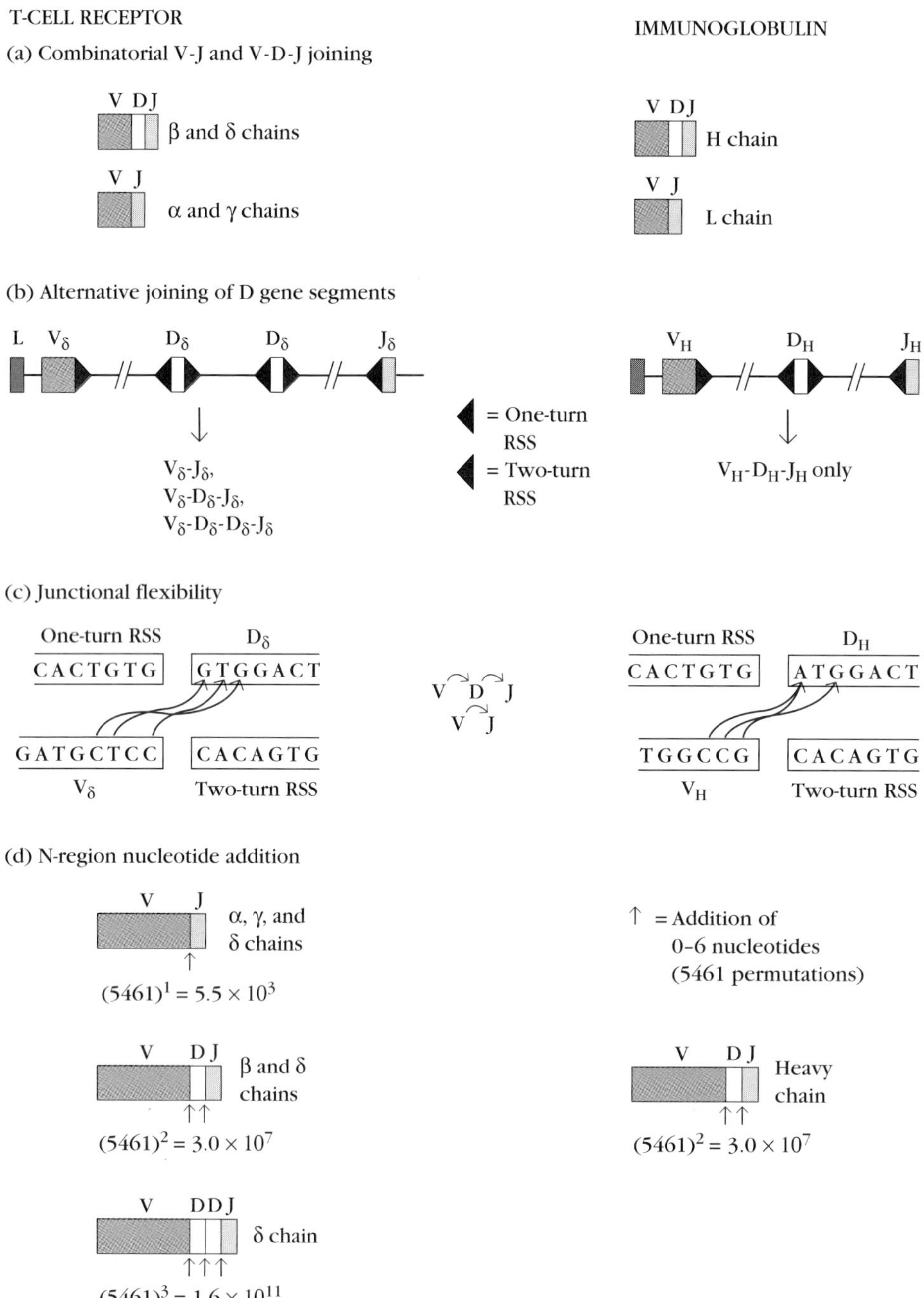

FIGURE 11-6 Comparison of mechanisms for generating diversity in TCR genes and immunoglobulin genes. In addition to the mechanisms shown, somatic mutation occurs in Ig genes. Combinatorial association of the expressed chains generates additional diversity among TCR and Ig molecules.

DNA, *alternative joining of D gene segments* can occur while the one-turn/two-turn joining rule is observed. Thus, it is possible for a V_β gene segment to join directly with a J_β or D_β gene segment, generating a $(VJ)_\beta$ or $(VDJ)_\beta$ unit. Alternative joining of δ-chain gene segments generates similar units; in addition, one D_δ can join with another, yielding $(VDDJ)_\delta$ and in humans $(VDDDJ)_\delta$. This mechanism, which cannot occur in Ig heavy-chain DNA, generates considerable additional diversity in TCR genes.

The joining of gene segments during TCR gene rearrangement exhibits *junctional flexibility*. As with the Ig genes, this flexibility can generate many nonproductive rearrangements, but it also increases diversity by encoding several alternative amino acids at each junction (see Figure 11-6c). *N-region nucleotide addition,* catalyzed by a terminal deoxynucleotidyl transferase, generates additional junctional diversity. Whereas N-region nucleotide addition occurs only in the Ig heavy-chain genes, it occurs in the genes encoding all the TCR chains. As many as six nucleotides can be added by this mechanism at each junction, generating up to 5461 possible combinations assuming random selection of nucleotides (see Figure 11-6d). Some of these combinations, however, lead to nonproductive rearrangements.

Although each junctional region in a TCR gene encodes only 10–20 amino acids, enormous diversity can be generated in these regions. Estimates suggest that the combined effects of N-region nucleotide addition and joining flexibility can generate as many as 10^{13} possible amino acid sequences in the TCR junctional regions alone. Unlike the Ig genes, the TCR genes do not seem to undergo somatic mutation. That is, the functional TCR genes generated during T-cell maturation in the thymus are the same as those found in the mature peripheral T-cell population. The absence of somatic mutation in T cells ensures that T-cell specificity does not change after thymic selection and therefore reduces any possibility that random mutation might generate a self-reactive T cell.

The T-cell receptor must function to recognize both a very large number of different processed antigens and a relatively small number of self-MHC molecules. It has been suggested that the limited number of germ-line V gene segments carried by T cells may generate the diversity needed for MHC recognition, whereas the enormous diversity generated at the junctional regions facilitates recognition of antigen.

T-Cell Receptor Complex: TCR-CD3

As discussed in Chapter 5, membrane-bound immunoglobulin on B cells associates with another membrane protein, the Ig-α/Ig-β heterodimer, to form the B-cell antigen receptor (see Figure 5-10). Similarly, the T-cell receptor associates with CD3, forming the TCR-CD3 membrane complex. In both cases, the accessory molecule is involved in signal transduction after interaction of a B or T cell with antigen.

The first evidence suggesting that the T-cell receptor is associated with another membrane molecule came from experiments in which fluorescent antibody to the receptor was shown to "co-cap" another membrane protein, designated CD3. Later experiments by J. P. Allison and L. Lanier demonstrated that the T-cell receptor and CD3 are located quite close together in the T-cell membrane. These researchers first treated a T-cell membrane preparation with a cross-linking agent that spans 12 Å, and then precipitated the T-cell receptor with anti-TCR monoclonal antibody. Analysis of the precipitated T-cell receptors showed that they were cross-linked to CD3 molecules, indicating that the two proteins must be positioned within 12 Å of each other in the membrane. Subsequent experiments demonstrated not only that CD3 is closely associated with the $\alpha\beta$ heterodimer but also that its expression is required for membrane expression of $\alpha\beta$ and $\gamma\delta$ T-cell receptors. Thus the $\alpha\beta$ and $\gamma\delta$ heterodimer each exist as a molecular complex with CD3 on the T-cell membrane. Mutation in either the CD3 or TCR genes results in loss of the entire molecular complex from the membrane, demonstrating the obligate requirement for coexpression of both CD3 and the T-cell receptor on the membrane.

As diagrammed in Figure 11-7, CD3 is a complex of five invariant polypeptide chains that associate to form three dimers: a heterodimer of gamma and epsilon chains ($\gamma\epsilon$), a heterodimer of delta and epsilon chains ($\delta\epsilon$), and a homodimer of two zeta chains ($\zeta\zeta$) *or* a heterodimer of zeta and eta chains ($\zeta\eta$). The ζ and η chains, which are encoded by the same gene, differ in their carboxyl-terminal ends due to differences in RNA splicing of the primary transcript. About 90% of the CD3 complexes examined to date incorporate the $\zeta\zeta$ homodimer; the remainder have the $\zeta\eta$ heterodimer. The T-cell receptor complex can thus be envisioned as four dimers: The $\alpha\beta$ or $\gamma\delta$ TCR heterodimer determines the ligand-binding specificity, whereas the CD3 dimers ($\gamma\epsilon$, $\delta\epsilon$, and $\zeta\zeta$ or $\zeta\eta$) are required for expression of the T-cell receptor and for signal transduction.

The γ, δ, and ϵ chains of CD3 are members of the immunoglobulin superfamily, each containing an immunoglobulin-like extracellular domain followed by a transmembrane region and a cytoplasmic domain of more than 40 amino acids. The ζ and η chains have a distinctly different structure: Both have a very short external region of only 9 amino acids, a transmembrane region, and a long cytoplasmic tail containing 113 amino acids in ζ and 155 amino acids in η. The transmembrane region of all the CD3 polypeptide chains contains a negatively charged aspartic acid residue. These negatively charged groups may enable the CD3 complex to interact with one or two positively charged amino acids that are present in the transmembrane region of each TCR chain. Another unusual feature of CD3 is the presence of a common sequence referred to as the *antigen recognition activation motif (ARAM).* The γ, δ, and ϵ cytoplasmic tails each contain a single copy of ARAM, whereas the ζ and η cytoplasmic tails contain three copies (see Figure 11-7).

CD3 has structural and functional similarities with several other receptors expressed by immune-system cells including the Ig-α/Ig-β heterodimer on B cells

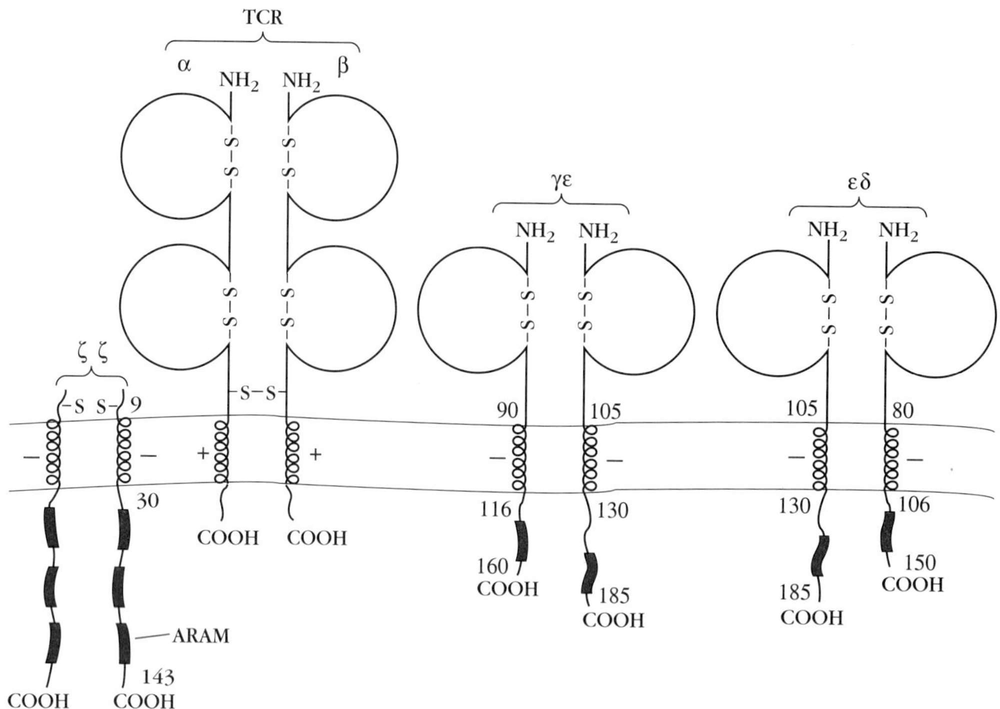

FIGURE 11-7 Schematic diagram of the TCR-CD3 complex, which constitutes the T-cell antigen-binding receptor. The figure shows the $\alpha\beta$ T-cell receptor and CD3 complex consisting of the $\zeta\zeta$ homodimer plus $\gamma\epsilon$ and $\epsilon\delta$ heterodimers. The external domains of the γ, δ, and ϵ chains of CD3 are similar to the immunoglobulin-fold structure, which may facilitate their interaction with the T-cell receptor and each other. Ionic interactions also may occur between the oppositely charged transmembrane regions in the TCR and CD3 chains. The long cytoplasmic tails of the CD3 chains contain a common sequence, the antigen recognition activation motif (ARAM), which functions in signal transduction.

and subunits of the Fc receptors for IgE and IgG (FcϵRI and FcγRIII). Each of these receptors is a complex of multiple chains and contains an ARAM in the cytoplasmic tail of at least one chain of the complex. These receptors are grouped together as *multichain immune recognition receptors (MIRRs).* Following receptor cross-linkage, each MIRR transduces an intracellular signal that involves several common steps in the signal-transduction pathway including the activation of various protein tyrosine kinases. The ARAM in the

TABLE 11-4 SELECTED T-CELL ACCESSORY MOLECULES

Name	Ligand	Adhesion	Signal transduction	Member of Ig superfamily
CD4	Class II MHC	+	+	+
CD8	Class I MHC	+	+	+
CD2 (LFA-2)	CD58 (LFA-3)	+	+	+
LFA-1 (CD11a/CD18)	ICAM-1 (CD54)	+	?	+/(−)
CD28	B7	?	+	+
CTLA-4	B7	?	+	−
CD45R	CD22	+	+	+
CD5	CD72	?	+	−

cytoplasmic domain of these receptors is thought to interact with protein tyrosine kinases during signal transduction. In addition each ARAM contains tyrosine residues that are phosphorylated by the protein tyrosine kinases following receptor stimulation. These events are discussed more fully in Chapter 12.

T-Cell Accessory Membrane Molecules

Although recognition of antigen-MHC complexes is mediated solely by the TCR-CD3 complex, a variety of other membrane molecules play an important accessory role in antigen recognition and T-cell activation (Table 11-4). Many of these accessory molecules function as adhesion molecules, strengthening the interaction between a T cell and antigen-presenting cell or target cell. In addition, several of these accessory molecules transduce signals from the T-cell receptor through the membrane to the cytoplasm. As indicated in Table 11-4, some of these accessory molecules belong to the immunoglobulin superfamily (see Figure 5-16). The association of the $\alpha\beta$ T-cell receptor with several accessory molecules is schematically depicted in Figure 11-8.

CD4 and CD8 Coreceptors

T cells can be subdivided based on their expression of CD4 or CD8 membrane molecules. As discussed in previous chapters, $CD4^+$ T cells recognize antigen in association with class II MHC molecules and largely function as helper cells, whereas $CD8^+$ T cells recognize antigen in association with class I MHC molecules and largely function as cytotoxic cells. Both CD4 and CD8 have dual functions as adhesion molecules and as co-signaling coreceptors. A number of experiments have demonstrated that CD4 and CD8 play a role in T-cell activation. For example, when T cells are incubated with monoclonal antibodies to CD4 or CD8, activation can be inhibited or enhanced.

CD4 is a 55-kDa monomeric membrane glycoprotein that contains four extracellular immunoglobulin-like domains, a hydrophobic transmembrane region, and a long cytoplasmic domain containing three serine residues, which can be phosphorylated. CD8 is present generally as a disulfide-linked $\alpha\beta$ heterodimer and less frequently as an $\alpha\alpha$ homodimer. Both the α and β

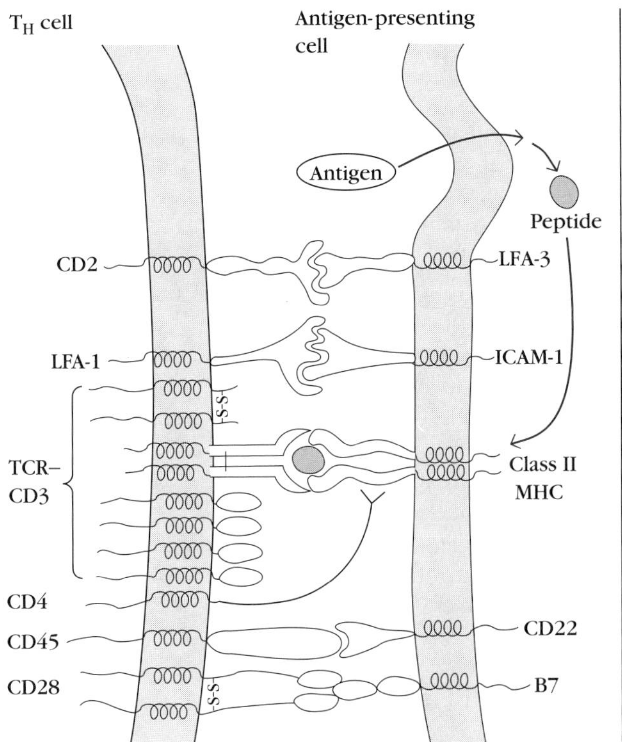

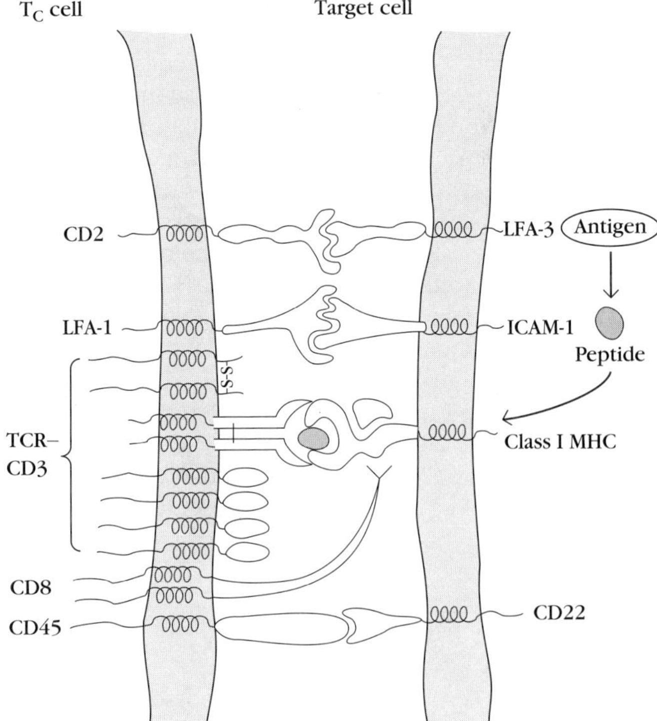

FIGURE 11-8 Schematic diagram of the association between the T-cell receptor and various accessory molecules that function to transduce signals and/or to strengthen the interaction between a T_H cell and antigen-presenting cell *(left)* or T_C cell and target cell *(right)*.

chains of CD8 are small glycoproteins of approximately 30–38 kDa. Each chain consists of a single extracellular immunoglobulin-like domain, a hydrophobic transmembrane region, and a cytoplasmic domain containing 25–27 residues, of which several can be phosphorylated.

As cell-adhesion molecules, CD4 binds to the membrane-proximal β_2 domain of the class II MHC molecule, and CD8 binds to the membrane-proximal α_3 domain of the class I MHC molecule (see Figure 9-5). The binding specificity of CD4 and CD8 was determined by experiments using chimeric MHC molecules, generated by exon shuffling (see Figure 9-17). In one such experiment a chimeric class I molecule consisting of human α_1 and α_2 domains and an α_3 domain of mouse origin was used. This chimeric molecule was shown to activate a $CD8^+$ T-cell response in mice, whereas a complete human class I MHC molecule was unable to do so. CD4 and CD8 apparently function to increase the avidity of the interaction between a T-cell receptor and an antigen-MHC complex. For example, binding of T-cell receptors to antigen-MHC complexes has been shown to be augmented about 100-fold by the presence of CD4 or CD8 on the membrane.

As coreceptors, CD4 and CD8 are thought to interact with the same MHC molecule that is recognized by the T-cell receptor. The evidence supporting coaggregation of CD4 with the TCR-CD3 complex is strong, but the evidence that this happens with CD8 is less convincing. When $CD4^+$ T cells are incubated with antigen-presenting cells, for example, a close membrane interaction, called conjugate formation, occurs between the two interacting cell types. If these conjugates are fixed with formaldehyde, CD4 and the TCR-CD3 complex are found to be closely associated at the juncture of the two interacting cells. The recent x-ray crystallographic analysis of a class II MHC molecule suggests that it may occur as a dimer of class II molecules on the membrane. If this turns out to be true, then T-cell recognition of antigen may involve a complex of two TCRs (and associated CD3), two CD4 molecules, and two class II MHC molecules (see Figure 9-9c). A complex of this sort may be crucial for signal transduction in T cells. This topic is presented in detail in Chapter 12.

Other Accessory Molecules

In addition to CD4 and CD8, T cells possess several other accessory membrane molecules including CD2, LFA-1, CD28, and CD45R. These molecules bind to ligands present on antigen-presenting cells or target cells (see Table 11-4) thereby strengthening the association between a T cell and an antigen-presenting cell or a target cell. As T cells are activated, the strength of adhesion between some of these accessory molecules and their respective ligands has been shown to increase. This increased avidity of a T cell for an antigen-presenting cell or target cell prolongs the association between the interacting cells, providing time for directed secretion of various cytokines or lytic enzymes (see Chapter 15). Some of these accessory molecules also function as signal-transducing molecules. The important role of these accessory molecules is demonstrated by the ability of monoclonal antibodies specific for these molecules to block T-cell activation.

TCR-Antigen-MHC Interaction

With the cloning and sequencing of the $\alpha\beta$ TCR heterodimer and the discovery of associated CD3, CD4, and CD8 molecules, researchers began to unravel the contribution of each of these molecules to recognition of antigen–MHC molecule complexes. The experiment of Kappler and Marrack outlined in Figure 11-1 supported the notion that a single receptor on the T cell recognizes antigen complexed to a self-MHC molecule. However, that experiment did not rule out the possibility that another membrane molecule, associated with the T-cell receptor, might contribute to the recognition of either antigen or MHC. A definitive experiment proving that the $\alpha\beta$ T-cell receptor alone recognizes both antigen and MHC molecules used an approach similar to that of the earlier Kappler and Marrack experiment but involved gene transfection instead of cell fusion. Functional TCR α- and β-chain genes from a T_C-cell clone specific for one hapten on H-2^d target cells were transfected into another T_C-cell clone specific for a second hapten on H-2^k target cells. The transfected cells expressed both their own T-cell receptor and the new transfected T-cell receptor. Cytolysis assays showed that the transfected cells recognized both hapten–MHC molecule complexes for which the original T_C clones were specific; however the transfected cells did not recognize either hapten when it was presented on target cells of a different MHC haplotype (Figure 11-9). In other words, transfection of the TCR genes alone transferred reactivity to both a particular antigen and particular MHC molecule.

Affinity of TCR for Antigen-MHC Complexes

Although the TCR-antigen-MHC interaction is central to development of both humoral and cell-mediated responses, very little is known about the nature of this

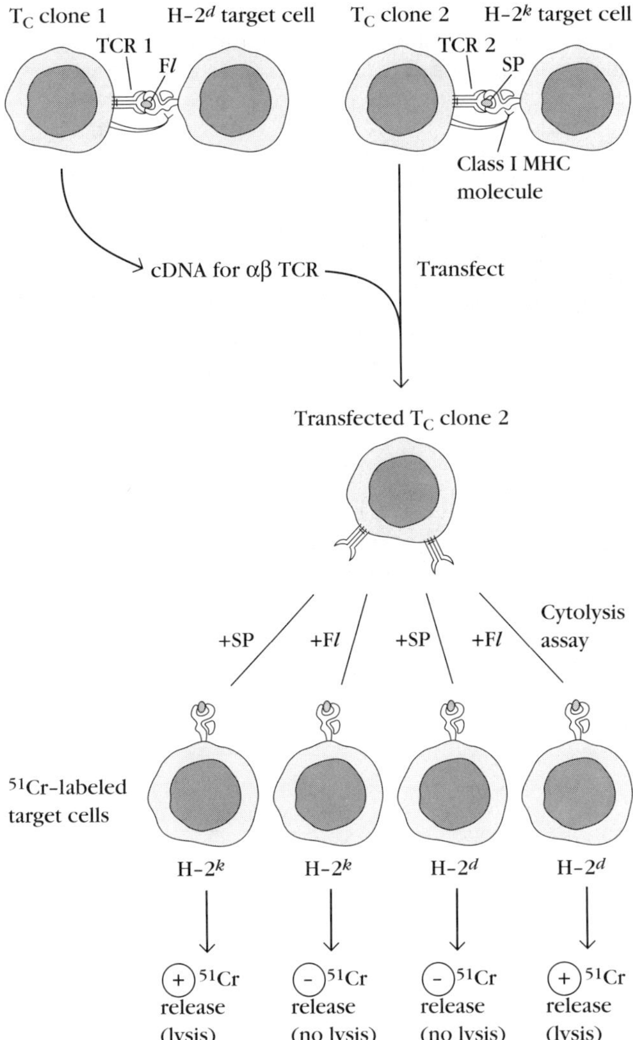

FIGURE 11-9 Experimental demonstration that the $\alpha\beta$ T-cell receptor alone recognizes both antigen and MHC molecules. cDNA corresponding to the $\alpha\beta$ T-cell receptor was prepared from T_C clone 1, which was specific for fluorescein (Fl) on H-2^d target cells. This cDNA was transfected into T_C clone 2, specific for 3-(*p*-sulphophenyldiazo)-4-hydroxy-phenylacetic acid (SP) on H-2^k target cells. The transfected cells were assayed for their ability to kill H-2^d or H-2^k target cells, labeled intracellularly with ^{51}Cr, in the presence of Fl or SP. The transfected cells could kill only those target cells presenting antigen associated with the original MHC restriction molecule.

trimolecular interaction. One obstacle to study of this interaction is that T-cell receptors and MHC molecules are membrane bound and are not expressed in a soluble form. An ingenious way of circumventing this obstacle is to engineer genes that encode glycolipid-anchored T-cell receptors or MHC molecules. Cells that contain such engineered genes express the glycolipid-anchored TCR or MHC molecules; both the T-cell receptors and MHC molecules can then be released in a soluble form by enzymatically cleaving them from their glycolipid membrane anchor.

K. Matsui, M. Davis, and their colleagues used this experimental approach to study the binding affinity of a T-cell receptor for a peptide-MHC complex. First they engineered a T_H-cell line with glycolipid-bound T-cell receptors specific for moth cytochrome *c* (MCC) bound to an IE^k MHC molecule. They demonstrated that the T-cell line could be activated by soluble MCC-IE^k complexes bound to a microtiter plate. (Activation was assayed by T-cell proliferation or IL-3 secretion.) The researchers then measured the ability of the MCC-IE^k complex to inhibit binding of a Fab fragment of a monoclonal antibody specific for the binding site of the T-cell receptor. From these competition studies they determined that the solubilized MCC-IE^k complex binds to the T-cell receptor with a K_d in the range of $4-6 \times 10^{-5}$ *M*. This is an incredibly weak interaction compared with the antigen-antibody interaction, which generally has a K_d ranging from 10^{-7} *M* to 10^{-11} *M*.

The low affinity of the T-cell receptor for antigenic peptide–MHC complexes suggests that binding of T cells to antigen-presenting cells and target cells does not depend solely on the TCR-peptide-MHC interaction. Instead, cell-adhesion molecules are thought to initiate the contact between a T cell and antigen-presenting cell or target cell. Once cell-to-cell contact is made, the T-cell receptor may scan the membrane for peptide-MHC complexes. During T-cell activation by a particular peptide-MHC complex, a transient increase in cell-adhesion molecules occurs, allowing close contact between the interacting cells so that cytokines or cytotoxic substances may be released at the junction between the cells. Within a short time of activation, the enhanced adhesion declines and the T cell detaches from the antigen-presenting cell or target cell.

TCR-Peptide Interaction

As discussed previously, a T-cell receptor recognizes a specific peptide only when it is bound to a specific MHC molecule. The high degree of TCR specificity for both antigenic peptides and MHC molecules must be achieved through the diversity of the variable region of the T-cell receptor. Although crystallographic analysis of the T-cell receptor has not been achieved as yet, the similarity between TCR and immunoglobulin genes suggests that the T-cell receptor resembles a Fab-like structure whose variable domains are folded in a β-pleated sheet structure with the CDRs facing outward. The most likely hypothesis is that the CDRs, the most diverse regions within the TCR variable domains, are involved in the TCR-peptide and TCR-MHC

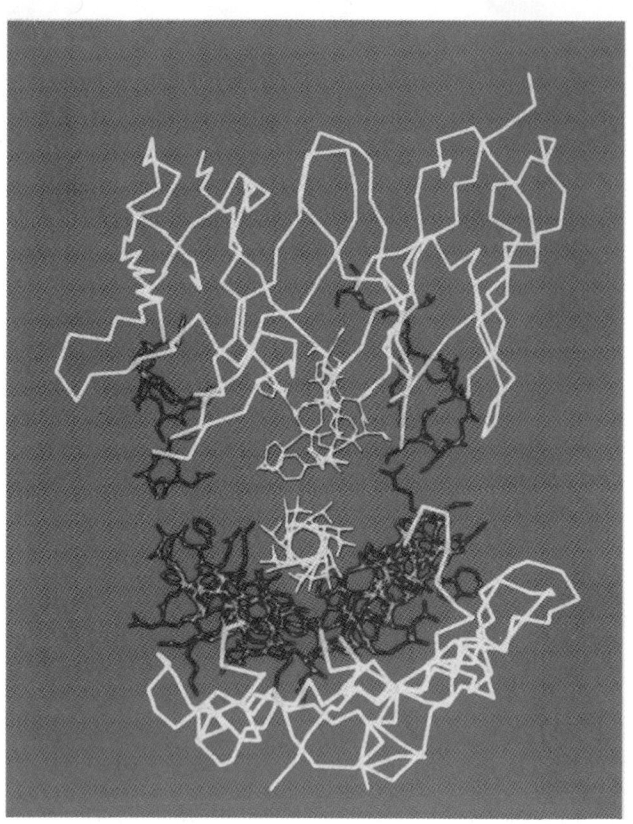

FIGURE 11-10 A computer model of the trimolecular complex involving a T-cell receptor, an antigenic peptide, and an MHC molecule. The foreign peptide *(middle)* contacts both the MHC molecule *(bottom)* and the T-cell receptor *(top),* which resembles the Fab portion of an antibody molecule. The T-cell receptor can be seen to contact amino acid residues in both the peptide and the MHC molecule. [Courtesy of M. M. Davis and P. J. Bjorkman, Stanford University.]

interactions (Figure 11-10). Evidence presented in this section and the next suggests that the two CDR3 loops interact with antigenic peptides, while the CDR1 and CDR2 loops are thought to interact with MHC molecules.

Various approaches have been used to determine which residues of a particular antigenic peptide are

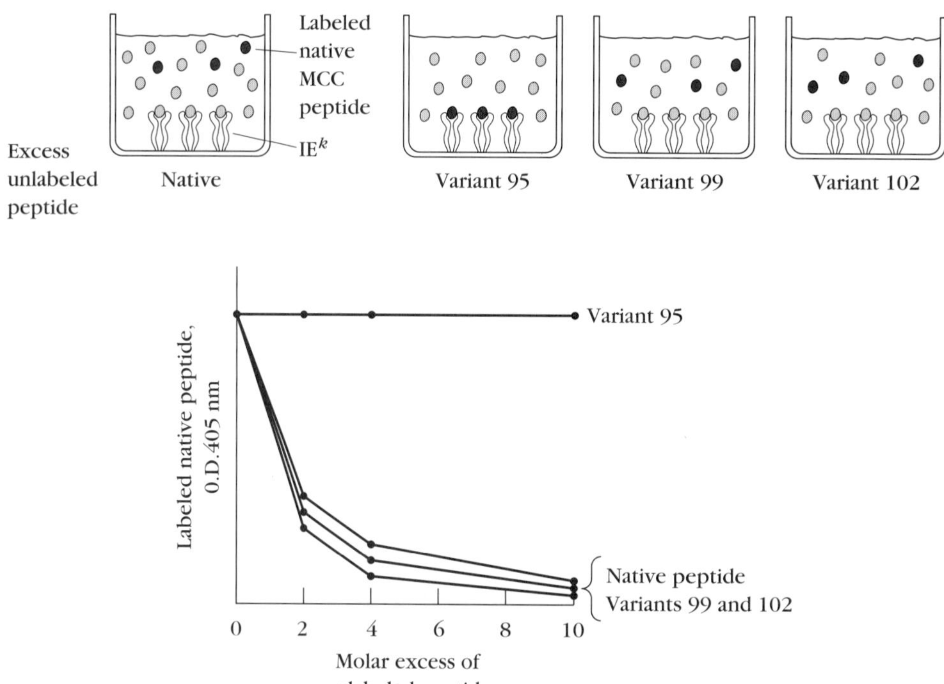

FIGURE 11-11 Binding competition experiments to identify amino acids in moth cytochrome *c* (MCC) that interact with the class II MHC molecule IE^k. The MCC peptide containing residues 88–103 activated an MCC-specific T_H-cell line. Labeled native MCC peptide (purple circles) was incubated, in microtiter wells containing bound IE^k, with excess amounts of three different unlabeled variant peptides containing single amino acid substitutions at position 95, 99, or 102 (grey circles). After the excess soluble peptides were removed, the amount of label bound to IE^k was determined. Variant 99 and 102 successfully competed with the native peptide, indicating that residues 99 and 102 are not involved in the MCC-IE^k interaction. In contrast, variant 95 did not compete with the native peptide; thus residue 95 is necessary for MCC binding to IE^k.

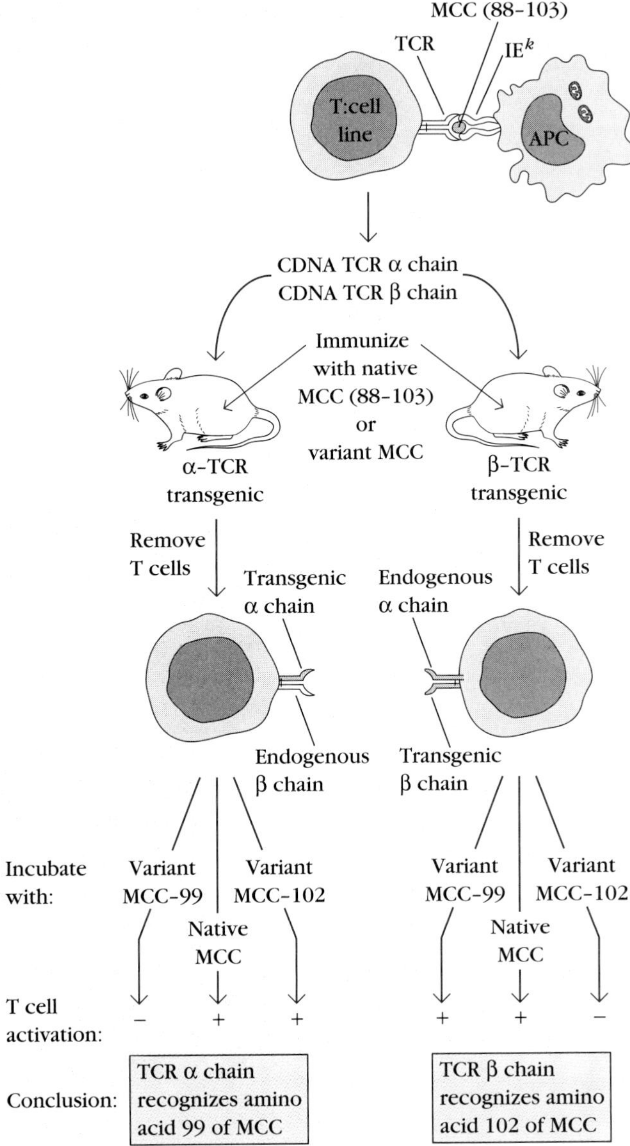

FIGURE 11-12 Experimental system for identifying which amino acids in moth cytochrome *c* (MCC) interact with the T-cell receptor. The variant MCC peptides contained a single amino acid substitution at either position 99 or 102. See text for discussion.

recognized by MHC molecules and by the T-cell receptor. To study this question, Matsui and co-workers first demonstrated that their T-cell line specific for moth cytochrome *c* (MCC) was activated by the MCC peptide containing residues 88–103 plus IE^k. They then synthesized several variants of this MCC peptide by substituting a negatively charged glutamic acid residue at position 95, 99, or 102. The native MCC peptide contained uncharged or positively charged residues at these positions. None of the three variant peptides was able to activate the MCC-specific T-cell line.

The binding studies illustrated in Figure 11-11 showed that the variant peptide with a substitution at position 95 was unable to bind to IE^k, whereas the variants with a substitution at position 99 or 102 were able to bind to IE^k. These findings suggest that position 95, but not positions 99 and 102, are critical in the interaction between MCC and the MHC molecule. Although the variant MCC peptides with substitutions at positions 99 and 102 could still bind to the MHC, they failed to activate the MCC-specific T-cell line, suggesting that these substitutions might interfere with binding to the T-cell receptor. To test this hypothesis, J. Jorgensen, M. Davis, and their colleagues used transgenic mice containing transgenes encoding either the TCR α chain or β chain from the MCC-specific T-cell line (Figure 11-12). More than 90% of the T cells in these transgenic mice expressed T-cell receptors containing one chain encoded by the transgene and the other chain encoded by the endogenous α or β gene. After the transgenic mice were immunized with the native MCC peptide or variant peptides, their spleen cells were isolated and assayed for T-cell activation. Both the α- and β-chain transgenics responded well to challenge with the native MCC, but their responses to the variant peptides differed. T cells from the α-chain transgenics proliferated in response to the peptide with a substitution at position 102 but not to the peptide with a substitution at position 99. In contrast, T cells from the β-chain transgenics showed the opposite response. These results suggest that the TCR α chain recognizes the amino acid at position 99 of the MCC peptide, whereas the β chain recognizes the amino acid at position 102.

The researchers next set out to determine the sequences of the endogenous TCR α and β chains expressed by the β-chain and α-chain transgenic mice, respectively. To do this, they prepared T-cell hybridomas using T cells isolated from the α- or β-chain transgenics that had been immunized with the native MCC peptide or with one of the variant peptides. After isolating the endogenous α- or β-chain mRNA, they converted it to cDNA, which was amplified by the polymerase chain reaction. Finally, they sequenced the variable regions of the α-chain and β-chain cDNA. The general picture to emerge from the sequencing data was that the TCR chains elicited in response to the native or variant MCC peptides often had reciprocally charged amino acid residues, and these residues were found to fall within the CDR3. These findings suggest that residues within the CDR3 loop of the T-cell receptor are specifically involved in interaction with antigenic peptides.

TCR-MHC Interaction

Although the evidence just discussed strongly suggests that CDR3 in the T-cell receptor makes direct contact with antigenic peptides, the interaction of the T-cell receptor and MHC molecules is less clearly defined. Several experimental approaches have been used to identify the interacting TCR and MHC residues. In one approach, P. Ajitkumar and co-workers carried out site-directed mutagenesis of a gene encoding a class I MHC molecule and transfected the resulting mutated MHC genes into target cells. The researchers then assessed the ability of T_C cells specific for the MHC molecule to kill the transfected cells. The results indicated that a single amino acid change in the exposed surface of the α helix the α_1 or α_2 domain directly affected the ability of T_C cells to lyse target cells for which they were specific. This finding suggests that the T-cell receptor recognizes amino acid residues of the α_1 and α_2 domains of class I MHC molecules (see Figure 9-6).

An ingenious study by Soon-Cheol Hong and his colleagues supports the hypothesis that CDR1 and CDR2 in the T-cell receptor interacts with MHC molecules. These researchers first cloned the TCR genes from two related T_H-cell clones whose T-cell receptors were shown to have identical β chains but to differ in all three CDRs of the α chain. They then engineered a chimeric TCR gene encoding an α chain whose amino-terminal half, which contains CDR1 and CDR2, was from clone 2 and whose carboxyl-terminal half, which contains CDR3, was from clone 1. This chimeric α-chain gene and the β-chain gene were then transfected into a TCR^- T-cell line, and the T-cell response of the transfected cells was compared with the response of clone 1 and clone 2. The results showed that a change in CDR1 or CDR2 (but not in CDR3) of the TCR α chain altered the specificity of MHC recognition by T cells.

E. W. Ehrlich and co-workers have obtained results suggesting that the TCR-MHC interaction may be quite fluid and that it can be influenced by the antigenic peptide. In their experiments they used T cells from transgenic mice expressing an $\alpha\beta$-TCR transgene that could cross-react with two peptides of moth cytochrome *c* differing from each other by a single amino acid substitution. They measured the responses of the transgenic T cells to each peptide presented by 13 mutant MHC molecules that differed from each other by a single amino acid predicted to be in the α helices of the MHC molecule and to point up toward the T-cell receptor. The results showed that the T-cell response to the mutant MHC molecules depended upon which peptide was being recognized. This finding suggests that the interaction between CDR3 and a peptide can affect the TCR-MHC interaction.

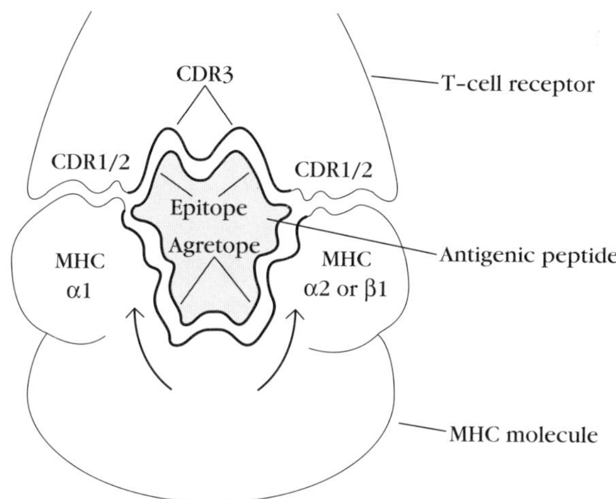

FIGURE 11-13 Schematic diagram showing the various sites in a T-cell receptor, antigenic peptide, and MHC molecule that interact in the TRC-peptide-MHC trimolecular complex. [Adapted from J. McCluskey et al., 1992, in *Antigen Processing and Recognition,* CRC Press.]

Model of TCR-Peptide-MHC Interaction

Figure 11-13 schematically illustrates the current model of the interaction between a T-cell receptor, antigenic peptide, and MHC molecule. The peptide-binding site of the T-cell receptor appears to map to CDR3, while CDR1 and CDR2 interact with MHC molecules. As discussed in Chapter 9, the peptide-binding site of the MHC molecule lies in a cleft between the α_1 and α_2 domains of class I molecules and between the α_1 and β_1 domains of class II molecules (see Figure 9-5). These same membrane-distal domains are involved in the interaction of MHC molecules with the T-cell receptor. The site on an antigenic peptide that interacts with a T-cell receptor is called the *epitope,* and the site that interacts with an MHC molecule is the *agretope.*

Alloreactivity of T Cells

So far the discussion of MHC molecules has focused on their role in antigen presentation. As noted in Chapter 9, however, MHC molecules were first identified because of their role in rejection of foreign tissue. Graft-rejection reactions result from the direct response of T cells to MHC molecules, which function as *histocompatibility antigens.* Because of the extreme polymorphism of the MHC, most individuals of the same species have a unique set of histocompatibility antigens.

Therefore, T cells respond even to allogeneic grafts *(alloreactivity),* and MHC molecules are considered *alloantigens.* Generally, $CD4^+$ T cells respond to class II alloantigens and $CD8^+$ T cells respond to class I alloantigens.

The alloreactivity of T cells is troubling for two reasons. First, the ability of T cells to respond to allogeneic histocompatibility antigens alone appears to contradict all the evidence indicating that T cells can respond only to foreign antigen plus self-MHC molecules. For example, in the Zinkernagle and Doherty experiment discussed in Chapter 10, T cells from a virus-infected mouse could kill syngeneic target cells infected with the same virus but not allogeneic target cells infected with the same virus (see Figure 10-2). The T cells were therefore shown to be self-MHC restricted. In responding to allogeneic grafts, however, T cells recognize a foreign MHC molecule directly, instead of responding to an antigen that has been processed and presented together with a self-MHC molecule. This would appear to contradict all that we have learned about T-cell specificity. A second problem posed by the T-cell response to allogeneic MHC molecules is that the frequency of alloreactive T cells is quite high; it has been estimated that 1–5% of all T cells are alloreactive, which is far higher than the frequency of T cells reactive with a particular foreign antigen plus self-MHC molecule. This finding is troubling because the high frequency of alloreactive T cells appears to contradict the basic tenet of clonal selection. If 1 T cell in 20 reacts with a given alloantigen and if one assumes there are on the order of 100 distinct H-2 haplotypes in mice, then there are not enough distinct T-cell specificities to cover all the unique H-2 alloantigens, let alone foreign antigens displayed by self-MHC molecules.

One possible biologically satisfying explanation for the high frequency of alloreactive T cells is that the T-cell receptor is indeed specific for foreign antigen plus a self-MHC molecule but that receptors can cross-react with certain allogeneic MHC molecules. In other words, if an allogeneic MHC molecule plus allogeneic peptide structurally resembles a processed foreign peptide plus self-MHC molecule, the same T-cell receptor may recognize both peptide-MHC complexes (Figure 11-14). Since allogeneic cells express on the order of 10^5 class I MHC molecules per cell, T cells bearing low-affinity cross-reactive receptors might be able to bind by virtue of the high density of membrane alloantigen. Foreign antigen, on the other hand, would be sparsely displayed on the membrane of an antigen-presenting cell or altered self-cell associated with class I or class II MHC molecules, limiting responsiveness to only those T cells bearing high-affinity receptors.

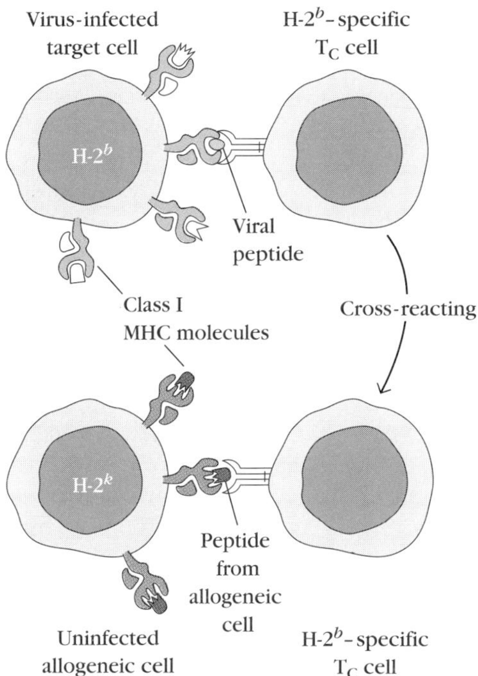

FIGURE 11-14 Possible mechanism of T-cell cross-reactivity that would explain the observed high incidence of alloreactive T cells. As schematically illustrated, a T-cell receptor specific for an H-2^b class I MHC molecule plus viral peptide cross-reacts with an allogeneic H-2^k class I molecule plus an allogeneic peptide.

Experimental evidence that antigen-specific T cells can also be alloreactive has come from studies with a number of T-cell clones. For example, after immunizing an H-2^a haplotype mouse with DNP-OVA, B. Sredni and R. H. Schwarz were able to obtain a T-cell clone that responded to DNP-OVA associated with a class II IA^a molecule. This same clone, however, also responded to allogeneic cells bearing IA^s in the absence of DNP-OVA. To determine the frequency of such antigen-specific and alloreactive T cells, Sredni and Schwarz immunized three congenic strains (B10.A, B10, and B10.S) with DNP-OVA and then isolated 20–40 antigen-specific clones from each strain. Each antigen-specific clone was then tested for alloreactivity against cells expressing different MHC haplotypes in the absence of antigen. Between 19 and 44% of the antigen-specific clones were able to respond to allogeneic cells. These findings support the hypothesis that the high percentage of alloreactive T cells reflects the existence of antigen-specific T cells whose receptor recognizes antigen plus a self-MHC molecule but can cross-react with various allogeneic MHC molecules.

Summary

1. T-cell receptors, unlike antibodies, do not react with soluble antigen but rather with processed antigen associated with a self-MHC molecule on an antigen-presenting cell or a target cell. T-cell receptors, first isolated by means of clonotypic monoclonal antibodies, are heterodimers consisting of an α and β chain or a γ and δ chain. Like the immunoglobulin heavy and light chains, the TCR chains have constant and variable regions.

2. TCR germ-line DNA is organized into multigene families corresponding to the α, β, γ, and δ chains. Each multigene family contains multiple variable-region gene segments (V and J in α- and γ-chain DNA and V, D, and J in β- and δ-chain DNA) and one or more constant-region C gene segments. By mechanisms similar to those used by B cells to rearrange immunoglobulin germ-line DNA, T cells rearrange the variable-region TCR gene segments to form functional genes encoding either the TCR α and β chains or γ and δ chains.

3. The mechanisms generating TCR diversity are generally similar to those generating antibody diversity. However, during rearrangement of TCR β- and δ-chain gene segments alternative joining of V, D, and J segments can occur and random nucleotides can be added at the junctions between gene segments encoding all the chains. Because of these mechanisms, the potential diversity of TCR genes is significantly greater than that of immunoglobulin genes, even though somatic mutation does not occur in TCR genes, as it does in immunoglobulin genes.

4. T-cell receptors are organized into variable and constant domains similar to those in immunoglobulins. The TCR variable-region domains are thought to be folded into the characteristic immunoglobulin-fold structure and contain three hypervariable complementarity-determining regions (CDRs), which appear to be equivalent to those in immunoglobulins. Each chain in a TCR molecule also contains a short membrane-proximal connecting region, a hydrophobic transmembrane segment, and a short cytoplasmic tail.

5. The T-cell receptor is closely associated with CD3, which is a complex of five different polypeptide chains that associate to form three dimers. Both the T-cell receptor and CD3 are coexpressed on the membrane of T cells. Following interaction of a T-cell receptor with an antigen-MHC complex, CD3 is thought to transduce the activation signal leading to T-cell proliferation and secretion of cytokines. The cytoplasmic tail of each CD3 chain contains a common sequence known as the antigen recognition activation motif (ARAM), which is involved in signal transduction. This same motif is present in the Ig-α/Ig-β heterodimer on B cells and in Fc receptors for IgE and IgG.

6. T cells possess several other membrane molecules that play accessory roles in antigen recognition and T-cell activation. These include the coreceptors CD4 and CD8, which bind to the membrane-proximal domains of MHC molecules, and strengthen the relatively weak interaction between the T-cell receptor and antigen-MHC complex. Other accessory membrane molecules include CD2, LFA-1, CD28, and CD45R.

7. Formation of the TCR-antigen-MHC complex, which is essential for an immune response, depends on several interactions. The antigen-binding site of the T-cell receptor maps to CDR3 and interacts with the epitope on the antigen. Sites in CDR1 and CDR2 of the T-cell receptor interact with the MHC membrane-distal domains. The antigen-binding cleft of the MHC molecule interacts with the agretope of the antigen.

8. T cells respond not only to foreign antigen–self-MHC complexes but also to foreign MHC molecules (histocompatibility antigens) alone. This T-cell response leads to rejection of allogeneic grafts. Some evidence suggests that this alloreactivity results from the ability of T cells specific for an antigen plus self-MHC molecule to cross-react with various allogeneic MHC molecules.

References

ALLISON, J. P., and W. L. HAVRAN. 1991. The immunobiology of T cells with invariant $\gamma\delta$ antigen receptors. *Annu. Rev. Immunol.* **9**:679.

DAVIS, M. M. 1990. T cell receptor gene diversity and selection. *Annu. Rev. Biochem.* **59**:475.

EHRLICH, E. W., B. DEVAUX, E. P. ROCK et al. 1993. T cell receptor interaction with peptide/major histocompatibility complex (MHC) and superantigen/MHC ligands is dominated by antigen. *J. Exp. Med.* **178**:713.

HEDRICK, S. M., D. I. COHEN, E. A. NIELSEN, and M. M. DAVIS. 1984. Isolation of cDNA clones encoding T cell-specific membrane associated proteins. *Nature* **308**:149.

HONG, S. C., A. CHELOUCHE, R. H. LIN et al. 1992. An MHC interaction site maps to the amino-terminal half of the T cell receptor α chain variable domain. *Cell* **69**:999.

JANEWAY, C. A. 1992. The T cell receptor as a multicomponent signalling machine: CD4/CD8 coreceptors and CD45 in T cell activation. *Annu. Rev. Immunol.* **10**:645.

JORGENSEN, J. L., U. ESSER, B. F. DE ST. GROTH et al. 1992. Mapping T-cell receptor-peptide contacts by variant peptide immunization of single-chain transgenics. *Nature* **355**:224.

JORGENSEN, J. L., P. A. REAY, E. W. EHRICH, and M. M. DAVIS. 1992. Molecular components of T-cell recognition. *Annu. Rev. Immunol.* **10**:835.

JULIUS, M., C. R. MAROUN, and L. HAUGH. 1993. Distinct roles for CD4 and CD8 as co-receptors in antigen receptor signalling. *Immunol. Today* **14**:177.

MALISSEN, M., J. TRUCY, E. JOUVIN-MARCHE et al. 1992. Regulation of TCR α and β gene allelic exclusion during T-cell development. *Immunol. Today* **13**:315.

MATIS, L. A. 1990. The molecular basis of T cell specificity. *Annu. Rev. Immunol.* **8**:65.

MATSUI, K., J. J. BONIFACE, P. A. REAY et al. 1991. Low affinity interaction of peptide-MHC complexes with T cell receptors. *Science* **254**:1788.

MOSS, P. A. H., W. M. C. ROSENBERG, and J. I. BELL. 1993. The human T cell receptor in health and disease. *Annu. Rev. Immunol.* **10**:71.

RAULET, D. H. 1989. The structure, function, and molecular genetics of the $\gamma\delta$ T cell receptor. *Annu. Rev. Immunol.* **7**:175.

Study Questions

1. Indicate whether each of the following statements is true or false. If you think a statement is false, explain why.
   a. Monoclonal antibody specific for CD4 will coprecipitate the T-cell receptor along with CD4.
   b. Subtractive hybridization can be used to enrich for mRNA that is present in one cell type but absent in another cell type within the same species.
   c. Clonotypic monoclonal antibody was used to isolate the T-cell receptor.
   d. The T cell uses the same set of V, D, and J gene segments as the B cell but uses different C gene segments.
   e. The $\alpha\beta$ TCR is bivalent and has two antigen-binding sites.

2. Describe the critical experiment that proved that the $\alpha\beta$ T-cell receptor alone recognizes both antigen and MHC molecules.

3. Draw the basic structure of the $\alpha\beta$ T-cell receptor indicating the polypeptide chains, domain structure, disulfide bonding, transmembrane region, cytoplasmic tails, variable region, and constant region.

4. Several membrane molecules, in addition to the T-cell receptor, are involved in antigen recognition and T-cell activation. Describe the properties and distinct functions of the following T-cell membrane molecules: (a) CD3, (b) CD4 and CD8, and (c) CD2.

5. Indicate whether each of the properties listed below applies to the T-cell receptor (TCR), B-cell immunoglobulin (Ig), or both (TCR/Ig).
   a. ____ Is associated with CD3
   b. ____ Is monovalent
   c. ____ Exists in membrane-bound and secreted forms
   d. ____ Contains domains with immunoglobulin fold
   e. ____ Is MHC restricted
   f. ____ Exhibits diversity generated by imprecise joining of gene segments
   g. ____ Exhibits diversity generated by somatic mutation

6. A major obstacle to identifying and cloning TCR genes is the low level of TCR mRNA in T cells.
   a. To overcome this obstacle, Hedrick and Davis made three important assumptions that proved to be correct. What were these assumptions and how did they facilitate identification of the genes encoding the T-cell receptor?
   b. Suppose, instead, that Hedrick and Davis wanted to identify the genes encoding IL-4. What changes in the three assumptions should they make?

7. Hedrick and Davis used the technique of subtractive hybridization to isolate cDNA clones encoding the T-cell receptor. You wish to use this technique to isolate cDNA clones encoding several gene products and have available clones of various cell types to use as the cDNA source or source of mRNA for hybridization. For each gene product (a–e), select the most appropriate cDNA source clone and corresponding mRNA source clone from the cell types listed below (1–8). More than one cell type may be correct in some cases.
   a. ____ IL-2
   b. ____ CD8
   c. ____ J chain
   d. ____ IL-1
   e. ____ CD3
   1) T_H1 cell line
   2) T_H2 cell line
   3) T_C cell line
   4) Macrophage
   5) IgA-secreting myeloma cell
   6) IgG-secreting myeloma cell
   7) Myeloid progenitor cell
   8) B cell line

8. Mice from different inbred strains listed in the *left* column of the table below have been infected with LCM virus. Spleen cells derived from these LCM-infected mice are then tested for their ability to lyse LCM-infected ^{51}Cr-labeled target cells from the strains *listed across the top of the table.* Indicate with (+) or (−) whether you would expect to see ^{51}Cr released from the labeled target cells.

For use with Question 8.

Source of spleen cells from LCM-infected mice	Release of ^{51}Cr from LCM-infected target cells			
	B10.D2 (H-2^d)	B10 (H-2^b)	B10.BR (H-2^k)	F_1 (BALB/c × B10) (H-$2^{b/d}$)
B10.D2(H-2^d)				
B10 (H-2^b)				
BALB/c (H-2^d)				
BALB/b (H-2^b)				

T-CELL MATURATION, ACTIVATION, AND DIFFERENTIATION

The attribute that distinguishes antigen recognition by T cells from that by B cells is MHC restriction. Both the maturation of progenitor T cells in the thymus and the activation of mature peripheral T cells are influenced by the involvement of MHC molecules. The potential antigenic diversity of T cells is reduced during maturation by a selection process that allows only MHC-restricted and nonself-reactive T cells to mature. The final stages in T-cell maturation proceed along two different developmental pathways, which generate functionally distinct $CD4^+$ and $CD8^+$ subpopulations that exhibit class II and class I MHC restriction, respectively.

Activation of mature peripheral T cells is initiated through the interaction of the T-cell receptor with an antigenic peptide displayed in the groove of an MHC molecule. The low affinity of this interaction necessitates the involvement of coreceptors and other accessory membrane molecules that function to strengthen the TCR-antigen-MHC interaction and to transduce the activating signal. Activation leads to the proliferation and differentiation of T cells into various types of effector cells and memory T cells. Because the vast majority of thymocytes and peripheral T cells express the $\alpha\beta$ T-cell receptor, all references to T cells and the T-cell receptor in this chapter denote the $\alpha\beta$ receptor unless otherwise indicated.

T-Cell Maturation

Progenitor T cells from the bone marrow begin to migrate to the thymus at about day 11 of gestation in mice and in the eighth or ninth week of gestation in humans. The progenitor cells are attracted to the thymus by a chemotactic factor secreted by thymic epithelial cells. In a manner similar to B-cell differentiation in the bone marrow, differentiation of progenitor T cells is correlated with rearrangements of the germ-line TCR genes and expression of various membrane markers. In contrast to B-cell development, however, thymocytes proliferate and differentiate along several different developmental pathways, these pathways generate functionally distinct subpopulations of mature T cells (Figure 12-1).

T-Cell Developmental Pathways

Changes in various membrane molecules and TCR-gene rearrangements during thymocyte development in the mouse have been studied with monoclonal antibodies and restriction-endonuclease analyses of genomic DNA. Upon entry into the thymus, progenitor T cells begin to express a membrane marker called Thy-1, which is a marker of all thymus-derived lymphocytes in the mouse. The earliest fetal thymocytes lack detectable CD4 and CD8 and are referred to as *double-negative* cells. These double-negative thymocytes differentiate along one of two developmental pathways. Those thymocytes that make productive rearrangements of both the γ- and δ-chain genes develop into double-negative, CD3$^+$ $\gamma\delta$ T cells, which account for

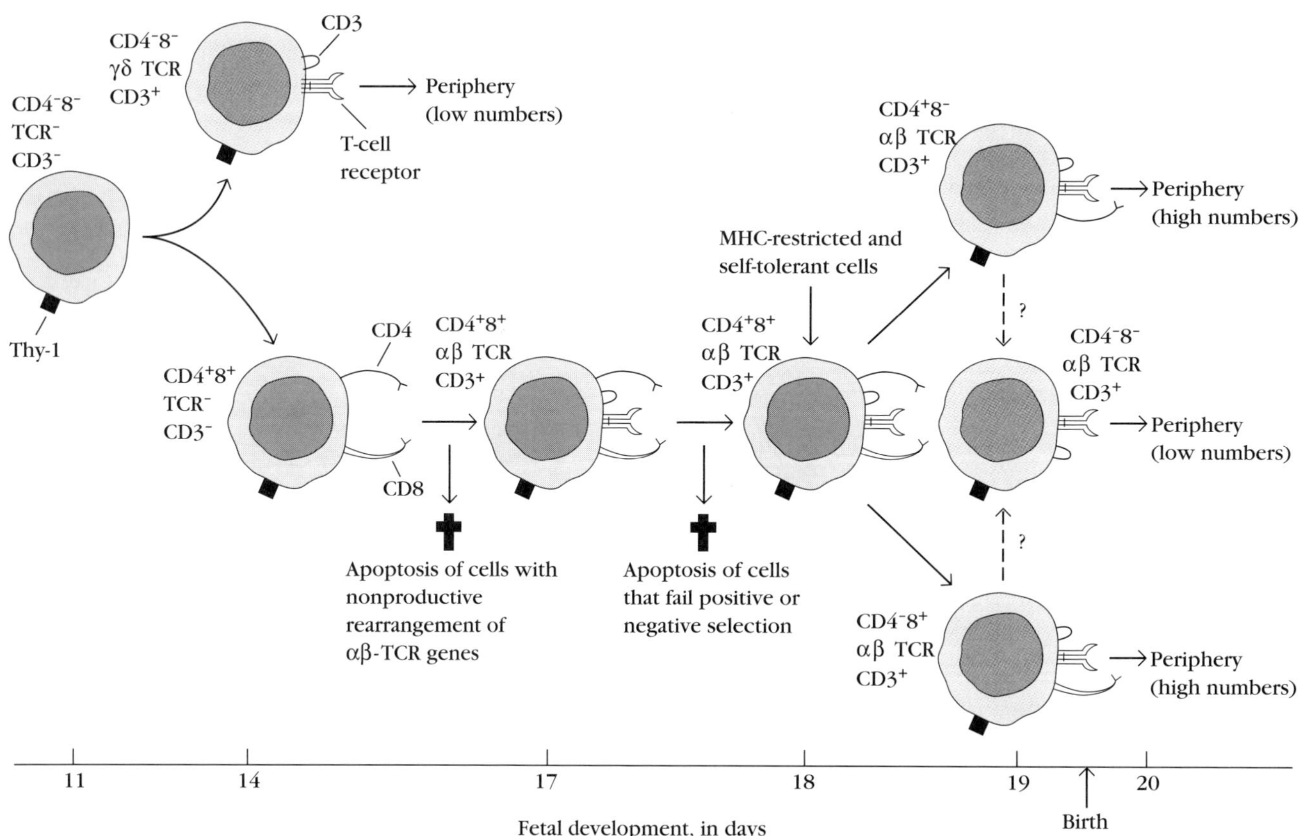

FIGURE 12-1 Proposed pathways for T-cell development in the thymus. Most of the immature thymocytes in the thymus die because they make an unproductive TCR-gene rearrangement or fail positive or negative selection. Four mature T-cell populations (purple) are produced and move to the peripheral lymphoid organs. The vast majority of peripheral T cells express the $\alpha\beta$ T-cell receptor and either CD4 or CD8. [Adapted from B. J. Fowlkes and D. M. Pardoll, 1989, *Adv. Immunol.* **44**:207.]

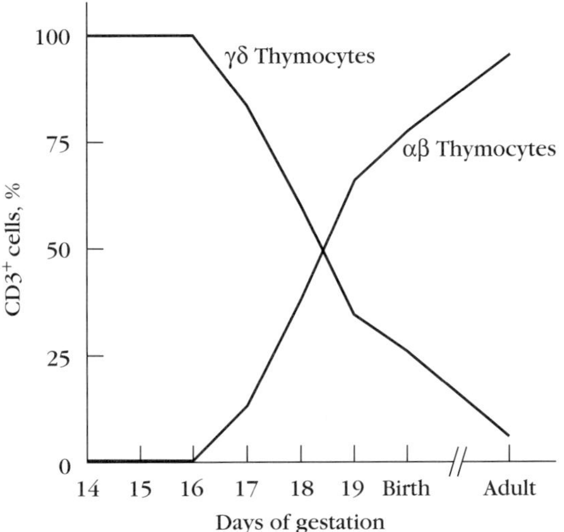

FIGURE 12-2 Time course of appearance of $\gamma\delta$ thymocytes and $\alpha\beta$ thymocytes during mouse fetal development. The graph shows the percentage of $CD3^+$ cells in the thymus that are double-negative ($CD4^-8^-$) and bear the $\gamma\delta$ T-cell receptor (black) or are double-positive ($CD4^+8^+$) and bear the $\alpha\beta$ T-cell receptor (purple).

only 0.5 – 1.0% of thymocytes. This thymocyte subpopulation can be detected by day 14 of gestation, reaches maximal numbers between days 17 and 18, and then declines until birth (Figure 12-2). The majority of double-negative thymocytes progress down a different developmental pathway. They begin to rearrange the TCR β-chain genes and to express both CD4 and CD8 membrane molecules. At day 16 of gestation, these *double-positive* cells can first be detected expressing both CD4 and CD8 but not CD3 or the $\alpha\beta$ T-cell receptor. The TCR α-chain genes are not expressed until day 16 or 17, and double-positive cells expressing both CD3 and the $\alpha\beta$ T-cell receptor begin to appear at day 17 and reach maximal levels about the time of birth.

An estimated 99% of all thymocytes do not mature and die by apoptosis within the thymus either because they fail to make a productive TCR-gene rearrangement or because they fail to survive thymic selection, which is discussed below. Double-positive thymocytes that express the $\alpha\beta$ TCR-CD3 complex and survive thymic selection develop into either single-positive $CD4^+$ thymocytes, representing 10% of the total thymocyte population, or single-positive $CD8^+$ thymocytes, representing 5% of the total thymocyte population (Table 12-1). In addition, a small population (0.5%) of double-negative thymocytes expressing the TCR-CD3 complex can also be detected. These cells appear late in development, usually within 5 days following birth. The origin of this population is uncertain, but it may develop from the single-positive populations through the loss of either CD4 or CD8.

Thymic Selection of the T-Cell Repertoire

As shown in Table 11-3, random gene rearrangement within TCR germ-line DNA combined with junctional diversity can potentially generate an enormous TCR repertoire with an estimated diversity exceeding 10^{15} for the $\alpha\beta$ receptor and 10^{18} for the $\gamma\delta$ receptor. The gene products encoded by the rearranged TCR genes do not generally have an inherent affinity for foreign antigen plus a self-MHC molecule, and theoretically should be capable of recognizing soluble antigen, self-MHC molecules, self-antigen, or antigen plus a nonself-MHC molecule. Nonetheless, the most distinctive property of mature T cells is that they only recognize foreign antigen associated with self-MHC molecules.

Clearly, in some way thymocytes that undergo productive TCR-gene rearrangement must be "selected" so that only a subset of thymocytes whose receptors are capable of binding antigen plus self-MHC molecules are permitted to mature. By processes discussed in detail later, *positive selection* eliminates thymocytes whose receptor fails to recognize self-MHC molecules. Also eliminated, by *negative selection,* are thymocytes bearing a high-affinity receptor for self-MHC molecules alone or self-antigen plus self-MHC molecules; such thymocytes would pose the threat of an autoimmune response if they matured. As noted already, some 99% of all thymocyte progeny die by apoptosis within the thymus. This high death rate is thought to reflect the weeding out of all thymocytes whose receptors do not specifically recognize foreign antigen plus self-MHC molecules.

Early evidence for the role of the thymus in selection of the T-cell repertoire came from chimeric mouse experiments by R. M. Zinkernagel and his colleagues (Figure 12-3). These researchers implanted

TABLE 12-1 DISTRIBUTION OF MOUSE THYMOCYTE SUBPOPULATIONS

Thymocyte subpopulations			Relative %
$CD4^-8^-$	TCR^-	$CD3^-$	4
$CD4^+8^+$	TCR^-	$CD3^-$	40
$CD4^-8^-$	$\gamma\delta$ TCR^+	$CD3^+$	0.5
$CD4^+8^+$	$\alpha\beta$ TCR^+	$CD3^+$	40
$CD4^+8^-$	$\alpha\beta$ TCR^+	$CD3^+$	10
$CD4^-8^+$	$\alpha\beta$ TCR^+	$CD3^+$	5
$CD4^-8^-$	$\alpha\beta$ TCR^+	$CD3^+$	0.5

thymectomized and lethally irradiated F_1 (A × B) mice with a B-type thymus and then reconstituted the animal's immune system with an intravenous infusion of F_1 bone marrow cells. To be certain that the thymus graft did not contain any mature T cells, it was irradiated before being transplanted. In such an experimental system, pre-T cells from the F_1 (A × B) bone marrow mature within a thymus expressing only B-haplotype MHC molecules on its stromal cells. Would these F_1 (A × B) T cells now be MHC-restricted for the haplotype of the thymus? To answer this question, the chimeric mice were infected with LCM virus and the mature T cells were then tested for their ability to kill LCM-infected target cells from strain A or strain B mice. As shown in Figure 12-3, T_C cells from the chimeric mice could lyse only LCM-infected target cells bearing the same MHC haplotype as the implanted thymus. Apparently the implanted thymus had selected for maturation only T cells having receptors capable of recognizing antigen in association with the MHC haplotype of the thymus.

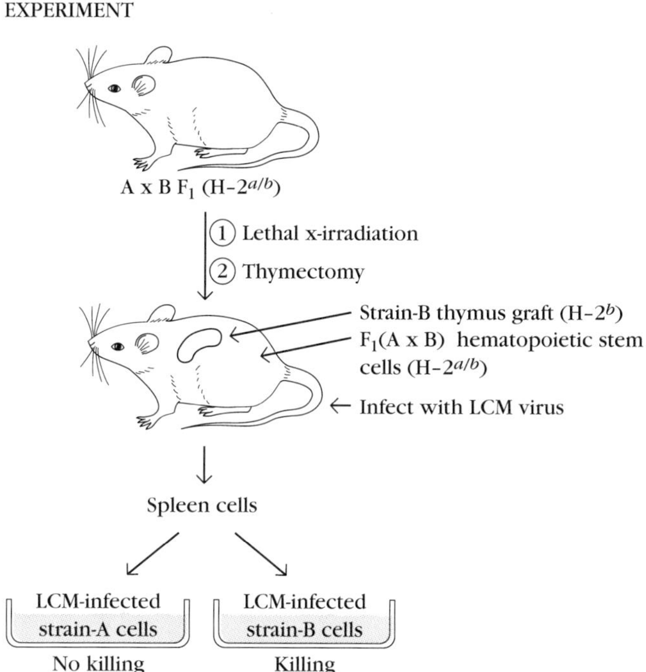

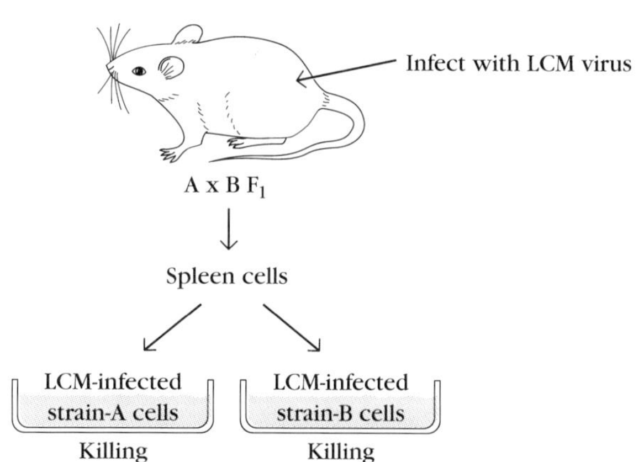

FIGURE 12-3 Experimental demonstration that the thymus selects only those T cells for maturation whose T-cell receptors recognize antigen presented on target cells with the haplotype of the thymus. Lethally irradiated and thymectomized F_1(A × B) mice were grafted with a strain-B thymus and reconstituted with F_1(A × B) bone marrow cells. Following infection with the LCM virus, the CTL cells were assayed for their ability to kill ^{51}Cr-labeled strain-A or strain-B target cells infected with the LCM virus. Only strain-B target cells were lysed, suggesting that the H-2^b grafted thymus had selected for maturation only those T cells that could recognize antigen in association with H-2^b MHC molecules.

Positive and Negative Thymic Selection

The selection of TCR specificity in the thymus is thought to involve two processes: (1) positive selection of thymocytes bearing receptors capable of binding self-MHC molecules, which results in *MHC restriction,* and (2) negative selection by elimination of thymocytes bearing high-affinity receptors for self-MHC molecules alone or self-antigen presented by self-MHC, which results in *self-tolerance* (Figure 12-4). Both processes are necessary to generate mature T cells that are self-MHC restricted and self-tolerant. Thymic stromal cells, including epithelial cells, macrophages, and dendritic cells, are thought to play a role in positive and negative selection. These thymic stromal cells express high levels of class I and class II MHC molecules. Immature thymocytes expressing the TCR-CD3 complex are thought to interact with these thymic stromal cells, leading to positive and negative selection by mechanisms that are not fully understood.

Positive selection appears to involve an interaction of immature thymocytes with epithelial cells in the cortex of the thymus. Electron micrographs reveal close contact between thymocytes and epithelial cells within the thymic cortex, and there is evidence that the T-cell receptors tend to cluster at sites of contact. Some researchers have suggested that the interaction of immature $CD4^+$, $CD8^+$ thymocytes with thymic epithelial cells, mediated by MHC-restricted T-cell receptors, might allow the cells to receive some kind of protective signal; cells whose receptors are not MHC restricted would not interact with the thymic epithelial

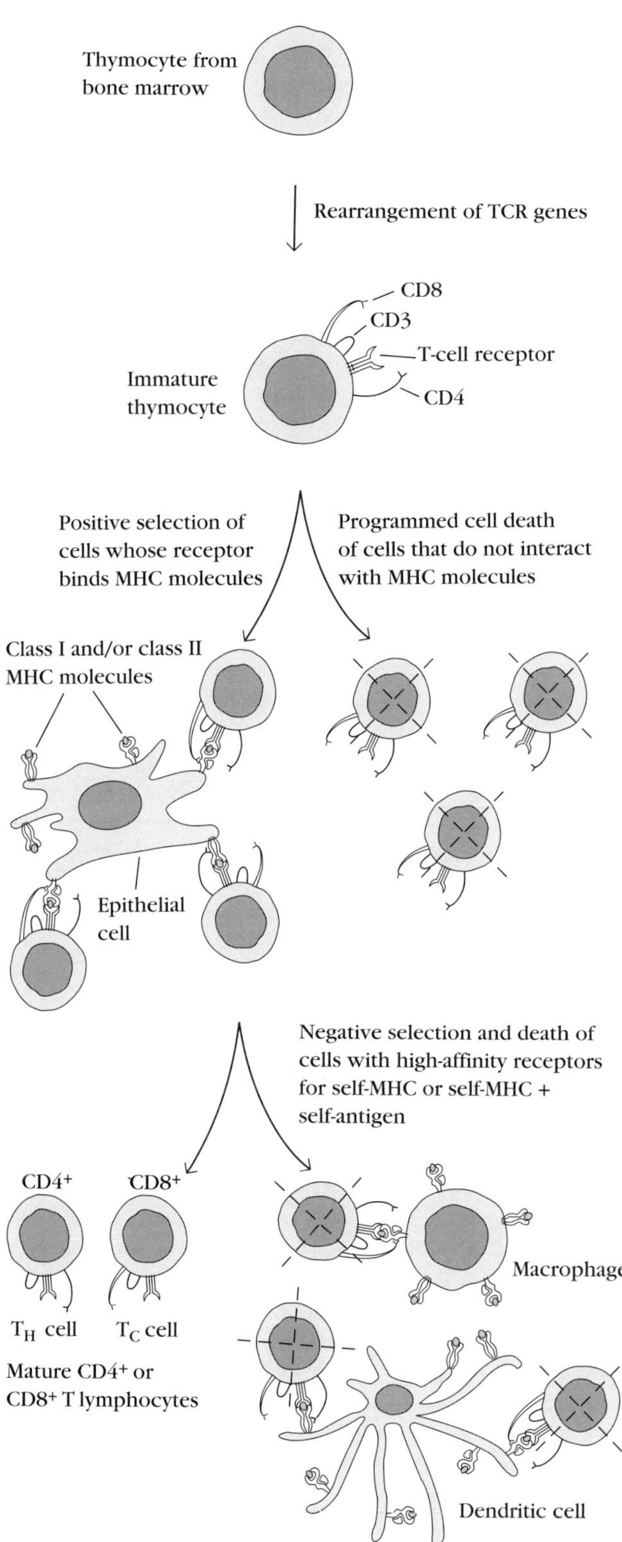

FIGURE 12-4 Positive and negative selection of thymocytes in the thymus. Because of thymic selection, which involves thymic stromal cells (epithelial cells, dendritic cells, and macrophages), mature T cells are both self-MHC restricted and self-tolerant.

cells and would consequently not receive the protective signal, leading to programmed cell death by apoptosis (see Figure 3-3).

The population of MHC-restricted thymocytes that survive positive selection comprises some cells with low-affinity receptors for self-antigen presented by self-MHC molecules and other cells with high-affinity receptors. The latter thymocytes undergo negative selection, which most probably occurs within the thymic medulla, although some evidence suggests it may also occur within the thymic cortex. During negative selection, bone marrow–derived cells (dendritic cells and macrophages) bearing class I and class II MHC molecules are thought to interact with thymocytes bearing high-affinity receptors for self-antigen plus self-MHC molecules or self-MHC molecules alone. Tolerance to self-antigens is thereby achieved by eliminating T cells that are self-reactive and only allowing maturation of T cells specific for foreign antigen plus self-MHC molecules *(altered self)*. The nature of the interaction leading to negative selection is not known, but the selected cells are observed to undergo death by apoptosis.

Experimental Evidence for Positive Selection

Ada Kruisbeek obtained experimental evidence suggesting that binding of thymocytes to class I or class II MHC molecules within the thymus leads to positive selection of MHC-restricted T cells. In her experiments, mouse fetal thymic tissue was grown in tissue-culture media containing high concentrations of monoclonal antibody to either the class I or class II MHC molecules expressed by the thymic cells (Figure 12-5). Analysis of the T cells from these fetal thymic organ cultures revealed the absence of $CD4^+$ T cells in cultures grown with anti-class II monoclonal antibody and the absence of $CD8^+$ T cells in cultures grown with anti-class I monoclonal antibody. Similarly, injection of neonatal mice with anti-class II antibody prevented the development of $CD4^+$ T cells and injection of anti-class I antibody prevented the development of $CD8^+$ T cells. Thus development of these two thymocyte subpopulations correlates with the ability to recognize either class I or class II MHC molecules in the thymus. Taken together, these experiments suggest that positive selection of the $CD4^+$ or $CD8^+$ cells requires interaction of thymocytes with class I or class II MHC molecules. If the class I or class II MHC molecules are blocked by antibody, developing thymocytes cannot bind to the self-MHC molecules on the thymic stromal cells and are not positively selected.

Further support that binding of thymocytes to class I or class II MHC molecules is required for positive selection in the thymus came from more recent experi-

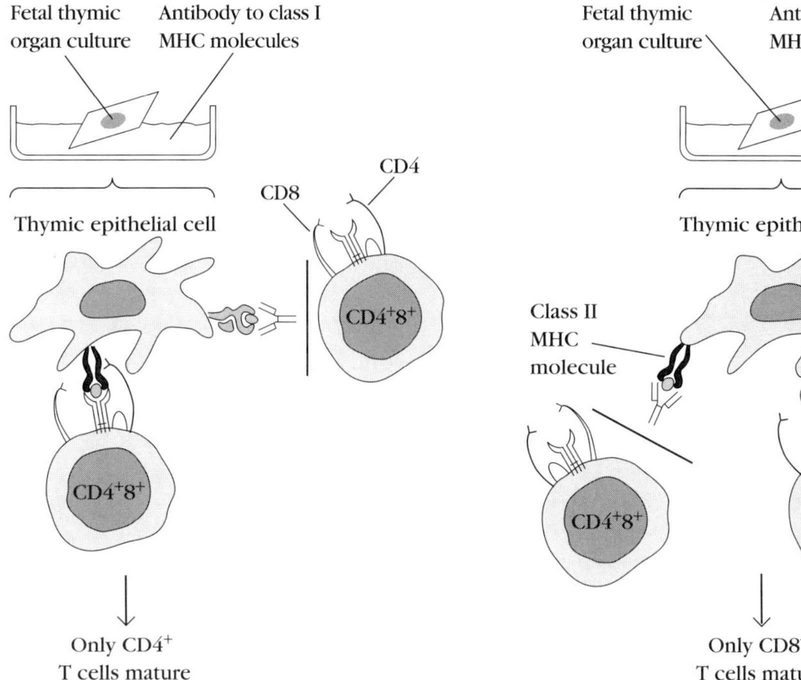

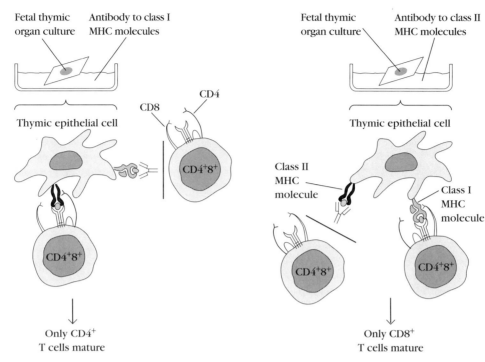

FIGURE 12-5 Experimental demonstration that acquisition of MHC restriction depends on interaction of immature thymocytes with class I or class II MHC molecules on thymic epithelial cells. See text for discussion.

mental studies with knock-out mice lacking a gene for class I or class II MHC molecules. Knock-out of the β_2-microglobulin gene resulted in class I–deficient mice. These mice were found to have a normal distribution of $\gamma\delta$ T cells and had double-positive ($CD4^+8^+$) $\alpha\beta$ thymocytes and $CD4^+$ T cells but failed to produce $CD8^+$ T cells. A similar technique was used to produce class II MHC–deficient mice. In this case, H-2^b haplotype mice were used because these mice have a deletion of the *IEβ* gene and therefore do not express class II IE molecules. Knock out of the *IAβ* gene thus rendered these mice class II deficient. FACS analysis revealed that the thymus of these class II–deficient mice had $CD4^+8^+$ and $CD8^+$ thymocytes but lacked $CD4^+$ thymocytes (Figure 12-6). Similarly, the lymph nodes of these class II–deficient mice lacked $CD4^+$ T cells. Thus the absence of class II MHC molecules prevented positive selection of $CD4^+$ T cells.

Additional evidence that interaction with MHC molecules plays a role in positive selection came from experiments with transgenic mice depicted in Figure 12-7. In these experiments rearranged $\alpha\beta$-TCR genes derived from a $CD8^+$ T-cell clone specific for influenza antigen plus H-2^k class I MHC molecules were injected into fertilized eggs from two different mouse strains, one with the H-2^k haplotype and one with the H-2^d haplotype. Since the receptor transgenes were already rearranged, other TCR-gene rearrangements were suppressed in the transgenic mice; therefore, a high percentage of the thymocytes in the transgenic mice

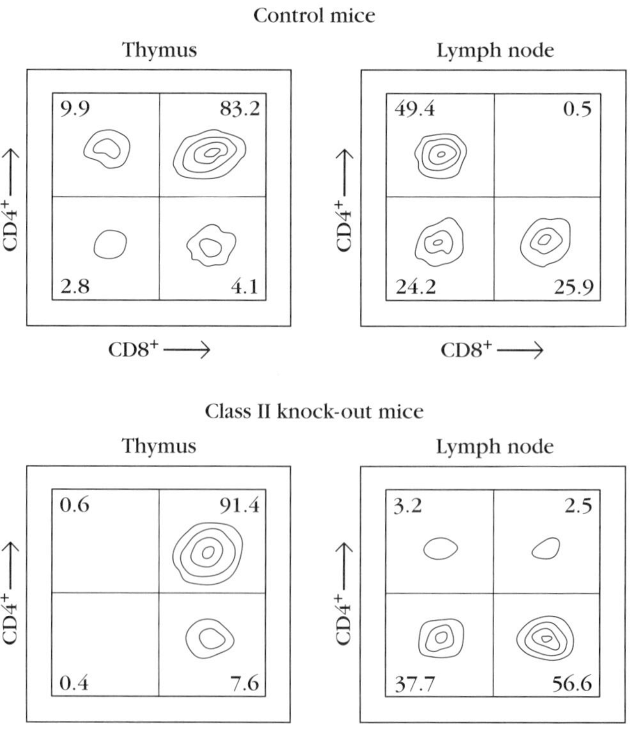

FIGURE 12-6 FACS analysis of thymocytes and peripheral lymph-node T cells from normal mice and knock-out mice lacking class II MHC molecules. Note the large decrease in $CD4^+$ cells in the knock-out mice. The percentage of staining cells is listed in each quadrant.

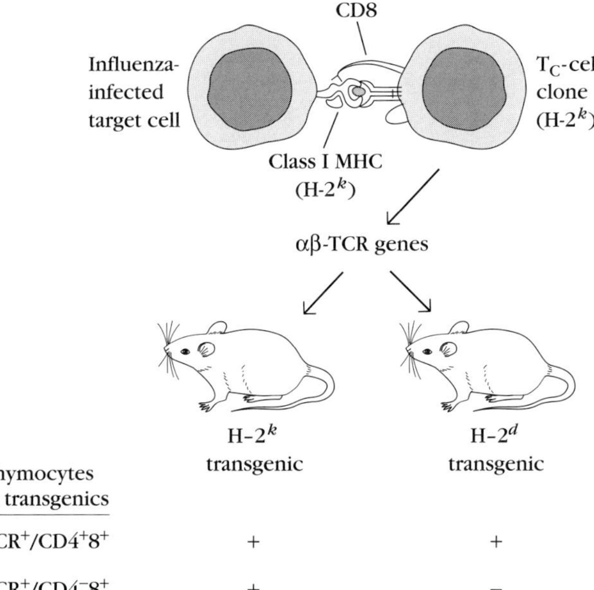

FIGURE 12-7 Effect of host haplotype on T-cell maturation in mice carrying transgenes encoding an H-2^k class I-restricted T-cell receptor specific for influenza virus. The presence of the rearranged TCR transgenes suppressed other gene rearrangements in the transgenics; therefore, most of the thymocytes in the transgenics expressed the $\alpha\beta$ T-cell receptor encoded by the transgene. Immature double-positive thymocytes matured into $CD8^+$ T cells only in transgenics with the haplotype (H-2^k) corresponding to the MHC restriction of the TCR transgene.

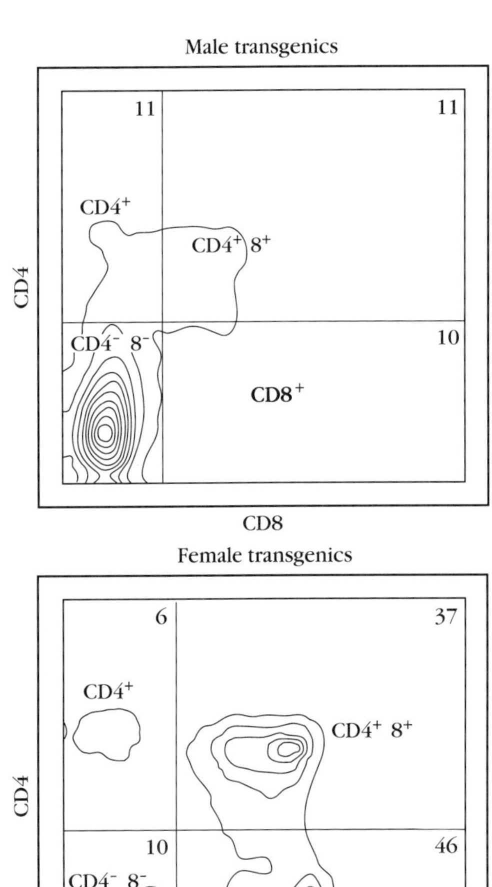

FIGURE 12-8 FACS analysis of thymocytes from H-2^b transgenic mice carrying a transgene that encodes an $\alpha\beta$ T-cell receptor specific for male H-Y antigen plus an H-2^b class I MHC molecule. As the plots show, mature $CD8^+$ T cells expressing the transgene were absent in the male mice but present in the female mice, suggesting that thymocytes reactive with a self-antigen (in this case, H-Y antigen in the male mice) are deleted during thymic selection. Numbers in quadrants refer to percentages of cells. [Adapted from H. von Boehmer and P. Kisielow, 1990, *Science* **248**:1370.]

expressed the T-cell receptor encoded by the transgene. Thymocytes expressing the TCR transgene were found to mature into $CD8^+$ T cells only in the transgenic mice with the H-2^k class I MHC haplotype (i.e., the haplotype for which the transgene receptor was restricted). In transgenic mice with a different MHC haplotype (H-2^d), immature, double-positive thymocytes expressing the transgene were present, but these thymocytes failed to mature into $CD8^+$ T cells. These findings also suggest that interaction between T-cell receptors on immature thymocytes and self-MHC molecules is required for positive selection. In the absence of self-MHC molecules, as in the H-2^d transgenic mice, positive selection and subsequent maturation do not occur.

Experimental Evidence for Negative Selection

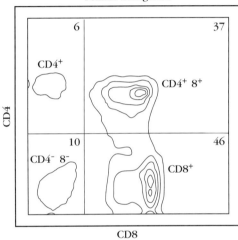

Evidence for deletion of thymocytes reactive with self-antigen plus MHC molecules has been accumulating in a number of diverse experimental systems. In one system thymocyte maturation was analyzed in transgenic mice bearing an $\alpha\beta$-TCR transgene specific for the H-Y antigen plus class I D^b MHC molecules. The H-Y antigen is encoded on the Y chromosome and therefore is expressed in male mice but not in female mice. In this experiment, the MHC haplotype of the transgenic mice was H-2^b, the same as the MHC restriction of the transgene-encoded receptor. Therefore any differences in the selection of thymocytes in male and female transgenics would be related to the presence or absence of H-Y antigen. Analysis of thymocytes in the transgenic mice revealed that female mice contained thymocytes expressing the H-Y–specific TCR transgene, but male mice did not (Figure 12-8). In other words, H-Y–reactive thymocytes were self-reactive in the male mice and were eliminated. However, in the female transgenics, which did not express the H-Y antigen, these cells were not self-reactive and thus were not eliminated. When thymocytes from these male transgenic mice were cultured in vitro with antigen-presenting cells expressing the H-Y antigen, the thymocytes were observed to undergo apoptosis, providing a striking example of this process.

Superantigen systems have also been quite useful in demonstrating negative selection. Superantigens are molecules that bind simultaneously to the V_β domain of the T-cell receptor and to a class II MHC molecule (see Figure 4-15). Because superantigens bind outside of the TCR antigen-binding cleft, any T cell expressing a particular V_β sequence will be activated by a particular superantigen. Mice have about 20 V_β gene segments and therefore, assuming equal frequency of expression, about 1 in 20 T cells (roughly 5%) will express a given V_β domain in their T-cell receptors and respond to a particular superantigen. If a superantigen is present during thymic processing, it should facilitate binding of all thymocytes bearing a TCR V_β domain corresponding to the superantigen specificity to thymic stromal cells, leading to deletion of those thymocytes. Such massive deletion creates what is commonly called "holes in the repertoire," characterized by the absence of all T cells whose receptors possess a particular V_β domain.

Both exogenous and endogenous superantigens have been identified. Exogenous superantigens include a variety of exotoxins secreted by gram-positive bacteria, such as staphylococcal enterotoxins, toxic-shock syndrome toxin, and exfoliative dermatitis toxin; mycoplasma arthritidis supernatant; and streptococcal pyrogenic exotoxins. Each of these exogenous superantigens binds particular V_β sequences in T-cell receptors (Table 12-2).

Evidence that an exogenous superantigen can induce negative selection of a subset of thymocytes expressing receptors with a particular V_β was obtained by injecting neonatal mice with staphylococcal enterotoxin B (SEB), which binds to virtually all T cells bearing receptors with $V_\beta 3$ or $V_\beta 8$. Thymocytes from SEB-injected mice and noninjected controls then were stained with monoclonal antibody specific for $V_\beta 3$ or $V_\beta 8$. These analyses revealed a slight reduction in immature (double-positive) thymocytes and a dramatic reduction in mature (single-positive) thymocytes bearing $V_\beta 3$ or $V_\beta 8$ in the injected mice compared with controls (Table 12-3).

Endogenous superantigens are produced by the animal, and the genes encoding them are carried within

TABLE 12-2 EXOGENOUS SUPERANTIGENS AND THEIR V_β SPECIFICITY

		V_β Specificity	
Superantigen	Disease*	Mouse	Human
Staphylococcal products			
Enterotoxins			
SEA	Food poisoning	1, 3, 10, 11, 12, 17	nd
SEB	Food poisoning	3, 8.1, 8.2, 8.3	3, 12, 14, 15, 17, 20
SEC1	Food poisoning	7, 8.2, 8.3, 11	12
SEC2	Food poisoning	8.2, 10	12, 13, 14, 15, 17, 20
SEC3	Food poisoning	7, 8.2	5, 12
SED	Food poisoning	3, 7, 8.3, 11, 17	5, 12
SEE	Food poisoning	11, 15, 17	5.1, 6.1–6.3, 8, 18
Toxic-shock syndrome toxin (TSST1)	Toxic-shock syndrome	15, 16	2
Exfoliative dermatitis toxin (ExFT)	Scalded-skin syndrome	10, 11, 15	2
Mycoplasma arthritidis supernatant (MAS)	Arthritis, shock	6, 8.1–8.3	nd
Streptococcal pyrogenic exotoxins (SPE-A, B, C, D)	Rheumatic fever, shock	nd	nd

* Disease results from infection by bacteria producing the indicated superantigens.

TABLE 12-3 NEGATIVE SELECTION OF $\alpha\beta$ THYMOCYTES BEARING $V_\beta 3$ AND $V_\beta 8$ FOLLOWING NEONATAL INJECTION OF AN EXOGENOUS SUPERANTIGEN (SEB)*

	Percentage of thymocytes expressing V_β								
	Immature thymocytes Day 15			Mature thymocytes Day 10			Mature thymocytes Day 15		
SEB (μg)	$V_\beta 3$	$V_\beta 6$	$V_\beta 8$	$V_\beta 3$	$V_\beta 6$	$V_\beta 8$	$V_\beta 3$	$V_\beta 6$	$V_\beta 8$
0	5.1	10.4	21.5	5.7	15.8	18.9	6.5	12.2	12.1
20	2.1	10.5	14.2	1.2	19.5	0.0	1.6	15.5	0.2
100	2.3	12.8	10.8	1.1	17.6	0.2	1.1	16.9	0.1

* Mice were injected intraperitoneally with a solution containing the indicated amounts of SEB on the day of birth and every other day thereafter. Mice given 20 μg of SEB grew and survived as well as those given none. Mice given 100 μg SEB were significantly smaller than their littermates and had higher mortality rates.

the genome. One endogenous superantigen, which has not yet been characterized, binds to the TCR $V_\beta 17a$ domain and the class II IE molecule in mice. J. Marrack and P. Kappler determined the percentage of $V_\beta 17a$-bearing T cells in normal mice that expressed IE and in mutant mice that were unable to express IE. They reasoned that the endogenous superantigen should induce negative selection of $V_\beta 17a$-bearing T cells only in the IE^+ mice. As shown in Figure 12-9, the percentage of immature thymocytes expressing $V_\beta 17a$ was only slightly lower in IE^+ than in IE^- mice. However, the percentage of mature thymocytes expressing $V_\beta 17a$ was dramatically lower in the IE^+ mice than in the IE^- mice. These results support the deletion by negative selection of self-reactive thymocytes during T-cell maturation in the thymus.

Another group of endogenous superantigens are the minor lymphocyte-stimulating (Mls) determinants. These superantigens were first identified by their ability to stimulate a mixed-lymphocyte reaction (MLR) between lymphocytes derived from mice of the *same* MHC haplotype. (Normally, an MLR only occurs between lymphocytes of different haplotypes, as illustrated in Figure 9-12 and Table 15-2.) Because such a same-haplotype MLR was unexpected and because the magnitude of the reaction was so large, the Mls superantigens have been the subject of intense investigation.

The Mls superantigens are actually encoded by a retrovirus, called mouse mammary tumor virus (MTV), that can integrate into the genome of certain inbred mouse strains. Four Mls superantigens, originating in different MTV strains, have been identified. These superantigens exhibit different V_β specificity, and the four *Mls* loci are located on different chromosomes (Table 12-4). The presence of a particular Mls allele in an inbred mouse strain is indicated with a superscript *a*, whereas the absence of a particular Mls allele is indicated with a superscript *b*. The AKR strain, for example, has MTV-7 integrated in chromosome 1 and is designated $Mls1^a$, $Mls2^b$, $Mls3^b$, and $Mls4^b$. The B10.BR strain, in contrast, contains no MTV strain and thus does not express any Mls superantigen. Since the Mls1 superantigen binds to the $V_\beta 6$, $V_\beta 7$, $V_\beta 8.1$, and $V_\beta 9$

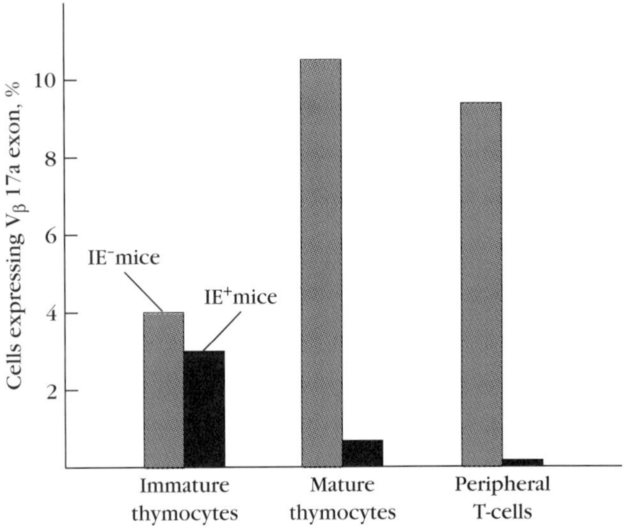

FIGURE 12-9 Expression of the $V_\beta 17a$ exon in immature and mature thymocytes and in mature peripheral T cells in IE^- and IE^+ mice. The dramatic reduction in mature thymocytes bearing T-cell receptors with the $V_\beta 17a$ domain in IE^+ mice suggests that these cells have been deleted by negative selection mediated by an endogenous superantigen specific for $V_\beta 17a$ plus IE.

TABLE 12-4 PROPERTIES OF MLS SUPERANTIGENS

Mls allele	Retroviral carrier	Chromosome location	V_β specificity
Mls1	MTV-7	1	6, 7, 8.1, 9
Mls2	MTV-13	4	3
Mls3	MTV-6	16	3, 5
Mls4	MTV-1	7	3

domains in T-cell receptors, negative selection would be expected to eliminate T cells expressing receptors with these V_β domains in AKR mice but not in B10.BR mice. As shown in Table 12-5, both mouse strains have immature thymocytes expressing the V_β domains to which Mls1 binds, but only B10.BR mice contain mature thymocytes bearing T-cell receptors with these V_β domains. Thus negative selection, mediated by the Mls1 superantigen, eliminates T cells bearing the $V_\beta6$, $V_\beta7$, $V_\beta8.1$, or $V_\beta9$ domain in the AKR strain.

Unsolved Questions Regarding Thymic Selection

Although the general process of T-cell maturation, which generates mature CD4$^+$ and CD8$^+$ T cells, is understood, several unsolved questions regarding thymic selection remain. For example, if positive selection selects for thymocytes reactive with self-MHC molecules and then negative selection eliminates the self-MHC–reactive thymocytes, how do any MHC-restricted T cells survive? What keeps these two processes from eliminating the entire repertoire of MHC-restricted T cells? As noted earlier, one hypothesis is that differences in the affinity of T-cell receptors for self-MHC molecules prevents the thymocyte population remaining after positive selection from being completely deleted by negative selection. According to this hypothesis, all thymocytes bearing receptors that can bind to self-MHC molecules are selected during positive selection, whereas subsequently only those thymocytes bearing high-affinity receptors for self-MHC (or self-antigen plus self-MHC) bind during negative selection and undergo death by apoptosis. In this way, only thymocytes bearing receptors with a low affinity for self antigen plus self-MHC molecules survive positive and negative selection, eventually leaving the thymus as mature T cells with self-MHC–restricted receptors (see Figure 12-4).

If this hypothesis is to explain why all MHC-restricted thymocytes are not eliminated during negative selection, then there must be some mechanism that increases the ability of cells bearing low-affinity receptors to bind with thymic stromal cells during positive selection and/or that decreases their binding ability during negative selection. One possibility is that differential expression of other membrane molecules influences the avidity of thymocytes for thymic stromal cells at different stages in thymic processing. For example, the coreceptors CD4 and CD8 are known to bind to class II and class I MHC molecules, respectively. Perhaps the expression of these or other unidentified membrane molecules sufficiently increases the avidity of thymocytes bearing low-affinity receptors so that they can bind to thymic epithelial cells during positive selection. The subsequent loss or decrease of these membrane molecules during development of thymocytes may lower their avidity, so that only thymocytes with high-affinity receptors for self-MHC (or self-MHC plus self-antigen) would be able to bind to thymic stromal cells during negative selection.

TABLE 12-5 EFFECT OF MLS1 SUPERANTIGEN ON V_β EXPRESSION IN MICE

		Expression of V_β					
Strain	Mls1	$V_\beta3$	$V_\beta5$	$V_\beta6$	$V_\beta7$	$V_\beta8.1$	$V_\beta9$
		Immature $\alpha\beta$ thymocytes					
AKR	Present	+	+	+	+	+	+
B10.BR	Absent	+	+	+	+	+	+
		Mature peripheral $\alpha\beta$ t cells					
AKR	Present	+	+	–	–	–	–
B10.BR	Absent	+	+	+	+	+	+

To test the possibility that differential expression of CD8 affects thymic selection, E. Robey, B. J. Fowlkes, and their colleagues experimentally manipulated the level of CD8 expression in mice and then analyzed the composition of the thymocyte population. Since the interaction of T cells with class I MHC molecules is strengthened by participation of CD8, these researchers predicted that increasing the level of CD8 expression would increase the avidity of thymocytes for class I molecules, leading to their negative selection. In their study, they first produced two types of transgenic mice: mice bearing a CD8 transgene and mice bearing an *αβ*-TCR transgene derived from a class I-restricted CTL clone. They then mated the two transgenic mice to produce double-transgenic mice expressing both the *αβ* T-cell receptor and CD8. The $CD8^+$ T cells in the double transgenics expressed both endogenous CD8 and transgenic CD8; thus these cells had twice the normal level of CD8. As predicted, FACS analyses of thymocytes from the three transgenics showed that the proportion of mature thymocytes expressing the transgenic T-cell receptor and CD8 was 13-fold lower in the double transgenics, which had elevated levels of CD8, than in the single transgenics (Figure 12-10).

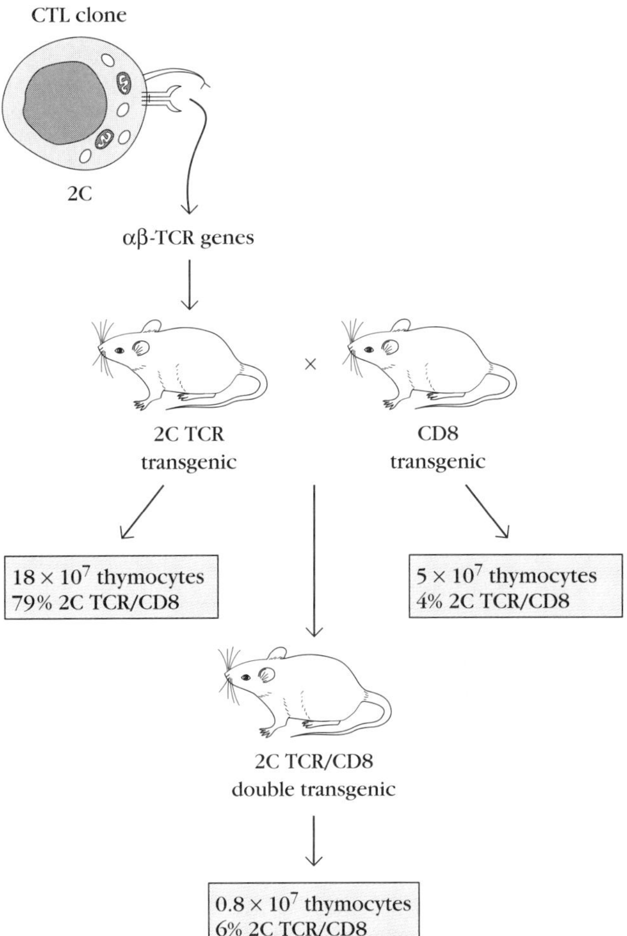

FIGURE 12-10 Experimental demonstration that elevated levels of CD8 stimulate negative selection. The double-transgenic mice (2C TCR/CD8) expressed elevated levels of CD8 and a T-cell receptor from a class I-restricted CTL clone called 2C. FACS analyses of thymocytes showed that a much higher proportion of thymocytes expressed the 2C TCR and CD8 in the single 2C TCR transgenics (79%) than in the double transgenics (6%). In addition, the double transgenics had a significantly lower number of total thymocytes than the single transgenics—a likely consequence of increased negative selection. [Data from: E. A. Robey et al. 1992. *Cell* **69**:1089.]

Differences in the populations of thymic stromal cells involved in positive and negative selection also may influence the avidity of the thymocyte-stromal cell interaction. As noted earlier, thymic cortical epithelial cells appear to be involved in positive selection, whereas most negative selection appears to involve bone marrow-derived dendritic cells and macrophages. Some researchers have suggested that thymic cortical epithelial cells express additional membrane molecules that facilitate their interaction with thymocytes bearing low-affinity receptors for self-MHC molecules. If these membrane molecules are not expressed on thymic macrophages or dendritic cells, then thymocytes bearing low-affinity receptors for self-MHC molecules might not bind and therefore would not be deleted.

Another unresolved question is how thymocyte recognition of self-MHC molecules is converted into a protective signal early in thymic processing (positive selection) and into a negative signal leading to apoptosis at a later stage (negative selection). One hypothesis is that the effect of TCR-mediated signal transduction may change during thymocyte maturation perhaps due to differences in coupling between the T-cell receptor and CD3. In one study, for example, cross-linking of the T-cell receptor with monoclonal antibodies induced a pronounced Ca^{2+} influx in mature single-positive thymocytes but only minimal Ca^{2+} influx in immature double-positive cells. In contrast, cross-linking of CD3 induced comparable Ca^{2+} influx in both mature and immature thymocytes. These results have led to speculation that in immature thymocytes the T-cell receptor and CD3 are not fully coupled and thus the signal generated by interaction with self-MHC molecules is incomplete; as a result such immature thymocytes undergo programmed cell death by apoptosis.

Although this proposed mechanism explains why immature thymocytes are susceptible to programmed cell death, it does not account for the different outcomes of positive and negative selection.

Accumulating evidence suggests that the proto-oncogene *bcl-2* may influence whether thymocytes receive a positive protective signal or negative deleting signal during thymic processing. *Bcl-2* was first identified as an oncogene associated with follicular B-cell lymphoma. Expression of *bcl-2,* which was shown to prevent programmed cell death by apoptosis, allows unregulated growth of the B-lymphoma cells. Further studies showed that *bcl-2* is expressed in surviving mature thymocytes of the medulla, whereas the majority of immature cortical thymocytes do not express *bcl-2.*

To assess the role of Bcl-2, the protein encoded by *bcl-2,* researchers generated transgenic mice in which the transgene consisted of *bcl-2* engineered with the promoter for the $p56^{lck}$ gene. Since $p56^{lck}$ is expressed in immature thymocytes prior to positive selection, *bcl-2* also will be expressed at this early stage in thymocyte development in these transgenic mice. The presence of Bcl-2 appeared to prevent apoptosis during positive thymic selection in these mice. Based on this finding, some have suggested that the interaction of cortical thymocytes with epithelial cells during positive selection may induce production of Bcl-2, thereby preventing apoptosis of the selected self-MHC–reactive thymocytes. All of the remaining cortical thymocytes, which do not interact with epithelial cells, would not express *bcl-2* and therefore would be subject to death by apoptosis. According to this hypothesis, interaction of MHC-reactive thymocytes with macrophages or dendritic cells during negative selection would not result in induction of Bcl-2; thus selected cells would not be protected and would undergo apoptosis. These hypotheses are still quite speculative and have not yet been confirmed experimentally.

T_H-Cell Activation

The central event in generation of both humoral and cell-mediated immune responses is the activation and clonal expansion of T_H cells. (Activation of T_C cells, which is generally similar to T_H-cell activation, is discussed in Chapter 15.) T_H-cell activation is initiated by the interaction of the TCR-CD3 complex with a processed antigenic peptide bound to a class II MHC molecule on the surface of an antigen-presenting cell. This interaction and the resulting activating signals also involve a variety of accessory membrane molecules on the T_H cell and antigen-presenting cell (see Table 11-4). Interaction of a T_H cell with antigen initiates a cascade of biochemical events that induces the resting T_H cell to enter the cell cycle (G_0 to G_1 transition) and culminates in expression of the high-affinity receptor for IL-2 and secretion of IL-2. In response to IL-2 (and in some cases IL-4), the activated T_H cell progresses through the cell cycle, proliferating and differentiating into memory cells or effector cells.

Following interaction of T_H cells with antigen, numerous genes are activated. The gene products that appear can be grouped into different categories depending on how early they can be detected following antigen recognition (Table 12-6). *Immediate genes,* which are expressed within half an hour of antigen recognition, encode a number of transcription factors including c-Fos, c-Myc, NF-AT, and NF-κB. *Early genes* are expressed within 1–2 h of antigen recognition and encode IL-2, IL-2R, IL-3, IL-6, IFN-γ, and numerous other proteins. *Late genes,* which are expressed more than 2 days after antigen recognition, encode various adhesion molecules.

TCR-Coupled Signaling Pathways

Although the precise molecular mechanisms that link antigen recognition by the T-cell receptor to gene activation are not fully understood, a number of signaling events common to many cells have been shown to occur in the T_H cell. These events include activation of inositol-lipid–specific phospholipase C (PLC); hydrolysis of plasma membrane inositol phospholipids; increase in intracellular Ca^{2+} levels; and activation of various protein kinases that subsequently phosphorylate a number of proteins involved in mediating the activation signal.

The T-cell receptor itself has short cytoplasmic domains, which are unable to mediate signal transduction. Instead, signal transduction is mediated by the cytoplasmic domains of the CD3 complex, by the coreceptor CD4 or CD8, and by various accessory molecules including CD2 and CD45. It appears that signal transduction is accomplished by a series of protein-phosphorylation events catalyzed by protein kinases and dephosphorylation events catalyzed by protein phosphatases (Figure 12-11). As discussed in Chapter 11, the cytoplasmic domains of each CD3 chain contain a sequence, called the antigen recognition activation motif (ARAM), that is thought to interact with protein tyrosine kinases during signal transduction (see Figure 11-7). Two protein tyrosine kinases ($p59^{fyn}$ and ZAP-70) have been shown to be associated with the cytoplasmic domains of the ϵ and ζ chains of CD3. In addition, the cytoplasmic domain of CD4 and CD8 is associated with the protein tyrosine kinase $p56^{lck}$. It is hypothesized that the simultaneous binding of a T-cell receptor and CD4 or CD8 coreceptor to an MHC molecule results in the juxtaposition of $p56^{lck}$ and the cytoplasmic domains of CD3, facilitating phosphorylation.

TABLE 12-6 TIME COURSE OF GENE EXPRESSION BY T_H CELLS FOLLOWING INTERACTION WITH ANTIGEN

Gene product	Function	Time mRNA expression begins	Location	Ratio of activated to nonactivated cells
		Immediate		
c-Fos	Cellular oncogene Nuclear-binding protein	15 min	Nucleus	>100
NF-AT	Nuclear-binding protein	20 min	Nucleus	50
c-Myc	Cellular oncogene	30 min	Nucleus	20
NF-κB	Nuclear-binding protein	30 min	Nucleus	>10
		Early		
IFN-γ	Cytokine	30 min	Secreted	>100
IL-2	Cytokine	45 min	Secreted	>1000
c-Abl	Cellular oncogene	1 h	Nuclear	10
Insulin receptor	Hormone receptor	1 h	Cell membrane	3
IL-3	Cytokine	1–2 h	Secreted	>100
TGF-β	Cytokine	<2 h	Secreted	>10
IL-2 receptor	Cytokine receptor	2 h	Cell membrane	>50
TNF-β	Cytokine	1–3 h	Secreted	>100
Cyclin	Cell cycle protein	4–6 h	Cytoplasmic	>10
IL-4	Cytokine	<6 h	Secreted	>100
IL-5	Cytokine	<6 h	Secreted	>100
IL-6	Cytokine	<6 h	Secreted	>100
c-Myb	Cellular oncogene	16 h	Nuclear	100
GM-CSF	Cytokine	20 h	Secreted	?
		Late		
HLA-DR	Class II MHC molecule	3–5 days	Cell membrane	10
VLA-4	Adhesion molecule	4 days	Cell membrane	>100
VLA-1, VLA-2, VLA-3, VLA-5	Adhesion molecules	7–14 days	Cell membrane	>100, ?, ?, ?

SOURCE: Adapted from G. Crabtree, 1989, *Science* **243**:357.

The requirement for CD4 in T_H-cell activation was demonstrated in an experiment by N. Glaichenhaus and his colleagues. These researchers isolated functional rearranged TCR α- and β-chain genes from a T-cell hybridoma that was specific for lysozyme together with the class II MHC molecule IA^b. The genes were transfected into a lymphoma cell line that lacked TCR, CD4, and CD8. The transfected lymphoma cell line expressed the $\alpha\beta$-TCR-CD3 complex but still could not respond to lysozyme presented by IA^b molecules. When this transfected lymphoma cell line was infected with a retrovirus carrying CD4 cDNA, the cell line became $CD4^+$ and was able to respond to lysozyme presented by IA^b by secreting IL-2. The experiment was taken one step further by later infecting the $\alpha\beta$-TCR^+ lymphoma cell line with a retrovirus carrying a mutant CD4 cDNA; the mutant CD4 was still able to bind to class II MHC molecules but was unable to

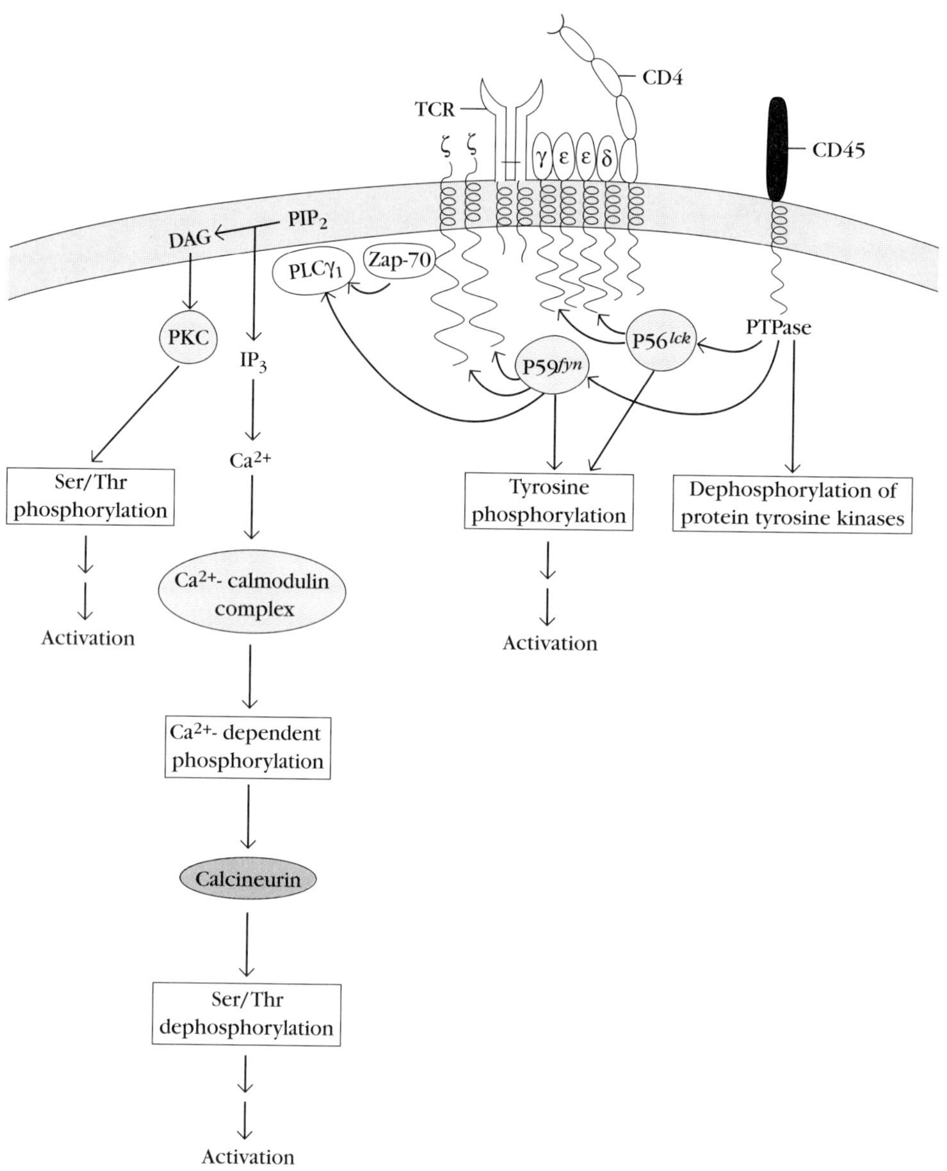

FIGURE 12-11 Role of protein phosphorylation and dephosphorylation steps in cytoplasmic pathways leading to T_H-cell activation. Protein phosphatases are shaded dark purple, and protein kinases are shaded light purple. PTPase = protein tyrosine phosphase; PLCγ1 = phospholipase C; PIP_2 = phosphatidylinositol 4,5-bisphosphate; IP_3 = inositol 1,4,5-trisphosphate; DAG = diacylglycerol; PKC = protein kinase C. See text for full discussion. Similar pathways are thought to operate in $CD8^+$ T cells. [Adapted from M. Izquierdo and D. A. Cantrell, 1992, *Trends in Cell Biol.* **2**:268.]

associate with $p56^{lck}$. The inability of the CD4 to associate with $p56^{lck}$ resulted in a significant reduction in the cell line's response to lysozyme plus IA^b.

Activation of these protein tyrosine kinases by CD3 and the CD4 or CD8 coreceptor appears to require the activity of CD45. This membrane molecule has a cytoplasmic tail with two protein tyrosine phosphatase domains, which are thought to catalyze dephosphorylation of a tyrosine residue of $p56^{lck}$ and $p59^{fyn}$. This dephosphorylation step is thought to activate the tyrosine kinases so that they begin to phosphorylate the ϵ and ζ chains of CD3, phospholipase C (PLCγ1), and other cellular substrates. Phosphorylation of PLCγ1 allows it to hydrolyze phosphatidylinositol 4,5-bisphosphate (PIP_2) into two important products, inositol 1,4,5-trisphosphate (IP_3) and diacylglycerol (DAG). These two products initiate two necessary signaling pathways (see Figure 12-11). In one pathway, IP_3 triggers an increase in intracellular Ca^{2+} and the subsequent activation of a calmodulin-dependent phosphatase called *calcineurin,* which dephosphorylates a cytoplasmic component of the nuclear factor of activated T cells designated NF-ATc. In the other pathway, DAG activates protein kinase C (PKC), which then phosphorylates various cellular substrates and mediates release of the nuclear factor NF-κB. Both nuclear factors enter the nucleus where they participate in activation of various genes (see Figure 12-13).

The Co-stimulatory Signal

In addition to the signals mediated by the T-cell receptor and its associated accessory molecules, activation of the T_H cell requires an additional *co-stimulatory signal* provided by the antigen-presenting cell. The co-stimulatory signal may be induced by cytokines released by the APC or it may involve the interaction of membrane molecules on the APC and T_H cell. The cytokines IL-1 and IL-6 have each been shown to provide co-stimulatory signals in T_H-cell activation. More recent evidence, however, suggests that a more potent co-stimulatory signal is provided by the interaction between the B7 molecule on the APC membrane and the CD28 or CTLA-4 molecule on the T_H-cell membrane. B7, which is expressed as a monomer by activated B cells, activated macrophages, and dendritic cells binds to both CD28 and CTLA-4 but with different affinities (Figure 12-12a). Both CD28 and CTLA-4 are expressed as homodimers on the T-cell membrane; like B7 they

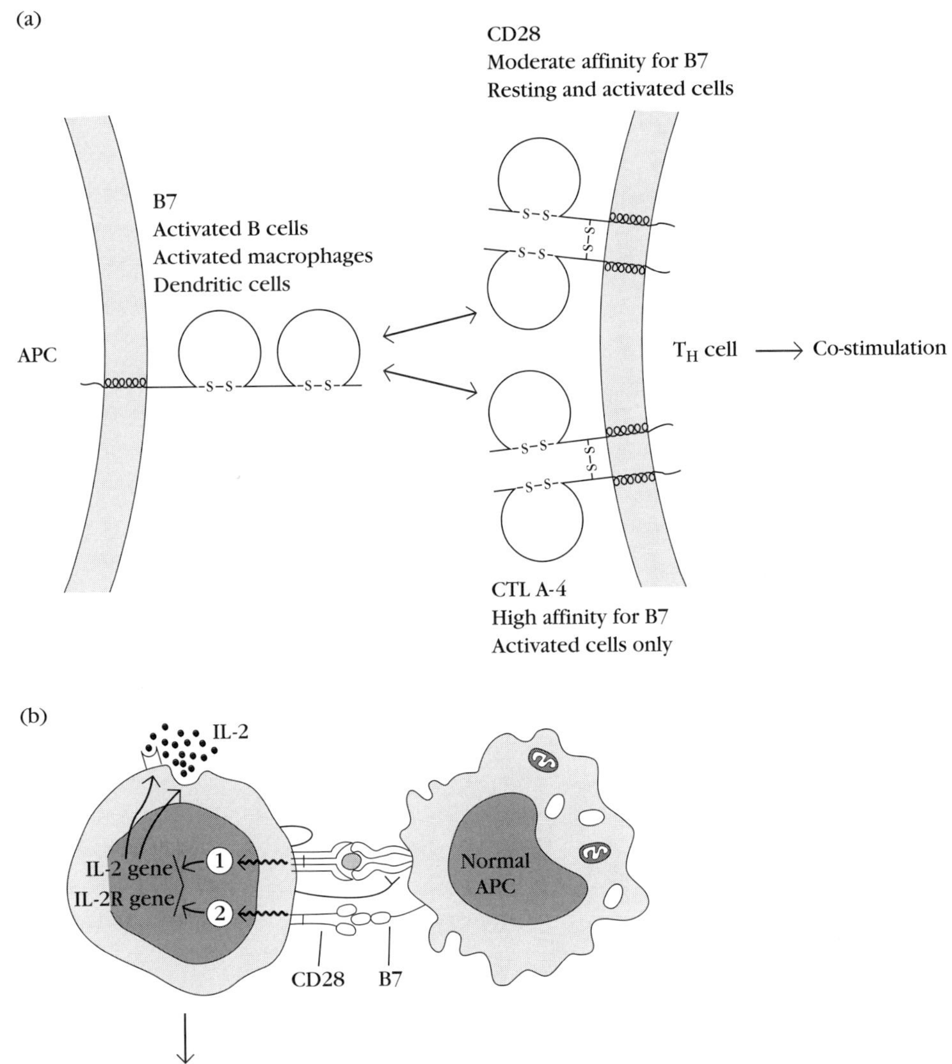

FIGURE 12-12 T_H-cell activation requires a co-stimulatory signal provided by antigen-presenting cells (APCs). (a) One co-stimulatory signal is generated by interaction of B7 on APCs with CD28 or CTLA-4 on T_H cells. (b) Activating signal 1, generated by antigen recognition, and a co-stimulatory signal 2, in this case generated by the B7-CD28 interaction, are both required for induction of IL-2 production and expression of the high-affinity IL-2 receptor. [Part (a) adapted from P. S. Linsley and J. A. Ledbetter, 1993, *Annu. Rev. Immunol.* **11**:191.]

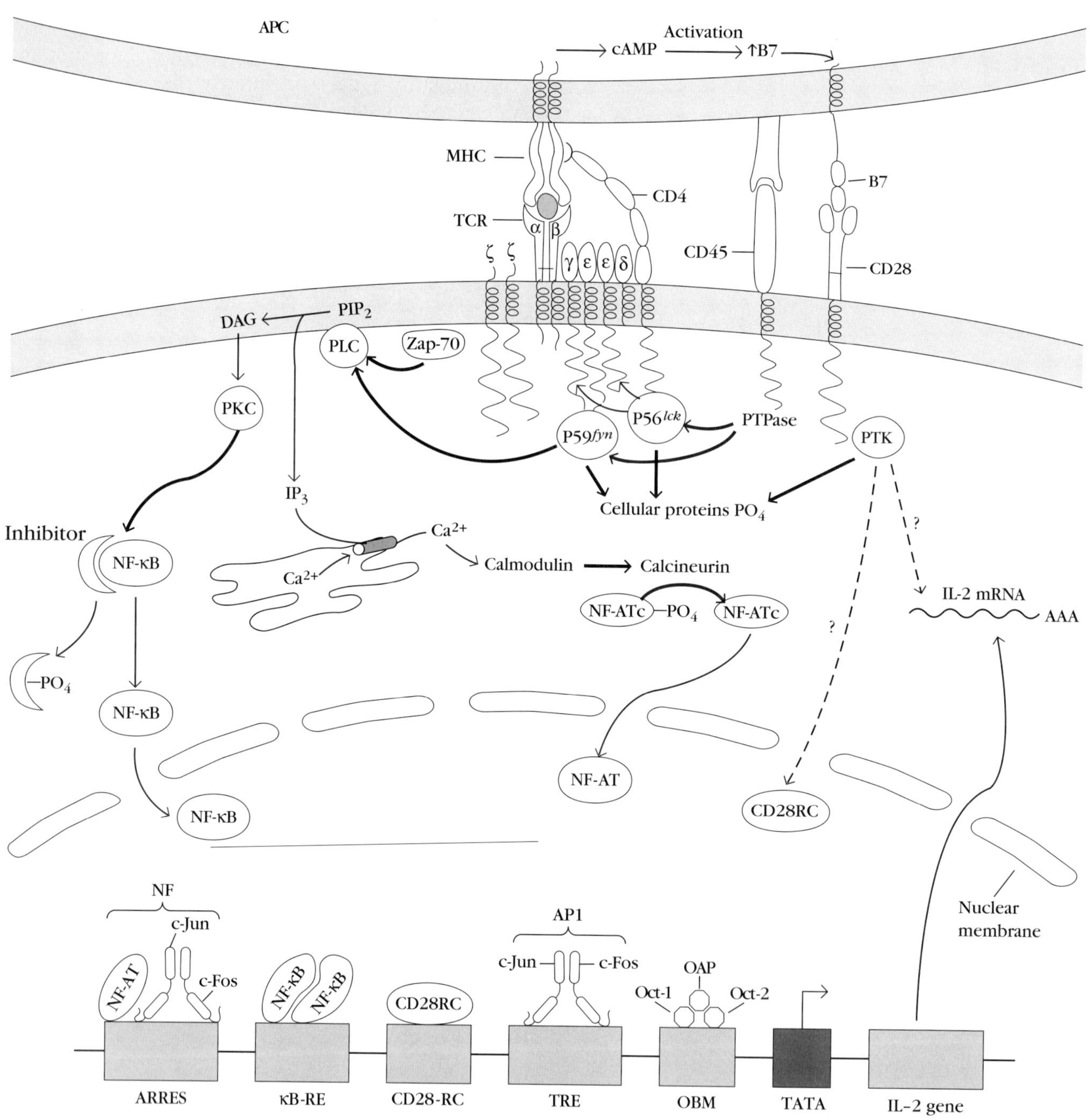

FIGURE 12-13 Overview of biochemical pathways thought to transduce the signals required for T_H-cell activation and the DNA-binding proteins that bind to the IL-2 enhancer region. The TCR-mediated signal results in production of two nuclear factors, NF-AT and NF-κB. The co-stimulatory signal, generated by the CD28-B7 interaction, results in production of a third nuclear factor, CD28RC. Binding of these and other nuclear factors to response elements in the IL-2 enhancer *(bottom)* stimulates transcription of the IL-2 gene, leading to increased secretion of IL-2 about 45 min after antigen recognition. Thick black arrows indicate protein phosphorylation steps; thick purple arrows indicate dephosphorylation steps. PTK = protein tyrosine kinase; see Figure 12-11 for other abbreviations.

are members of the immunoglobulin superfamily. CD28 is expressed by both resting and activated T cells and binds B7 with moderate affinity. In contrast, CTLA-4 binds B7 with a 20-fold higher affinity, but it is expressed only on activated T cells and at much lower levels (only 3% of CD28 levels).

As discussed in detail later, T cells can be activated experimentally in such a way that only the TCR-coupled signaling pathways operate. In this case, activation results in very little production of IL-2 compared with normal activation in which the CD28-B7 co-stimulatory signal also operates. The co-stimulatory signal appears to synergize with the TCR-coupled signals to augment IL-2 production and T-cell proliferation (Figure 12-12b). Very little is known about how signal transduction is mediated via the CD28-B7 interaction. This interaction is known to result in activation of a protein tyrosine kinase, which then phosphorylates phospholipase C and other cellular substrates. Thus the co-stimulatory signal augments the Ca^{2+}-dependent calmodulin-calcineurin pathway and a transcription factor called CD28RC is induced. Two hypotheses have been proposed to explain how the co-stimulatory signal enhances expression of IL-2. One hypothesis suggests that the CD28RC transcription factor binds to the IL-2 enhancer along with NF-AT and NF-κB, leading to increased transcription of the IL-2 gene. The second hypothesis suggests that the signal mediated through CD28 increases the half-life of IL-2 mRNA.

Gene Activation by DNA-Binding Proteins

The expression of both IL-2 and the IL-2 receptor (IL-2R) are necessary for the clonal expansion of the activated T_H cell. A number of DNA-binding proteins have been shown to bind to enhancer or promoter regions of the genes encoding IL-2 and IL-2R. The enhancer region of the IL-2 gene, for example, contains sequences that bind the AP1 complex (a dimer of c-Fos and c-Jun), NF-κB, NF-AT, and a complex of Oct-1, Oct-2, and OAP (Figure 12-13). Of these DNA-binding proteins, only NF-AT is T-cell specific; the others are found in many types of cells.

NF-AT, which is expressed by activated T_H cells within 20 min of antigen recognition, is actually a complex of two subunits: a cytosolic subunit (NF-ATc) and a nuclear subunit (AP1). Following antigen recognition by T_H cells the phosphorylated form of the cytosolic subunit (NF-ATc-PO_4) is dephosphorylated by calcineurin. NF-ATc then translocates to the nucleus where it dimerizes with AP1; the resulting complex then binds to the IL-2 enhancer. If dephosphorylation of NF-ATc-PO_4 is inhibited, as it is by cyclosporin A and FK506, then T_H-cell activation is blocked and the immune response is reduced (Figure 12-14). Because of their potent immunosuppressive capabilities, cyclosporin A and FK506 have proven to be extremely effective in prolonging graft survival in transplant recipients (see Chapter 24).

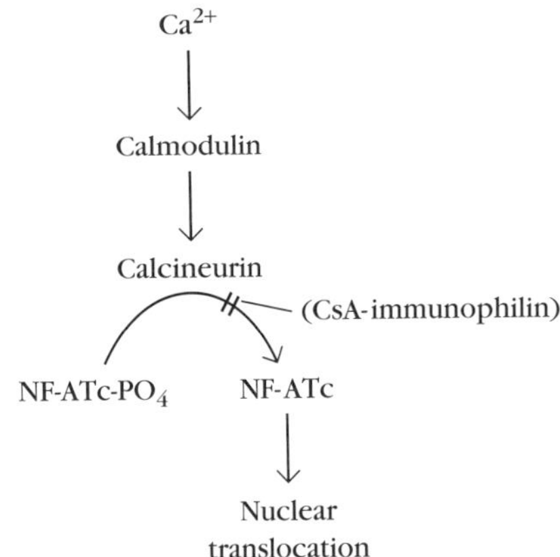

FIGURE 12-14 Mechanism of immunosuppression by cyclosporin A (CsA), which binds to cytoplasmic proteins called immunophilins. This complex blocks the phosphatase activity of calcineurin, thereby preventing production of NF-ATc, which is necessary for T-cell activation. Another drug, designated FK506, acts in the same manner. The immunophilins are *cis-trans* peptidyl-prolyl isomerase enzymes. CsA binds to an immunophilin called cyclophilin, and FK506 binds to one called FKBP.

In addition to its role in regulating expression of IL-2, NF-AT may also be involved in regulating the expression of several other cytokine genes including those encoding IL-3, IL-4, IL-5, and IFN-γ. Evidence for the role of NF-AT in regulating these additional cytokine genes comes from a child born with a combined immunodeficiency due to a structural defect in NF-AT. T-cell proliferation in this child was severely impaired, and the child could not produce IL-2, IL-3, IL-4, IL-5, and IFN-γ, suggesting that NF-AT was necessary for expression of each of these cytokines.

Clonal Expansion Versus Clonal Anergy

T_H-cell recognition of an antigenic peptide–MHC complex on an antigen-presenting cell results either in activation and *clonal expansion* or in a state of nonresponsiveness called *clonal anergy*. Anergy is a state of inactivation marked by the inability of T cells to proliferate in response to an antigen-MHC complex. Whether clonal expansion or clonal anergy ensues is determined by the presence or absence of a co-stimulatory signal (signal 2), such as that provided by interaction of CD28 on T_H cells with B7 on antigen-presenting cells. If a resting T_H cell receives the TCR-mediated signal (signal 1) in the absence of a suitable co-stimulatory signal, then the T_H cell will become anergic.

One way of inducing clonal anergy is to incubate resting T_H cells with glutarldehyde-fixed APCs, which do not express B7 (Figure 12-15a). The fixed APCs are able to present peptides together with class II MHC molecules, thereby providing signal 1, but they are unable to provide the necessary co-stimulatory signal 2. In the absence of a co-stimulatory signal, there is minimal production of cytokines, especially of IL-2. That the anergic state is not simply the absence of a response, but rather an active state of unresponsiveness, can be demonstrated by incubating anergic T_H cells with normal APCs. In this case, the anergic T_H cells cannot be activated by the antigenic peptides displayed on the normal APCs (Figure 12-15c).

The systems illustrated in Figure 12-15d,e have shown that the co-stimulatory signal 2 is distinct from signal 1 provided by TCR recognition of an antigen-MHC complex. In these systems, T_H cells are incubated with fixed APCs and either normal, unfixed APCs expressing allogeneic MHC molecules or anti-CD28. Clonal expansion occurs in both systems because the T_H cells receive signal 1 by interacting with the fixed APCs and signal 2 by interacting with the unfixed allogeneic APCs or anti-CD28. As noted already, the co-stimulatory signal normally is provided by the same APC that presents antigen (see Figure 12-12b).

The demonstration of T-cell anergy and the role of accessory membrane molecules in providing the co-stimulatory signal necessary for T_H-cell activation opens possibilities for immune intervention. For example, treatment with monoclonal antibodies to CD28 or CTLA-4 might increase the T-cell response to infectious agents or tumors. Alternatively, blocking of CD28, CTLA-4, or B7 might provide a means of inducing clonal anergy. For example, CTLA-4Ig, a soluble fusion protein consisting of the extracellular domain of CTLA-4 and the constant region of the IgGl heavy chain, has been shown to completely block T-cell

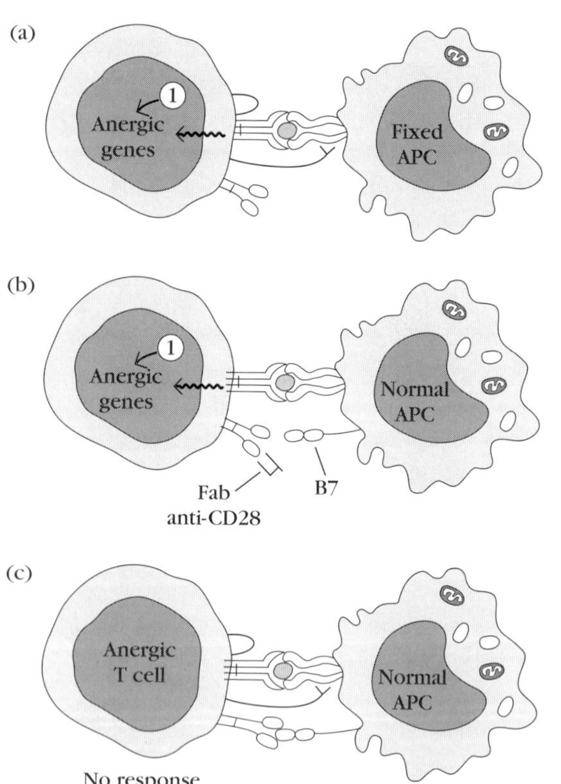

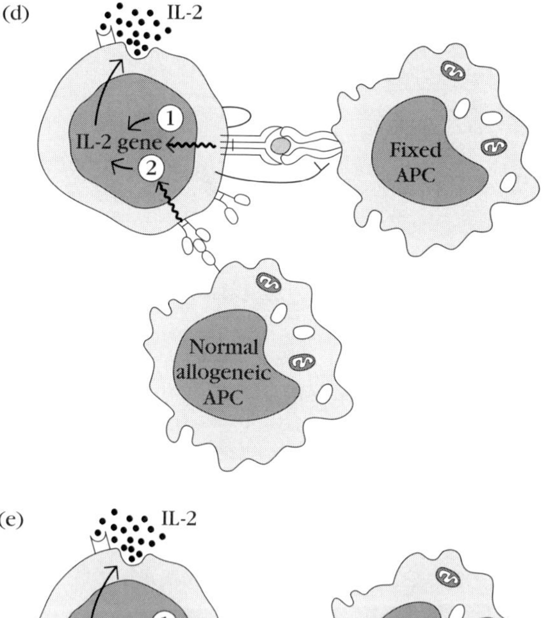

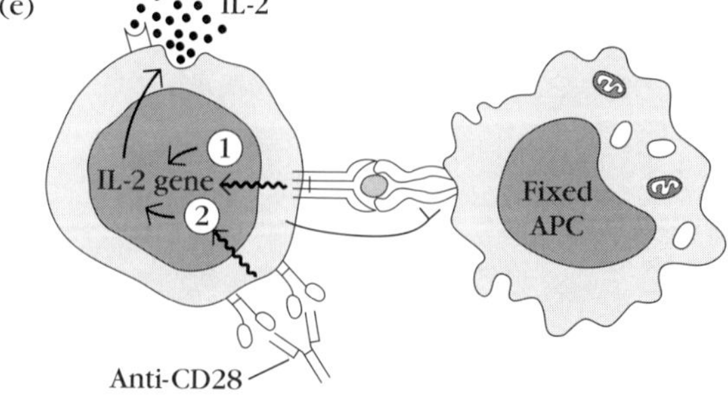

FIGURE 12-15 Experimental demonstration of clonal anergy versus clonal expansion. (a) Glutaraldehyde-fixed antigen-presenting cells (APCs), which lack B7, induce T cells to become anergic. (b) Anergy also is induced if T cells are incubated with normal APCs and anti-CD28. (c) Anergic T cells cannot respond to normal APCs. (d,e) In the presence of normal allogeneic APCs or anti-CD28, both of which interact with CD28, T cells are activated by fixed APCs. These systems demonstrate that the TCR-mediated signal 1 is distinct from the co-stimulatory signal 2. Normally, the co-stimulatory signal is provided by the same APC that presents antigen (see Figure 12-12b).

activation. In a recently reported study this reagent completely abolished graft rejection in mice transplanted with human pancreatic islet cells (see Chapter 24).

Mature Peripheral T-Cell Populations

$\alpha\beta$ T Cells

As has been indicated earlier, an estimated 90–95% of peripheral T cells express the $\alpha\beta$ T-cell receptor–CD3 complex. These cells express either CD4 or CD8 membrane markers; there are about twice as many $CD4^+$ T cells as $CD8^+$ T cells in the periphery. In general $CD4^+$ cells function as T helper cells and $CD8^+$ cells function as cytotoxic cells. Since both populations express the $\alpha\beta$ T-cell receptor, a question that arises is whether the T cytotoxic and T helper cells express different V_α and V_β gene segments. The available evidence seems to suggest that both populations can use the same pool of V_α and V_β gene segments; in one case, indeed, the same V_β gene product was identified on both class I MHC–restricted T_C cells and class II MHC–restricted T_H cells.

The peripheral T-cell population consists of *naive, effector,* and *memory* T cells. Following antigenic challenge, naive T cells proliferate and differentiate into effector and memory cells. The properties of these three classes of T cells are summarized in Table 12-7.

Naive T Cells

$CD4^+$ and $CD8^+$ T cells leave the thymus and enter the circulation as resting cells in the G_0 stage of the cell cycle. These naive T cells, which have not yet encountered antigen, are characterized by expression of low levels of most cell-adhesion molecules but high levels of the homing receptor L-selectin, which is called

Table 12-7 Properties of peripheral $\alpha\beta$ T cells

Property	Naive T cells	Effector T cells	Memory T cells
Definition	Resting cells that have migrated from thymus and have not encountered Ag	Cells, derived from Ag-activated naive or memory cells, that carry out effector functions	Resting cells, derived from Ag-activated naive cells or effector cells, that are easily activated by subsequent Ag challenge
Effector functions	None	Helper, cytotoxic, or DTH activity	None
Life span	5–7 weeks	2–3 days	Years (up to 30); some may be maintained by continual Ag exposure
Antigen-presenting cell	Dendritic cells	Dendritic cells, B cells, macrophages	Dendritic cells, B cells, macrophages
CD45R isoform	CD45RA (high-MW isoform)	Variable levels of CD45RA and CD45RO	CD45RO (low-MW isoform)
L-selectin*	Present	Absent	Absent
Other adhesion molecules	Low levels of a few	High levels of many†	High levels of many†
Recirculation	Migrate from tissues into lymph nodes at HEVs; continually recirculate between blood and lymph	Disperse from lymph nodes to sites where Ag is present and tend to remain there; exhibit little recirculation	Migrate from blood into tissues and return to lymph nodes via afferent lymphatic vessels

* L-selection (MEL-14 in mice; LAM-1 in humans) functions as a peripheral lymph-node homing receptor.
† Include ICAM-1, VLA-4, LFA-1, and CD44 (Pgp-1).

MEL-14 in mice and LAM-1 in humans. The expression of this homing receptor allows naive T cells to bind to a vascular addressin that is present only on high-endothelial venules (HEVs) of the peripheral lymph nodes. This binding is required for extravasation, enabling naive T cells to migrate through the endothelial layer into the node (see Figure 3-25). Naive T cells also express high levels of the high-molecular-weight isoform of CD45 (designated CD45RA), which is involved in transducing the activation signal. Thus, if a naive T cell recognizes an antigen-MHC complex on an appropriate antigen-presenting cell or target cell, it will be activated, initiating a *primary response.*

If a naive T cell does not encounter appropriate antigen, it leaves the node through the efferent lymphatic vessel and becomes part of the recirculating lymphocyte pool, continually recirculating between the blood and lymph (see Figure 3-23). It is estimated that naive T cells recirculate from the blood to the lymph and back again every 12–24 h. Because only about 1 in 10^5 naive T cells is specific for any given antigen, this large-scale recirculation increases the chances of a naive T cell encountering appropriate antigen. In the absence of antigen activation, a naive T cell has a relatively short life span and dies within 5–7 weeks.

Effector T Cells

About 48 h after activation, a T cell enlarges into a blast cell and begins to proliferate in the lymph node. Within about 5–7 days the activated T cell will differentiate into an effector cell that is specialized to carry out a particular function such as cytotoxicity (T_C cells), secretion of cytokines (T_H cells), or participation in delayed-type hypersensitivity responses (T_{DTH} cells).

Effector and naive T cells can be distinguished by differences in their expression of certain membrane molecules (see Table 12-7). Effector T cells exhibit increased expression of cell-adhesion molecules (e.g., ICAM-1, the integrins VLA-4 and LFA-1, and CD44); these molecules may initially serve to keep the activated cells at the site of activation. Indeed, antigen-activated T cells are known to be depleted from the recirculating lymphocyte pool for a few days following antigen activation. The cell-adhesion molecules specifically expressed by effector T cells enable these cells to disperse to sites of inflammation in "tertiary" or "extralymphoid" tissue where they may again encounter the original activating antigen. Here, after restimulation, activated effector T cells carry out a variety of effector functions. Effector T cells are short-lived with a life span of only 2–3 days. In one study, effector T cells were shown to die by apoptosis as IL-2 levels decreased.

As discussed in more detail in Chapter 13, $CD4^+$ effector T cells form two subpopulations characterized by the panel of cytokines that they secrete. One population, called the *T_H1 subset,* secretes IL-2, IFN-γ, and TNF-β. The T_H1 subset is responsible for classical cell-mediated functions, such as delayed-type hypersensitivity and the activation of cytotoxic T lymphocytes. The other subset, called the T_H2 subset, secretes IL-4 IL-5 and functions more effectively as a helper for B cell activation.

Because of their functional differences, the effector $CD4^+$ and $CD8^+$ T-cell populations can be distinguished by various in vitro functional assays. The most common functional assay for $CD8^+$ cytotoxic T cells is a cell-mediated cytotoxicity assay using ^{51}Cr-labeled target cells; the amount of ^{51}Cr released is a measure of target-cell killing by the T cells. Because the functions of $CD4^+$ cells are diverse, this subpopulation can be assayed in various ways including activation of B cells, stimulation of delayed-type hypersensitivity, induction of T cytotoxic cells, suppression of antibody production, secretion of distinct cytokines, and in some cases cytolytic activity. The various T-cell assay systems are described in other chapters.

Memory T Cells

In the course of a primary response, memory T cells also are generated, either from effector cells themselves or from a separate naive T-cell population (Figure 12-16). Memory T cells are thought to be long-lived, antigen-activated T cells that respond with heightened reactivity to a subsequent challenge with the same antigen *(secondary response).* An expanded population of memory T cells appears to remain long after the population of effector T cells has declined. In general, memory T cells express the same membrane molecules as effector cells (see Table 12-7). Like naive T cells, most memory T cells are resting cells in the G_0 stage of the cell cycle, but they appear to have less stringent requirements for activation than do naive T cells. For example, naive T_H cells are only activated by dendritic cells, whereas memory T_H cells can be activated by macrophages, dendritic cells, and B cells. It is thought that the expression of high levels of numerous adhesion molecules by memory T_H cells enables these cells to adhere to a broad spectrum of antigen-presenting cells.

Like naive T cells, memory T cells recirculate in the blood and lymph. However, because memory T cells lack L-selectin homing receptors and express increased levels of other adhesion molecules, they exhibit a different pattern of recirculation. Because they lack L-selectin, memory T cells do not bind to the HEVs of lymph nodes. Thus, naive T cells account for most of the cells entering the lymph nodes from the

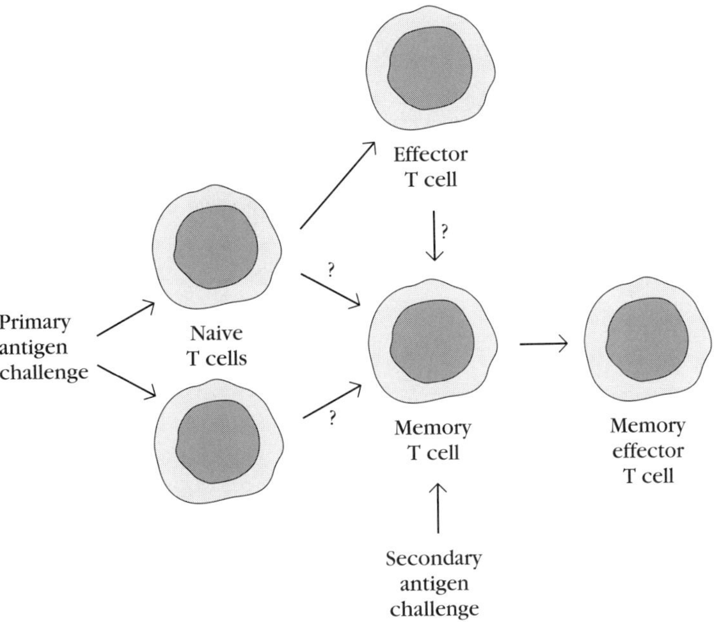

FIGURE 12-16 Memory T cells are generated during a primary response either from effector T cells or from naive T cells directly.

blood through the HEVs. In contrast, memory cells tend to migrate to "tertiary" or nonlymphoid tissue including the lamina propria of the gut, the epithelial surfaces of the lung, and the skin. In general, memory T cells tend to return to the tissue in which they were originally stimulated. Memory T cells are also the predominant cell type present within inflammatory lesions.

$\gamma\delta$ T Cells

In 1986 a small population of peripheral-blood T cells was discovered that expressed CD3 but failed to stain with monoclonal antibody specific for the $\alpha\beta$ T-cell receptor, indicating an absence of the $\alpha\beta$ heterodimer. These cells eventually were found to express the $\gamma\delta$ receptor. Such $\gamma\delta$ T cells constitute 5–10% of peripheral blood lymphocytes and 1–3% of the T-cell population in lymphoid organs of the mouse, but surprisingly they appear to represent a major T-cell population in the skin, intestinal epithelium, and pulmonary epithelium. Up to 1% of the epidermal cells in the skin of mice are $\gamma\delta$ T cells, called "dendritic epidermal cells" (DEC). These cells express the Thy-1 T-cell marker and the $\gamma\delta$ T-cell receptor associated with the CD3 membrane complex but fail to express either CD4 or CD8. A second population of $\gamma\delta$ T cells has recently been identified in the intestinal epithelium of the mouse. These "intestinal epithelial lymphocytes" (IEL) also express the $\gamma\delta$ receptor associated with the CD3 complex; unlike DEC, these cells express CD8. Another unusual characteristic of intestinal epithelial lymphocytes is that 25–50% of them fail to express Thy-1. Whether these cells lose the Thy-1 marker and acquire CD8 after thymic processing or whether they differentiate at a site other than the thymus remains to be determined.

Unlike $\alpha\beta$ T cells, which recirculate extensively, $\gamma\delta$ T cells in these epithelial tissues appear not to circulate and instead remain fixed in these tissue sites. The $\gamma\delta$ T cells in different epithelial tissue sites appear to express different V_γ and V_δ gene segments. Comparison of a number of DEC clones, for example, has revealed an unusual limitation in TCR diversity. Each of the DEC clones was shown to express a restricted repertoire encoded by $V_\gamma 3J_\gamma 1$ and $V_\delta 1D_\delta 2J_\delta 2$ gene segments, with essentially no N-region diversification. In contrast, IELs were found to express $V_\gamma 5J_\gamma 1C_\gamma 1$. This selective expression of different V gene segments in different epithelial tissues may make these T cells specialized to respond to certain types of antigens that tend to be found at these sites.

The function of $\gamma\delta$ T cells is a matter of intense speculation. There are indications that some $\gamma\delta$ T cells can mediate cytotoxicity, but it is not clear whether their recognition of antigen is MHC restricted. Several research reports have shown that $\gamma\delta$ T cells can mediate tumor-cell lysis in a non-MHC-restricted manner, suggesting that they may function like natural killer cells. The finding that $\gamma\delta$ T cells respond to a mycobacterial antigen called purified protein derivative (PPD) may be an important clue regarding their function. The PPD antigen belongs to a group of highly conserved proteins, found in all organisms, called heat-shock proteins, which were so named following the observation that they are produced by cells in response to sudden increases in temperature or other environmental stresses. But heat-shock proteins are also induced by other stresses such as inflammatory responses, viral infections, and cancer. Mycobacterial PPD shows sequence homology with a mammalian heat-shock protein that is a normal component of the mitochondrial matrix. This has led to the speculation that $\gamma\delta$ T cells may be uniquely suited to respond to mammalian heat-shock proteins and may have evolved to eliminate damaged cells as well as microbial invaders.

C. A. Janeway has suggested that the $\gamma\delta$ T cell may represent the most primitive and earliest cell-mediated immune system, uniquely specialized to recognize epithelial-cell alterations outside the basement-membrane barrier. One proposal is that these $\gamma\delta$ T cells, which may be especially suited to combat epidermal or intestinal antigens, form a surveillance system monitoring the integrity of the external epithelial cell milieu. These cells may be able to recognize heat-shock proteins or alterations caused by ultraviolet irradiation in the outer epidermal layer. DECs may be activated by epidermal keratinocytes, which have been shown to be both effective antigen-presenting cells and secretors of IL-1. Such a system would protect the epithelial-cell surfaces, preventing the spread of infection or cancer across the basement membrane into the internal milieu.

Summary

1. T-cell maturation occurs in the thymus as progenitor T cells from the bone marrow enter the thymus and rearrange the TCR genes. The earliest thymocytes lack detectable CD4 and CD8 and are referred to as double-negative cells. These double-negative thymocytes differentiate along two developmental pathways: Those thymocytes that make a productive rearrangement of the $\gamma\delta$-TCR genes develop into $CD4^-$, $CD8^-$, $CD3^+$ $\gamma\delta$ T cells, which account for only 0.5–1.0% of thymocytes. The majority of double-negative thymocytes rearrange the $\alpha\beta$-TCR genes and develop into $CD4^+$, $CD3^+$ $\alpha\beta$ T cells or $CD8^+$, $CD3^+$ $\alpha\beta$ T cells.

2. Rearrangement of germ-line TCR genes during T-cell maturation in the thymus appears to produce many functional genes encoding receptors that are not specific for foreign antigen plus self-MHC molecules. Thymocytes with unwanted TCR specificities are deleted in a two-step selection process. First, positive selection of all thymocytes bearing receptors that can bind a self-MHC molecule confers MHC restriction. Second, negative selection and elimination of thymocytes bearing high-affinity receptors for self-MHC molecules alone or self-antigen plus self-MHC confers self-tolerance. As a result of this thymic selection, only thymocytes that are both self-MHC restricted and self-tolerant develop into mature T cells.

3. T_H-cell activation is initiated by the interaction of the TCR-CD3 complex with a peptide-MHC complex on an antigen-presenting cell. The activating signal is not transduced solely by the TCR-CD3 complex but also is mediated and regulated by a variety of accessory molecules including the coreceptors CD4 or CD8, CD2, and CD45. Signal transduction is accomplished by a series of protein phosphorylation events catalyzed by protein kinases and dephosphorylation events catalyzed by protein phosphatases.

4. In addition to the signals mediated by the T cell receptor and its associated accessory molecules (signal 1), activation of the T_H cell requires an additional co-stimulatory signal (signal 2) provided by the antigen-presenting cell. The co-stimulatory signal can be mediated by the cytokines IL-1 and IL-6 secreted by the APC and by an interaction between the B7 molecule on the membrane of the APC with CD28 (or CTLA-4) on the membrane of the T_H cell.

5. T_H-cell recognition of an antigenic peptide–MHC complex on an antigen-presenting cell results either in activation and clonal expansion or in a state of nonresponsiveness called clonal anergy. The presence or absence of the co-stimulatory signal (signal 2) determines whether activation results in clonal expansion or clonal anergy.

6. Some 90–99% of the peripheral T cells express the $\alpha\beta$ T-cell receptor. Those T cells that express CD4 recognize antigen associated with a class II MHC molecule and generally function as T_H cells; those T cells that express CD8 recognize antigen associated with a class I MHC molecule and generally function as T_C cells. The peripheral $CD4^+$ and $CD8^+$ T cells consist of naive, effector, and memory T cells. Naive T cells are resting cells (G_0) that have not encountered antigen; effector T cells are derived from antigen-activated naive or memory cells and perform helper, cytotoxic, or delayed-type hypersensitivity functions; memory cells either have a long life span or are maintained by continual antigen exposure.

7. T cells expressing the $\gamma\delta$ T-cell receptor constitute only a small percentage of the total T-cell population, but they are concentrated in several epithelial tissues and may represent a primitive cell-mediated immune system that evolved to protect the integrity of external epithelial surfaces.

References

ABRAHAM, R. T., L. M. KARNITZ, J. PAUL SECRIST, and P. J. LEIBSON. 1992. Signal transduction through the T-cell antigen receptor. *Trends Biol. Sci.* **17** (Oct.):434.

ARNAIZ-VILLENA, A., M. TIMON, C. RODRIGUEZ-GALLEGO, et al. 1992. Human T-cell activation deficiencies. *Immunol. Today* **13**:259.

BEYERS, A. D., L. L. SPRUYT, and A. F. WILLIAMS. 1993. Multimolecular associations of the T-cell antigen receptor. *Trends in Cell Biol.* **2**:253.

BRADLEY, L. M., M. CROFT, and S. L. SWAIN. 1993. T-cell memory: new perspectives. *Immunol. Today* **14**:197.

CLIPSTONE, N. A., and G. R. CRABTREE. 1992. Identification of calcineurin as a key signalling enzyme in T-lymphocyte activation. *Nature* **357**:695.

HERMAN, A., J. W. KAPPLER, P. MARRACK, and A. M. PULLEN. 1991. Superantigens: mechanism of T-cell stimulation and role in immune responses. *Annu. Rev. Immunol.* **9**:745.

IZQUIERDO, M., and D. A. CANTRELL. 1992. T-cell activation. *Trends in Cell Biol.* **2**:268.

JANEWAY, C. A. 1992. The T cell receptor as a multicomponent signalling machine: CD4/CD8 coreceptors and CD45 in T cell activation. *Annu. Rev. Immunol.* **10**:645.

JENKINS, M. K. 1992. The role of cell division in the induction of clonal anergy. *Immunol. Today* **13**:69.

JENKINS, M. K., and R. A. MILLER. 1992. Memory and anergy: challenges to traditional models of T lymphocyte differentiation. *The FASEB J.* **6**:2428.

LINSLEY, P. S., and J. A. LEDBETTER. 1993. The role of the CD28 receptor during T cell responses to antigen. *Annu. Rev. Immunol.* **11**:191.

O'KEEFE, S. J., J. TAMURA, R. L. KINCAID, M. J. TOCCI, and E. A. O'NEILL. 1992. FK506-, and CsA-sensitive activation of the interleukin-2 promoter by calcineurin. *Nature* **357**:692.

PEREIRA, P., and S. TONEGAWA. 1993. Gamma/delta cells. *Annu. Rev. Immunol.* **11**:637.

PERLMUTTER, R. W., S. D. LEVIN, M. W. APPLEBY, S. J. ANDERSON, and J. ALBEROLA-ILA. 1993. Regulation of lymphocyte function by protein phosphorylation. *Annu. Rev. Immunol.* **11**:451.

ROBEY, E. A., F. RAMSDELL, D. KIOUSSIS et al. 1992. The level of CD8 expression can determine the outcome of thymic selection. *Cell* **69**:1089.

SCHREIBER, S. L., and G. R. CRABTREE. 1992. The mechanism of action of cyclosporin A and FK506. *Immunol. Today* **13**:136.

SCHWARZ, R. H. 1992. Costimulation of T lymphocytes: the role of CD28, CTLA-4 and B7/BB1 in interleukin-2 production and immunotherapy. *Cell* **72**:1066.

SIGAL, N. H., and F. J. DUMONT. 1992. Cyclosporin A, FK506 and rapamycin: pharmacologic probes of lymphocyte signal transduction. *Annu. Rev. Immunol.* **10**:519.

VON BOEHMER, H., and P. KISIELOW. 1993. Lymphocyte lineage commitment: instruction versus selection. *Cell* **73**:207.

WEISS, A. 1993. T cell antigen receptor signal transduction: a tale of tails and cytoplasmic protein-tyrosine kinases. *Cell* **73**:209.

Study Questions

1. You have a $CD8^+$ CTL clone (from an H-2^k mouse) that has a T-cell receptor specific for the H-Y antigen. You clone the $\alpha\beta$-TCR genes from this clone and use them to prepare transgenic mice with the H-2^k or H-2^d haplotype.
   a. How can you distinguish the immature thymocytes from the mature $CD8^+$ thymocytes in the transgenic mice?
   b. For each transgenic mouse listed in the table below, indicate whether the mouse would (+) or would not (−) have immature double-positive and mature $CD8^+$ thymocytes bearing the transgenic T-cell receptor.

Transgenic mouse	Immature thymocytes	Mature $CD8^+$ thymocytes
H-2^k female		
H-2^k male		
H-2^d female		
H-2^d male		

   c. Explain your answers for the H-2^k transgenics.
   d. Explain your answers for the H-2^d transgenics.

2. Cyclosporin A is a powerful immunosuppressive drug that now is given to transplant recipients. Describe how this drug suppresses the immune response.

3. Antigen activation of T_H cells leads to the release or induction of various nuclear factors that activate gene transcription.
   a. Which two transcription factors required for proliferation of activated T_H cells are present in the cytoplasm of resting T_H cells in inactive forms.
   b. To which enhancer do these transcription factors bind?

4. You have fluorescein-labeled anti-CD4 and rhodamine-labeled anti-CD8. You use these antibodies to stain thymocytes and lymph-node cells from normal mice and from *RAG-1* knock-out mice. In the accompanying diagrams, draw the FACS plots that you would expect.

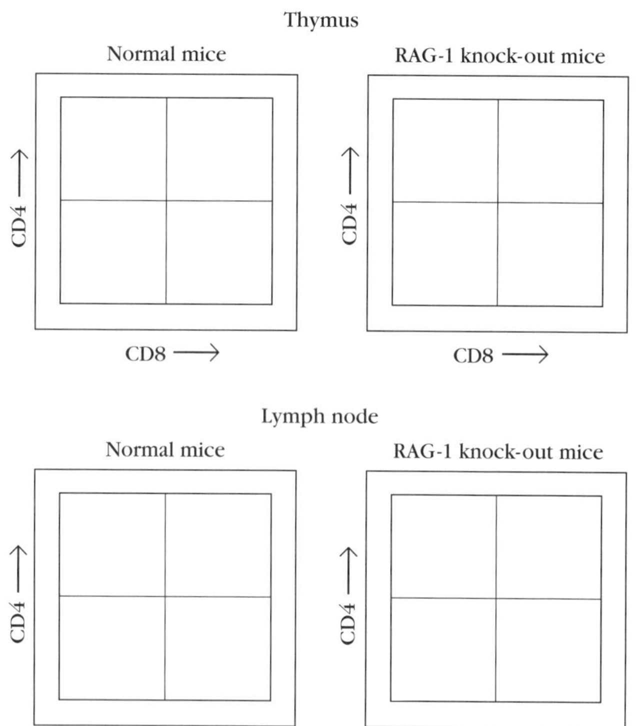

5. In order to demonstrate positive thymic selection experimentally, researchers analyzed the thymocytes from H-2^b mice, which have a deletion of the class II *IEβ* gene, and from H-2^b mice in which the *IAβ* gene had been knocked out.

a. What MHC molecules would you find on antigen-presenting cells from the H-2^b mice?

b. What MHC molecules would you find on antigen-presenting cells from the *IAβ* knock-out H-2^b mice.

c. Would you expect to find CD4$^+$ T cells, CD8$^+$ T cells, or both in each type of mouse. Why?

6. In his classic chimeric-mouse experiments, Zinkernagel took bone marrow from mouse 1 and a thymus from mouse 2 and transplanted them into mouse 3, which was thymectomized and lethally irradiated. He then challenged the reconstituted mouse with LCM virus and removed its spleen cells. These spleen cells were then incubated with LCM-infected target cells with different MHC haplotypes, and the lysis of the target cells was monitored. The results of two such experiments are shown in the accompanying table. The haplotype of strain C57BL/6 is H-2^b and that of strain BALB/c is H-2^d.

a. What was the haplotype of the thymus-donor strain in experiment A and experiment B?

b. Why were the H-2^b target cells not lysed in experiment A but were lysed in experiment B?

c. Why were the H-2^k target cells not lysed in either experiment?

7. You wish to determine the percentage of various types of thymocytes in a sample of cells from mouse thymus using the indirect immunofluorescence method.

a. You first stain the sample with goat anti-CD3 (primary antibody) and then with rabbit FITC-labeled anti-goat Ig (secondary antibody), which emits a green color. Analysis of the stained sample by flow cytometry indicates that 70% of the cells are stained. Based on this result, how many of the thymus cells in your sample are expressing antigen-binding receptors on their surface? Explain your answer. What are the remaining unstained cells likely to be?

b. You then separate the CD3$^+$ cells with the fluorescent-activated cell sorter (FACS) and restain them. In this case, the primary antibody is hamster anti-CD4 and the secondary antibody is rabbit PE-labeled anti-hamster-Ig, which emits a red color. Analysis of the stained CD3$^+$ cells shows that 80% of them are stained. Based on this result, can you determine how many T_C cells are present in this sample? If you can, then how many T_C cells are there? If you cannot, what additional experiment would you perform in order to determine the number of T_C cells that are present?

For use with Question 6.

Experiment	Bone marrow donor	Thymectomized, x-irradiated recipient	Lysis of LCM-infected target cells H-2^d	H-2^k	H-2^b
A	C57BL/6 × BALB/c	C57BI/6 × BALB/c	+	–	–
B	C57BL/6 × BALB/c	C57BI/6 × BALB/c	–	–	+

CYTOKINES

The development of an effective immune response involves lymphoid cells, inflammatory cells, and hematopoietic cells. The complex interactions among these cells are mediated by a group of secreted low-molecular-weight proteins that are collectively designated *cytokines* to denote their role in cell-to-cell communication. Cytokines assist in regulating the development of immune effector cells, and some cytokines possess direct effector functions of their own. Just as hormones serve as messengers of the endocrine system, so cytokines serve as messengers of the immune system; however, unlike endocrine hormones, which exert their effects over large distances, the cytokines generally act locally. This chapter focuses on the biological activity and structure of cytokines, their interaction with specific receptors, their role in the inflammatory response and certain diseases, and possible therapies that alter cytokine activity.

General Properties of Cytokines

Cytokines are a group of low-molecular-weight regulatory proteins secreted by white blood cells and a variety of other cells in the body in response to a number of inducing stimuli. Cytokines bind to specific receptors on the membrane of target cells, eliciting biochemical changes responsible for signal transduction that results in an altered pattern of gene expression in the target cells (Figure 13-1a). The nature of the target cell for a particular cytokine is determined by the presence of specific membrane receptors. In general, the cytokines and their receptors exhibit very high affinity for each other with dissociation constants ranging from 10^{-10} to 10^{-12} *M*. Because of this high affinity, picomolar concentrations of cytokines can mediate a biological effect.

A particular cytokine may exhibit *autocrine* action, binding to receptors on the membrane of the same cell that secreted it; it may exhibit *paracrine* action, binding to receptors on a target cell in close proximity to the producer cell; in a few cases it may exhibit *endocrine* action, binding to target cells in distant parts of the body (Figure 13-1b). Cytokines regulate the intensity and duration of the immune response by stimulating or inhibiting the activation, proliferation, and/or differentiation of various cells and by regulating their secretion of antibodies or other cytokines. As discussed later, binding of a given cytokine to responsive target cells generally stimulates expression of cytokine receptors and of other cytokines, which in turn affect other target cells. Thus, the cytokines secreted by a single lymphocyte following antigen-specific activation can influence the activity of various cells involved in the immune response. For example, cytokines produced by activated T_H cells can influence the activity of B cells, T_C cells, natural killer cells, macrophages, granulocytes, and hematopoietic stem cells, thereby activating an entire network of interacting cells.

Cytokines exhibit the attributes of pleiotropy, redundancy, synergy, and antagonism, which permit them to regulate cellular activity in a coordinated interactive way (Figure 13-2). A given cytokine that has different biological effects on different target cells has a *pleiotropic* action. Two or more cytokines that mediate similar functions are said to be *redundant;* this property makes it difficult to ascribe a particular activity to a single cytokine. Cytokine *synergism* occurs when the combined effect of two cytokines on cellular activity is greater than the additive effects of the individual cytokines. In some cases cytokines exhibit *antagonism;* that is, the effects of one cytokine inhibit or offset the effects of another cytokine.

The term *cytokine* encompasses those cytokines secreted by lymphocytes, formerly known as *lymphokines,* and those cytokines secreted by monocytes and macrophages, formerly known as *monokines.* Although the terms lymphokine and monokine continue to be used in the literature, they are misleading because many lymphokines and monokines are secreted by a broad spectrum of cells and not simply by lym-

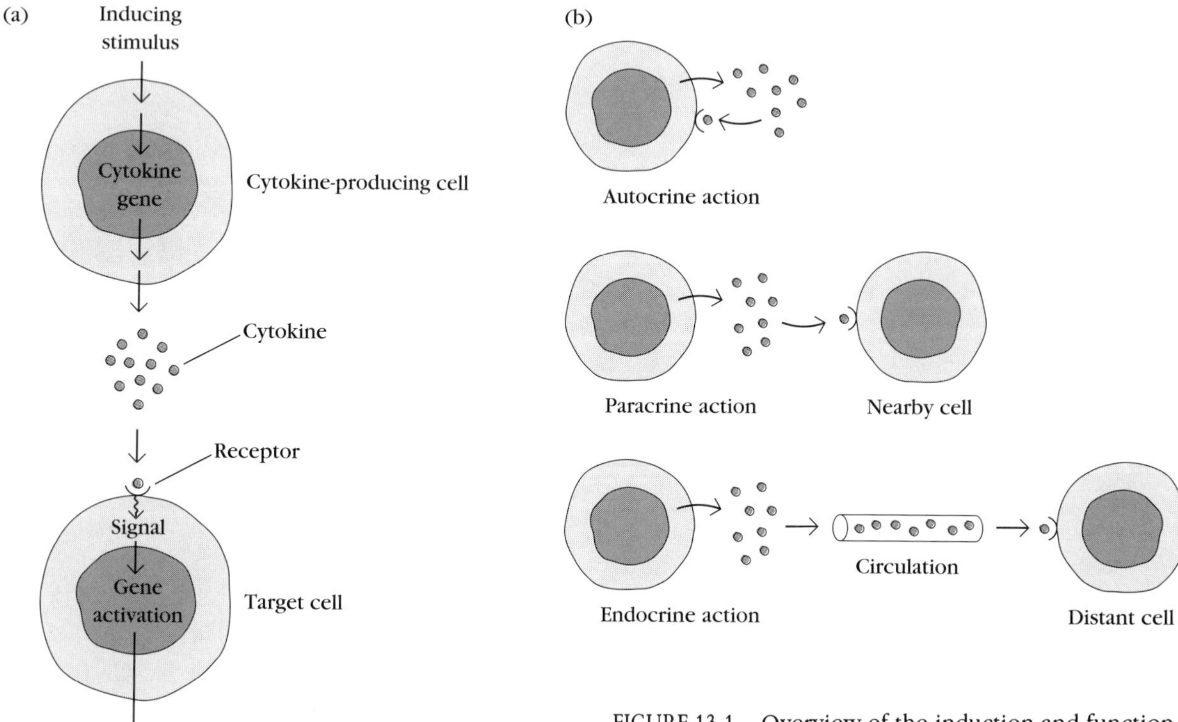

FIGURE 13-1 Overview of the induction and function of cytokines. Most cytokines exhibit autocrine and/or paracrine action.

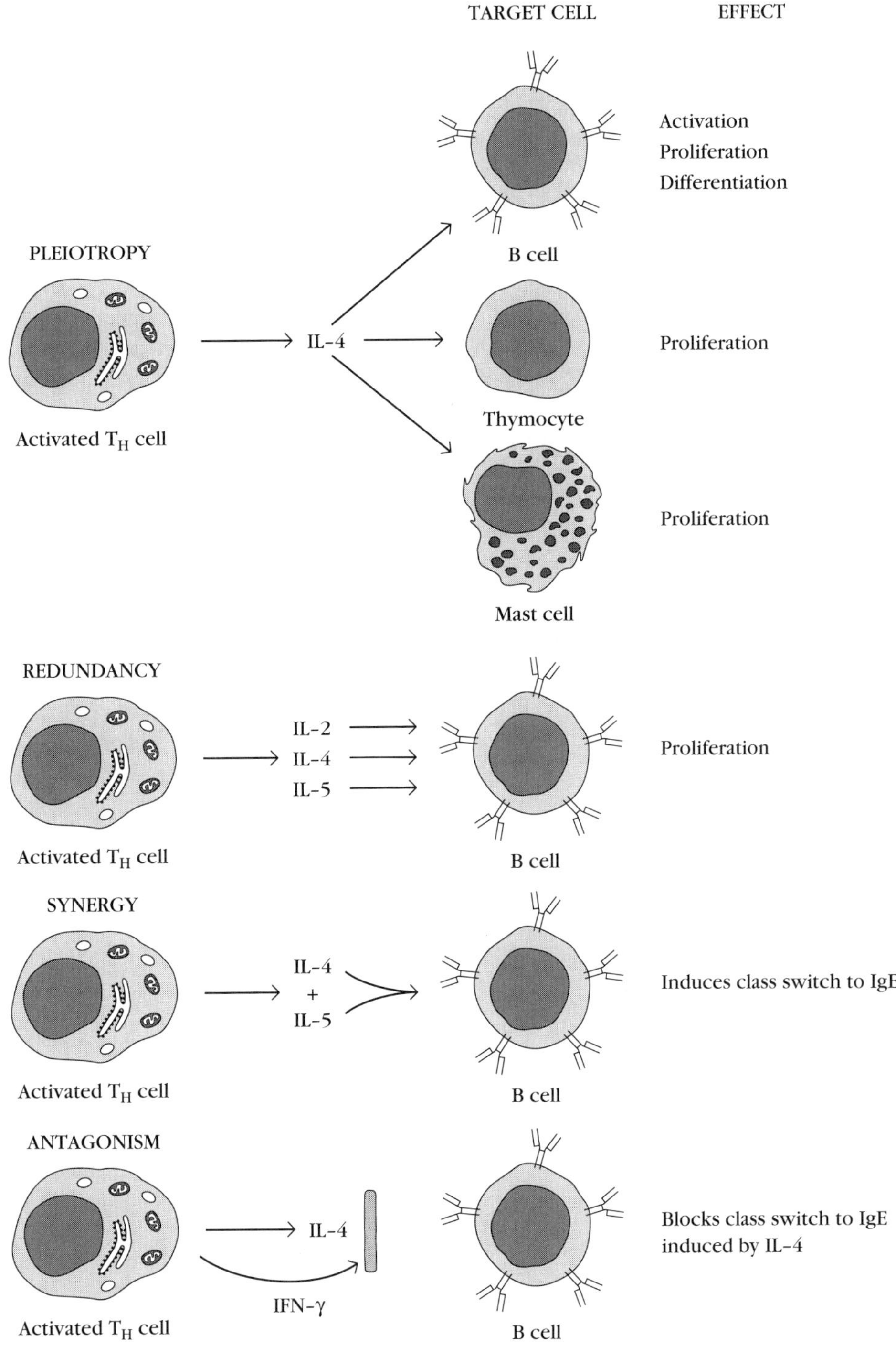

FIGURE 13-2 Examples of the cytokine attributes of pleiotropy, redundancy, synergy (synergism), and antagonism.

phocytes and monocytes as their name would imply. For this reason the more inclusive term cytokine is preferred.

Many of the properties of cytokines are shared by hormones and growth factors, and the distinction between these three classes of mediators often is blurred. All three classes of mediators are secreted soluble factors that elicit their biological effects at picomolar concentrations by binding to receptors on target cells. While growth factors tend to be produced constitutively, cytokine production is carefully regulated. Unlike hormones, which generally act long range in an endocrine fashion, most cytokines act over a short distance in an autocrine or paracrine fashion. In addition, most hormones are produced by specialized glands and tend to have a unique action on one or a few target cells. In contrast, cytokines are often produced by a variety of cells and bind to receptors present on numerous types of cells.

Discovery and Purification of Cytokines

Recognition of the activity of cytokines began in the mid-1960s, when culture supernatants derived from in vitro cultures of allogeneic lymphocytes were found to contain biologically active factors that could regulate proliferation, differentiation, and maturation of various types of lymphoid cells and accessory cells. Soon after, it was discovered that production of these factors by cultured lymphocytes could be induced by activation with antigen or with nonspecific mitogens.

Functional Identification

Following these early discoveries, reports of various biologically active factors generated by different in vitro culture systems rapidly accumulated. Because of slight differences in assay conditions, numerous functional responses were observed, each of which was initially attributed to a unique factor. As a consequence, the literature soon was filled with reports about different factors, each named for its biological activity and given its own acronym.

The formidable list of factors reported during this period included the following: lymphocyte-activating factor (LAF), T-cell growth factor (TCGF), B-cell growth factor (BCGF), T-cell replacing factor (TRF), B-cell differentiation factor (BDF), B-cell activating factor (BAF), mitogenic protein (MP), and thymocyte mitogenic factor (TMF). The numerous reports appearing in the literature left even experts in the field engulfed in a bewildering sea of factors and acronyms. Once cytokines were purified and eventually cloned, this vast array of factors generated in different biological systems was shown to represent the activities of a limited number of cytokines.

Biochemical Purification

Biochemical isolation of cytokines was hampered by several obstacles. For one thing, a culture supernatant often contained mixtures of cytokines rather than a single cytokine, making it difficult to assign a given function to a single substance. Coupled with this was the problem that the early systems available for assaying cytokine function involved heterogeneous populations of lymphocytes, and their various responses to the cytokine being tested often gave ambiguous results. A further difficulty was that culture supernatants contained extremely low concentrations of the cytokines, with subnanomolar concentrations (10^{-10} – 10^{-15} *M*) being biologically active.

Two developments provided a way around these obstacles and led to the biochemical characterization of cytokines. The first development was the discovery of tumor-cell lines that secreted cytokines. These tumor-cell lines provided researchers with homogeneous populations of cells that in some cases secreted much higher concentrations of a given cytokine than did cultures of lymphoid cells. The second development was the discovery of cell lines whose growth depended on the presence of a particular cytokine. These cell lines provided researchers with a simple assay system—a homogeneous population of cells capable of proliferating in response to a given growth factor.

When the cytokines previously identified by a variety of different functions were assessed for biological activity in these defined assay systems, it soon became clear that what had seemed to be a great many cytokines, each named for its biological activity, were often just different activities of the same factor. A standardized nomenclature was developed, with most of the cytokines designated *interleukins* in reference to their role in cellular communication among leukocytes. The first to be named were interleukins 1 and 2. Interleukin 1 (IL-1) was shown to account for the biological activities previously ascribed to at least eight factors, and interleukin 2 (IL-2) accounted for the activities ascribed to four factors. In the past decade the list of defined cytokines has increased to 13 interleukins and several other cytokines still named for their biological activity, and the correspondence between these purified cytokines and previously identified factors has been clarified.

Biochemical purification of the interleukins involved a number of protein purification techniques, and usually began with cytokine-containing supernatants from cell lines producing high levels of a given cytokine. For example, leukemic monocyte lines were chosen for their production of IL-1 and various T-cell lymphomas for their production of IL-2. The cell lines were grown in large-scale cultures and were induced to produce cytokines with mitogens, phorbol esters, or other appropriate inducing agents. The secreted cytokine was then purified from several liters of culture supernatant. However, even with cell lines that produce high levels of cytokines, biochemical purification yielded only small quantities of highly purified cytokines, amounts too small for subsequent research on their structure and function.

Cloning of Cytokine Genes

The frustrations of attempting to purify cytokines with standard biochemical techniques were overcome when the various cytokine genes were cloned using recombinant DNA techniques. The general approach used was to generate a cDNA library from appropriate cytokine-producing cell lines and then express the DNA in COS cells (Figure 13-3). COS cells are a monkey kidney cell line that contains an integrated portion of the SV40 genome. When COS cells are transfected with an expression plasmid consisting, for example, of a cytokine gene together with an SV40 replication origin, the plasmid will be massively replicated, allowing the COS cells to express high yields of the desired cytokine. Identification of COS cells expressing a

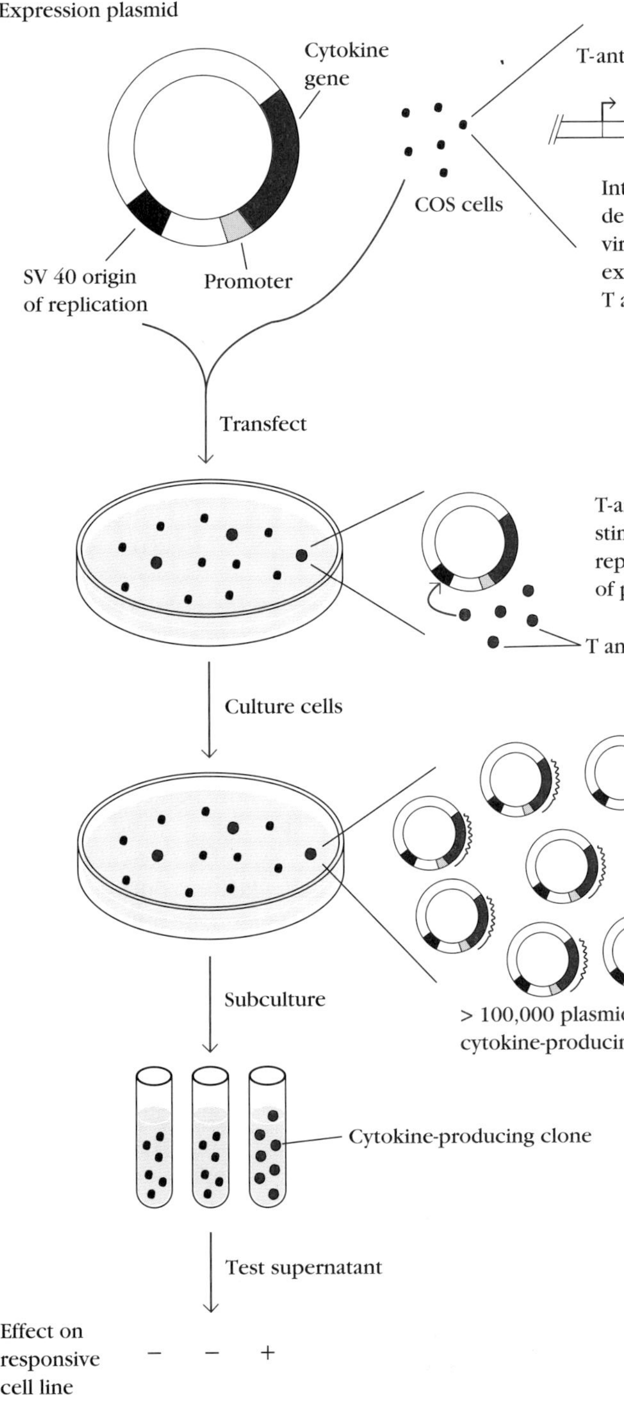

FIGURE 13-3 Experimental procedure for high-level expression of cloned cytokine genes. The cytokine gene of interest (purple) is incorporated into a plasmid that contains the SV40 replication origin. The plasmid is then transfected into COS cells, which contain an integrated portion of the SV40 genome and express T antigen, a protein that stimulates viral replication. The transfected COS cells express high levels of the cytokine encoded by the gene on the plasmid. A biological assay or monoclonal antibody is used to identify the cytokine-secreting clones. A similar system is used to express cytokine receptors.

desired cytokine is generally achieved with a biological assay. Since cells are sensitive to picomolar levels of cytokines, it is possible to identify the cytokine-secreting clones by adding the culture supernatant from the COS cells to a cytokine-responsive cell line. Alternatively, monoclonal antibodies can be used to identify the cytokine in the COS cell-culture supernatant in an ELISA or RIA assay.

To date genes encoding thirteen interleukins (IL-1 through IL-13), three interferons (IFN-α, IFN-β, and IFN-γ), two tumor necrosis factors (TNF-α and TNF-β), transforming growth factor β (TGF-β), leukemia inhibitory factor (LIF), and oncostatin M (OSM) have been cloned and expressed, providing researchers with homogenous preparations of the individual cytokines.

Structure of Cytokines

Once the genes encoding various cytokines had been cloned, sufficient quantities of purified preparations became available for detailed studies on the structure and function of these important proteins. Cytokines are proteins or glycoproteins that generally have a molecular weight less than 30 kDa. Structural predictions based on sequence analyses, in some cases confirmed by x-ray crystallographic analysis, suggest that many of the cytokines belong to a family of structurally related proteins. Included in this family are IL-2, IL-3, IL-4, IL-5, IL-6, IL-7, IFN-β, GM-CSF, M-CSF, G-CSF, and oncostatin M. Despite a lack of similarity in their amino acid sequences, all of these cytokines have a high degree of α-helical structure and little or no β-sheet structure. The molecules share a similar polypeptide fold with four α-helical bundles. The structure of IL-2, a prototype member of this family, is shown in Figure 13-4.

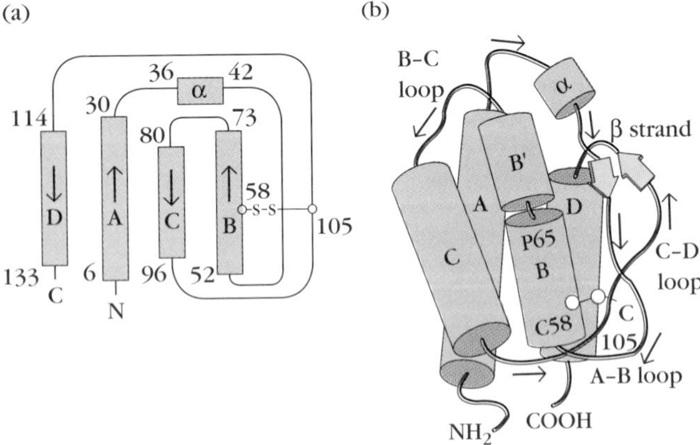

FIGURE 13-4 Structure of interleukin 2. (a) Topographical representation of the α-helical bundles (A–D) and connecting chains of the molecule. (b) Proposed structural model of IL-2. The structure of many other cytokines is thought to be generally similar.

Function of Cytokines

Cytokines generally function as intercellular messenger molecules that evoke particular biological activities after binding to a receptor on a responsive target cell. Although a variety of cells can secrete cytokines, the two principal producers are the T_H cell and the macrophage. Cytokines released from these two cells activate an entire network of interacting cells (Figure 13-5). The binding of a cytokine to its receptor induces numerous physiologic responses including the development of cellular and humoral immune responses, induction of the inflammatory response, regulation of hematopoiesis, control of cellular proliferation and differentiation, and induction of wound healing.

Table 13-1 summarizes the main biological activities of the most important cytokines. It should be kept in mind that most of the listed functions have been identified from analysis of the effects of recombinant cytokines in in vitro systems and often at nonphysiologic concentrations. However, cytokines rarely, if ever, act alone in vivo. Instead a target cell is exposed to a milieu containing a mixture of cytokines, whose combined synergistic or antagonistic effects can have very different consequences. In addition, cytokines often induce the synthesis of other cytokines, resulting in cascades of cytokine activity in which later cytokines may influence the activity of earlier cytokines.

It is difficult to reconcile the nonspecificity of cytokines with the established specificity of the immune system. What keeps the nonspecific cytokines from activating cells in a nonspecific fashion during the immune response? Clearly some mechanisms must operate to ensure that the specificity of the immune response is maintained. One way in which specificity is maintained is by careful regulation of the expression of cytokine receptors on cells. Often cytokine receptors are expressed on a cell only after that cell has interacted with antigen. In this way nonspecific cytokine activation is limited to antigen-primed lymphocytes. Another means of maintaining specificity may be a requirement for cell-to-cell interaction to generate effective concentrations of a cytokine at the juncture of interacting cells. In the case of the T_H cell, a major producer of cytokines, close cellular interaction occurs when the T-cell receptor recognizes an antigen-MHC complex on an appropriate antigen-presenting cell, such as a macrophage, dendritic cell, or B

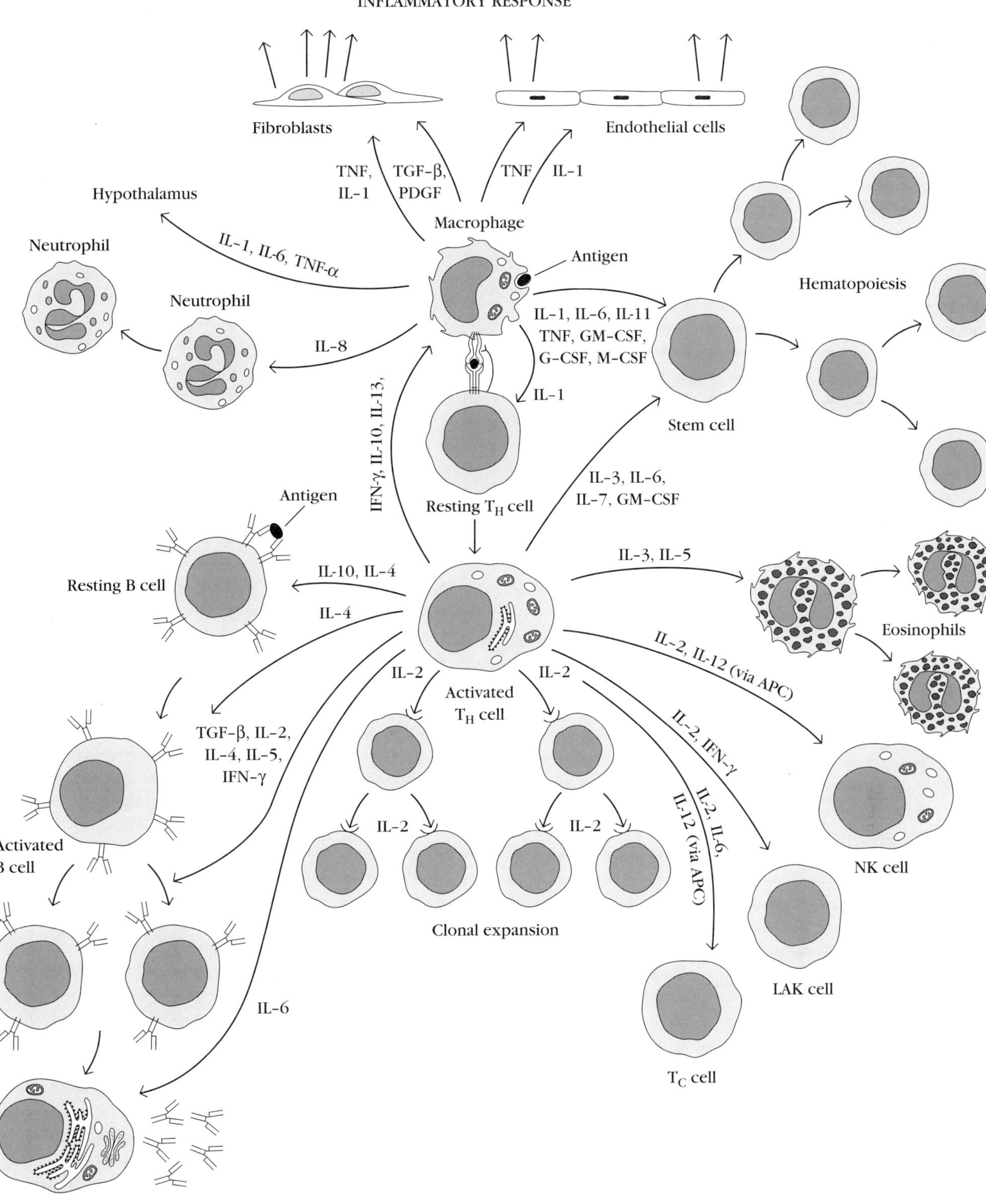

FIGURE 13-5 Interaction of antigen (purple) with macrophages and the subsequent activation of resting T_H cells leads to release of numerous cytokines, generating a complex network of interacting cells in the immune response.

TABLE 13-1 SELECTED FUNCTIONS OF SOME CYTOKINES

Cytokine	Secreted by*	Major biological functions	
		Target cells/tissues	Activity
Interleukin 1 (IL-1α, IL-1β)	Monocytes, macrophages, B cells, dendritic cells, endothelial cells, and other cell types	T_H cells	Co-stimulates activation
		B cells	Promotes maturation and clonal expansion
		NK cells	Enhances activity
		Vascular endothelial cells	Increases expression of ICAMs
		Macrophages and neutrophils	Chemotactically attracts
		Hepatocytes	Induces synthesis of acute-phase proteins
		Hypothalamus	Induces fever
Interleukin 2 (IL-2)	T_H1 cells	Antigen-primed T_H and T_C cells	Induces proliferation
		Antigen-specific T-cell clones	Supports long-term growth
		NK cells (some) and T_C cells	Enhances activity
Interleukin 3 (IL-3)	T_H cells, NK cells, and mast cells	Hematopoietic cells	Supports growth and differentiation
		Mast cells	Stimulates growth and histamine secretion
Interleukin 4 (IL-4)	T_H2 cells	Antigen-primed B cells	Co-stimulates activation
		Activated B cells	Stimulates proliferation and differentiation; induces class switch to IgG1 and IgE
		Resting B cells	Up-regulates class II MHC expression
		Thymocytes and T cells	Induces proliferation
		Macrophages	Up-regulates class II MHC expression; increases phagocytic activity
		Mast cells	Stimulates growth
Interleukin 5 (IL-5)	T_H2 cells	Activated B cells	Stimulates proliferation and differentiation; induces class switch to IgA
		Eosinophils	Promotes growth and differentiation
Interleukin 6 (IL-6)	Monocytes, macrophages, T_H2 cells and bone-marrow stromal cells	Proliferating B cells	Promotes terminal differentiation into plasma cells
		Plasma cells	Stimulates antibody secretion
		Myeloid stem cells	Helps promote differentiation
		Hepatocytes	Induces synthesis of acute-phase proteins
Interleukin 7 (IL-7)	Bone-marrow and thymic stromal cells	Lymphoid stem cells	Induces differentiation into progenitor B and T cells
		Resting T cells	Increases expression of IL-2 and its receptor

(Continued)

TABLE 13-1 (CONTINUED) SELECTED FUNCTIONS OF SOME CYTOKINES

Cytokine	Secreted by*	Major biological functions	
		Target cells/tissues	Activity
Interleukin 8 (IL-8)	Macrophages and endothelial cells	Neutrophils	Chemotatically attracts; induces adherence to vascular endothelium and extravasation into tissues
Interleukin 9 (IL-9)	T_H cells	Some T_H cells	Acts as mitogen, supporting proliferation in absence of antigen
Interleukin 10 IL-10)	T_H2 cells	Macrophages	Suppresses cytokine production and thus indirectly reduces cytokine production by T_H1 cells
		Antigen-presenting cells	Down-regulates class II MHC expression
Interleukin 11 (IL-11)	Bone-marrow stromal cells	Plasmacytomas	Supports growth
		Progenitor B cells	Promotes differentiation
		Megakaryocytes	Promotes differentiation
		Hepatocytes	Induces synthesis of acute-phase proteins
Interleukin 12 (IL-12)	Macrophages and B cells	Activated T_C cells	Acts synergistically with IL-2 to induce differentiation into CTLs
		NK and LAK cells and activated T_H1 cells	Stimulates proliferation
Interleukin 13 (IL-13)	T_H cells	Macrophages	Inhibits activation and release of inflammatory cytokines; important regulator of inflammatory response
Interferon alpha (IFN-α)	Leukocytes	Uninfected cells	Inhibits viral replication
Interferon beta (IFN-β)	Fibroblasts	Uninfected cells	Inhibits viral replication
Interferon gamma (IFN-γ)	T_H1, T_C, and NK cells	Uninfected cells	Inhibits viral replication
		Macrophages	Enhances activity
		Many cell types	Increases expression of class I and class II MHC molecules
		Proliferating B cells	Induces class switch to IgG2a; blocks IL-4–induced class switch to IgE and IgG1
		T_H2 cells	Inhibits proliferation
		Inflammatory cells	Mediates various effects important in delayed-type hypersensitivity

(Continued)

TABLE 13-1 (CONTINUED) SELECTED FUNCTIONS OF SOME CYTOKINES

		Major biological functions	
Cytokine	Secreted by*	Target cells/tissues	Activity
Leukemia inhibitory factor (LIF)	Thymic epithelial cells and bone-marrow stromal cells	Hepatocytes	Induces synthesis of acute-phase proteins
		Embryonic stem (ES) cells	Supports proliferation
		Hematopoietic cells	Regulates proliferation and differentiation
Oncostatin M (OSM)	Macrophages and T cells	Tumor cells	Inhibits growth
		Hepatocytes	Induces synthesis of acute-phase proteins
		Kaposi's sarcoma	Stimulates growth
Transforming growth factor β (TGF-β)	Platelets, macrophages, and lymphocytes	Monocytes and macrophages	Chemotactically attracts
		Activated macrophages	Induces increased IL-1 production
		Epithelial, endothelial, lymphoid, and hematopoietic cells	Inhibits proliferation, thus limiting inflammatory response and promoting wound healing
		Proliferating B cells	Induces class switch to IgA
Tumor necrosis factor α (TNF-α)	Macrophages	Tumor cells	Has cytotoxic effect
		Inflammatory cells	Induces cytokine secretion and is responsible for extensive weight loss (cachexia) associated with chronic inflammation
Tumor necrosis factor β (TNF-β)	T_H1 and T_C cells	Tumor cells	Has cytotoxic and other effects similar to TNF-α
		Macrophages and neutrophils	Enhances phagocytic activity

* Activated cells generally exhibit greater cytokine secretion than unactivated cells.

lymphocyte (see Figure 14-9). Cytokines secreted at the junction of these interacting cells reach concentrations high enough to affect the target cell. In addition, the half-life of cytokines in the bloodstream or other extracellular fluids into which they are secreted is usually very short, ensuring that they act for only a limited period of time.

CYTOKINE RECEPTORS

The cytokines exert their biological effects through specific receptors expressed on the membrane of responsive target cells. Because these receptors are expressed by many types of cells, the cytokines can affect a diverse array of cells. Biochemical characterization of cytokine receptors initially progressed at a very slow pace because their levels on the membrane of responsive cells is quite low. As in the case of the cytokines themselves, cloning of the genes encoding cytokine receptors has led to rapid advances in the identification and characterization of these receptors. High-level expression of cytokine receptors has been achieved by transfection of a cDNA library into COS cells and subsequent detection of receptor-producing cells with fluorescent antibodies against the cytokine receptor or with radiolabeled cytokine ligands.

General Structure of Cytokine Receptors

Once the genes encoding the various cytokine receptors were cloned, research on the structure of these receptors accelerated. Sequence analysis of the cloned cytokine receptor cDNAs and characterization of the recombinant receptor proteins have revealed some common structural features. All the cytokine receptors have an extracellular domain, a single membrane-spanning domain, and a cytoplasmic domain. Conserved amino acid sequence motifs have been identified in the extracellular domain of many cytokine receptors; these motifs can be used to define the *cytokine-receptor family* (Figure 13-6). The shared motifs are four conserved cysteine residues (CCCC) and a conserved sequence of Trp-Ser-X-Trp-Ser and sometimes γ chain. Generally the α subunit is cytokine specific, and the β or γ subunits are required for high-affinity binding of the cytokine and/or signal transduction. The IL-2Rα subunit has a different structure and is not a member of this receptor family. [Adapted from D. Cosman, 1993, *Cytokine* **5**:95.]

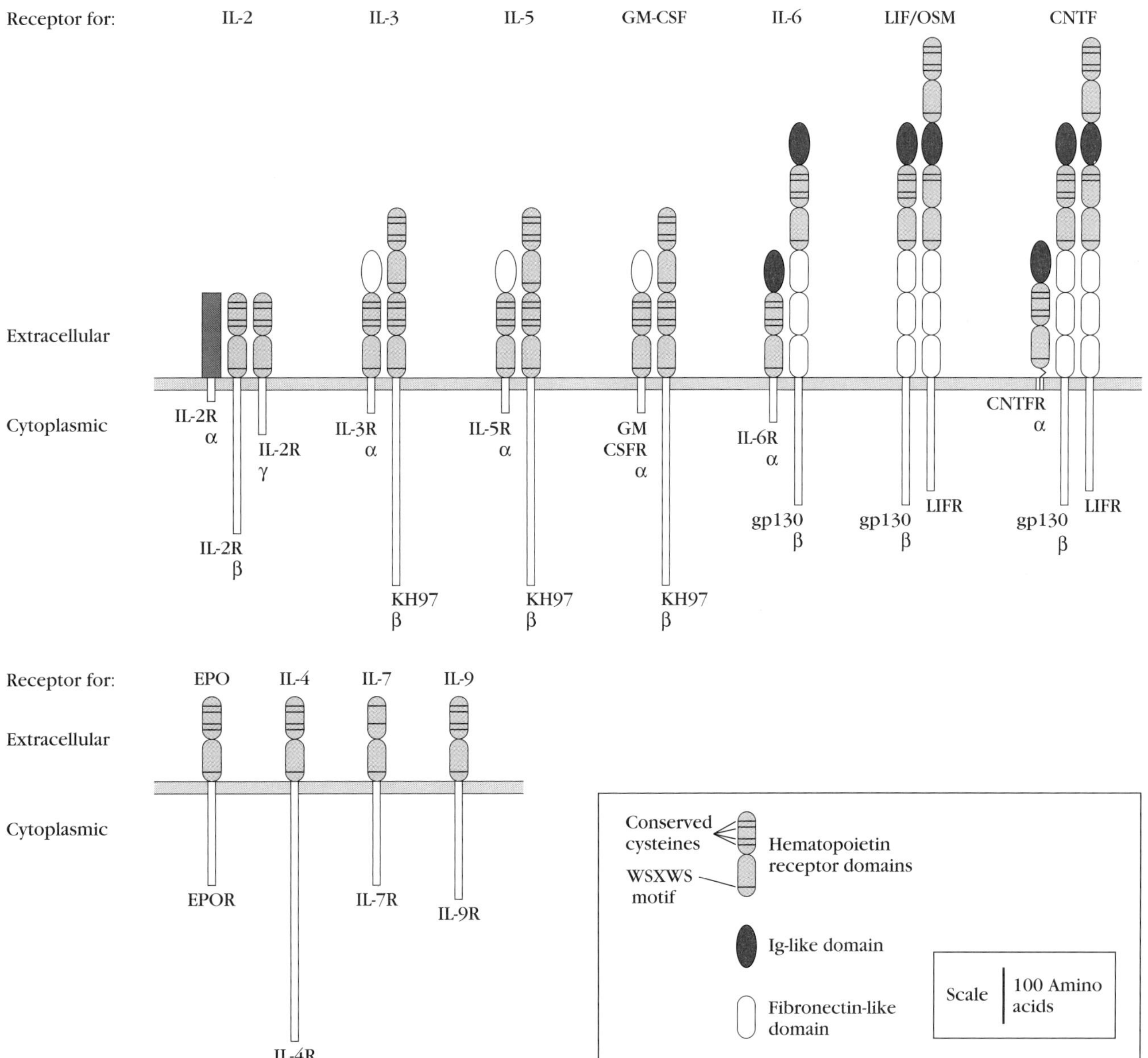

FIGURE 13-6 Schematic diagram of members of the cytokine-receptor family illustrating conserved motifs (CCCC and WS) in their extracellular domains. In some cases additional immunoglobulin-like domains or fibronectin-like domains are also present. The cytokine receptors are generally dimeric or trimeric molecules, consisting of an α, β,

(W-S-X-W-S), where X is a nonconserved amino acid, that is designated the WS motif.

Another common feature found in many cytokine receptors is the presence of two polypeptide chains: a cytokine-specific α subunit and a signal-transducing β subunit, which often is not specific for the cytokine. The β subunit is required for high-affinity binding of a cytokine as well as for transduction of an activating signal across the membrane. The transducing β subunits of all the cytokine receptors studied to date have been shown to induce tyrosine phosphorylation, although none has tyrosine kinase activity. This finding suggests that the transmembrane or cytoplasmic domain of the transducing subunit is closely associated with an intracellular protein kinase.

Some cytokine receptors have been found to share a common signal-transducing subunit, a phenomenon that explains the redundancy and antagonism exhibited among some cytokines. For example, IL-3, IL-5, and GM-CSF each bind to a unique low-affinity, cytokine-specific receptor consisting of an α subunit only. All three low-affinity α subunits can associate noncovalently with a common β subunit, designated KH97, which increases the affinity of the α subunit for the cytokine and functions to transduce the signal across the membrane (Figure 13-7). Interestingly, IL-3, IL-5, and GM-CSF exhibit considerable redundancy. Both IL-3 and GM-CSF act upon hematopoietic stem cells and progenitor cells, activate monocytes, and induce megakaryocyte differentiation. All three of these cytokines induce eosinophil proliferation and basophil degranulation with release of histamine.

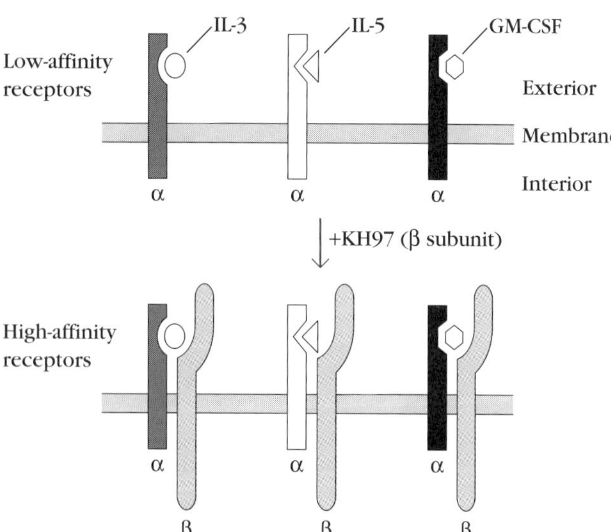

FIGURE 13-7 Schematic diagram of the low-affinity and high-affinity receptors for IL-3, IL-5, and GM-CSF. The cytokine-specific α subunits exhibit low-affinity binding and cannot transduce an activation signal. Noncovalent association of each α subunit with a common β subunit (KH97) yields a high-affinity dimeric receptor that can transduce a signal across the membrane. [Adapted from T. Kishimoto et al., 1992, *Science* **258**:593.]

Since the receptors for IL-3, IL-5, and GM-CSF share a common signal-transducing β subunit, each of these cytokines would be expected to induce a similar activation signal, accounting for the redundancy among their biological effects. In fact, all three cytokines induce the same patterns of protein phosphorylation and phosphorylate the protein kinase Raf. Furthermore, IL-3 and GM-CSF exhibit antagonism; IL-3 binding has been shown to be inhibited by GM-CSF, and conversely, the binding of GM-CSF has been shown to be inhibited by IL-3. Since the signal-transducing β subunit is shared among these two cytokines, their antagonism is due to competition for a limited number of β subunits by the cytokine-specific α subunits.

A similar situation has been discovered among the receptors for IL-6, leukemia inhibitory factor (LIF), oncostatin M (OSM), and ciliary neurotrophic factor (CNTF). In this case, a common signal-transducing β subunit, called gp130, associates with one or two different cytokine-specific α subunits (see Figure 13-6). LIF and OSM, which must share certain structural features, both bind to the same α subunit. As expected, these four cytokines display overlapping biological activities: IL-6, OSM, and LIF induce synthesis of acute-phase proteins by liver hepatocytes; IL-6, OSM, and LIF induce differentiation of myeloid leukemia cells into macrophages; IL-6, LIF, and CNTF affect neuronal development; IL-6 and OSM stimulate megakaryocyte maturation and platelet production; and IL-6 and OSM stimulate proliferation of Kaposi's sarcoma cells. The presence of gp130 in all four receptors explains their common signaling pathways as well as the binding competition that is observed among these cytokines.

As illustrated in Figure 13-6, the receptors for IL-4, IL-7, IL-9, and erythropoietin (EPO) consist of only one polypeptide chain. This single chain contains the conserved cysteines and WS motif typical of cytokine receptors and is generally similar to the β chain in the IL-2 receptor. Presumably, ligand binding and signal transduction are both mediated by the single chain of these monomeric receptors.

Signal Transduction by Cytokine Receptors

Little is known about the mechanism by which the interaction between a cytokine and its receptor is transduced into an intracellular signal that activates the genes responsible for cellular proliferation, differentiation, and other biological activities. Phosphorylation of protein tyrosine residues is induced by many cytokines, including interleukins 2–7, G-CSF, GM-CSF, LIF, CNTF, and erythropoietin (EPO). However, the receptors for all of these cytokines lack any domains with tyrosine kinase activity. Rather, these receptors appear to be closely associated with intracellular protein kinases that participate in a signaling cascade. For example, the large cytoplasmic domain of the β subunit of the IL-2 receptor has been shown to associate with the Src-like protein tyrosine kinases $p56^{lck}$ and $p59^{fyn}$. This association is similar to that found between $p56^{lck}$ and CD4 or CD8 molecules on T cells (see Figure 12-11). The signal-transduction cascade initiated by binding of a cytokine to its receptor eventually results in the production of DNA-binding proteins that influence transcription of various genes. The cytokine-mediated signals involved in the activation and proliferation of lymphocytes are discussed in Chapters 14 and 15.

In some cases the binding of a cytokine to its receptor has been shown to activate expression of another cytokine, leading to cascades of cytokines that sometimes display synergistic or antagonistic activities. Following cloning of genes encoding cytokines, researchers began to identify nuclear factors that bind to promoter and enhancer sequences in these genes. The promoter in the IL-6 gene, for instance, has been shown to contain several regulatory regions to which DNA-binding proteins bind (Figure 13-8). Three such proteins are the nuclear factor IL-6 (NF-IL6), the multiresponse element (MRE), and nuclear factor κB (NF-κB). The finding that each of these DNA-binding proteins can be induced by IL-1 and TNF-α accounts for the observation that IL-1, TNF-α, and IL-6 are expressed together. Both TNF-α and IL-1 have been shown to induce expression of each other as well as expression of IL-6. The coordinated expression of these three cytokines plays an important role in generating an inflammatory response.

IL-2 Receptor

Because of the central role of IL-2 and its receptor in the clonal proliferation of T cells, the IL-2 receptor is the most studied of the cytokine receptors. Three distinct membrane subunits—the α chain, β chain, and recently discovered γ chain—compose the IL-2 receptor. The β and γ chains are members of the cytokine-receptor family, contain the characteristic CCCC and WS motifs, and mediate signal transduction. The α chain has a quite different structure and is not a member of the cytokine-receptor family. The IL-2 receptor may be present in three forms that exhibit different affinities for IL-2: the low-affinity monomeric IL-2Rα, the intermediate-affinity dimeric IL-2R$\beta\gamma$, and the high-affinity trimeric IL-2R$\alpha\beta\gamma$ (Figure 13-9). Because the α chain is expressed by activated but not resting T cells, it is often referred to as the TAC (T-cell activation) antigen. A monoclonal antibody, designated anti-TAC, which binds to the 55-kDa α chain, is often used to identify IL-2Rα on cells.

Signal transduction requires expression of both the β and γ chains, but only when the α chain also is

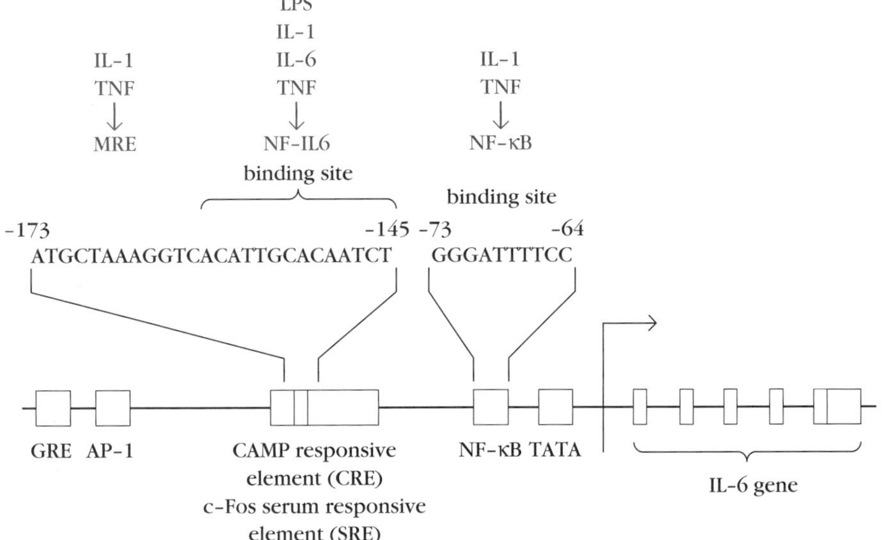

FIGURE 13-8 The promoter region of the gene encoding IL-6 contains regulatory sequences to which MRE, NF-IL6 and NF-κB bind. These DNA-binding proteins, which are induced by IL-1 and TNF-α, stimulate transcription of the IL-6 gene. Thus, as IL-1 and TNF-α levels increase, production of IL-6 also increases.

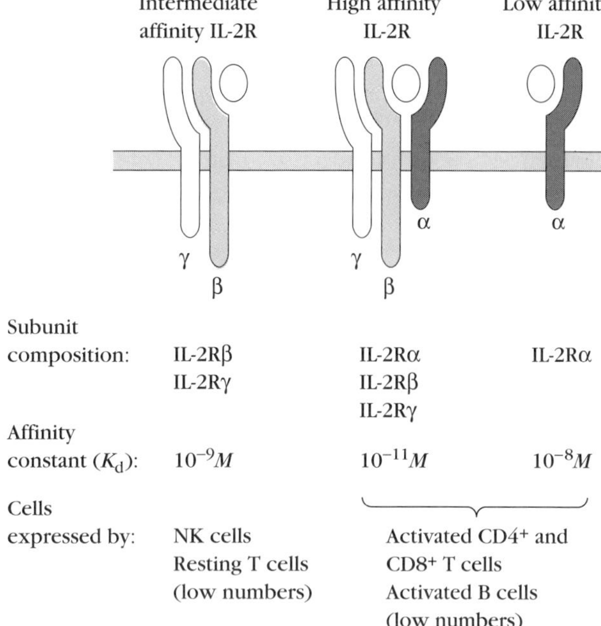

FIGURE 13-9 Comparison of the three forms of the IL-2 receptor. Signal transduction is mediated by the β and γ chains, but all three chains are required for high-affinity binding of IL-2.

expressed can a T cell bind IL-2 with high affinity. Although the γ chain appears to be constitutively expressed on most lymphoid cells, expression of the α and β chains is more restricted and is markedly enhanced following antigen activation of resting cells. This phenomenon ensures that only antigen-activated $CD4^+$ and $CD8^+$ T cells will express the high-affinity IL-2 receptor and proliferate in response to physiologic levels of IL-2. Activated T cells express both high-affinity and low-affinity IL-2 receptors; there are approximately 5×10^3 high-affinity receptors and ten times as many low-affinity receptors. NK cells express the $\beta\gamma$ subunits constitutively accounting for their ability to bind IL-2 with an intermediate affinity and to be activated by IL-2.

Like other members of the cytokine-receptor family, the IL-2 receptor lacks domains with tyrosine kinase activity. However, when IL-2 binds to the IL-2 receptor, rapid tyrosine phosphorylation occurs. Signaling is mediated by interaction of the long cytoplasmic domain of the β chain with Src-family tyrosine kinases ($p56^{lck}$, $p59^{fyn}$, $p53/56^{lyn}$), leading to the phosphorylation of cellular proteins and expression of c-Fos, c-Jun, and c-Myc. The IL-2R γ chain also appears to play a role in signal transduction, and it is thought that the cytoplasmic domain of the γ chain interacts with the β chain to transduce the activating signal. When certain mutations are introduced into the cytoplasmic domain of the γ chain, IL-2–mediated signaling is abolished. The γ chain of IL-2R also may be required for T-cell maturation in the thymus. This possibility is suggested by the finding that three patients with X-linked severe combined immunodeficiency, which is characterized by the absence of mature T cells, have a nonsense mutation in the gene encoding the IL-2R γ chain.

Cytokine Antagonists

A number of proteins that inhibit the biological activity of cytokines have been reported. These proteins act in one of two ways: Either they bind directly to a cytokine receptor but fail to activate the cell, or they bind directly to a cytokine inhibiting its activity. The best characterized inhibitor is the IL-1 receptor antagonist (IL-1Ra), which binds to the IL-1 receptor but has no activity. Binding of IL-1Ra to the IL-1 receptor blocks binding of IL-1α or IL-1β, thus accounting for the antagonistic properties of IL-1Ra. Production of IL-1Ra appears to play a role in regulating the intensity of the inflammatory response. IL-1Ra has been cloned and is currently being investigated as a potential treatment for chronic inflammatory diseases.

A second group of cytokine inhibitors are soluble cytokine receptors that are able to bind to the cytokine and neutralize its activity. Enzymic cleavage of the extracellular domain of a cytokine receptor releases a soluble fragment that retains its cytokine-binding properties. Among the soluble cytokine receptors that have been detected are those for IL-2, IL-4, IL-6, IL-7, IFN-γ, TNF-α, TNF-β, and LIF. Of these, the soluble IL-2 receptor, which is released following chronic T-cell activation, is the best characterized. The amino-terminal 192 amino acids of the α subunit is released by proteolytic cleavage, forming a 45-kDa soluble IL-2 receptor (sIL-2R). The shed receptor can bind IL-2 and prevent its interaction with the membrane-bound IL-2R. The presence of sIL-2R has been used as a clinical marker of chronic T-cell activation and is observed in a number of diseases including autoimmunity, transplant rejection, and AIDS.

Viruses have also been shown to produce cytokine-binding proteins. The poxviruses, for example, have been shown to encode a soluble TNF-binding protein and a soluble IL-1–binding protein. Since both TNF and IL-1 exhibit a broad spectrum of activities in the inflammatory response, these soluble cytokine-binding proteins may prohibit or diminish the inflammatory effects of the cytokine, thereby conferring upon the virus a selective advantage.

Cytokine Secretion and Biological Activity of T_H1 and T_H2 Subsets

The immune response to a specific antigen must induce an appropriate set of effector functions that can eliminate the particular pathogen involved in the infection. For example, the neutralization of a soluble bacterial toxin requires antibodies, whereas the response to an intracellular virus or bacterial cell requires cell-mediated cytotoxicity or delayed-type hypersensitivity. In the last few years a large body of evidence has accumulated suggesting that differences in cytokine-secretion patterns among T-cell subsets play a major role in regulating the choice of immune functional modality.

$CD4^+$ T cells exert most of their helper functions through secreted cytokines, which either act on the cells that produce them in an autocrine fashion or modulate the responses of other cells through paracrine pathways. Although $CD8^+$ CTLs also secrete cytokines, their array of cytokines generally is more restricted than that of $CD4^+$ T_H cells. As discussed in previous chapters, two mouse $CD4^+$ T_H-cell subsets can be distinguished in vitro by the cytokines they secrete. As shown in Table 13-2, these two subsets, designated T_H1 and T_H2, both secrete IL-3 and GM-CSF, but otherwise they differ in the cytokines they secrete. The difference in the cytokines secreted is thought to reflect different biological functions of these two subsets. The T_H1 subset is responsible for classical cell-mediated functions such as delayed-type hypersensitivity and activation of T_C cells, whereas the T_H2 subset functions more effectively as a helper for B-cell activation. The T_H1 subset may be particularly suited to respond to viral infections and intracellular pathogens because it secretes IL-2 and IFN-γ, which activate T_C cells. The T_H2 subset may be more suited to respond to freeliving bacteria and helminthic parasitics and may mediate allergic reactions, since IL-4 and IL-5 are known to induce IgE production and eosinophil activation, respectively. In humans, there is now considerable evidence for T_H1-like and T_H2-like subsets, although the expression of a few cytokines such as IL-2 and IL-10 do not show such a clear segregation as seen in the mouse.

Because the T_H1 and T_H2 subsets were originally identified in long-term in vitro cultures, some researchers have doubted that they represent true in vivo subpopulations and have suggested instead that they represent different maturational stages of a single lineage. Nevertheless, numerous reports in both mice and humans suggest that the in vivo outcome of the immune response depends on the relative levels of T_H1-like or T_H2-like activity: T_H1 cytokines are generally elevated in responses to intracellular pathogens, and T_H2 cytokines are elevated in allergic diseases and helminthic infections.

Table 13-2 Cytokine secretion and principal functions of mouse T_H1 and T_H2 subsets

Cytokine/function	T_H1	T_H2
Cytokine secretion		
IL-2	+	−
IFN-γ	++	−
TNF-β	++	−
GM-CSF	++	+
IL-3	++	++
IL-4	−	++
IL-5	−	++
IL-10	−	++
IL-13	−	++
Functions		
Help for total antibody production	+	++
Help for IgE production	−	++
Help for IgG2a production	++	+
Eosinophil and mast-cell production	−	++
Macrophage activation	++	−
Delayed-type hypersensitivity	++	−
T_C-cell activation	++	−

SOURCE: Adapted from F. Powrie and R. L. Coffman, 1993, *Immunol. Today* **14**:270.

The cytokines produced by the T_H1 and T_H2 subsets exhibit *cross-regulation;* that is, the cytokines secreted by one subset can block the production and/or activity of the cytokines secreted by the other subset (Figure 13-10). For instance, IFN-γ (secreted by the T_H1 subset) preferentially inhibits proliferation of the T_H2 subset, and IL-10 (secreted by the T_H2 subset) down-regulates secretion of IFN-γ and IL-2 by the T_H1 subset. Similarly, IFN-γ and IL-2 (secreted by the T_H1 subset) promote IgG2a production by B cells but inhibit IgG1 and IgE production. On the other hand, IL-4 (secreted by the T_H2 subset) promotes production of IgG1 and IgE and suppresses production of IgG2a. The phenomenon of cross-regulation provides an explanation

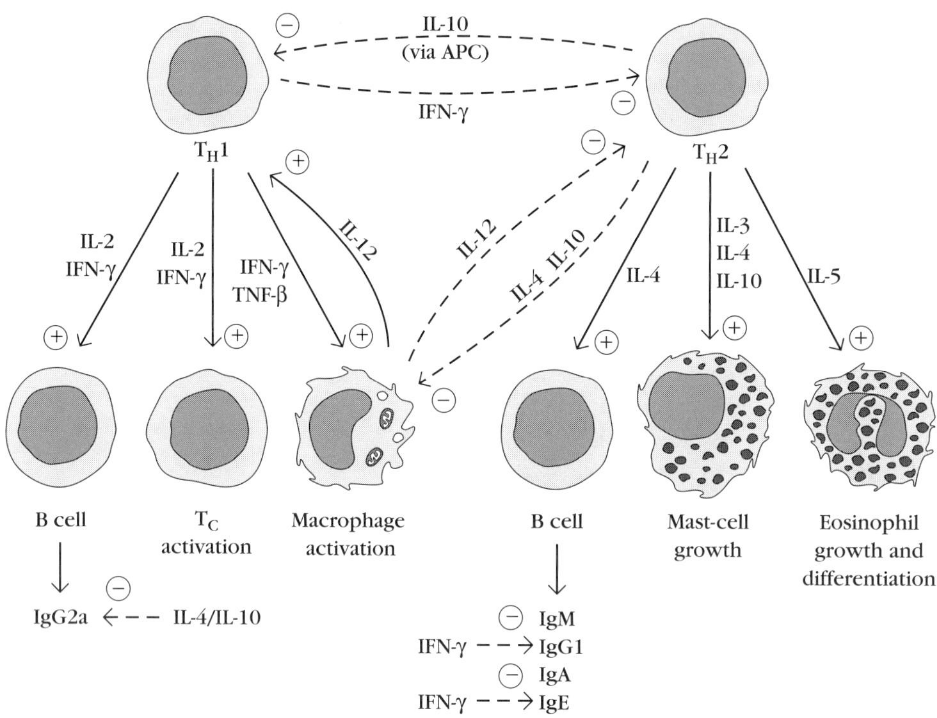

FIGURE 13-10 Cross-regulation by cytokines secreted from T_H1 and T_H2 subsets. Solid arrows indicate stimulatory effects; dashed arrows indicate inhibitory effects.

for the earlier observation that there is an inverse relationship between antibody production and delayed-type hypersensitivity; that is, when antibody production is high, delayed-type hypersensitivity is low and vice versa.

Interleukin 10 does not inhibit T_H1 cells directly, instead, it acts on monocytes and macrophages and interferes with their ability to activate the T_H1 subset. This interference is thought to result from the demonstrated ability of IL-10 to dramatically down-regulate the expression of class II MHC molecules on these antigen-presenting cells. IL-10 has other potent immunosuppressant effects on the monocyte/macrophage lineage: It suppresses the production of nitrogen oxides and other bactericidal metabolites involved in the destruction of pathogens and the production of various inflammatory mediators (e.g., IL-1, IL-6, IL-8, GM-CSF, G-CSF, and TNF-α). These suppressive effects on the macrophage serve to further diminish the biologic consequences of T_H1 activation.

Macrophages and other antigen-presenting cells also produce cytokines that regulate immune effector functions. A newly discovered cytokine, interleukin 12 (IL-12), is secreted by activated macrophages in response to bacterial or protozoan infections. IL-12 induces proliferation of NK cells and T_H1 cells resulting in increased IFN-γ production. Since IFN-γ activates macrophages, it has a positive feedback effect inducing even more IL-12. Cross-regulation also influences cytokine production by macrophages; the T_H2-derived cytokines IL-4 and IL-10 have both been shown to inhibit IL-12 production.

The cytokine environment that is present as T_H cells differentiate may influence the subset that develops. For example, when T_H cells are activated in vitro by an antigen together with IL-4, they develop into the T_H2 subset; in contrast, activation with the same antigen in the presence of IFN-γ results in the development of the T_H1 subset. The effect of the cytokine environment has also been shown to regulate T_H-cell subset development in vivo. When transgenic mice expressing a T-cell receptor specific for ovalbumin were challenged with the ovalbumin antigen in the presence of IL-12, they produced a T_H1 response; in contrast, immunization with ovalbumin in the presence of IL-4 produced a T_H2 response.

The activity of the T_H subsets may also be influenced by some pathogens. The Epstein-Barr virus, for instance, produces a protein that has been shown to have sequence homology with IL-10. This viral protein, designated vIL-10 in reference to this homology, has IL-10–like activity and tends to suppress T_H1 activity. Some researchers have speculated that vIL-10 may reduce the cell-mediated response to the virus, thus conferring a survival advantage to the Epstein-Barr virus. There is also evidence for changes in T_H-subset activity in AIDS. Early in the disease T_H1 activity is high, but as AIDS progresses, there is a shift from a T_H1-like to a T_H2-like response that correlates with disease progression (see Chapter 22).

Role of Cytokines in the Inflammatory Response

Inflammation is a physiologic response to a variety of stimuli such as infections and tissue injury. In general, an acute inflammatory response exhibits rapid onset and is of short duration. Acute inflammation is generally accompanied by a systemic response, known as the acute-phase response, which is characterized by a rapid alteration in the levels of several plasma proteins. In some diseases persistent immune activation can result in chronic inflammation resulting in pathologic consequences.

Acute Inflammatory Response

Infection or tissue injury induces a complex cascade of nonspecific events, known as the inflammatory response, that provides early protection by restricting the tissue damage to the site of infection or tissue injury. The acute inflammatory response involves both localized and systemic responses. The localized inflammatory response develops as plasma clotting factors are produced, resulting in activation of the clotting, kinin-forming, and fibrinolytic pathways. A local acute inflammatory response can occur without the overt involvement of the immune system. Often, however, cytokines released at the site of inflammation facilitate both the adherence of immune-system cells to vascular endothelial cells and their migration through the vessel into the tissue spaces. The result is an influx of lymphocytes, neutrophils, monocytes, eosinophils, basophils, and mast cells to the site of tissue damage, where these cells participate in clearance of the antigen and healing of the tissue.

The local inflammatory response is accompanied by a systemic response known as the *acute-phase response.* This response includes the induction of fever, increased synthesis of hormones such as ACTH and hydrocortisone, increased production of white blood cells (leukocytosis), and production of a large number of hepatocyte-derived acute-phase proteins including C-reactive protein (CRP) and serum amyloid A (SAA). The increase in body temperature inhibits the growth of a number of pathogens and appears to enhance the immune response to the pathogen. C-reactive protein is a prototype acute-phase protein whose serum level increases by 1000-fold during an acute-phase response. It is composed of five identical polypeptides held together by noncovalent interactions. C-reactive protein binds to a wide variety of microorganisms and activates complement, resulting in deposition of a complement component (C3b) on the surface of the microorganism. Phagocytic cells, which express C3b receptors, can then readily phagocytose the C3b-coated microorganisms.

The acute inflammatory reaction is initiated following activation of tissue macrophages and release of TNF-α, IL-1, and IL-6, which induce many of the localized and systemic changes observed in the acute response (Table 13-3). All three cytokines act locally on fibroblasts and endothelial cells inducing coagulation and an increase in vascular permeability. Both TNF-α and IL-1 induce increased expression of adhesion molecules on vascular endothelial cells. TNF-α stimulates expression of ELAM-1, an endothelial leukocyte adhesion molecule that selectively binds neutrophils. IL-1 induces increased expression of ICAM-1 and VCAM-1, the intercellular adhesion molecules for

Table 13-3 Redundant and pleiotropic effects of IL-1, TNF-α, and IL-6

Effect	IL-1	TNF-α	IL-6
Endogenous pyrogen fever	+	+	+
Synthesis of acute-phase proteins by liver	+	+	+
Increased vascular permeability	+	+	+
Increased adhesion molecules on vascular endothelium	+	+	−
Fibroblast proliferation	+	+	−
Platelet production	+	−	+
Induction of IL-8	+	+	−
Induction of IL-6	+	+	−
T-cell activation	+	+	+
B-cell activation	+	+	+
Proliferation of Kaposi's sarcoma	+	−	+
Increased immunoglobulin synthesis	−	−	+

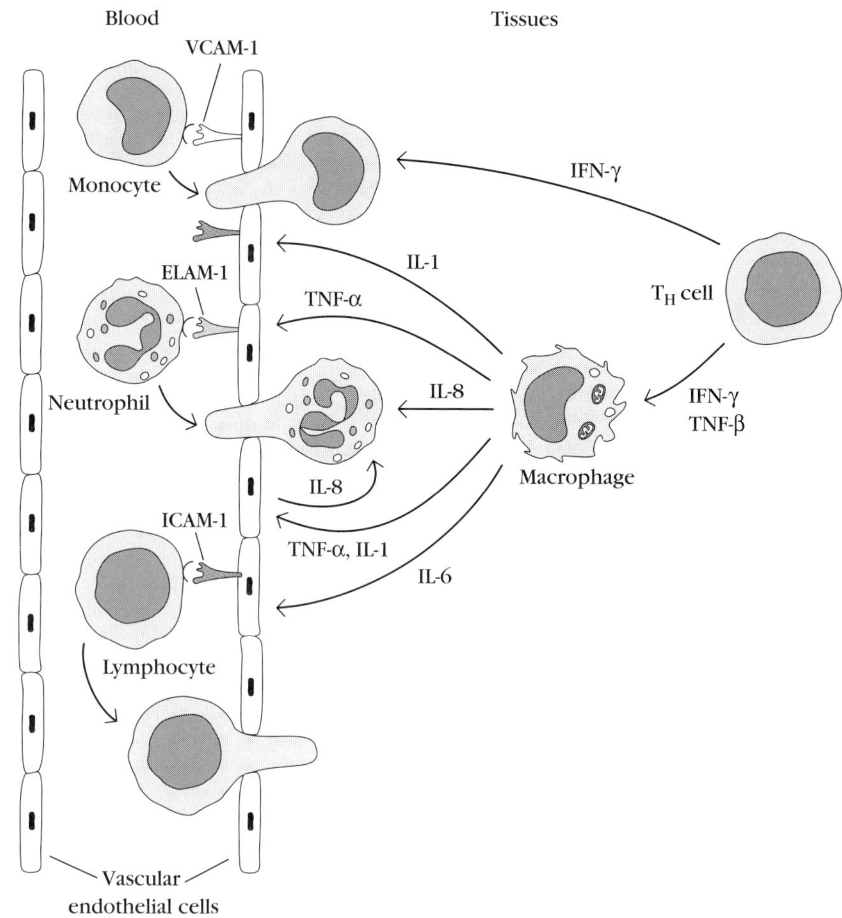

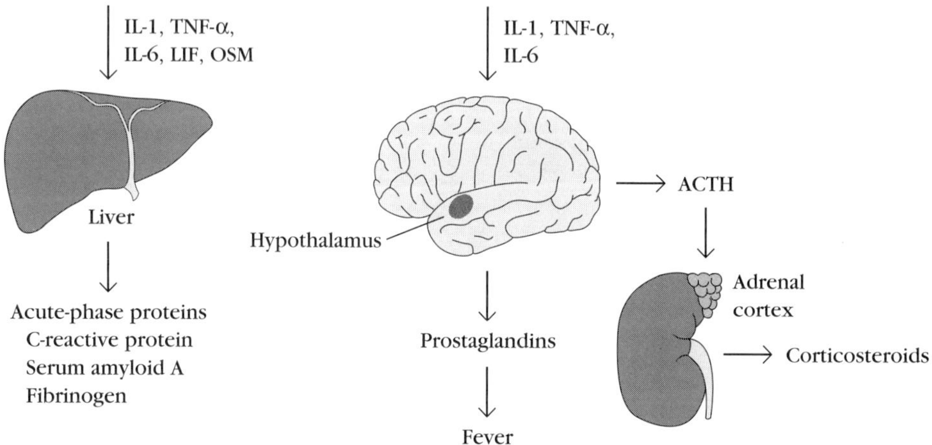

FIGURE 13-11 The acute inflammatory response is mediated primarily by TNF-α, IL-1, and IL-6. (a) Localized effects include increased adherence of circulating white blood cells to vascular endothelial cells and their extravasation into the tissue spaces. Both IL-1 and TNF-α induce increased expression of cell-adhesion molecules (CAMs) on endothelial cells. These two cytokines also induce production of IL-8 by macrophages and endothelial cells. IL-8 chemotactically attracts neutrophils and promotes their adherence to endothelial cells; IFN-γ chemotactically attracts macrophages. Both IFN-γ and TNF-β enhance the phagocytic activity of macrophages and neutrophils and their release of lytic enzymes. (b) Systemic acute-phase response includes increased production of acute-phase proteins by liver hepatocytes. Fever and increased production of corticosteroids are induced by the action of cytokines on the hypothalamus.

lymphocytes and monocytes. Circulating neutrophils, monocytes, and lymphocytes adhere to the wall of a blood vessel by recognizing these adhesion molecules and then move through the vessel wall into the tissue spaces (Figure 13-11a). IL-1 and TNF-α also act on macrophages and endothelial cells inducing production of IL-8. IL-8 contributes to the influx of neutrophils by increasing their adhesion to vascular endothelial cells and by acting as a potent chemotactic factor. Other cytokines also serve as chemotactic factors for various leukocyte populations. For example, IFN-γ has been shown to chemotactically attract macrophages, bringing increased numbers of phagocytic cells to a site where antigen is localized. In addition, IFN-γ and TNF-α activate macrophages and neutrophils, promoting increased phagocytic activity and increased release of lytic enzymes into the tissue spaces.

The combined action of IL-1, TNF-α, and IL-6 are also responsible for many of the systemic acute-phase effects that occur during an acute inflammatory response (Figure 13-11b). Each of these cytokines acts on the hypothalamus to induce a fever response. Within 12–24 h of an acute-phase inflammatory response, increased levels of IL-1, TNF-α, and IL-6 (as well as LIF and OSM) induce production of acute-phase proteins by hepatocytes. TNF-α also acts on vascular endothelial cells and macrophages to induce secretion of colony-stimulating factors (M-CSF, G-CSF, and GM-CSF). These CSFs stimulate hematopoiesis, resulting in transient increases in the necessary white blood cells to fight the infection.

Several of the events associated with the acute-phase response are mediated by more than one cytokine. For example, at least five cytokines (TNF-α, IL-1, IL-6, LIF and OSM) can induce production of acute-phase proteins by the liver. This redundancy is due to the induction of a common DNA-binding protein, NF-IL6, following interaction of each of these cytokines with its receptor. Amino acid sequencing of cloned NF-IL6 revealed that it has a high degree of sequence homology with a liver-specific DNA-binding protein called C/EBP (Figure 13-12a). Both NF-IL6 and C/EBP contain a leucine-zipper domain and a basic DNA-binding domain, and both proteins bind to the same nucleotide sequence in the promoter or enhancer of the genes encoding various acute-phase proteins. C/EBP, which stimulates production of albumin and transthyretin, is expressed constitutively by liver hepatocytes. As an inflammatory response develops and the cytokines interact with their respective receptors on liver hepatocytes, expression of NF-IL6 increases and that of C/EBP decreases (Figure 13-12b). The inverse relationship between these two DNA-binding proteins accounts for the observation that serum levels of proteins such as albumin and transthyretin decline while those of acute-phase proteins increase during an inflammatory response.

(a)

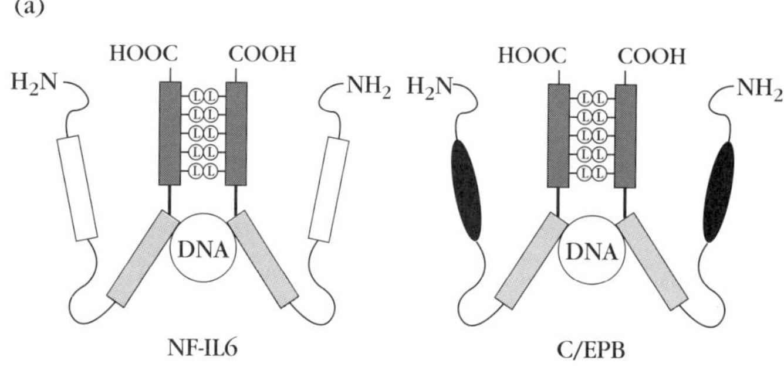

(b)

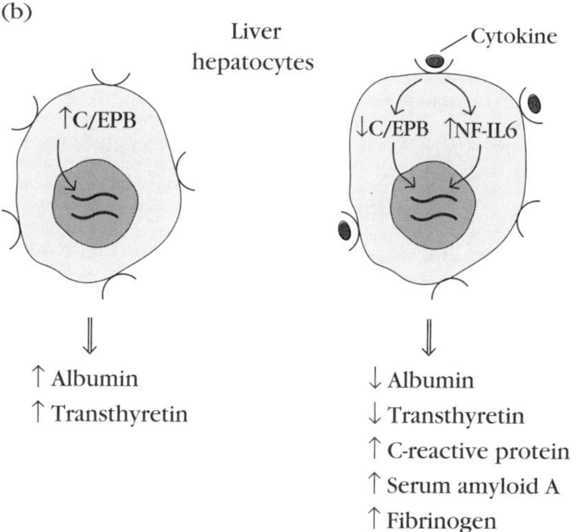

FIGURE 13-12 Comparison of structure and function of C/EBP and NF-IL6. (a) Both transcription factors are dimeric proteins containing a leucine-zipper domain (gray) and basic DNA-binding domain (purple). (b) C/EBP is expressed constitutively in liver hepatocytes and promotes transcription of albumin and transthyretin genes. During an inflammatory response, binding of IL-1, IL-6, TNF-α, LIF, or OSM to receptors on liver hepatocytes induces production of NF-IL6, which promotes transcription of the genes encoding various acute-phase proteins. Concurrently, C/EBP levels decrease and in turn the levels of albumin and transthyretin also decrease.

It is important that the duration and intensity of the inflammatory response be carefully regulated to control tissue damage and facilitate the tissue-repair mechanisms that are necessary for wound healing. TGF-β has been shown to play an important role in limiting the inflammatory response. It also promotes accumulation and proliferation of fibroblasts and the deposition of an extracellular matrix that is required for proper tissue repair.

Chronic Inflammatory Response

Chronic inflammation develops following prolonged persistence of an antigen. Some microorganisms, for example, have cell-wall components that enable them to resist phagocytosis. Such organisms often induce a chronic inflammatory response, resulting in significant tissue damage. Chronic inflammation also occurs in a number of autoimmune diseases in which self-antigens continually activate T cells. Finally, chronic inflammation also contributes to the tissue damage and wasting associated with many types of cancer. Two cytokines in particular, IFN-γ and TNF-α, produced by T_H1 cells and macrophages, respectively, play a central role in the development of chronic inflammation.

Interferon gamma is a member of the interferon family of glycoproteins. All three members of this family (IFN-α, IFN-β, and IFN-γ) are released from virus-infected cells and confer antiviral protection on neighboring cells. However, IFN-γ has a number of pleiotropic activities that distinguish it from IFN-α and IFN-β and contribute to the inflammatory response (Figure 13-13). One of the most striking effects of IFN-γ is its effect on macrophages. IFN-γ activates macrophages resulting in increased expression of class II MHC molecules, increased cytokine production, and increased microbicidal activity. Once activated, the macrophage serves as a more effective antigen-presenting cell and is more effective at killing intracellular microbial pathogens. In a chronic inflammatory response, the accumulation of large numbers of activated macrophages is responsible for much of the tissue damage. These cells release various hydrolytic enzymes and reactive oxygen and nitrogen intermediates resulting in damage to the surrounding tissue (see Tables 3-4 and 3-5).

One of the principal cytokines secreted by activated macrophages is TNF-α. The activity of this cytokine was first observed around the turn of the century by a surgeon, William Coley. He noted that when cancer patients developed certain bacterial infections, the tumors would become necrotic. In the hope of providing a cure for cancer, Coley began to inject cancer patients with supernatants derived from various bacterial cultures. These culture supernatants, called "Coley's toxins," induced hemorrhagic necrosis in the tumor but had numerous undesirable side-effects, making them unsuitable for cancer therapy. Decades later the active component of Coley's toxin was shown to be a lipopolysaccharide (endotoxin) component of the bacterial cell wall. Endotoxin does not itself induce tumor necrosis but instead induces macrophages to produce TNF-α. This cytokine has a direct cytotoxic effect on tumor cells but not on normal cells (Figure

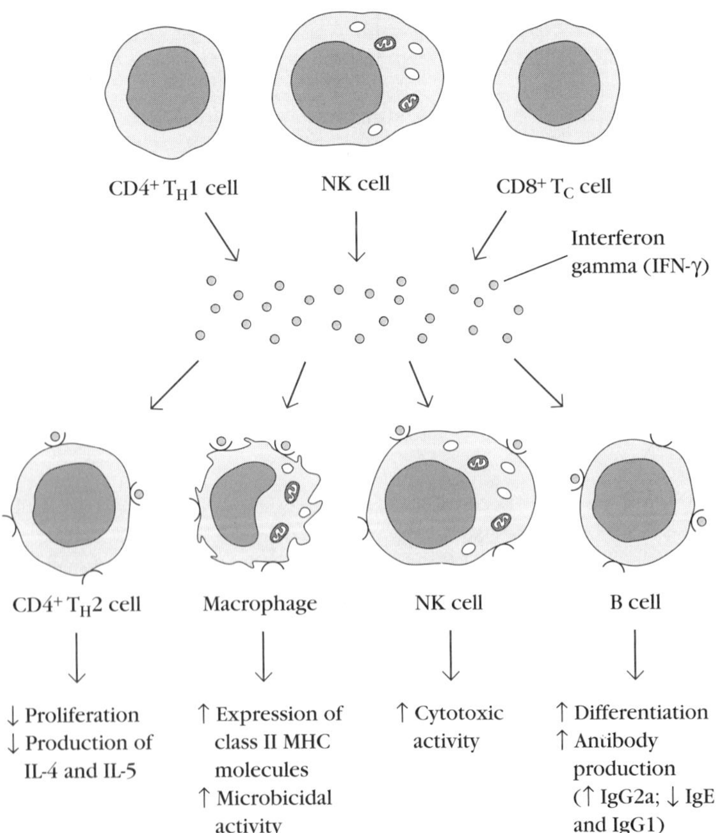

FIGURE 13-13 Summary of pleiotropic activity of interferon gamma (IFN-γ). [Adapted from Research News, 1993, *Science* **259**:1693.]

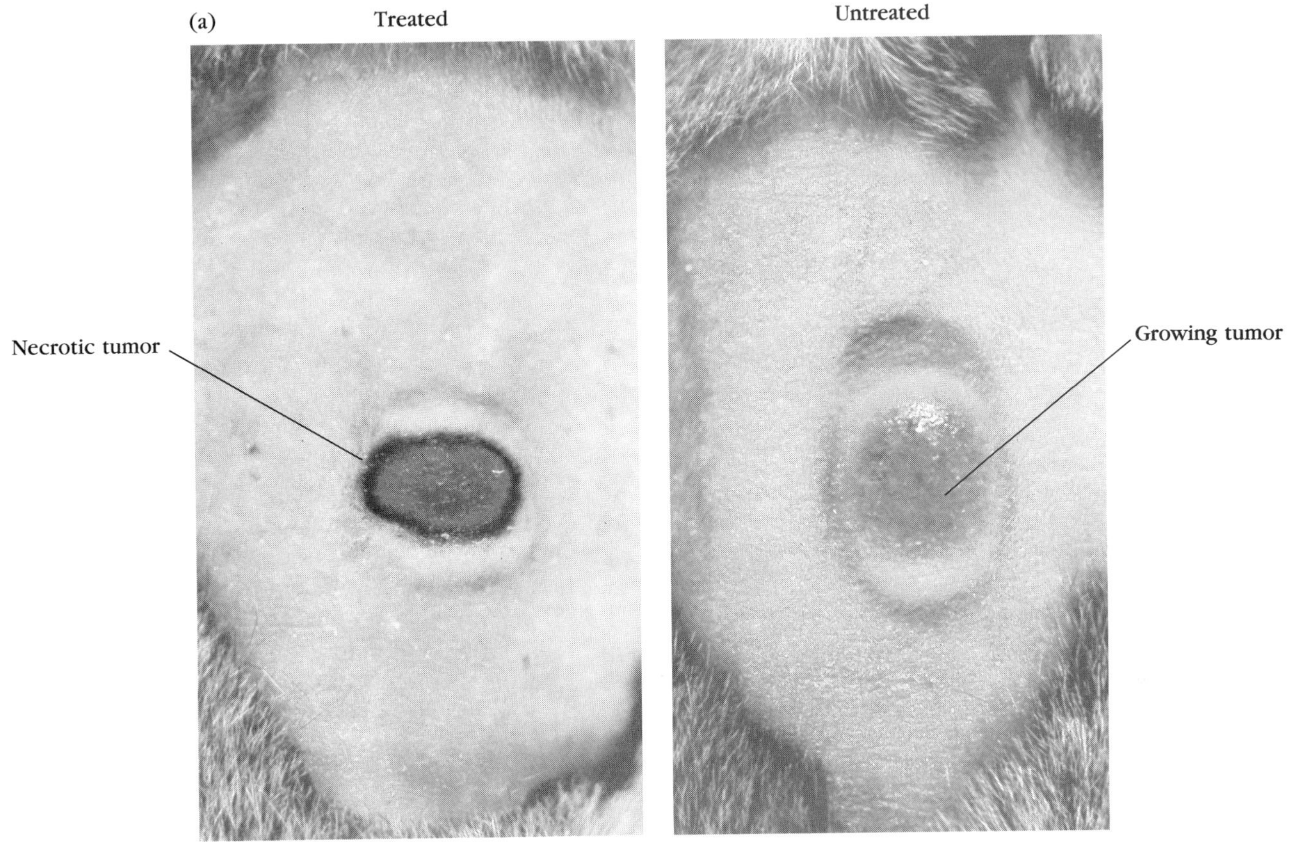

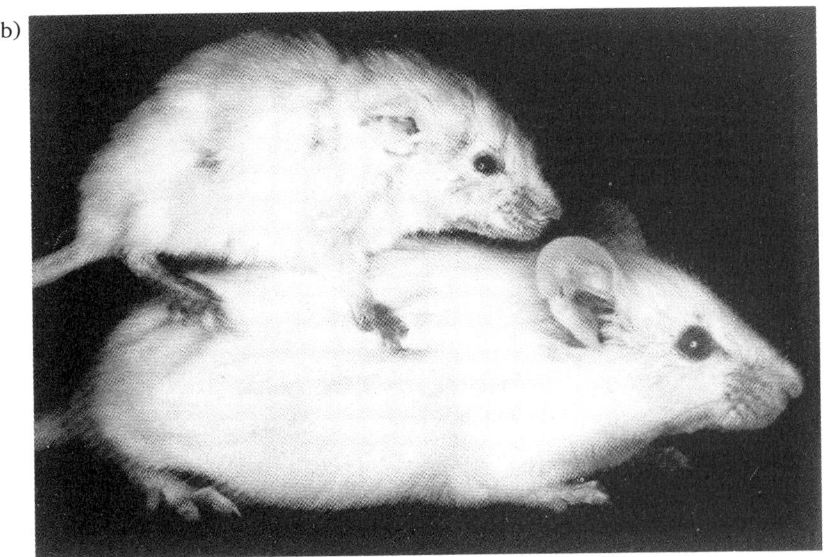

FIGURE 13-14 Biological activities of TNF-α. (a) A cancerous tumor in a mouse injected with endotoxin *(left)* shows hemorrhagic necrosis compared with a tumor in an untreated mouse *(right)*. Endotoxin induces production of TNF-α, which then acts to destroy the tumor. (b) Transgenic mouse *(top)* bearing a TNF-α transgene becomes anorectic and severely wasted. Normal mouse is on the bottom. [Part (a) from L. J. Old, 1988, *Sci. Am.* **258**:59; part (b) from B. Beutler, 1993, *Hosp. Prac.* (April 15):45.]

13-14a). Potential immunotherapeutic approaches using TNF-α for the treatment of cancer are examined in Chapter 25.

TNF-α also contributes to much of the tissue wasting that characterizes chronic inflammation (Figure 13-14b). In the 1980s A. Cerami and co-workers noted that within two months after infecting rabbits with trypanosomes, the animals lost nearly half of their body mass. Cerami set out to determine why some parasitic and bacterial infections and tumors induced a catabolic state leading to extensive weight loss (cachexia), sometimes resulting in shock and death. They discovered that a macrophage-derived factor was responsible for the profound wasting and called the factor cachetin. Subsequent cloning of the genes for TNF-α and cachetin revealed that they were the same protein.

Activation of macrophages by IFN-γ promotes increased transcription of the TNF-α gene and increases the stability of TNF-α mRNA. Both effects result in increased TNF-α production. TNF-α acts synergistically with IFN-γ to initiate an inflammatory response. Both cytokines together were shown to induce dramatic increases in ICAM-1, ELAM-1, and class I MHC molecules compared to either cytokine alone. The increase in intercellular adhesion molecules facilitates the recruitment of large numbers of cells in a chronic inflammatory response.

Cytokines and Disease

Defects in the complex regulatory networks governing the expression of cytokines and cytokine receptors have been implicated in a number of diseases. Overexpression or underexpression of an appropriate or inappropriate cytokine or cytokine receptor may contribute to a disease process. In this section, several examples of diseases resulting from cytokine abnormalities are described and the possible therapeutic uses of cytokines are discussed.

Bacterial Septic Shock

The role of cytokine overproduction in pathogenesis can be illustrated by bacterial septic shock. This condition may develop within a few hours following infection by certain gram-negative bacteria including *E. coli, Klebsiella pneumoniae, Pseudomonas aeruginosa, Enterobacter aerogenes,* and *Neisseria meningitidis.* The symptoms of bacterial septic shock, which often is fatal, include a drop in blood pressure, fever, diarrhea, and widespread blood clotting in various organs. This condition afflicts about 500,000 Americans annually and causes more than 70,000 deaths. The annual cost for treating bacterial septic shock is an estimated $5–10 billion.

Bacterial septic shock appears to develop when bacterial cell-wall endotoxins stimulate macrophages to overproduce IL-1 and TNF-α. It is the increased levels of IL-1 and TNF-α that cause septic shock. In one study, for example, higher levels of TNF-α were found in patients who died of meningitis than in those who recovered. Furthermore, a condition resembling bacterial septic shock can be produced by injection of recombinant TNF-α in the absence of gram-negative bacterial infection. Several studies offer some hope that neutralization of TNF-α or IL-1 activity with monoclonal antibodies or antagonists may prevent this fatal shock from developing in these bacterial infections. In one study, monoclonal antibody to TNF-α was shown to prevent an otherwise fatal endotoxin-induced shock in animal models. And another study has shown that injection of recombinant IL-1 receptor antagonist, (IL-1Ra), which prevents binding of IL-1 to the IL-1 receptor, reduced the mortality due to septic shock in humans from 45 to 16%. It is hoped that these experimental results will have therapeutic benefit for the treatment of bacterial septic shock in humans.

Bacterial Toxic Shock and Related Diseases

A variety of microorganisms produce toxins that act as superantigens. As discussed in previous chapters, superantigens bind simultaneously to a class II MHC molecule and to the V_β domain of the T-cell receptor, activating all T cells bearing a particular V_β domain. Unlike conventional antigens, superantigens are not internalized, processed, and presented by antigen-presenting cells. Instead they bind directly to class II MHC molecules, apparently outside of the antigen-binding cleft. Likewise, the interaction of a superantigen with the T-cell receptor appears to involve regions well away from the sites that interact with normal antigenic peptides. Rather superantigens are thought to bind to an exposed region of the β pleated sheet on the side of the T-cell receptor (see Figure 4-15). Because of their unique binding ability, superantigens can activate large numbers of T cells irrespective of their antigenic specificity. Moreover, T cells can be activated by superantigens bound to allogeneic or even xenogeneic MHC molecules, in contrast to the response to conventional antigens, which is self-MHC restricted.

Although less than 0.01% of T cells respond to a given conventional antigen, between 5% and 25% of T cells can respond to a given superantigen. The large proportion of T cells responsive to a particular superantigen results from the limited number of TCR V_β genes carried in the germ line. Mice, for example, have about 20 V_β genes. Assuming that each V_β gene is expressed with equal frequency, then each superantigen would be expected to interact with 1 in 20 T cells, or 5% of the total T-cell population.

A number of bacterial superantigens have been implicated as the causative agent of several diseases such as bacterial toxic shock and food poisoning (see Table 12-2). Included among these bacterial superantigens are several enterotoxins, exfoliating toxins, and toxic-shock syndrome toxin (TSST1) from *Staphylococcus aureus;* pyrogenic exotoxins from *Streptococcus pyrogenes;* and *Mycoplasma arthritidis* supernatant (MAS). The large number of T cells activated by these superantigens results in excessive production of cytokines. The toxic-shock syndrome toxin, for example, has been shown to induce extremely high levels of TNF and IL-1. As discussed for bacterial septic shock, these cytokines can induce systemic reactions including fever, widespread blood clotting, and shock.

Lymphoid and Myeloid Cancers

Abnormalities in the production of cytokines or their receptors have been associated with some types of cancer. For example, abnormally high levels of IL-6 are secreted by cardiac myxoma (a benign heart tumor) cells, myeloma and plasmacytoma cells, and cervical and bladder cancer cells. In the case of myeloma cells, IL-6 appears to operate in an autocrine manner to stimulate cell proliferation. When monoclonal antibodies to IL-6 are added to in vitro cultures of myeloma cells, their growth is inhibited. In addition, transgenic mice that express high levels of IL-6 have been found to exhibit a massive, fatal plasma-cell proliferation, called plasmacytosis. Although these plasma cells were not malignant, the high rate of plasma-cell proliferation possibly contributes to the development of cancer.

Perhaps the strongest case for an association between malignancy and inappropriate expression of a cytokine and/or its receptor comes from the often-fatal adult T-cell leukemia associated with the HTLV-1 retrovirus. The leukemic T cells express IL-2 and the high-affinity IL-2 receptor in the absence of activation by antigen or mitogen. An HTLV protein called Tax has been shown to induce expression of a cellular transcription factor (or factors) that binds to the promoter regions of the genes encoding IL-2 and IL-2R, thus activating these genes (see Figure 25-4). As a result, a cell infected with HTLV-1 expresses IL-2 and its receptor constitutively, rendering the cell responsive to IL-2–induced proliferation in the absence of antigen activation. The role of cytokine abnormalities in the pathogenesis of various cancers is examined more fully in Chapter 25.

Chagas' Disease

The protozoan *Trypanosoma cruzi* is the causative agent of Chagas' disease, which is characterized by severe immune suppression. The ability of *T. cruzi* to mediate immune suppression can be observed by culturing peripheral-blood T lymphocytes in the presence and in the absence of *T. cruzi* and then evaluating their immune reactivity. Antigen, mitogen, or anti-CD3 monoclonal antibody normally can activate peripheral T lymphocytes, but in the presence of *T. cruzi* T lymphocytes are not activated by any of these agents. The defect in these lymphocytes has been traced to a dramatic reduction in the expression of the 55-kDa α subunit of the IL-2 receptor. Co-culturing of T lymphocytes with *T. cruzi* and subsequent staining with fluorescein-labeled anti-TAC, which binds to the α subunit, revealed a 90% decrease in the level of the α subunit. As noted earlier, the high-affinity IL-2 receptor contains the α, β and δ subunits (see Figure 13-9). Although the mechanism by which *T. cruzi* suppresses expression of the α subunit is still unknown, the suppression can be induced across a filter that prevents contact between the lymphocytes and protozoa. This finding suggests that a diffusible factor mediates suppression. Such a factor, once isolated, might have numerous clinical applications for regulating the level of activated T cells in leukemias and autoimmune diseases.

Cytokine-Related Therapies

The availability of purified cloned cytokines and soluble cytokine receptors offers the prospect of specific clinical therapies to modulate the immune response selectively. For example, activation and proliferation of T_H cells in response to alloantigens on organ transplants initiates activation of T_C cells and subsequent graft rejection. Various approaches that have been tried experimentally to suppress T_H-cell activation and proliferation, thereby prolonging graft survival, are illustrated in Figure 13-15.

A cloned soluble form of the IL-1 receptor, which lacks the transmembrane and cytoplasmic domains, blocks activation of T_H cells in response to alloantigens and has prolonged heart transplants in animal models. Binding of IL-1, which is a co-stimulator of T_H-cell activation, also can be inhibited with the recombinant IL-1 receptor antagonist; this agent binds to the IL-1 receptor but does not induce activation. Proliferation of activated T_H cells and activation of T_C cells can be blocked by anti-TAC, which binds to the α subunit of the high-affinity IL-2 receptor. Administration of anti-TAC, for example, has prolonged the survival of heart transplants in rats. Similar results have been obtained

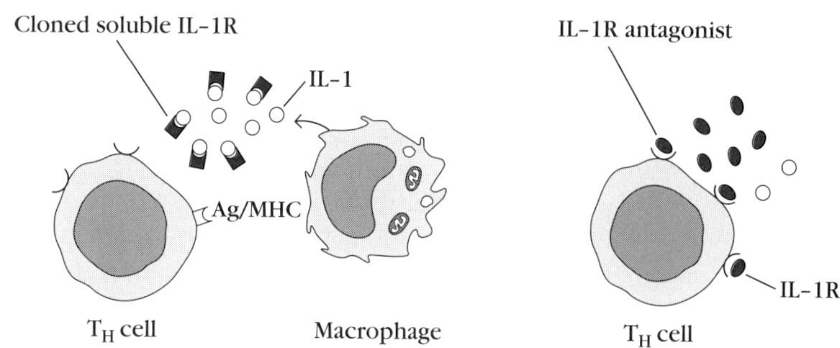

FIGURE 13-15 Experimental cytokine-related therapeutic agents offer the prospect of selectively modulating the immune response. (a,b) The agents (purple) bind either to the cytokine (open circles) or to the cytokine receptor, thereby preventing interaction of the cytokine with its receptor. (c) Conjugation of a toxin with a cytokine results in destruction of cells expressing the cytokine receptor.

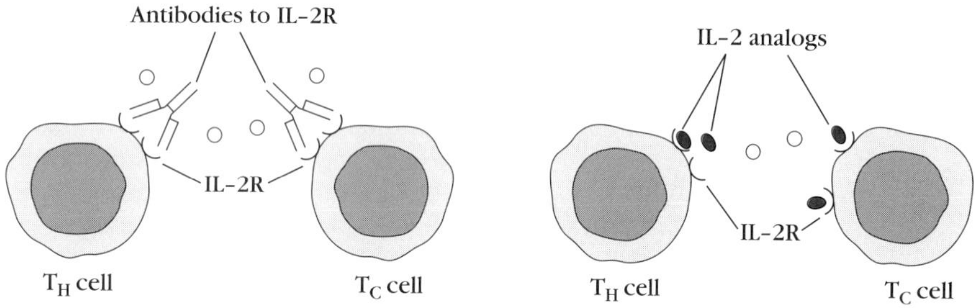

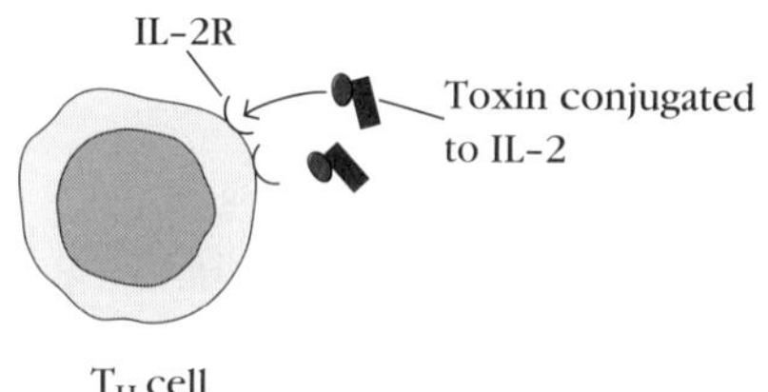

with IL-2 analogs that retain their binding ability but have lost their biological activity. Such analogs have been produced by site-directed mutagenesis of cloned IL-2 genes. Finally, cytokines conjugated to various toxins (e.g., the β chain of diphtheria toxin) have been shown to diminish rejection of kidney and heart transplants in animals. Such conjugates containing IL-2 selectively bind to and kill activated T_H cells.

In immunodeficiency diseases and in cancer, enhanced—rather than diminished—T-cell activation is desirable. Intervention with cloned IL-2, IFN-γ, and TNF-α have each had some degree of clinical success. Culturing of various populations of NK cells or T_C cells in the presence of high concentrations of IL-2 has been shown to generate cells with effective antitumor properties. The role of such cells, referred to as *lymphokine-activated killer (LAK)* cells, in tumor therapy is examined in Chapter 25.

Cytokine therapy may also prove to be effective in the treatment of allergies. Given the opposing effects of IL-2 and IL-4 on isotype production, it may be possible to enhance production of a desired isotype selectively. Selective inhibition of IgE may benefit patients with allergies. In animal models, for example, monoclonal antibody to IL-4 has been used to decrease IgE production. Clearly these approaches have enormous clinical applications for the millions of people who suffer from allergies.

Cytokine-related therapy does have limitations, however. During an immune response, cytokines produced locally by interacting cells may reach relatively high local concentrations that cannot be mimicked by clinical administration. In addition, cytokines often have a very short half-life, so that repeated administration may be required in order to maintain effective levels. For example, recombinant human IL-2 has a half-life of only 7–10 min when administered intraveneously. Finally, the pleiotropic effects of many cytokines can cause unpredictable and undesirable side effects. The side effects from administration of recombinant IL-2, for instance, range from mild ones (e.g., fever, chills, diarrhea, and weight gain) to anemia, thrombocytopenia, shock, respiratory distress, and coma.

Summary

1. The complex cellular interactions involving cells of the immune, inflammatory, and hematopoietic systems are mediated by a group of secreted low-molecular-weight proteins collectively called cytokines. Most cytokines act on nearby target cells, although in some cases a cytokine can act on the cell that secretes it or on a distant cell. The biological activities of cytokines exhibit pleiotropy, redundancy, synergy, and antagonism, which contribute to the complexity of cytokine networks.

2. Biochemical purification of cytokines and subsequently the cloning of cytokine genes revealed that many activities previously attributed to different cytokines in fact were mediated by a relatively small number of multifunctional proteins. These discoveries brought some simplification to a field that was plagued by an overwhelming array of supposedly single-function factors. Today, the most important recognized cytokines include IFN-γ, interleukins 1–13, TNF-α, TNF-β, and TGF-β.

3. A particular cytokine can act on any target cell that expresses receptors for that cytokine. An important way in which the activity of cytokines is directed toward specific cells is by regulation of the expression of their receptors. For example, a T_H cell does not express the high-affinity IL-2 receptor until it has interacted with an antigen-MHC complex and a co-stimulatory signal. As long as the antigen-MHC-TCR interaction continues, the high-affinity IL-2 receptor is expressed, but once this interaction ceases, expression of the IL-2 receptor stops as well.

4. Cytokine-binding receptors share several structural features. All these receptors contain an extracellular domain, a transmembrane domain, and a cytoplasmic domain. Many cytokine receptors possess conserved sequences in the extracellular domain. Many receptors, including those that bind IL-2, IL-3, IL-5, IL-6, and GM-CSF, contain a cytokine-specific α chain and a signal-transducing β chain. In some cases, a common β chain occurs in the receptors for several different cytokines, accounting for the redundancy among the biological effects of these cytokines.

5. Development of an effective inflammatory response depends on the action of numerous cytokines. These include IL-1, IL-8, and IFN-γ, which aid in the movement of leukocytes to tissue sites where antigen is located. The phagocytic activity of macrophages and neutrophils is promoted by IFN-γ and TNF-α. The inflammatory response is, in part, limited by TGF-β, which also promotes wound healing.

6. Abnormalities in the expression of cytokines or their receptors may result in various diseases including bacterial toxic shock, certain lymphoid and myeloid cancers, and Chagas' disease. Cytokine-related therapies that either increase or decrease the immune response offer promise of reducing graft rejection, treating certain cancers and immunodeficiency diseases, and reducing allergic reactions.

References

AKIRA, S., and T. KISHIMOTO. 1992. IL-6 and NF-IL6 in acute-phase response and viral infection. *Immunol. Rev.* **127**:25.

ARAI, K., F. LEE, A. MIYAJIMA et al. 1990. Cytokines: coordinators of immune and inflammatory responses. *Annu. Rev. Biochem.* **59**:783.

BALKWILL, F. R., and F. BURKE. 1989. The cytokine network. *Immunol. Today* **10**:299.

BARON, S., S. K. TYRING, W. R. FLEISCHMANN et al. 1991. The interferons: mechanism of action and clinical applications. *JAMA* **266**:1375.

BAZAN, J. F. 1992. Unraveling the structure of IL-2. *Science* **257**:410.

BEUTLER, B. 1990. The tumor necrosis factors: cachectin and lymphotoxin. *Hospital Practice* (February 15):45.

COSMAN, D. 1993. The hematopoietin receptor superfamily. *Cytokine* **5**:95.

DALTON, D. K., S. PITTS-MEEK, S. KESHAV et al. 1993. Multiple defects of immune cell function in mice with disrupted interferon-γ genes. *Science* **259**:1739.

DI GIOVINE, F. S., and G. W. DUFF. 1990. Interleukin 1: the first interleukin. *Immunol. Today* **11.**

FARRAR, W. L., D. K. FERRIS, and A. HAREL-BELLAN. 1990. Lymphokine-induced molecular signal transduction. In *Immunophysiology.* Oxford Press, p. 67.

HERMAN, A., J. W. KAPPLER, P. MARRACK, and A. M. PULLEN. 1991. Superantigens: mechanism of T-cell stimulation and role in immune responses. *Annu. Rev. Immunol.* **9**:745.

HOWARD, M., and A. O'GARRA. 1992. Biological properties of interleukin 10. *Immunol. Today* **13**:198.

HUANG, S., W. HENDRIKS, A. ALTHAGE et al. 1993. Immune response in mice that lack the interferon-γ receptor. *Science* **259**:1742.

KIERSZENBAUM, F., M. B. SZTEIN, and L. A. BELTZ. 1989. Decreased human IL-2 receptor expression due to a protozoan pathogen. *Immunol. Today* **10**:129.

KISHIMOTO, T., S. AKIRA, and T. TAGA. 1992. Interleukin-6 and its receptor: a paradigm for cytokines. *Science* **258**:593.

MIYAJIMA, A., T. HARA, and T. KITAMURA. 1992. Common subunits of cytokine receptors and the functional redundancy of cytokines. *Trends Biol. Sci.* **17.**

MIYAJIMA, A., T. KITAMURA, N. HARADA et al. 1992. Cytokine receptors and signal transduction. *Annu. Rev. Immunol.* **10**:295.

MOORE, K. W., A. O'GARRA, R. DE WAAL MALEFYT et. al. 1993. Interleukin-10. *Annu. Rev. Immunol.* **11**:165.

PARRY, D. A., E. MINASISN, and S. J. LEACH. 1988. Conformational homologies among cytokines: interleukins and colony-stimulating factors. *J. Mol. Recog.* **1**:107.

POWRIE, F., and R. L. COFFMAN. 1993. Cytokine regulation of T-cell function: potential for therapeutic intervention. *Immunol. Today* **14**:270.

SCHOENHAUT, D. S., A. O. CHAU, A. G. WOLITZKY et al. 1992. Cloning and expression of murine IL-12. *J. Immunol.* **148**:3433.

SMITH, K. 1988. Interleukin-2: inception, impact and implications. *Science* **240**:1169.

SMITH, K. 1990. Interleukin-2. *Sci. Am.* **262**:50.

TANAGUCHI, T. 1988. Regulation of cytokine expression. *Annu. Rev. Immunol.* **6**:439.

TRINCHIERI, G. 1993. Interleukin-12 and its role in the generation of T_H1 cells. *Immunol. Today* **14**:335.

VASSALLI, P. 1992. The pathophysiology of tumor necrosis factors. *Annu. Rev. Immunol.* **10**:411.

WALDMANN, T. A. 1993. The IL-2/IL-2 receptor system: a target for rational immune intervention. *Immunol. Today* **14**:264.

Study Questions

1. Indicate whether each of the following statements is true or false. If you think a statement is false, explain why.
   a. The high-affinity IL-2 receptor consists of two transmembrane proteins.
   b. The anti-TAC monoclonal antibody recognizes the IL-1 receptor on T cells.
   c. All members of the cytokine-receptor family contain two or three subunits.
   d. Expression of the β subunit of the IL-2 receptor is indicative of T-cell activation.
   e. Cytokine receptors possess domains with tyrosine kinase activity that function in signal transduction.

2. When IL-2 is secreted by one T cell in a peripheral lymphoid organ, do all the T cells in the vicinity proliferate in response to the IL-2 or only some of them? Explain.

3. An infection usually elicits both an immune response and a localized inflammatory response at the site of the infection. An effective inflammatory response requires differentiation and proliferation of various nonlymphoid white blood cells. Explain how hematopoiesis in the bone marrow is induced by an infection.

4. The discovery of two general types of cell lines paved the way for biochemical isolation and purification of cytokines and the subsequent cloning of cytokine genes.
   a. What are the unique properties of these cell lines?
   b. Why have these cell lines been so important in cytokine research?

5. Briefly describe the similarities and differences among cytokines, growth factors, and hormones.

6. Which subunits of the IL-2 receptor are expressed by the following types of cells.
   a. Resting T_H cells
   b. Activated T_H cells
   c. Activated T_H cells + cyclosporin A
   d. Resting T_C cells
   e. CTLs
   f. NK cells

7. Superantigens have been implicated in several diseases and have been useful as research tools.
   a. What properties of superantigens distinguish them from conventional antigens?
   b. By what mechanism are bacterial superantigens thought to cause symptoms associated with food poisoning and toxic-shock syndrome?

8. IL-3, IL-5, and GM-CSF exhibit considerable redundancy in their effects. What structural feature of the receptors for these cytokines might explain this redundancy.

GENERATION OF THE HUMORAL IMMUNE RESPONSE

The humoral immune response, which is uniquely adapted to the elimination of extracellular pathogens, is characterized by the production of large numbers of antibody molecules specific for antigenic determinants (epitopes) on a foreign pathogen. The potential diversity generated by this branch of the immune system can provide $\sim 10^8 - 10^{11}$ different antigen-binding specificities. This enormous antigen-binding diversity is coupled with conservation of constant-region sequences, which confer biological effector functions on antibody molecules. These effector functions facilitate effective elimination of foreign pathogens from a host animal in a variety of ways discussed in other chapters. Antibodies can activate the complement system, resulting in lysis of the microorganism; antibodies serve as opsonins, enhancing phagocytosis of the microorganism; antibodies bind to bacterial toxins and neutralize their toxicity; antibodies bind to viruses and inhibit their ability to infect host cells; antibodies at mucous membrane surfaces bind to potential pathogens and prevent colonization; antibodies bind to Fc receptors on NK cells or macrophages in ADCC, conferring specificity for antigen on these otherwise nonspecific cells.

The significant role of humoral immunity in host defense is highlighted by individuals born with humoral immunodeficiencies. Such individuals suffer recurrent bacterial infections, which can become so severe that bacteremia, meningitis, or cellulitis develop, often with life-threatening consequences. Recurrent or chronic gastrointestinal infection is also common in patients with humoral immunodeficiencies; these can result in malabsorption of nutrients, leading to malnutrition.

The primary focus of this chapter is the cellular interactions involved in generation of an effective immune response. As discussed briefly in previous chapters, this process requires the participation of macrophages, activated T_H cells, and, of course, B cells (see Figure 1-14). Interaction between an antigen-specific naive T_H cell and an antigen–class II MHC complex on a macrophage leads to activation and proliferation of the T cell. B cells also serve as antigen-presenting cells (APCs). However, unlike macrophages, which phagocytose antigen nonspecifically, B cells interact with antigen via their antigen-specific B-cell receptor (BCR), a complex of membrane-bound immunoglobulin and a disulfide-linked heterodimer (see Figure 5-10). Following antigen recognition, a B cell internalizes the antigen via receptor-mediated endocytosis, processes it into antigenic peptides, and then presents these together with a class II MHC molecule on the membrane (see Figure 10-8). An activated antigen-specific T_H cell can then interact with the B cell via a trimolecular complex involving the T-cell receptor and antigenic peptide–class II MHC complex on the membrane of the B cell (see Figure 11-13). This interaction releases cytokines from the T_H cell in localized concentrations necessary for the activation, proliferation, and differentiation of the B cell into antibody-secreting plasma cells and memory B cells.

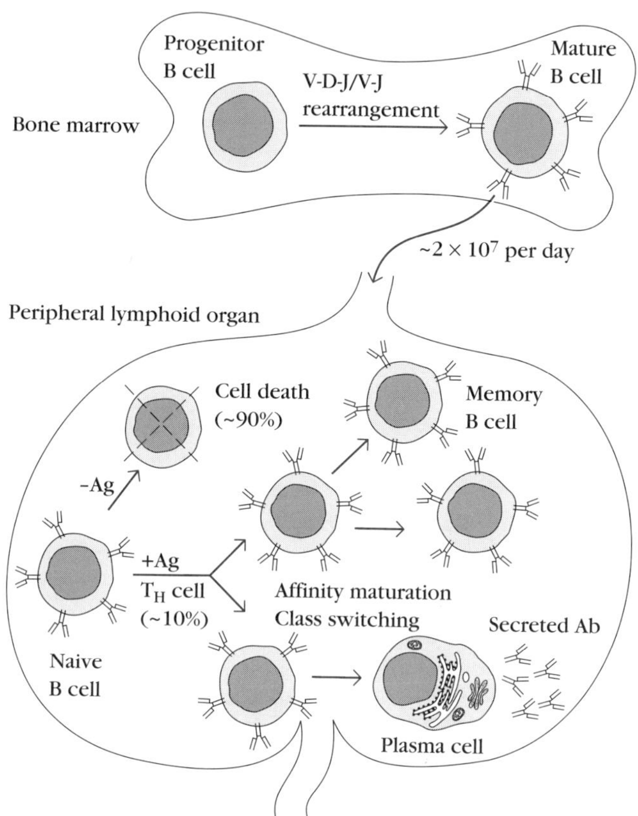

FIGURE 14-1 Schematic diagram of possible fate of B cells. Random gene rearrangements of the immunoglobulin genes occurs during B-cell maturation in the bone marrow. Approximately 2×10^7 mature, naive B cells leave the bone marrow each day. These cells are carried to various peripheral lymphoid organs. In the absence of antigen activation, peripheral B cells have a short life span and die within days. In the presence of antigen and activated T_H cells, those B cells expressing high-affinity membrane antibody differentiate into plasma cells and memory B cells. As discussed later, affinity maturation drives the response toward production of higher-affinity antibodies.

Kinetics of the Humoral Response

The maturation of B cells during hematopoiesis in the bone marrow is marked by the ordered progression of immunoglobulin variable-region gene rearrangements. The outcome of this process is the generation of mature, immunocompetent B cells, all expressing IgM and IgD membrane-bound antibodies specific for a single epitope. These mature, immunocompetent B cells migrate from the bone marrow to the peripheral lymphoid organs. If a B cell encounters the antigen for which its membrane IgM and IgD are specific, the cell will be activated and will undergo clonal proliferation and differentiation. Within 24 h of activation, a B cell enlarges into a lymphoblast (see Figure 3-8), replicates its DNA, and then divides. Eight or nine rounds of cell division follow, each with an average cell-cycle time of about 12–15 h. Either direct T_H-cell interaction or indirect T_H-cell participation in the form of soluble cytokines is required for these successive rounds of cell division, which culminate in differentiation of the activated B cell into plasma and memory cells. If a B cell does not encounter the antigen for which it is specific, the cell dies within a few days. Of the ~ 10^8 B cells in mouse peripheral lymphoid organs, nearly 90% die within a few days (Figure 14-1). These cells are continuously replaced by new virgin (or naive) B cells produced in the bone marrow at the rate of about 2×10^7 immunocompetent B cells per day.

Primary Response

The first contact of an individual with an exogenous antigen generates a primary humoral immune response, characterized by the production of antibody-secreting plasma cells and memory B cells. The kinetics of the primary response, as measured by serum antibody level, vary depending on the nature of the antigen, the route of antigen administration, the presence or absence of adjuvants, and the species or strain being immunized. The response is characterized by a lag phase, during which the B cells undergo clonal selection in response to the antigen and differentiate into plasma cells and memory cells (Figure 14-2). The lag phase is followed by a logarithmic increase in serum antibody level, which reaches a peak, plateaus for a variable time, and then declines. In the case of an antigen such as sheep red blood cells (SRBCs), the lag phase lasts 3–4 days; peak plasma-cell levels are attained within 4–5 days; and peak serum antibody levels are attained by 5–7 days. Eight or nine successive cell divisions occur within the 4- to 5-day period, generating plasma and memory cells. For soluble protein antigens the lag phase is a little longer, often lasting about a week, and peak plasma-cell levels are attained by 9–10 days. During a primary humoral response, IgM is secreted initially, often followed by IgG. Depending on the persistence of the antigen, a primary response can last for varying periods, sometimes only a few days and sometimes several weeks.

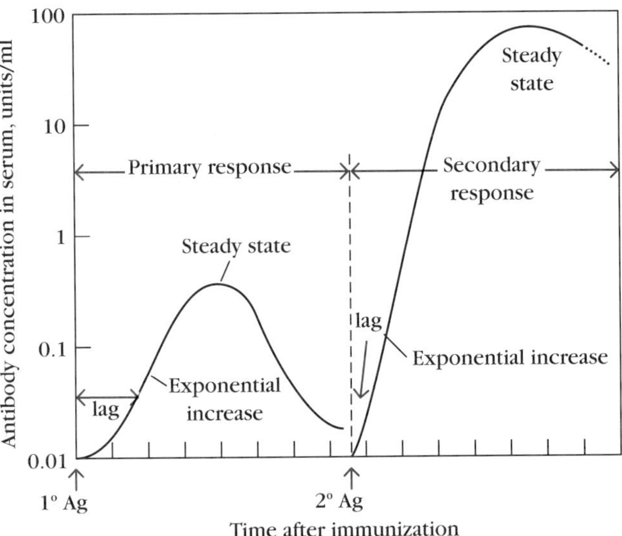

FIGURE 14-2 Serum antibody concentrations following primary (1°) or secondary (2°) immunization with antigen. The antibody concentrations are plotted on a logarithmic scale. The time units are not specified because the kinetics differ with the type of antigen, the route of administration, the presence or absence of adjuvants, and the species or strain of animal.

Secondary Response

The memory B cells formed during a primary response stop dividing and enter the G_0 phase of the cell cycle. These cells have variable life spans, and some persist for the life of the individual. The existence of long-lived memory B cells accounts for a phenomenon called "original antigenic sin," which was first observed when the antibody response to influenza vaccines was monitored. Monitoring revealed that immunization with an influenza vaccine of one strain elicited an antibody response to that strain but, paradoxically, also elicited an antibody response of greater magnitude to another influenza strain that the individual had been exposed to during childhood. It was as if the memory of the first antigen exposure had left a life-long imprint on the immune system. This phenomenon can be explained by the presence of a memory-cell population, elicited by the influenza strain encountered in childhood, that is activated by cross-reacting epitopes on the vaccine strain. This process then generates a secondary response, characterized by antibodies with higher affinity for the earlier viral strain.

The capacity to develop a secondary response depends on the existence of a population of memory B cells and memory T cells. Antigen activation of these memory cells results in a secondary antibody response that can be distinguished from the primary response in several ways: The response occurs more rapidly, reaches a greater magnitude, and lasts for a longer duration (see Figure 14-2). In addition, the secondary response is characterized by secretion of antibody with a higher affinity for the antigen and includes a variety of isotypes in addition to IgM (Table 14-1). The fact that there are more memory B cells specific for the given antigen than there were naive B cells in the primary response accounts, in part, for some of these differences. It is not uncommon for a secondary response to generate antibody levels 100 to 1000 times higher than the levels attained in the primary response. The higher levels of antibody coupled with the overall higher affinity provide an effective host defense against reinfection. In addition, the change in isotype that occurs in the secondary response provides antibodies whose biological effector functions are particularly suited to eliminate a given pathogen.

TABLE 14-1 COMPARISON OF PRIMARY AND SECONDARY ANTIBODY RESPONSES

Property	Primary response	Secondary response
Responding B cell	Naive (virgin) B cell	Memory B cell
Lag period following antigen administration	Generally 4–7 days	Generally 1–3 days
Time and magnitude of peak antibody response	7–10 days Varies depending on antigen	3–5 days Generally 100–1000 times higher than primary response
Isotype produced	IgM predominates early in the response	IgG predominates
Antigens	Thymus-dependent and thymus-independent	Thymus-dependent
Antibody affinity	Lower	Higher

EXPERIMENTAL SYSTEMS

Studies of the cellular interactions required to generate a humoral immune response and of various factors that influence the response have depended on in vitro systems for generating the response and assay methods for measuring it.

In Vitro Generation of the Humoral Response

Analysis of the cellular interactions involved in the generation of the humoral response advanced with the development of in vitro culture systems by R. Mishell and R. Dutton and by J. Marbrook in the 1960s. In the Mishell-Dutton system, spleen cells are grown under low oxygen tension and with gentle agitation in tissue-culture media supplemented with fetal bovine serum to provide essential growth factors. Addition of SRBC antigen to the culture induces B-cell proliferation and differentiation into plasma cells. As will be seen, this system played an important role in clarifying the cellular interactions involved in the humoral response. Today the Mishell-Dutton culture technique continues to be used with minor modifications including the use of small microcultures.

In the Marbrook system, as in the Mishell-Dutton system, spleen cells are cultured in tissue-culture medium supplemented with fetal bovine serum. The culture conditions, however, differ from those of the Mishell-Dutton system in that the cells and antigen are placed in a tube that is separated from a larger flask containing the tissue-culture medium by a semipermeable membrane. The membrane enables nutrients to diffuse into the tube containing the cells and allows waste and metabolites to diffuse out where they are diluted in the larger volume of medium.

Hemolytic Plaque Assay

For many years the humoral immune response could be monitored only by quantifying antibody production. Development of the hemolytic plaque assay, by N. K. Jerne, A. A. Nordin, and C. Henry, permitted researchers to determine the number of plasma cells. This assay and its various modifications have played a significant role in studies of the humoral response.

The hemolytic plaque assay is similar in principle to the viral plaque assay. The original direct assay is used to measure plasma-cell numbers in mice primed with SRBCs. Spleen cells from primed mice are mixed in warm, melted agar with an excess of SRBCs (Figure 14-3a). The agar containing the cell suspension is poured into a Petri dish, whose bottom is covered with a layer of hard agar, and allowed to cool and solidify. The splenic lymphocytes thus are immobilized in the agar, surrounded by a sea of SRBCs. The Petri dish is incubated for 1 h at 37° C, during which time antibody secreted by plasma cells diffuses into the agar matrix and binds to the SRBCs in the vicinity of each antibody-secreting plasma cell. Guinea pig serum containing complement is then added. The complement reacts with the antibody bound to the SRBCs and mediates their lysis, leaving each plasma cell surrounded

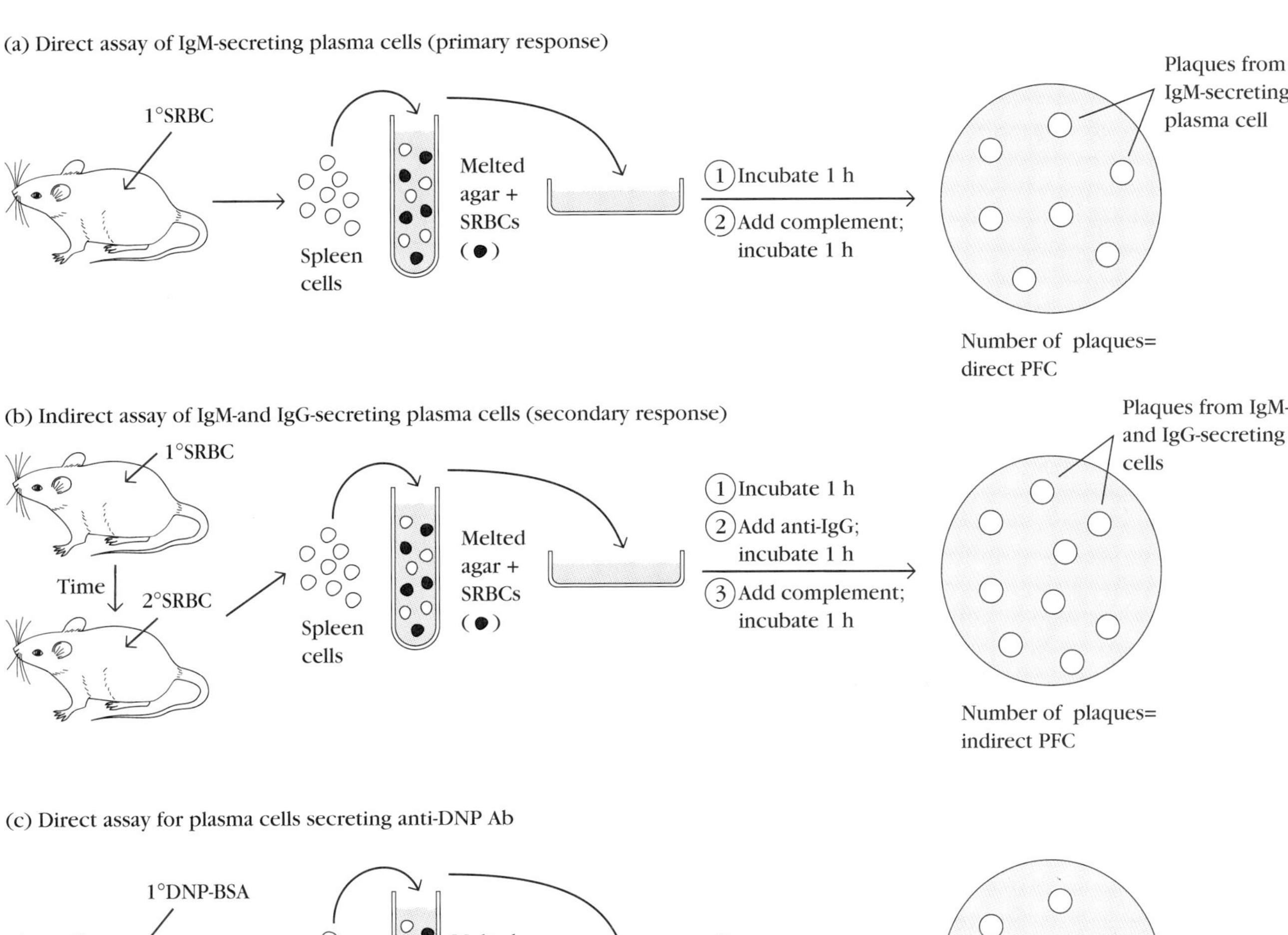

FIGURE 14-3 Hemolytic plaque assays. (a) A direct assay detects IgM-secreting plasma cells, which are predominant in a primary response. (b) In an indirect assay, which detects both IgM- and IgG-secreting plasma cells, antibodies against mouse IgG are added so that complement-mediated lysis of IgG-SRBC complexes will occur. By subtracting the direct PFC from the indirect PFC, the number of IgG-secreting plasma cells can be determined. In a secondary response, the indirect PFC is high and the direct PFC is low. (c) The response to immunization with antigens other than SRBCs can be determined with the hemolytic plaque assay if the immunizing protein or hapten is coupled with SRBCs.

by a clear plaque devoid of cells. The plaques are counted, and their number is the number of plaque-forming plasma cells specific for the SRBC antigen, referred to as the direct plaque-forming count (PFC).

The hemolytic plaque assay can be adapted to determine the number of IgM-secreting plasma cells and IgG-secreting plasma cells. In the case of IgM, complement-mediated lysis is triggered by the binding of a single pentameric IgM molecule to an SRBC. However, in the case of IgG, which exists as a monomer, complement-mediated lysis does not occur unless the Fc regions from two IgG molecules are located within 30–40 nm of each other on the membrane of an SRBC. (As discussed in Chapter 17, complement binds to the

Fc region of antibody molecules.) Such close proximity of two IgG molecules does not normally result from the random binding of IgG secreted by a single plasma cell. Therefore a secondary anti-isotype antibody that reacts with the bound IgG is added to the Petri dish after the first hour of incubation and the complement is added after another hour (Figure 14-3b). This procedure, called the indirect hemolytic plaque assay, results in lysis of SRBCs to which IgM or IgG are bound. Subtraction of the number of plaques formed in the direct assay from the number formed in the indirect assay gives the number of IgG-secreting plasma cells, or indirect PFC. Since most of the antibody secreted during a primary response is IgM, the direct PFC is high and the indirect PFC is low. In contrast, a secondary response leads to a low direct PFC and a high indirect PFC, reflecting the switch from IgM to IgG secretion.

The hemolytic plaque assay also can be modified to quantitate plasma cells secreting antibodies specific for proteins, polysaccharides, or small haptens. In this case, the animal is immunized with the desired antigen, but before the SRBCs are mixed with the isolated spleen cells, they are coated with the immunizing antigen. The induced antibody binds to these antigen-coated SRBCs, which are lysed after the complement is added (Figure 14-3c). Uncoated SRBCs can serve as a control, since they do not lyse in response to antibody secreted from the antigen-specific plasma cells.

A modification of the Jerne plaque-forming assay, called the "Elispot assay," allows plasma cells to be quantitated without requiring SRBCs. In this modification the antigen-primed lymphocytes are incubated on a Petri dish to which antigen has been bound. As the plasma cells secrete antibody, it binds to antigen in the vicinity of the plasma cell. The bound antibody is then visualized after removal of the cells by an ELISA assay in which the dish is first incubated with enzyme-labeled anti-Ig followed by an appropriate substrate. The enzyme-substrate reaction produces a colored spot, allowing enumeration of the plasma cells.

Identification of Cells Required for Induction of Humoral Immunity

Most antigens that elicit a humoral immune response are thymus dependent; that is, participation of T_H cells is required for such antigens to activate B cells. Some antigens, however, can activate B cells in the absence of T_H cells; these are termed thymus-independent antigens.

Response to Thymus-Dependent Antigens

Experiments conducted in the 1960s and 1970s demonstrated that several types of cells must cooperate to generate a humoral immune response. Even before B and T cells were clearly defined, evidence that distinct subpopulations are required to generate an antibody response came from adoptive-transfer experiments done by H. Claman and his co-workers in 1966. Lethally x-irradiated mice were reconstituted with syngeneic thymus cells alone, with bone marrow cells alone, or with a mixture of thymus and bone marrow cells. The mice were then immunized with SRBCs and their serum anti-SRBC levels were determined. Mice reconstituted with either thymus cells or bone marrow cells alone failed to produce any anti-SRBC antibodies, but mice reconstituted with both thymus and bone marrow cells generated a response. This early experiment demonstrated that both bone marrow cells and thymus cells were necessary for induction of the humoral response.

The development of the Mishell-Dutton in vitro culture system allowed D. Mosier to identify still another cell population required for induction of the humoral response. When spleen cells are grown in the Mishell-Dutton system, the macrophages adhere to the surface of the culture dish, whereas the lymphocytes do not. Mosier thus was able to separate macrophages from lymphocytes by carefully decanting the culture medium containing the nonadherent cells into a separate culture dish. He then determined the response of the adherent and nonadherent cells to SRBCs in the direct hemolytic plaque assay. Neither the adherent nor the nonadherent cells alone exhibited a plaque-forming response to SRBCs, but when the two populations were combined, the plaque-forming response was evident. This experiment gave the first indication that macrophages, as well as lymphocytes, are involved in generation of the humoral response.

Claman's experiments showed that both thymus and bone marrow cells are necessary to generate a humoral antibody response, but they did not identify which population produced antibodies. A now classic experiment by G. Mitchell and J. F. A. P. Miller in 1968 demonstrated that bone marrow cells were the source of antibody-producing cells. Using an adoptive-transfer system similar to that of Claman, these researchers reconstituted lethally x-irradiated and thymectomized mice with various populations of cells. (Instead of thymus cells, Mitchell and Miller used thoracic-duct thymocytes as an enriched source of T cells.) The reconstituted mice were immunized with SRBCs, after which the spleen cells were tested in a direct hemolytic plaque assay for plasma cells secreting anti-SRBC antibodies. They found that only mice reconstituted with thoracic-duct cells and bone marrow cells in combination were able to generate SRBC-specific plasma cells, confirming Claman's findings.

Mitchell and Miller then sought to identify the source of the antibody-producing population of cells by repeating their experiments using thoracic-duct cells expressing one MHC haplotype and bone marrow cells expressing another MHC haplotype. By incubating the isolated spleen cells with antisera specific for each MHC molecule, they could selectively remove the thoracic duct-derived or marrow-derived cells. When reconstitution was tried initially with cells from two different allogeneic strains, no SRBC-specific plasma cells were generated. Although this finding was puzzling at the time, it made sense once the self-MHC restriction of T_H cells was demonstrated (see Figure 10-1). Mitchell and Miller then tried using semi-allogeneic cells to reconstitute thymectomized and lethally irradiated CBA (H-2^k) mice, as outlined in Figure 14-4. The mice were then reconstituted with CBA (H-2^k) bone marrow and F_1 (CBA × C57BL) (H-$2^{k/b}$) thoracic-duct cells. The reconstituted mice were challenged with SRBCs, and after 5 days the spleen cells were assayed. The spleen cells from these reconstituted mice exhibited a high PFC specific for SRBCs. Treatment of the isolated spleen cells with antibody to H-2^k MHC molecules in the presence of complement, which removed both the thoracic duct-derived and marrow-derived cells, abolished the plaque-forming response. However, removal of the H-$2^{k/b}$ thoracic duct-derived cells with H-2^b antibody did not affect the response. These results demonstrated that the bone marrow population, now known to contain B cells, supplied the antibody-forming cells and that the thoracic-duct population provided helper cells for generating the humoral response.

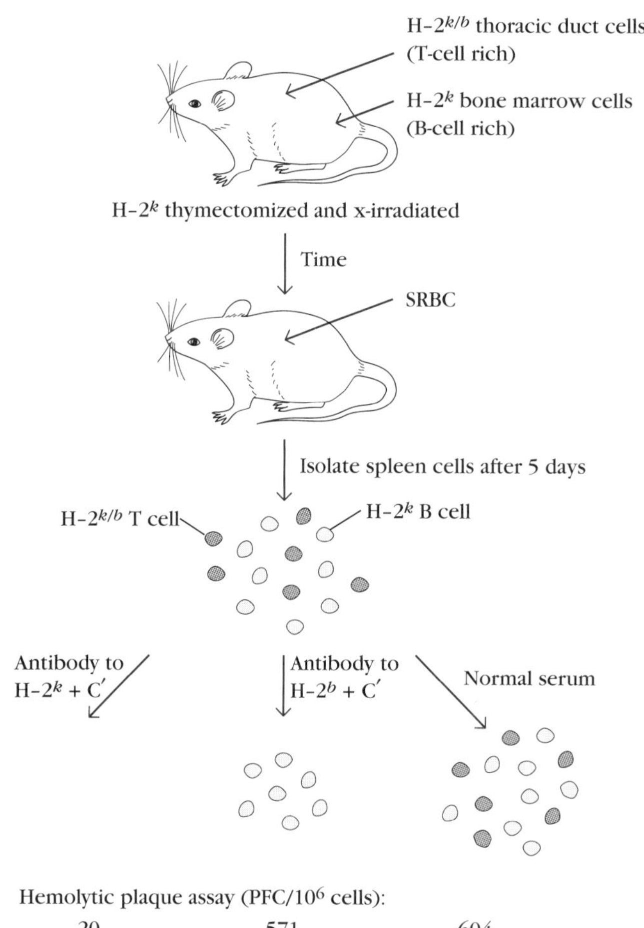

FIGURE 14-4 In the experimental system of Miller and Mitchell H-2^k thymectomized and x-irradiated mice were reconstituted with F_1 H-$2^{k/b}$ thoracic-duct lymphocytes and H-2^k bone marrow cells. The mice were challenged with SRBCs, and 5 days later the spleen cells first were treated with antibody to H-2^k or H-2^b MHC antigens, and then complement (C′) was added. Removal of H-2^k-bearing cells eliminated the PFC response, whereas removal of H-2^b-bearing cells had no significant effect. This experiment demonstrated that bone marrow cells contain the antibody-forming population now known to be B cells.

Response to Thymus-Independent Antigens

Those antigens that can activate B cells without the assistance of T_H cells include polymerized bacterial flagellin, lipopolysaccharide (LPS) derived from gram-negative bacterial cell walls, dextran, pneumococcal capsular polysaccharide, levan, polyvinylpyrrolidone, and ficoll.

Thymus-independent antigens have various properties in common. Many are polysaccharides and therefore cannot be displayed as peptides together with class II MHC molecules on the membrane of the B cell. In addition, many have a polymeric structure with repeating epitopes, and many are resistant to degradation. Their polymeric structure may facilitate the cross-linkage of antigen-binding receptors on the B-cell membrane that is required for activation. Some thymus-independent antigens, at high doses, act as mitogens and are able to induce nonspecific B-cell activation, giving rise to a polyclonal response that bypasses the normal T_H-cell requirement for activation. A possible explanation of this phenomenon is that at high doses enough nonspecific binding occurs to result in polyclonal activation, whereas at lower doses only those B cells with specific receptors for a thymus-independent antigen bind enough of the antigen to be activated. These bacterial antigens induce a humoral antibody response characterized primarily by the production of IgM. Because the response to these bacterial antigens is independent of T cells, individuals born with various T-cell deficiencies generally are immune to many bacterial pathogens. Instead these individuals succumb to infection by viruses, fungi, or other pathogens capable of intracellular growth (see Chapter 22).

The humoral immune response to thymus-independent antigens is different from the response to thymus-dependent antigens. The response is generally weaker, no memory cells are formed, and only IgM is secreted. These differences highlight the important role played by the T_H cell in generating memory B cells and in class switching to other isotypes.

TABLE 14-2 COMMON HAPTEN-CARRIER CONJUGATES USED IN IMMUNOLOGIC RESEARCH

Hapten-carrier acronym	Hapten	Carrier protein
DNP-BGG	Dinitrophenol	Bovine gamma-globulin
TNP-BSA	Trinitrophenyl	Bovine serum albumin
NIP-KLH	5-Nitrophenyl acetic acid	Keyhole limpet hemocyanin
ARS-OVA	Azophenylarsonate	Ovalbumin
LAC-HGG	Phenyllactoside	Human gamma-globulin

Use of Hapten-Carrier Conjugates to Study Cellular Interactions

The discovery of haptens and their use in studying antigenicity was described in Chapter 4. When animals are immunized with small organic compounds *(haptens)* conjugated to large proteins *(carriers),* the conjugate induces a humoral immune response with antibodies formed both to hapten epitopes and to unaltered epitopes on the carrier protein. Since the chemical conjugation allows multiple molecules of a single hapten to be coupled to the carrier protein and since the position of the hapten is easily accessible to the B cell's membrane-bound antibody, the hapten functions as the immunodominant B-cell epitope (see Figure 4-12). Such hapten-carrier conjugates provided immunologists with an ideal system for studying cellular interactions involved in the humoral response. Unlike complex proteins, whose B-cell epitopes are often conformational sequences dependent on the tertiary structure of the protein, a hapten constitutes a defined B-cell epitope that can be presented to B cells on different protein carriers. Studies with hapten-carrier conjugates demonstrated that the generation of a humoral antibody response requires associative recognition by T_H cells and B cells, each recognizing different epitopes on the same antigen.

A variety of different hapten-carrier conjugates have been used in immunologic research (Table 14-2). After an animal has been immunized with a hapten-carrier conjugate, the humoral response to the hapten is assessed with a modified hemolytic plaque assay, with hapten-conjugated SRBCs as the indicator cells (see Figure 14-3c). A direct hemolytic plaque assay is used to quantitate plasma cells secreting IgM antihapten antibody and an indirect assay is used to quantitate plasma cells secreting IgG antihapten antibody, an indicator of a secondary response.

Recognition of Carrier Epitopes by T_H Cells

The results of early experiments using hapten-carrier conjugates to study induction of the humoral immune response were puzzling. Eventually, however, a model of T-cell and B-cell collaboration was formulated, providing a framework in which the results could be understood.

One of the earliest findings with hapten-carrier conjugates was that a hapten had to be chemically coupled to a larger carrier molecule to induce a humoral response to the hapten. If an animal was immunized with both hapten and carrier separately, no plasma cells specific for the hapten were generated. A second important observation was that in order to generate a secondary antibody response to a hapten, the animal had to be immunized with the same hapten-carrier conjugate used for the primary immunization. If the secondary immunization was with the same hapten but conjugated to a different, unrelated carrier, no secondary antihapten response occurred. This phenomenon,

TABLE 14-3 SECONDARY HUMORAL RESPONSE TO DNP IN MICE IMMUNIZED WITH VARIOUS COMBINATIONS OF DNP AND CARRIER PROTEIN*

Primary immunization	Secondary immunization	Secondary anti-DNP PFC
DNP-BSA	DNP-BSA	+
DNP + BSA	DNP + BSA	−
DNP-BSA	DNP + BSA	−
DNP-BSA	DNP-BGG	−
DNP-BSA + BGG	DNP-BGG	+

* Following the secondary immunization, spleen cells were isolated and an indirect hemolytic plaque assay was performed to determine the secondary anti-DNP PFC, using DNP-SRBCs as the indicator cells.

called the *carrier effect,* could be circumvented by priming the animal separately with the unrelated carrier (Table 14-3).

Similar experiments conducted with an adoptive-transfer system showed that hapten-primed cells and carrier-primed cells were distinct populations (Figure 14-5). In these experiments one mouse was primed with the DNP-BSA conjugate and another was primed with the unrelated carrier BGG, which was not conjugated to the hapten. Spleen cells from both mice were mixed and injected into a lethally irradiated syngeneic recipient. When this mouse was now challenged with DNP conjugated to the unrelated carrier BGG, there was a secondary antihapten response, as indicated by a positive hemolytic plaque assay to DNP. Spleen cells from the BGG-immunized mice then were treated with anti-T-cell antiserum (anti-Thy-1) and complement to remove the T cells. When this T-cell–depleted sample was mixed with the DNP-BSA–primed spleen cells and injected into an irradiated mouse, no secondary antihapten response was observed. However, similar treatment of the DNP-BSA–primed spleen cells did not abolish the secondary antihapten response (see Figure 14-6b,c). Later experiments, in which antisera were used to specifically deplete $CD4^+$ or $CD8^+$ T cells, showed that the removal of the $CD4^+$ T-cell subpopulation primed with the second carrier abolished the carrier effect. These experiments demonstrate that the response of hapten-primed B cells to the hapten-carrier conjugate requires the presence of carrier-primed $CD4^+$ T_H cells specific for carrier epitopes. (It is important to keep in mind that the B-cell response is

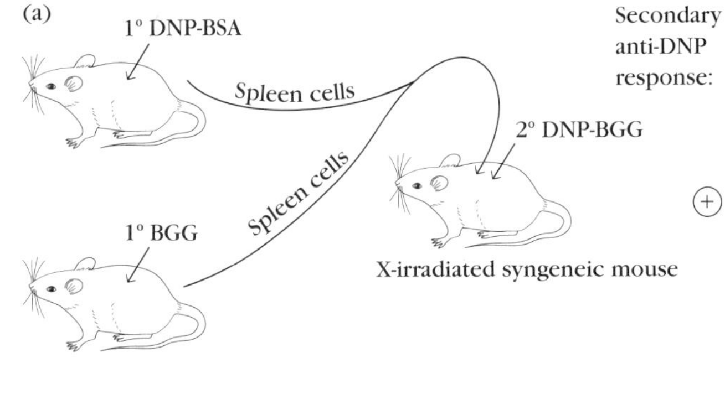

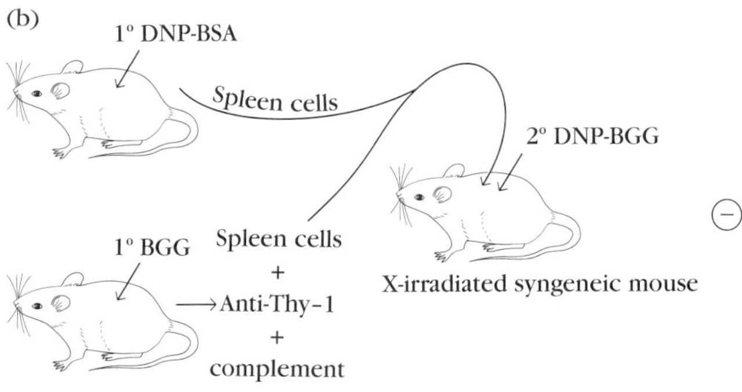

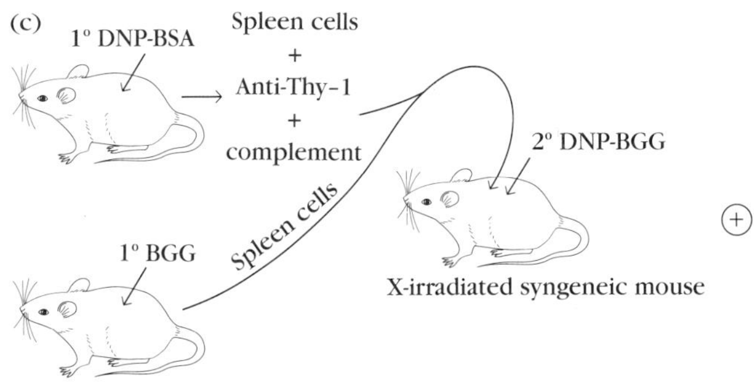

FIGURE 14-5 Adoptive-transfer experiments demonstrating that hapten-primed and carrier-primed cells are separate populations. (a) X-irradiated syngeneic mice reconstituted with spleen cells from both DNP-BSA–primed mice and BGG-primed mice and challenged with DNP-BGG generated a secondary anti-DNP response. (b) Removal of T cells from the BGG-primed spleen cells, by treatment with anti-Thy-1 antiserum, abolished the secondary anti-DNP response. (c) Removal of T cells from the DNP-BSA–primed spleen cells had no effect on the secondary response to DNP. These experiments show that carrier-primed cells are T cells and hapten-primed cells are B cells. The secondary anti-DNP response was measured with an indirect hemolytic plaque assay.

not limited to the hapten determinant; in fact some B cells do react to epitopes on the carrier, but because the assay system uses hapten-conjugated SRBCs, it measures only the antihapten response.)

Because of the carrier effect, a secondary antihapten response normally occurs only if an animal has previously been primed both to the hapten and to the carrier epitopes. Under unusual experimental conditions it is possible to bypass the carrier effect by using allogeneic T cells in place of carrier-primed T cells. The allogeneic T cells recognize the MHC molecules displayed on B cells as foreign, enabling the allogeneic T cells to bind to B cells, resulting in localized cytokine production. These cytokines enable a B cell to be activated in the absence of a carrier-primed T cell. This phenomenon is called the *allogeneic effect.*

MHC Restriction in the Interaction between T_H and B Cells

Hapten-carrier systems enabled immunologists to explore various parameters affecting the collaborative response of hapten-primed B cells and carrier-primed T_H cells. Experiments by D. H. Katz and B. Benacerraf were designed to explore the influence of the MHC on the collaboration of T_H and B cells in a hapten-carrier system. The basic question they sought to answer was whether carrier-primed T cells of one MHC haplotype could cooperate with hapten-primed B cells of another MHC haplotype. To answer this question they carried out adoptive transfer of BGG-primed T cells from strain A mice into an (A × B) F_1 recipient, followed by the transfer of DNP-KLH–primed B cells derived from strain A or strain B mice. The mice then were immunized with DNP-BGG, and the secondary response to DNP was assessed.

One complication of this experimental design, which initially made the experiment unworkable, was the allogeneic effect. The transferred strain-A T cells recognized the strain-B allogeneic MHC antigens of the F_1 host as foreign and therefore activated the host B cells nonspecifically, making it impossible to assess the response to DNP-BGG. In order to circumvent this complication, Katz and Benacerraf exploited a previous observation that primed T cells were less susceptible to x-irradiation than unprimed T cells. Irradiation of the F_1 A × B recipient 24 h after the transfer of the BGG-primed strain-A T cells eliminated the alloreactive T cells but not the BGG-primed T cells. Strain A or strain B B cells from DNP-KLH–primed mice could now be transferred into the F_1 recipient, and the secondary response to DNP-BGG could be measured (Figure 14-6).

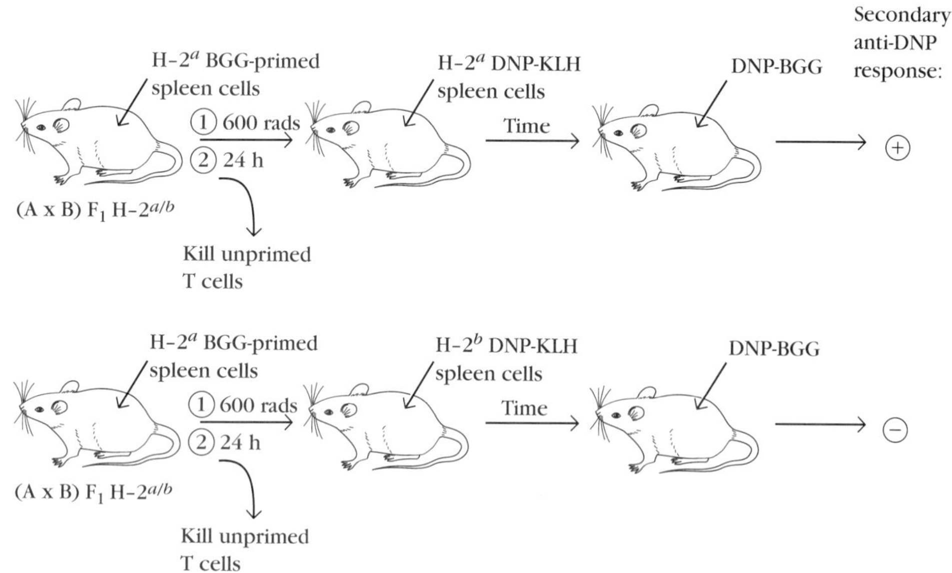

FIGURE 14-6 Experimental system of Katz and Benacerraf for studying effect of MHC haplotype on collaboration of T_H cells and B cells. F_1 (A × B) mice were reconstituted with strain A spleen cells from a BGG-primed animal. In order to reduce nonspecific T-cell activation by allogeneic MHC molecules expressed by the F_1 host, the adoptive recipients were x-irradiated with 600 rads. This amount of radiation had previously been shown to kill unprimed T cells but not primed T cells. In this way only the BGG-primed T cells survived. The mice were then reconstituted with strain A or strain B spleen cells from a DNP-KLH–primed mouse, and the antibody response to DNP-BGG was measured. The results revealed that the carrier-primed T_H cell and hapten-primed B cell must share the same MHC haplotype.

The results revealed that carrier-primed T_H cells could assist only hapten-primed B cells sharing the same MHC haplotype. Later experiments with congenic recombinant strains revealed that allelic identity at either the IA or IE class II MHC subregions was necessary for collaboration between T_H and B cells.

Associative Recognition

The experiments with hapten-carrier conjugates revealed that both T_H cells and B cells must recognize antigenic determinants on the same molecule for B-cell activation to occur. This feature of the T- and B-cell interaction in the humoral response is called *associative,* or *linked, recognition.* The conclusions drawn from hapten-carrier experiments apply generally to the humoral response. In the case of a protein such as BSA, for example, a B-cell response to epitopes on the BSA molecule takes place only if there is associative recognition by a T_H cell that is specific for distinctly different epitopes on the BSA molecule.

Early models of associative recognition based on hapten-carrier experiments envisioned a B cell binding to the hapten and a T cell binding to carrier epitopes, with the hapten-carrier conjugate serving to bridge the two cells (Figure 14-7a). Activation of the B cell was hypothesized to result from membrane interactions between the T_H and B cell and/or from the high localized concentrations of cytokines released by the T_H cell at the junction of the interacting cells. The discovery of MHC restriction in this process meant that this simple hapten-carrier bridge model was not sufficient and that any model of associative recognition must include a role for class II MHC molecules. That role was made clear with the discovery that B cells, like macrophages, are antigen-presenting cells. Unlike the macrophage, the B cell is antigen-specific and binds a hapten-carrier conjugate via its membrane-bound antibody. After binding, the hapten-carrier conjugate is internalized, processed in the endocytic processing pathway, and presented as a processed peptide together with a class II MHC molecule on the membrane of the B cell (Figure 14-7b). Because MHC molecules bind small peptides, often with amphipathic properties, internal peptides of the carrier are generally presented. An activated T_H cell then recognizes the processed peptide together with the class II MHC molecule.

The hapten-carrier systems highlight the important differences in epitope recognition by B and by T cells. B cells recognize the hapten determinant because it is accessible and hydrophilic, because it is of a size comparable to that of the antigen-binding sites on B cells, and because it is also present in multiple copies that

(a) Early model

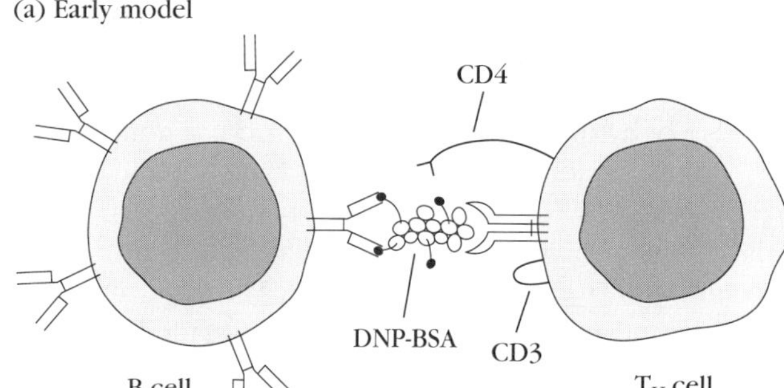

(b) Current model

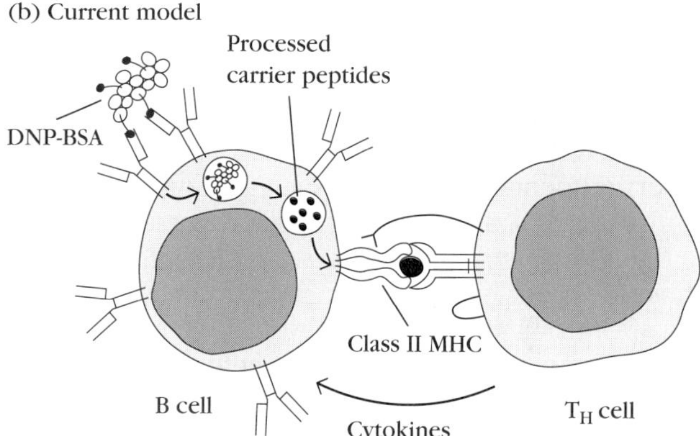

FIGURE 14-7 (a) Early models of associative recognition envisioned the B cell binding to hapten determinants (black circles) and the T cell binding to carrier determinants (open circles). In this model, MHC molecules were not involved. (b) The current model of associative recognition proposes that the B cell binds the hapten-carrier conjugate, internalizes and processes it, and presents carrier peptides (purple circles) together with a class II MHC molecule on its membrane. The T_H cell recognizes this processed peptide together with the class II MHC molecule.

make it the immunodominant B-cell epitope. T cells in contrast, recognize certain internal, hydrophobic residues of the carrier that are displayed following antigen processing (together with class II MHC molecules) on the membrane of an antigen-presenting cell. B-cell activation results from membrane-mediated events and the localized release of cytokines, which together drive the B cell to proliferate and differentiate.

Steps in B-Cell Activation, Proliferation, and Differentiation

Activation of a B cell requires a number of sequential processes: (1) presentation of processed antigen plus a class II MHC molecule by the B cell to an activated T_H

cell specific for that antigen; (2) formation of a T_H-cell/B-cell conjugate, which induces expression of CD40L on the T_H-cell membrane and the directional release of cytokines by the T_H cell; and (3) generation of signals, by membrane-mediated events and localized cytokines, that are transduced in the B cell, causing changes in gene expression that lead to proliferation and differentiation of the B cell. The experimental demonstration of these processes and the mechanisms involved are described in this section.

Antigen Presentation by B Cells

The first experimental evidence demonstrating that B cells were major antigen-presenting cells came from an experiment of R. Chesnut and H. Grey in 1981. Up to that time, it had been impossible to compare the antigen-presenting capabilities of macrophages with those of B cells because macrophages take up antigen nonspecifically through phagocytosis, whereas B cells take up antigen specifically by receptor-mediated endocytosis. Less than 1 B cell in 10,000 is specific for a given antigen, and it was not possible to study the response of such a small minority of antigen-presenting cells.

Chestnut and Grey bypassed this difficulty by using as the antigen rabbit antibody against mouse immunoglobulin (anti-mouse Ig). This antigen binds to the Fc portion of the membrane-bound immunoglobulin (mIg) on B cells, not to specific antigen-binding sites in the Fab portion, which are present on only a few B cells. Nonetheless, rabbit anti-mouse Ig is endocytosed and processed by mouse B cells like any antigen, and the processed peptides are presented with class II MHC molecules on the B-cell membrane (Figure 14-8). Using this experimental system, Chesnut and Grey showed that B cells were just as effective as macrophages in presenting antigen to T_H cells.

Experiments with other systems involving antigen-specific B-cell lines have confirmed the results of Chesnut and Grey and have extended these results by showing that internalization of antigen by B cells generally requires binding of the antigen to the membrane-bound Ig. In some cases, however, this requirement for antigen binding can be bypassed by incubating B cells in extremely high (nonphysiologic) concentrations of a particular antigen. Such *antigen-pulsed* B cells take up the antigen nonspecifically by pinocytosis (see Figure 1-3), allowing antigen processing and presentation to occur.

In all of these B-cell experimental systems it takes 30–60 min following internalization for the processed antigen to be displayed on the membrane with class II MHC molecules. Presumably this is the time required

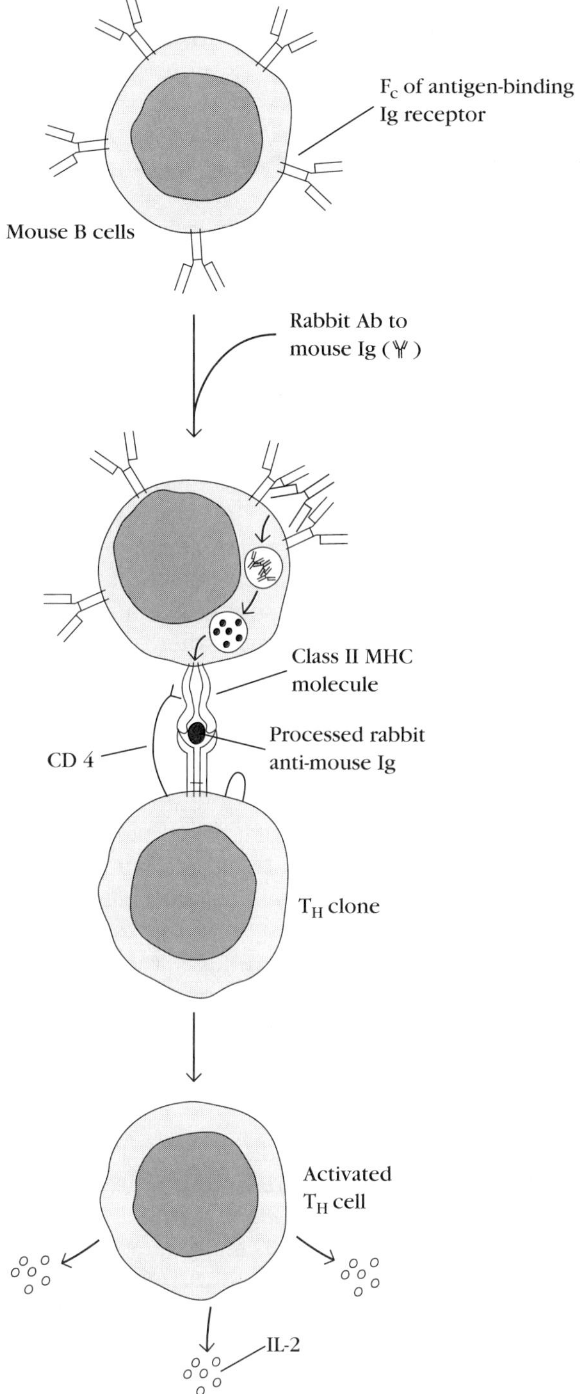

FIGURE 14-8 Unique experimental system of Chesnut and Grey used to demonstrate antigen-presentation by B cells. Rabbit antibody against mouse immunoglobulin binds to the Fc region of membrane-bound antibodies (Ig receptors) on all B cells, not to specific antigen-binding sites present on just a few B cells. The rabbit anti-mouse Ig (purple) is internalized, processed, and presented like other antigens by the B cells. Addition of T_H cells specific for the rabbit antibody results in T_H-cell activation as measured by production of IL-2.

for antigen processing and binding to MHC molecules within B cells. Antigen processing in B cells, as in macrophages, can be inhibited by chloroquine, suggesting that the processing pathways may be similar in the two cell types. Because a B cell recognizes antigen specifically, by way of its membrane-bound Ig, a B cell is able to present antigen to T_H cells at antigen concentrations that are 100- to 10,000-times lower than what is required for macrophage presentation. When antigen concentrations are high, therefore, the macrophage serves as an effective antigen-presenting cell, but as antigen levels drop, the B cell takes over as the major presenter of antigen to T_H cells.

Formation of T_H-Cell/B-Cell Conjugate

Once a T_H cell recognizes a processed antigen displayed by a class II MHC molecule on the membrane of a B cell, the two cells interact, forming a T-B conjugate (Figure 14-9). Events occurring during this interaction were studied by observing the interaction of an antigen-specific T_H-cell line with antigen-pulsed B-cell hybridomas. Controls using B-cell hybridomas pulsed with a nonspecific antigen were also included. The question asked was whether an antigen-specific T-B cell interaction would be qualitatively different from a nonspecific T-B interaction. Micrographs of the T-B conjugates revealed that the antigen-specific conjugates had a greater area of membrane contact than nonspecific conjugates. What was most interesting was that the T_H cells in antigen-specific conjugates exhibited a reorganization of the Golgi apparatus and the microtubular-organizing center toward the junction with the B cell, whereas T_H cells in nonspecific conjugates exhibited random orientation of the Golgi apparatus and microtubular-organizing centers. This reorganization of the Golgi apparatus may provide a mechanism for the directed release of cytokines toward the antigen-specific B cell.

Another qualitative difference between antigen-specific T-B conjugates and nonspecific ones is that the TCR, CD4, and LFA-1 molecules on the T_H-cell membrane become redistributed along the B-cell junction in antigen-specific conjugates. This clustering is seen only if the B cells are presenting both the antigen and the MHC molecule for which the T_H cell is specific. Thus antigen-specific recognition, mediated by the T-cell receptor, influences the distribution of two important T_H-cell membrane proteins—LFA-1 and CD4—both of which are involved in cellular adhesion. As discussed in Chapter 3, LFA-1 is a member of the integrin family of receptors, which bind to intercellular adhesion molecules (ICAMs). In a T-B conjugate, LFA-1 and CD4 molecules on the T_H cell bind to ICAM and class II MHC molecules, respectively, on the B-cell membrane. It has been suggested that clustering of TCR, CD4, and LFA-1 molecules at the junction of an antigen-specific T-B conjugate may increase the avidity of the cellular interaction. This increased avidity would prolong the association between the T_H cell and B cell, providing time for additional membrane signaling events and for the directed secretion of various cytokines.

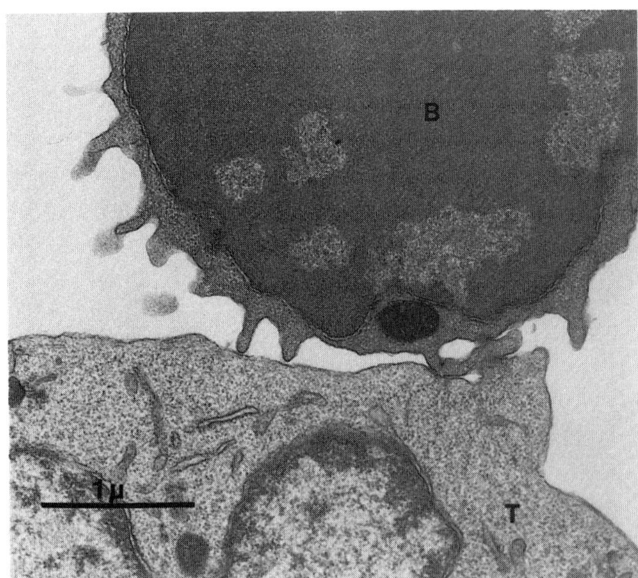

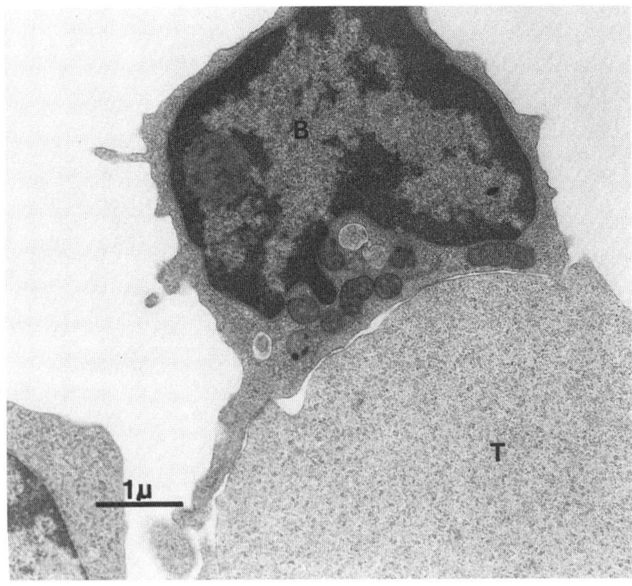

FIGURE 14-9 Transmission electron micrographs of initial contact between a T cell and B cell *(left)* and of a T-B conjugate *(right)*. Note the broad area of membrane contact between the cells following conjugate formation. The bar = 1 μm. [From V. M. Sanders et al., 1986, *J. Immunol.* **137**:2395.]

Contact-Dependent Help Mediated by CD40-CD40L Interaction

Formation of a T-B conjugate not only leads to the directional release of T_H-cell cytokines, but also to the activation-dependent expression of a new T_H-cell membrane protein that is necessary for B-cell activation. This phenomenon was revealed by incubating naive B cells with antigen and plasma membranes prepared either from activated T_H-cell clones or from resting T_H-cell clones. Only the membranes from the activated T cells induced B-cell proliferation, suggesting that one or more molecules expressed on the membrane of an activated T_H cell engage receptors on the B cell to provide contact-dependent help. Likely mediators of such contact-dependent help are CD40, which is expressed on the membrane of all B cells, and its newly discovered ligand, designated CD40L, which is expressed on the membrane of activated T_H cells (Figure 14-10).

Evidence in support of this hypothesis comes from the observation that antibodies to CD40 can induce proliferation of antigen-stimulated B cells in the absence of T_H cells. Indeed, if cytokines are provided, then anti-CD40 also induces B-cell differentiation into plasma cells. Further evidence for the role of the CD40-CD40L interaction comes from experiments with an engineered soluble form of CD40 consisting of the extracellular domains of CD40 with the Fc region of IgG. (The IgG Fc region often is used to produce soluble forms of membrane proteins and to prolong the serum half-life of the fusion product.) The CD40-IgG fusion protein was found to inhibit the activation of B cells mediated by plasma membranes from activated T_H cells. Presumably, the soluble CD40 binds to CD40L on activated T_H cells, thus preventing them from providing contact-dependent help to B cells.

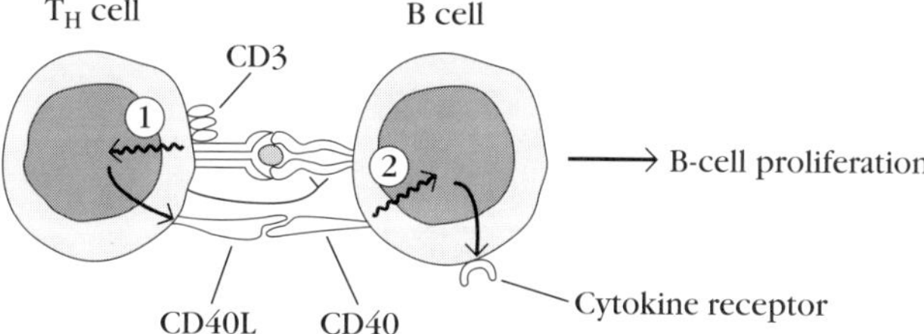

FIGURE 14-10 Contact-dependent help mediated by CD40-CD40L interaction. Formation of a T-B conjugate generates a signal (1) that leads to expression of CD40L on the T-cell membrane. This membrane molecule can interact with CD40 on the B-cell membrane, generating a signal (2) that induces expression of cytokine receptors. In some, but not all, experimental systems, these interactions are sufficient to fully activate B cells and induce their proliferation. [Based on P. D. Hodgkin and M. R. Kehry, 1993, *The Immunologist* **1**:5.]

Directional Release of Cytokines from T_H Cells

Although B cells stimulated with membranes from activated T_H cells are able to proliferate, they fail to differentiate unless cytokines also are present; this finding suggests that both a membrane contact signal and cytokine signal are necessary to induce B-cell proliferation and differentiation. As noted already, electron micrographs of T-B conjugates suggest that an antigen-specific interaction between T_H and B cells induces a redistribution of T-cell membrane proteins and cytoskeletal elements that may result in the polarized release of cytokines toward the interacting B cell. In a simple, yet ingenious experiment, W. J. Poo and C. A. Janeway sought to determine whether cytokines are released from T_H cells in a directional manner. They worked with a T_H-cell clone that secreted IL-4 in response to binding of a clonotypic monoclonal antibody specific for the idiotype of the T-cell receptor. This T_H clone was centrifuged onto a nucleopore membrane having 3-μm pores. Since the cells were larger than 3 μm, they completely plugged the pores. The cell-packed membrane was then suspended between two chambers, and the anti-TCR monoclonal antibody was added to one chamber. Measurement of IL-4 in both chambers showed that IL-4 was released toward the chamber containing the activating monoclonal antibody (Figure 14-11). These findings suggest that formation of specific T-B conjugates results in directional release of cytokines toward the interacting B cell.

Signal Generation by Membrane Events and Cytokines

Naive, or resting, B cells are noncycling cells in the G_0 stage of the cell cycle. Activation drives the resting cell into the cell cycle, progressing through G_1 into the S phase, in which DNA is replicated. The G_1-to-S transition represents a critical restriction point in the cell cycle. Once a cell has reached S, it completes the cell cycle, moving through G_2 and into mitosis (M). After analyzing the events involved in the progression of lymphocytes from G_0 to the S phase, Ken Ichi Arai noted a number of similarities with events that had been identified in fibroblast cells. He divided these signals into *competence* and *progression* signals.

(a)

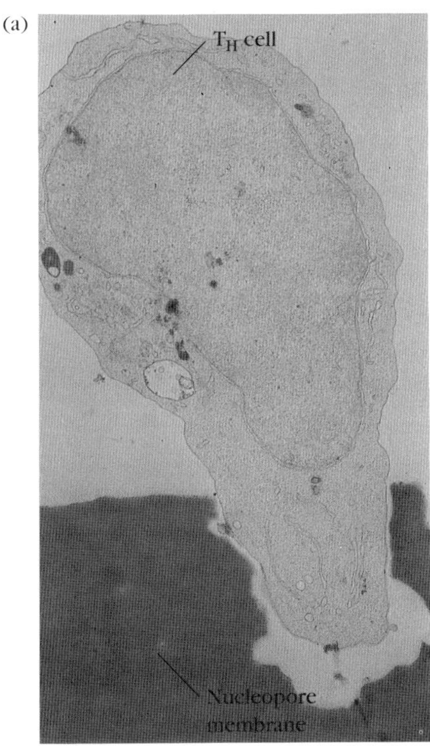

(b)

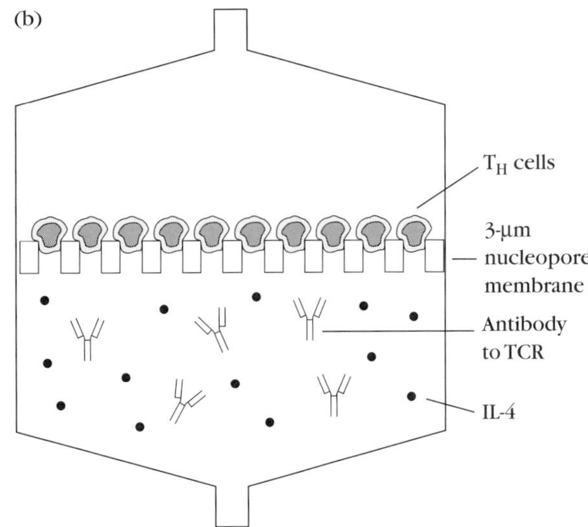

FIGURE 14-11 Experimental demonstration of directional release of cytokines from T_H cells. (a) Electron micrograph of T_H cell centrifuged onto nucleopore membrane. Note how cell completely blocks the pore. (b) Diagram of culture system. Addition of monoclonal antibody specific for the idiotype of the T-cell receptors resulted in T_H-cell activation and release of IL-4 on one side of the membrane only. [From W. J. Poo et al., 1988, *Nature* **332**:378.]

Competence signals are envisioned to drive the B cell from G_0 into early G_1, rendering the cell competent to receive the next level of signals. Progression signals then drive the cell from G_1 into S and ultimately to cell division and differentiation.

Membrane Signals

As shown in Figure 14-12a, several competence signals are generated by interactions involving membrane-bound immunoglobulin (mIg) or other molecules on the B-cell membrane. Antigen-mediated cross-linkage of membrane-bound IgM or IgD molecules on B cells has been shown to trigger a complex cascade of biochemical and cellular responses. Within minutes of cross-linkage, tyrosine kinase and tyrosine phosphatase activities are released; tyrosine phosphorylation can be detected by 30 s and peaks within 3–5 min of cross-linkage. As tyrosines are phosphorylated and dephosphorylated, a number of more-or-less parallel activation pathways are activated. One pathway leads to activation of phospholipase C and the subsequent hydrolysis of phosphatidylinositols, leading to generation of inositol 1,4,5-trisphosphate (IP_3) and diacylglycerol (DAG). By a pathway probably similar to that involved in T-cell activation (see Figure 12-13), IP_3 and DAG act as second messengers that either individually or synergistically induce a number of biochemical events including mobilization of Ca^{2+} from intracellular stores, activation of protein kinase C (PKC), and activation of the Ca^{2+}/calmodulin-dependent kinase. These events ultimately result in changes in B-cell gene expression.

Both mIgM and mIgD on B cells extend into the cytoplasm by only three amino acids and therefore are ineffective in transducing an activation signal following interaction with antigen. However, membrane Ig is associated with a disulfide-linked heterodimer (Ig-α/Ig-β) forming the B-cell receptor (BCR) (see Figure 5-10). The cytoplasmic tails of Ig-α/Ig-β function to transduce the cross-linking of mIg molecules into an effective signal. These tails contain tyrosine residues that have been shown to be phosphorylated or dephosphorylated after mIg cross-linkage. Recent evidence also suggests that three members of the *src* family of tyrosine kinases ($p55^{blk}$, $p59^{fyn}$, and $p56^{lyn}$) are associated with the BCR and are activated following mIg cross-linkage. Interestingly, some differences have been observed in tyrosine phosphorylation induced by cross-linkage with anti-IgM or anti-IgD, which may reflect a qualitative difference in the signals mediated by these two membrane immunoglobulins.

Other B-cell membrane molecules probably play a role in generating competence signals. For example,

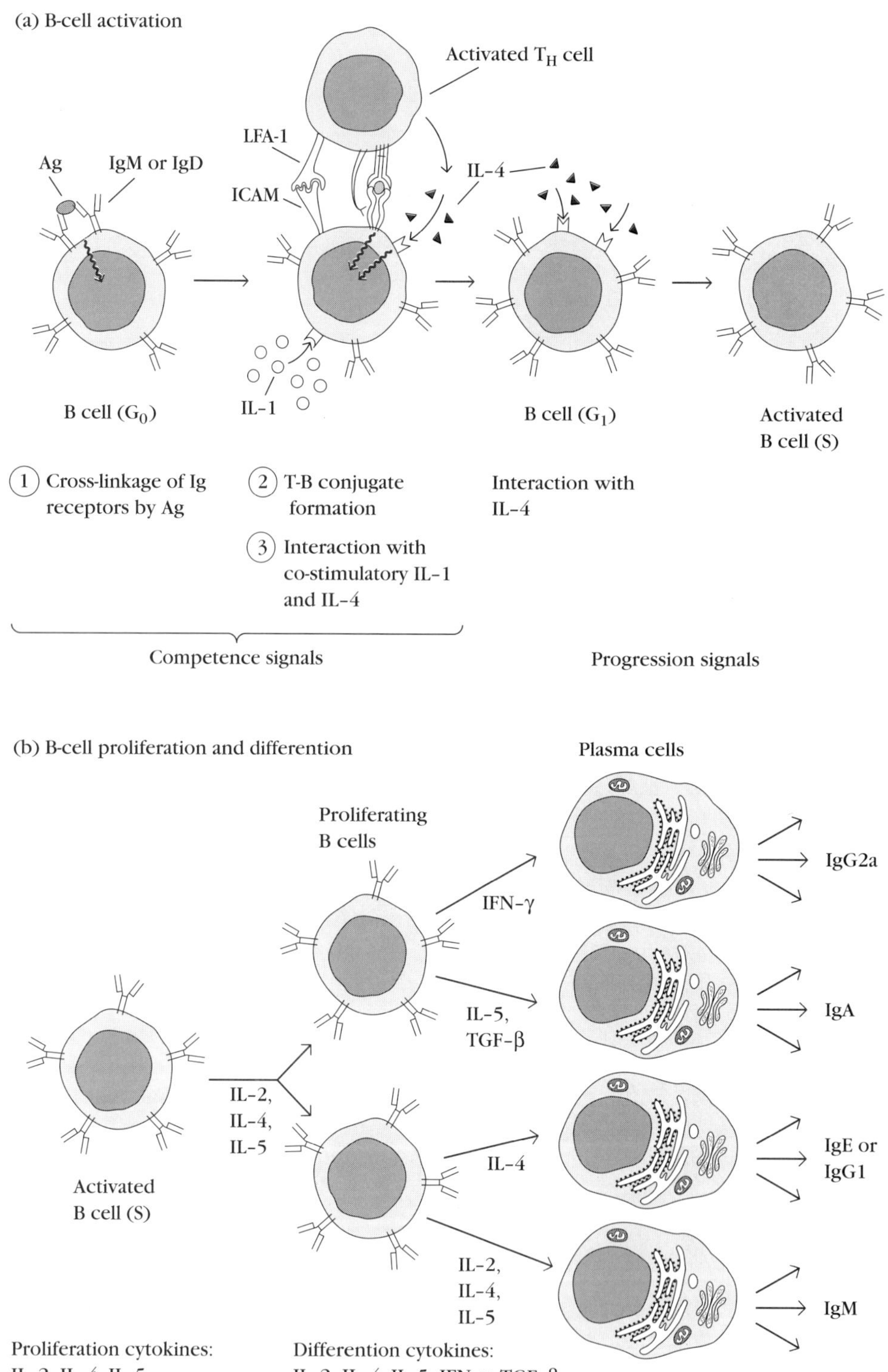

FIGURE 14-12 Overall pathways of B-cell activation, proliferation, and differentiation. (a) Antigen cross-linkage of mIg molecules and interactions with IL-1 and IL-4 generate intracellular signals that ultimately result in gene activation. Not shown is the CD40-CD40L interaction (see Figure 14-11), which also generates a required competence signal. (b) Numerous cytokines participate in B-cell proliferation and differentiation. The indicated cytokine effects have been demonstrated; however, similar or identical effects may be mediated by other cytokines.

the interaction of CD40 on B cells with CD40L on activated T cells, discussed previously, is now known to generate a signal that activates expression of cytokine receptors. In addition, cross-linkage of class II MHC molecules on the membrane of B cells has been shown to induce second messengers similar to those induced following mIg cross-linkage. Thus a membrane signal may be transmitted through the class II MHC molecule as it presents antigen to a T_H cell during conjugate formation. The nature of these signals and the relation of one signaling pathway to another will be an exciting area of research in the coming years.

Cytokine Signals

In most experimental systems, cross-linkage of mIg molecules and interactions involving other membrane molecules cannot support B-cell proliferation and differentiation. Instead, other signals mediated by cytokines also are required. About 12 h following mIg cross-linkage, a B cell enlarges into a blast cell and moves from the resting G_0 stage of the cell cycle into the G_1 stage. At this point the B cell begins to express increased levels of membrane receptors for various cytokines secreted by T_H cells. Binding of these cytokines to their receptors drives the B cell from G_1 into S and then on through mitosis.

A variety of cytokines have been shown to act at various stages of B-cell activation, proliferation, and differentiation (see Figure 14-12). Both redundancy and pleiotropy are exhibited in these effects. Binding of IL-1 and IL-4 to their respective receptors serves as a competence signal driving the resting B cell from G_0 into the G_1 phase of the cell cycle. IL-4 also generates a progression signal driving the B cell from G_1 into S and then on into mitosis. Proliferation of activated B cells then is induced by IL-2, IL-4, or IL-5. Finally, differentiation into plasma cells producing different immunoglobulin isotypes is induced by IL-2, IL-4, IL-5, IFN-γ, or TGF-β.

Studies with the T_H1 and T_H2 subsets, which produce distinct profiles of cytokines (see Table 13-2), have helped to demonstrate the effect of these various cytokines. Both subsets, for example, can induce proliferation and differentiation of activated B cells. However, in general, T_H2 cell lines are more effective helper cells for activating resting B cells than are T_H1 cell lines. This finding probably reflects the important role of IL-4, which is produced only by T_H2 cells, as a competence and progression signal.

T_H1- and T_H2-supported humoral responses also exhibit some consistent differences in the isotype of the antibody secreted. T_H1 cells induce IgG2a, whereas only T_H2 cells induce IgG1 and IgE. This difference is due to the different patterns of cytokines produced by these subsets. Only T_H1 cells produce IFN-γ, which inhibits IgG1 production and enhances Ig2a production. In contrast, only T_H2 cells produce IL-4, which induces IgG1 or IgE. Current evidence supports the view that cytokines promote class switching by inducing rearrangement of the heavy-chain constant region genes (see Figure 8-18). Cytokines also stimulate antibody secretion by plasma cells. For example, secretion of IgM and IgG antibody by cultured plasma cells is inhibited by more than 90% in the presence of monoclonal antibody to IL-6, suggesting that this cytokine stimulates secretion of these isotypes.

Induction of the Humoral Response In Vivo

In vivo the humoral response is generated in defined anatomic sites whose structure places certain restrictions on the kinds of cellular interactions that can take place. When an antigen is introduced into the body, it becomes concentrated in various peripheral lymphoid organs. Blood-borne antigen is filtered by the spleen, whereas tissue antigen is filtered by regional lymph nodes or lymph nodules. This discussion focuses on the generation of the humoral response in lymph nodes. A lymph node is an extremely efficient filter capable of trapping more than 90% of any antigen carried into the node by the afferent lymphatics. As antigen percolates through the cellular architecture of a node, it will encounter one of three types of antigen-presenting cells: interdigitating dendritic cells in the paracortex, macrophages scattered throughout the node, or specialized follicular dendritic cells in the follicles and germinal centers. Antigenic challenge leading to a humoral immune response involves a complex series of events, which take place in distinct microenvironments within a lymph node (Figure 14-13a). Slightly different pathways may operate during a primary and secondary response because much of the tissue antigen is complexed with circulating antibody during a secondary response.

Antigen or antigen-antibody complexes enter the lymph nodes via afferent lymphatics, either alone or associated with antigen-transporting cells (e.g., Langerhans cells or dendritic cells) and macrophages. Lymphocytes enter the lymph nodes either through the afferent lymphatic vessels or from the blood by extravasation through high-endothelial cells in the postcapillary venules. The initial activation of both B

(a)

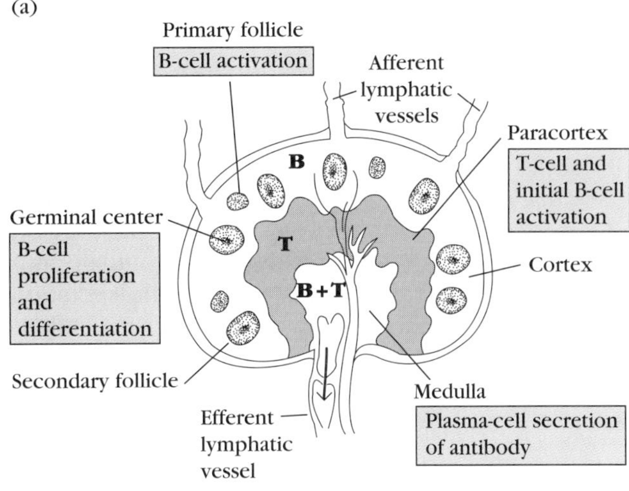

(b)

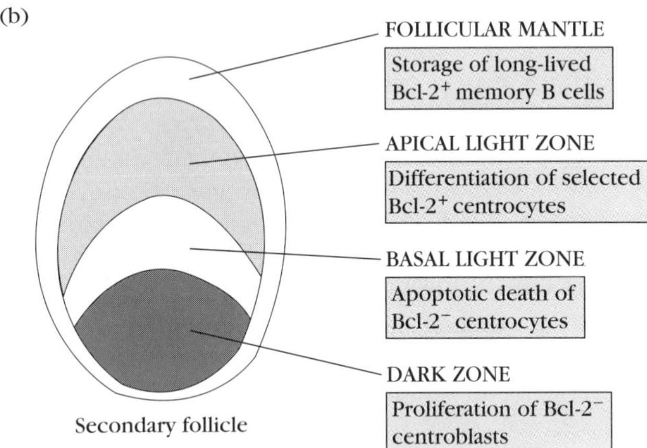

FIGURE 14-13 Schematic diagram of (a) peripheral lymph node and (b) secondary follicle within a node showing anatomic sites at which various steps in B-cell activation, proliferation, and differentiation occur. The cortex is rich in B cells, and the paracortex in T cells; both B and T cells are present in the large numbers in the medulla. A secondary follicle comprises the follicular mantle and germinal center, which contains three distinct zones.

and T cells is thought to take place in the paracortex, a region heavily populated with T cells, macrophages, and interdigitating dendritic cells. The interdigitating dendritic cells in the paracortex express high levels of class II MHC molecules and have long processes that have been shown to contact upwards of 200 T_H cells. Within 1–2 days of antigenic challenge, extensive T_H-cell activation and proliferation occurs within the paracortex. Once activated, the T_H cells interact with B cells, inducing initial B-cell activation. The activated T_H and B cells then migrate to *primary follicles* located in the cortex, which is rich in B cells. As lymphocytes are activated by antigen, the primary follicle develops into a *secondary follicle,* characterized by a central region of proliferating cells called a *germinal center.*

A secondary follicle provides a specialized microenvironment favorable for interactions between B cells, activated T_H cells, and follicular dendritic cells. Follicular dendritic cells have long processes, along which are arrayed Fc receptors that bind antigen-antibody complexes effectively and retain the complexes for months to years on the cell membrane (see Figure 3-14). Because follicular dendritic cells bind antigen that has been complexed to antibody, they are thought to be particularly important in the secondary response, when circulating antibody levels are significant. The periodicity of these immune complexes along the long dendritic processes of these cells is thought to provide an optimum cross-linking matrix favoring B-cell activation. In addition, follicular dendritic cells express ICAM-1 and VCAM-1 adhesion molecules, which would serve to further strengthen the interaction between a follicular dendritic cell and B cell. Follicular dendritic cells release small membrane-derived particles, 0.3–0.4 μm in diameter, which appear to originate from the beaded structures of the dendritic processes. These particles, which are heavily coated with immune complexes, are called *iccosomes,* for immune-complex coating. Especially during a secondary response, iccosomes released from follicular dendritic cells bind to mIg on B cells and are endocytosed by B cells. The endocytosed antigen is then processed and presented together with class II MHC molecules, allowing the B cells to function as effective antigen-presenting cells for activated T_H cells. T-B conjugate formation may then occur, resulting in B-cell activation and proliferation. As cell proliferation continues, the activated B cells (together with some activated T_H cells) migrate towards the center of the secondary follicle, forming the germinal center.

A germinal center, which provides a specialized microenvironment essential for the proliferation and subsequent differentiation of activated B cells, can be divided into several zones (Figure 14-13b). In the *dark zone* of a germinal center, activated B cells (called *centroblasts*) divide into small lymphocytes (called *centrocytes*). Centrocytes have been observed making close contact with the long processes of follicular dendritic cells within germinal centers; thus these cells continue to present antigen to B cells within germinal centers. The majority of centrocytes die by apoptosis within the *basal light zone* of germinal centers and are phagocytosed by an unusual type of macrophage, the *tingible-body macrophage,* that specializes in phagocytosis of lymphoid cells (Figure 14-14). The high rate of cell death by apoptosis is thought

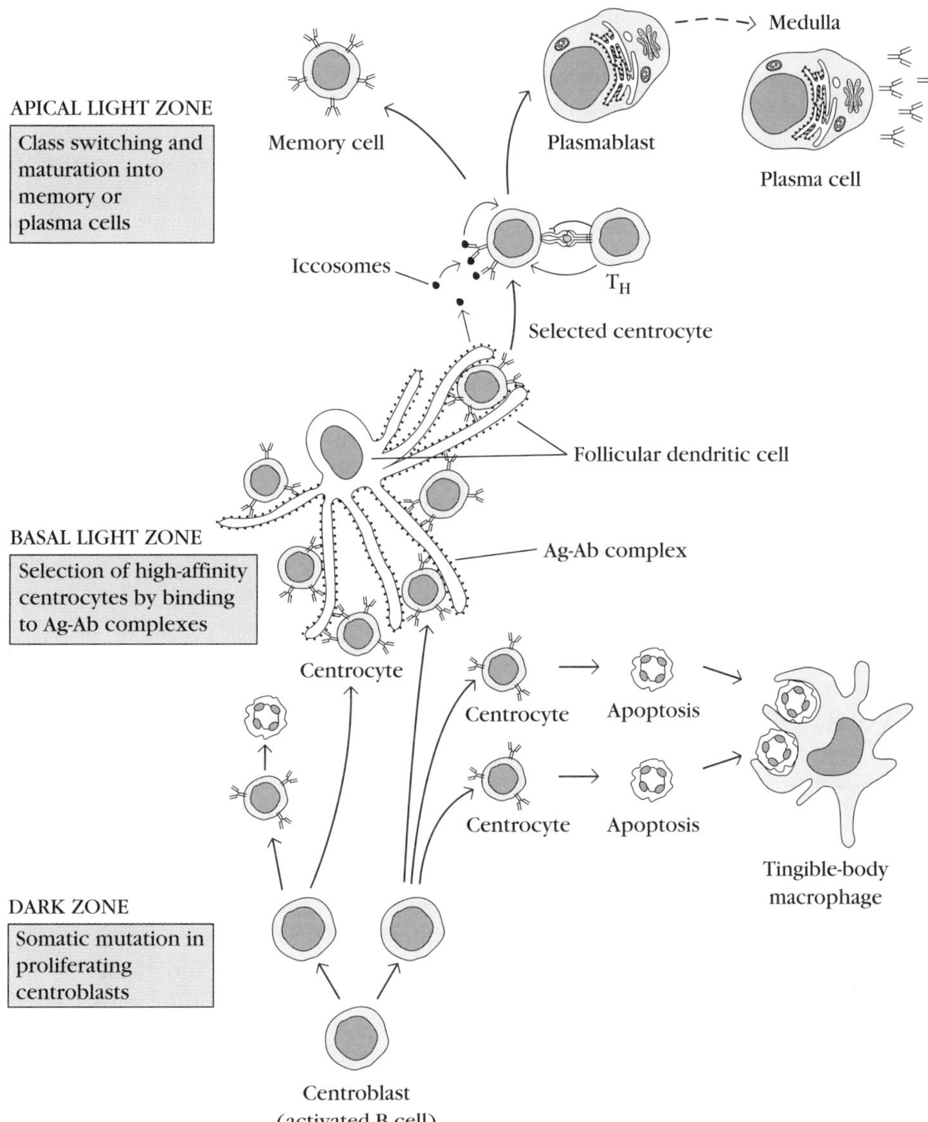

FIGURE 14-14 Schematic diagram of cellular events within secondary follicles of peripheral lymph nodes. Follicular dendritic cells bind antigen-antibody complexes along their long processes. Small B cells (centrocytes) bearing high-affinity membrane immunoglobulin (mIg) are thought to interact with antigen presented on the follicular dendritic cells; unselected centrocytes bearing low-affinity mIg die by apoptosis and the debris is phagocytosed by tingible-body macrophages. Selected centrocytes, which may undergo class switching, then mature into memory B cells or plasmablasts; the latter migrate to the medulla where they develop into plasma cells.

to be a means of eliminating those B cells that fail to recognize antigen presented by follicular dendritic cells.

Some evidence suggests that the proto-oncogene *bcl-2* may play a role in this process by suppressing apoptosis. The follicular mantle, for example, contains long-lived recirculating memory B cells, which have been shown to express high levels of Bcl-2 and therefore are protected from programmed cell death. In contrast, the majority of centroblasts and centrocytes within a germinal center are short lived and fail to express Bcl-2. Some have proposed that within a germinal center B cells expressing mIg molecules with high affinity for the antigen present on the follicular dendritic cells in some way receive a signal that induces production of Bcl-2, thereby protecting these B cells from apoptotic death. B cells lacking such high-affinity antigen-binding receptors thus would not express Bcl-2 and would undergo apoptosis.

The Bcl-2^+ centrocytes that survive selection undergo differentiation within the *apical light zone,* forming two types of progeny: small memory B cells and large plasmablasts. The plasmablasts leave the germinal center and migrate to the medulla of the node, where they develop into plasma cells and begin to secrete antibody molecules. Some memory B cells remain in the *follicular mantle,* while others leave the lymph node through the efferent lymphatic vessel and recirculate to other parts of the body.

Three important processes—affinity maturation, isotype switching, and formation of memory B cells—occur in the different zones of a germinal center (see Figure 14-14). These are discussed in the remainder of this chapter.

TABLE 14-4 EFFECT OF IMMUNIZING DOSE AND TIME ON AVERAGE AFFINITY OF INDUCED ANTI-DNP ANTIBODIES IN RABBITS

Group	DNP-BGG immunizing dose (mg per animal)	*K* of anti-DNP antibodies* (L/mol × 10^6)		
		2 weeks	5 weeks	8 weeks
I	5	0.86	14	120
II	250	0.18	0.13	0.15

* Values are averages for five animals per group and are based on binding of DNP-L-lysine with serum antibody samples obtained at indicated times after immunization.

SOURCE: Adapted from H. N. Eisen and G. W. Siskind, 1964, *Biochemistry* **3**:966.

Affinity Maturation

In the course of a humoral immune response, the average affinity of the antibodies produced in response to an antigen increases as much as 100- to 10,000-fold. This *affinity maturation* is the result of two processes: *somatic hypermutation* and *antigen selection of high-affinity clones.*

As discussed in Chapter 8, somatic mutation acts on the V, D, and J gene segments in rearranged immunoglobulin genes, introducing point mutations, deletions, and insertions. The majority of mutations occur within the three complementarity-determining regions (CDRs). It is not known whether targeting to CDRs occurs because the enzymes involved in somatic mutation preferentially recognize the CDRs or whether mutations within the CDRs are selected over other mutations because of their impact on antigen-binding affinity. Because somatic mutation is random, it potentially can generate antibodies of higher affinity, lower affinity, or the same affinity. Contact with antigen, however, selects for those clones bearing higher-affinity antibodies. Somatic mutation can first be detected late in the primary response, and it increases after a secondary contact with antigen (see Figure 8-17). The molecular basis of somatic mutation remains to be determined. The finding that somatic mutations are found predominantly in secondary antibodies and in isotypes resulting from class switching, may indicate that the mutation process is influenced by events in B-cell differentiation. Some workers have suggested that the observed increase in somatic mutation during a secondary response may result from an error-prone DNA-repair process, which would be heightened during the additional cell divisions required to generate a secondary response. The role of somatic mutation in affinity maturation has been assessed by comparing the H- and L-chain mRNA sequences of antigen-specific B-cell hybridomas at various times after antigen exposure. In one study, the secondary antibody differed from the primary antibody by 13 replacement mutations and exhibited a 100-fold higher affinity for antigen.

The role played by antigen in the selection of high-affinity B-cell clones was clarified in an early experiment by H. N. Eisen and G. W. Siskind, who immunized two groups of rabbits with two different doses of DNP-BGG. Group I was immunized with 5 mg, and group II with 250 mg of DNP-BGG. The affinity of the serum anti-DNP antibodies produced in response to the antigen was then measured at 2 weeks, 5 weeks, and 8 weeks following immunization. As the data in Table 14-4 show, the average affinity of the group I anti-DNP antibodies increased about 140-fold from 2 weeks to 8 weeks, whereas the affinity of the group II antibodies was initially lower and did not increase.

The affinity of antibody secreted by differentiated plasma cells corresponds to that of the membrane-bound antibody on the B cell from which they derive. Therefore, the nearly fivefold lower average affinity of the group II antibodies at 2 weeks suggests that at high immunizing doses, B cells expressing both high-affinity and low-affinity membrane antibody are activated and clonally expanded. In contrast, when the immunizing dose is low, only B cells with high-affinity membrane antibody are activated and clonally expanded (Figure 14-15). As antigen levels decline over time following immunization, competition for the available antigen increases. Now only those B cells possessing high-affinity membrane antibody are able to bind

(a) Low immunizing dose

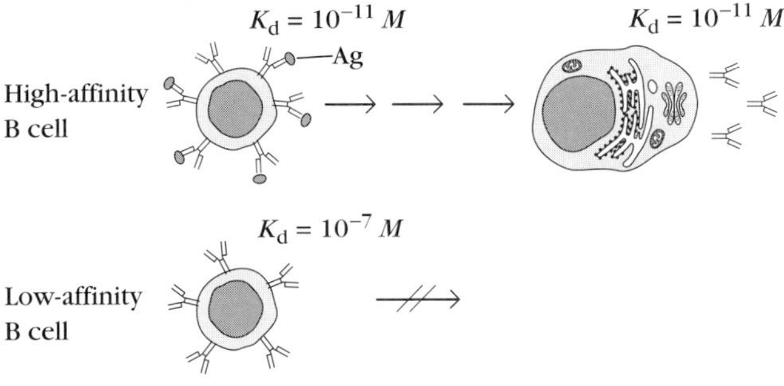

(b) High immunizing dose

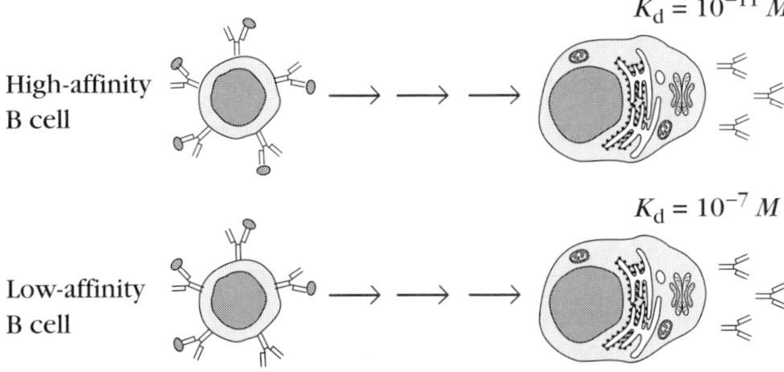

FIGURE 14-15 The immunizing dose determines whether B cells bearing high-affinity membrane antibody (purple) or low-affinity antibody are selected for activation. The average affinity of the antibodies secreted by plasma cells derived from the B cells reflects this selection process.

sufficient antigen to be activated and clonally expanded. Thus, with time, the average affinity of the secreted antibody increases. In the experimental system of Eisen and Siskind, antigen concentration was never limited in group II; therefore, low-affinity B cells never had to compete with the high-affinity cells for available antigen, and the response never showed an increase in antibody affinity.

As described already, when activated B cells (centroblasts) first migrate into the dark zone of a germinal center, they begin to proliferate. It is at this point that somatic hypermutation is thought to occur (see Figure 14-15). The centroblasts give rise to a large population of centrocytes that cease dividing. These cells are thought to be selected for their ability to bind to antigen retained on follicular dendritic cells by the mechanism discussed previously. Only high-affinity cells are selected, and the majority of centrocytes (~90%), which bear low-affinity membrane antibodies, undergo programmed cell death. As a result, the antibodies expressed by memory B cells and plasma cells exhibit an increase in average affinity as a humoral response progresses.

Class Switching

In the primary humoral response to thymus-dependent antigens, the first antibody to be secreted is IgM, followed by IgG later in the response. With secondary antigen challenge very little IgM is produced and instead IgG, IgA, or IgE appear. As noted already, T_H-cell cytokines play an important role in regulating class switching. As discussed in Chapter 8, class switching involves rearrangements of C gene segments in immunoglobulin heavy-chain genes. The data shown in Figure 8-18 suggest that IL-4–mediated class switching in B cells is a sequential process going from C_μ to $C_\gamma 1$ to C_ε. The first switch results in replacement of IgM expression with IgG1 expression; the second switch, in loss of IgG1 and appearance of IgE. Thus activation of IgG1-positive memory B cells might give rise to IgE-secreting plasma cells. Other T_H-cell cytokines also have been implicated in class switching. For example, IFN-γ induces LPS-activated B cells to secrete IgG2a, and TGF-β and IL-5 have been associated with IgA secretion.

Generation of Memory B Cells

A secondary humoral response is dependent on a population of memory B cells. Characterization of the memory B-cell population is dependent on the identification of unique cell-membrane molecules to distinguish them from naive B cells. Except for membrane-bound immunoglobulins, few membrane molecules have been identified that distinguish naive B cells from memory B cells. While naive B cells only express IgM and IgD, memory B cells express additional isotypes, including IgG, IgA, and IgE. In addition, the level of IgD often appears to be reduced on memory B cells. Another membrane marker that appears to distinguish naive and memory B cells is an antigen designated J11d. Naive B cells express high levels of J11d, whereas memory B cells express little or no J11d. In addition, memory B cells express higher levels of various adhesion molecules (e.g., ICAM-1) than do naive B cells. Some characteristics of naive and memory B cells are compared in Table 14-5.

Memory B cells are generated from centrocytes in the apical light zone of germinal centers. Because memory B cells arise from cells that have undergone affinity maturation, they express high-affinity membrane antibody, enabling them to be activated by lower levels of antigen than virgin B cells. For reasons that are not understood, some antigens induce a long-lasting memory response, whereas others do not. This difference may result from inherent variation in the life span of memory B cells induced by different antigens.

TABLE 14-5 COMPARISON OF NAIVE AND MEMORY B CELLS

Properties	Naive B cell	Memory B cell
Membrane markers		
Immunoglobulin	IgM, IgD	IgM, IgD(?), IgG, IgA, IgE
Jlld	High	Low
Complement receptor	Low	High
Anatomic location	Spleen	Bone marrow, lymph node, spleen
Life span	Short-lived	May be long-lived
Recirculation	Yes	Yes
Receptor affinity	Lower average affinity	Higher average affinity due to affinity maturation*
Adhesion molecules	Low ICAM-1	High ICAM-1

*Affinity maturation results from somatic mutation during proliferation of centroblasts and subsequent antigen selection of centrocytes bearing high-affinity mIg.

In some cases, perhaps, memory B-cell levels may be maintained by continuous low-level activation. Some have suggested that antigen trapped by follicular dendritic cells may continue to activate memory B cells for months to years, thus maintaining memory-cell numbers regardless of whether the cells have a long life span or not.

Little is known about the process of memory-cell formation and three models have been proposed: The most widespread model is that memory B cells and plasma cells develop from "unequal" division of a common precursor cell. A second model is that cytokines produced from T cells or various accessory cells may influence the differentiation of a common precursor cell into a memory cell or a plasma cell. A third model, which is gaining support, is that memory cells and plasma cells arise from different lineages, each of which clonally expands following primary antigen exposure. Support for this last model comes from analysis of the primary and secondary antibodies induced by certain antigens. Phosphorylcholine, for example, induces antibodies characterized by a single idiotype in the primary response, whereas the antibodies produced in the secondary response completely lack this idiotype. This finding suggests that the memory cells generated in the primary response arose from a different lineage than did the plasma cells.

SUMMARY

1. Primary and secondary humoral responses show different kinetics of antibody formation. The primary response is characterized by a long lag period, a logarithmic rise in antibody formation, a short plateau, and then a relatively rapid decline. IgM is the first antibody class to be secreted, followed by IgG later in the primary response. The secondary response has a shorter lag period, a more rapid logarithmic phase, a longer plateau, and a slower decline than the primary response. Little IgM is produced in the secondary response, which is characterized by production of IgG or other isotypes.

2. Early adoptive-transfer experiments revealed that both B cells and T cells are required to generate a humoral immune response. The B cell was shown to be the antibody-producing cell, and the T cell was shown to function as a necessary helper cell. In vitro experiments in which adherent macrophages and nonadherent lymphocytes were separated demonstrated that macrophages also are required participants in induction of humoral immunity.

3. Studies of the humoral response to hapten-carrier conjugates revealed that both B cells and T_H cells recognize epitopes on the same conjugate molecule. The hapten serves as the immunodominant B-cell epitope, while carrier epitopes are recognized by T_H cells. These T-cell epitopes tend to be internal peptides that are exposed during antigen processing in the B cell and are presented together with class II MHC molecules on the B-cell membrane.

4. The activation, proliferation, and differentiation of B cells involves several sequential processes, starting with the uptake, processing, and presentation of antigen plus class II MHC molecules by naive B cells. Interaction of an activated antigen-specific T_H cell with an antigen-primed B cell leads to formation of a specific T-B conjugate, which exhibits close membrane interaction. The T_H cells in these conjugates undergo reorganization of the Golgi apparatus and microtubular-organizing center as well as clustering of several membrane proteins near the junction of the two cells. This redistribution of T_H-cell components may aid in the directional release of cytokines from the T_H cell toward the interacting B cell. Conjugate formation also induces expression of CD40L on the T-cell membrane; interaction of CD40L with CD40 on the B-cell membrane mediates a contact-dependent help signal, which is necessary for B-cell activation.

5. Signals generated by membrane events and cytokines are transduced into the B cell, ultimately leading to changes in gene expression. Relatively little is known about membrane-signaling events in B-cell activation, proliferation, and differentiation, but the roles of several cytokines have been demonstrated. Both IL-1 and IL-4 function as activation signals; IL-4 and numerous other T_H-cell lymphokines function as proliferation and differentiation signals (e.g., by inducing secretion of pentameric IgM and class switching to other isotypes).

6. Generation of the humoral response to antigens in vivo occurs primarily in regional lymph nodes. Intense proliferation of activated B cells (centroblasts) takes place in the dark zone of germinal centers in secondary follicles and may be accompanied by somatic mutation. About 90% of the resulting centrocytes undergo death by apoptosis within the basal light zone. The remainder, which express mIg with high affinity for antigen, are protected by interacting with antigen on follicular dendritic cells. Selected centrocytes undergo class switching and differentiation within the apical light zone, generating memory B cells and plasmablasts. The latter migrate to the medulla and develop into antibody-secreting plasma cells.

7. As the humoral immune response proceeds, the average affinity of the induced serum antibodies increases. Such affinity maturation results from somatic mutation and antigen selection of high-affinity cells within a lymph node. Affinity maturation and class switching, which results in expression of antibodies with different isotypes, lead to more effective elimination of pathogens.

References

ALES-MARTINEZ, J. E., E. CUENDE, C. MARTINEZ et al. 1991. Signalling in B cells. *Immunol. Today* **12**:201.

ARMITAGE, R. J., W. C. FANSLOW, L. STROCKBINE et al. 1992. Molecular and biological characterization of a murine ligand for CD40. *Nature* **357**:80.

CLARK, E. A., and P. J. L. LANE. 1991. Regulation of human B-cell activation and adhesion. *Annu. Rev. Immunol.* **9**:97.

FINKELMAN, F. D., J. HOLMES, I. M. KATONA et al. 1990. Lymphokine control of in vivo immunoglobulin isotype selection. *Annu. Rev. Immunol.* **8**:303.

GRAY, D. 1993. Immunological memory. *Annu. Rev. Immunol.* **11**:49.

HODGKIN, P. D., and M. R. KEHRY. 1993. B cell activation by T cells—the "TICCL" model. *The Immunologist* **1**:5.

KLINMAN, N. R., and P. J. LINTON. 1990. The generation of B-cell memory: a working hypothesis. *Curr. Top. Microbiol. Immunol.* **159**:19.

KUPFER, A., and S. J. SINGER. 1991. The specific interaction of helper T cells and antigen-presenting B cells. IV. Membrane and cytoskeleton reorganizations in the bound T cell as a function of antigen dose. *J. Exp. Med.* **170**:1697.

KUPFER, A., S. J. SINGER, C. A. JANEWAY, and S. L. SWAIN. 1987. Coclustering of CD4 (L3T4) molecule with the T-cell receptor is induced by specific direct interaction of helper T cells and antigen-presenting cells. *Proc. Nat'l. Acad. Sci. USA* **84**:5888.

NOELLE, R. J., J. DAUM, W. C. BARTLETT et al. 1991. Cognate interactions between helper T cells and B cells. V. Reconstitution of T helper cell function using purified plasma membranes from activated T_H1 and T_H2 T helper cells and lymphokines. *J. Immunol.* **146**:1118.

PARKER, D. C. 1993. T cell-dependent B cell activation. *Annu. Rev. Immunol.* **11**:331.

RETH, M., J. HOMBACH, J. WIENANDS et al. 1991. The B-cell antigen receptor complex. *Immunol. Today* **12**:196.

ROUSSET, F., E. BARCIA, and J. BANCHEREAU. 1991. Cytokine-induced proliferation and immunoglobulin production of human B lymphocytes triggered through their CD40 antigen. *J. Exp. Med.* **173**:705.

SNAPPER, C. M., and J. J. MOND. 1993. Towards a comprehensive view of immunoglobulin class switching. *Immunol. Today* **14**:15.

SZAKAL, A. K., M. H. KOSCO, and J. G. TEW. 1989. Microanatomy of lymphoid tissue during humoral immune responses: structure-function relationships. *Annu. Rev. Immunol.* **7**:91.

VITETTA, E. S., M. T. BERTON, C. BURGER et al. 1991. Memory B and T cells. *Annu. Rev. Immunol.* **9**:193.

VITETTA, E. S., R. FERNANDEZ-BOTRAN, C. D. MYERS, and V. M. SANDERS. 1989. Cellular interactions in the humoral immune response. *Adv. Immunol.* **45**:1.

Study Questions

1. Indicate whether each of the following statements is true or false. If you believe a statement is false, explain why.
   a. The indirect hemolytic plaque assay detects only IgG-secreting plasma cells.

b. The B cell serves as an antigen-presenting cell to the T_H cell.
c. IL-4 decreases IgE production by plasma cells.
d. Immunoglobulin class switching from IgM to IgE usually is mediated by DNA rearrangements with loss of intervening DNA.
e. Immunization with a hapten-carrier conjugate results in production of antibodies to both hapten and carrier epitopes.
f. All the antibodies secreted by a single plasma cell have the same idiotype and isotype.

2. Four mice are immunized with antigen under the conditions listed below (a–d). In each case, indicate whether the induced serum antibodies will be heterogeneous or relatively homogeneous; have high affinity or low affinity; and be largely IgM or IgG.
   a. A primary response to a low antigen dose.
   b. A secondary response to a low antigen dose.
   c. A primary response to a high antigen dose.
   d. A secondary response to a high antigen dose.

3. Three groups of mice were immunized according to the schedule shown in the table above. Spleen cells were isolated from the immunized mice, and the number of plaque-forming cells were determined; the direct and indirect PFC for each group are listed in the table.

Immunization schedule	Direct PFC/10^6 spleen cells	Indirect PFC/10^6 spleen cells
(A) 1° DNP-BSA	310	343
(B) 1° DNP-BSA 2° DNP-BSA	62	4060
(C) 1° DNP-BSA 2° DNP-BGG	366	386

a. Which assays are used to measure a primary (1°) and secondary (2°) plaque-forming response? Describe each assay.
b. Calculate the number of IgM-secreting and IgG-secreting plasma cells/10^6 spleen cells for each group of mice.
c. Why is the indirect PFC so much higher than the direct PFC for group B but not for group A or C?

4. Describe the primary signals required to activate naive B cells. What additional signals, if any, are needed to stimulate proliferation and differentiation of activated B cells?

15

CELL-MEDIATED IMMUNITY

The cell-mediated branch of the immune system confers immunity primarily through the generation of various effector immune cells. Although antibody sometimes is involved, it plays only a secondary role. Both antigen-specific and nonspecific cells contribute to the cell-mediated immune response. Specific cells include $CD4^+$ T-lymphocyte subsets and $CD8^+$ T lymphocytes; nonspecific cells include macrophages, neutrophils, eosinophils, and natural killer cells. The activity of both the specific and nonspecific component is dependent on high localized concentrations of various cytokines. Unlike the humoral branch of the immune system, which serves mainly to eliminate extracellular bacteria and bacterial products, the cell-mediated branch is responsible for the clearance of intracellular pathogens, virus-infected cells, tumor cells, and foreign grafts. The system is adapted to recognizing altered self-cells and eliminating them from the body.

The importance of cell-mediated immunity becomes evident when the system is defective. Children with DiGeorge syndrome, who are born without a thymus and therefore lack the T-cell component of the cell-mediated immune system, generally are able to cope with infections of extracellular bacteria, but they cannot effectively eliminate intracellular pathogens. Their lack of functional cell-mediated immunity results in repeated infections with viruses, intracellular bacteria, and fungi. The severity of the cell-mediated immunodeficiency in these children is such that even attenuated vaccines, capable of only limited growth in normal individuals, can produce life-threatening infections.

Cell-mediated immune responses can be divided into two major categories involving different effector populations. One group involves effector cells having direct cytotoxic activity. The second group involves a subpopulation of effector $CD4^+$ cells that mediate delayed-type hypersensitivity reactions. This chapter examines the cells and effector mechanisms involved in each type of cell-mediated immune response.

Direct Cytotoxic Response

One way the immune system eliminates foreign cells and altered self-cells is to mount a cytotoxic reaction that results in lysis of target cells. The various cell-mediated cytotoxic effector mechanisms can be subdivided into two general categories: (1) cytotoxicity involving antigen-specific cytotoxic T lymphocytes (CTLs) and (2) cytotoxicity involving nonspecific cells, such as natural killer (NK) cells and macrophages. The target cells to which these effector mechanisms are directed include allogeneic cells, malignant cells, virus-infected cells, and chemically conjugated cells.

CTL-Mediated Cytotoxicity

Immune activation of T cytotoxic (T_C) cells generates a population of effector cells with lytic capability called cytotoxic T lymphocytes, or CTLs. These effector cells have important roles in the recognition and elimination of altered self-cells, including virus-infected cells and malignant cells, and in graft-rejection reactions. In general, CTLs are $CD8^+$ and are therefore class I MHC restricted, although in rare instances $CD4^+$ class II–restricted T cells have been shown to function as CTLs. Since virtually all nucleated cells in the body express class I MHC molecules, CTLs can recognize and eliminate almost any altered body cell.

The CTL-mediated immune response can be divided into two phases, reflecting different aspects of the cytotoxic T-cell response. The first phase involves the activation and differentiation of T_C cells into functional effector CTLs. In the second phase, CTLs recognize antigen–class I MHC complexes on specific target cells, initiating a sequence of events that culminates in target-cell destruction.

Phase I: Activation and Differentiation of CTL Precursors

Resting T_C cells are incapable of killing target cells and are therefore referred to as *CTL precursors (CTL-Ps)* to denote their functionally immature state. Only after a CTL-P has been activated will the cell differentiate into a functional CTL possessing cytotoxic activity. Generation of CTLs from CTL-Ps appears to require several signals: one signal is provided when the T-cell receptor and CD8 on the CTL-P interact with an antigenic peptide–class I MHC complex on the membrane of a target cell; a second signal is usually provided by cytokines produced by activated $CD4^+$ T_H cells. IL-2 is the principal cytokine required for the differentiation of CTL-Ps into effector CTLs, but a number of other cytokines (e.g., IL-4, IL-6, and IFN-γ) have also been shown to play a role in this process.

Unactivated CTL-Ps do not express IL-2 receptors, do not proliferate, and do not display cytotoxic activity (Figure 15-1). Antigen activation induces a CTL-P to increase its expression of the IL-2 receptor. IL-2 produced by proliferating T_H cells binds to the IL-2 receptors on the CTL-P, inducing it to proliferate and differentiate into effector CTLs. The fact that the IL-2 receptor is not expressed until after a CTL-P has been activated by antigen plus a class I MHC molecule ensures that only antigen-specific CTL-Ps are clonally expanded by IL-2 and acquire cytotoxicity. After antigen activation, both T_H cells and CTLs are dependent on IL-2 for their proliferation. In IL-2 knock-out mice, for example, the absence of IL-2 has been shown to abolish CTL-mediated cytotoxicity. Following antigen clearance, the levels of IL-2 decline. This decline in IL-2 induces activated T_H cells and CTLs to undergo programmed cell death by apoptosis, ensuring that the immune response is rapidly terminated and lessening the likelihood of nonspecific tissue damage from the inflammatory response.

Activated CTL-Ps have been shown to secrete a number of cytokines including IL-4, IL-6, IFN-γ, TNF-β, and, to a lesser degree, IL-2. However, the levels of these cytokines are not sufficient to support the differentiation of CTL-Ps into functional CTLs. Thus, in general, cytokine secretion by activated $CD4^+$ T_H cells is necessary for generation of the full CTL effector function; this constraint may not apply to memory T_C cells, which are more readily activated. The role of the $CD4^+$ T_H cell in the activation of the CTL-P is not completely understood. It is unlikely that the two cells interact directly. Some have suggested that activation of both T_H and CTL-P populations occurs at sites of organized lymphoid tissue such as regional lymph nodes. In a primary response to a virus, for example, naive T cells are unable to respond to the virus except in organized lymphoid tissues. Within the organized lymphoid

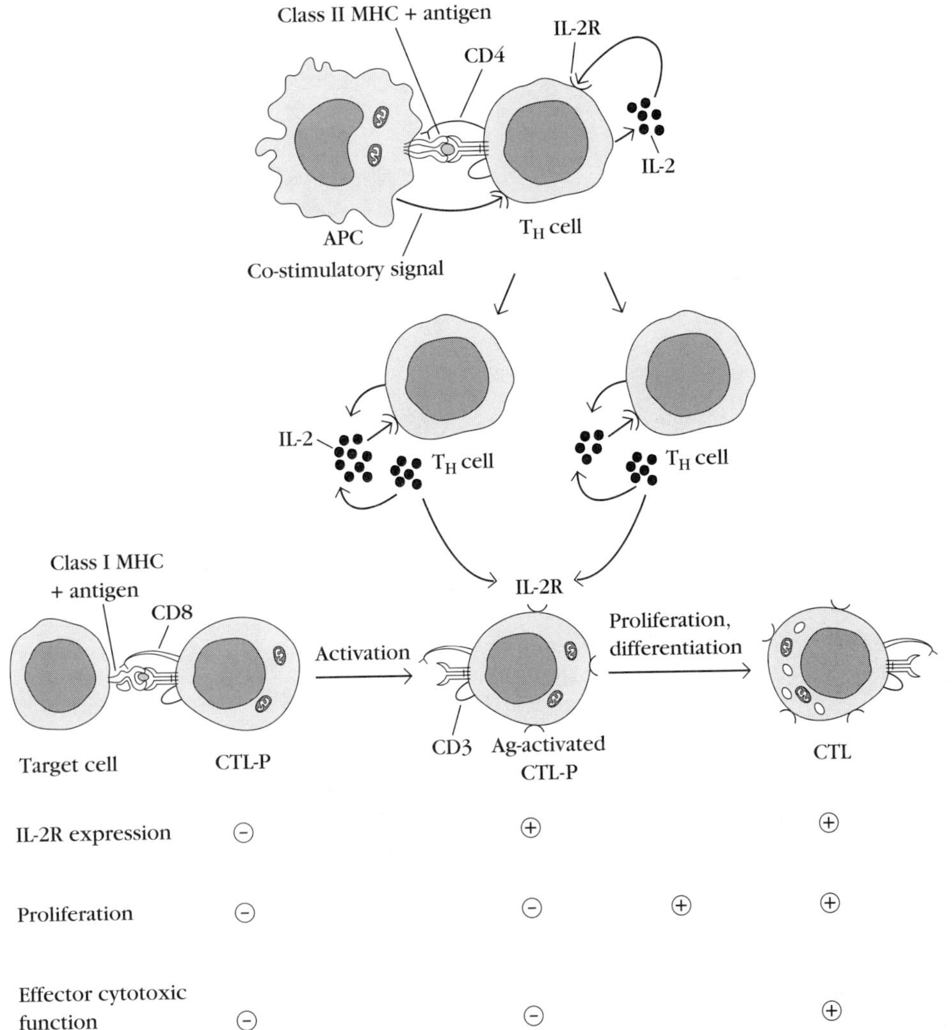

FIGURE 15-1 Activation and differentiation of CTL precursors (CTL-Ps) into effector CTLs. Antigen-mediated activation and subsequent proliferation of T_H cells leads to localized increases in IL-2. Upon interaction with antigen–class I MHC complexes on appropriate target cells, CTL-Ps begin to express IL-2 receptors (IL-2R). In the presence of IL-2 secreted by activated T_H cells, activated CTL-Ps proliferate and differentiate into CTLs. In the subsequent effector phase, CTLs destroy specific target cells.

tissues, $CD4^+$ T_H cells and $CD8^+$ CTL-Ps may interact with common antigen-presenting cells that have internalized and processed the virus in the endocytic pathway and also have been infected by the virus. Such cells would present antigenic viral peptides associated with both class I and class II MHC molecules and thus would be recognized by both $CD4^+$ and $CD8^+$ T cells. Another possibility is that organized lymphoid tissue forms an anatomic niche rich in cytokines, providing an ideal milieu for CTL-P activation.

Various experimental results indicate that the requirement for $CD4^+$ T_H cells in CTL-P activation is not absolute. For example, depletion of $CD4^+$ T_H cells with monoclonal anti-CD4 produces variable effects (ranging from slight to substantial) on the magnitude of the CTL response in mice. In some experimental systems, interaction of accessory membrane molecules has been shown to provide a sufficient co-stimulatory signal to permit proliferation and differentiation of antigen-activated CTL-Ps in the absence of cytokines secreted by $CD4^+$ T_H cells. For example, when CTL-Ps are incubated with melanoma cells in vitro, antigen recognition occurs, but in the absence of a co-stimulatory signal, the CTL-Ps do not proliferate and differentiate. However, when melanoma cells transfected with the gene encoding the cell-surface ligand B7 are

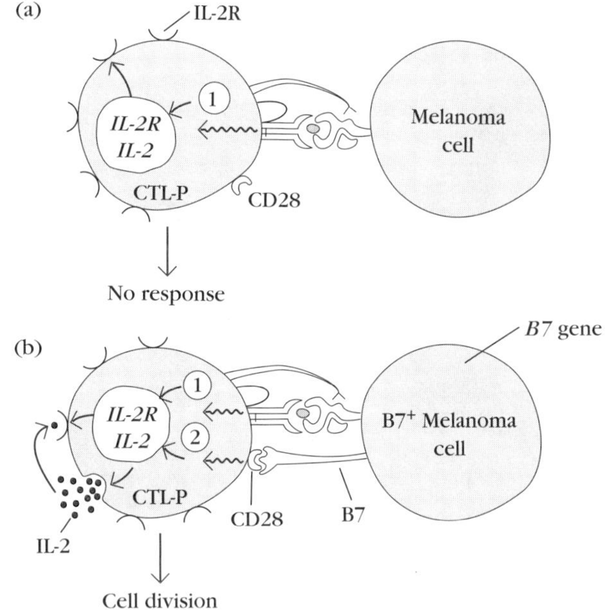

FIGURE 15-2 Demonstration of alternative co-stimulatory signal in generation of CTL activity. (a) Incubation of CTL-Ps with melanoma cells in vitro generates an activating signal (1) that induces transcription of the gene encoding the IL-2 receptor *(IL-2R)*. In the absence of IL-2, however, no co-stimulatory signal is produced and the CTL-Ps fail to proliferate and differentiate. (b) When melanoma cells transfected with the gene encoding B7, a cell-surface ligand, are incubated with CTL-Ps, CTL activity is generated. Interaction of CD28 and B7 is thought to produce a co-stimulatory signal (2) that induces transcription of the *IL-2* gene. Autostimulation by IL-2 then leads to the proliferation and differentiation of the CTL-Ps into CTLs.

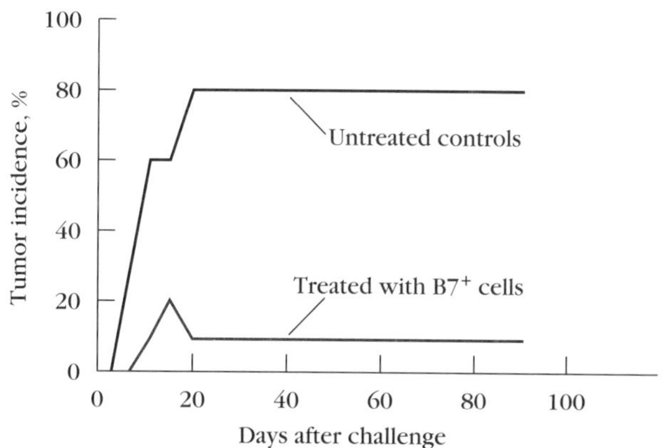

FIGURE 15-3 Protective effect of vaccination with B7$^+$ melanoma cells. Normal mice were treated with melanoma cells that had been transfected with the *B7* gene. Subsequently, treated mice and untreated controls were challenged with unaltered malignant melanoma cells. Only about 11% of the treated mice developed tumors, whereas 80% of the controls did. [Adapted from S. Townsend and J. Allison, 1993, *Science* **259**:368.]

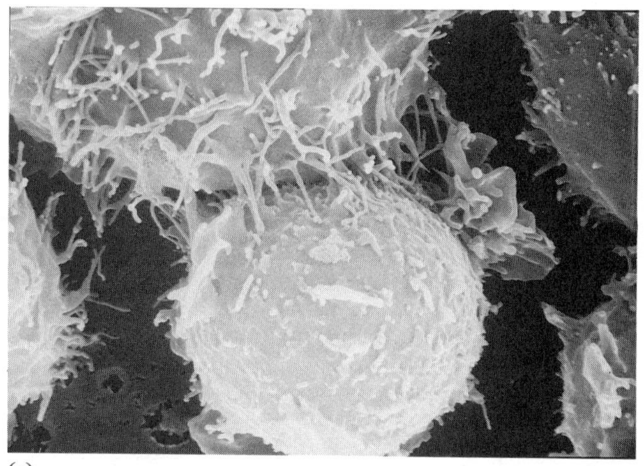
(a)

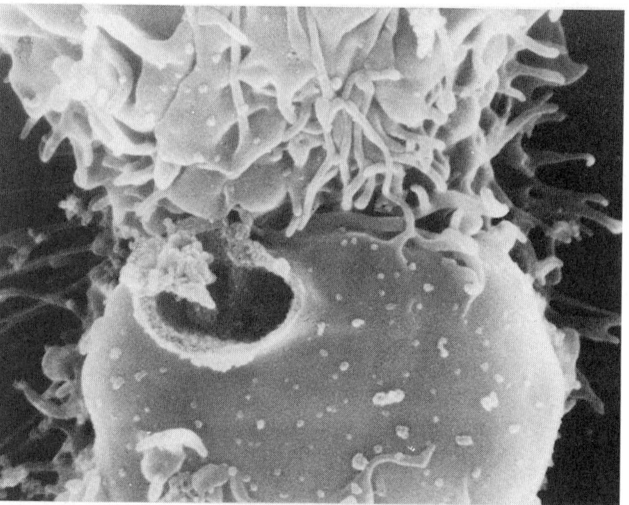
(b)

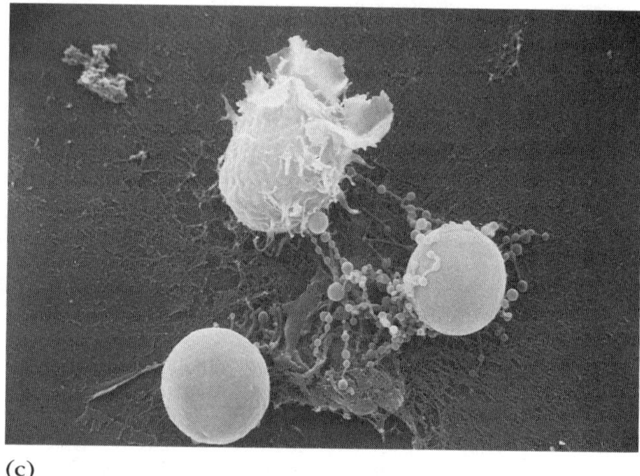
(c)

FIGURE 15-4 Scanning electron micrographs of tumor-cell destruction by a CTL. (a) A CTL *(top left)* makes contact with a smaller tumor cell. (b) Membrane damage to the tumor cell results in a visible cavity and allows an influx of water, resulting in cell swelling. (c) Lysis of the tumor cell has occurred leaving only cell debris and the nucleus *(right)*. [From J. D. E. Young and Z. A. Cohn, 1988, *Sci. Am.* **258**(Jan.):38.]

incubated with CTL-Ps, functional CTLs are generated (Figure 15-2). It is thought that interaction of B7 with CD28 on the CTL-Ps serves as a strong co-stimulatory signal that induces the CTL-Ps to express sufficient IL-2 to autostimulate their own proliferation and differentiation. The resulting CTLs can then kill melanoma cells without requiring a further co-stimulatory B7-CD28 signal.

Experiments conducted by several research groups suggest that B7-transfected tumor cells might be used to induce a CTL response in vivo. For instance, when P. Linsley, L. Chen, and their colleagues injected melanoma-bearing mice with $B7^+$ melanoma cells, the melanomas completely regressed in more than 40% of the mice. S. Townsend and J. Allison used a similar approach to vaccinate mice against malignant melanoma. Normal mice were first immunized with transfected $B7^+$ melanoma cells and then later challenged with unaltered malignant melanoma cells. The "vaccine" was found to protect a high percentage of the mice (Figure 15-3). It is hoped that a similar vaccine might prevent metastasis after surgical removal of a primary melanoma in human patients.

Phase 2: CTL-Mediated Destruction of Target Cells

The effector phase of a CTL-mediated response involves a carefully orchestrated sequence of events culminating in target-cell lysis by CTLs (Figure 15-4). Long-term cultures of CTL clones have been used to identify many of the membrane molecules and membrane events involved in CTL-mediated target-cell destruction. These clones are produced by removing lymphocytes from immunized mice and culturing them with the original immunizing target cells; the differentiated CTLs are cloned in microwell cultures at limiting dilutions in the presence of high concentrations of IL-2. These cloned CTL lines provide immunologists with large numbers of homogeneous T cells with identical receptor specificity for a given target cell.

PERFORIN-MEDIATED TARGET-CELL LYSIS. The primary events in CTL-mediated cytotoxicity are conjugate formation, membrane attack, CTL dissociation, and target-cell destruction (Figure 15-5). When

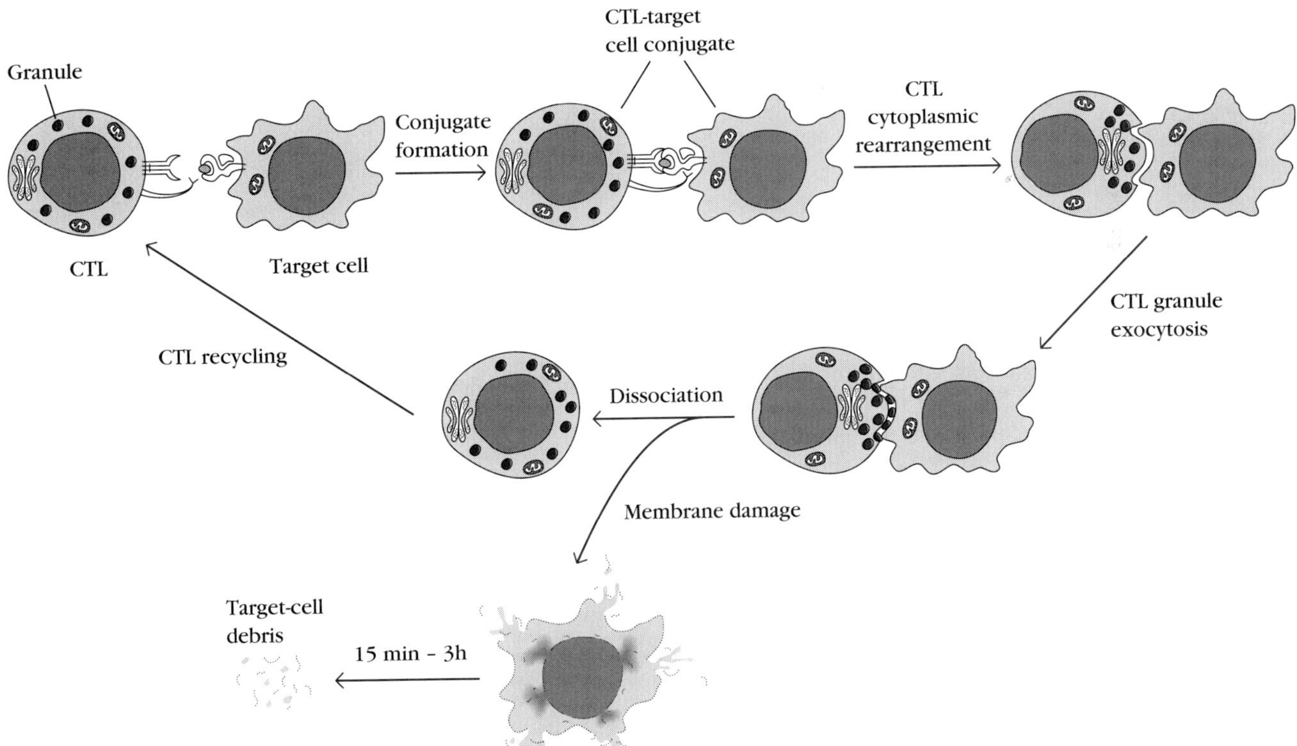

FIGURE 15-5 Stages in CTL-mediated killing of target cells. T-cell receptors on a CTL interact with processed antigen–class I MHC complexes on an appropriate target cell, leading to formation of a CTL/target-cell conjugate. The Golgi stacks and granules in the CTL reorient toward the point of contact with the target cell, and the granules' contents are released by exocytosis. Following dissociation of the conjugate, the CTL is recycled and the target cell is destroyed in time as the result of damage to its membrane. [Adapted from P. A. Henkart, 1985, *Annu. Rev. Immunol.* **3**:31.]

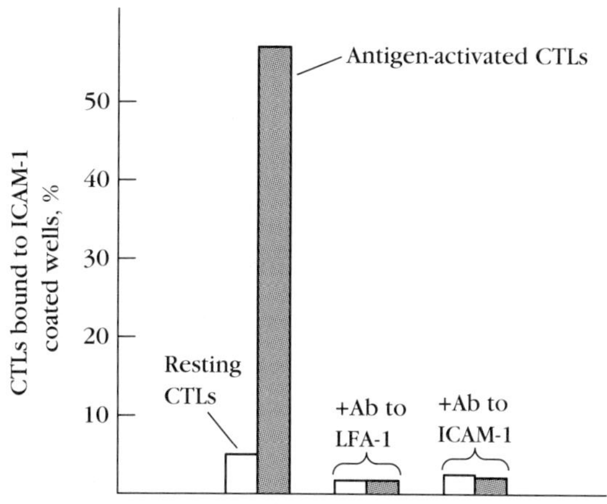

FIGURE 15-6 Effect of antigen activation on ability of CTLs to bind to the intercellular cell-adhesion molecule ICAM-1. Resting mouse CTLs were first incubated with anti-CD3 antibodies. Cross-linkage of CD3 molecules on the CTL membrane by anti-CD3 has the same activating effect as interaction with antigen–class I MHC complexes on a target cell. Adhesion was assayed by binding of radiolabeled CTLs to microwells coated with ICAM-1. Antigen activation increased CTL binding to ICAM-1 more than 10-fold. The presence of excess monoclonal antibody to LFA-1 or ICAM-1 in the microwells abolished binding, demonstrating that both molecules are necessary for adhesion to occur. [Based on M. L. Dustin and T. A. Springer, 1989, *Nature* **341**:619.]

antigen-specific CTLs are incubated with appropriate target cells, the two cell types interact and undergo conjugate formation. Formation of a CTL–target-cell conjugate is followed within several minutes by a Ca^{2+}-dependent, energy-requiring step in which the CTL inflicts membrane damage on the target cell. Following this step the CTL dissociates from the target cell and goes on to bind to another target cell. Within a variable period of time (from 15 min to 3 h) after CTL dissociation, the target cell lyses. Each of the steps involved in this process have been studied in more detail with cloned CTLs.

The TCR-CD3 membrane complex on a CTL recognizes antigen in association with class I MHC molecules on a target cell. Following this antigen-specific recognition, the integrin receptor LFA-1 on the CTL membrane binds to intercellular cell-adhesion molecules (ICAMs) on the target-cell membrane. This adhesion process appears to require prior activation of the CTL resulting from interaction of its TCR-CD3 complex with the antigen-MHC complex on the target cell. M. L. Dustin and T. A. Springer found that antigen-mediated CTL activation converts LFA-1 from a low-avidity state to a high-avidity state (Figure 15-6). Because of this phenomenon, CTLs adhere to and form conjugates only with appropriate target cells that display antigenic peptides associated with class I MHC molecules. LFA-1 persists in the high-avidity state for only 5–10 min after antigen-mediated activation, and then it returns to the low-avidity state. This downshift in LFA-1 avidity is thought to facilitate CTL dissociation from the target cell.

Electron microscopy of cultured CTL clones reveals the presence of intracellular electron-dense storage granules. These granules have been isolated by fractionation and shown to mediate target-cell damage by themselves. Characterization of isolated CTL storage granules has shown that they contain some high-molecular-weight proteoglycans, various toxic cytokines (e.g., TNF-β), a pore-forming protein called *perforin,* and a family of seven esterases *(granzymes A–G).* Although CTL precursors lack cytoplasmic granules and perforin, CTL-P activation results in the appearance of these cytoplasmic granules and expression of 70-kDa perforin monomers within them.

Immediately following formation of a CTL–target-cell conjugate, the Golgi stacks and storage granules reorient within the cytoplasm of the CTL, becoming concentrated near the junction with the target cell (Figure 15-7). Perforin monomers then are released from the granules by exocytosis into the junctional space between the two cells. As the perforin monomers contact the target-cell membrane, they undergo a conformational change, exposing an amphipathic domain that inserts into the target-cell membrane; the monomers then polymerize (in the presence of Ca^{2+}) to form a cylindrical pore with an internal diameter of 5–20 nm (Figure 15-8a). A large number of perforin pores are visible on the target-cell membrane in the region of conjugate formation (Figure 15-8b). These pores are thought to facilitate entry of various lytic substances (also released from CTL granules) that destroy the target cell. Interestingly, perforin exhibits some sequence homology with the terminal C9 component of the complement system (see Chapter 17), and the membrane pores formed by perforin are similar to those observed in complement-mediated lysis.

One unanswered question in CTL-mediated target-cell killing is why the CTL cell itself is not killed by its own secreted perforin molecules. A single CTL cell is capable of killing multiple target cells, and yet it is not damaged in the process. Several hypotheses have been proposed to account for CTL protection. One proposal, advanced by J. D. E. Young and Z. A. Cohn, is that

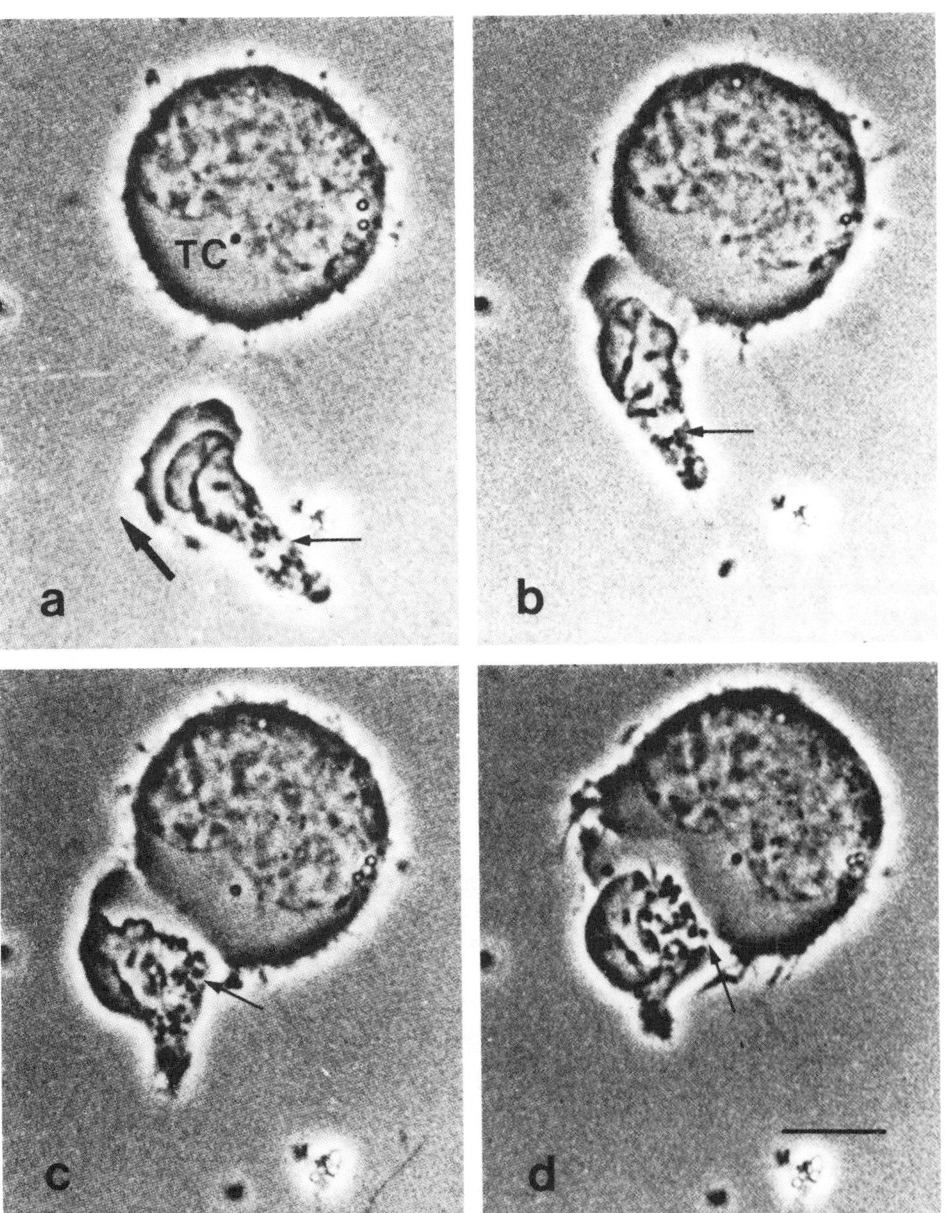

FIGURE 15-7 Formation of a conjugate between a CTL and target cell and reorientation of CTL cytoplasmic granules as seen by time-lapse cinematography. (a) A motile mouse CTL *(bottom)* approaches an appropriate target cell (TC). Thick arrow indicates direction of movement. (b) Initial contact of the CTL and target cell has occurred. (c) Within 2 min of initial contact, the membrane-contact region has broadened and the rearrangement of dark cytoplasmic granules (thin arrows) is under way. (d) Further movement of dark granules toward the target cell is evident 10 min after initial contact. [From J. R. Yanelli et al., 1986, *J. Immunol,* **136**:377.]

the CTL has a membrane protein ("protectin") that inactivates perforin either by preventing its insertion into the CTL membrane or by preventing its polymerization there. So far, however, no evidence has been adduced for such a protective protein.

A second hypothesis, proposed by P. J. Peters and coworkers, is that perforin is not released in a soluble form but rather is released within small membrane-bounded vesicles that in turn are housed in the electron-dense CTL granules. Such vesicles have in fact been observed by electron microscopy and have been shown by antibody conjugated with colloidal gold to express the TCR, CD3, and CD8 molecules of the CTL membrane (Figure 15-9). According to this hypothesis, the vesicles released from CTL granules exhibit specificity for the target cell via interaction of the TCR and CD8 with the antigen-MHC complexes on the target-cell membrane. Once the vesicles bind to the specific target cell, perforin is released and forms pores as described already. This mechanism not only would

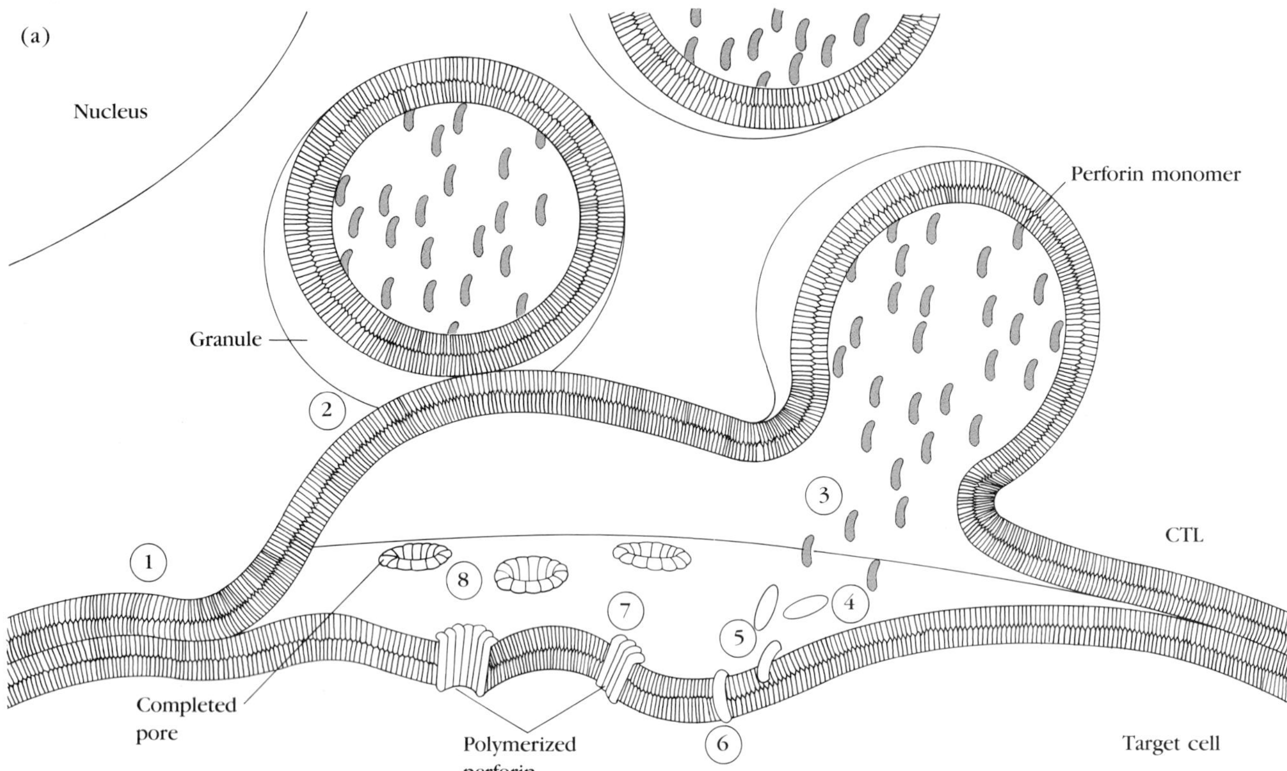

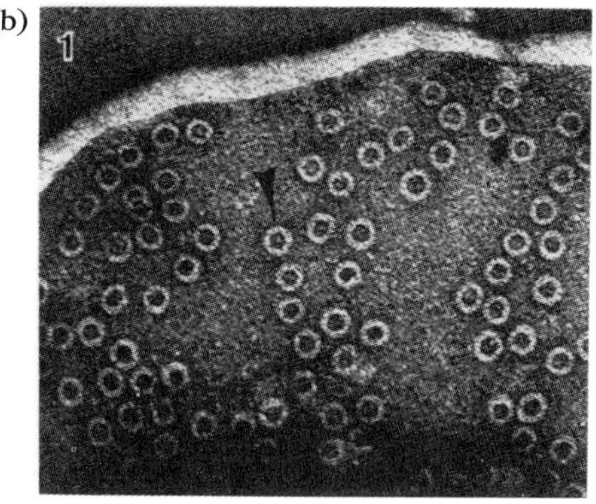

FIGURE 15-8 CTL-mediated pore formation in target-cell membrane. (a) In this model, a rise in intracellular Ca^{2+} triggered by CTL–target-cell interaction (1) induces exocytosis, in which the granules fuse with the CTL cell membrane (2) and release monomeric perforin into the small intracellular space between the two cells (3). The released perforin monomers undergo a Ca^{2+}-induced conformational change (4) and then bind to the target-cell membrane (5) and insert into it (6). In the presence of Ca^{2+}, the monomers polymerize within the membrane (7), forming cylindrical pores (8). (b) Electron micrograph of perforin pores on the surface of a rabbit erythrocyte target cell. [Part (a) adapted from J. D. E. Young and Z. A. Cohn, 1988, *Sci. Am.* **258**(Jan.):38; part (b) from E. R. Podack and G. Dennert, 1983, *Nature* **301**:442.]

prevent self-killing of CTLs but also would prevent accidental killing of inappropriate target cells by perforin molecules that move away from the site of conjugate formation.

TARGET-CELL DESTRUCTION BY APOPTOSIS. Some investigators have questioned whether perforin-mediated lysis is really the primary mechanism of CTL-mediated killing. One of the problems with the CTL lines in which cytotoxicity is studied is that they are obtained by culturing cells with high levels of IL-2. It has been suggested that such high levels of IL-2 might convert CTLs into NK-like cells exhibiting perforin-mediated killing that may not necessarily be the normal mechanism of CTL killing. A number of unexplained observations sharpen the controversy. Some CTL lines have been isolated that are potent target-cell killers but lack detectable perforin. Moreover, target-cell killing is accomplished by some CTL lines in the complete absence of Ca^{2+}; since Ca^{2+} is required for perforin polymerization, some other mechanism of killing must be operative in these cell lines. These findings suggest that other cytolytic mechanisms, in addition to perforin-mediated lysis, may be employed by the CTL to assure rapid and complete destruction of the target cell.

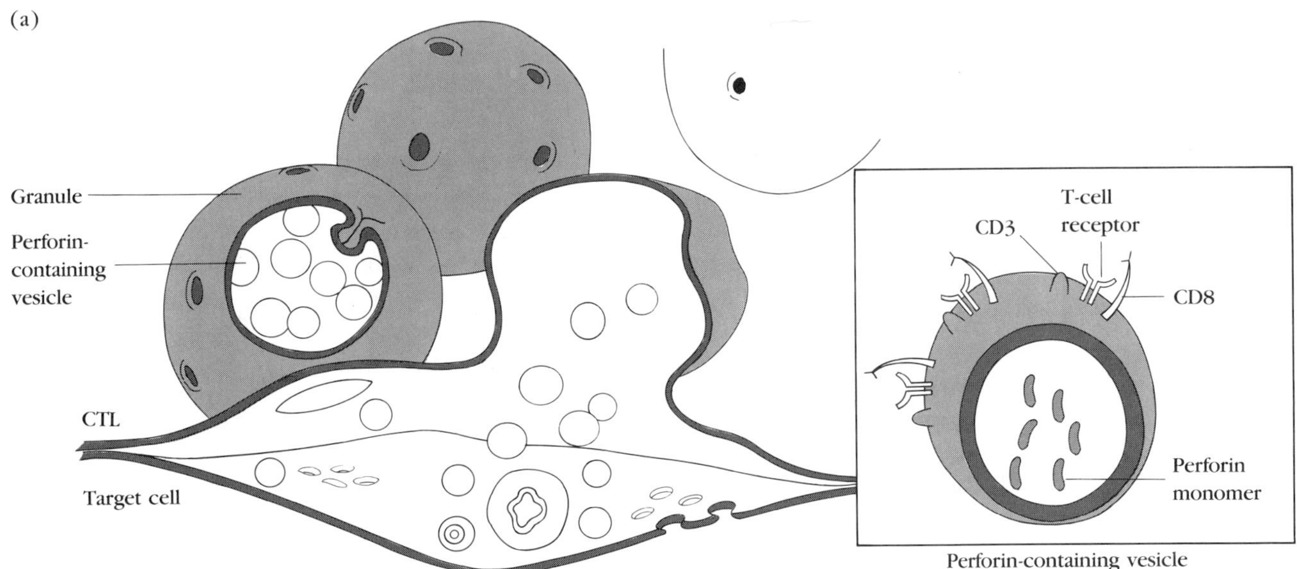

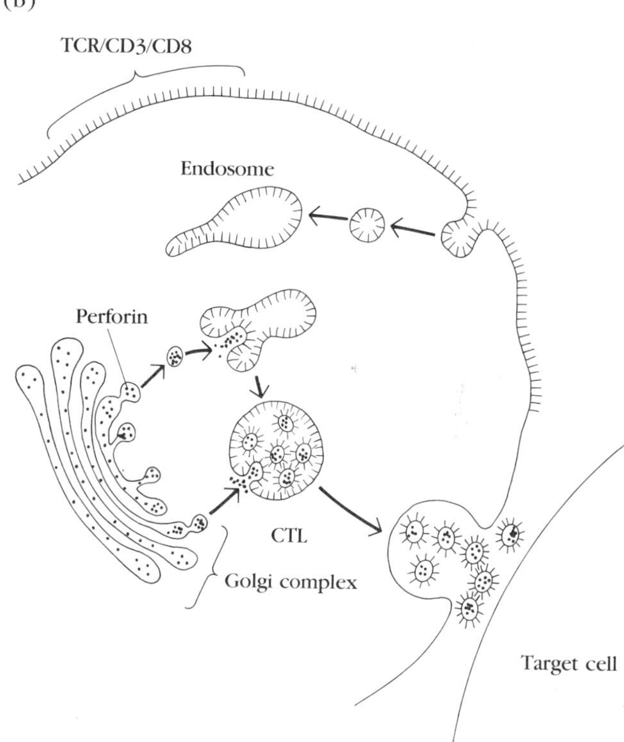

FIGURE 15-9 Alternative model of CTL-mediated killing in which perforin is released in small membrane-bounded vesicles. (a) Exocytosis of perforin-containing vesicles is depicted. The membrane molecules on the outer surface of these vesicles *(inset)* direct them toward the target cell where the TCR-CD3 complex and CD8 interact with antigen-class I MHC on the target-cell membrane. (b) A more schematic illustration showing the perforin-containing vesicles thought to be derived by endocytosis of the CTL plasma membrane. Initial endocytosis results in TCR/CD3/CD8 facing inward, but subsequent membrane invagination produces smaller vesicles with TCR/CD3/CD8 facing outward. [Adapted from P. J. Peters et al., 1990, *Immunol. Today* **11**:28.]

Several researchers have recently reported that interaction of CTLs with target cells results in a killing process in which the target cells show all the morphologic hallmarks of apoptosis (see Figure 3-3). Within 5 min following CTL contact, target cells begin to exhibit DNA fragmentation. Interestingly, viral DNA within infected target cells has also been shown to be fragmented during this process. This observation has led to the speculation that the rapid onset of DNA fragmentation following CTL contact may prevent continued viral replication and assembly during the time prior to target-cell destruction. This apoptotic process does not require mRNA or protein synthesis in either the CTL or target cell. Some have suggested that either the CTL secretes a factor that induces DNA fragmentation or else the CTL–target cell interaction induces a transmembrane signal that results in apoptosis. One CTL-derived factor that has been implicated in apoptosis is TNF-β. TNF receptors are expressed on virtually all nucleated cells. There are two TNF receptors (55-kDa TNF-R1 and 75-kDa TNF-R2), both of which bind TNF with comparable affinities. Cross-linkage of TNF receptors by TNF has been shown to induce apoptosis in some cell types, most notably tumor cells. It is not known why receptor cross-linkage leads to apoptosis in tumor cells but generally not in other types of cells that express the TNF receptor. Perhaps other apoptosis-inducing factors are involved or perhaps a signal-transduction mechanism is involved.

NK-Cell–Mediated Cytotoxicity

Natural killer cells were discovered quite by accident when immunologists were measuring tumor-specific CTL activity in mice with tumors. Normal unimmunized mice and mice with unrelated tumors served as negative controls. Much to the consternation of the researchers, the controls showed significant tumor lysis in a cell-mediated lympholysis (CML) assay. Characterization of the cells responsible for this nonspecific tumor-cell killing revealed that a population of large, granular lymphocytes was responsible. The cells, which were named natural killer (NK) cells for their nonspecific cytotoxicity, make up 5–10% of the recirculating lymphocyte population. These cells have been implicated in viral immunity and in defense against tumors.

NK-Cell Lineage

The lineage of NK cells remains uncertain, as they express some membrane markers of T lymphocytes and some markers of monocytes and granulocytes. Moreover, different NK cells express different sets of membrane molecules. It is not known whether this heterogeneity reflects subpopulations of NK cells or different stages in their activation or maturation. Among the membrane molecules expressed by NK cells are Thy-1, CD2, the 75-kDa β subunit of the IL-2 receptor, and CD16 (or FcγRIII)—a receptor for the Fc region of IgG (see Figure 3-9c). Monoclonal antibody to CD16 has been shown to remove almost all NK-cell activity from peripheral blood, and this reagent can be used to separate NK cells from other cell types.

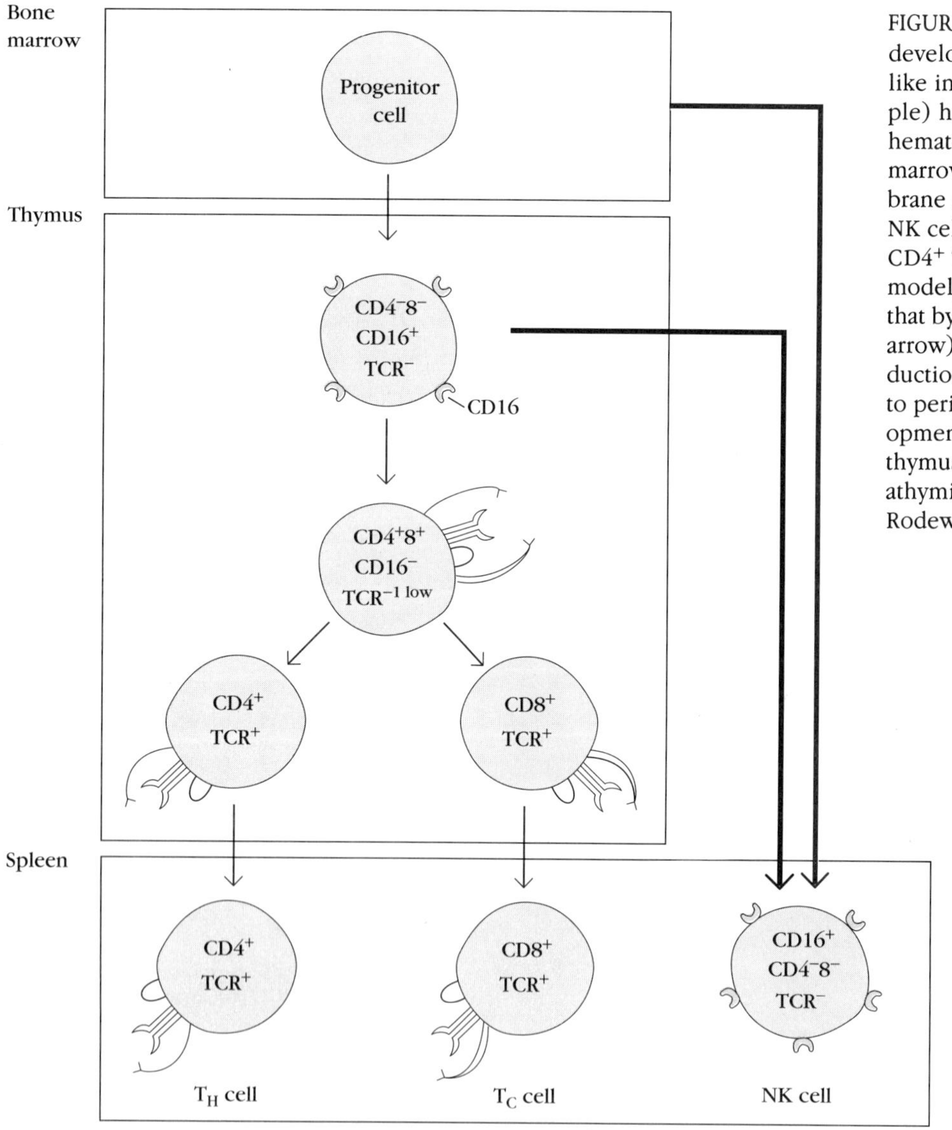

FIGURE 15-10 Model of thymocyte development involving a CD16$^+$, NK-like intermediate. CD16 (light purple) has been identified on hematopoietic cells in the bone marrow and fetal thymus. This membrane molecule is present on mature NK cells but is absent from CD8$^+$ and CD4$^+$ T cells. According to this model, bone marrow progenitor cells that bypass the thymus (thick purple arrow) or fail to undergo thymic induction (thick black arrow) give rise to peripheral NK cells. NK-cell development clearly can bypass the thymus, since NK cells are found in athymic mice. [Adapted from H. R. Rodewald et al., 1992, *Cell* **69**:139.]

TABLE 15-1 COMPARISON OF NK CELLS AND CTLS

Characteristic	CTL	NK cell
TCR-CD3 expression	Yes	No
MHC restriction	Yes	No
Membrane molecules	Thy-1$^+$ CD2$^+$ CD8$^+$ CD16$^-$	Thy-1$^+$ CD2$^+$ CD8$^-$ CD16$^+$ (FcRγIII$^+$)
Effector function	Requires antigen activation	Does not require antigen activation
Effect of IL-2	Increases activity	Increases activity
Possesses perforin-containing granules	Yes	Yes
Exhibits immunologic memory	Yes	No

A population of CD16$^+$ cells has been identified in the bone marrow and fetal thymus with anti-CD16. At day 14.5 of gestation, a major fetal thymocyte population bears the phenotype CD16$^+$, CD4$^-$, CD8$^-$, and TCR$^-$. Interestingly, if these fetal thymocytes are isolated and injected into the thymus of an irradiated adult mouse, they differentiate into double-positive TCR$^+$, CD4$^+$, CD8$^+$, CD16$^-$ cells and later mature into the single-positive CD4$^+$ or CD8$^+$ subpopulations, expressing the T-cell receptor. However, if the CD16$^+$, CD4$^-$, CD8$^-$ fetal thymocytes are grown in tissue culture in the presence of exogenous IL-2, then the cells maintain their CD16$^+$ phenotype and acquire the functional cytotoxic properties of NK cells. This has led to the suggestion that both CD4$^+$ and CD8$^+$ T cells and NK cells may be derived from a common lineage (Figure 15-10). However, the observation that NK cells can develop in *scid* mice suggests that either NK cells develop from a lineage distinct from T cells or else that they develop from a common early progenitor cell prior to the rearrangement of the TCR genes.

Mechanism of NK-Cell Killing

Natural killer cells appear to kill tumor cells and virus-infected cells by a process similar to CTL-mediated lysis. After an NK cell adheres to a target cell, degranulation of perforin-containing granules occurs. The released perforin appears to damage the target cell in the same way described for the CTL. NK cells have also been shown to mediate target-cell destruction by apoptosis. A number of toxic molecules, including TNF-α, secreted by NK cells may initiate the process of apoptosis. Despite these similarities, NK cells differ from CTLs in several significant ways (Table 15-1). First, NK cells do not express antigen-specific T-cell receptors or CD3. In addition, target-cell recognition by NK cells is not MHC restricted; that is, the same levels of NK-cell activity are observed with syngeneic and allogeneic tumor cells. Also, although prior priming enhances CTL activity, no increase in NK-cell activity occurs after a second injection with the same tumor cells; thus the NK-cell response generates no immunologic memory. The nature of the NK cell's receptor and of the tumor-cell structures with which it interacts remain unknown.

Natural killer cells play an important role in eliminating virus-infected cells during the first few days of many viral infections. This activity appears early in the response and appears to provide protection during the time required for activation, proliferation, and differentiation of T_C cells into functional CTLs. The importance of NK cells in defense against viral infections is illustrated by the case report of a young woman who completely lacked NK cells. Even though this patient had normal T- and B-cell counts, she suffered severe varicella virus infections and a life-threatening cytomegalovirus infection.

Regulation of NK-Cell Cytotoxicity

Since NK cells do not express antigen-specific receptors, some mechanism must prevent them from attacking normal body cells. In other words, why do NK cells preferentially attack tumor cells and virus-infected cells? One clue is the observation that tumor cells and virus-infected cells generally express *lower* levels of class I MHC molecules than do normal cells. K. Karre has suggested that NK cells have membrane receptors for class I MHC molecules and that interaction of these receptors with class I molecules on target cells inhibits target-cell destruction. In contrast, if target cells lack class I molecules or express only low levels, then the NK cell's receptor will not be fully engaged and target-cell killing will proceed.

Support for this hypothesis has come from studies demonstrating an inverse relationship between the level of class I MHC molecules expressed on a cell and its susceptibility to NK-mediated killing. For example, mouse cells from a class I–deficient cell line were shown to be readily killed by NK cells. However, when this cell line was transfected with genes for class I MHC molecules, the cells became resistant to NK-mediated lysis. One proposal is that the NK cell recognizes conserved self-peptides displayed by class I MHC molecules. If the self-peptide–MHC complex is present on a target cell, then NK-mediated killing is blocked; if the conserved self-peptide is replaced by an exogenous (nonself) peptide, then killing proceeds.

Support for this hypothesis comes from the RMA-S mouse cell line. As discussed in Chapter 10, this cell line is unable to assemble class I MHC molecules on the membrane because of a defect in the peptide transporter. Therefore, RMA-S cells have much lower levels of class I molecules on their membrane than do normal RMA cells. RMA-S cells have been shown to be much more sensitive to NK-cell-mediated killing than normal RMA cells. This difference suggests that the class I molecules on the membrane of normal RMA cells inhibit their destruction by NK cells. If RMA-S cells are incubated with exogenous (nonself) peptide, they can load the peptide and express peptide–class I complexes on their membrane. The finding that these cells still are killed by NK cells suggests that only when the NK cell's receptor interacts with certain self-peptides presented by class I MHC molecules is NK-mediated killing inhibited. Possible self-peptides that might function in this capacity are those derived from heat-shock proteins, histones, or elongation factor.

Antibody-Dependent Cell-Mediated Cytotoxicity

A number of cells that have cytotoxic potential express membrane receptors for the Fc region of the antibody molecule. When antibody is specifically bound to a target cell, these receptor-bearing cells can bind to the antibody Fc region, and thus to the target cells, and subsequently cause lysis of the target cell. Although the cytotoxic cells involved are nonspecific, the specificity of the antibody directs them to specific target cells. This type of cytotoxicity is referred to as *antibody-dependent cell-mediated cytotoxicity* (ADCC). A variety of cells have been shown to exhibit ADCC including NK cells, macrophages, monocytes, neutrophils, and eosinophils. Antibody-dependent cell-mediated killing of cells infected with the measles virus can be observed in vitro by adding antimeasles antibody together with macrophages to a culture of measles-infected cells. Similarly, cell-mediated killing of helminths, such as schistosomes or blood flukes, can be observed in vitro by incubating newly infected larvae (schistosomules) with antibody to the schistosomules together with eosinophils.

Target-cell killing by ADCC, which does not involve complement-mediated lysis, appears to involve a number of different cytotoxic mechanisms (Figure 15-11). When macrophages, neutrophils, or eosinophils bind to a target cell by way of the Fc receptor, they become more active metabolically; as a result, the lytic components in their cytoplasmic lysosomes or granules increase. Release of these lytic components at the site of the Fc-mediated contact may result in damage to the target cell. In addition, activated monocytes, macrophages, and NK cells have been shown to secrete

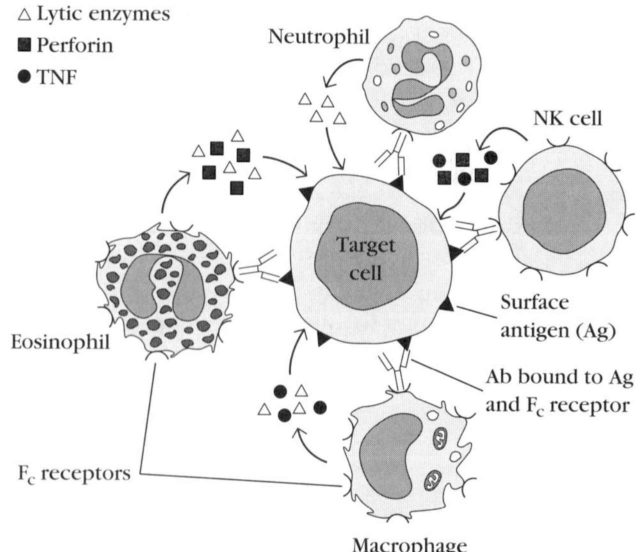

FIGURE 15-11 Antibody-dependent cell-mediated cytotoxicity (ADCC). Nonspecific cytotoxic cells are directed to specific target cells by binding to the Fc region of antibody bound to surface antigens on the target cells. Various substances (e.g., lytic enzymes, TNF, perforin) secreted by the nonspecific cytotoxic cells then mediate target-cell destruction.

tumor necrosis factor, which may have a cytotoxic effect on the bound target cell. Since both NK cells and eosinophils contain perforin in cytoplasmic granules, their target-cell killing may result from perforin-mediated membrane damage similar to the mechanism described for CTL-mediated cytotoxicity.

Experimental Assessment of Cell-Mediated Cytotoxicity

Three experimental systems have been particularly useful for measuring the activation and effector phases of cell-mediated cytotoxicity. The mixed-lymphocyte reaction is an in vitro system for assaying T_H-cell proliferation in a cell-mediated response; cell-mediated lympholysis is an in vitro assay of effector cytotoxic function; and the graft-versus-host reaction in experimental animals provides an in vivo system for studying cell-mediated cytotoxicity.

Mixed-Lymphocyte Reaction (MLR)

In 1965, X. Ginsburg and D. H. Sachs observed that when rat lymphocytes were cultured on a monolayer of mouse fibroblast cells, the rat lymphocytes proliferated and destroyed the mouse fibroblasts. In 1970 it was discovered that functional CTLs could also be generated by co-culturing allogeneic spleen cells in a system termed the mixed-lymphocyte reaction (MLR). The T lymphocytes in an MLR undergo extensive blast transformation and cell proliferation. The degree of proliferation can be assessed by adding [^{3}H]thymidine to the culture medium and monitoring uptake of label into DNA in the course of repeated cell divisions. Both populations of allogeneic T lymphocytes proliferate in an MLR unless one population is rendered unresponsive by treatment with mitomycin C or lethal x-irradiation (see Figure 9-12). In the latter system, called a one-way MLR, the unresponsive population provides stimulator cells that express alloantigens foreign to the responder T cells. Within 24–48 h the responder T cells begin dividing in response to the alloantigens of the stimulator cells, and by 72–96 h a population of functional CTLs is generated. With this experimental system functional CTLs can be generated entirely in vitro, after which their activity can be assessed with various effector assays.

The significant role of T_H cells in the one-way MLR can be demonstrated by use of antibodies to the T_H-cell membrane marker CD4. In a one-way MLR, responder T_H cells recognize allogeneic class II MHC molecules on the stimulator cells and proliferate in response to these differences. Removal of the CD4$^+$ T_H cells from the responder population with anti-CD4 plus complement abolishes the MLR and prevents generation of CTLs (Table 15-2). In addition to T_H cells, accessory cells such as macrophages also are necessary for the MLR to proceed. When adherent cells (largely macrophages) are removed from the stimulator population,

TABLE 15-2 DEPENDENCE OF ONE-WAY MLR ON CLASS II MHC DIFFERENCES AND THE PRESENCE OF T_H CELLS AND MACROPHAGES

Responder population			Stimulator population			
MHC haplotype			MHC haplotype			
Class I	Class II	Treatment	Class I	Class II	Treatment	Stimulation index*
s	*k*	None	*s*	*k*	None	1.0
s	*k*	None	*k*	*k*	None	1.2
s	*k*	None	*s*	*s*	None	18.0
s	*k*	$-T_H$ cells†	*s*	*s*	None	1.0
s	*k*	None	*s*	*s*	−Macrophages‡	1.0

* Stimulation index is directly related to the uptake of [^{3}H]thymidine and is a measure of cell proliferation.

† T_H cells removed by treatment with anti-CD4 and complement.

‡ When spleen cells are cultured, most of the macrophages adhere to the wall of the culture vessel; they can be removed from the stimulator population simply by decantation.

the proliferative response in the MLR is abolished and functional CTLs are no longer generated. Now it is known that the function of these macrophages is to activate class II MHC–restricted T_H cells whose proliferation is measured in the MLR. In the absence of T_H-cell activation, there is no proliferation.

The requirement for T_H cells in the generation of functional CTL activity in the MLR was demonstrated in a now-classical experiment by H. Cantor and E. A. Boyse. They performed one-way mixed-lymphocyte reactions with various populations of splenic lymphocytes and then assayed the cytotoxic activity generated with cell-mediated lympholysis (see Figure 9-11). The lymphocyte populations were obtained by treating spleen-cell aliquots with complement plus antibodies against subpopulation membrane molecules (equivalent to CD4 or CD8) to remove T_H cells and T_C cells, respectively. Their experiment, outlined in Figure 15-12, confirmed that $CD8^+$ T cells are responsible for functional cytotoxicity, which had been demonstrated previously. In addition, they found that removal of $CD4^+$ T cells from the MLR abolished the cytotoxicity of the $CD8^+$ T cells. These results provided the first evidence that T_C cells, like B cells, require T_H cells for their activation.

Cell-Mediated Lympholysis (CML)

Development of the cell-mediated lympholysis (CML) assay was a major experimental advance that contributed to understanding of the mechanism of target-cell killing by CTLs. In this assay suitable target cells are labeled intracellularly with chromium-51 (^{51}Cr) by incubating the target cells in with $Na_2{}^{51}CrO_4$. After the ^{51}Cr diffuses into a cell, it binds to cytoplasmic proteins, reducing its ability to passively diffuse out of the labeled target cell. When specific activated CTLs are incubated for 1–4 h with such labeled target cells, the cells lyse and the ^{51}Cr is released. The amount of ^{51}Cr released is directly related to the number of target cells lysed by the CTLs. By means of this assay the specificity of CTLs for allogeneic cells, tumor cells, virus-infected cells, and chemically modified cells has been demonstrated.

The T cells responsible for CML were identified by selectively depleting different T-cell subpopulations by means of antibody-plus-complement lysis. The experiment depicted in Figure 15-12 shows that removal of $CD8^+$ T cells eliminates lysis of target cells, whereas removal of $CD4^+$ T cells has no effect on CML. In general, the activity of CTLs exhibits class I MHC

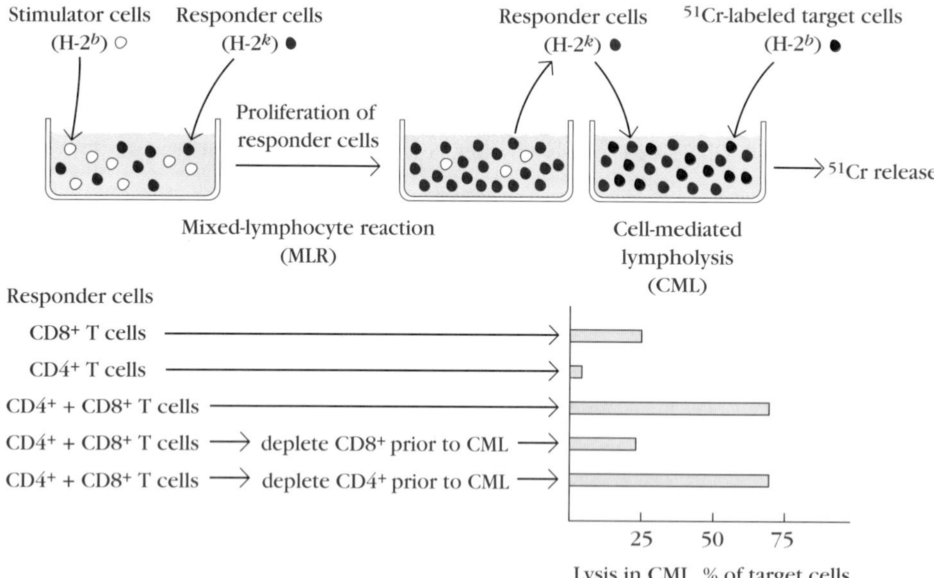

FIGURE 15-12 Experimental demonstration that $CD4^+$T cells are necessary to generate CTLs in an MLR reaction and that $CD8^+$T cells mediate target-cell lysis. The responder-cell population was first treated with antibodies plus complement to remove the T_H cells or T_C cells, respectively. The responder cells were then cultured with allogeneic x-irradiated stimulator cells. The cytotoxic activity of the generated CTLs was measured in a cell-mediated lympholysis (CML) assay using target cells labeled with chromium-51 (^{51}Cr). The amount of ^{51}Cr released is proportional to the number of CTLs. [Based on H. Cantor and E. A. Boyse, 1975, *J. Exp. Med.* **141**:1390.]

TABLE 15-3 EFFECT OF CTL HAPLOTYPE ON ABILITY TO LYSE H-2^k TARGET CELLS*

Spleen cells from LCM-primed mice						
	Haplotype†				^{51}Cr released from LCM-infected H-2^k target cells (%)‡	
Strain	*K*	*IA*	*IE*	*D*		Interpretation
CBA	*k*	*k*	*k*	*k*	86	Syngeneic combination works
BALB/c	*d*	*d*	*d*	*d*	18	Allogeneic combination does not work
ATL	*s*	*k*	*k*	*d*	18	Identity at class II loci does not work
B10.A	*k*	*k*	*k*	*d*	65	Identity at class I *K* locus works
C3H.OH	*d*	*d*	*d*	*k*	57	Identity at class I *D* locus works

* Spleen cells containing CTLs were isolated from mice with the indicated haplotypes that had been infected with the LCM virus. Lytic ability of the spleen cells was determined in a CML assay using ^{51}Cr-labeled H-2^k target cells.

† The indicated alleles are for the following H-2 loci in sequence: *K, IA, IE,* and *D. K* and *D* are class I MHC loci; *IA* and *IE* are class II MHC loci.

‡ Controls with uninfected target cells had ^{51}Cr release ranging from 17 to 22%.

SOURCE: Adapted from J. W. Kimball, 1983, *Introduction to Immunology,* Macmillan Publishing Co.

restriction. That is, CTLs can only kill target cells that present antigen associated with syngeneic class I MHC molecules (Table 15-3). Occasionally, however, CD4$^+$, class II–restricted T cells have been shown to function as CTLs.

Graft-versus-Host Reaction

The graft-versus-host (GVH) reaction is an in vivo indication of cell-mediated cytotoxicity. The reaction develops when immunocomponent lymphocytes are injected into an allogeneic recipient whose immune system is compromised. The grafted lymphocytes begin to attack the host, and the host's compromised state prevents an immune response against the graft. In humans, GVH reactions often develop following transplantation of bone marrow into patients who have had radiation exposure or who have leukemia, immunodeficiency diseases, or autoimmune anemias. The clinical manifestations of the GVH reaction include diarrhea, skin lesions, jaundice, spleen enlargement, and death. Epithelial cells of the skin and gastrointestinal tract often become necrotic, causing the skin and intestinal lining to be sloughed.

Experimentally, GVH reactions develop when immunocompetent lymphocytes are transferred into a neonatal or an x-irradiated animal. The recipients, especially neonatal ones, often exhibit weight loss. The grafted lymphocytes generally are carried to a number of organs, including the spleen, where they begin to proliferate in response to the allogeneic MHC antigens of the host. This proliferation induces an influx of host cells, which in turn undergo intense proliferation that results in visible spleen enlargement, or splenomegaly. The intensity of a GVH reaction can be assessed by calculating the spleen index as follows:

$$\text{Spleen index} = \frac{\text{Weight of exp. spleen/Total body weight}}{\text{Weight of control spleen/Total body weight}}$$

A spleen index of 1.3 or greater is considered to be indicative of a positive GVH reaction. Spleen enlargement results from proliferation of both CD4$^+$ and CD8$^+$ T-cell populations. NK cells also have been shown to play a role in the GVH reaction, and these cells may contribute to some of the skin lesions and intestinal wall damage observed.

Delayed-Type Hypersensitivity Response

When some subpopulations of activated T_H cells encounter certain types of antigens, they secrete cytokines that induce a localized inflammatory reaction called *delayed-type hypersensitivity* (DTH). The reaction is characterized by large influxes of nonspecific inflammatory cells, in which the macrophage is a major participant. Historically, this type of reaction was first described in 1890 by Robert Koch, who observed that individuals infected with *Mycobacterium tuberculosis* developed a localized inflammatory response when injected intradermally with a filtrate derived from a mycobacterial culture. He called this localized skin reaction a "tuberculin reaction." Later, as it became apparent that a variety of other antigens could induce this response, its name was changed to delayed-type hypersensitivity in reference to the delayed onset of the reaction and to the extensive tissue damage (hypersensitivity) that is often associated with the reaction. The term *hypersensitivity* is somewhat misleading for it suggests that a DTH response is always detrimental. Although in some cases a DTH response does cause extensive tissue damage and is in itself pathologic, in many cases tissue damage is limited, and the response plays an important role in defense against intracellular pathogens and contact antigens.

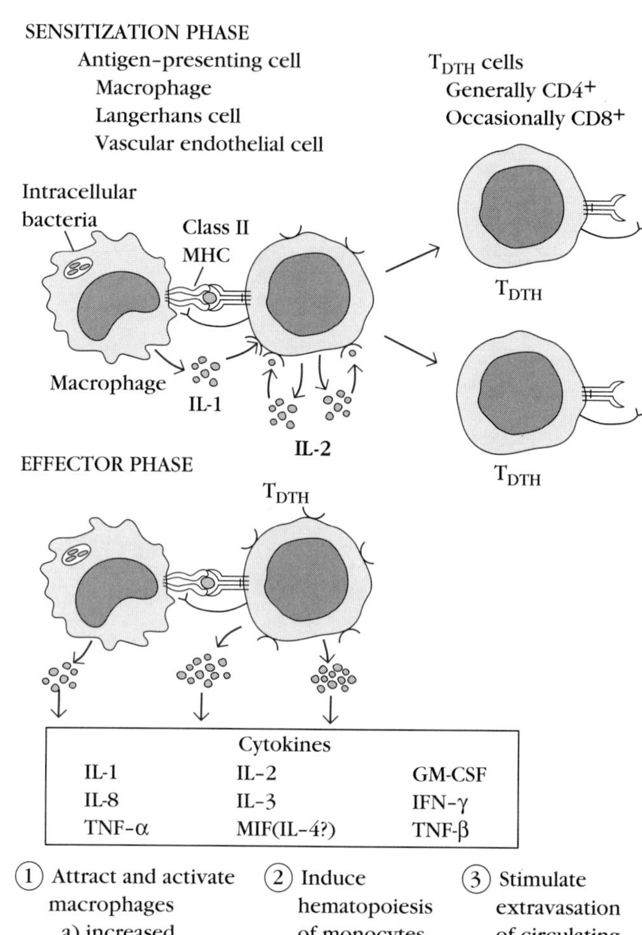

FIGURE 15-13 Overview of the DTH response. In the sensitization phase following primary contact with antigen, T_H cells proliferate and differentiate into T_{DTH} cells. This phase takes about 1–2 weeks. In the effector phase following a secondary contact with antigen, T_{DTH} cells secrete a variety of cytokines, which have three primary functions. This phase peaks about 2–3 days after secondary contact with antigen.

Phases of the DTH Response

The development of the DTH response requires an initial sensitization period of 1–2 weeks following primary contact with the antigen. During this period T_H cells are activated and clonally expanded by antigen presented together with the requisite class II MHC molecule on an appropriate antigen-presenting cell (Figure 15-13). A variety of antigen-presenting cells have been shown to be involved in the activation of a DTH response, including Langerhans cells and macrophages. Langerhans cells are dendritic cells found in the epidermis. These cells are thought to pick up antigen that enters through the skin and transport the antigen to regional lymph nodes where T cells are activated by the antigen. In some species, including humans, the vascular endothelial cells express class II MHC molecules and also function as antigen-presenting cells in the development of the DTH response.

A secondary contact with antigen induces the effector phase of the response. In the effector phase the activated T cells secrete a variety of cytokines that are responsible for the recruitment and activation of macrophages and other nonspecific inflammatory cells. Generally, the activated T cells are $CD4^+$ (primarily of the T_H1 subtype), but in a few cases $CD8^+$ cells have also been shown to induce a DTH response. The activated T cells are often designated as T_{DTH} cells to denote their function in the DTH response, although in reality they are simply a subset of T_H cells (or in some cases T_C cells).

A DTH response normally does not become apparent until an average of 24 h following secondary contact with the antigen; the response generally peaks 48–72 h after secondary contact. The delayed onset of this response reflects the time required for the cytokines to induce localized influxes of macrophages and activation of these cells. Once a DTH response begins, a complex interplay of nonspecific cells and mediators is set in motion that can result in tremendous amplification. By the time the DTH response is fully developed, only about 5% of the participating cells are antigen-specific T_{DTH} cells and the remainder are macrophages and other nonspecific cells. The macrophage functions as the principal effector cell of the DTH response. Cytokines elaborated by the T_{DTH} cell induce blood monocytes to adhere to vascular endothelial cells and migrate from the blood into the surrounding tissues. During this process the monocytes differentiate into *activated macrophages.* These activated macrophages exhibit increased levels of phagocytosis and an increased ability to kill microorganisms. In addition, activated macrophages express increased levels of class II MHC molecules and cell-adhesion molecules and therefore function as more effective antigen-presenting cells.

The influx and activation of macrophages in the DTH response provides an effective host defense against intracellular pathogens. Generally the pathogen is rapidly cleared with little tissue damage. However, in some cases, especially if the antigen is not easily cleared, a prolonged DTH response can itself become destructive to the host as the intense inflammatory response develops into a visible *granulomatous reaction*. A granuloma develops when continuous activation of macrophages induces the macrophages to adhere closely to one another, assuming an epitheloid shape and sometimes fusing to form multinucleated giant cells. These giant cells displace the normal tissue cells, forming palpable nodules, and release high concentrations of lytic enzymes, which destroy the surrounding tissue. In these cases the response can lead to blood-vessel damage and extensive tissue necrosis.

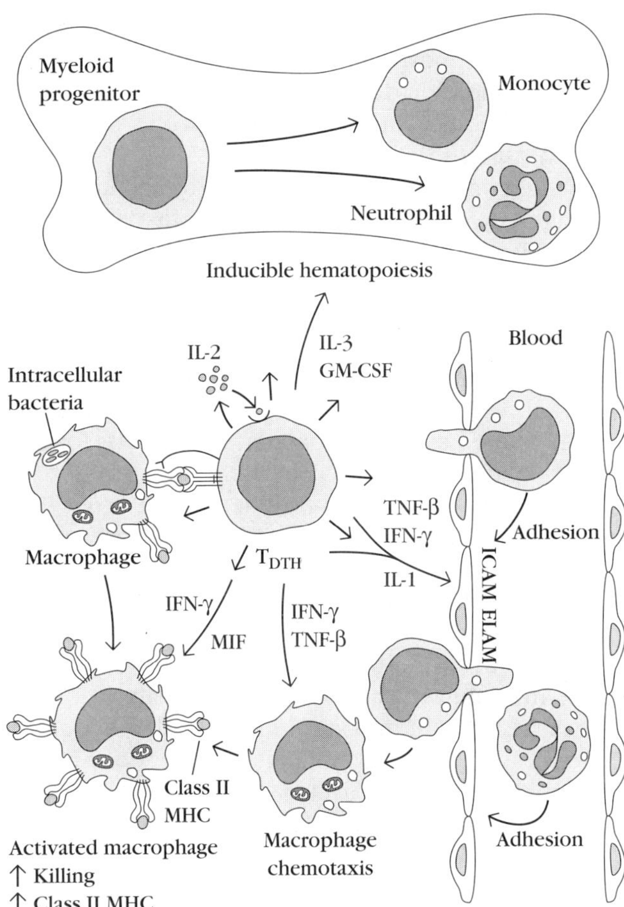

FIGURE 15-14 Role of cytokines secreted by T_{DTH} cells in mediating a DTH tissue reaction. These cytokines (shown in purple) act to (1) induce hematopoiesis of monocytes and neutrophils, (2) increase the expression of cell-adhesion molecules (ICAM, VCAM, and ELAM) on nearby vessel endothelial cells, (3) attract monocytes and macrophages by chemotaxis, and (4) activate macrophages. Migration-inhibition factor (MIF) inhibits the motility of macrophages, thereby confining them to the site of tissue activation.

Cytokines Involved in DTH Reaction

Numerous cytokines play a role in generating a DTH reaction (Figure 15-14). The pattern of cytokines implicated in a DTH response suggest that T_{DTH} cells may be primarily of the T_H1 subset (see Table 13-2). IL-2 functions in an autocrine manner to amplify the population of cytokine-producing T cells. Among the cytokines produced by these cells are a number that serve to activate and attract macrophages to the site of T_H1 activation. IL-3 and GM-CSF induce localized hematopoiesis of the granulocyte-monocyte lineage. IFN-γ and TNF-β (together with macrophage-derived TNF-α and IL-1) act on nearby endothelial cells, inducing a number of changes that facilitate extravasation of monocytes and other nonspecific inflammatory cells. Among the changes induced are increases in the expression of cellular-adhesion molecules including ICAMs, VCAMs, and ELAMs; changes in the shape of the vascular endothelial cells to facilitate extravasation; and secretion of IL-8 and monocyte chemotactic factor. Circulating neutrophils and monocytes adhere to the adhesion molecules displayed on the vascular endothelial cells and extravasate into the tissue spaces. Neutrophils appear early in the reaction, peaking by about 6 h and then declining in numbers. The monocyte infiltration occurs between 24 and 48 h after antigen exposure.

As the monocytes enter the tissues to become macrophages, they are chemotactically drawn to the site of the DTH response by factors such as monocyte chemotactic and activating factor (MCAF) and IFN-γ. Another cytokine, called *migration-inhibition factor* (MIF), inhibits further macrophage migration and thus prevents the macrophages from migrating beyond the site of a DTH reaction. As discussed later, production of MIF is the basis for a common in vitro test for the ability of an individual to generate a DTH reaction.

As macrophages accumulate at the site of a DTH reaction, they are activated by cytokines, particularly IFN-γ. Compared with unactivated macrophages, activated macrophages are larger, contain higher levels of lytic enzymes, have greater phagocytic ability, and are more effective in killing intracellular pathogens. Because macrophages activated by IFN-γ also express more class II MHC molecules and IL-1, they are more effective antigen-presenting cells than unactivated macrophages. Such activated macrophages can efficiently mediate activation of more T_{DTH} cells, which in turn secrete more cytokines that recruit and activate even more macrophages. This self-perpetuating response, however, is a double-edged sword, with a fine line existing between a beneficial, protective response and a detrimental response characterized by extensive tissue damage.

A 1993 report of experiments with knock-out mice that could not produce IFN-γ demonstrated the importance of this cytokine in the DTH response. When these knock-out mice were infected with an attenuated (nonpathogenic) strain of *Mycobacterium bovis* (BCG), nearly all the animals died within 60 days, whereas wild-type mice survived (Figure 15-15). Macrophages from the IFN-γ knock-out mice were shown to have reduced levels of class II MHC molecules and of bactericidal metabolites such as nitric oxide and superoxide anion.

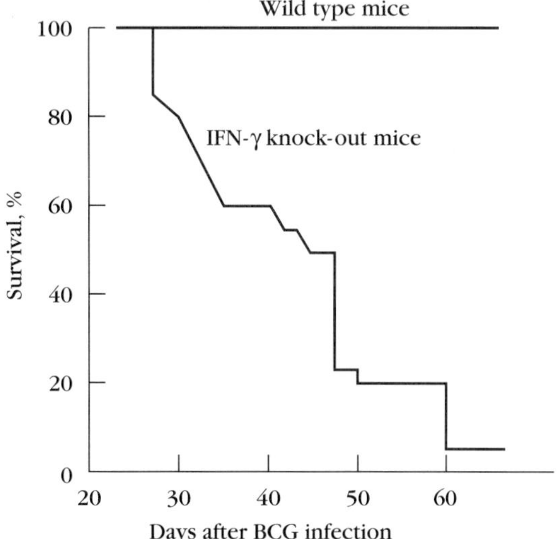

FIGURE 15-15 Experimental demonstration of role of IFN-γ in host defense against intracellular pathogens. Knock-out mice were produced by introducing a targeted mutation in the gene encoding IFN-γ. The mice were then infected with 10^7 colony-forming units of attenuated *Mycobacterium bovis* (BCG) and their survival monitored. [Adapted from D. K. Dalton et al., 1993, *Science* **259**:1739.]

Protective Role of the DTH Response

A variety of intracellular pathogens and contact antigens can induce a DTH response (Table 15-4). Cells harboring intracellular pathogens are rapidly destroyed by lytic enzymes released by macrophages that accumulate at the site of a DTH reaction (Figure 15-16). The initial response, however, is nonspecific and often results in significant damage to healthy tissue. Generally this is the price the body pays for successful elimination of cells harboring intracellular and fungal pathogens. The response to *Mycobacterium tuberculosis* illustrates the double-edged nature of the DTH response. Immunity to this intracellular bacterium involves a DTH response in which activated macrophages wall-off the organism and contain it within a cluster of activated macrophages, called a *granuloma.* Often, however, the activation of these macrophages results in the concentrated release of lytic enzymes leading to tissue damage within the lung.

The vitally important role of the DTH response in protecting the host against various intracellular pathogens is illustrated by AIDS. In this disease, $CD4^+$ T cells are severely depleted, resulting in a loss of the DTH response. Often patients suffering with AIDS develop life-threatening infections from intracellular bacteria, fungi, or protozoans that would not threaten an individual whose DTH response was intact. The immune response in AIDS patients is discussed in more depth in Chapter 23.

Another example in which delayed-type hypersensitivity plays an important role in host defense is infection by *Leishmania major,* an intracellular protozoan that causes leishmaniasis, an often fatal disease in Third World countries. An animal model of this disease has been developed in mice. Various inbred strains

TABLE 15-4 INTRACELLULAR PATHOGENS AND CONTACT ANTIGENS THAT INDUCE DELAYED-TYPE HYPERSENSITIVITY

Intracellular bacteria	Intracellular viruses
Mycobacterium tuberculosis	Herpes simplex virus
Mycobacterium leprae	Variola (smallpox)
Listeria monocytogenes	Measles virus
Brucella abortus	
	Contact antigens
Intracellular fungi	Poison oak and ivy
Pneumocystis carinii	Picrylchloride
Candida albicans	Hair dyes
Histoplasma capsulatum	Nickel salts
Cryptococcus neoformans	
Intracellular parasites	
Leishmania sp.	
Schistosoma sp.	

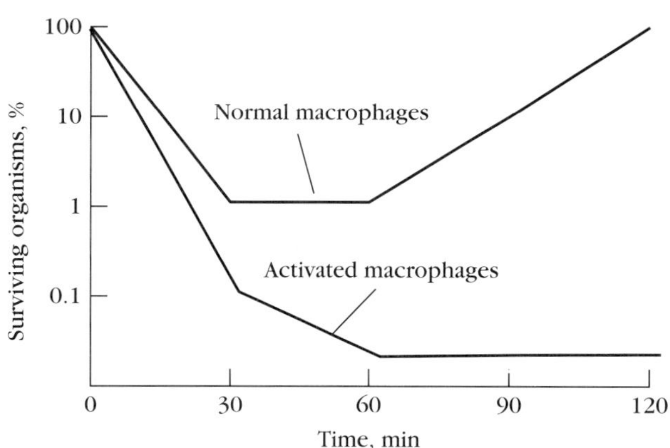

FIGURE 15-16 Survival of the intracellular pathogen *Listeria monocytogenes* when mixed with normal macrophages (not activated by IFN-γ) or activated macrophages in vitro. Note the logarithmic scale. The much greater ability of activated macrophages to destroy intracellular pathogens is evident.

infected with *L. major* show genetic differences in susceptibility to the pathogen. For example, CBA-strain mice develop small lesions at the site of inoculation and progress to a self-limited infection that renders the animals immune to further infection. Analysis of the immune response in these mice has revealed that $CD4^+$ T cells are responsible for the immune state; the transfer of $CD4^+$ T cells from immune CBA mice was shown to confer immunity on normal syngeneic recipients. The subpopulation of $CD4^+$ T cells that confers immunity in CBA mice was shown by cytokine analysis to resemble the T_H1 subset, a subpopulation of T_H cells that secrete IL-2, IL-3, GM-CSF, and IFN-γ. As described previously, these cytokines help mediate the DTH reaction, which results in elimination of intracellular pathogens by activated macrophages. Inbred strains of mice that do not develop immunity to *Leishmania* (e.g., BALB/c), and consequently progress to a fatal infection, mount an immune response characterized by lower levels of T_H1 cells than found in immune mice. These experiments suggest that variations in the levels and activity of T_H1 cells among inbred strains determine the degree of immune protection against *Leishmania*. It has been suggested that this animal model reflects possible differences in T_H-cell subpopulations that may exist in humans and may determine why some individuals are immune to certain intracellular pathogens, whereas others are susceptible. The next chapter will examine this topic in more detail.

Detection of the DTH Reaction

The presence of a DTH reaction can be measured experimentally by injecting antigen intradermally into an animal and observing whether a characteristic skin lesion develops at the injection site. A positive skin-test reaction indicates that the individual has a population of sensitized T_{DTH} cells specific for the test antigen. In the skin test to determine whether an individual has been exposed to *Mycobacterium tuberculosis,* the person is given an intradermal injection of PPD, a protein derived from the cell wall of this mycobacterium. Development of a red, slightly swollen, firm lesion at the site between 48 and 72 h later indicates that the individual has been exposed to *M. tuberculosis* antigens, either through direct exposure to the organism or through immunization—a procedure that is performed in some parts of the world. Development of a skin lesion in a previously sensitized individual results from the intense infiltration of cells to the site of injection during a DTH reaction; 80–90% of these cells are macrophages.

An in vitro DTH response can be detected by the presence of various cytokines whose level of activity gives some indication of the intensity of the response. For example, the secretion of migration-inhibition factor (MIF) by lymphocytes from a sensitized animal has been shown to correlate well with the animal's ability to mount a DTH response. As mentioned earlier, MIF is thought to be secreted by sensitized T_{DTH} cells.

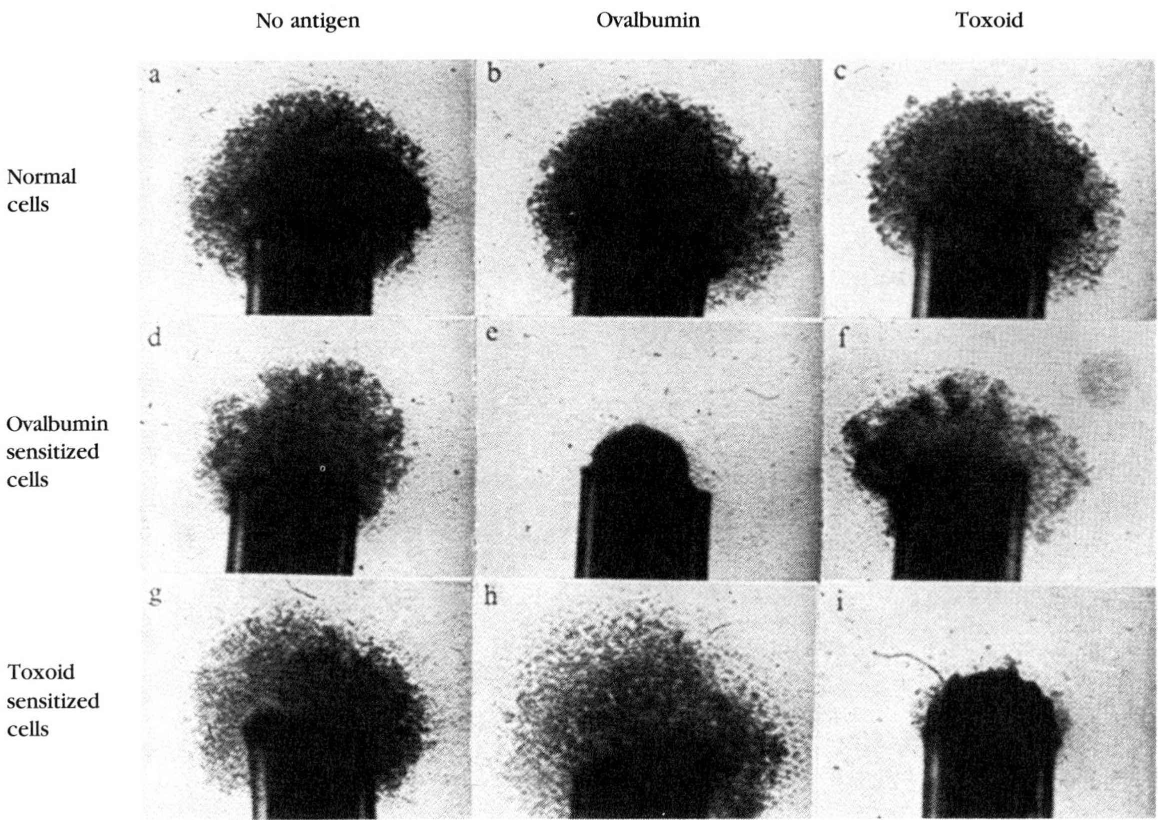

FIGURE 15-17 Assay for the production of migration-inhibition factor (MIF) by sensitized T_{DTH} cells on second exposure to the sensitizing antigen. Lymphocytes are first cultured in the presence of antigen and appropriate antigen-presenting cells. The culture supernatant then is added to macrophages in a glass capillary tube, which is placed horizontally on a surface bathed in culture medium. If MIF is present in the supernatant, the macrophages remain in the tube (+ reaction); if MIF is absent, the macrophages migrate out of the tube (− reaction). A + reaction indicates the presence of T_{DTH} cells sensitized to the antigen used in the assay. [From J. R. David, 1970, *Immunology,* The Upjohn Company, Kalamazoo, Mich.]

Production of MIF by cultured lymphocytes exposed to antigen thus can serve as an in vitro assay for the DTH response (Figure 15-17).

Pathologic DTH Responses

In some cases the DTH response to an intracellular pathogen can cause such extensive tissue damage that the response itself is pathologic and constitutes a truly hypersensitive condition. Much of the tissue damage to the lung in tuberculosis results from the accumulation of activated macrophages whose lysosomal enzymes destroy healthy lung tissue. Delayed-type hypersensitive reactions can also develop to inappropriate antigens such as poison oak and skin-contact sensitizers. Such examples, of truly hypersensitive conditions, in which tissue damage far outweighs any beneficial effects, are discussed in Chapter 18.

Summary

1. Cell-mediated immune reactions involving direct cytotoxicity are mediated by antigen-specific cytotoxic T lymphocytes (CTLs) and nonspecific effector cells such as natural killer cells and macrophages.

2. Phase I of the CTL-mediated immune response involves the activation and differentiation of CTL precursors (CTL-Ps). Interaction of a CTL-P with an antigen–class I MHC complex leads to expression of IL-2 receptors on the activated CTL-P. IL-2 produced by proliferating T_H cells than binds to the IL-2 receptors, inducing proliferation and differentiation of the CTL-P into an effector CTL.

3. Phase II of the CTL-mediated immune response begins with recognition of specific target cells bearing antigen and class I MHC molecules and formation of CTL/target-cell conjugates. Following conjugate formation, cytoplasmic granules within the cytoplasm of the CTL concentrate in the region of close membrane interaction with the target cell. Granule exocytosis in the zone of cellular adhesion releases the granular contents, including the protein perforin, which polymerizes and forms pores in the target-cell membrane. The CTL then dissociates from the target cell, which eventually is destroyed by the membrane damage. Target-cell killing by some CTLs may depend on a slower process involving apoptosis.

4. Various nonspecific cells can kill target cells without having to interact with antigen-MHC complexes. NK cells, for example, mediate lysis of tumor cells and virus-infected cells by perforin-induced pore formation similar to the mechanism employed by CTLs. The presence of relatively high levels of class I MHC molecules plus certain self-peptides on normal cells appears to protect them against NK-cell–mediated killing. Several types of nonspecific cytotoxic cells can bind to the Fc region of antibody on target cells and subsequently release lytic enzymes, perforin, or TNF, which damage the target-cell membrane. This process, called antibody-dependent cell-mediated cytotoxicity (ADCC), thus directs nonspecific cytotoxic cells to specific target cells.

5. Cell-mediated immunity involving delayed-type hypersensitivity plays an important role in host defense against intracellular pathogens. T_{DTH} cells, which differentiate from activated T_H cells, secrete a number of cytokines that cause macrophages to accumulate and to become activated. The activated macrophages are more effective killers of intracellular pathogens.

References

DUSTIN, M. L., and T. A. SPRINGER. 1989. T cell receptor cross-linking transiently stimulates through LFA-1. *Nature* **341**:619.

GROMO, G., L. INVERARDI, R. L. GELLER et al. 1987. Signal requirements in the stepwise functional maturation of cytotoxic T lymphocytes. *Nature* **327**:424.

MULLER, I., T. PEDRAZZINI, J. P. FARRELL, and J. LOUIS. 1989. T cell responses and immunity to experimental infection with *Leishmania major. Annu. Rev. Immunol.* **7**:561.

PETER, P. J., H. J. GEUZE, H. A. VAN DER DONK et al. 1989. Molecules relevant for T cell-target cell interaction are present in cytolytic granules of human T lymphocytes. *Eur. J. Immunol.* **19**:1469.

PETER, P. J., H. J. GEUZE, H. A. VAN DER DONK, and J. BORST. 1990. A new model for lethal hit delivery by cytotoxic T cells. *Immunol. Today* **11**:28.

POBER, J. S., and R. S. COTRAN. 1990. Cytokines and endothelial cell biology. *Physiol. Rev.* **70**:427.

RAHEMTULLA, A., W. P. FUNG-LEUNG, M. W. SCHILHAM et al. 1991. Normal development and function of CD8+ cells but markedly decreased helper cell activity in mice lacking CD4. *Nature* **353**:180.

RODEWALD, H. R., P. MOINGEON, J. L. LUCICH et al. 1992. A population of early fetal thymocytes expressing FcγRII/III contains precursors of T lymphocytes and natural killer cells. *Cell* **69**:139.

SHER, A., and R. L. COFFMAN. 1992. Regulation of immunity to parasites by T cells and T cell-derived cytokines. *Annu. Rev. Immunol.* **10**:385.

TARTAGLIA, L. A., M. ROTHE, Y. F. HU, and D. V. GOEDDEL. 1993. Tumor necrosis factor's cytotoxic activity is signaled by the p55 TNF receptor. *Cell* **73**:213.

TAUB, D. D., K. CONLON, A. R. LLOYD, J. J. OPPENHEIM, and D. J. KELVIN. 1993. Preferential migration of activated CD4+ and CD8+ T cells in response to MIP-1α and MIP-1β. *Science* **260**:355.

TSCHOPP, J., and M. NABHOLZ. 1990. Perforin mediated target cell lysis by cytolytic T lymphocytes. *Annu. Rev. Immunol.* **8**:279.

VERSTEEG, R. 1992. NK cells and T cells: mirror images? *Immunol. Today* **13**:244.

YOUNG, J. D. E., and Z. A. COHN. 1988. How killer cells kill. *Sci. Am.* **258**(Jan):38.

Study Questions

1. You have a monoclonal antibody specific for LFA-1. You perform CML assays of a CTL clone, using target cells for which the clone is specific, in the presence and absence of this antibody. Predict the relative amounts of ^{51}Cr released in the two assays. Explain your answer.

2. You decide to co-culture lymphocytes from the strains listed in the table below in order to observe the mixed-lymphocyte reaction (MLR). In each case, indicate which lymphocyte population(s) you would expect to proliferate.

Population 1	Population 2	Proliferation
C57BL/6 (H-2^b)	CBA (H-2^k)	
C57BL/6 (H-2^b)	CBA (H-2^k) mitomycin C-treated	
C57BL/6 (H-2^b)	F_1 (CBA × C57BL/6)	
C57BL/6 (H-2^b)	C57L (H-2^b)	

3. In the mixed-lymphocyte reaction (MLR), the uptake of [^{3}]thymidine often is used to assess cell proliferation.
   a. Which cell type proliferates in the MLR?
   b. How could you prove the identity of the proliferating cell?
   c. Explain why production of IL-2 also can be used to assess cell proliferation in the MLR.

4. Indicate whether each of the properties listed below is exhibited by T_H cells, CTLs, both T_H cells and CTLs, or neither cell type.
   a. _____ Can make IL-1
   b. _____ Can make IL-2
   c. _____ Is class I MHC restricted
   d. _____ Expresses CD8
   e. _____ Is required for B-cell activation
   f. _____ Is cytotoxic for target cells
   g. _____ Is the main proliferating cell in an MLR
   h. _____ Is the effector cell in a CML assay
   i. _____ Is class II MHC restricted
   j. _____ Expresses CD4
   k. _____ Can respond to IL-1
   l. _____ Expresses CD3
   m. _____ Adheres to target cells via LFA-1
   n. _____ Can express the IL-2 receptor
   o. _____ Expresses the $\alpha\beta$ T-cell receptor
   p. _____ Is the principal target of HIV
   q. _____ Responds to soluble antigens alone
   r. _____ Produces perforin

5. Mice from several different inbred strains were infected with LCM virus, and several days later their spleen cells were isolated. The ability of the primed spleen cells to lyse LCM-infected, ^{51}Cr-labeled target cells from various strains was determined. In the table below, indicate with a + or − whether the spleen cells listed in the left column would cause ^{51}Cr release from the target cells listed across the top of the table.

6. A mouse is infected with influenza virus. How could you assess whether the mouse has T_H and T_C cells specific for influenza?

For use with Question 5.

Source of primed spleen cells	^{51}Cr release from LCM-infected target cells: B10.D2 (H-2^d)	B10 (H-2^b)	B10.BR (H-2^k)	F_1 (BALB/c × B10) (H-2$^{b/d}$)
B10.D2 (H-2^d)				
B10 (H-2^b)				
BALB/c (H-2^d)				
(BALB/c × B10)				

IMMUNE REGULATION AND TOLERANCE

Upon encountering an antigen the immune system can either develop an immune response or enter a state of unresponsiveness called *tolerance.* The development of immunity or tolerance, both of which involve specific recognition of antigen by antigen-reactive T or B cells, needs to be carefully regulated since an inappropriate response — whether it be immunity to self-antigens or tolerance to a potential pathogen — can have serious and possibly life-threatening consequences.

Regulation of the immune response takes place in both the humoral and the cell-mediated branch. Every time an antigen is introduced, important regulatory decisions determine the branch of the immune system to be activated, the intensity of the response, and its duration. Unfortunately, very little is yet known about these regulatory events; this lack of knowledge has made it difficult for immunologists to selectively up-regulate or down-regulate immune reactivity when such fine-tuning would be desirable. This chapter examines the regulation immune responsiveness by antigen, antibody, cytokines, T cells, and the neuroendocrine system and also examines the conditions under which tolerance is induced.

Regulation of Immune Responsiveness

The nature, intensity, and duration of both the humoral and cell-mediated immune responses is influenced by prior host exposure to antigen, the nature and concentration of antigen, circulating antibodies and immune complexes, cytokines, the development of anti-idiotype antibodies, and certain T cells. Each of these factors is discussed in this section; the induction of tolerance is examined later in this chapter.

Effect of Prior Antigen Exposure

The immunologic history of an animal influences the quality and quantity of its immune response. A naive animal responds very differently than a previously primed animal to antigen challenge. Previous antigen encounter may have rendered the animal tolerant to the antigen or may have resulted in the formation of memory cells. These memory cells include distinct T_H-cell subpopulations having distinct cytokine patterns, T_C cells, and B cells, which may have class-switched to various isotypes.

Antigen-Mediated Regulation

The nature of the antigen exerts a major effect on the type of immune response generated. Bacteria, bacterial products, and soluble protein antigens tend to induce the production of humoral antibody; intracellular bacteria and viruses induce cell-mediated immunity. Since antigen is required for immune activation, it is obvious that the clearance of antigen will diminish further immune activation and the immune response will decline.

In some cases the presence of a competing antigen can regulate the immune response to an unrelated antigen. This *antigenic competition* is illustrated by injecting mice with a competing antigen a day or two before immunization with a test antigen. As Table 16-1 reveals, the response to horse red blood cells (HRBCs) is severely reduced by prior immunization with sheep red blood cells (SRBCs) and vice versa. At the cellular level, a competing antigen may interfere with antigen presentation to and activation of T_H cells; alternatively, the immune response to the competing antigen may generate various cytokines that down-regulate a subsequent response.

Although antigen concentration is the primary regulator of the intensity of an immune response, other regulators operate at a coarse or fine level to contribute to the intensity and duration of the response. An early finding suggesting that a decline in antigen level is not solely responsible for immune regulation came from experiments of C. G. Romball and W. O. Weigle. They injected rabbits with a single dose of human IgG and then determined the number of plaque-forming plasma cells at various times. Although antigen concentrations declined in a linear fashion, the number of plasma cells generated in response to the antigen showed a cyclical response, peaking, declining, and peaking again several times (Figure 16-1). This cyclical response indicates that something other than antigen concentration must be regulating the response.

TABLE 16-1 Antigenic competition between SRBCs and HRBCs

Immunizing antigen		Hemolytic plaque assay (day 8)*	
Ag1 (day 0)	Ag2 (day 3)	Test Ag	PFC/10^6 spleen cells
None	HRBC	HRBC	205
SRBC	HRBC	HRBC	13
None	SRBC	SRBC	626
HRBC	SRBC	SRBC	78

* See Figure 14-3 for assay details.

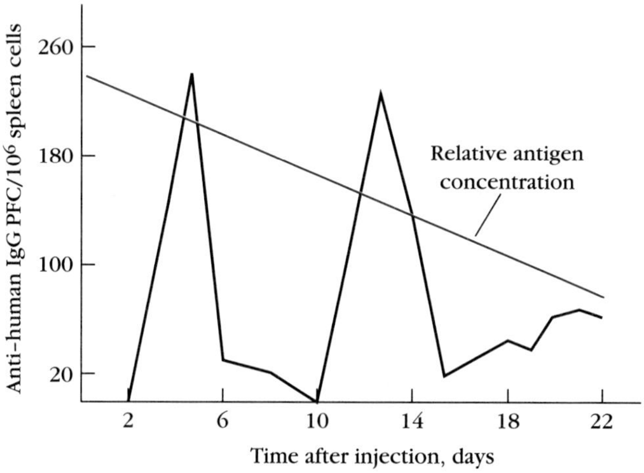

FIGURE 16-1 Following a single primary immunization of rabbits with human IgG, the number of splenic plasma cells secreting anti-human IgG antibodies showed a cyclical pattern despite the linear decrease in serum antigen concentration. This finding indicates that the immune response is not regulated solely by antigen concentration. [Adapted from C. G. Romball and W. O. Weigle, 1973, *J. Exp. Med.* **138**:1426.]

Antibody-Mediated Suppression

As in so many biochemical reactions subject to feedback inhibition by the end product, antibody exerts feedback inhibition on its own further production. If an animal is immunized with a specific antigen and is injected with preformed antibody to that same antigen just before or within 5 days after antigen priming, the immune response to the antigen is reduced as much as 100-fold. That this *antibody-mediated suppression* is not simply due to more rapid clearance of the antigen can be demonstrated if the antigen is a protein conjugated with two different haptens. For example, administration of preformed antibody to azobenzenearsonate (ABA) suppressed only the antibody response to ABA even though both ABA and DNP were presented on the same carrier and thus should have been cleared at the same rate (Figure 16-2).

One explanation for antibody-mediated suppression is that the passively administered antibody competes with antigen-reactive B cells for antigen, so that the B cells do not clonally expand. Evidence for such competition between passively administered antibody and antigen-reactive B cells comes from studies in which it took more than 10 times more low-affinity anti-DNP antibody than high-affinity anti-DNP antibody to induce comparable suppression. Furthermore, the competition for antigen between passively administered antibody and antigen-reactive B cells drives the response toward higher affinity. Only the high-affinity antigen-reactive cells can compete successfully with the passively administered antibody for the available antigen. This process is similar to affinity maturation, which occurs in the course of an immune response as the antibody formed early in the response begins to bind to the antigen, decreasing its concentration so that only the high-affinity antigen-reactive cells are stimulated later in the response (see Table 14-4).

Because of antibody-mediated suppression, certain vaccines (e.g., those for measles and mumps) are not administered to infants before the age of 1 year. The level of naturally acquired maternal IgG that the fetus acquires by transplacental transfer remains high for about 6 months after birth. If an infant is immunized with the measles or mumps vaccine while this maternal antibody is still present, the humoral response is low and the production of memory cells is inadequate to confer long-lasting immunity.

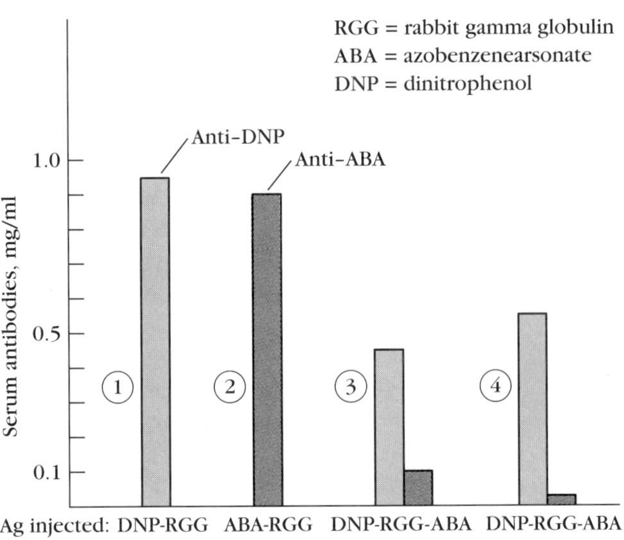

FIGURE 16-2 Experimental demonstration that antibody-mediated suppression is not caused only by more rapid antigen clearance. After animals were immunized with the indicated hapten-carrier conjugates, the serum concentrations of antibodies to the haptens DNP and ABA were determined. The suppression of anti-ABA production, but not of anti-DNP production, in experiment 4 indicates that antibody-mediated antigen clearance is not the sole cause of antibody-mediated suppression. [Based on data from N. I. Brody et al., 1967, *J. Exp. Med.* **126**:81.]

Immune Complexes as Regulators

Preformed antigen-antibody complexes have been shown in some experiments to enhance and in others to suppress the immune response. These immune complexes may exert their effect by binding to Fc receptors on various cells. It has not yet been possible to predict the effect of immune-complex size on immune responsiveness. There is evidence suggesting that patients with malignant tumors often develop circulating immune complexes in which antibody is complexed with tumor antigens. These complexes have been shown to suppress the immune response in these patients.

Cytokine-Mediated Regulation

The pleiotropic, synergistic, and antagonistic effects of cytokines enable them to function as regulators of both the humoral and cell-mediated branches of the immune system. Since the early 1970s, it has been observed that antibody production and the activity of T_{DTH} cells are inversely related. More recent evidence suggests that the pattern of cytokines produced during an immune response may explain the distinction between these two functional activities.

TABLE 16-2 EFFECTS OF IL-4 AND IFN-γ ON ISOTYPE PRODUCTION IN VITRO

	Supernatant* levels (ng/ml)	
Cytokine added to culture	IgE	IgG1
None	1.3	1,340
IL-4	171	20,000
IL-4 + IFN-γ	4.1	3,700

* Determined after culturing LPS-activated B cells for 7 days.

As discussed in previous chapters, mouse T_H-cell clones derived from long-term cultures can be divided into T_H1 and T_H2 subsets, distinguished by the patterns of cytokines they secrete (see Table 13-2). The T_H1 subset functions better at mediating cell-mediated immunity than activating B cells, whereas the T_H2 subset exhibits the reverse activity pattern. Furthermore, cytokines secreted by these two subsets have been shown to regulate each other. Interferon γ (IFN-γ), produced by T_H1 cells, inhibits proliferation of T_H2 cells; similarly, interleukin 10 (IL-10), produced by T_H2 cells, inhibits cytokine production by T_H1 cells. These experimental systems illustrate the important role that the cytokine balance plays in the regulation of antibody and T_{DTH} responses, although it remains to be seen whether T cells with the T_H1 and T_H2 cytokine patterns exist as distinct subpopulations within the normal animal.

In addition to influencing whether a humoral or cell-mediated response predominates, the cytokine balance may influence susceptibility to infection by certain pathogens. For example, as noted in the last chapter, BALB/c mice are susceptible to infection by the intracellular protozoan *Leishmania major,* whereas CBA mice are resistant. Analysis of the cytokine mRNAs from these two strains showed that the level of IFN-γ mRNA was 50- to 100-fold higher in resistant CBA mice than in susceptible BALB/c mice. Since IFN-γ plays a vital role in mediating the DTH reaction, particularly macrophage recruitment and activation (see Figure 15-14), macrophages in CBA mice would be more effective than those in BALB/c mice in killing *L. major.* These results strengthen the hypothesis that T_H1-like or T_H2-like cytokine activities may regulate which branch of the immune system is activated by various antigens.

The regulatory functions of cytokines also extend to the selection of immunoglobulin isotypes. The opposing effects of IL-4 and IFN-γ illustrate how the balance of cytokines produced during an immune response can contribute to the production of very different isotypes. Class switching of LPS-activated B cells to IgG1 and IgE is induced by IL-4, but in the presence of IFN-γ the IL-4 effect is blocked (Table 16-2). In contrast, if LPS-activated B cells are cultured in the presence of IFN-γ, they secrete IgG2a; however, this effect is blocked if IL-4 is added to the culture. Thus the balance of IL-4 and IFN-γ produced during an immune response can regulate the levels of the IgG1, IgE, and IgG2a isotypes.

Idiotype Regulation: The Network Theory

The enormous diversity of antibody and T-cell receptor (TCR) specificities that can be generated by the immune system is mind-boggling. Current estimates suggest that the immune system is capable of generating on the order of 10^{11} distinct antibody specificities and $10^{15}-18^{18}$ distinct TCR specificities. Since a mouse produces only 10^8 lymphocytes per day, only a fraction of the potential repertoire is expressed during the lifetime of a mouse. Because antigen-specific antibodies and T-cell receptors are not expressed during fetal development of the immune system, their variable-region sequences can be recognized as non-self by the immune system.

In 1973 Niels Jerne proposed a conceptual theory, called the *network theory,* that predicted the consequences of immune-system recognition of self-antibody; for this work, Jerne was awarded a Nobel prize in 1985. According to the network theory, as antibody is produced in response to an antigen, it in turn induces the formation of antibodies to its unique variable-region sequences. Jerne referred to each individual antigenic determinant of the variable region as an *idiotope.* Each antibody contains multiple idiotopes, and the sum of the individual idiotopes is called the *idiotype* of the antibody. In some cases, a particular idiotope and the actual antigen-combining site, which Jerne called the *paratope,* are identical; in other cases the idiotopes consist of variable-region sequences outside the antigen-binding site (Figure 16-3a). The network theory proposes that during an antibody response the antibodies formed in response to the antigen in turn induce the formation of secondary antibodies to the individual idiotopes of the first (primary) antibody. The idiotype of the primary antibody (Ab-1) activates a network of B cells whose receptors recognize the individual idiotopes of Ab-1. These B cells then differentiate into plasma cells that secrete anti-idiotype antibody (Ab-2). The individual idiotopes of Ab-2 can then further extend the network by inducing production of an anti-anti-idiotype, or Ab-3 (Figure 16-3b). This

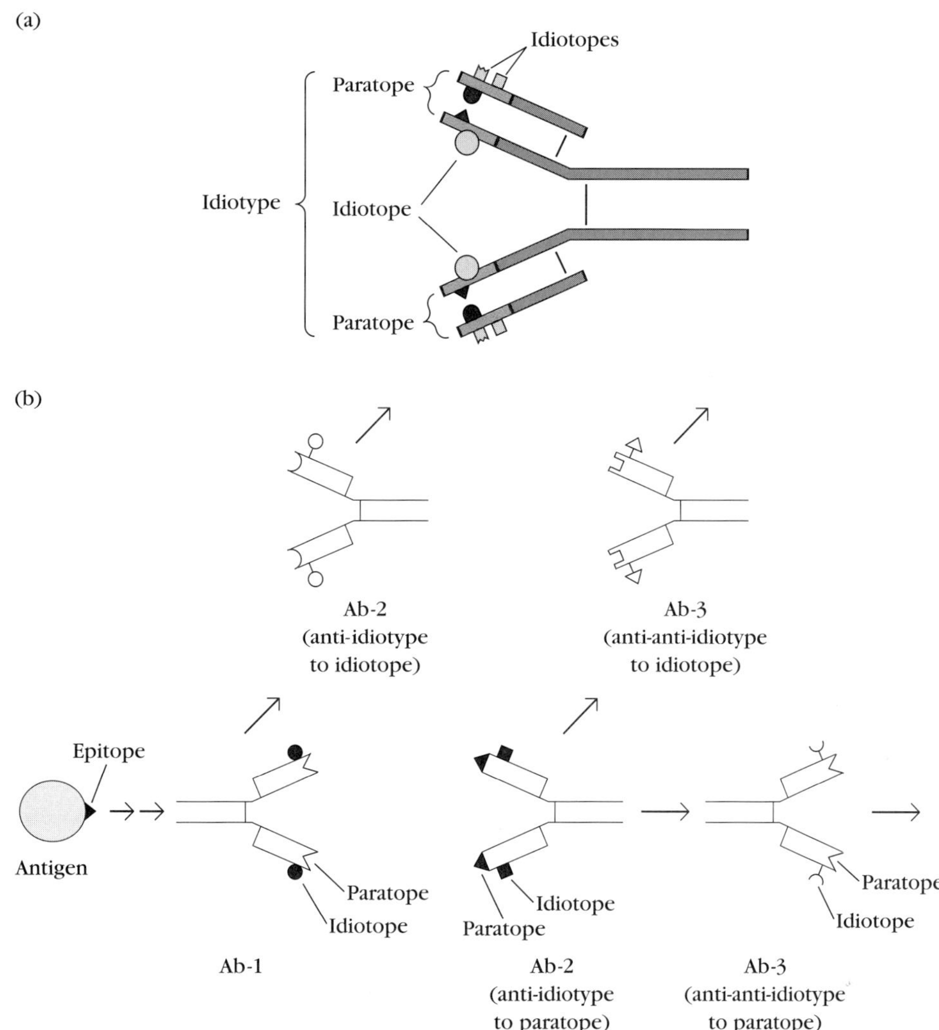

FIGURE 16-3 Network theory proposed by Niels Jerne. (a) Each antibody molecule expresses unique variable-region epitopes called idiotopes; the sum of the idiotopes is its idiotype. Idiotopes may coincide with the antigen-binding site, or paratope. (b) According to the network theory, the immune response to an antigen results in the formation of anti-idiotype antibodies specific for the individual idiotopes of the primary antibody (Ab-1). These anti-idiotype antibodies (Ab-2) in turn induce the formation of anti-anti-idiotype antibodies (Ab-3). A network of interacting antibodies is thus formed that serves to regulate the immune response. Note that the anti-idiotype antibody to the paratope of Ab-1 is an internal image of the original epitope on the antigen.

antibody often resembles idiotopes of Ab-1, and the network begins to limit itself as decreased levels of antibody are produced in each successive activation. Anti-idiotype regulation can also function within the T-cell branch of the immune system, since the $\alpha\beta$ and $\gamma\delta$ T-cell receptors have variable regions and are therefore capable of expressing idiotopes that can be recognized by other T or B cells. The idiotype network involving B and T cells represents a complex circuitry of interacting cells that functions either to enhance or to suppress immune activation. The complexity of the idiotype network has made it difficult to predict whether administration of anti-idiotype antibodies or T cells bearing anti-idiotype receptors will up-regulate or down-regulate immune responsiveness.

A central principle of the network theory is that some anti-idiotype antibody will be directed against the paratope and therefore will appear as the *internal image* of the original epitope on the antigen. For example, if mice are immunized with anti-insulin antibody (Ab-1), they produce anti-idiotype antibody (Ab-2) to Ab-1. Some of this anti-idiotype antibody will bind to the insulin-binding paratope of Ab-1. This anti-paratope antibody thus mimics the original insulin ligand; indeed this molecular mimicry is evidenced by the ability of the anti-paratope antibody to bind to the insulin receptor and induce glycolysis, just as insulin would. By re-expressing the image of the original epitope in the form of anti-paratope antibody, the immune system will continue to be activated even after the original antigen has been cleared; this may ensure that sufficient clonal proliferation and memory-cell production occurs in response to the original epitope.

The regulatory activity of anti-idiotype antibody was first observed in vivo with a system involving a myeloma protein designated TEPC-15 from BALB/c mice. Prior to the development of monoclonal antibodies immunologists depended on spontaneously occurring myelomas as sources of homogeneous antibodies. The limitation with these myeloma proteins was that the antigenic specificity was unknown and therefore researchers took on the tedious task of attempting to characterize the antigenic specificity of various myelomas. One of the myelomas characterized during this period was a BALB/c IgA myeloma designated TEPC-15, which was found to be an IgA antibody specific for phosphorylcholine (PC). Since phosphorylcholine is the major component of the pneumococcal cell-wall C polysaccharide, TEPC-15 could therefore serve as an antigen to assess anti-idiotype antibody production in mice that had been immunized with pneumococci. When BALB/c mice were immunized with pneumococci, the number of plaque-forming plasma cells was determined in two hemolytic plaque assays (see Figure 14-3). The first assay detected plasma cells secreting antibody to PC by use of sheep red blood cells coated with PC as the test antigen; the second assay detected plasma cells secreting anti-idiotype antibody by use of SRBCs coated with TEPC-15. As Figure 16-4 reveals, a peak anti-PC PFC was reached about 4 days after immunization followed by a peak anti-idiotype PFC 4 days later.

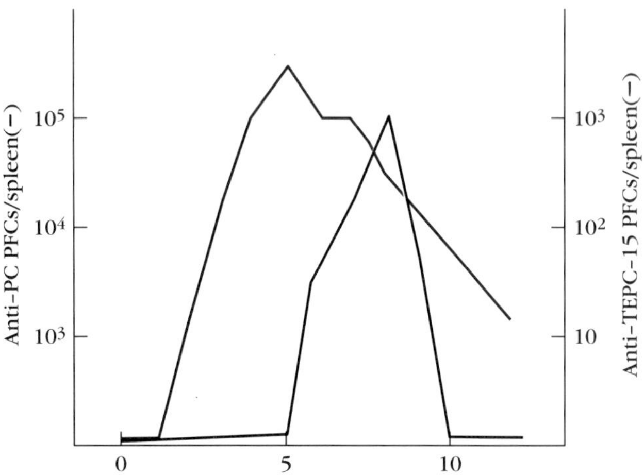

FIGURE 16-4 Production of anti-idiotype antibodies following immunization of BALB/c mice with pneumococci. Splenic plasma cells secreting antibody to the phosphorylcholine (PC) component of the pneumococcal cell wall (black curve) were detected in a hemolytic plaque assay using PC-coated SRBCs. Splenic plasma cells secreting anti-idiotype antibody (purple curve) were detected using SRBCs coated with the myeloma protein TEPC-15, which is specific for PC. [Adapted from H. Cozenza, 1976, *Eur. J. Immunol.* **6**:114.]

Anti-idiotype antibody representing the internal image of the original antigen can potentially serve as a vaccine to induce an immune response to a pathogenic antigen, thus avoiding immunization with the pathogen itself. For example, if mice are immunized with anti-idiotype antibody specific for the binding site of TEPC-15, they will be immune when they are later challenged with live pneumococci. Anti-idiotype vaccines have been shown to induce protective immunity in mice against hepatitis B virus (Figure 16-5), as well as rabies virus, Sendai virus, *Streptococcus pneumoniae, Listeria monocytogenes, Trypanosoma rhodesiense,* and *Schistosoma mansoni.* The development of anti-idiotype vaccines for humans holds much promise, particularly when immunization with a killed or attenuated vaccine would pose an unacceptable risk to the patient.

T-Cell–Mediated Suppression

When animals are immunized with large doses of certain antigens, they become unresponsive, or tolerant, to those antigens. In the early 1970s, R. Gershon and K. Kondo discovered that the unresponsive state could be transferred from tolerant mice to normal syngeneic mice simply by the transfer of T cells. Their experiments led to the hypothesis that there exists a population of regulatory T cells that are capable of mediating suppression of the immune response. The cells were called T suppressor (T_S) cells.

T. Tada and T. Takemori confirmed the results of Gershon and Kondo using high doses of keyhole limpet hemocyanin (KLH) to induce suppression. When KLH-primed spleen cells from suppressed mice were transferred to normal syngeneic recipients, the recipients' response to an injection of DNP-KLH, measured by a hemolytic plaque assay, was nearly abolished. However, spleen cells from mice suppressed with an unrelated antigen (BGG) had no effect on the recipients' response to DNP-KLH, demonstrating that the suppressive effect is antigen specific (Table 16-3).

Experiments with the A/J strain of mice revealed that the suppressive effect of T_S cells can be idiotype specific in some cases. When A/J mice are immunized with KLH conjugated to the hapten azobenzenearson-

(a)

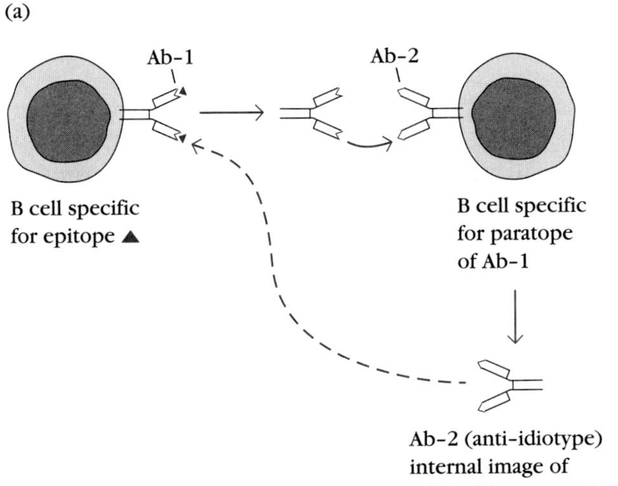

(b)

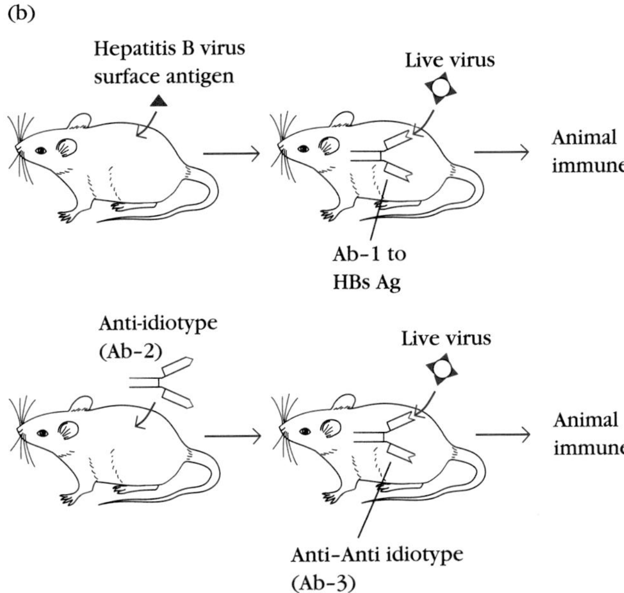

FIGURE 16-5 Use of anti-idiotype antibody as a vaccine. (a) The binding site on some anti-idiotype antibodies (Ab-2) resembles the structure of the epitope on the original antigen. Such anti-paratope antibody can interact with B cells specific for the original antigen, thus inducing production of more antibody against the antigen. (b) Immunization with anti-idiotype antibody has been shown experimentally to protect mice against hepatitis B virus without exposing the animal to the virus. HBsAg = hepatitis B surface antigen.

ate (ABA), they exhibit a limited antibody response, with most of the induced antibody expressing a single anti-ABA idiotype designated CRI_A. When A/J mice were pretreated with anti-idiotype (anti-CRI_A) serum and then were immunized with ABA-KLH, they no longer produced anti-ABA antibodies with the CRI_A idiotype. This suppressive effect also occurred when T cells from A/J mice treated with the anti-idiotype serum were transferred to normal A/J mice. When these recipient mice were immunized with ABA-KLH, they did not express anti-ABA antibody with the CRI_A idiotype, demonstrating that in this system the T_S cells are idiotype specific.

In some experimental systems T suppressor cells have been shown to release suppressor factors. Unlike cytokines, which are not antigen specific, some suppressor factors have been shown to be antigen specific, some have been shown to be idiotype specific, and some have been shown to be MHC restricted, suggesting that they may be soluble released forms of the T cell's receptor. There is speculation that suppressor factors might bind to peptide-MHC complexes displayed on antigen-presenting cells, serving to block the interaction of the antigen-presenting cells with other T cells.

TABLE 16-3 TRANSFER OF IMMUNE SUPPRESSION BY ANTIGEN-SPECIFIC T CELLS*

	Immune response of recipient	
Donor spleen cells*	Immunogen	Anti-DNP PFC
None	DNP-KLH	11,000
KLH-primed	DNP-KLH	89
KLH-primed with T cells removed	DNP-KLH	20,600
BGG-primed	DNP-KLH	11,600

* Donor mice were immunized with high doses of KLH or BGG, and their spleen cells were transferred to normal syngeneic mice. The recipients were then injected with DNP-KLH, and the immune response was determined in a hemolytic plaque assay using DNP-coated SRBCs as the test antigen.

SOURCE: Data from T. Tada and T. Takemori, 1974, *J. Exp. Med.* **140**:239.

Lack of Evidence for Distinct T_S-Cell Subpopulation

Although immune suppression mediated by T cells is a very real phenomenon that has been reproduced in several experimental systems, little solid evidence has supported the hypothesis that this suppression is mediated by a distinct T_S-cell subpopulation. Indeed, the lack of supporting evidence suggests that this hypothesis is not a tenable explanation for T-cell–mediated suppression.

For example, so far, no membrane marker unique to the putative T_S cells has been demonstrated. In most experimental systems, the cells mediating suppression have been identified as $CD8^+$ T cells. These presumed T_S cells were initially distinguished from $CD8^+$ T_C cells by MHC restriction to I-J, which purportedly mapped between the IA and IE loci. When the MHC was mapped by chromosome walking, however, no *I-J* locus was demonstrated—a finding that called into question the existence of the supposed I-J membrane marker. To date, despite the development of a large number of monoclonal antibodies specific for cell-membrane molecules, no unique membrane marker for a T_S-cell population has been identified.

The inability to maintain stable T-cell clones capable of transferring suppression in vivo or to clone antigen-specific suppressor factors also raises doubt about their existence. This limitation is in stark contrast to the large number of stable T_H and T_C clones that have been produced and the many factors that have been characterized and shown to mediate helper or cytotoxic activities in vivo. The antigen receptor on putative T_S cells has also not been characterized. S. Hedrick and co-workers evaluated rearrangements of the gene encoding the β chain of the $\alpha\beta$ T-cell receptor in T-cell lines that had been defined functionally as T_H cells, T_C cells, and T_S cells. Whereas each of the different T_H and T_C lines showed unique β-chain gene rearrangements, the T_S lines did not show functional rearrangements of the β chain, suggesting that suppressor cells do not utilize the $\alpha\beta$ heterodimer as their antigen-binding receptor (Figure 16-6).

Possible Explanations for T-Cell–Mediated Suppression

The inability to characterize a T-cell subpopulation functioning as the effector cell in immune suppression has led many immunologists to question whether a distinct T_S-cell lineage actually exists. They suggest that immune suppression may be generated by existing lymphocyte subpopulations, not by a separate cell lineage. For example, in one experimental system T cells activated by Con A had been shown to suppress a mixed-lymphocyte reaction (MLR). This suppression had been attributed to T_S cells. Later experiments revealed that the suppression resulted from the absorption of IL-2 by activated T_C cells, which depleted the level of IL-2 in the culture supernatant; since IL-2 is required for the MLR, this depletion of IL-2 effectively blocked the MLR in this system. This finding suggests that some of the suppressive effects observed in other experimental systems that have been attributed to putative T_S cells may, in fact, result from depletion of IL-2, an essential cytokine in both humoral and cell-mediated immune responses.

In some experimental systems the activities attributed to T_S cells may actually result from the antagonistic effects of cytokines produced by different subpopulations of antigen-specific T_H cells. For example, IL-10 is secreted by the T_H2 subset and functions to inhibit cytokine production by the T_H1 subset. If a

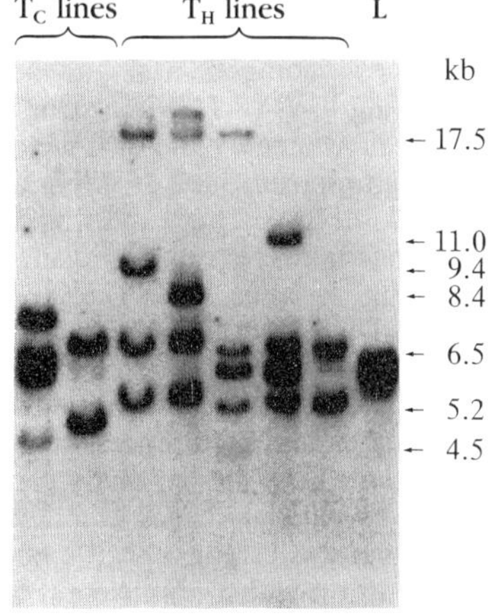

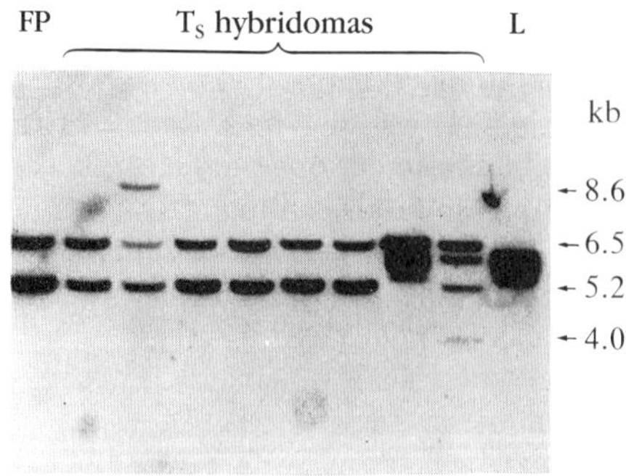

FIGURE 16-6 Evaluation of gene rearrangements in β-chain DNA by Southern blot analysis of TCR genes in T-cell lines functionally defined as T_H, T_C, and T_S cells. DNA from each cell line was digested with restriction endonucleases; the fragments were electrophoresed, blotted onto nitrocellulose, and then identified with radiolabeled β-chain cDNA. The liver-cell DNA (L) represents unrearranged, germ-line β-chain DNA. The blot patterns for all the T_H and T_C lines were different from one another and from liver-cell DNA, indicating that β-chain gene rearrangement had occurred in these lines. In contrast, the T_S hybridomas exhibited the same blot patterns as liver cells and the fusion partner (FP) indicating that no rearrangement of the β-chain gene DNA had occurred. [Adapted from S. Hedrick et al., 1985, *Proc. Nat'l Acad. Sci.* **82**:531.]

particular immune response depended on IL-2–mediated activation, the production of IL-10 would suppress that response. Similarly, IL-4 has been shown to block the IL-2 signal for proliferation in a B-cell line. In an experimental system that monitors B-cell activation by IL-2, production of IL-4 by antigen-specific T_H cells might lead to the erroneous conclusion that T_S cells had suppressed the response. Similar antagonistic effects between IL-4 and IFN-γ, discussed earlier in this chapter, might also be interpreted as suppression mediated by T_S cells.

In most experimental systems, only a single response is monitored (e.g., production of IL-2; generation of plasma cells secreting a particular isotype). For this reason, what appear to be suppressive effects may, in some cases, represent diversion from one isotype to another or diversion from one type of immune response to another. For example, if an experimental system is measuring IgE production and if IFN-γ is produced, then the IgE response would be suppressed and the production of IgG2a, induced by the IFN-γ, would go undetected. In such a system, a change in the nature of the immune response would be misinterpreted as suppression.

In some cases, T-cell–mediated suppression may be mediated by a population of T cells with cytotoxic activity. Recent evidence has demonstrated the existence of class II MHC–restricted cytotoxic T cells that are able to selectively kill antigen-presenting cells. These cytotoxic T cells have been shown to kill antigen-specific B cells, which capture antigen by means of their membrane-bound immunoglobulin and display a processed peptide together with the class II MHC on their membrane. In humans activated T_H cells also display class II MHC molecules, and there is some intriguing evidence suggesting that some of the depletion of $CD4^+$ T cells in AIDS may be due to selective killing by a population of class II–restricted cytotoxic T cells. Chapter 23 covers this topic in more detail.

The considerations discussed in this section and the previous section call into question the T_S cell as a distinct subpopulation. The observed suppression of particular immune responses in various experimental systems may, in fact, result from cytokine-mediated regulation of immune responsiveness or merely reflect changes in the pattern of cytokines present in the system, or changes in the population of effector cells that have been generated.

Neuroendocrine Regulation (Neuroimmunomodulation)

For centuries clinical observations have implicated psychosocial factors in susceptibility to disease. Reports abound suggesting a relationship between stress and immune function. Large numbers of popular books have appeared suggesting that psychoneuroimmune interactions could provide a biological mechanism for resistance or susceptibility to disease. Research in this area has been hampered by several limitations: The interdisciplinary nature of this area requires a breadth of expertise in immunology, neurobiology, and endocrinology that few people have, and the quantification of stress in general is fraught with numerous methodological difficulties. Nevertheless the past decade has witnessed a virtual explosion of interdisciplinary research that has documented the effects of the neural and endocrine systems on the activity of the immune system. The interaction appears to be two directional; that is, neuroendocrine mechanisms regulate the immune response and an active immune response induces changes in both neural and endocrine functions (Figure 16-7).

The central nervous system interacts with the immune system through autonomic innervation of lymphoid organs and through neuroendocrine mediators. The autonomic nervous system consists of motor neurons that conduct nerve impulses from the brain stem or spinal cord to heart muscle tissue and to various smooth muscles and glandular epithelial tissue. The autonomic nervous system, composed of the sympathetic and parasympathetic systems, serves to regulate the body's involuntary functions. Often both parasympathetic and sympathetic systems innervate an organ, exerting opposite effects on the organ. For example, the parasympathetic system slows down the heartbeat, whereas the sympathetic system accelerates the heartbeat; the ratio between sympathetic and para-

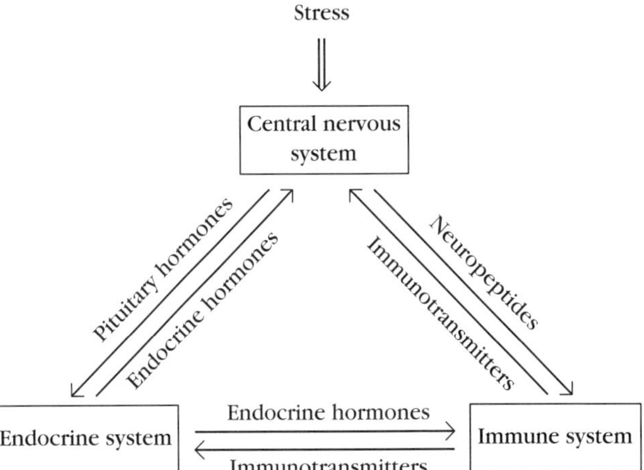

FIGURE 16-7 Schematic overview of the relationships between the neuroendocrine system and the immune system. See text for discussion. [Adapted from D. N. Khansari et al., 1990, *Immunol. Today* **11**:170.]

sympathetic impulses therefore determines the rate of heartbeat. During periods of stress (when strong emotions such as anger or fear are elicited), the sympathetic nervous system predominates. The sympathetic system releases neurotransmitter substances: Cholinergic fibers release acetylcholine and adrenergic fibers release norepinephrine (also known as noradrenaline).

Both primary and secondary lymphoid organs are innervated by the autonomic nervous system, particularly by adrenergic sympathetic nerve fibers, which often end in regions where lymphocytes are clustered. For example, adrenergic sympathetic nerve fibers crisscross the stromal-cell matrix of the bone marrow and are scattered throughout the cortex and medulla of the thymus. Similarly, a variety of compartments within lymph nodes and spleen are innervated by adrenergic nerve fibers. In some regions, such as the periarteriolar lymphatic sheath (PALS), these nerve fibers have been shown to form intimate anatomic associations with T lymphocytes and interdigitating dendritic cells.

During periods of stress the close functional relationship between the nervous system and the endocrine system is highlighted. For example, a number of neuroendocrine responses are commonly observed during periods of stress, regardless of the nature of the stress. During a stress response the hypothalamus acts on the anterior pituitary gland to secrete adrenocorticotropin (ACTH), which then acts upon the adrenal cortex inducing secretion of glucocorticoids (including hydrocortisone). In addition, the sympathetic nervous system and adrenal medulla are stimulated, resulting in production of the neurotransmitters acetylcholine and norepinephrine, and release of epinephrine from the adrenal medulla. Other neuroendocrine mediators (e.g., growth hormones, prolactin, melatonin, endorphins, and enkephalins) also are associated with the stress response.

Many of the neuroendocrine and neurotransmitter substances that are released during a stress response have been shown to either enhance or suppress the immune response (Table 16-4). Lymphocytes have receptors for a variety of neuroendocrine substances including ACTH, acetylcholine, epinephrine, vasoactive intestinal peptide (VIP), substance P, prolactin, growth hormone, stomatostatin, β-endorphin, and enkephalin. Perhaps the best-studied neuroendocrine substance is the glucocorticoid hydrocortisone, which has been shown to exhibit pronounced immunosuppressive effects on the immune response. Other neuroendocrine substances have been shown to have various effects on the immune system ranging from marked immunosuppression to immunopotentiation.

The immune system is also able to modulate the neural and endocrine systems. A number of thymic hormones, including thymosin and thymopoietin, have been shown to induce increased production of ACTH by the pituitary. Furthermore, a number of cytokines have been shown to modulate neural or endocrine responses. IL-1, for example, induces a constellation of effects that modulate the hypothalamus fever response, ACTH production by the pituitary, and glucocorticoid production by the adrenal cortex. In addition, some evidence indicates that cells of the immune system can produce a variety of neuropeptides and neuroendocrine hormones. Thus an interacting network exists between the nervous system, endocrine system, and immune system and changes in any one system can modulate the activity of the other systems.

The evidence that the neural and endocrine systems regulate the immune system raises the possibility that psychologic factors may also impact on immune function. A number of studies have suggested that a positive mental state is associated with a longer survival time for both cancer and AIDS. In contrast, patients hospitalized for major depression were found to have significantly reduced immune responses to various mitogens. Perhaps the most provocative experiments indicating a relationship between psychological factors and immune function comes from the work of R. Ader and N. Cohen indicating that behavorial conditioning can modify the immune response. Rats were injected with the immunosuppressive drug cyclophosphamide and at the same time were fed saccharin-flavored water (a conditioning stimulus). The rats were subsequently immunized with sheep red blood cells and antibody titers were later measured. As expected, the antibody response was suppressed by the cyclophosphamide. However, when the animals were later fed saccharin-flavored water (the conditioning stimulus) and were then reimmunized with SRBC, the immune response was suppressed compared with that of control animals which had received the initial treatment but had not been re-exposed to the conditioning stimulus at the time of the secondary injection.

A few studies suggest that conditioning also may be able to modify the immune response in humans. In one study the immune function of 20 ovarian cancer patients undergoing chemotherapy was assessed. A blood sample was drawn from each patient at home several days before each chemotherapy visit and a second sample was drawn at the hospital just prior to chemotherapy. Cell counts were the same in both blood samples, but the proliferative response to mitogen stimulation in the sample taken just prior to chemotherapy was significantly reduced. Thus, anticipation of chemotherapy in the hospital setting appears to have reduced the immune function in these women. In another study healthy volunteers received the tuberculin skin test once a month for 6 months. The test was administered by injecting PPD from a green vial

TABLE 16-4 NEUROENDOCRINE FACTORS WITH IMMUNOMODULATORY PROPERTIES

Factor	Action*	Immune response affected
Glucocorticoids (hydrocortisone)	S	Antibody production, NK-cell activity, cytokine production
Catecholamines (epinephrine)	S	Lymphocyte proliferation in response to mitogens
Acetylcholine	E	Number of lymphocytes and macrophages in bone marrow
β-Endorphin	E/S	Antibody production, activation of macrophages and T cells
Enkephalin	E/S	T-cell activation (enhanced at low dose; suppressed at high dose)
Prolactin	E	Macrophage activation, IL-2 production
Growth hormone	E	Antibody production, macrophage activation, IL-2 modulation
VIP	S/E	Cytokine production
Melatonin	E	Mixed-lymphocyte reaction (MLR), antibody production
ACTH	E/S	Cytokine production, NK-cell activity, antibody production, macrophage activation
Somatostatin	S/E	Plaque-forming count, response to mitogens
Sex hormones	S/E	Lymphocyte transformation, mixed-lymphocyte reaction

* E = enhancement; S = suppression.

SOURCE: Adapted from D. N. Khansari, 1990, *Immunol. Today* **11**:170.

into one arm and saline from a red vial into the other arm. Each volunteer was skin-test positive, developing a positive skin test only in the arm receiving the PPD. After 6 months the colored vials were switched, so that the PPD was now in the red vial and the saline was in the green vial; neither the experimenter nor the subject was aware of the switch. The results revealed a significant reduction in swelling and redness elicited by the PPD compared to the six previous times.

TOLERANCE

Why does the immune system not respond to self-antigens? Clearly there is nothing that uniquely distinguishes self-antigens from foreign antigens. And certainly the random V-J and V-D-J gene rearrangements of the immunoglobulin genes and TCR genes are capable of generating self-reactive specificities. Therefore the immune system must become nonresponsive to self-antigens. This active state of specific immunologic nonresponsiveness induced by prior exposure to an antigen is called *tolerance.* Tolerance can develop naturally, as it does when the developing animal becomes unresponsive to self-antigens, or tolerance can be induced experimentally. Experimentally induced tolerance is defined as a state in which an animal will fail to respond to an antigen that would normally be immunogenic. It is not known whether similar mechanisms generate both naturally acquired self-tolerance and experimentally induced tolerance. What is clear, however, is that the induction of tolerance depends on a number of variables and may proceed by a number of mechanisms. If tolerance to self-antigens fails to develop, then the consequences are autoimmunity.

Immunologic tolerance does not simply reflect the absence of an immune response, but rather an active response of the immune system that exhibits *antigenic specificity* and *memory*—the hallmarks of any immune response. Recognition of antigen by a lymphocyte can lead either to the cell's activation or to a nonresponsive (tolerant) state. Those antigens that induce lymphocyte activation are called *immunogens,* whereas those that induce a state of tolerance are called *tolerogens.* In naturally acquired tolerance, self-antigens serve as the tolerogens. In experimentally induced tolerance, a variety of foreign antigens can function as tolerogens provided that they are administered under certain conditions that promote a state of tolerance rather than immune activation.

Properties of Tolerance Induction

Tolerance is an acquired state that is induced most readily in immature lymphocytes and requires the persistence of antigen to be maintained.

Tolerance is learned or acquired. In 1945 R. Owen noted some interesting characteristics of nonidentical (dizygotic) twins born to cows whose twin placentas had fused at an early developmental stage, resulting in mixing of the circulating cells and antigens of the two calves. Owen observed that such twins are chimeras expressing two genetically distinct types of blood cells. Each calf was found to accept the genetically dissimilar blood cells of its twin without mounting an immune response against the cells; in other words these calves were tolerant to each other's blood cells. In 1951 P. B. Medawar extended these observations by showing that such dizygotic twins could also accept skin grafts from each other. On the basis of these observations, F. M. Burnet postulated in 1954 that "recognition of self is something that needs to be learned and is not an inherent genetic quality of an organism." He suggested that this learning takes place during embryonic development of the immune system when interaction of immune cells with self-antigens would lead to the elimination or inactivation of self-reactive lymphocyte clones. In the dizygotic twin cows, Burnet hypothesized, exposure to the blood-cell antigens during fetal development had resulted in elimination of reactive lymphocytes, allowing the nonself–blood cells to be viewed as self-cells by the immune system.

To test the hypothesis that tolerance is learned by the immune-system cells during early development of the immune system, R. Billingham, L. Brent, and P. B. Medawar injected strain A mice at birth with allogeneic strain B spleen cells. They discovered that as adults the neonatally injected strain A mice accepted skin grafts from the same strain B allogeneic mice while retaining the ability to reject skin grafts from other strains of mice. Exposure to strain B alloantigens when the immune system was immature had created a specific state of tolerance to these antigens. Since the immune system normally responds to alloantigens with an active response, the state of tolerance, or nonresponsiveness, had been acquired by exposure to these antigens during lymphocyte maturation.

Tolerance is induced more readily in immature lymphocytes than in mature ones. Burnet proposed that the immune system normally learns not to respond to self-antigens because of their presence during fetal development. Triplett tested this hypothesis by removing the pituitary gland from embryonic tree frog larvae. He reasoned that if the pituitary gland was absent during embryonic life, the frog's immune system would not acquire self-tolerance to the antigens of the pituitary. He allowed the larvae to mature in the absence of the pituitary (maintaining the pituitary glands by implanting them in the dermis of other tadpoles until the larvae had matured). When the pituitary gland was reimplanted in its original donor, the frog rejected its own pituitary, suggesting that in the absence of the pituitary antigens self-tolerance to the pituitary had not been acquired. If, however, only one half of the pituitary was removed and later reimplanted, the reimplanted part of the pituitary was accepted, suggesting that exposure of the immune system to pituitary antigens during early development had induced tolerance.

These experiments suggest that exposure to self-antigens during lymphocyte maturation leads to self-tolerance. It is much more difficult to induce a state of tolerance in adult animals. Tolerance is induced by 100-fold lower concentrations of protein antigens in neonatal mice than in adult mice, suggesting that immature lymphocytes are more readily tolerized than mature lymphocytes.

Maintenance of tolerance depends on the persistence of antigen. Tolerance induced by injecting animals with allogeneic cells lasts longer than that induced by injection of protein antigens. It appears that this difference is due to the persistence of the antigen. When neonatal animals are injected with allogeneic cells, the foreign cells survive within the neonatal host creating a chimera in which the antigen persists. When tolerance is induced to protein antigens, on the other hand, the antigen is gradually cleared and the tolerant state reverts to normal immune responsiveness.

F. Ramsdell and B. J. Fowlkes designed an experimental system to study the role of antigen persistence in the maintenance of tolerance. The system that they used made use of the previous finding that an endogenous superantigen binds simultaneously to $V_\beta17$ or $V_\beta6$ T-cell receptors and to the class II IE MHC molecule (see Table 12-4). Bone marrow cells from a strain lacking both the superantigen and the class II IE molecule were injected into lethally irradiated, MHC-compatible mice, which expressed the superantigen and class II IE molecule. The T cells expressing $V_{\beta}17$ or $V_{\beta}6$ TCRs that developed in these mice became tolerant and could no longer respond to this superantigen. However, when the tolerant T cells were removed and transferred back to mice that lacked both the superantigen and IE, the tolerant T cells reverted to a state of normal responsiveness. These results suggest that antigen is required to maintain the tolerant state.

Factors Affecting Experimentally Induced Tolerance

Antigen structure, dosage, and route of administration and the lymphocytes themselves determine whether the response of the immune system to a given foreign antigen will lead to immunity or tolerance. Experimental evidence demonstrating the role of these factors is reviewed briefly in this section.

Antigen Structure, Dosage, and Route of Administration

Generally, antigens introduced by an oral route lead to a state of tolerance. This phenomenon—called *oral tolerance*—may have evolved to prevent systemic immune reactions to ingested proteins that are necessary for nutrition. A number of folk remedies take advantage of oral tolerance. For example, American Indians used to eat deer liver to induce tolerance to poison oak. Since deer often feed upon poison oak, eating deer liver introduces the antigenic component of poison oak by an oral route. However, this method is not recommended because ingestion of the poison oak antigen may induce a potentially fatal hypersensitivity reaction along the mucous membranes of the gut.

Experimentally, antigens are usually introduced by subcutaneous or intravenous injection. In general, intravenous administration of an antigen is more likely to induce tolerance than administration by subcutaneous routes. Soluble antigens, in which aggregates have been removed, are also more likely to induce a state of tolerance. Recent evidence suggests that the ability of soluble antigens to induce tolerance may be due to the absence of a co-stimulatory signal. When soluble antigens are internalized by APCs, they fail to activate the cell and therefore fail to induce significant expression of the co-stimulatory B7 ligand. T-cell recognition of this antigen, in the absence of the co-stimulatory signal, may lead to a state of anergy (see Figure 12-15). This observation has led to several clinical trials in which soluble (deaggregated) antigens are being administered with the hope of inducing a specific state of tolerance. Clinical trials in humans are presently underway with soluble forms of allergens (cat dander and ragweed pollen) and autoantigens (myelin basic protein) to see if clinical tolerance can be induced in patients with allergies or autoimmune diseases.

The effect of antigen dosage on tolerogenicity was first discovered in mice when a potential vaccine for pneumococcal pneumonia was tested at two different doses. Mice were injected with 0.5 mg or 0.5 μg of the pneumococcal polysaccharide antigen and then were challenged with live pneumococci. Much to the surprise of the researchers, the mice given a high dose of the polysaccharide antigen all died after being challenged with live pneumococci, whereas the mice given the low dose were immune and survived challenge with the live organism. When this experiment was repeated, this time giving the mice an initial high dose of the polysaccharide followed by the low dose, the mice continued to show an absence of immunity and died following injection of the live organism. In other words, the high antigen dose had created a state of tolerance in these mice, so that they were no longer responsive to the 0.5-μg antigen dose that had previously induced immunity.

The relation of antigen dose to tolerance induction was studied more fully by N. A. Mitchison. He immunized groups of mice with various dosages of BSA over a 16-week period, waited 2 weeks, and then challenged the mice with a dose of BSA previously shown to be immunogenic. Serum antibody to BSA was measured, expressed as a percentage of that in control animals that had received only the final, immunogenic BSA challenge, and plotted against the BSA doses in the priming immunizations (Figure 16-8). Mitchison was surprised to find two zones of tolerance in which prior immunization inhibited the response to the immunogenic dose: a high zone above 10^{-2} g of BSA and a low zone that peaked at about 10^{-9} g of BSA. Between these two zones was an immunogenic zone, ranging from about 10^{-6} to 10^{-3} g of BSA, in which prior immunization produced immunity, evidenced by a secondary response to the final immunogenic dose of BSA. From these results Mitchison concluded that very high or very low doses of antigen are most likely to lead to a tolerant state. This principle has been applied in vaccine production, where the dosage has been shown to be critical for induction of immune status, and in allergy desensitization, where repeated low-dose injections of allergens have been shown to induce a state of tolerance to normal allergen levels (see Chapter 18).

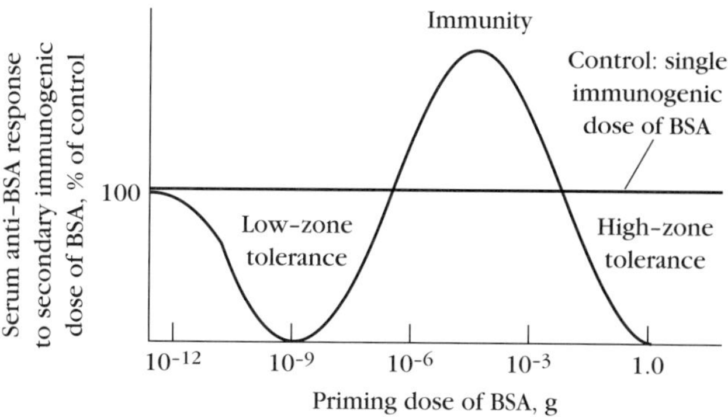

FIGURE 16-8 Experimental induction of tolerance at low and high doses of antigen. Mice were primed with various doses of BSA and then challenged with a known immunogenic dose. The serum anti-BSA level was less than that of controls at priming doses above 10^{-2} g (high-zone tolerance) and at low doses centered at 10^{-9} g (low-zone tolerance). Between these tolerance zones was a zone of immunity, characterized by a heightened secondary antibody response. [Adapted from N. A. Mitchison, 1964, *Proc. Royal Society (B)* **161**:275.]

Susceptibility of T and B Cells

Tolerance can be induced in both B and T cells, but the two lineages differ substantially in the quantity of antigen needed to induce tolerance and in the duration of the tolerant state. In order to compare tolerance induction in T cells and B cells, J. Chiller and co-workers injected mice with deaggregated human gamma globulin (deHGG) and then removed thymus (T) and bone marrow (B) cells at various times after injection. The tolerant cells were combined with normal bone marrow or thymus cells and then injected into x-irradiated syngeneic recipients, which were later challenged with an immunogenic dose of HGG. Mice receiving either tolerant thymus cells plus normal bone marrow cells or tolerant bone marrow cells plus normal thymus cells were tolerant to the immunogenic dose of HGG. However, the kinetics of tolerance induction was fundamentally different for T cells and B cells (Figure 16-9). The thymus cells became tolerant sooner after injection of deHGG and remained tolerant longer than the bone marrow cells, indicating that immunologic tolerance is maintained more effectively by T cells than by B cells. However, since most B-cell responses require T-cell help, even if a B cell is responsive to a given antigen, antibody production will be determined by the state of responsiveness of the T cells.

Mechanisms of Tolerance Induction

The ability of the immune system to discriminate between self- and nonself-antigen implies that the system must be able to make a qualitative distinction between contact with self-antigen and contact with nonself-antigen. Just how this distinction is achieved is a matter of a great deal of speculation. Presently two hypotheses have been suggested that provide a qualitative basis by which tolerogenicity versus immunogenicity can be achieved. The first long-standing hypothesis suggests that the qualitative distinction of what constitutes a self-antigen is achieved temporally, that is, by the maturational state of a T or B cell when it contacts antigen. Immature T and B cells would be expected to contact only self-antigens and therefore would enter a state of immunologic tolerance. A second hypothesis suggests that differences in signaling may regulate whether a state of immune activation or a state of tolerance is achieved. For example, activation in the absence of the co-stimulatory signal may lead to tolerance, whereas activation together with the co-stimulatory signal may lead to immunity.

A functional state of tolerance can be achieved either by eliminating the reactive cells *(clonal deletion)* or by inactivating them *(clonal anergy),* so that while the cells are present they are functionally nonresponsive. Tolerance induction in immature B and T cells occurs in the primary lymphoid organs (bone marrow and thymus) during the process of maturation. Since T and B-cell maturation is an ongoing process, occurring throughout the life of the animal, this type of tolerance, known as *central tolerance,* must also be an ongoing process.

It is difficult to imagine, however, that all possible self-antigens have access to the bone marrow and thymus during T- and B-cell maturation. Instead, it seems likely that some immunocompetent T and B cells are generated with receptors specific for self-antigens that were not present in the primary lymphoid organ during their maturation. To account for tolerance to such antigens, some have suggested that tolerance to self-antigens also may be induced in mature peripheral lymphocytes. This tolerance, which may be achieved through different means than central tolerance, is referred to as *peripheral tolerance.* Both B and T cells can be tolerized in the periphery. Peripheral tolerance is thought to be particularly important in the case of the B-cell system because a B cell's antigen-binding receptor does not remain constant following maturation but is diversified in mature peripheral B cells through the process of somatic mutation. It is therefore possible that self-reactive B cells might be generated by random mutational events in mature B

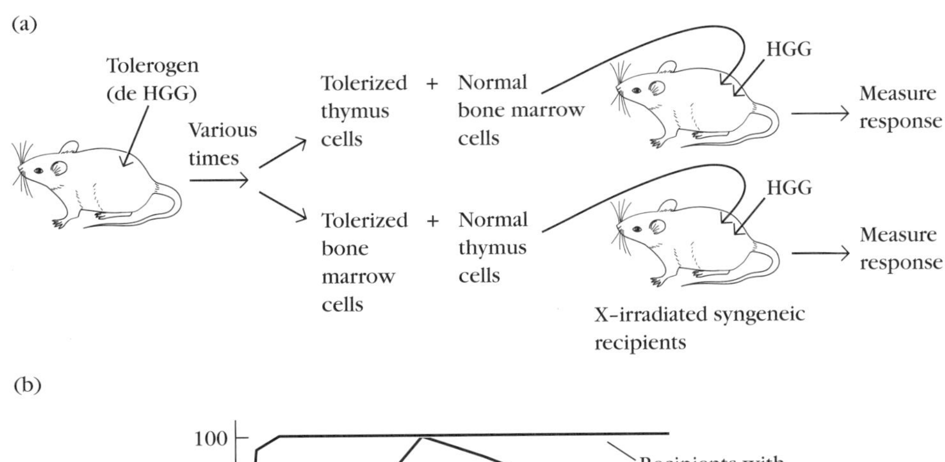

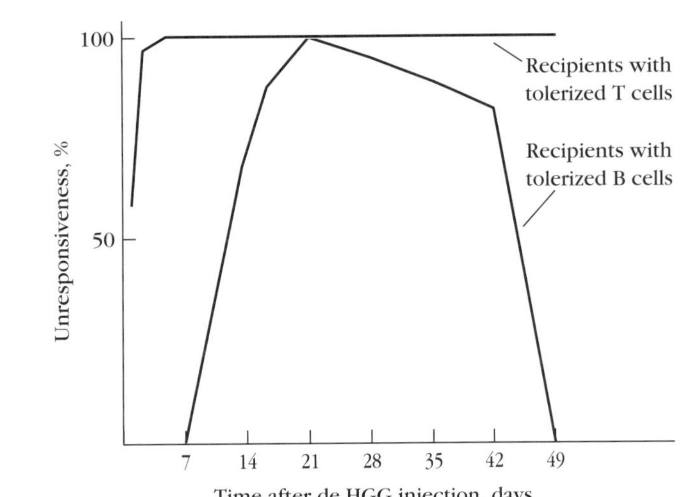

FIGURE 16-9 Experimental demonstration that T cells and B cells differ in their susceptibility to tolerance induction. (a) Outline of experimental protocol. At the time of this experiment there was no way to separate B cells from T cells; therefore, the thymus was used as a source of T cells and bone marrow as a source of B cells. After transfer of tolerized cells plus normal cells into syngeneic, x-irradiated recipients, the response of the recipients to an immunizing dose of HGG was determined. (b) Plot of unresponsiveness of the recipients versus time after tolerogen injection when tolerance-induced cells were removed. Note that T cells became tolerant sooner and remained tolerant longer than B cells. [Adapted from J. Chiller et al., 1971, *Science* **171**:813.]

cells. Peripheral tolerance would serve to regulate these potentially self-reactive cells.

Experimental Induction of B-Cell Tolerance

A variety of transgenic systems have been developed to study tolerance induction in B cells. These systems have shown that self-reactive B cells can be rendered tolerant either through clonal deletion of self-reactive B cells or through clonal anergy in which self-reactive B cells continue to be present but are functionally inactivated. Induction of B-cell tolerance can occur either in the bone marrow (central tolerance) or in the peripheral lymphoid tissue (peripheral tolerance).

Detection of self-reactive B cells in central or peripheral lymphoid tissue of tolerant animals is technically very difficult owing to the rarity of these cells within the animal. Transgenic mice expressing an immunoglobulin transgene have provided a way to resolve the technical difficulties. Because the immunoglobulin transgene is already productively rearranged, the transgene will inhibit further rearrangement of the endogeneous immunoglobulin genes; consequently a high percentage of the B cells in these mice will express the transgene as their membrane-bound immunoglobulin (mIg).

EVIDENCE FOR CLONAL ANERGY OF B CELLS. Although demonstrating antigen-specific tolerant B cells in vivo is difficult, some researchers have done so successfully by administering radioactively labeled antigen and quantitating the number of antigen-binding B cells in tolerant mice and in normal immune mice. Most such experiments have shown that antigen-reactive B cells are not deleted in animals in which tolerance has been induced experimentally. Even in normal animals, B cells reactive with self-antigens can be shown to be present, but their activity is regulated either by the tolerant state of the T_H cell or by an anergic state of the B cell itself.

A transgenic system developed by C. Goodnow and his co-workers has served to clarify the process of tolerance induction in B cells. Goodnow's experimental system included two groups of transgenic mice (Figure 16-10a). One carried a hen egg lysozyme (HEL) transgene linked to a metallothionine promoter, which placed transcription of the HEL gene under the control of zinc levels. The other group of transgenic mice carried rearranged immunoglobulin heavy- and light-chain transgenes encoding anti-HEL antibody. In normal mice the frequency of HEL-specific B cells is on the order of 1 in 10^3, but in these transgenic mice the rearranged anti-HEL transgene is expressed by 60–90% of the B cells. Goodnow mated the two groups of transgenics to produce "double-transgenic" offspring carrying both the HEL and anti-HEL transgenes. The question Goodnow then asked was whether the expression of HEL early in development would regulate development of the B cells expressing the anti-HEL transgene.

The Goodnow double-transgenic system has yielded several interesting findings concerning tolerance induction in B cells (Table 16-5). He found that double-transgenic mice expressing high levels of HEL (10^{-9} *M*) continued to have peripheral B cells bearing anti-HEL membrane antibody, but these B cells were functionally anergic. The concentration of HEL in these double transgenic mice was estimated to be sufficient to occupy 45% of the anti-HEL antibodies on the B cells. A second group of double transgenics, expressing ten times lower levels of HEL (10^{-10} *M*) also was obtained from the matings. In this case HEL occupied less than 5% of the anti-HEL antibodies on the B cells, and under these conditions the B cells were shown to be functionally active. Thus the concentration of HEL and receptor occupancy appeared to

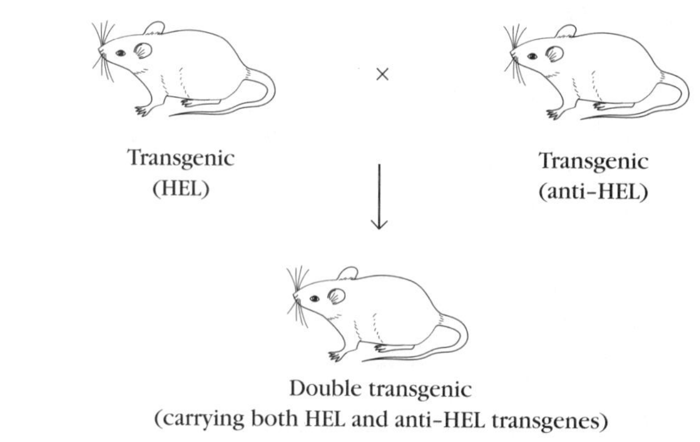

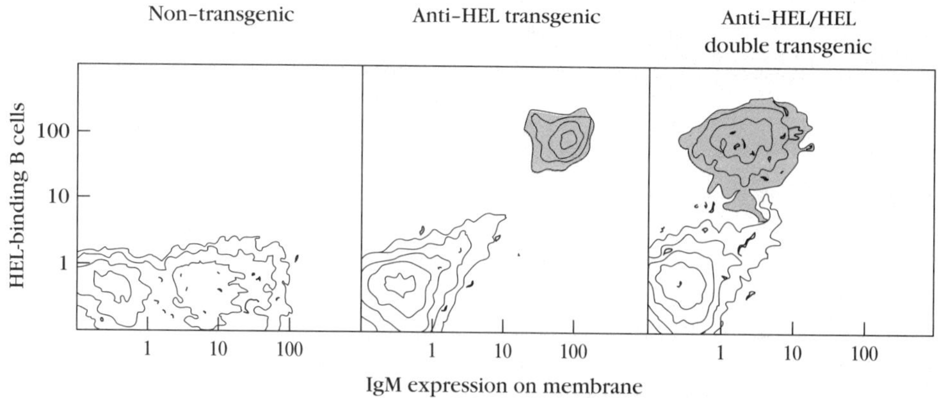

FIGURE 16-10 Goodnow's experimental system for studying B-cell tolerance. (a) Production of double-transgenic mice carrying transgenes encoding HEL (hen egg lysozyme) and anti-HEL antibody. (b) FACS analysis of B-cell binding to HEL compared with membrane IgM levels. Nontransgenics had no B cells that bound HEL *(left)*. Both anti-HEL transgenics *(middle)* and anti-HEL/HEL double transgenics *(right)* had B cells that bound HEL (purple), although the level of membrane IgM was somewhat lower in the double transgenics.

TABLE 16-5 EXPRESSION OF ANTI-HEL TRANSGENE BY MATURE PERIPHERAL B CELLS IN SINGLE AND DOUBLE-TRANSGENIC MICE

Experimental group	HEL level	Membrane anti-HEL	Anti-HEL PFC/spleen*	Anti-HEL serum titer*
Anti-HEL single transgenics	None	+	High	High
Anti-HEL/HEL double transgenics				
Group 1	High (10^{-9} *M*)	+	Low	Low
Group 2	Low (10^{-10} *M*)	+	High	High
Group 2 + Zn^{2+}	High (>10^{-9} *M*)	+	Low	Low

* Experimental animals were immunized with hen egg lysozyme (HEL). Several days later hemolytic plaque assays were conducted to determine the PFC/spleen, and the serum anti-HEL titer was determined.

SOURCE: Adapted from C. C. Goodnow, 1992, *Annu. Rev. Immunol.* **10**:489.

determine whether the B cell became anergic or not. To determine whether the mature HEL-reactive B cells in the low-HEL double transgenics could later be rendered anergic, Goodnow fed the mice zinc water to elevate the serum HEL concentration. Within 4 days, the previously responsive anti-HEL B cells became functionally anergic. Thus tolerance could be restored in low-HEL animals by elevating the level of HEL.

Analysis of B cells from the double transgenics showed that the tolerant cells expressed twenty-fold lower levels of membrane IgM than reactive cells but about the same levels of membrane IgD. Goodnow has suggested that reduction in the mIgM level might cause quantitative differences in signal transduction, leading to the anergic state. The observation that the anergic B cells in this system express both IgM and IgD indicates that anergy is being induced in mature B cells rather than in immature B cells.

EVIDENCE FOR CLONAL DELETION OF B CELLS. Transgenic experiments also have provided evidence that B cells can be rendered tolerant by clonal deletion. D. A. Nemazee and K. Burki used transgenic mice carrying a transgene encoding an IgM antibody specific for an H-2^k class I MHC molecule. Since class I molecules are expressed on the membrane of all nucleated cells, the H-2^k class I MHC molecule would be present on bone marrow cells. The presence of B cells expressing the anti-class I^k transgene was determined in H-2^d and H-$2^{d/k}$ transgenics. In the H-2^d mice 25–50% of the peripheral B cells expressed the transgene both as membrane-bound antibody and as secreted antibody. In the H-$2^{d/k}$ mice, in contrast, the transgene was not expressed by peripheral B cells either as membrane antibody or as secreted antibody (Table 16-6). This study suggests that the presence of the H-2^k class I MHC molecules in the H-$2^{d/k}$ transgenic mice induced

TABLE 16-6 EXPRESSION OF TRANSGENE ENCODING IgM ANTIBODY TO H-2^k CLASS I MHC MOLECULES

		Expression of transgene	
Experimental animal	No. animals tested	As membrane Ab	As secreted Ab (μg/ml)
Nontransgenic	13	(−)	<0.3
H-2^d Transgenics	7	(+)	93.0
H-$2^{d/k}$ Transgenics	6	(−)	<0.3

SOURCE: Adapted from D. A. Nemazee and K. Burki, 1989, *Nature* **337**:562.

clonal deletion of those B cells expressing the transgene-encoded IgM specific for H-2^k class I MHC molecules. Deletion in this case appears to occur during B-cell maturation in the bone marrow.

Nemazee and Burki then asked what would happen if the class I MHC molecule was expressed only in the periphery. To determine this, they produced a transgene consisting of the class I K^b locus linked to a liver-specific promoter, so that the transgene could be expressed only in the liver. Transgenic mice expressing an anti-K^b antibody on their B cells also were produced, and the two groups of transgenic mice were then mated. FACS analysis of the B cells in the resulting double-transgenic mice showed that immature B cells expressing the transgene product (anti-K^b) were present in the bone marrow but not in the peripheral lymphoid organs (Figure 16-11). In the first experiments of Nemazee and Burki, the class I MHC transgene was expressed on all nucleated cells, and B-cell deletion occurred in the bone marrow. In their second system, however, the class I MHC transgene was expressed only in the liver, and B-cell deletion occurred in the periphery.

A modification of the Goodnow HEL/anti-HEL double-transgenic system (see Figure 16-10) has provided additional evidence that B-cell tolerance can be achieved through clonal deletion. In this modified system the HEL transgene was engineered to include the extracellular spacer, transmembrane sequence, cytoplasmic tail, and promoter sequence of the class I K^b gene. This allowed HEL to be expressed in a membrane-bound form, whereas in the original system HEL was secreted. Analysis of double-transgenic mice carrying the modified HEL transgene showed that immature B cells expressing the anti-HEL transgene were present in the bone marrow but mature B cells expressing anti-HEL, were deleted. In the original system in which HEL was secreted, however, mature B cells expressing anti-HEL membrane-bound antibody were shown to be present but functionally anergic (see Table 16-5, group 1).

The process of clonal deletion appears to involve two separate sequential events: developmental arrest and cell death. Developmental arrest appears to occur after B-cell binding to the self-antigen (HEL). The arrested B cells exhibit several changes: They express membrane markers of immature cells, they fail to express high levels of homing receptors and adhesion molecules, and they also appear to lack certain signal-transduction membrane molecules. In the presence of the tolerogen (membrane-bound HEL) the arrested B cells will die by apoptosis within 1–3 days. However, if the arrested B cells are purified by flow cytometry and cultured with thymocytes (as a source of T cells) in the absence of tolerogen, then developmental arrest can be reversed.

Experimental Induction of T-Cell Tolerance

Experiments studying tolerance induction in T cells have been difficult to perform because T cells bind antigen associated with MHC molecules rather than soluble antigen. Therefore, the number of antigen-specific T cells cannot be determined by the binding of radioactively labeled antigen, as is possible with B cells. Antigen-specific T cells can be assessed with clonotypic monoclonal antibody specific for the binding site of the T-cell receptor.

EVIDENCE FOR CLONAL DELETION OF T CELLS. The most effective way to ensure self-tolerance of T cells is by the process of intrathymic deletion (negative selection) of self-reactive thymocytes discussed in Chapter 12 (see Figure 12-4). Most probably, exogenous (secreted) proteins synthesized in peripheral tissue outside the thymus circulate through the thymus where they can be internalized, processed, and presented by antigen-presenting cells to immature, double-positive $CD4^+8^+$ thymocytes, resulting in deletion of any self-reactive thymocytes. However, thymic deletion of thymocytes reactive with endogenous (nonsecreted) self-proteins synthesized outside the thymus seems more unlikely because such self-proteins would not be presented to the developing thymocytes. Therefore, self-tolerance to extrathymic endogenous proteins may need to be induced in mature $CD8^+$ T cells in peripheral tissues.

Two transgenic systems have been used to analyze induction of tolerance to endogenous self-proteins, which are recognized by $CD8^+$ T cells. These analyses have revealed that the occurrence of central or peripheral tolerance induction depends on whether the antigen is synthesized within the thymus or outside of it. In one of these systems transgenic mice were prepared carrying an $\alpha\beta$-TCR transgene derived from an H-2^b CTL clone that cross-reacted with allogeneic L^d class I MHC molecules. T cells expressing this transgene could be identified with a clonotypic monoclonal antibody. The presence of mature T cells expressing the transgene was compared in H-2^b and H-$2^{b/d}$ transgenic mice (Figure 16-12). In the H-2^b mice the TCR transgene product was present on 20–95% of the peripheral T cells. Most of these T cells were $CD8^+$ cells and were functionally capable of lysing target cells expressing L^d molecules. In the H-$2^{b/d}$ transgenic mice, functional CTLs capable of lysing L^d target cells were absent. The results indicate that expression of the L^d molecule within the thymus had resulted in intrathymic

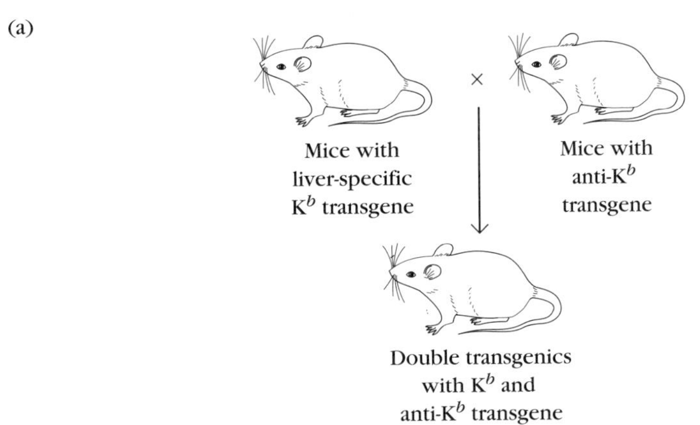

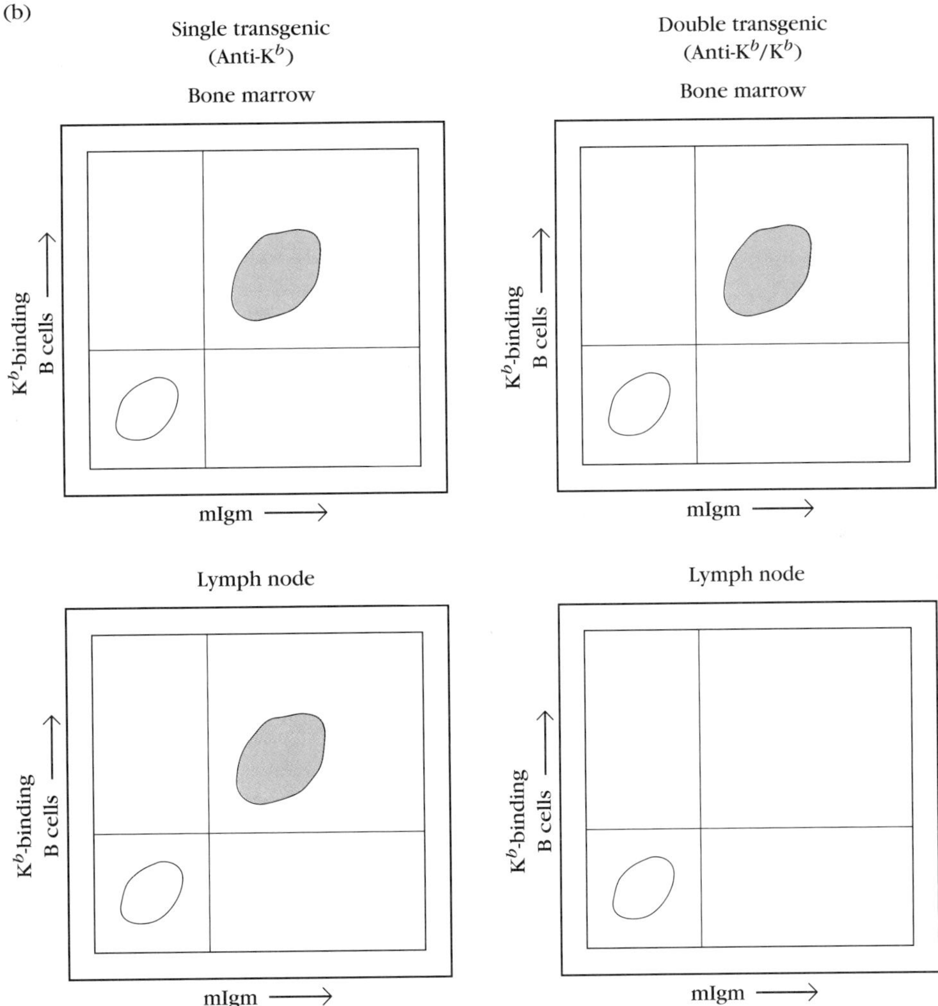

FIGURE 16-11 Experimental demonstration of clonal deletion of self-reactive mature peripheral B cells. (a) Production of double-transgenic mice expressing the class I K^b molecule and anti-K^b antibody. Because the K^b transgene contained a liver-specific promoter, K^b was not expressed in the bone marrow in the double transgenics. (b) FACS analysis of B-cell binding to K^b in anti-K^b single transgenics and anti-K^b/K^b double transgenics versus level of membrane IgM (mIgM). In the double transgenics, the absence of B cells expressing anti-K^b in the lymph nodes and their presence in the bone marrow indicates that mature self-reactive B cells were deleted in the periphery.

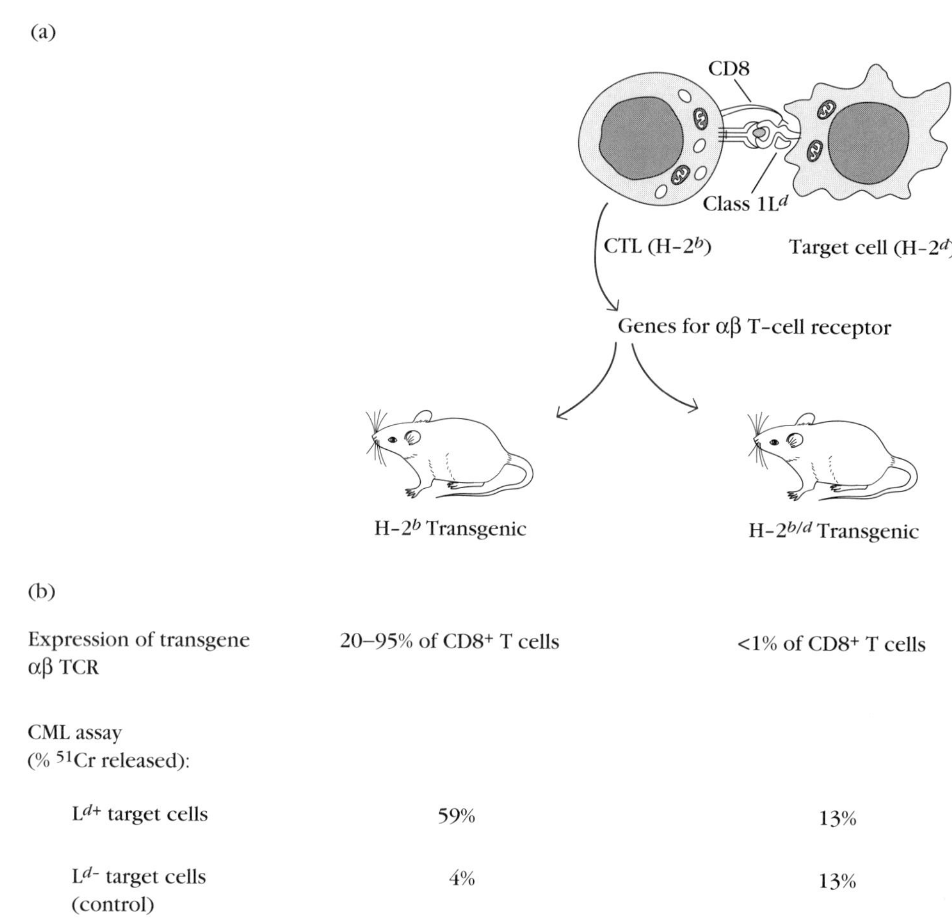

FIGURE 16-12 Experimental demonstration of clonal deletion of self-reactive T cells. (a) H-2^b and H-$2^{b/d}$ transgenic mice were produced carrying transgenes for an $\alpha\beta$ T-cell receptor derived from an H-2^b CTL. Although this particular transgene must have been specific for foreign peptides presented with self-class I MHC molecules, it cross-reacted with allogeneic L^d class I MHC molecules. (b) Peripheral T cells from the transgenic mice were analyzed by FACS to determine the presence of $CD8^+$ T cells expressing the transgenic $\alpha\beta$ T-cell receptor. The functional activity of the $CD8^+$ T cells was determined by CML assays using ^{51}Cr-labeled target cells that expressed L^d molecules. The expression of L^d in the H-$2^{b/d}$ transgenics induced clonal deletion of T cells expressing L^d-specific receptors. [Adapted from W. C. Sha et al., 1988, *Nature* **336**:73.]

(central) deletion of thymocytes bearing the transgene-encoded TCR specific for L^d molecules.

The second transgenic system consisted of H-2^k mice carrying a transgene for the K^b class I molecule linked to an insulin promoter, which limited expression of K^b to pancreatic β cells. These transgenic mice were tolerant to K^b and could not reject allogeneic K^b skin grafts. In this system thymocytes specific for K^b were shown to be present in the thymus, whereas mature peripheral $CD8^+$ T cells specific for K^b were absent, suggesting that clonal deletion of mature T cells had occurred in the periphery.

EVIDENCE FOR CLONAL ANERGY OF T CELLS. Recent experiments suggest that T-cell tolerance also can be induced in mature T cells by clonal anergy. As discussed in Chapter 12, when a T cell is activated in the absence of a suitable co-stimulatory signal, the cell may become anergic (see Figure 12-15). L. C. Burkly and co-workers asked what would happen if class II MHC molecules were inappropriately expressed on peripheral cells that were not antigen-presenting cells (APCs) and therefore could not generate the requisite co-stimulatory signal. The experimental system that Burkly used involved an endogenous superantigen specific for the class II IE molecule and T-cell receptors with the $V_\beta17a$ domain. As discussed in Chapter 4, superantigens bind to specific V_β sequences in the T-cell receptor and to MHC molecules outside their normal antigen-binding sequences (see Figure 4-15). Kappler and Marrack showed that this particular superantigen can cross-link all thymocytes expressing $V_\beta17a$

to IE molecules on thymic stromal cells, resulting in clonal deletion of these thymocytes within the thymus (see Figure 12-9).

Burkly modified this system so that T cells did not encounter the class II IE molecule in the thymus but instead encountered it only in the periphery on non-APCs. To do this, he inserted an IE transgene linked to an insulin promoter into IE^- mice. These transgenics expressed IE molecules only on their pancreatic β cells. Analysis of these transgenic mice revealed the presence of mature T cells expressing V_β17a TCRs in the periphery; however, these T cells were functionally anergic. Thus it appears that when the superantigen cross-linked the mature V_β17a T cells to IE molecules on pancretic β cells, the lack of a co-stimulatory signal led to clonal anergy rather than immunity.

Summary

1. Antigen, antibody, and immune complexes have each been shown to play a role in regulation of immune responsiveness. A decline in antigen levels ultimately results in diminished clonal proliferation and a decline in further humoral or cell-mediated responses. That antigen concentration is not the only regulating factor is indicated by the cyclical appearance of plasma cells that are specific for a given antigen despite a linear decline in the levels of that antigen. Antibody has been shown to suppress the immune response, possibly by binding to antigen and preventing further B-cell activation. Immune complexes have been shown to both increase and decrease the immune response to an antigen.

2. Cytokines are also important regulators of the immune response. In some cases they act synergistically, so that two cytokines together have more than an additive effect. In other cases cytokines act antagonistically, so that the presence of one cytokine blocks the activity of another. Cytokines may also influence the type of immune response that occurs. Some cytokines have been shown to preferentially activate a cell-mediated response, such as delayed-type hypersensitivity, and other cytokines are more likely to activate a humoral antibody response.

3. The unique variable-region amino acid sequences of antibodies and T-cell receptors are recognized as antigenic determinants by the immune system. Thus the secreted antibodies and clonally expanded T-cell receptors generated in an immune response in turn elicit anti-idiotype antibodies. According to the network theory, a series (or network) of anti-idiotype antibodies are induced during an immune response; these anti-idiotype antibodies act to up-regulate the immune response in some cases and to down-regulate it in other cases.

4. The observed suppression of immune responsiveness by T cells, which can be transferred from a suppressed animal to a nonsuppressed one, was originally attributed to a distinct subpopulation of T cells called T_S cells. However, T_S cells expressing unique membrane markers and secreting suppression factors have not been cloned. Many researchers now believe that T-cell–mediated suppression can be explained by shifts in cytokine patterns and/or consumption in various experimental systems, resulting in changes in the nature or intensity of the immune response.

5. Immunologic tolerance is a specific state of nonresponsiveness to an antigen. Tolerance develops more easily in fetal and neonatal animals than in adults, suggesting that immature T and B cells are more susceptible to the induction of tolerance. Induction of tolerance in adult animals, which can be achieved under certain circumstances, is influenced by the route of antigen administration, the dosage of antigen, and the ability of the antigen to be phagocytosed. In general, T cells are more susceptible to tolerance induction than B cells, and the tolerance of an animal probably is determined by the state of responsiveness of its T cells.

6. Induction of tolerance in both T and B cells appears to occur by two mechanisms—clonal deletion and clonal anergy—both of which have been demonstrated experimentally. Immature lymphocytes are eliminated by clonal deletion during T-cell and B-cell maturation in the thymus and bone marrow, respectively. Mature peripheral T and B cells reactive with endogenous self-antigens expressed only in peripheral tissues also are eliminated by clonal deletion. In clonal anergy, mature lymphocytes present in the peripheral lymphoid organs become functionally inactivated possibly by the interaction with antigen in the absence of the co-stimulatory signals necessary for generation of an immune response.

References

ADER, R., and N. COHEN. 1993. Psychoneuroimmunology: conditioning and stress. *Annu. Rev. Psychol.* **44**:53.

ADER, R., D. FELTEN, and N. COHEN. 1990. Interactions between the brain and the immune system. *Annu. Rev. Pharmacol. Toxicol.* **30**:561.

BATCHELOR, J. R., G. LOMBARDI, and R. I. LECHLER. 1989. Speculations on the specificity of suppression. *Immunol. Today* **10**:37.

BURKLY, L. C., D. LO, and R. A. FLAVELL. 1990. Tolerance in transgenic mice expressing major histocompatibility molecules extrathymically on pancreatic cells. *Science* **248**:1364.

DAVIE, J. M., M. V. SEIDEN, N. S. GREENSPAN et al. 1986. Structural correlates of idiotopes. *Annu. Rev. Immunol.* **4**:147.

FINKELMAN, F. D., J. HOLMES, J. F. URBAN et al. 1990. Lymphokine control of in vivo immunoglobulin isotype secretion. *Annu. Rev. Immunol.* **8**:303.

FIORENTINO, D. F., M. W. BOND, and T. R. MOSMANN. 1989. Two types of mouse T helper cells: T_H2 clones secrete a factor that inhibits cytokine production by T_H1 clones. *J. Exp. Med.* **170**:2081.

GOODNOW, C. C. 1992. Transgenic mice and analysis of B-cell tolerance. *Annu. Rev. Immunol.* **10**:489.

HARTLEY, S. B., M. P. COOKE, D. A. FULCHER et al. 1993. Elimination of self-reactive B lymphocytes proceeds in two stages: arrested development and cell death. *Cell* **72**:325.

HERMANN, G. E., and M. S. O'DORISIO. 1991. Modulation of IgA synthesis by neuroendocrine peptides. *Trends Endocrinol. Metab.* **2**:68.

JERNE, N. K. 1974. Towards a network theory of the immune system. *Annals of Immun.* (Institute Pasteur) **125C**:373.

KHANSARI, D. N., A. J. MURGO, and R. E. FAITH. 1990. Effects of stress on the immune system. *Immunol. Today* **5**:170.

MILLER, J. F. A. P., G. MORAHAN, J. ALLISON et al. 1989. T cell tolerance in transgenic mice expressing major histocompatibility class I molecules in defined tissues. *Immunol. Rev.* **107**:109.

MILLER, J. F. A. P., and G. MORAHAN. 1992. Peripheral T cell tolerance. *Annu. Rev. Immunol.* **10**:51.

NIO, D. A., R. N. MOYLAN, and J. K. ROCHE. 1993. Modulation of T lymphocyte function by neuropeptides. *J. Immunol.* **150**:5281.

RAMSDELL, F., and B. J. FOWLKES. 1992. Maintenance of in vivo tolerance by persistence of antigen. *Science* **257**:1130.

ROSER, B. J. 1989. Cellular mechanisms in neonatal and adult tolerance. *Immunol. Rev.* **107**:179.

SCHWARZ, R. H. 1989. Acquisition of immunologic self-tolerance. *Cell* **57**:1073.

SCHWARZ, R. H. 1990. A cell culture model for T lymphocyte clonal anergy. *Science* **248**:1349.

VON BOEHMER, H., and P. KISIELOW. 1990. Self-nonself discrimination by T cells. *Science* **248**:1369.

Study Questions

1. Indicate whether each of the following statements is true or false. If you think a statement is false, explain why.
   a. The mature B cell is made tolerant more easily than the immature B cell.
   b. Tolerance can be induced more easily in neonatal animals than in adult animals.
   c. If mice are immunized with HRBC and then are immunized a day later with SRBC, the antibody response to the SRBC will be much higher than that achieved in control mice immunized only with SRBC.
   d. IFN-γ and IL-4 act antagonistically.
   e. Cytokines can regulate which branch of the immune system is activated.
   f. Anti-idiotype antibody appears as the internal image of the original antigen.
   g. TEPC-15 monoclonal antibody is an anti-idiotype antibody induced in the immune response to the phosphorylcholine determinant of pneumococcal polysaccharide.
   h. The idiotype of an antibody molecule is composed of multiple idiotopes.
   i. A state of tolerance can be induced more readily with aggregated than with deaggregated protein.
   j. Following tolerance induction by clonal anergy, antigen-binding lymphocytes are present in the tolerant animal.
   k. All T-cell tolerance occurs via clonal deletion.

2. If you wanted to use the idiotype principle to vaccinate against hepatitis B virus, what would you use to immunize the animals?

3. You have been given a mouse that is tolerant to a protein antigen A and does not produce anti-A antibodies when immunized with antigen A. How could you determine whether this tolerance results from failure of the animal's T_H cells or B cells to respond to antigen A.

4. Define the following terms: (a) paratope, (b) epitope, (c) idiotope, and (d) agretope.

5. In the Goodnow experiment demonstrating clonal anergy of B cells, transgenic mice carrying a transgene encoding antibody against hen egg lysozyme (HEL) were compared with double transgenics containing the anti-HEL gene and a HEL gene linked to the zinc-activated metallothionine promoter.
   a. In both the single and double transgenics, 60–90% of the B cells expressed anti-HEL membrane-bound antibody. Explain why.

b. How could you show that the membrane antibody on these B cells is specific for HEL and how could you determine its isotype?
c. Why was the metallothionine promoter used in constructing the HEL transgene?
d. Design an experiment to prove that the B cells, not the T_H cells, from the double transgenics were anergic.

6. Experiments in which expression of the TCR β-chain exon $V_{\beta}17a$ was assessed have provided evidence for both clonal deletion and clonal anergy of T cells. What was the major difference between these experiments that would explain why clonal deletion occurred in the Kapplar and Marrack experiment and clonal anergy in the Burkly experiment?

7. As discussed in Chapter 12, both positive and negative selection of thymocytes occurs during T-cell maturation in the thymus.
a. What would be the consequences if a mouse strain were unable to carry out positive thymic selection?
b. What would be the consequences if a mouse strain were unable to carry out negative thymic selection?

8. Experiments in the early 1970s led to the hypothesis that T suppressor cells, a distinct T-cell subpopulation, mediates immune suppression.
a. Describe the experimental findings that led to this hypothesis.
b. Describe four experimental findings that have called into question the existence of a distinct T_S subpopulation.
c. Assuming that a distinct T_S-cell lineage does not exist, what other mechanisms could account for the T-cell–mediated suppression observed in vitro?

9. In the transgenic experiment depicted in Figure 16-12, H-2^b and H-$2^{b/d}$ transgenic mice were produced carrying genes for the $\alpha\beta$ T-cell receptor of a H-2^b CTL clone that cross-reacted with the L^d class I MHC molecule.
a. Why did a high percentage of mature $CD8^+$ T cells express this transgene in the H-2^b mice but not in H-$2^{b/d}$ mice?
b. Why were H-$2^{b/d}$ mice used instead of H-2^d mice in this experiment?
c. What assay was used to assess the functional activity of the $CD8^+$ T cells?

THE COMPLEMENT SYSTEM

The complement system, the major effector of the humoral branch of the immune system, consists of nearly 30 serum and membrane proteins. Following initial activation, the various complement components interact, in a highly regulated enzymatic cascade, to generate reaction products that facilitate antigen clearance and generation of an inflammatory response. There are two pathways of complement activation: the classical pathway and the alternative pathway. The two pathways share a common terminal reaction sequence that generates a macromolecular membrane-attack complex (MAC), which lyses a variety of cells, bacteria, and viruses. The complement reaction products amplify the initial antigen-antibody reaction and convert that reaction into a more effective defense mechanism. A variety of small, diffusible reaction products that are released during complement activation induce localized vasodilation and attract phagocytic cells chemotactically, leading to an inflammatory reaction. As antigen becomes coated with complement reaction products, it is more readily phagocytosed by phagocytic cells that bear receptors for these complement products. In addition, some of the complement products have been shown to play a role in the activation of B lymphocytes. Finally, the terminal components of the complement system generate the membrane-attack complex.

This chapter describes the similarities and differences in the two pathways, the regulation of the complement system, the effector functions of various complement components, and the consequences of hereditary deficiencies in some components.

The Complement Components

The proteins and glycoproteins composing the complement system are synthesized largely by liver hepatocytes, although significant amounts of complement components are also produced by blood monocytes, tissue macrophages, and epithelial cells of the gastrointestinal and genitourinary tracts. These components constitute 15% (by weight) of the serum globulin fraction and circulate in the serum in functionally inactive forms, many of them as proenzymes in which the enzymatically active site is masked. Activation of the proenzyme cleaves the molecule, removing an inhibitory fragment and exposing the active site. Activation of the complement system involves a sequential enzyme cascade in which the proenzyme product of one step becomes the enzyme catalyst of the next step. Each activated component has a short half-life before being inactivated.

Each complement component is designated by numerals (C1–C9), by letter symbols, or by trivial names (Table 17-1). After a component is activated, the peptide fragments are denoted by small letters, with the smaller fragment designated "a" and the larger fragment designated "b" (e.g., C3a, C3b). The larger "b" fragments bind to the target near the site of activation, and the smaller "a" fragments diffuse from the site and play a role in initiating a localized inflammatory response. The complement fragments interact with one another to form functional complexes. Those complexes that have enzymatic activity are designated by a bar over the number or symbol (e.g., $\overline{\text{C4b2a}}$, $\overline{\text{C3bBb}}$).

Table 17-1 Characteristics of the complement proteins

Protein	Molecular weight	Serum conc. (μg/ml)	Immunologic function
		Early components	
Classical pathway			
C1q	410,000	70	Collagen-like protein: binds to Fc region of IgM and IgG antibodies
C1r	85,000	50	Serine protease: enzymatically activates C1s
C1s	85,000	50	Serine protease: enzymatically activates C4 and C2
C4	210,000	300	Thioester-containing protein: C4b binds C2a; C4a is an anaphylatoxin
C2	110,000	25	Serine protease: C2a bound to C4b acts as a convertase to enzymatically activate C3 and C5
Alternative pathway			
Factor D	25,000	1	Serine protease: enzymatically activates factor B
Factor B	93,000	200	Serine protease: Bb subunit bound to C3b acts as a convertase to activate C3 and C5
Properdin	220,000	25	Binds to $\overline{\text{C3bBb}}$ convertase and stabilizes it
Both pathways			
C3	190,000	1200	Thioester-containing protein; C3b binds to $\overline{\text{C4b2a}}$ or $\overline{\text{C3bBb}}$ to form C5 convertase; C3a is an anaphylotoxin
		Terminal components	
C5	190,000	70	Structural protein: C5b is a component of MAC that binds C6; C5a is an anaphylatoxin
C6	120,000	60	Structural protein: component of MAC that binds C7
C7	110,000	55	Structural protein: component of MAC that binds C8
C8	150,000	55	Structural protein: component of MAC that binds C9
C9	70,000	60	Structural protein: polymerizes to form MAC pore

Initial Steps in Complement Activation

The early steps in complement activation, culminating in formation of C5b, can occur via two pathways—the classical and the alternative. The final steps leading to formation of a membrane-attack complex are the same in both pathways. The complement components involved in each pathway, and the sequence in which they take part, are outlined in Figure 17-1.

Classical Pathway

Complement activation via the classical pathway is commonly initiated by the formation of soluble antigen-antibody complexes or by the binding of antibody to antigen on a suitable target, such as a bacterial cell. IgM and certain subclasses of IgG (IgG1, IgG2, and IgG3) can activate the classical complement pathway, as can certain nonimmunologic activators. The initial stage of activation involves C1, C2, C3, and C4, which are present in plasma in functionally inactive forms. The components were named in order of their discovery and before their functional roles had been determined, so that their names do not reflect the sequence in which they react.

The complexing of antibody with antigen induces conformational changes in the Fc portion of the antibody molecule that exposes a binding site for the C1 component of the complement system. C1 exists in serum as a macromolecular complex consisting of C1q and two molecules each of C1r and C1s, held together in a complex ($C1qr_2s_2$) stabilized by Ca^{2+} ions. The C1q molecule is composed of 18 polypeptide chains that associate to form 6 collagen-like triple helical arms, the tips of which bind to exposed C1q-binding sites in the C_H2 domain of the antibody molecule (Figure 17-2a,b). The $C1r_2s_2$ complex can exist in two

Protein	Molecular weight	Serum conc. (μg/ml)	Immunologic function
		Regulatory components	
C1 inhibitor (C1Inh)	105,000	200	Acts as serine protease inhibitor by dissociating $C1r_2S_2$ from C1
Factor H	150,000	560	Blocks formation of C3 convertase in alternative pathway; serves as cofactor for factor I–mediated inactivation
C4b-binding protein (C4bBP)	560,000	250	Blocks formation of C3 convertase in classical pathway; serves as cofactor for factor I–mediated inactivation
Membrane cofactor protein (MCP [CD46])	60,000	Cell-bound	Blocks C3 convertase formation in classical and alternative pathways; serves as cofactor for factor I–mediated inactivation
Factor I	90,000	35	Cleaves C4b or C3b using MCP, CR1, factor H_2 or C4bBP as cofactors
Anaphylatoxin inactivator	310,000	35	Blocks anaphylatoxin activity
S protein	85,000	505	Binds soluble C5b67 and prevents membrane insertion
Homologous restriction factor (HRF)	65,000	Cell-bound	Binds to C5b678 and blocks C9 binding to autologous cells
Membrane inhibitor of reactive lysis (MIRL [CD59])		Cell-bound	Binds to C5b678 and blocks C9 binding to autologous cells

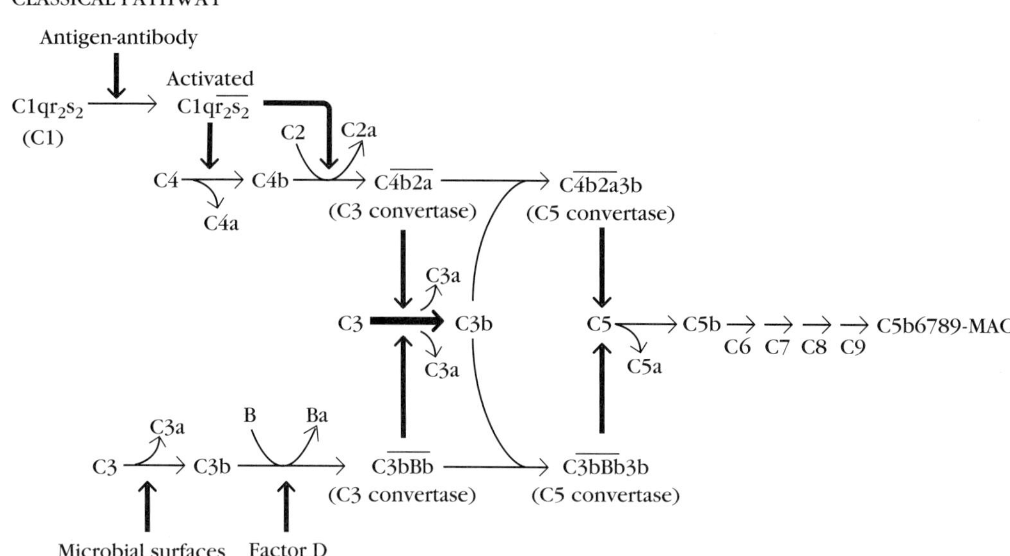

FIGURE 17-1 Overview of the complement activation pathways. The classical pathway is initiated by binding of C1 to antigen-antibody complexes. The alternative pathway is initiated by binding of C3b to activating surfaces such as microbial cell walls. Both pathways generate C3 and C5 convertases and bound C5b, which is converted into a membrane-attack complex (MAC) by a common sequence of terminal reactions. Hydrolysis of C3 is the major amplification step in both pathways, generating large amounts of C3b, which forms part of C5 convertase. C3b also can diffuse away from the activating surface and bind to immune complexes or cell surfaces, where it functions as an opsonin. Purple arrows indicate reaction steps; black arrows indicate enzymatic or activating activity.

configurations. When it is free and not bound to C1q, it assumes an S-shaped form; on binding to C1q, $C1r_2s_2$ assumes a shape similar to a figure 8 (Figure 17-2c–e). Each C1r and C1s monomer contains a catalytic domain and an interaction domain; the latter facilitates interaction with C1q or with each other.

Each C1 molecule must bind, via its C1q globular heads, to at least two Fc sites for a stable C1-antibody interaction to occur. When pentameric IgM is bound to antigen on a target surface, at least three binding sites for C1q are exposed. Circulating IgM, however, assumes a planar configuration in which the C1q-binding sites are not exposed (Figure 17-3). For this reason, circulating IgM cannot activate the complement cascade by itself. An IgG molecule, on the other hand, contains only a single C1q-binding site in its Fc portion, so that firm C1q binding is achieved only when two IgG molecules are within 30–40 nm of each other on a target surface or in a complex, providing two attachment sites for C1q. This difference in the structure of IgM and IgG accounts for the observation that a single molecule of IgM bound to a red blood cell is enough to activate the classical complement pathway and lyse the red blood cell, whereas some 1000 molecules of IgG are required if two molecules, randomly distributed, are to end up close enough to each other to initiate C1q binding.

The intermediates in the classical activation pathway are depicted schematically in Figure 17-4. Binding of C1q to its Fc binding sites induces a conformational change in C1r that autocatalytically converts C1r to an active serine protease enzyme. The $C\overline{1r}$ then cleaves the C1s to a similar active enzyme $C\overline{1s}$. $C\overline{1s}$ has two substrates, C4 and C2 (see Figure 17-1). The C4 component is a glycoprotein containing three polypeptide chains (α, β, and γ). C4 is activated when $C\overline{1s}$ hydrolyzes a small fragment (C4a) from the amino terminus of the α chain, exposing a binding site on the larger fragment (C4b). The C4b fragment attaches to the target surface in the vicinity of C1, and the C2 proenzyme then attaches to the exposed binding site on C4b, where it too is cleaved by the neighboring $C\overline{1s}$; the

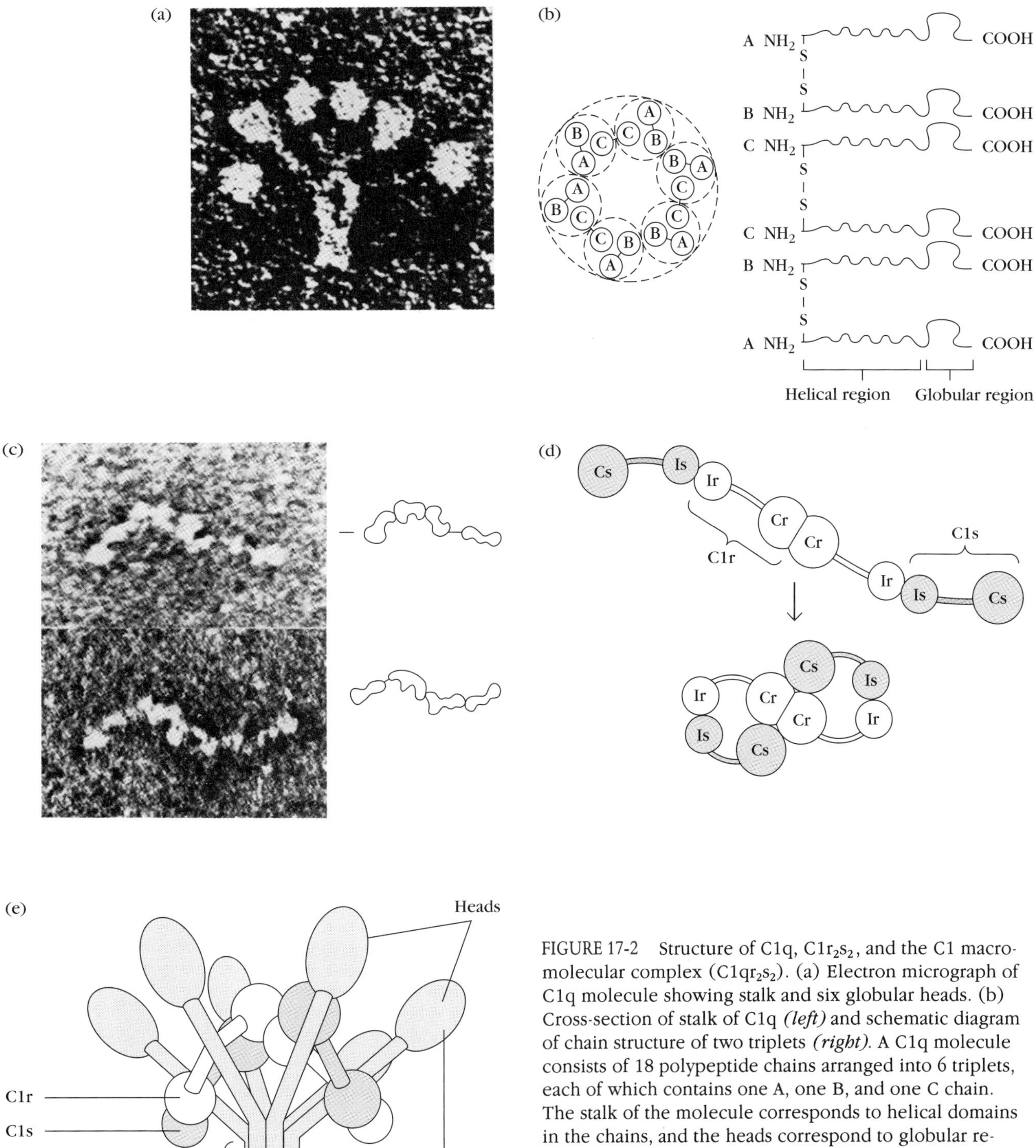

(a)

(b)

A NH_2 — S — S — B NH_2 COOH COOH

C NH_2 — S — S — C NH_2 COOH COOH

B NH_2 — S — S — A NH_2 COOH COOH

Helical region Globular region

(c)

(d)

Cs Is Ir Cr Cr C1r Ir Is Cs C1s

Cs Is Ir Cr Cr Ir Is Cs

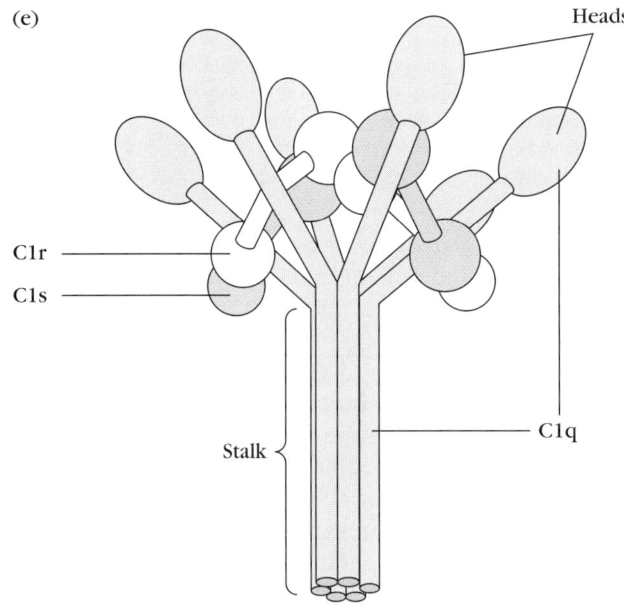

FIGURE 17-2 Structure of C1q, $C1r_2s_2$, and the C1 macromolecular complex ($C1qr_2s_2$). (a) Electron micrograph of C1q molecule showing stalk and six globular heads. (b) Cross-section of stalk of C1q *(left)* and schematic diagram of chain structure of two triplets *(right)*. A C1q molecule consists of 18 polypeptide chains arranged into 6 triplets, each of which contains one A, one B, and one C chain. The stalk of the molecule corresponds to helical domains in the chains, and the heads correspond to globular regions. (c) Electron micrograph of free $C1r_2s_2$ complex showing characteristic S shape. (d) Diagram of $C1r_2s_2$ complex in S-shaped form *(top)* and figure-8 form *(bottom),* which it assumes on binding with C1q. Each C1r (white) and C1s (purple) monomer contains a catalytic domain (C) with enzymatic activity and an interaction domain (I), which facilitates binding with C1q or with each other. (e) Diagram of $C1qr_2s_2$ complex. [Part (a) from H. R. Knobel et al., 1975, *Eur. J. Immunol.* **5**:78; part (c) from J. Tschopp et al., 1980, *Proc. Nat'l. Acad. Sci. USA* **77**:7014.]

(a)

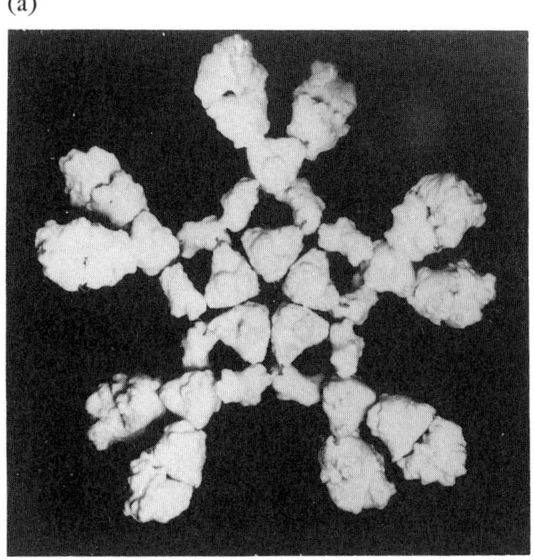

(b)

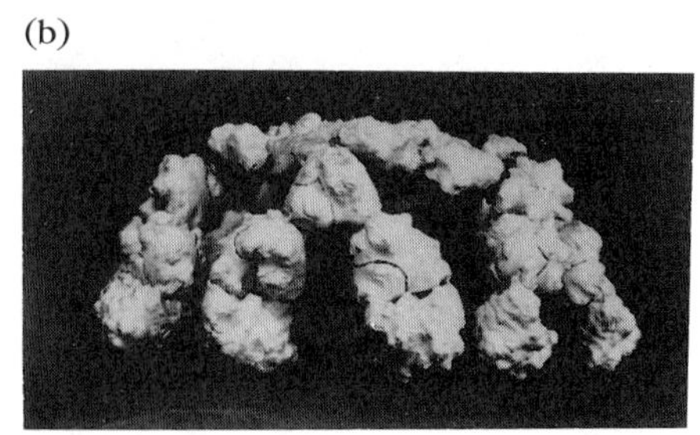

(c) (d)

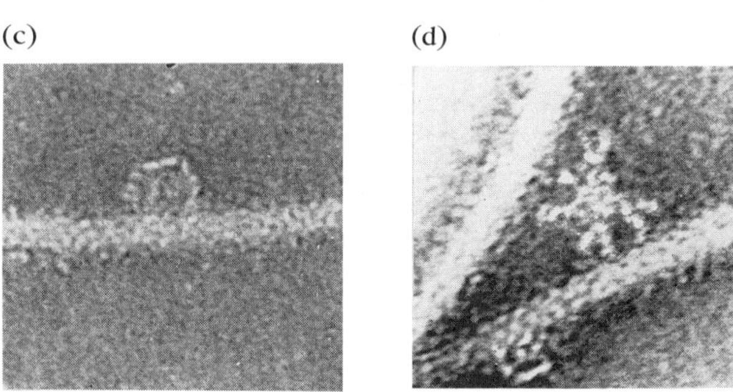

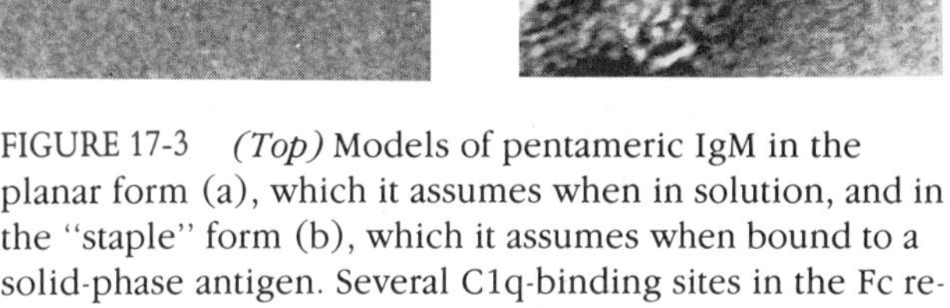

(e)

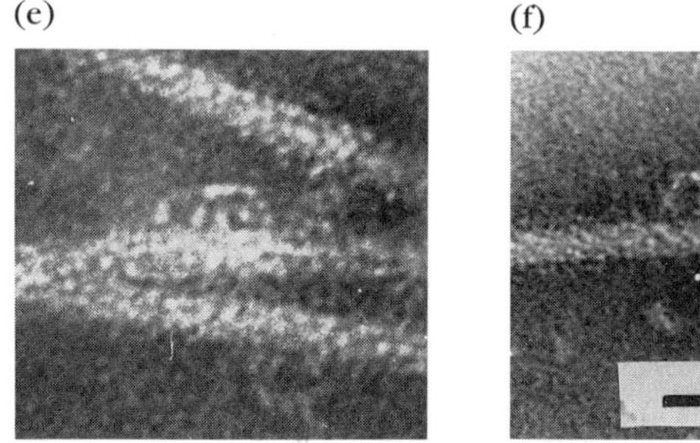

(f)

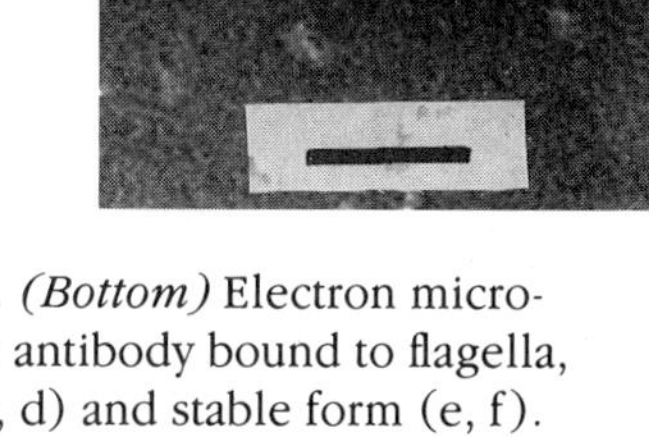

FIGURE 17-3 *(Top)* Models of pentameric IgM in the planar form (a), which it assumes when in solution, and in the "staple" form (b), which it assumes when bound to a solid-phase antigen. Several C1q-binding sites in the Fc region are accessible in the staple form, whereas none are exposed in the planar form. *(Bottom)* Electron micrographs of IgM antiflagellum antibody bound to flagella, showing the planar form (c, d) and stable form (e, f). [From A. Feinstein et al., 1981, *Monogr. Allergy* **17**:28 and, 1981, *Ann. N. Y. Acad. Sci.* **190**:1104.]

smaller fragment (C2b) diffuses away. The resulting C$\overline{4b2a}$ complex* is called C3 convertase, referring to its role in converting the C3 proenzyme into an enzymatically active form. The native C3 component consists of two polypeptide chains, α and β. Hydrolysis of a short fragment (C3a) from the amino terminus of the α chain by the C3 convertase generates C3b (Figure 17-5). A single C3 convertase molecule can generate over 200 molecules of C3b, resulting in tremendous amplification at this step of the sequence. Some of the C3b binds to C$\overline{4b2a}$ to form a trimolecular complex (C$\overline{4b2a3b}$) called C5 convertase. The C3b component of this complex binds C5 and alters its conformation so that the C$\overline{4b2a}$ component can cleave C5 into C5a, which diffuses away, and C5b, which attaches to the antigenic surface. The bound C5b initiates formation of the membrane-attack complex in a sequence described later. Some of the C3b generated by C3 convertase activity does not associate with C$\overline{4b2a}$; instead it coats immune complexes and particulate antigens, functioning as an opsonin as discussed in a later section.

* The larger fragment of C2 is designated as C2a and the smaller fragment is designated as C2b. It was reported that the C2 nomenclature was changed to bring it in line with the convention of designating the larger fragment as "b" and the smaller fragment as "a." The first edition of this text used the new nomenclature. However, at a recent meeting the change in nomenclature was not approved. Therefore the second edition is using the original nomenclature.

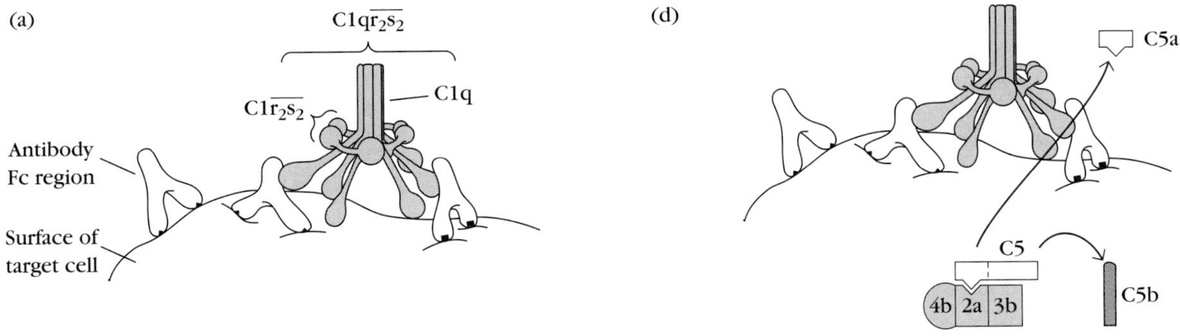

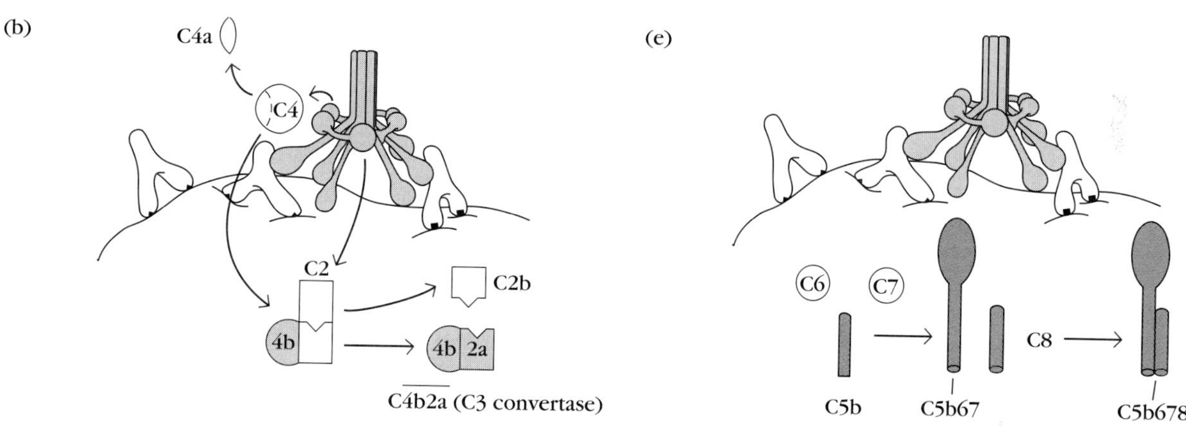

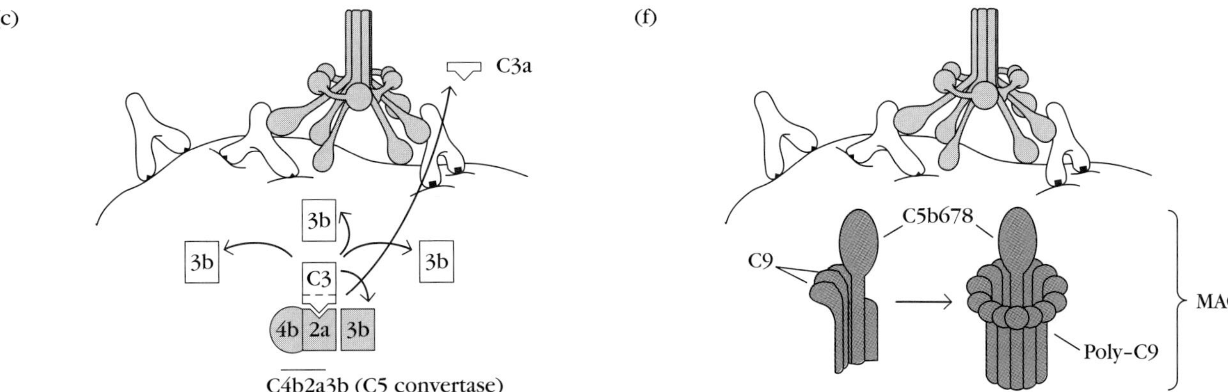

FIGURE 17-4 Schematic diagram of intermediates in classical pathway of complement activation. Complement complexes shaded gray are bound to the antigenic surface but do not penetrate it; those shaded purple can insert into the cell membrane; and free diffusible components are white. The completed membrane-attack complex (MAC) forms a large pore in the membrane. See text for details.

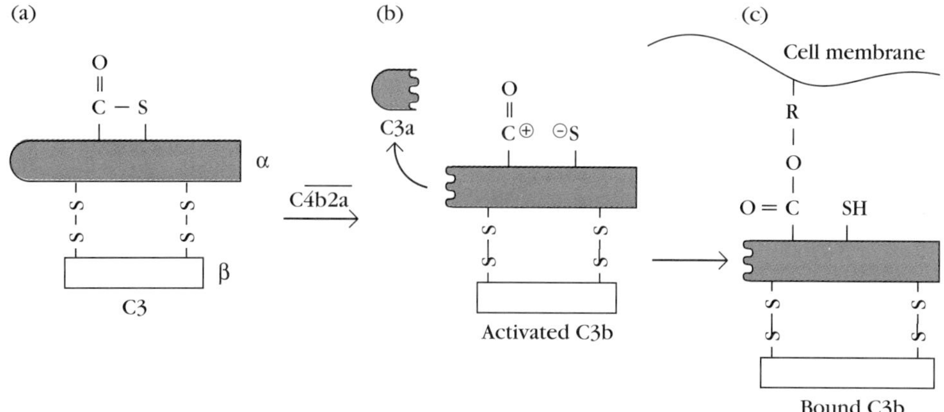

FIGURE 17-5 Hydrolysis of C3 by C3 convertase (C4b2a). (a) Native C3. (b) Activated C3 showing site of cleavage by C4b2a, resulting in production of the C3a and C3b fragments. (c) C3 has a labile internal thioester bond that is activated as C3b is formed, allowing the C3b fragment to bind to free hydroxyl or amino groups (R) on a cell membrane. Bound C3b exhibits various biological activities including binding of C5 and binding to C3b receptors on phagocytic cells.

TABLE 17-2 INITIATORS OF THE ALTERNATIVE PATHWAY OF COMPLEMENT ACTIVATION

Pathogens and particles of microbial origin	Nonpathogens
Many strains of gram-negative bacteria	Human IgG, IgA, and IgE in complexes
Lipopolysaccharides from gram-negative bacteria	Rabbit and guinea pig IgG in complexes
Many strains of gram-positive bacteria	Cobra venom factor
Teichoic acid from gram-positive cell walls	Heterologous erythrocytes (rabbit, mouse, chicken)
Fungal and yeast cell walls (zymosan)	Anionic polymers (dextran sulfate)
Some viruses and virus-infected cells	Pure carbohydrates (agarose, inulin)
Some tumor cells (Raji)	
Parasites (trypanosomes)	

SOURCE: M. K. Pangburn, 1986, in *Immunobiology of the Complement System,* Academic Press.

Alternative Pathway

Bound C5b can also be generated by a second major pathway of complement activation called the alternative pathway (see Figure 17-1). The alternative pathway involves four serum proteins: C3, factor B, factor D, and properdin. Unlike the classical pathway, which generally requires antibody to be initiated, the alternative pathway is initiated in most cases by various cell-surface constituents that are foreign to the host (Table 17-2). For example, both gram-negative and gram-positive bacteria have cell-wall constituents that can activate the alternative pathway. The intermediates in the alternative pathway are depicted schematically in Figure 17-6.

Serum C3, which contains an unstable thioester bond, is subject to slow spontaneous hydrolysis into C3a and C3b. The C3b component can bind to foreign surface antigens (such as those on bacterial cells or viral particles) or even to the host's own cells (see Figure 17-5c). The membranes of most mammalian cells have high levels of sialic acid, which contributes to the rapid inactivation of bound C3b molecules on host cells. Because foreign antigenic surfaces (e.g., bacterial cell walls, yeast cell walls, and certain viral envelopes) have only low levels of sialic acid, C3b bound to these surfaces remains active for a longer time. Bound C3b can bind another serum protein called factor B by way of a Mg^{2+}-dependent bond. Binding to C3b exposes a site on factor B that serves as

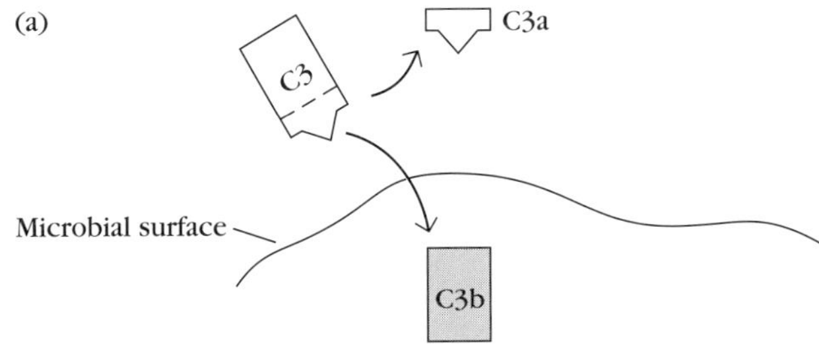

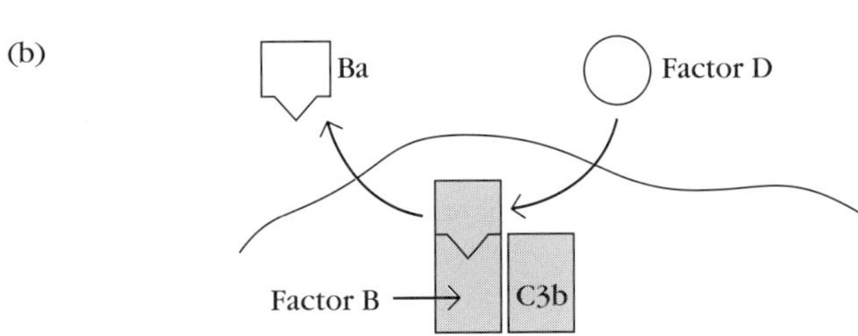

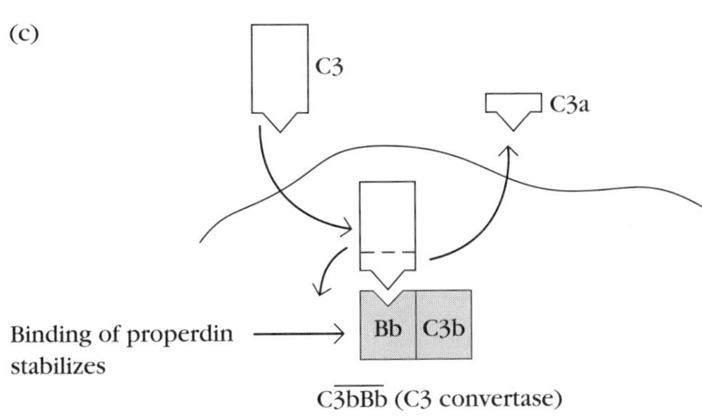

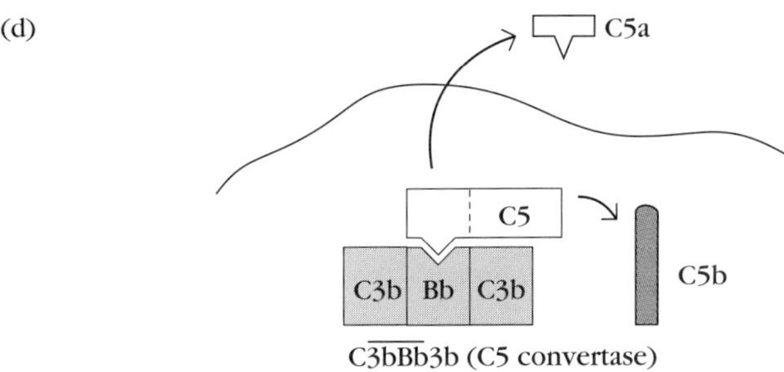

FIGURE 17-6 Schematic diagram of intermediates in formation of bound C5b by alternative pathway of complement activation. The C$\overline{3bBb}$ complex is stabilized by binding of properdin. Membrane-bound intermediates are shaded gray; those that can penetrate the membrane are shaded purple; free diffusible components are white. Conversion of bound C5b to the membrane-attack complex occurs by the same sequence of reactions as in the classical pathway (see Figure 17-4e,f). See text for details.

TABLE 17-3 COMPLEMENT COMPONENTS IN THE FORMATION OF C3 AND C5 CONVERTASES

	Classical pathway	Alternative pathway
Precursor proteins	C4 + C2	C3 + factor B
Activating protease	C$\overline{1s}$	Factor D
C3 convertase	C$\overline{4b2a}$	C$\overline{3bBb}$
C5 convertase	C$\overline{4b2a}$3b	C$\overline{3bBb}$3b
C5-binding component	C3b	C3b

the substrate for an enzymatically active serum protein called factor D. Factor D cleaves the C3b-bound factor B, releasing a small fragment (Ba), which diffuses away, and generating C$\overline{3bBb}$. The C$\overline{3bBb}$ complex has C3 convertase activity and thus is analogous to the C$\overline{4b2a}$ complex in the classical pathway. The C3 convertase activity of C$\overline{3bBb}$ has a half-life of only 5 min unless the serum protein properdin binds to it, stabilizing it and extending the half-life of its convertase activity to 30 min.

The C$\overline{3bBb}$ generated in the alternative pathway can activate unhydrolyzed C3 to generate more C3b autocatalytically. As a result, the initial steps are repeated and amplified, so that more than 2×10^6 molecules of C3b can be deposited on an antigenic surface in less than 5 min. The C3 convertase activity of C$\overline{3bBb}$ generates the C$\overline{3bBb}$3b complex, which exhibits C5 convertase activity, analogous to the C$\overline{4b2a}$3b complex in the classical pathway. The nonenzymatic C3b component binds C5, and the C$\overline{3bBb}$ component subsequently hydrolyzes the bound C5 to generate C5a and C5b; the latter binds to the antigenic surface. Table 17-3 summarizes the components involved in formation of the C3 and C5 convertases in the classical and alternative pathways.

FORMATION OF MEMBRANE-ATTACK COMPLEX

The terminal sequence of complement activation involves C5b, C6, C7, C8, and C9, which interact sequentially to form a macromolecular structure called the *membrane-attack complex (MAC)*. This complex displaces the membrane phospholipids, forming a large transmembrane channel that disrupts the membrane and enables ions and small molecules to diffuse through it freely.

As noted in the previous section, in both the classical and alternative pathways, a C5 convertase cleaves C5, which contains two protein chains (α and β). Following binding of C5 to the nonenzymatic C3b component of the convertase, the amino terminus of the α chain is cleaved, generating the small C5a fragment, which diffuses away, and the large C5b fragment, which provides a binding site for the subsequent components of the membrane-attack complex (see Figure 17-4d). The C5b component is extremely labile and is inactivated within 2 min unless C6 binds with it and stabilizes its activity.

Up to this point all the complement reactions take place on the hydrophilic surface of membranes or on immune complexes in the fluid phase. As the C5b6 complex binds to C7, it undergoes a hydrophilic-amphiphilic structural transition exposing hydrophobic regions, which serve as binding sites for membrane phospholipids. If the reaction is on a target-cell membrane, the hydrophobic binding site enables the C5b67 complex to insert into the phopholipid bilayer (see Figure 17-4e). If, however, the reaction occurs on an immune complex or other noncellular activating surface, then the hydrophobic binding site cannot anchor the complex and it is released. This released C5b67 complex can bind to nearby cells and bring about "innocent-bystander" lysis. In a number of diseases in which immune complexes are produced, tissue damage results from such innocent-bystander lysis. This autoimmune process will be discussed in Chapter 19.

Binding of C8 to membrane-bound C5b67 induces a conformational change in C8, so that it too undergoes a hydrophilic-amphiphilic structural transition exposing a hydrophobic region, which interacts with the plasma membrane. The C5b678 complex creates a small pore 10 Å in diameter; formation of this pore can lead to lysis of red blood cells but not of nucleated cells. The final step in formation of the MAC is the binding and polymerization of C9, a perforin-like molecule, to the C5b678 complex. As many as 10–16 molecules of C9 can be bound and polymerized by a single C5b678 complex. During polymerization the C9 molecules undergo a hydrophilic-amphiphilic transition, so that they also can insert into the membrane (see Figure 17-4f). The completed MAC, which has a tubular form and functional pore size of 70–100 Å, consists of a C5b678 complex surrounded by a poly-C9 complex (Figure 17-7). Since ions and small molecules can diffuse freely through the central channel of the MAC, the cell cannot maintain its osmotic stability and is lysed by an influx of water and loss of electrolytes.

Regulation of the Complement System

Because the complement system is nonspecific and thus capable of attacking host cells as well as microorganisms, elaborate regulatory mechanisms are

(a)

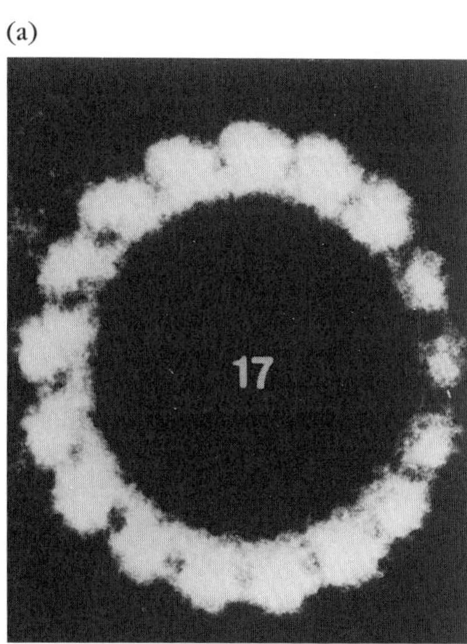

(b)

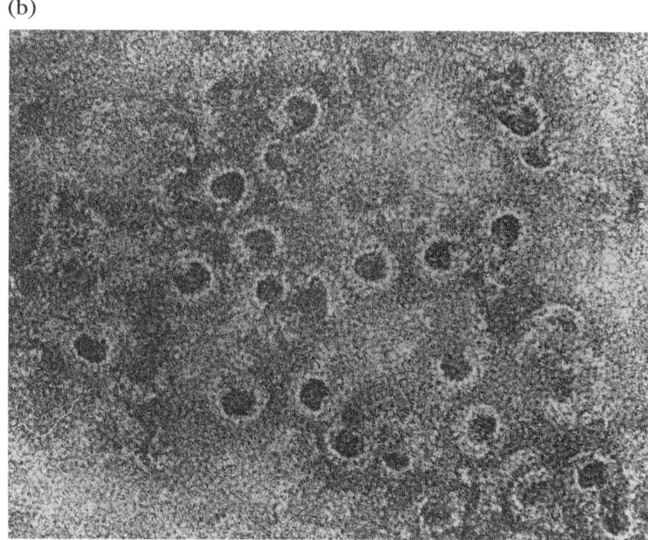

FIGURE 17-7 (a) Photomicrograph of poly-C9 complex formed by in vitro polymerization of C9. (b) Photomicrograph of complement-induced lesions on the membrane of a red blood cell. These lesions result from formation of membrane-attack complexes. [Part (a) from E. R. Podack, 1986, in *Immunobiology of the Complement System,* Academic Press; part (b) from J. Humphrey and R. Dourmashkin, 1969, *Adv. Immunol.* **11**:75.]

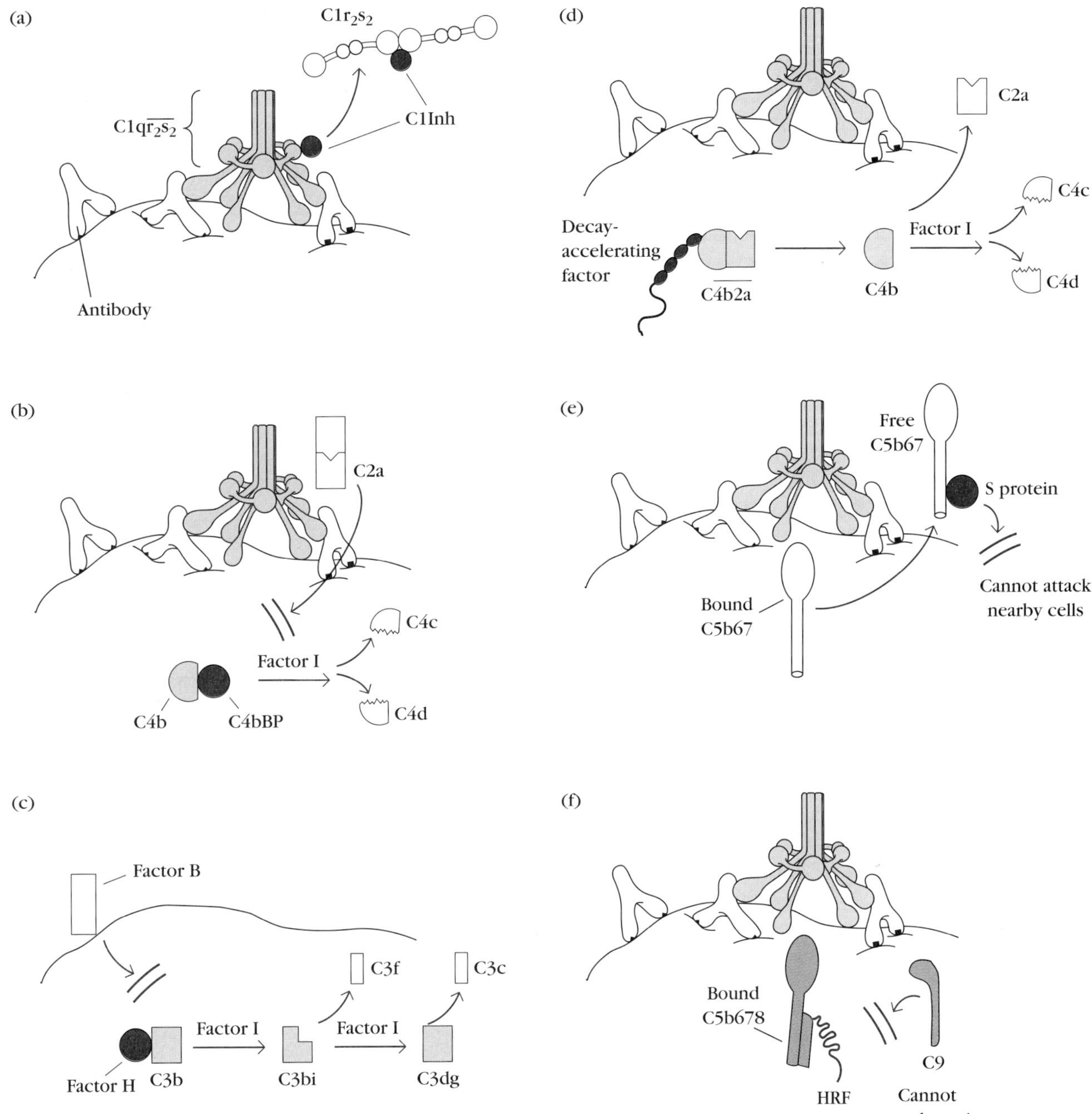

FIGURE 17-8 Schematic diagram of regulation of complement system by regulatory proteins (dark purple), which either cause dissociation of various intermediates or block their formation. Membrane-bound intermediates are shaded gray; those that can penetrate the membrane are shaded light purple; free diffusible components are white. C1Inh = C1 inhibitor; C4bBP = C4b-binding protein; HRF = homologous restriction factor. See text for details.

required to confine the reaction to designated targets. Both the classical and alternative pathways include a number of extremely labile components, which undergo spontaneous inactivation as they diffuse away from target cells. For example, the target-binding site on C3b undergoes spontaneous hydrolysis by the time it has diffused 40 nm away from the $\overline{C4b2a}$ or $\overline{C3bBb}$ convertase enzymes. This rapid hydrolysis limits binding of C3b to nearby host cells. In addition, both pathways include a series of regulatory proteins that inactivate various complement components (see Table 17-1). A glycoprotein called C1 inhibitor (C1Inh) can form a complex with $C1r_2s_2$, causing it to dissociate from C1q and preventing further activation of C4 or C2 (Figure 17-8a).

The reaction catalyzed by the C3 convertase enzymes of the classical and alternative pathways is the major amplification step in complement activation, generating hundreds of molecules of C3b. The C3b generated by these enzymes can bind to nearby cells, mediating damage to the healthy cells by opsonization to phagocytic cells bearing C3b receptors or by induction of the membrane-attack complex. It is estimated that circulating red blood cells are exposed to thousands of molecules of C3b molecules each day. In order to prevent C3b-mediated damage to healthy cells, a family of regulatory proteins has evolved to regulate C3 convertase activity in the classical and alternative pathways. This family of C3 convertase regulatory proteins are related structurally by the presence of short 60–amino acid repeating sequences (or motifs) termed *short consensus repeats (SCRs),* and they are related genetically, as they are encoded at a single chromosomal location on chromosome 1, known as the *regulators of complement activation (RCA)* gene cluster. Included within the RCA gene cluster are membrane cofactor protein (CD46), decay-accelerating factor (CD55), complement receptor type 1 (CD35), complement receptor type 2 (CD21), C4b-binding protein, and factor H.

A number of RCA proteins prevent assembly of C3 convertase. In the classical pathway three structurally different proteins act similarly to prevent assembly of C3 convertase (Figure 17-8b). These regulatory proteins include soluble C4b-binding protein (C4bBP) and two membrane-bound proteins, type 1 complement receptor (CR1) and membrane cofactor protein (MCP). Each of these regulatory proteins binds to C4b and prevents its association with C2a. Once C4bBP, CR1, or MCP is bound to C4b, another regulatory protein, factor I, cleaves the C4b into bound C4d and soluble C4c (Figure 17-9a). A similar regulatory sequence occurs in the alternative pathway. In this case CR1, MCP, or a regulatory component called factor H binds to C3b and prevents its association with factor B (Figure 17-8c). Once CR1, MCP, or factor H is bound to C3b, factor I cleaves the C3b into a bound C3bi fragment and a soluble C3f fragment. Further cleavage of C3bi by factor I releases C3c and leaves C3dg bound to the membrane (Figure 17-9b).

RCA proteins also act on the assembled C3 convertase, causing it to dissociate. Included among these regulatory proteins are the previously mentioned C4bBP, CR1, and factor H, as well as an additional protein, decay-accelerating factor (DAF). DAF is a glycoprotein that is anchored covalently to a glycophospholipid membrane protein. Each of these RCA proteins accelerates decay (dissociation) of C3 convertase, releasing the component with enzymatic activity (C2a or Bb) from the cell-bound component (C4b or C3b). Once dissociation of the C3 convertase occurs, then factor I cleaves the remaining membrane-bound C4b or C3b component to irreversibly inactivate the convertase (Figure 17-8d).

Regulatory proteins also operate at the level of the membrane-attack complex. The ability of the C5b67 complex to be released and then bind to nearby cells poses a threat of innocent-bystander lysis of healthy cells. A number of serum proteins can counter this threat by binding to released C5b67 and preventing its insertion into the membrane of nearby cells. A serum protein called S protein can bind to C5b67, inducing a hydrophilic transition and thereby preventing insertion of C5b67 into the membrane of nearby cells (Figure 17-8e). The binding of the S protein to C5b67 also keeps C9 from binding to the soluble C5b67 and polymerizing, and thereby prevents the futile consumption of C9.

Complement-mediated lysis of cells is more effective if the complement is from a different species than the cells being lysed. This unusual phenomenon, which remained unexplained for several years, is now known to depend on two membrane proteins that block MAC formation. These two proteins, present on the membrane of many cell types, are homologous restriction factor (HRF) and membrane inhibitor of reactive lysis (MIRL), or CD59. Both HRF and MIRL protect cells from nonspecific complement-mediated lysis by binding to C8, preventing assembly of poly-C9 and its insertion into the plasma membrane (Figure 17-8f). However, this inhibition occurs only if the complement components are from the same species as the target cells. For this reason, MIRL and HRF are said to display homologous restriction, for which the latter was named.

Complement-Binding Receptors

Each of the circulating red and white blood cells express cell-membrane receptors for complement fragments. These complement receptors mediate many of the biological activities of the complement system. In addition, some complement receptors play an important role in regulating complement activity by binding biologically active complement components and degrading them into inactive products. The complement receptors and their primary ligands, which include various complement components and their proteolytic breakdown products, are listed in Table 17-4.

Type 1 Complement Receptor (CR1)

The type 1 complement receptor (CD35) is a glycoprotein having a high affinity for C3b, although it can also bind C3bi, C4b, and C4bi with lower affinity. This receptor is expressed on red blood cells, monocytes, macrophages, neutrophils, eosinophils, B cells, and

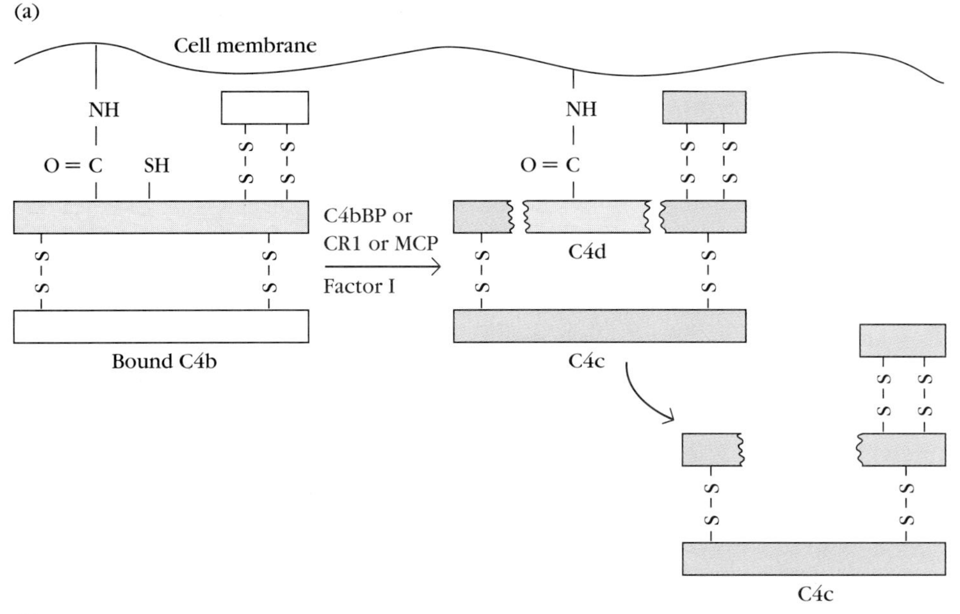

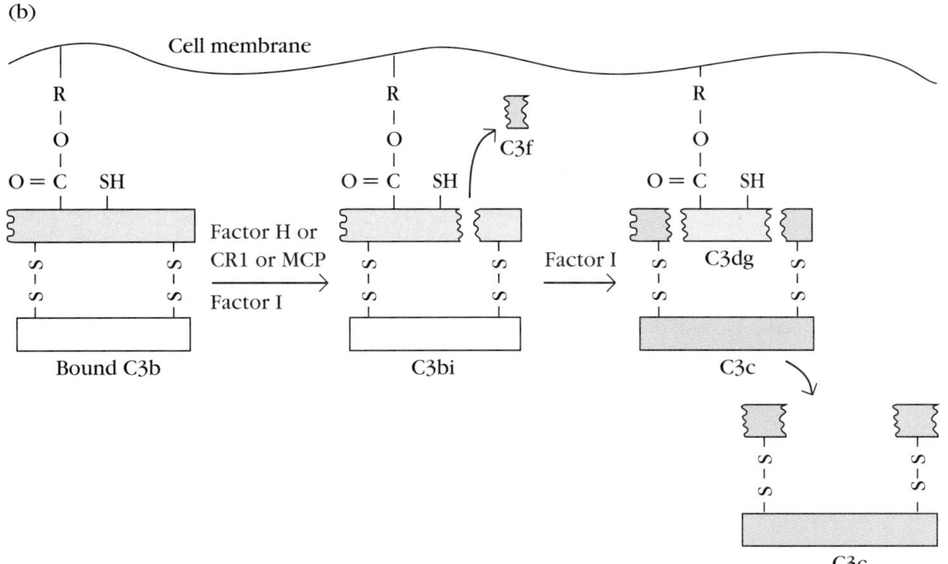

FIGURE 17-9 Inactivation of bound C4b and C3b by regulatory proteins of the complement system. (a) In the classical pathway, C4bBP (C4b-binding protein), CR1 (complement receptor type 1), or MCP (membrane cofactor protein) bind to C4b and act as cofactors for factor I–mediated cleavage of C4b. (b) In the alternative pathway, factor H, CR1, or MCP bind to C3b and act as cofactors for factor I–mediated cleavage of C3b. Free diffusible fragments are shaded purple. See text for details.

TABLE 17-4 LIGANDS AND CELLULAR DISTRIBUTION OF COMPLEMENT-BINDING RECEPTORS

Receptor	Major ligands	Cellular distribution
CR1 (CD35)	C3b, C4b	Erythrocytes, neutrophils, monocytes, macrophages, B cells, some T cells, eosinophils, follicular dendritic cells
CR2 (CD21)	C3d, C3dg*, C3bi	B cells, some T cells
CR3 (CD11b/CD18) CR4 (CD11c/CD18)	C3bi	Integrin adhesion molecule found on monocytes, macrophages, neutrophils, natural killer cells, some T cells
C3a/C4a receptor	C3a, C4a	Mast cells, basophils, granulocytes
C5a receptor	C5a	Mast cells, basophils, granulocytes, monocytes, macrophages, platelets, endothelial cells

* Cleavage of C3dg by serum proteases generates C3d and C3g.

some T cells. Because activation of C3 into C3a and C3b represents the major amplification step in both the classical and alternative pathways, immune complexes and particulate antigens generally become coated with C3b during complement activation. Cells expressing CR1 are able to bind both immune complexes and particulate antigens to which C3b is attached, facilitating antigen clearance. The expression of CR1 on follicular dendritic cells may enable these cells to trap C3b-coated immune complexes in the lymph nodes and spleen, enabling the antigen to persist longer in these sites so that a more effective immune response can be generated.

As mentioned previously, CR1 also plays an important role in regulating the complement cascade. The binding of C3b or C4b to CR1 has been shown to enable proteolytic degradation by factor I (see Figure 17-9). This regulatory activity is thought to be important in limiting the complement cascade so that extensive tissue damage does not occur. The biological role of CR1 is examined in more detail in the next section.

Type 2 Complement Receptor (CR2)

The type 2 complement receptor (CD21) is a glycoprotein that binds several degradation products of C3b including C3d, C3dg, and C3bi. Unlike CR1, which is present on all types of circulating blood cells, CR2 expression is limited to B cells and some T cells. Interestingly, the Epstein-Barr virus, which has amino acid sequence homology with C3dg, can bind to CR2. For this reason, B cells are susceptible to infection by this virus. The function of CR2 on B cells remains unknown, although some evidence suggests that cross-linking of C3dg bound to CR2 may play a role in B-cell activation.

Type 3 and Type 4 Complement Receptor (CR3 and CR4)

The type 3 complement receptor (CD11b/CD18) and type 4 complement receptor (CD11c/CD18) primarily bind the C3b degradation product C3bi. CR3 and CR4 are found on monocytes, macrophages, neutrophils, natural killer cells, and some subpopulations of T cells. These receptors are heterodimers consisting of two noncovalently associated glycoproteins: an α and a β chain. CR3 is also known as Mac-1, and CR4 is also known as p150,95. Both are members of the integrin family of receptors along with LFA-1; these receptors generally bind cell-adhesion molecules. Each of these integrin receptors has a unique α chain but a common β chain (CD18). The α chain of CR3 and CR4 can bind C3bi. Some evidence suggests that CR3 may also bind to ICAMs and may facilitate extravasation of neutrophils from the capillary into the tissue spaces during an inflammatory reaction. Binding of complement-coated particles to CR3 triggers phagocytosis by phagocytic cells.

Receptors for C3a, C4a, and C5a

C3a, C4a, and C5a are low-molecular-weight complement fragments that diffuse away from the site of complement activation. Receptors for these fragments are present on basophils, mast cells, and granulocytes. Binding of C3a, C4a, or C5a to its receptor on a mast cell or basophil induces the cell to degranulate, releasing pharmacologically active mediators.

Biological Consequences of Complement Activation

Complement serves as an important mediator of the humoral response by amplifying the response and converting it into an effective defense mechanism to destroy invading microorganisms and viruses. The MAC mediates cell lysis, while other complement components or split products participate in the inflammatory response, opsonization of antigen, viral neutralization, and clearance of immune complexes (Table 17-5).

Table 17-5 Summary of biological effects of complement activation

Effect	Mediated by
Cell lysis	C5b–9 (membrane-attack complex)
Degranulation of mast cells and basophils	C3a, C4a, and C5a (anaphylatoxins)
Extravasation and chemotaxis of neutrophils and monocytes	C3a, C5a*, and C5b67
Opsonization of antigen	C3b*, C4b, C3bi
Viral neutralization	C3b and C5b–9
Clearance of immune complexes	C3b

* Indicates component that is most important in mediating a particular effect.

Cell Lysis

The membrane-attack complex formed by complement activation is capable of lysing a broad spectrum of microorganisms, viruses, erythrocytes, and nucleated cells. Because the alternative pathway of activation generally occurs without an initial antigen-antibody interaction, this pathway serves as an important innate system of nonspecific defense against infectious microorganisms. The requirement for an initial antigen-antibody reaction in the classical pathway supplements the nonspecific innate defense of the alternative pathway with a more specific defense mechanism.

Up to this point this text has stressed the role of cell-mediated immunity in host defense against viral infections. Nevertheless antibody and complement do play a role in host defense against viruses and are often crucial in containing viral spread during acute infection and in protecting against reinfection. Most—perhaps all—enveloped viruses are susceptible to complement-mediated lysis. The viral envelope is largely derived from the plasma membrane of the infected host cell and is therefore susceptible to pore formation via the membrane-attack complex. Among the pathogenic viruses shown to be lysed by complement-mediated lysis are herpes virus, myxoviruses, paramyxoviruses, and retroviruses.

The complement system is generally quite effective in lysing gram-negative bacteria (Figure 17-10). However, some gram-negative bacteria and most gram-positive bacteria have mechanisms for evading complement-mediated damage (Table 17-6). For example, a few gram-negative bacteria can develop resistance to complement-mediated lysis that correlates with the virulence of the organism. In *Escherichia coli* and *Salmonella,* resistance to complement is associated with the smooth bacterial phenotype, which is characterized by the presence of long polysaccharide side chains in the cell-wall lipopolysaccharide (LPS) component. It has been proposed that the increased LPS in the wall of resistant strains may prevent insertion of the MAC into the bacterial membrane, so that the complex is released from the bacterial cell rather than forming a pore. Strains of *Neisseria gonorrhoeae* resistant to complement-mediated killing have been associated with disseminated gonococcal infections in humans. Some evidence suggests that the membrane proteins of resistant *Neisseria* strains undergo noncovalent interactions with the MAC that prevent its insertion into the outer membrane of the bacterial cells. These examples of resistant gram-negative bacteria are the exception; most gram-negative bacteria are susceptible to complement-mediated lysis.

In contrast, gram-positive bacteria are generally resistant to complement-mediated lysis because the thick peptidoglycan layer in their cell wall prevents insertion of the MAC into the inner membrane. Although complement activation can occur on the cell membrane of encapsulated bacteria such as *Streptococcus pneumoniae,* the capsule prevents interaction between C3b deposited on the membrane and the CR1 on phagocytic cells. Some bacteria possess an elastase that inactivates C3a and C5a, preventing these split products from inducing an inflammatory response. In addition to these mechanisms of evasion, various bacteria, viruses, fungi, and protozoans contain proteins

(a)

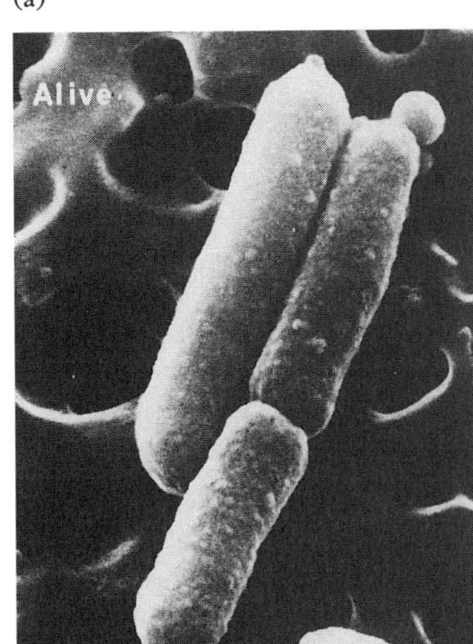

(b)

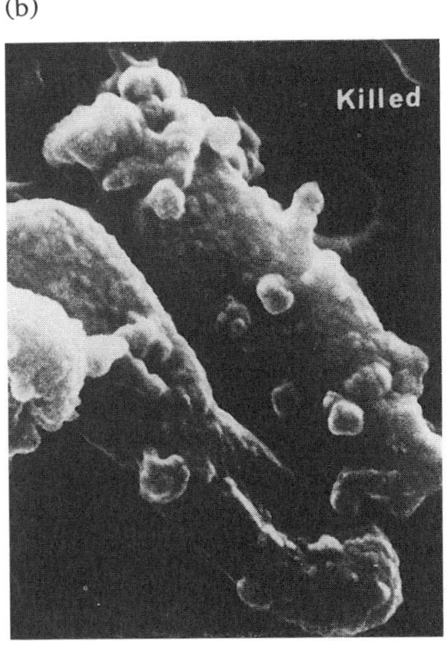

(c)

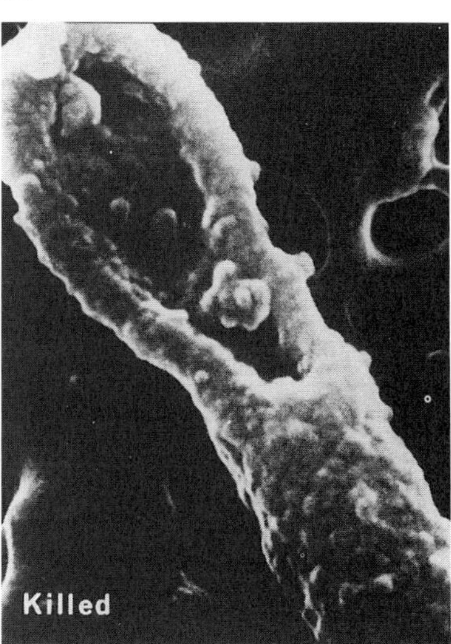

FIGURE 17-10 Scanning electron micrographs of *E. coli* showing (a) intact cells and (b, c) cells killed by complement-mediated lysis. Note membrane blebbing on lysed cells. [From R. D. Schreiber et al., 1979, *J. Exp. Med.* **149**:870.]

TABLE 17-6 MICROBIAL EVASION OF COMPLEMENT-MEDIATED DAMAGE

Microbial component	Mechanism of evasion	Examples
Gram-negative bacteria		
Long polysaccharide chains in cell-wall LPS	Side chains prevent insertion of MAC in bacterial membrane	Resistant strains of *E. coli* and *Salmonella* sp.
Outer membrane protein	MAC interacts with membrane protein and fails to insert into bacterial membrane	Resistant strains of *Neisseria gonorrhoeae*
Elastase	Anaphylotoxins C3a and C5a are inactivated by microbial elastase	*Pseudomonas aeruginosa*
Gram-positive bacteria		
Peptidoglycan layer of cell wall	Insertion of MAC into bacterial membrane is prevented by thick layer of peptidoglycan	*Streptococcus* sp.
Bacterial capsule	Capsule provides physical barrier between C3b deposited on bacterial membrane and CR1 on phagocytic cells	*Streptococcus pneumoniae*
Other microbes		
Proteins that mimic complement regulatory proteins	Proteins present in various bacteria, viruses, fungi, and protozoans inhibit the complement cascade	Vaccinia virus, herpes simplex, Epstein-Barr virus, *Trypanosoma cruzi, Candida albicans*

KEY: CR1 = type 1 complement receptor; LPS = lipopolysaccharide; MAC = membrane-attack complex (C5b–9).

TABLE 17-7 ROLE OF COMPLEMENT SPLIT PRODUCTS IN AN INFLAMMATORY RESPONSE

Substance	Biological effect
C3a	Degranulation of mass cells and basophils* Degranulation of eosinophils Aggregation of platelets
C3b	Opsonization of particulate antigens and solubilization of immune complexes, which facilitate subsequent phagocytosis
C3c	Release of neutrophils from bone marrow resulting in leukocytosis
C4a	Degranulation of mast cells and basophils*
C5a	Degranulation of mast cells and basophils* Degranulation of eosinophils Aggregation of platelets Chemotaxis of basophils, eosinophils, neutrophils, and monocytes Release of hydrolytic enzymes from neutrophils Increased expression of type 1 and type 3 complement receptors (CR1 and CR3) on neutrophils
Bb	Inhibition of monocyte/macrophage migration and induction of their spreading

* Degranulation leads to release of histamine and other mediators that induce contraction of smooth muscle and an increase in vascular permeability.

that can interrupt the complement cascade on their surfaces; thus mimicing the effects of the normal complement regulatory proteins C4bBP, CR1, and DAF.

Nucleated cells tend to be more resistant to complement-mediated lysis than red blood cells. Lysis of nucleated cells requires formation of multiple membrane-attack complexes, whereas a single MAC can lyse a red blood cell. Many nucleated cells, including the majority of cancer cells, can endocytose MAC. If the complex is removed soon enough, the cell can repair any membrane damage and restore its osmotic stability. This is the reason why complement-mediated lysis by monoclonal antibody specific for tumor-cell antigens is often not effective; rather, such monoclonal antibodies must be conjugated with toxins or radioactive isotopes to be effective tumor-killing agents.

Inflammatory Response

The complement cascade is often viewed in terms of the final outcome of cell lysis, but various peptides generated during formation of the MAC play a decisive role in the development of an effective inflammatory response (Table 17-7). As noted already, the complement "split products" C3a, C4a, and C5a, called *anaphylatoxins,* bind to receptors on mast cells and blood basophils and induce degranulation with release of histamine and other pharmacologically active mediators. The mediators induce smooth-muscle contraction and increases in vascular permeability. C3a, C5a, and C5b67 act together to induce monocytes and neutrophils to adhere to vascular endothelial cells, extravasate through the endothelial lining of the capillary, and migrate toward the site of complement activation in the tissues. C5a is most potent in mediating these processes, with picomolar quantities being effective. Activation of the complement system thus results in influxes of fluid that carries antibody and phagocytic cells to the site of antigen entry.

Opsonization of Antigen

C3b is the major opsonin of the complement system. The amplification that occurs with C3 activation results in a coating of C3b on immune complexes and particulate antigens. Each of the phagocytic cells expresses complement receptors (CR1, CR3, and CR4) that bind C3b, C4b, or C3bi (see Table 17-4). When antigen has been coated with C3b during complement activation by either pathway, the coated antigen binds to cells bearing CR1. If the cell is a phagocyte (e.g., a neutrophil, monocyte, or macrophage), phagocytosis will be enhanced (Figure 17-11). Activation of phagocytic cells by various agents including C5a anaphylatoxin has been shown to increase the number of CR1s from 5000 on resting phagocytes to 50,000 on activated

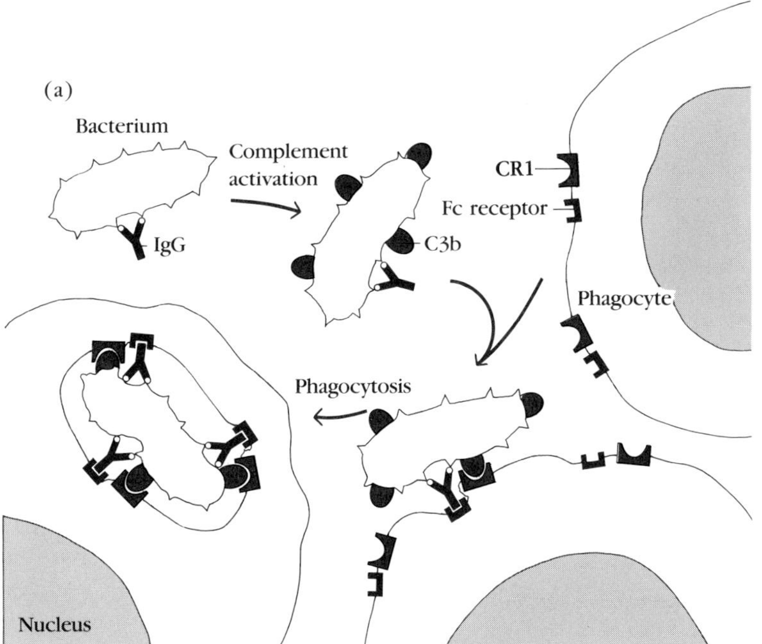

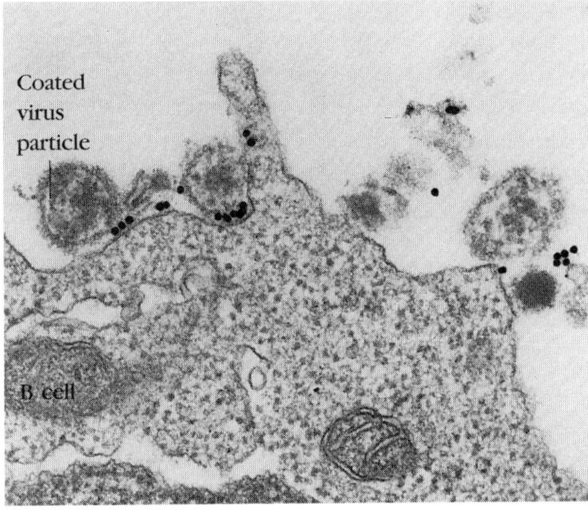

FIGURE 17-11 (a) Schematic representation of the role of C3b in opsonization. (b) Electron micrograph of Epstein-Barr virus coated with antibody and C3b and bound to the C3b receptors (CR1) on a B lymphocyte. [From N. R. Cooper and G. R. Nemerow, 1986, in *Immunobiology of the Complement System,* Academic Press.]

cells, greatly facilitating their phagocytosis of C3b-coated antigen. Once C3b-coated antigen has bound to CR1, some of the C3b is degraded into C3bi and C3f. This enables the antigen to bind to CR3, which triggers phagocytosis more effectively than CR1.

Viral Neutralization

The complement system plays an important role in host defense by neutralizing viral infectivity. Some viruses (e.g., retroviruses, Epstein-Barr virus, Newcastle disease virus, and rubella virus) can activate the alternative or even the classical pathway in the absence of antibody. For most viruses, the binding of serum antibody to the repeating subunits of the viral structural proteins creates particulate immune complexes ideally suited for complement activation by the classical pathway.

The complement system mediates viral neutralization by a number of mechanisms (Table 17-8). Some degree of neutralization is achieved through the formation of larger viral aggregates, simply because these aggregates reduce the net number of infectious viral particles. Although antibody does play a role in the formation of viral aggregates, in vitro studies show that the C3b component facilitates aggregate formation in the presence of as little as two molecules of antibody per virion. For example, polyoma virus coated with antibody is neutralized when serum is added containing activated C3. The binding of antibody and/or complement to the surface of a viral particle creates a thick protein coating that can be visualized by electron microscopy (Figure 17-12). This coating neutralizes viral infectivity by blocking attachment to susceptible host cells. The deposits of antibody and complement on viral particles also facilitate binding of the viral particle to cells possessing Fc or type 1 complement receptors (CR1). In the case of phagocytic cells, such binding can be followed by phagocytosis and intracellular destruction of the ingested viral particle. Finally, complement is effective in lysing most, if not all, enveloped viruses, resulting in fragmentation of the envelope and disintegration of the nucleocapsid.

TABLE 17-8 MECHANISMS OF COMPLEMENT-MEDIATED NEUTRALIZATION OF VIRUSES

Process	Mechanism	Requirements	Example
Aggregation of viruses by Ab and/or C*	Cross-linking by bivalent Ab and/or C reduces net number of viral particles	High levels of virus and C (and/or Ab), high density of binding sites on virus, and high-affinity virus-C or virus-Ab interactions must occur concurrently	Polyoma virus
Coating of viruses with Ab and/or C†	Coating interferes with viral attachment to, or perforation of, host cell	Only low levels of Ab and/or C are needed; complement cascade must generate C3b but later steps not necessary	Influenza, Epstein-Barr, and Newcastle disease viruses
Binding of viruses to inflammatory cells via Fc and/or C receptors†	Interaction leads to viral destruction by released mediators or by phagocytosis and intracellular digestion	Ab and/or C must coat viral particles and sufficient numbers of inflammatory cells must be present	Influenza and Epstein-Barr viruses
Viral lysis by MAC‡	Disruption of viral structure causes irreversible loss of infectivity	Potent C-activation stimulus and accessibility of envelope for MAC insertion are needed	Enveloped viruses only: influenza, Newcastle disease, Epstein-Barr, and human immunodeficiency viruses

KEY: Ab = antibody; C = complement; MAC = membrane-attack complex (C5b–9).

SOURCE: N. R. Cooper and G. R. Nemerow, 1986, in *Immunology of the Complement System*, Academic Press.

* Mechanism of minor biological importance.

† Mechanism of major biological importance.

‡ Mechanism of minor biological importance, except for retroviruses.

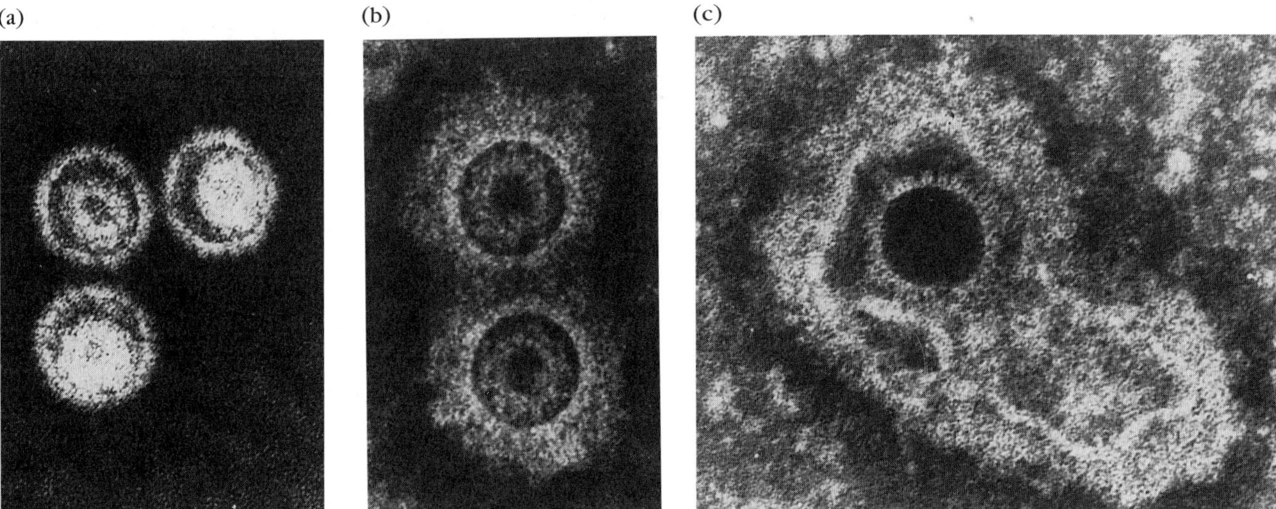

FIGURE 17-12 Electron micrographs of negatively stained preparations of Epstein-Barr virus. (a) Control without antibody. (b) Antibody-coated particles. (c) Particles coated with antibody and complement. [From N. R. Cooper and G. R. Nemerow, 1986, in *Immunobiology of the Complement System,* Academic Press.]

Solubilization of Immune Complexes

The role of the complement system in clearing immune complexes can be seen in patients with the autoimmune disease systemic lupus erythematosus (SLE). These individuals produce large quantities of immune complexes and suffer tissue damage as a result of complement-mediated lysis and the induction of type II or type III hypersensitivity (see Chapter 19). Although complement plays a significant role in the development of tissue damage in SLE, the paradoxical finding is that deficiencies in C1, C2, C4, and CR1 predispose an individual to SLE; indeed, 90% of the individuals who completely lack C4 develop SLE. The complement deficiencies are thought to interfere with effective solubilization and clearance of immune complexes; the result is the persistence of these complexes and subsequent tissue damage by the very system whose deficiency was to blame.

The coating of soluble immune complexes with C3b is thought to facilitate their binding to CR1 on erythrocytes. Although red blood cells express lower levels of CR1 ($\sim 5 \times 10^2$ per cell) than granulocytes ($\sim 5 \times 10^4$ per cell), there are about 10^3 red blood cells for every white blood cell; therefore, erythrocytes account for about 90% of the CR1 in the blood. For this reason, erythrocytes play an important role in binding C3b-coated immune complexes and carrying these complexes to the liver and spleen. In these organs, immune complexes are stripped from the red blood cells and are phagocytosed, thereby preventing their deposition in tissues. In SLE patients, deficiencies in C1, C2, and C4 each contribute to reduced levels of C3b on immune complexes and hence inhibit their clearance. The lower levels of CR1 expressed on the erythrocytes of SLE patients also may interfere with the proper binding and clearance of immune complexes.

Complement Deficiencies

Genetic deficiencies have been described for each of the complement components with the exception of factor B (Table 17-9). Homozygous deficiencies in any of the early components of the classical pathway (C1q, C1r, C1s, C4, and C2) manifest similar clinical presentations, notably a marked increase in such immune-complex diseases as systemic lupus erythematosus, glomerulonephritis, and vasculitis. These deficiencies highlight the important role of the early complement reactions in generating C3b, which is critical for solubilization and clearance of immune complexes. In addition to immune-complex diseases, some of these individuals suffer from recurrent infections by such pyogenic bacteria as streptococci and staphylococci. These organisms are gram-positive and therefore resistant in any case to the lytic effects of the MAC. Nonetheless, the early complement components ordinarily prevent recurrent infection by mediating a localized inflammatory response and opsonizing the bacteria. Deficiencies in factor D and properdin—early components of the alternative pathway—appear to be associated with *Neisseria* infections but not with immune-complex disease.

TABLE 17-9 INHERITED COMPLEMENT DEFICIENCIES AND ASSOCIATED DISEASES

Deficient protein	Individuals with homozygous deficiencies	Clinical manifestations: Immune-complex diseases*	Clinical manifestations: Other symptoms
Early components			
Classical pathway			
C1q	15	14	Many with pyogenic infections
C1r/C1s	8	6	
C4	16	14	
C2	66	38	Few with pyogenic infections
Alternative pathway			
Factor B	None known	None	None
Factor D	2	None	2 (Pyogenic infections)
Properdin	3	None	3 (Severe *Neisseria* infections)
Both pathways			
C3	11	8	10 (Pyogenic infections)
Membrane-attack complex			
C5	12	1	9 (*Neisseria* infections)
C6	17	2	10 (*Neisseria* infections)
C7	14	1	6 (*Neisseria* infections)
C8	14	1	8 (*Neisseria* infections)
C9	Many	None	None
Regulatory components			
C1 Inhibitor	>500	10	Hereditary angioedema
Factor I	5	1	4 (Pyogenic infections)
Factor H	2	1	Hemolytic uremia syndrome
DAF and HRF	NR	NR	Paroxysmal nocturnal hemoglobinuria (PNH)

KEY: DAF = decay-accelerating factor; HRF = homologous restriction factor; NR = not reported.

* Immune-complex diseases include systemic lupus erythematosus (SLE), various SLE-like syndromes, glomerulonephritis, and vasculitis.

SOURCE: Adapted from J. A. Schifferti and D. K. Peters, 1983, *Lancet* **2**:957.

C3 deficiencies have the most severe clinical manifestations, reflecting the central role of C3 in activation of C5 and formation of the MAC. The first patient identified with a C3 deficiency was a child who suffered from frequent severe bacterial infections and was erroneously thought to have agammaglobulinemia. When tests revealed normal immunoglobulin levels, a deficiency in C3 was discovered. This case highlights the critical function of the complement system in converting a humoral antibody response into an effective host-defense mechanism. The majority of patients with C3 deficiency have recurrent bacterial infections and manifest immune-complex diseases.

Individuals with homozygous deficiencies in the components involved in the MAC manifest recurrent meningococcal and gonococcal infections caused by *Neisseria* species. In normal individuals these gram-negative bacteria are generally susceptible to complement-mediated lysis or are cleared by the opsonizing activity of C3b. Few of these individuals manifest immune-complex disease, so generally they must produce enough C3b to clear immune complexes. Interestingly, a deficiency in C9 results in no clinical symptoms, suggesting that in some cases the entire MAC is not necessary for complement-mediated lysis to occur.

Congenital deficiencies of complement regulatory proteins have also been reported. The C1 inhibitor (C1Inh) regulates activation of the classical pathway by preventing excessive C4 and C2 activation by C1. Deficiency of C1Inh is an autosomal dominant condition with a frequency of 1 in 1000. The deficiency gives rise to a disease called hereditary angioedema, which manifests clinically as localized edema of the tissue, often following trauma but sometimes with no known cause. The edema can be in subcutaneous tissues or within the bowel or upper respiratory tract, where it causes abdominal pain or obstruction of the airway.

A number of the membrane-bound regulatory components including decay-accelerating factor (DAF) and homologous restriction factor (HRF) are anchored to the plasma membrane by glycosyl phosphatidylinositol membrane anchors. In paroxysmal nocturnal hemoglobinuria the glycosyl phosphatidylinositol membrane anchor is defective, resulting in an absence of DAF and HRF from the cell membrane. As a consequence of this defect, much lower levels of complement are able to lyse the red blood cells, and the individual suffers from chronic hemolytic anemia.

Summary

1. Activation of the complement system, which consists of a large group of serum proteins, generates a sequential enzymatic cascade of interacting components that play an important role in antigen clearance. The two pathways of complement activation, the classical pathway and the alternative pathway, involve different complement proteins and are initiated differently. The two pathways converge in a common terminal reaction sequence that generates a membrane-attack complex (MAC) responsible for cell lysis.

2. The classical pathway, initiated by binding of certain subclasses of IgG and by IgM, involves C1, C4, C2, and C3 components. The reaction sequence generates a complex of $\overline{C4b2a}$ (C3 convertase), which is able to convert C3 into C3a and C3b, and a $\overline{C4b2a3b}$ complex with C5 convertase activity. The alternative pathway is most commonly initiated by a variety of microorganisms (bacteria, fungi, some viruses, and some parasites); however, this pathway also can be initiated by IgG-, IgA-, and IgE-antigen complexes. This pathway involves C3, factor D, and properdin. The reaction sequence generates $\overline{C3bBb}$ (C3 convertase) and $\overline{C3bBb3b}$ (C5 convertases) analogous to the convertases in the classical pathway. Both the classical and alternative pathways generate bound C5b. This component reacts sequentially with C6, C7, C8, and C9 to produce the membrane-attack complex, which mediates cell lysis by forming a large pore in the cell membrane.

3. Because of its nonspecific nature, the complement system requires elaborate regulatory mechanisms to control reactions and prevent damage to normal tissues. Both pathways have a number of extremely labile components that lose their activity as they diffuse from the site of activation. In addition both pathways have a number of regulatory components that function to inactivate complement products and prevent excessive buildup of enzymatically active components.

4. The complement system serves as an important effector of the humoral immune response. It destroys foreign cells through the process of MAC-mediated lysis. The complement system also induces a localized inflammatory response with a buildup of fluid and inflammatory cells, and it facilitates phagocytosis of antigen through its effect as an opsonin. Complement also acts to neutralize viral infectivity by several mechanisms and aids in solubilizing immune complexes.

5. Inherited deficiencies of most of the complement components have been described. The consequences of these conditions depend on which complement component is deficient. C3 deficiencies, which are clinically the most severe, are often associated with immune-complex disease and susceptibility to recurrent bacterial infections. These effects reflect the central role of C3 in both the classical and alternative pathways of complement activation. Deficiency of the regulatory protein C1 inhibitor is fairly common and is associated with a localized edema called hereditary angioedema.

References

AHEARN, J. M., and D. T. FEARON. 1989. Structure and function of the complement receptors, CR1 (CD35) and CR2 (CD21). *Adv. Immunol.* **46**:183.

COOPER, N. R. 1991. Complement evasion strategies of microorganisms. *Immunol. Today* **12**:327.

COOPER, N. R., and G. R. NEMEROW. 1986. Complement-dependent mechanisms of virus neutralization. In *Immunobiology of the Complement System.* Academic Press.

DAVIS, A. E. 1988. C1 inhibitor and hereditary angioneurotic edema. *Annu. Rev. Immunol.* **6**:595.

ERDEI, A., G. FUST, and J. GERGELY. 1991. The role of C3 in the immune response. *Immunol. Today* **12**:332.

FEARSON, D. T. 1988. Complement, C receptors and immune complex disease. *Hosp. Pract.* (Aug. 15):63.

FRANK, M. M., and L. F. FRIES. 1991. The role of complement in inflammation and phagocytosis. *Immunol. Today* **12**:322.

HOURCADE, D., M. HOLERS, and J. P. ATKINSON. 1989. The regulators of complement activation (RCA) gene cluster. *Adv. Immunol.* **45**:381.

JOINER, K. 1986. Role of complement in infectious diseases. In *Immunobiology of the Complement System*. Academic Press.

KINOSHITA, T. 1991. Biology of complement: the overture. *Immunol. Today* **12**:291.

LACHMANN, P. J., and M. J. WALPORT. 1986. Genetic deficiency diseases of the complement system. In *Immunobiology of the Complement System*. Academic Press.

LISZEWSKI, M. K., T. W. POST, and J. P. ATKINSON. 1991. Membrane cofactor protein (MCP or CD46): newest member of the regulators of complement activation gene cluster. *Annu. Rev. Immunol* **9**:431.

MORGAN, B. P., and M. J. WALPORT. 1991. Complement deficiency and disease. *Immunol. Today* **12**:301.

MULLER-EBERHARD, H. 1986. The membrane attack complex of complement. *Annu. Rev. Immunol.* **4**:503.

MULLER-EBERHARD, H. J. 1988. Molecular organization and function of the complement system. *Annu. Rev. Biochem.* **57**:321.

PERLMUTTER, D. H., and H. R. COLTEN. 1986. Molecular immunobiology of complement biosynthesis. *Annu. Rev. Immunol.* **4**:231.

PODACK, E. R. 1986. Assembly and functions of the terminal components. In *Immunobiology of the Complement System*. Academic Press.

REID, K. B. M., and A. J. DAY. 1989. Structure-function relationships of the complement components. *Immunol. Today* **10**:177.

WILSON, J. G., W. W. WONG, E. E. MURPHY et al. 1987. Deficiency of the C3b/C4b receptor (CR1) of erythrocytes in systemic lupus erythematosus *J. Immunol.* **138**:2706.

Study Questions

1. Indicate whether each of the following statements is true or false. If you think a statement is false, explain why.
   a. A single molecule of bound IgM can activate the C1q component of the classical complement pathway.
   b. C3a and C3b are fragments of C3.
   c. All complement components are present in the serum in a functionally inactive proenzyme form.
   d. Nucleated cells tend to be more resistant to complement-mediated lysis than red blood cells.
   e. Enveloped viruses cannot be lysed by complement because their outer envelope is resistant to pore formation by the membrane-attack complex.
   f. C4-deficient individuals have difficulty eliminating immune complexes.

2. Explain why serum IgM cannot activate complement by itself.

3. Would you expect a C1 or C3 complement deficiency to be more serious clinically. Why?

4. Some microorganisms produce enzymes that can degrade the Fc portion of antibody molecules. Why would such enzymes be advantageous for the survival of microorganisms that possess them?

5. Complement activation can occur via the classical or alternative pathway.
   a. How do the two pathways differ in the substances required for the initial activation step.
   b. How do the reaction sequences differ in the two pathways?
   c. What important biological functions do the classical and the alternate pathways share?

6. Which complement complex mediates innocent-bystander lysis? When is such lysis likely to occur? How is the threat of such lysis reduced?

7. Match each complement component(s) or reaction (a–l) with the appropriate activity or description listed below (1–12). The numbers may be used once, more than once, or not at all.

   a. ______ C3b
   b. ______ C1, C4, C2, and C3
   c. ______ C9
   d. ______ C3, factor B, and factor D
   e. ______ $\overline{\text{C1q}}$
   f. ______ $\overline{\text{C4b2a3b}}$
   g. ______ C5b, C6, C7, C8, and C9
   h. ______ C3 → C3a + C3b
   i. ______ C3a, C5a, and C5b67
   j. ______ C3a, C4a, and C5a
   k. ______ $\overline{\text{C4b2a}}$
   l. ______ C3b + B → $\overline{\text{C3bBb}}$ + Ba

   1. Major amplification step
   2. Early components of alternative pathway
   3. Components of the membrane-attack complex
   4. Mediates opsonization
   5. Early components of classical pathway

6. Has perforin-like activity
7. Binds to Fc region of antibodies
8. Chemotatic factors
9. Has C3 convertase activity
10. Anaphylatoxins
11. Has C5 convertase activity
12. Reaction catalyzed by factor D

8. Indicate whether each of the following statement is true or false. If you think a statement is false, explain why.
 a. C1 inhibitor (C1Inh) prevents binding of C1q to the Fc region of an antibody.
 b. C4b-binding protein (C4bBP) binds to C4 and prevents binding of C2.
 c. Decay-accelerating factor is a membrane-bound regulatory component.
 d. C4bBP is a membrane-bound regulatory component.
 e. Homologous restriction factor (HRF) induces dissociation of C4b2a.
 f. S protein limits innocent-bystander lysis.

9. You have prepared knock-out mice with mutations in the genes that encode various complement components. Each knock-out strain cannot express one of the complement components listed across the top of the table below. Predict the effect of each mutation on the steps in complement activation and on the complement effector functions indicated in the facing table using the following symbols: NE = no effect; D = process/function decreased but not abolished; A = process/function abolished.

For use with Question 9.

	Component knocked out						
	C1q	C4	C3	C5	C6	C9	Factor B
Complement Activation							
Formation of C3 convertase in classical pathway							
Formation of C3 convertase in alternative pathway							
Formation of C5 convertase in classical pathway							
Formation of C5 convertase in alternative pathway							
Effector Functions							
C3b-mediated opsonization							
Neutrophil chemotaxis							
Cell lysis							

HYPERSENSITIVE REACTIONS

An immune response evokes a battery of effector molecules that act to remove antigen by various mechanisms. Generally, these effector molecules induce a subclinical, localized inflammatory response that eliminates antigen without extensive tissue damage to the host. Under certain circumstances, however, this inflammatory response can have deleterious effects, resulting in significant tissue damage or even death. These reactions have been termed *hypersensitive,* or *allergic,* reactions. Although hypersensitivity denotes an increased response, the response is not always heightened but may, instead, reflect an inappropriate immune response to an antigen. Hypersensitive reactions may develop in the course of either humoral or cell-mediated responses.

Reactions within the humoral branch are initiated by antibody or antigen-antibody complexes and are termed *immediate hypersensitivity reactions* because the symptoms manifest within minutes or hours following an encounter with antigen by a sensitized recipient. Three types of such reactions are commonly recognized.

Reactions within the cell-mediated branch are initiated by T_{DTH} cells and are referred to as *delayed-type hypersensitivity* (DTH) reactions in reference to the delay of symptoms for days following antigen exposure. Although DTH reactions, as discussed in Chapter 15 provide an important line of defense against intracellular pathogens, they sometimes cause extensive tissue damage that is pathologic and truly hypersensitive. This chapter examines the mechanisms and consequences of the four primary types of hypersensitive reactions.

Gell and Coombs Classification

Several types of hypersensitive reactions can be distinguished, reflecting differences in the effector molecules generated in the course of the reaction. In immediate hypersensitive reactions, different antibody isotypes induce different immune effector molecules. IgE antibodies, for example, induce mast-cell degranulation with release of histamine and other biologically active molecules. IgG and IgM antibodies, on the other hand, induce hypersensitive reactions by activating complement. The effector molecules in these reactions are the membrane-attack complex and such complement split products as C3a, C4a, and C5a. In delayed hypersensitive reactions, the effector molecules are various cytokines secreted by T_{DTH} cells.

As it became clear that different immune mechanisms can give rise to hypersensitive reactions, P. G. H. Gell and R. R. A. Coombs proposed a classification scheme in which hypersensitive reactions are divided into four types (I, II, III, and IV), each involving distinct mechanisms, cells, and mediator molecules. These are summarized in Table 18-1. This classification scheme has served an important function in identifying the mechanistic differences among various hypersensitive reactions. But it is important to point out that a great deal more complexity exists due to a vast array of secondary effects that cross the boundaries of the classification scheme.

Table 18-1 Gell and Coombs classification of hypersensitive reactions

Type	Descriptive name	Initiation time	Mechanism	Typical manifestations
		Immediate reactions		
Type I	IgE-mediated hypersensitivity	2–30 min	Ag induces cross-linkage of IgE bound to mast cells and basophils with release of vasoactive mediators	Systemic anaphylaxis Localized anaphylaxis: Hay fever Asthma Hives Food allergies Eczema
Type II	Antibody-mediated cytotoxic hypersensitivity	5–8 h	Ab directed against cell-surface antigens mediates cell destruction via complement activation or ADCC	Blood-transfusion reactions Erythroblastosis fetalis Autoimmune hemolytic anemia
Type III	Immune complex–mediated hypersensitivity	2–8 h	Ag-Ab complexes deposited in various tissues induce complement activation and an ensuing inflammatory response	Localized Arthus reaction Generalized reactions: Serum sickness Glomerulonephritis Rheumatoid arthritis Systemic lupus erythematosus
		Delayed reactions		
Type IV	Cell-mediated hypersensitivity	24–72 h	Sensitized T_{DTH} cells release cytokines that activate macrophages or T_C cells, which mediate direct cellular damage	Contact dermatitis Tubercular lesions Graft rejection

IgE-Mediated (Type I) Hypersensitivity

A type I hypersensitive reaction is induced by certain types of antigens, referred to as *allergens,* and has all the hallmarks of a normal humoral response. That is, an allergen induces a humoral antibody response by the same mechanisms as described previously for other soluble antigens, resulting in generation of antibody-secreting plasma cells and memory cells (see Figure 14-12). What distinguishes a type I hypersensitive response from a normal humoral response is that the plasma cells secrete IgE. This class of antibody binds with high affinity to Fc receptors on the surface of tissue mast cells and blood basophils. Such IgE-coated mast cells and basophils are said to be *sensitized.* A later exposure to the same allergen cross-links the membrane-bound IgE on sensitized mast cells and basophils, causing degranulation of these cells (Figure 18-1). The pharmacologically active mediators released from the granules exert biological effects on the surrounding tissues. The principal effects—vasodilation and smooth-muscle contraction—may be either systemic or localized, depending on the extent of mediator release.

Consequences of Type I Reactions

Type I reactions can produce conditions ranging from serious life-threatening reactions, such as systemic anaphylaxis and asthma, to hay fever and eczema, which are merely annoying.

Systemic Anaphylaxis

Systemic anaphylaxis is a shock-like and often fatal state whose onset occurs within minutes of a type I hypersensitive reaction. This type of response was first reported in 1839 by Magendie, who noted the sudden death of dogs following repeated injections of egg albumin. This report went unnoticed until 1902 when two French physicians, Paul J. Portier and Charles R. Richet, observed a similar phenomenon. During a cruise on the yacht of the Prince of Monaco, the two physicians had been asked to develop an antitoxin to

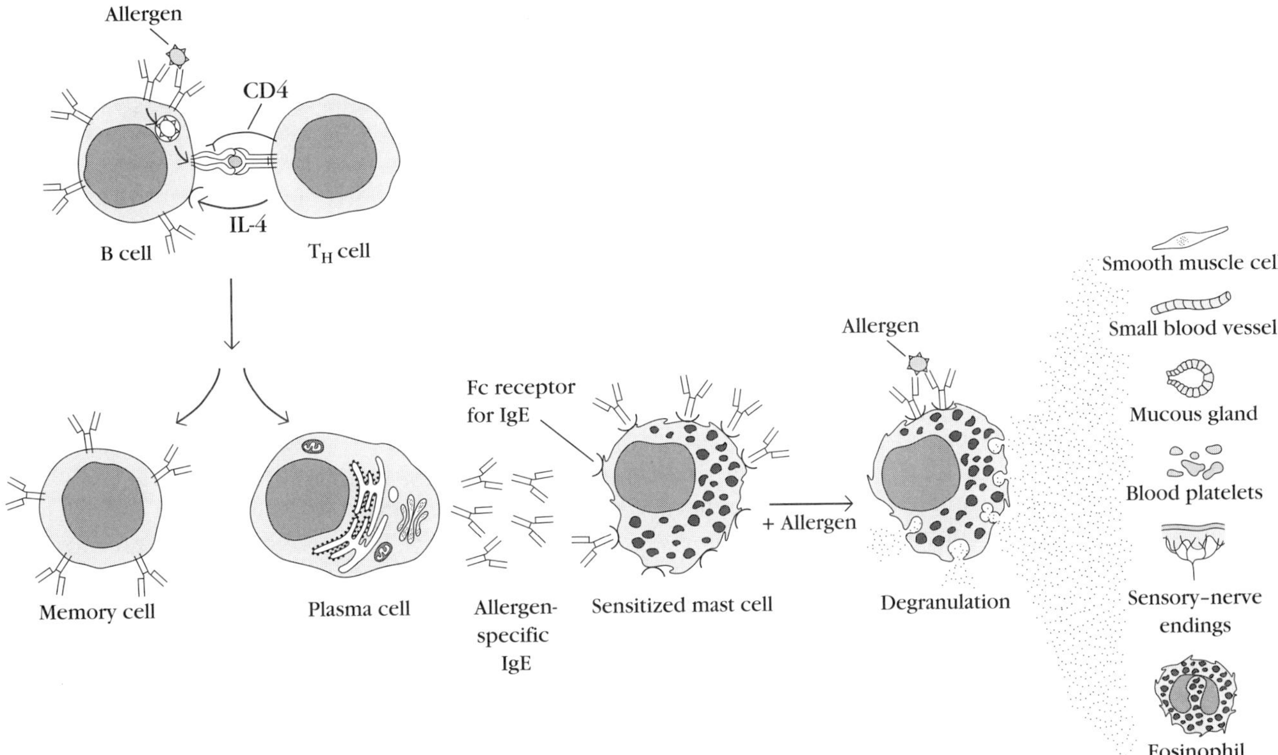

FIGURE 18-1 General mechanism underlying a type I hypersensitive reaction. Exposure to an allergen activates B cells to form IgE-secreting plasma cells. The secreted IgE molecules bind to IgE-specific Fc receptors on mast cells and blood basophils. Upon a second exposure to the allergen, the bound IgE is cross-linked, triggering the release of pharmacologically active mediators (purple) from mast cells and basophils. The mediators cause smooth-muscle contraction, increased vascular permeability, and vasodilation.

protect swimmers from the painful stings of the jellyfish, the Portuguese man-of-war. When they returned home, jellyfish were not available for their project, so they decided to use sea anemones because they also caused painful stings. While attempting to immunize dogs with a sublethal extract of sea anemone tentacles, they observed that a secondary challenge several weeks later with the same sublethal extract brought on a rapid sequence of symptoms including vomiting, bloody diarrhea, asphyxia, unconsciousness, and death. They called the response *anaphylaxis* (from Greek *ana,* against, and *phylaxis,* protection) to denote that this was an inappropriate response, counter to host protective mechanisms. For his work on anaphylaxis, Richet was awarded a Nobel prize in medicine in 1913.

Systemic anaphylaxis can be induced in a variety of experimental animals and is seen occasionally in humans. Each species exhibits characteristic symptoms of anaphylaxis, which reflect differences in the distribution of mast cells as well as differences in the biologically active mediators in their mast-cell granules. The animal model of choice for studying systemic anaphylaxis has been the guinea pig. Anaphylaxis can be induced in guinea pigs with relative ease, and its symptoms closely parallel those observed in humans. Active sensitization in guinea pigs is induced by a single injection of a foreign protein such as egg albumin. After an incubation period of about 2 weeks, the animal is usually challenged with an intravenous injection of the same protein. Within 1 min the animal becomes restless, its respiration becomes labored, and its blood pressure drops. As the smooth muscles of the gastrointestinal tract and bladder contract, the guinea pig defecates and urinates. Finally bronchiole constriction results in death by asphyxiation within 2–4 min of the injection. These events all stem from the systemic vasodilation and smooth-muscle contraction brought on by mediators released during the course of the reaction. Postmortem examination reveals that massive edema, shock, and bronchiole constriction are the major cause of death. The sequence of events is similar in systemic anaphylaxis in humans. A wide range of antigens have been shown to trigger this reaction in susceptible humans, including bee, wasp, hornet, and ant stings; drugs, such as penicillin, insulin, and antitoxins; and seafood and nuts. If not treated quickly, these reactions can be fatal.

Localized Anaphylaxis

In localized anaphylaxis the reaction is limited to a specific target tissue or organ, often involving epithelial surfaces at the site of allergen entry. The tendency to manifest localized anaphylactic reactions is inherited and is referred to as *atopy.* Several common conditions are associated with localized anaphylactic reactions. The most common, affecting 10% of the U.S. population, is allergic rhinitis, commonly known as *hay fever.* This results from airborne allergens reacting with sensitized mast cells in the conjunctivae and nasal mucosa to induce the release of pharmacologically active mediators from mast cells; these mediators then cause localized vasodilation and increased capillary permeability. The symptoms include watery exudation of the conjunctivae, nasal mucosa, and upper respiratory tract as well as sneezing and coughing. Asthma, another common manifestation of localized anaphylaxis, also is triggered by mast-cell degranulation and mediator release but in the lower respiratory tract. The resulting constriction of the bronchioles and obstruction of the airway cause difficulty in breathing, often with wheezing. In some cases airborne or blood-borne allergens trigger an asthmatic attack (allergic asthma); in other cases an asthmatic attack can be induced by exercise or cold, apparently independent of allergen stimulation (intrinsic asthma).

Food allergens can also play a role in localized anaphylaxis. Allergen cross-linking of IgE on mast cells along the upper or lower gastrointestinal tract can induce localized smooth-muscle contraction and vasodilation and thus such symptoms as vomiting or diarrhea. Mast-cell degranulation along the gut can also increase the permeability of mucous membranes, so that the allergen enters the bloodstream. Various symptoms can ensue, depending on where the allergen is deposited. For example, some individuals develop asthmatic attacks after ingesting certain foods. Others develop atopic urticaria, commonly known as hives, when a food allergen is carried to sensitized mast cells in the skin causing swollen (edematous), red (erythematous) eruptions; this response is known as a *wheal and flare* reaction. In atopic dermatitis (allergic eczema), which is observed most frequently in young children, the skin eruptions are filled with pus and are erythematous.

As a type I hypersensitivity reaction begins to subside, mediators released during the course of the reaction often induce a localized inflammatory reaction, called the *late-phase reaction.* The late-phase reaction begins to develop 4–6 h following the initial type I reaction and persists for 1–2 days. The reaction is characterized by infiltration of neutrophils, eosinophils, macrophages, lymphocytes, and basophils. Of these cells, the eosinophil plays a principal role, accounting for some 30% of the cells that accumulate in the late-phase reaction. As mast cells degranulate, they release eosinophil chemotactic factor, which serves to attract large numbers of eosinophils to the site. Various cytokines released at the site, including IL-3, IL-5, and GM-CSF, contribute to the growth and differentiation of the eosinophils. Eosinophils express Fc receptors for IgG and IgE isotypes and bind directly to antibody-coated allergen. As the eosinophils are activated, they degranulate, releasing a number of inflammatory mediators including leukotrienes, major basic protein, platelet-activation factor, cationic protein, and eosinophil-derived neurotoxin. The release of these eosinophil-derived mediators may play a protective role in parasitic infections. However, in response to allergens, these mediators contribute to extensive tissue damage in the late-phase reaction. Neutrophils are another major participant in late-phase reactions, accounting for 30% of the inflammatory cells. Neutrophils are attracted to the area of a type I reaction by neutrophil chemotactic factor, released from degranulating mast cells. In addition, a variety of cytokines released at the site, including IL-8, have been shown to activate neutrophils resulting in release of their granule contents including lytic enzymes, platelet-activating factor, and leukotrienes.

TABLE 18-2 COMMON ANTIGENS ASSOCIATED WITH TYPE I HYPERSENSITIVITY

Proteins	*Foods*
Foreign serum	Nuts
Vaccines	Seafood
	Eggs
Plant pollens	Peas, beans
Rye grass	
Ragweed	*Insect venoms*
Timothy grass	Bee
Birch trees	Wasp
	Ant
Drugs	
Penicillin	*Mold spores*
Sulfonamides	
Local anesthetics	*Animal hair and dander*
Salicylates	

Components of Type I Reactions

Allergens

The vast majority of humans mount significant IgE responses only as a defense against parasitic infections. After an individual is exposed to a parasite, serum IgE levels increase and remain high until the parasite is successfully cleared from the body. Atopic persons, however, appear to have a genetic defect affecting regulation of the IgE response. These regulatory defects allow nonparasitic antigens to stimulate inappropriate IgE production, leading to tissue-damaging type I hypersensitivity. The term *allergen* refers specifically to nonparasitic antigens capable of stimulating type I hypersensitive responses in allergic individuals.

Most allergic IgE responses occur on mucous membrane surfaces and thus in response to allergens that enter the body either by inhalation or ingestion. Of the common allergens listed in Table 18-2, relatively few have been purified and characterized. Those that have include the allergens from rye grass pollen, ragweed pollen, codfish, birch pollen, timothy grass pollen, and bee venom. Each of these allergens has been shown to be a multiallergen system containing a number of allergenic components. Ragweed pollen, a major pollen allergen in the United States, is a case in point. It has been reported that a square mile of ragweed yields 16 tons of pollen in a single season. The pollen particles are inhaled, and their tough outer wall is dissolved by enzymes in the mucous secretions, releasing the allergenic substances. Chemical fractionation of ragweed has revealed a variety of substances, most of which are not allergenic but are capable of eliciting an IgM or IgG response. Of the five fractions that are allergenic (i.e., able to induce an IgE response), two evoke allergenic reactions in about 95% of ragweed-sensitive individuals and are called major allergens; these are designated the E and K fractions. The other three, called Ra3, Ra4, and Ra5, are minor allergens that induce an allergic response in only 20–30% of sensitive subjects.

What makes these agents allergens? Why are some pollens (e.g., ragweed) highly allergenic, whereas other equally abundant pollens (e.g., nettle) are rarely allergenic? No single physicochemical property seems to distinguish the highly allergenic E and K fractions of ragweed from the less allergenic Ra3, Ra4, and Ra5 fractions and from the nonallergenic fractions. Rather, allergens as a group appear to possess diverse properties. Some allergens, including foreign serum and egg albumin, are potent antigens; others, such as plant pollens, are weak antigens. Although most allergens are proteins or protein-bound substances having a molecular weight between 15,000 and 40,000, attempts to identify some common chemical property of these antigens, one that would render them all allergenic, have failed. It appears that allergenicity is a consequence of a complex series of interactions involving not only the allergen but also the dose, the sensitizing route, sometimes an adjuvant, and—most importantly—the genetic constitution of the recipient.

Reaginic Antibody (IgE)

The first indication that some component of serum was responsible for hypersensitive reactions was C. R. Reichert's finding that he could transfer systemic anaphylaxis from primed dogs to unprimed dogs with an injection of serum from the primed dogs. As discussed in Chapter 5, the existence of human serum components that reacted with allergens was first demonstrated by K. Prausnitz and H. Kustner in 1921. The local wheal and flare response that occurs when an allergen is injected into a sensitized individual is referred to as the *P-K reaction.* Because the serum components responsible for the P-K reaction displayed specificity for allergen, they were assumed to be antibodies, but the nature of these P-K, or *reaginic,* antibodies was not demonstrated until the mid-1960s. Experiments by K. and T. Ishizaka showed that the biological activity of reaginic antibody in a P-K test could be neutralized by rabbit antisera against whole atopic human sera but not by rabbit antisera specific for the four known human immunoglobulin classes (IgA, IgG, IgM, and IgD) (Table 18-3). And when rabbits were immunized with sera from ragweed-sensitive individuals, the rabbit antiserum could inhibit (neutralize) a positive ragweed P-K test even after precipitation of the rabbit antibodies specific for the known human IgG, IgA, IgM, and IgD isotypes. The Ishizakas called this new isotype IgE in reference to the E antigen of ragweed that they used to characterize it.

Serum IgE levels in normal individuals fall within the range of 0.1–0.4 μg/ml; even the most severely allergic individuals rarely have IgE levels greater than 1 μg/ml. These low levels made physiochemical studies of IgE difficult, and it was not until the discovery of an IgE myeloma by S. G. O. Johansson and H. Bennich in 1967 that extensive chemical analysis of IgE could be undertaken. IgE was found to be composed of two heavy (ϵ) and two light chains with a combined molecular weight of 190,000. The increase in molecular weight over that of IgG (150,000) is due to the presence of an additional constant-region domain (see Figure 5-13). This additional domain (C_H4) contributes to an altered conformation of the Fc portion of the molecule that enables it to bind to glycoprotein receptors on the surface of basophils and mast cells. Although the half-life of IgE in the serum is only 2–3 days, once IgE is bound to its receptor on mast cells and basophils, it is stable in the bound state for a number of weeks.

Mast Cells and Basophils

The cells that bind IgE were identified by incubating human leukocytes and tissue cells with either ^{125}I-labeled IgE myeloma protein or ^{125}I-labeled anti-IgE. In both cases autoradiography revealed that the labeled probe bound to blood basophils and tissue mast cells. Basophils are granulocytes that circulate in the

TABLE 18-3 IDENTIFICATION OF IGE BASED ON REACTIVITY OF ATOPIC SERUM IN P-K TEST

Serum	Treatment	Allergen added	P-K reaction at skin site
Atopic	None	−	−
Atopic	None	+	+
Nonatopic	None	+	−
Atopic	Rabbit antiserum to human atopic serum*	+	−
Atopic	Rabbit antiserum to human IgM, IgG, IgA, and IgD†	+	+

* Serum from an atopic individual was injected into rabbits to produce antiserum against human atopic serum. When this antiserum was reacted with human atopic serum, it neutralized the P-K reaction.

† Serum from an atopic individual was reacted with rabbit antiserum to the known classes of human antibody (IgM, IgA, IgG, and IgD) to remove these isotypes from the atopic serum. The treated atopic serum continued to give a positive P-K reaction, indicating that a new immunoglobulin isotype was responsible for this reactivity.

SOURCE: Based on K. Ishizaka and T. Ishizaka, 1967, *J. Immunol.* **99**:1187.

blood of most vertebrates; in humans they account for 0.5–1.0% of the circulating white blood cells. Their granulated cytoplasm stains with basic dyes, hence the name basophil. Electron microscopy reveals a multilobed nucleus, few mitochondria, numerous glycogen granules, and electron-dense membrane-bounded granules scattered throughout the cytoplasm.

The mast cell was first described by Paul Ehrlich in 1877. The name in German means "fattening feed," a reference to the numerous granules, which were erroneously thought to have been engulfed by the cell. Mast-cell precursors are formed in the bone marrow during hematopoiesis and are carried to virtually all vascularized peripheral tissues where they differentiate into mature cells. Mast cells are found throughout connective tissue, particularly near blood and lymphatic vessels. Some tissues, including the skin and mucous membrane surfaces of the respiratory and gastrointestinal tract, contain high concentrations of mast cells; skin, for example, contains 10,000 mast cells per mm^3. Electron micrographs of mast cells reveal numerous membrane-bounded granules, which contain pharmacologically active mediators, distributed throughout the cytoplasm (Figure 18-2). After activation, these mediators are released from the granules, resulting in the clinical manifestations of the type I hypersensitive reaction.

Mast-cell populations in different anatomic sites exhibit significant variation in the types and amounts of allergic mediators they contain and in their sensitivity to activating stimuli and cytokines. Mast cells also secrete a variety of cytokines including IL-1, IL-2, IL-3, IL-5, IL-6, GM-CSF, TGF-β, and TNF-α. Because these cytokines exert diverse biological effects (see Table 13-1), mast cells contribute to a broad spectrum of physiologic, immunologic, and pathologic processes.

IgE-Binding Fc Receptors

The reaginic activity of IgE depends on its ability to bind to a receptor specific for the Fc region of the ϵ heavy chain. Two classes of FcϵR have been identified: FcϵRI and FcϵRII, which are expressed by different cell types and differ by 1000-fold in their affinity for IgE.

HIGH-AFFINITY RECEPTOR (FCϵRI). Mast cells and basophils express FcϵRI, which binds IgE with a high affinity ($K_d = 1-2 \times 10^{-9}$ M). The high affinity of this receptor enables it to bind IgE despite the low serum concentration of IgE (1×10^{-7} M). Between 40,000 and 90,000 FcϵRI molecules have been shown to be present on a human basophil.

The FcϵRI receptor contains four polypeptide chains: an α and a β chain and two identical disulfide-linked γ chains (Figure 18-3a). The α chain has an external region, a transmembrane segment, and a short cytoplasmic tail. The external region of the α chain contains two 90-aa domains that exhibit homology with the immunoglobulin-fold structure (see Figure 5-5), placing the molecule in the immunoglobulin superfamily. FcϵRI interacts with the C_H2/C_H2 domain of the IgE molecule via these two Ig-like domains of the α chain. The β chain spans the plasma membrane four times and is thought to link the α chain to the γ homodimer. The two γ chains are disulfide-linked and extend a considerable distance into the cytoplasm. They bear considerable sequence homology to the CD3 ζ

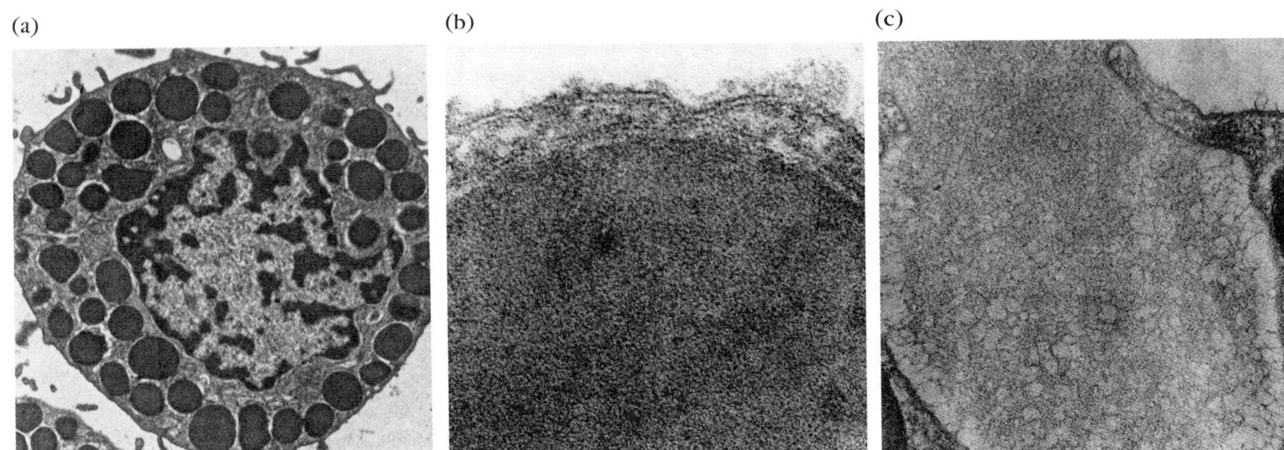

FIGURE 18-2 (a) Electron micrograph of a typical mast cell reveals numerous electron-dense membrane-bounded granules prior to degranulation. (b) Close-up of intact granule underlying the plasma membrane of a mast cell. (c) Granule releasing its contents during degranulation. [From S. Burwen and B. Satir, 1977, *J. Cell Biol.* **73**:662.]

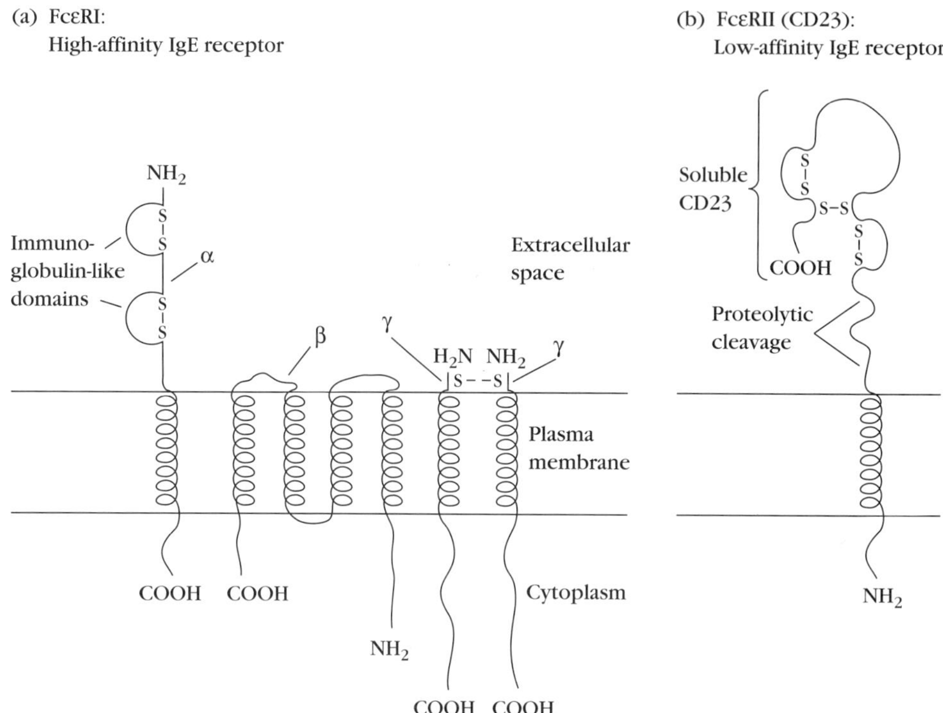

FIGURE 18-3 Schematic diagrams of the high-affinity and low-affinity receptors that bind the Fc region of IgE.

chains expressed by T cells. Like the CD3 ζ chains, the FcεRI γ chains are members of a group of membrane receptors, the multichain immune recognition receptors, which are characterized by a motif in their cytoplasmic domain called the antigen recognition activation motif (ARAM) (see Figure 11-7). The ARAM motif is thought to interact with protein tyrosine kinases during signal transduction. Allergen-mediated cross-linkage of the bound IgE results in aggregation of the FcεRI receptors and rapid tyrosine phosphorylation, which initiates the process of mast-cell degranulation.

LOW-AFFINITY RECEPTOR (FCεRII). The other IgE receptor, designated FcεRII (or CD23), is specific for the C_H3/C_H3 domain of IgE and has a lower affinity for IgE ($K_d \approx 1 \times 10^{-6}\ M$) than does FcεRI. This low-affinity receptor is unusual because it is oriented in the membrane with its N-terminus directed toward the cell interior and its C-terminus directed toward the extracellular space (Figure 18-3b). Two forms of FcεRII have been identified; these differ by only six amino acid residues in the N-terminus and are generated by differential RNA splicing of the same transcript. FcεRIIa is constitutively expressed on B cells, whereas expression of FcεRIIb is induced by IL-4 on B cells, macrophages, some T cells, and eosinophils. The FcεRII receptor appears to play a variety of roles in regulating the intensity of the IgE response. Allergen cross-linkage of IgE bound to FcεRII has been shown to activate B cells, alveolar macrophages, and eosinophils. When this receptor is blocked with monoclonal antibodies, IgE secretion by B cells is diminished. A soluble form of FcεRII (or sCD23), which is generated by autoproteolysis of the membrane receptor, has been shown to enhance IgE production by B cells. Interestingly, atopic individuals have higher levels of CD23 on their lymphocytes and macrophages and higher levels of sCD23 in their serum than nonatopic individuals.

Mechanism of IgE-Mediated Degranulation

The biochemical events mediating degranulation of mast cells and blood basophils have many features in common. For simplicity this section presents a general overview of mast-cell degranulation mechanisms without calling attention to the slight differences between mast cells and basophils. Although mast-cell degranulation generally is initiated by allergen cross-linkage of bound IgE, a number of other stimuli can also initiate the process including the anaphylatoxins (C3a, C4a, and C5a); various drugs such as synthetic ACTH, codeine, and morphine; and compounds such as the calcium ionophore. This section focuses on the biochemical events following allergen cross-linkage of bound IgE.

Receptor Cross-Linkage

IgE-mediated degranulation begins when an allergen cross-links receptor-bound (fixed) IgE on the surface of a mast cell or basophil. In itself, the binding of IgE to FcεRI apparently has no effect on a target cell. It is only after cross-linkage by allergen of the fixed IgE-receptor complex that degranulation proceeds. The importance of cross-linkage is indicated by the inability of monovalent allergens, which cannot cross-link the fixed IgE, to trigger degranulation. Experimental studies with preformed IgE-allergen complexes, in which the ratio of IgE to allergen was carefully monitored, revealed that only complexes having IgE-allergen ratios of 2 : 1 or greater could induce degranulation. Complexes in antigen excess (having an IgE-allergen ratio of 1 : 2) failed to induce degranulation because the requisite cross-linkage of receptors did not occur.

Other experiments have revealed that it is actually the cross-linkage of two or more FcεRI molecules—with or without IgE—that is essential for degranulation. Although cross-linkage is normally effected by the interaction of fixed IgE with divalent or multivalent allergen, it also can be effected by a variety of experimental means that bypass the need for allergen and in some cases even for IgE (Figure 18-4). For example, anti-IgE antibody can directly cross-link fixed IgE and induce degranulation. Chemical cross-linkage of IgE also can induce degranulation. Most significant, antibodies to the receptor itself can induce degranulation in the absence of both allergen and fixed IgE, demonstrating the crucial role of cross-linkage of FcεRI in initiating the subsequent biochemical events that culminate in degranulation. These events are diagrammed in Figure 18-5 and described in the following sections.

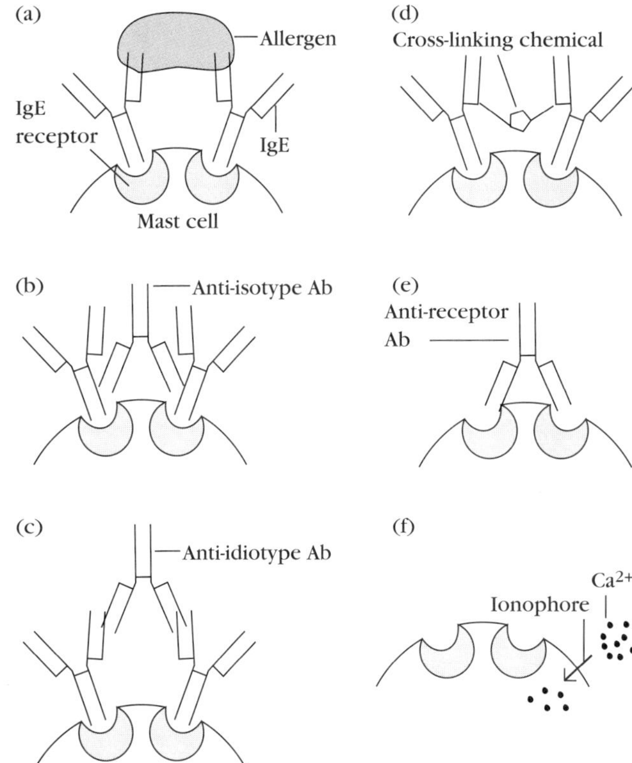

FIGURE 18-4 Schematic diagrams of mechanisms that can trigger mast-cell degranulation. (a) Allergen cross-linkage of cell-bound IgE molecules. (b, c) Antibody cross-linkage of IgE. (d) Chemical cross-linkage of IgE. (e) Cross-linkage of IgE receptors by antireceptor antibody. (f) Enhanced Ca^{2+} influx stimulated by an ionophore that increases membrane permeability to Ca^{2+} ions. Note that mechanisms (b), (c), and (d) do not require allergen; mechanisms (e) and (f) require neither allergen nor IgE; and mechanism (f) does not even require receptor cross-linkage.

Activation of Protein Tyrosine Kinases

The cytoplasmic domains of the β and γ chains of FcεRI are associated with protein tyrosine kinases (PTKs). After receptor aggregation the associated kinases are activated, resulting in the phosphorylation of a number of tyrosine residues including residues on the FcεRI β and γ chains and residues on phospholipase C. These phosphorylation events induce the production of a number of second messengers that induce the process of degranulation.

Methylation of Membrane Phospholipids

Within 15 s after cross-linkage of FcεRI by anti-IgE antibody, methylation of various membrane phospholipids can be observed (Figure 18-6). The cross-linkage of the IgE receptors is thought to activate a serine proesterase to form serine esterase, an enzyme that converts phosphatidylserine (PS) into phosphatidylethanolamine (PE). The cross-linkage of the IgE receptors also activates two other membrane-bound enzymes, phospholipid methyltransferase I and II (PMT I and II). PMT I faces the cytoplasmic side of the plasma membrane, and PMT II faces the exterior side. Methylation of PE to form phosphatidylcholine (PC) is achieved in two steps by the PMT enzymes. The accumulation of PC on the exterior surface of the plasma membrane causes an increase in membrane fluidity and is thought to facilitate the formation of Ca^{2+} channels. The finding that an inhibitor of methyltransferase activity (*S*-isobutyl-3-deazoadenosine) could inhibit both Ca^{2+} influx and the subsequent degranulation suggests that both effects depend on phospholipid methylation.

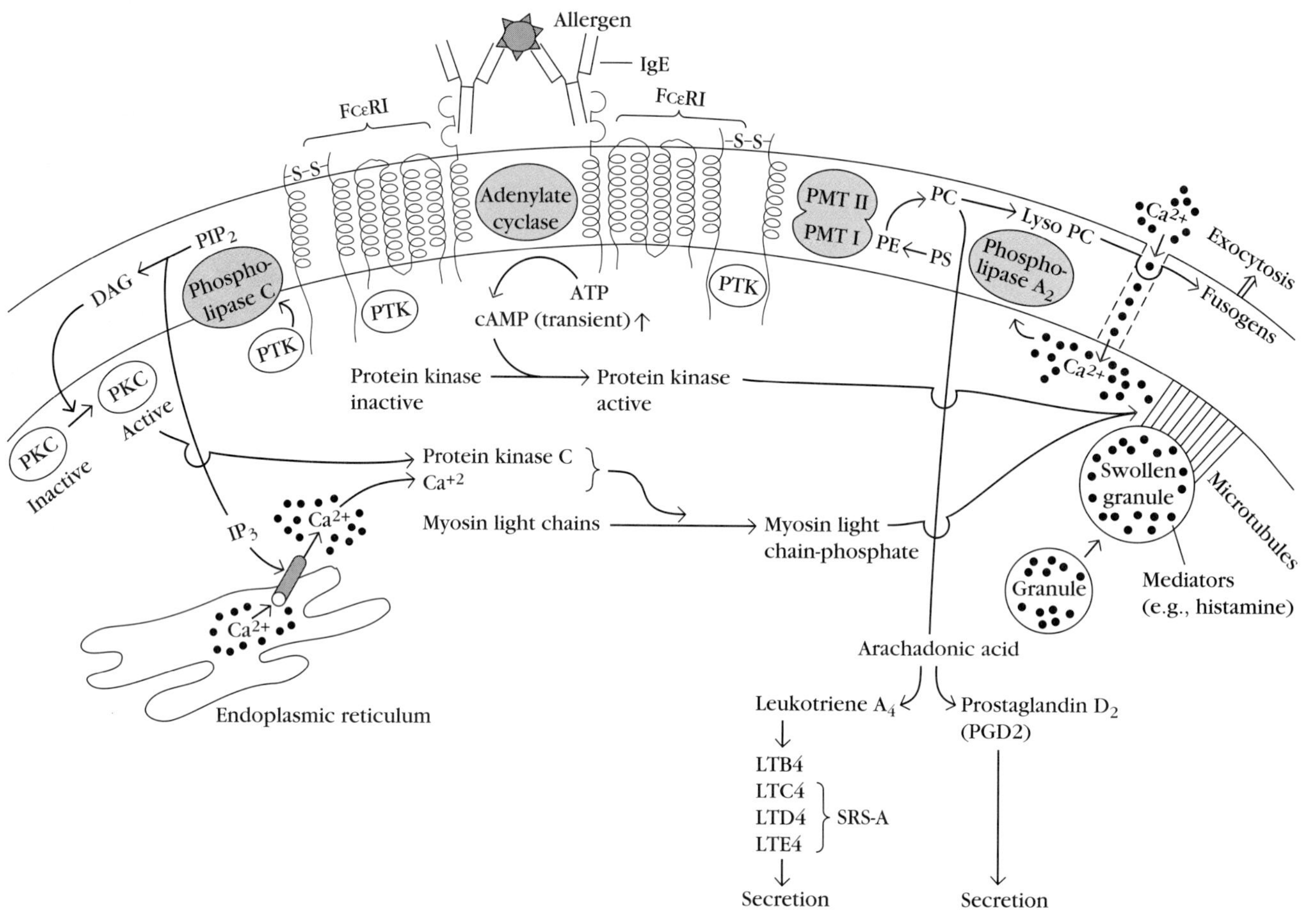

FIGURE 18-5 Diagrammatic overview of biochemical events in mast-cell activation and degranulation. Allergen cross-linkage of bound IgE activates protein tyrosine kinase (PTK), adenylate cyclase, and phospholipid methyltransferase I and II (PMT I and II). The action of these enzymes initiate several pathways that together lead to mast-cell degranulation. See text for discussion. PS = phosphatidylserine; PE = phosphatidylethanolamine; PC = phosphatidylcholine; PIP$_2$ = phosphatidylinositol-4,5-bisphosphate; DAG = diacylglycerol; IP$_3$ = inositol triphosphate; PKC = protein kinase C.

Influx of Ca^{2+}

The methylation of membrane phospholipids and subsequent conversion of PE to PC facilitates the opening of Ca^{2+} channels. The influx of Ca^{2+} reaches a peak within 2 min after receptor cross-linkage (see Figure 18-6). If mast cells are incubated with a receptor cross-linking agent in a medium lacking Ca^{2+}, degranulation does not occur unless the cells are rapidly returned to a medium containing Ca^{2+}. Moreover, degranulation can be experimentally induced, in the absence of receptor cross-linkage, by fusion of Ca^{2+}-containing phospholipid vesicles with the mast-cell plasma membrane. Both of these findings demonstrate the importance of Ca^{2+} uptake in degranulation.

The influx of Ca^{2+} has a number of effects on the mast cell. It activates the enzyme phopholipase A_2, which promotes the breakdown of PC to form lysophosphatidylcholine and arachidonic acid. Lysophosphatidylcholine further increases membrane fluidity, facilitating further Ca^{2+} influx (see Figure 18-5). The arachidonic acid is converted into two classes of potent mediators, the prostaglandins and the leukotrienes, which play a vital role in allergic manifestations. The influx of Ca^{2+} also promotes the assembly of microtubules and the contraction of microfilaments, both of which are necessary for the movement of granules to the plasma membrane.

Changes in cAMP Levels

Concomitant with phospholipid methylation and Ca^{2+} influx, there is a transient increase in membrane-bound adenylate cyclase activity, with a rapid peak of cAMP reached at 15 s after cross-linkage of FcεRI. The effects of cAMP are exerted through the activation of cAMP-dependent protein kinases. These are thought to phosphorylate the granule-membrane proteins, thereby changing the granules' permeability to water and Ca^{2+}. The consequent swelling of the granules appears to facilitate their fusion to the plasma membrane in degranulation. The increase in cAMP is transient: By the time Ca^{2+} influx and histamine release reach a peak after 2–3 min, the levels of intracellular cAMP have dropped to below the baseline level (see Figure 18-6). This drop in cAMP appears to be necessary for degranulation to proceed. When cAMP levels are increased by certain drugs, the degranulation process is blocked. Several of these drugs are often given to treat allergic disorders and are discussed later in the chapter.

Fusion of Granules with Plasma Membrane

As outlined in Figure 18-5, cross-linkage of FcεRI also leads to mobilization of intracellular Ca^{2+} stores, activation of protein kinase C, and phosphorylation of myosin light chains. As a result of these events and those described previously, the granules swell, microtubular assembly and contraction occurs, and the granules fuse with the plasma membrane, releasing their contents.

Mediators of Type I Reactions

The clinical manifestations of type I hypersensitive disorders are related to the biological effects of the mediators released during mast-cell or basophil degranulation. These mediators are pharmacologically active agents that act on local tissues as well as on populations of secondary effector cells including eosinophils, neutrophils, T lymphocytes, monocytes, and platelets. The mediators thus serve as an amplifying terminal effector mechanism, much as the complement system serves as an amplifier and effector of an antigen-antibody interaction. When generated in response to parasitic infection, these mediators initiate a beneficial defense process. Localized smooth-muscle contraction and the consequent vasodilation and increased vascular permeability bring an influx of plasma and inflammatory cells to attack the pathogen. On the other hand, mediator release induced by inappropriate antigens, such as allergens, results in unnecessary increases in vascular permeability and inflammation whose detrimental effects far outweigh any beneficial effect.

The mediators can be classified as either primary or secondary (Table 18-4). The primary mediators are produced before degranulation and are stored in the granules. The most significant primary mediators are

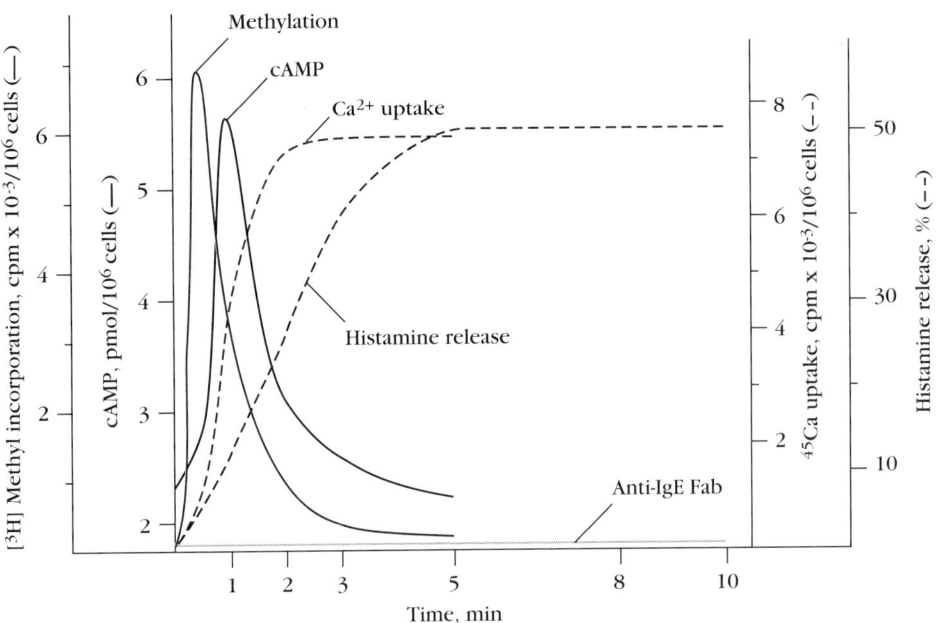

FIGURE 18-6 Kinetics of major biochemical events following cross-linkage of bound IgE on cultured human basophils with $F(ab')_2$ fragments of anti-IgE. Curves are shown for phospholipid methylation (solid purple), cAMP production (solid black), Ca^{2+} influx (dashed purple), and histamine release (dashed black). In control experiments with anti-IgE Fab fragments, no significant changes were observed. [Adapted from T. Ishizaka et al., 1985, *Int. Arch. Allergy Appl. Immunol.* **77**:137.]

TABLE 18-4 PRINCIPAL MEDIATORS INVOLVED IN TYPE I HYPERSENSITIVITY

Mediator	Effects
Primary	
Histamine	Increased vascular permeability; smooth-muscle contraction
Serotonin	Increased vascular permeability; smooth-muscle contraction
Eosinophil chemotactic factor (ECF-A)	Eosinophil chemotaxis
Neutrophil chemotactic factor (NCF-A)	Neutrophil chemotaxis
Proteases	Bronchial mucus secretion; degradation of blood-vessel basement membrane; generation of complement split products
Secondary	
Platelet-activating factor	Platelet aggregation and degranulation; contraction of pulmonary smooth muscles
Leukotrienes (slow reactive substance of anaphylaxis, SRS-A)	Increased vascular permeability; contraction of pulmonary smooth muscles
Prostaglandins	Vasodilation; contraction of pulmonary smooth muscles; platelet aggregation
Bradykinin	Increased vascular permeability; smooth-muscle contraction
Cytokines	
IL-1 and TNF-α	Systemic anaphylaxis; increased expression of CAMs on venular endothelial cells
IL-2, IL-3, IL-4, IL-5, IL-6, TGF-β and GM-CSF	Various effects (see Table 13-12)

histamine, proteases, eosinophil chemotactic factor, neutrophil chemotactic factor, and heparin. The secondary mediators either are synthesized after target-cell activation or are released by the breakdown of membrane phospholipids during the degranulation process. The secondary mediators include platelet-activating factor, leukotrienes, prostaglandins, bradykinin, and various cytokines. The differing manifestations of type I hypersensitivity in different species or different tissues partly reflect variations in the primary and secondary mediators present. The main biological effects of several of these mediators are discussed briefly in the following sections.

Histamine

Histamine is a major component of mast-cell granules, accounting for about 10% of the granule weight. Because it is stored—preformed—in the granules, its biological effects are observed within minutes of mast-cell activation. Once released from mast cells, histamine initially binds to specific receptors on various target cells. Three types of histamine receptors—designated H_1, H_2, and H_3—have been identified; these receptors have different tissue distributions and mediate different effects when they bind histamine. The binding of histamine to H_1 receptors induces contraction of intestinal and bronchial smooth muscles, increased permeability of venules, and increased mucous secretion by goblet cells. Interaction of histamine with H_2 receptors increases vasopermeability and dilation and stimulates exocrine glands. Binding of histamine to H_2 receptors on mast cells and basophils suppresses degranulation; thus histamine exerts negative-feedback control on mediator release. The function of the most recently discovered histamine receptor, H_3, is under investigation.

Leukotrienes

As secondary mediators, the leukotrienes are not formed until the mast cell undergoes degranulation and its plasma membrane is broken down. An ensuing enzymatic cascade generates the prostaglandins and the leukotrienes. It therefore takes a longer time for the biological effects of these mediators to become apparent. Their effects are more pronounced and longer-lasting, however, than those of histamine. Nanomole levels of the leukotrienes are as much as 1000 times more potent as bronchoconstrictors than histamine, and they are also more potent stimulators of vascular permeability and mucous secretion. In humans the leukotrienes are thought to contribute to the prolonged bronchospasm and buildup of mucus seen in asthmatics.

Cytokines

Adding to the complexity of the type I reaction are a variety of cytokines released from mast cells and eosinophils. Some of these may contribute to the clinical manifestations of a type I hypersensitivity. For example, the high concentrations of TNF-α and IL-1 secreted by mast cells may contribute to shock in systemic anaphylaxis. (This effect may parallel the role of TNF-α and IL-1 in bacterial septic shock and toxic-shock syndrome discussed in Chapter 13.) The localized late-phase response also may be partly mediated by cytokines released from mast cells. Both TNF-α and IL-1 increase the expression of cell-adhesion molecules on venular endothelial cells, thus facilitating the buildup of neutrophils, eosinophils, and monocytes that characterizes the late-phase response. The influx of eosinophils in the late-phase response has been shown to contribute to the chronic inflammation of the bronchial mucosa that characterizes persistent asthma.

Regulation of the Type I Response

As noted earlier, the genetic constitution of an animal, the antigen dose, and the mode of antigen presentation influence the level of the IgE response (i.e., the allergenicity of an antigen). For example, inbred strains of mice have been shown to differ in their tendency to mount an IgE response. Some strains (e.g., SJL) fail to produce an IgE response to appropriate allergens, whereas other strains (e.g., BDF1) have an increased propensity for IgE production. Breeding experiments have shown that this genetic variation is not linked to the MHC. A genetic component also has been shown to influence susceptibility to type I hypersensitive reactions in humans. When both parents are allergic, there is a 50% chance that a child will also be allergic; when only one parent is allergic, there is a 30% chance that a child will manifest some kind of type I reaction.

The effect of antigen dosage on the IgE response is illustrated by immunization of BDF1 mice. Repeated low doses of an appropriate antigen induce a persistent IgE response in these mice, but higher antigen doses result in transient IgE production and a shift toward IgG. The mode of antigen presentation also influences the development of the IgE response. For example, immunization of Lewis-strain rats with keyhole limpet hemocyanin (KLH) plus aluminum hydroxide gel or *Bordetella pertussis* as an adjuvant induces a strong IgE response, whereas injection of KLH with complete Freund's adjuvant produces a largely IgG response. Similar experimental findings have been reported in mice. Infection with the nematode *Nippostrongylus brasiliensis* (Nb), like certain adjuvants, preferentially induces an IgE response. For example, Nb-infected mice develop higher levels of IgE specific for an unrelated antigen than do uninfected control mice (Table 18-5).

TABLE 18-5 EFFECT OF INFECTION WITH *NIPPOSTRONGYLUS BRASILIENSIS* (NB) AND OF IL-4 ON SERUM IGE LEVELS IN MICE*

Treatment	Serum IgE (ng/ml)
None	0.24
N. brasiliensis	33.8
N. brasiliensis + anti-Nb antibody	35.4
N. brasiliensis + anti-IL-4 antibody	0.48

* Mice treated as indicated were immunized with TNP-KLH, and after an appropriate time the serum IgE level was determined.

SOURCE: F. D. Finkelman et al., 1988, *J. Immunol.* **141**:2335.

Cytokine-Mediated Regulation of Type I Response

The type I hypersensitivity response appears to be regulated by the relative levels of the T_H1 and T_H2 subsets: T_H1 cells reduce the response, whereas T_H2 cells enhance the response. Cytokines secreted by T_H2 cells —namely, IL-3, IL-4, IL-5, and IL-10—stimulate the type I response in several ways. IL-4 enhances class switching to IgE and regulates the clonal expansion of IgE-committed B cells; IL-3, IL-4, and IL-10 enhance mast-cell production; and IL-3 and IL-5 enhance eosinophil maturation, activation, and accumulation. T_H1 cells, in contrast, appear to inhibit the type I response through the effects of IFN-γ.

The pivotal role of IL-4 in regulating the type I response was demonstrated in experiments by W. E. Paul and co-workers. When these researchers activated normal, unprimed B cells in vitro with LPS, only 2% of the cells expressed membrane IgG1 and only 0.05% expressed membrane IgE. However, when unprimed B cells were incubated with LPS plus IL-4, the percentage of cells expressing IgG1 increased to 40–50% and the percentage expressing IgE increased to 15–25%. In an attempt to determine whether IL-4 plays a role in vivo in regulating IgE production, Paul primed Nb-infected mice with TNP-KLH in the presence or in the absence of monoclonal antibody to IL-4. The antibody to IL-4 inhibited the production of IgE specific for TNP-KLH by 99% in these Nb-infected mice compared with controls (see Table 18-5). Further support for the role of IL-4 in the IgE response comes from the experiments of K. Rejewski and co-workers with IL-4 knockout mice. These IL-4–deficient mice were unable to mount an IgE response to helminthic antigens. Increased levels of $CD4^+$ T_H2 cells and increased levels of IL-4 also have been detected in atopic individuals. When allergen-specific $CD4^+$ T cells from atopic individuals are cloned and added to an autologous B-cell culture, the B cells synthesize IgE, whereas allergen-specific $CD4^+$ T cells from nonatopic individuals do not support IgE production.

As discussed in Chapter 8, IL-4 has been shown to induce class switching from IgM to IgG1 and IgE isotypes in the mouse and from IgM to IgG4 and IgE in humans. More recent experiments suggest that class switching may involve two distinct signals: an IL-4–mediated signal and a second signal provided by physical contact of B cells with activated T cells. Although IL-4 is necessary to initiate class switching to IgG1 and IgE, a second signal, provided by formation of a T-cell/B-cell conjugate is necessary to complete the process. This second signal is thought to be mediated by CD40 on the B-cell membrane, which interacts with its ligand, CD40L, expressed on the membrane of activated T cells. This effect of the CD40-CD40L interaction appears to be distinct from its role as a co-stimulatory signal in B-cell activation discussed in Chapter 14.

In contrast to IL-4, IFN-γ decreases IgE production, suggesting that the balance of IL-4 and IFN-γ may determine the amount of IgE produced (Figure 18-7). Since IFN-γ is secreted by the T_H1 subset and IL-4 by the T_H2 subset, the relative activity of these subsets may influence an individual's response to allergens. According to this proposal, atopic and nonatopic individuals would exhibit qualitatively different type I responses to an allergen: The response in atopic individuals would involve the T_H2 subset and result in production of IgE; the response in nonatopic individuals would involve the T_H1 subset and result in production of IgM or IgG. To test this hypothesis, allergen-specific T cells were cloned from atopic and nonatopic individuals. The cloned T cells from the atopic individuals were predominantly of the T_H2 phenotype (IL-4 secreting), whereas the cloned T cells from nonatopic individuals were predominantly of the T_H1 phenotype (IFN-γ secreting). Needless to say, there is keen interest in down-regulating IL-4 as a possible treatment for allergic individuals.

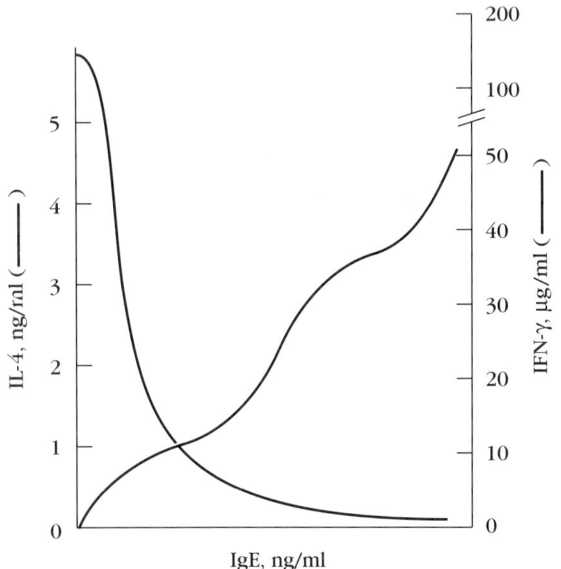

FIGURE 18-7 Effect of IL-4 and IFN-γ on in vitro production of IgE. Plasma cells were cultured in the presence of various concentrations of IL-4 or IFN-γ, and the amount of IgE produced was determined. [Adapted from G. Del Prete, 1988, *J. Immunol.* **140**:4193.]

Regulation of IgE Production by IgE-Binding Factors

In a series of experiments, the Ishizakas identified factors secreted by T cells that enhance or suppress IgE production by IgE-committed B cells. This regulatory mechanism thus operates after class switching has occurred. The Ishizakas first cultured mesenteric lymph nodes from Nb-infected mice and isolated IgE-binding factors from the culture supernatant. These factors had an affinity for IgE and were later shown to be derived from a subset of antigen-primed T cells. Subsequent experiments also revealed that some IgE-binding factors (IgE-PF) selectively potentiate IgE production and that others (IgE-SF) suppress it. The levels of potentiating and suppressing factors account in large part for the strain differences and adjuvant differences associated with the IgE response. T cells in the SJL strain, a low-IgE producer, secrete IgE-SF in response to antigen, whereas T cells in the BDF1 strain, a high-IgE producer, secrete IgE-PF. Similarly, adjuvants that potentiate the IgE response induce formation of IgE-PF, and adjuvants that suppress the IgE response induce IgE-SF. T-cell–derived IgE-binding factors that suppress or potentiate IgE production have also been detected in humans.

The Ishizakas were able to isolate the mRNA encoding an IgE-binding factor from a rat T-cell hybridoma stimulated with IgE. The mRNA was used to prepare a cDNA library and the cloned DNA was transfected into COS-1 monkey kidney cells (Figure 18-8). The transfected cells produced a potentiating IgE-binding factor (IgE-PF). However, when the transfected cells were grown in tunicamycin, an inhibitor of N-linked glycosylation, the cells produced a suppressing IgE-

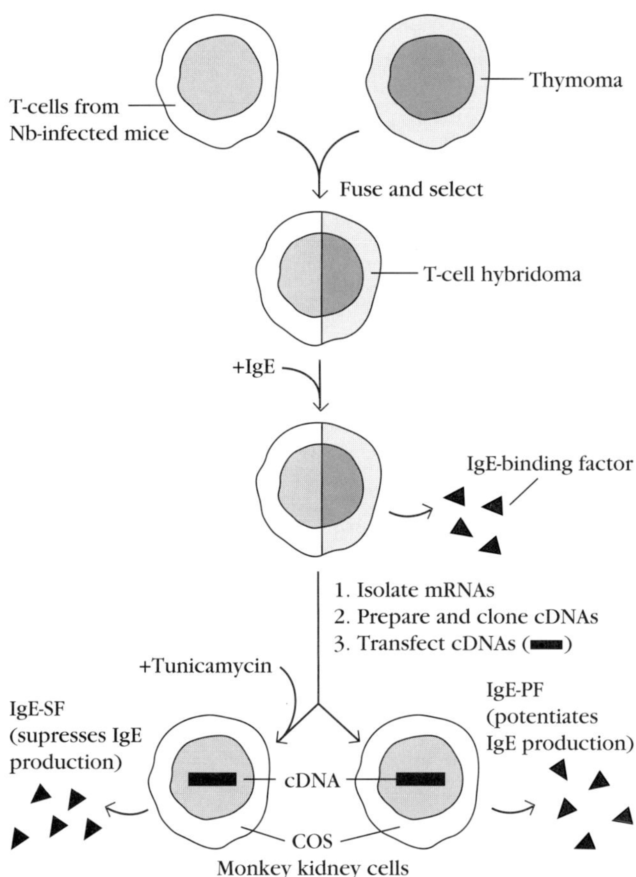

FIGURE 18-8 Experimental production of IgE-binding factors that either potentiate (IgE-PF) or suppress (IgE-SF) production of IgE by antigen-primed spleen cells in culture. In the presence of tunicamycin, an inhibitor of glycosylation, the transfected COS cells secreted IgE-SF, whereas in the absence of this inhibitor the same cells secreted IgE-PF. Thus a single gene appears to encode both factors, and differences in glycosylation of the initial gene product generate the two factors.

binding factor (IgE-SF). The IgE potentiating and suppressing factors therefore appear to be encoded by the same gene and to share a common polypeptide chain. Differences in post-translational glycosylation appear to determine whether the gene product functions as a potentiating or as a suppressing factor. Glycosylation-inhibiting factors (GIFs) inhibit the assembly of N-linked oligosaccharides to the IgE-binding factor, thereby generating IgE-SF, whereas glycosylation-enhancing factors (GEFs) promote the assembly of the oligosaccharides, thereby generating IgE-PF. The relative production of GIFs and GEFs ultimately determines whether a T cell produces IgE-SF or IgE-PF (Table 18-6).

The work of the Ishizakas suggests that some T-cell subpopulations produce glycosylation-enhancing factors (GEF), whereas others produce glycosylation-inhibiting factors (GIF). Adjuvants such as *Bordetella pertussis* and alum induce $CD4^+$ T cells to produce GEF, and complete Freund's adjuvant induces $CD8^+$ cells to produce GIF (Figure 18-9). As understanding of GEF and GIF increases, it may be possible to selectively down-regulate IgE production in allergic individuals.

Human B cells and monocytes also have been shown to secrete IgE-binding factors that regulate the IgE response. These IgE-binding factors appear to be unrelated to those secreted by T cells. The B-cell–derived IgE-binding factor appears to be a cleavage fragment of the low-affinity IgE receptor (CD23); this fragment is released from the cell by autoproteolytic cleavage. Release of these IgE-binding factors is induced by IL-4 and suppressed by IgE. Experiments are presently under way to determine the role of the B-cell–derived IgE-binding factor in regulation of the IgE response.

TABLE 18-6 CORRELATION OF IgE-BINDING FACTORS AND GLYCOSYLATION FACTORS WITH IgE RESPONSE

Experimental procedure	IgE-binding factor present	Glycosylation factor present	IgE response
Nb-infection (2 weeks)	IgE-PF	GEF	↑
Bordetella pertussis vaccine	IgE-PF	GEF	↑
KLH + alum priming	IgE-PF	GEF	↑
BDF1 mice immunized with OVA*	IgE-PF	GEF	↑
Complete Freund's adjuvant (CFA)	IgE-SF	GIF	↓
KLH + CFA priming	IgE-SF	GIF	↓
SJL mice immunized with OVA*	IgE-SF	GIF	↓

* Mice were immunized with alum-absorbed ovalbumin after ovalbumin immunization.

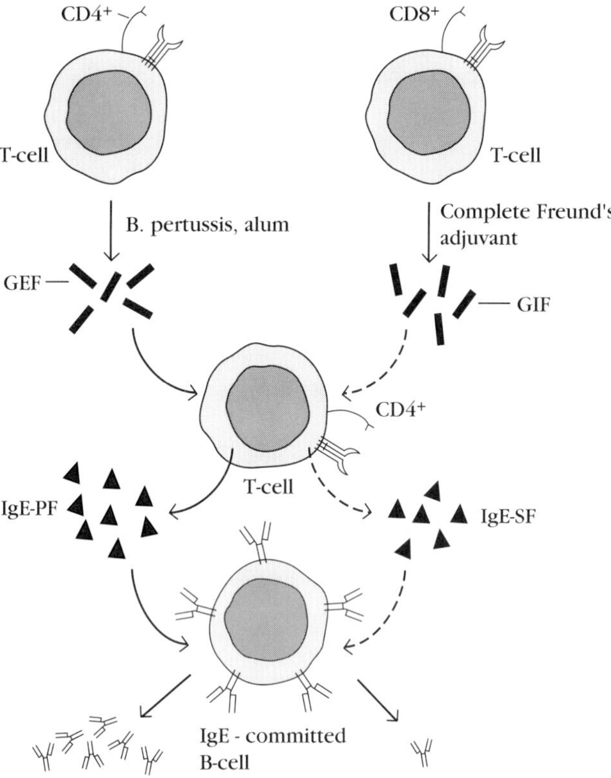

FIGURE 18-9 Different T-cell subpopulations produce glycosylation-enhancing factors (GEFs) or glycosylation-inhibiting factors (GIFs). These factors act on $CD4^+$ T_H cells, directing production of IgE-potentiating factor (IgE-PF) or IgE-suppressing factor (IgE-SF). The action of these factors on IgE-committed B cells leads to increased or decreased IgE production.

Detection of Type I Hypersensitivity

Type I hypersensitivity is commonly identified and assessed by skin testing. Small amounts of potential allergens are introduced at specific skin sites by either intradermal injection or superficial scratching. A number of tests can be applied to sites on the forearm or back of an individual at one time. If a person is allergic to the allergen, local mast cells will degranulate and the release of histamine and other mediators produces a wheal and flare within 30 min. The advantage of skin testing is that it is relatively inexpensive to perform and allows screening of a large number of allergens in a single sitting. The disadvantage of skin testing is that it sometimes sensitizes the allergic individual to new allergens and in some rare cases may induce systemic anaphylactic shock. A few individuals also manifest a late-phase reaction, which comes 4–6 h after testing and sometimes lasts for up to 24 h. A late-phase reaction site contains an increase in eosinophils, which constitute up to 30% of the cells at the site. Release of eosinophil-granule contents contributes to the tissue damage in a late-phase reaction.

Another method of assessing type I hypersensitivity is to determine the serum level of total IgE antibody by the radioimmunosorbent test (RIST). This highly sensitive technique, based on the radioimmunoassay, can determine nanogram levels of total IgE. The patient's serum is reacted with agarose beads or paper disks coated with rabbit anti-IgE. After the beads or disks are washed, ^{125}I-labeled rabbit anti-IgE is added. The beads or disks are counted in a gamma counter, and the radioactivity count is proportional to the level of IgE in the patient's serum (Figure 18-10a).

The similar radioallergosorbent test (RAST) detects the serum level of IgE specific for a given allergen. The allergen is coupled to beads or disks, the patient's serum is added, and unbound antibody is washed away. The amount of specific IgE bound to the solid-phase allergen is then measured by adding ^{125}I-labeled rabbit anti-IgE, washing the beads, and counting the bound radioactivity (Figure 18-10b).

Therapy for Type I Hypersensitivities

Clearly the obvious first step in controlling type I hypersensitivities is to identify the offending allergen and avoid contact if possible. Often the removal of house pets, dust-control measures, or avoidance of offending foods can eliminate a type I response. Elimination of inhalant allergens (such as pollens) is a physical impossibility, however, and other means of intervention must be pursued.

Immunotherapy involving repeated injections of increasing doses of allergens (hyposensitization) has been known for some time to reduce the severity of type I reactions, or even eliminate them completely, in a significant number of individuals suffering from allergic rhinitis. Such repeated introduction of allergen by subcutaneous injections appears to cause a shift toward IgG production or to induce T-cell–mediated suppression that turns off the IgE response (Figure 18-11). The IgG antibody is referred to as *blocking antibody* because it competes for the allergen, binds to it, and forms a complex that can be removed by phagocytosis; as a result, the allergen is not available to cross-link the fixed IgE on the mast-cell membrane and allergic symptoms decrease.

Another approach for treating allergies stems from the finding that soluble antigens tend to induce a state of anergy by activating T cells in the absence of the necessary co-stimulatory signal (see Figure 12-12). Presumably a soluble antigen is internalized by endocytosis, processed, and presented with class II MHC

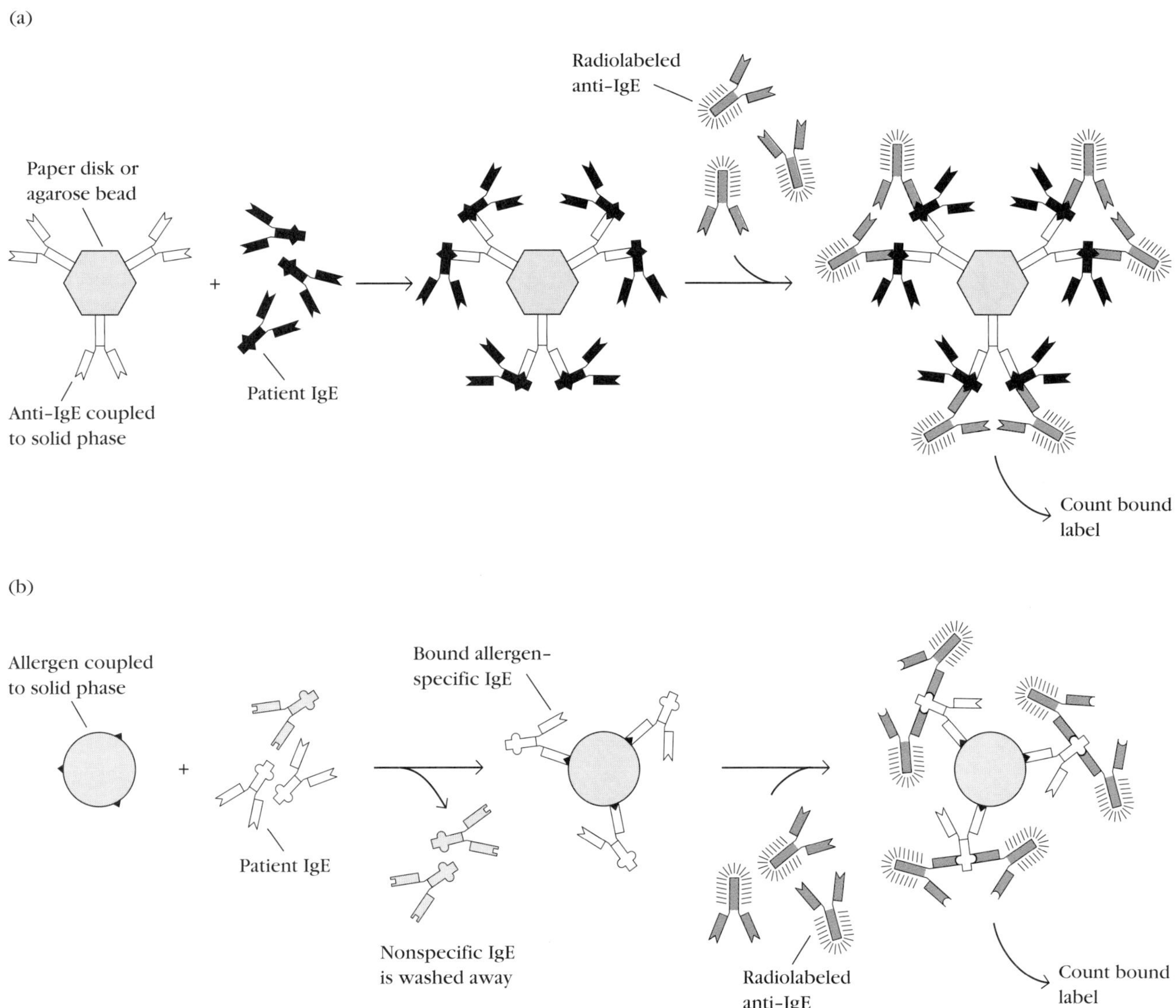

FIGURE 18-10 Procedures for assessing type I hypersensitivity. (a) Radioimmunosorbent test (RIST) can quantify nanogram amounts of total serum IgE. (b) Radioallergosorbent test (RAST) can quantify nanogram amounts of serum IgE specific for a particular allergen.

molecules, but fails to induce expression of the requisite co-stimulatory ligand (B7) on antigen-presenting cells. Immunologic Pharmaceuticals has reported the identification of the T-cell epitopes of ragweed pollen, cat hair, and house dust mites. When animals were injected with soluble antigens containing these T-cell epitopes, the animals became anergic to the corresponding allergen. Phase I clinical trials in humans are under way to determine if the soluble antigens will induce a similar allergen-specific state of nonresponsiveness in atopic individuals.

Knowledge of the mechanism of mast-cell degranulation and the mediators involved in type I reactions opened the way to drug therapy for allergy. Antihistamines have been the most useful drugs in alleviating allergic rhinitis symptoms. These drugs act by binding to the histamine receptors on target cells and blocking the binding of histamine. The H_1 receptors are blocked by the classical antihistamines, and the H_2 receptors by a newer class of antihistamines.

Several drugs block release of allergic mediators by interfering with various biochemical steps in mast-cell activation and degranulation (Table 18-7). Disodium cromoglycate (cromolyn sodium) prevents Ca^{2+} influx into mast cells. Theophylline, which is commonly administered orally or through inhalers to asthmatics, blocks phosphodiesterase, which catalyzes conversion of cAMP to 5′-AMP. The resulting prolonged increase

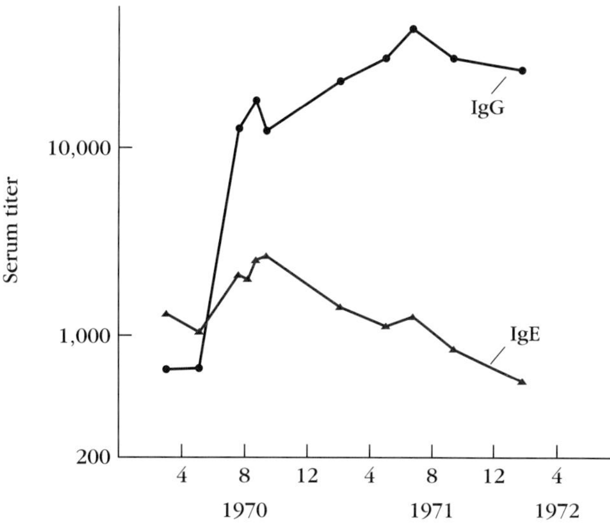

FIGURE 18-11 Injection of ragweed antigen periodically for 2 years into a ragweed-sensitive individual induced a gradual decrease in IgE levels and a dramatic increase in IgG. Both antibodies were measured by a radioimmunoassay. [From K. Ishizaka and T. Ishisaka, 1973, in *Asthma Physiology, Immunopharmacology and Treatment,* K. F. Austen and L. M. Lichtenstein (eds.), Academic Press.]

TABLE 18-7 MECHANISM OF ACTION OF SOME DRUGS USED TO TREAT TYPE I HYPERSENSITIVITY

Drug	Action
Antihistamines	Block H_1 and H_2 receptors on target cells
Cromolyn sodium	Blocks Ca^{2+} influx into mast cells
Theophylline	Prolongs high cAMP levels in mast cells by inhibiting phosphodiesterase, which cleaves cAMP to 5′-AMP*
Epinephrine (adrenalin)	Stimulates cAMP production by binding to β-adrenergic receptors on mast cells*
Cortisone	Reduces histamine levels by blocking conversion of histidine to histamine and stimulates mast-cell production of cAMP*

* Although cAMP rises transiently during mast-cell activation, degranulation is prevented if cAMP levels remain high.

in cAMP levels blocks degranulation. A number of drugs stimulate the β-adrenergic system by stimulating β receptors. Epinephrine (also known as adrenalin) is commonly administered during anaphylactic shock. It acts by binding to β receptors on bronchial smooth muscles and mast cells, elevating the cAMP levels within these cells. The increased levels of cAMP lead to relaxation of the bronchial muscles and decreased mast-cell degranulation. A number of altered versions of epinephrine have been developed that bind to select β receptors and induce cAMP increases with fewer side effects than epinephrine. Cortisone and various other anti-inflammatory drugs also have been used to reduce type I reactions.

Antibody-Mediated Cytotoxic (Type II) Hypersensitivity

Type II hypersensitive reactions involve antibody-mediated destruction of cells. This type of reaction is best characterized by blood-transfusion reactions in which host antibodies react with foreign antigens expressed by the incompatible transfused blood cells and mediate destruction of these cells. Antibody can mediate cell destruction by activating the complement system to create pores in the membrane of the foreign cell (see Figure 17-1). Antibody can also mediate cell destruction by antibody-dependent cell-mediated cytotoxicity (ADCC). In this process, cytotoxic cells with Fc receptors bind to the Fc region of antibodies on target cells and promote killing of the cells (see Figure 15-11). Antibody bound to a foreign cell also can serve as an opsonin, enabling phagocytic cells with Fc or C3b receptors to bind and phagocytose the antibody-coated cell. Several examples of type II hypersensitive reactions are examined.

Transfusion Reactions

A large number of proteins and glycoproteins on the membrane of red blood cells are encoded by different genes, each of which has a number of alternative alleles. An individual possessing one allelic form of a blood-group antigen can recognize other allelic forms on transfused blood as foreign and mount an antibody response. In some cases the antibodies are acquired by natural exposure to similar antigenic determinants on a variety of microorganisms thought to be normal flora of the gut. This is the case with the ABO blood-group antigens (Figure 18-12a). Antibodies to the A, B, and O antigens, called *isohemagglutinins,* are usually of the IgM class. An individual with blood type A, for example, recognizes B-like epitopes on intestinal microorganisms and produces isohemagglutinins to the B-like epitopes. This same individual does not respond to A-like epitopes on the same intestinal microorganisms because these A-like epitopes are too similar to self and a state of self-tolerance to these epitopes should exist (Figure 18-12b). If a type A individual is accidentally transfused with blood containing type B cells, the anti-B isohemagglutinins will bind to the B blood cells and mediate their destruction by means of complement-mediated lysis. Antibodies to other blood-group antigens are acquired through repeated blood transfusions because minor allelic differences in these antigens can stimulate antibody production. These antibodies are usually of the IgG class.

Transfusion of blood into a recipient possessing antibodies to one of the blood-group antigens can result in a transfusion reaction. The clinical manifestations of transfusion reactions result from massive intravascular hemolysis of the transfused red blood cells by antibody plus complement. The clinical manifestations may have immediate or delayed onset. Reactions having immediate onset are most commonly associated with ABO blood-group incompatibilities, which lead to complement-mediated lysis triggered by the IgM isohemagglutinins. Within hours free hemoglobin can be detected in the plasma; it is filtered through the kidneys, resulting in hemoglobinuria. Some of the hemoglobin gets converted to bilirubin, which at high levels is toxic. Typical symptoms include fever, chills, nausea, clotting within blood vessels, pain in the lower back, and hemoglobin in the urine. Treatment involves prompt termination of the transfusion and maintenance of urine flow with a diuretic because the accumulation of hemoglobin in the kidney can cause acute tubular necrosis.

Delayed hemolytic transfusion reactions generally occur in individuals who have received repeated transfusions of ABO-compatible blood that is incompatible for other blood-group antigens. The reactions develop between 2 and 6 days following transfusion and reflect the secondary nature of these reactions. The transfused blood induces clonal selection and production of IgG against a variety of blood-group membrane antigens. The most common blood-group antigens inducing delayed transfusion reactions are ABO, Rh, Kidd, Kell, and Duffy. The predominant isotype involved in these reactions is IgG, which is less effective than IgM in

(a)

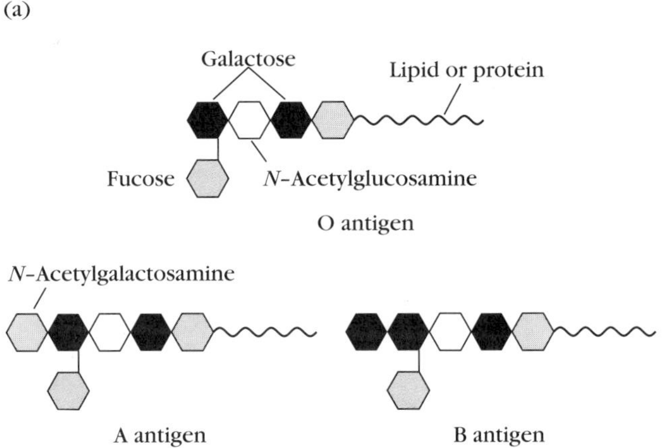

(b)

Genotype	Blood-group phenotype	Antigens on erythrocytes (*agglutinins*)	Serum antibodies (*isohemagglutinins*)
AA or AO	A	A	Anti-B
BB or BO	B	B	Anti-A
AB	AB	A and B	None
OO	O	None	Anti-A and anti-B

FIGURE 18-12 ABO blood group. (a) Structure of terminal sugars, which constitute the distinguishing epitopes, in the A, B, and O blood antigens. (b) ABO genotypes and corresponding phenotypes, agglutinins, and isohemagglutinins.

activating complement. For this reason, complement-mediated lysis of the transfused red blood cells is incomplete, and many of the transfused cells are destroyed at extravascular sites by agglutination, opsonization, and subsequent phagocytosis by macrophages. Symptoms include fever, low hemoglobin, increased bilirubin, mild jaundice, and anemia. Free hemoglobin is usually not detected in the plasma or urine in these reactions because RBC destruction occurs in extravascular sites. Blood-transfusion reactions can be prevented by proper cross-matching between the donor's and the recipient's blood. Cross-matching can reveal the presence of the antibodies in donor or recipient sera that can cause these reactions.

Hemolytic Disease of the Newborn

Hemolytic disease of the newborn develops when maternal IgG antibodies specific for fetal blood-group antigens cross the placenta and destroy fetal red blood cells. The consequences of such transfer can be minor, serious, or lethal. Severe hemolytic disease of the newborn, called *erythroblastosis fetalis,* is commonly caused by Rh incompatibility, which develops in Rh^- mothers who carry an Rh^+ fetus.

During pregnancy, fetal red blood cells are separated from the mother's circulation by a layer of cells in the placenta called the trophoblast. During her first pregnancy, a woman is usually not exposed to enough of these fetal red blood cells to activate Rh-specific B cells. At the time of delivery, however, separation of the placenta from the uterine wall allows larger amounts of fetal umbilical-cord blood to enter the mother's circulation. These fetal red blood cells activate Rh-specific B cells resulting in production of Rh-specific plasma cells and memory cells. The secreted IgM antibody clears the Rh^+ fetal red cells from the mother's circulation, but the memory cells remain, a threat to any subsequent pregnancy with an Rh^+ fetus. Activation of these memory cells in a subsequent pregnancy results in the formation of IgG anti-Rh

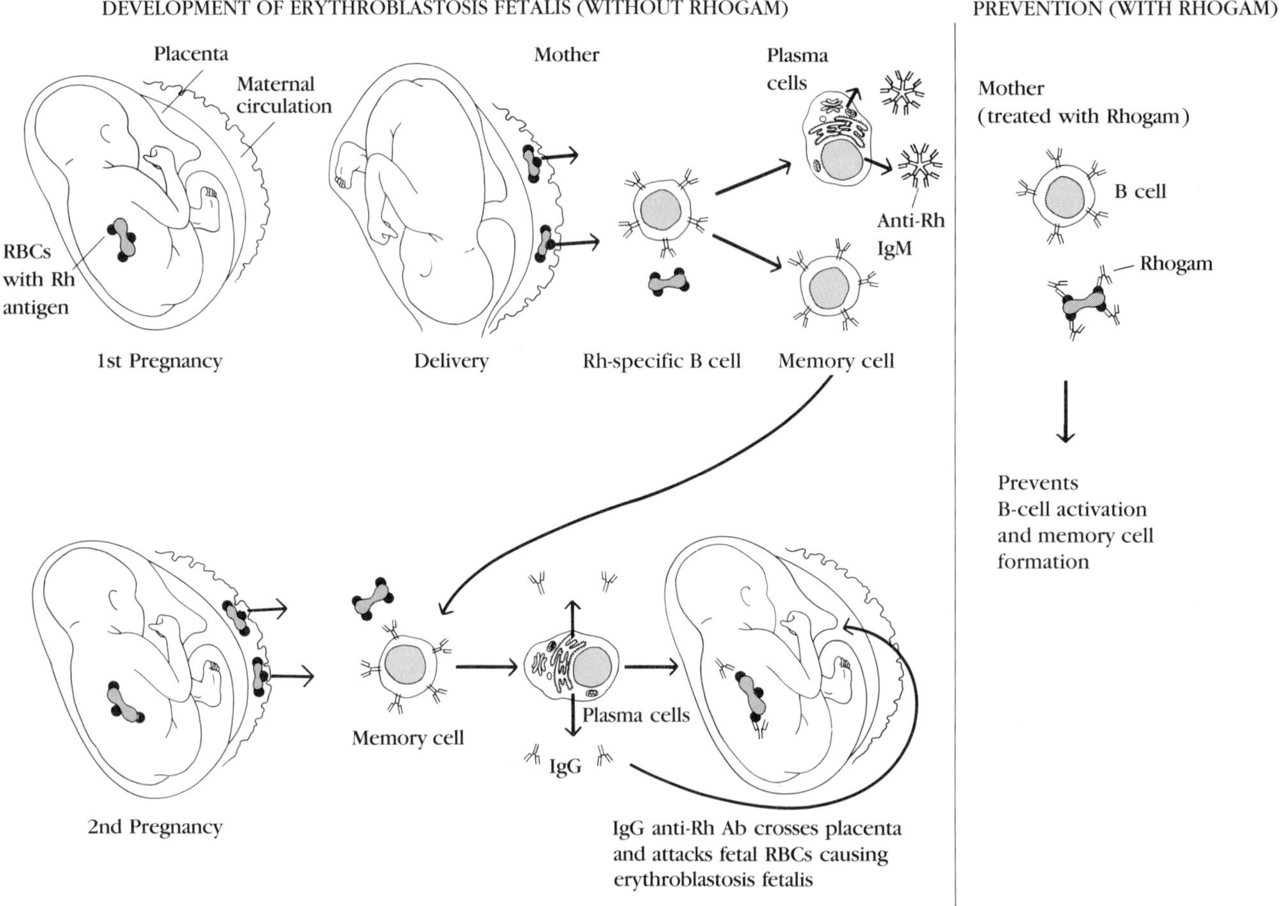

FIGURE 18-13 Development of erythroblastosis fetalis (hemolytic disease of the newborn) caused by an Rh^- mother carrying an Rh^+ fetus *(left)* and effect of treatment with anti-Rh antibody, or Rhogam *(right).* See text for details.

antibodies, which cross the placenta and damage the fetal red blood cells (Figure 18-13). Mild to severe anemia can develop, sometimes with fatal consequences. In addition, conversion of hemoglobin to bilirubin can present an additional threat to the newborn because the lipid-soluble bilirubin may accumulate in the brain and cause brain damage.

Hemolytic disease of the newborn caused by Rh incompatibility can be almost entirely prevented by the administration of antibodies to the Rh antigen (Rhogam) within 24–48 h after delivery. These antibodies bind to any fetal red blood cells that enter the mother's circulation at the time of delivery and facilitate their clearance before B-cell activation and ensuing memory-cell production can take place. In a subsequent pregnancy with an Rh^+ fetus, a Rhogam-treated mother is unlikely to produce IgG anti-Rh antibodies; thus the fetus is protected from the damage that occurs when these antibodies cross the placenta.

The development of hemolytic disease of the newborn caused by Rh incompatibility can be detected by testing maternal serum at intervals during pregnancy for antibodies to the Rh antigen. A rise in the titer of these antibodies as pregnancy progresses indicates that the mother has been exposed to Rh antigens and is producing increasing amounts of antibody. The presence of maternal IgG on the surface of fetal red blood cells can be detected by a *Coombs test.* Isolated fetal red cells are incubated with goat antibody to human IgG antibody (the Coombs reagent). If maternal IgG is bound to the fetal red cells, the cells agglutinate with the Coombs reagent.

Treatment of hemolytic disease caused by Rh incompatibility depends on the severity of the reaction. If the reaction is severe, the fetus can be given an intrauterine blood-exchange transfusion with Rh^- red blood cells. These transfusions are given every 10–21 days until delivery. In less severe cases a blood-exchange transfusion is not given until after birth, primarily to remove bilirubin; the infant is also exposed to low levels of UV light to break down the bilirubin and prevent any cerebral damage. The mother can also be treated during the pregnancy by plasmapheresis. In this procedure a cell-separation machine is used to separate the mother's blood into two fractions, cells and plasma. The plasma containing the anti-Rh antibody is discarded, and the cells are reinfused into the mother in an albumin or fresh plasma solution.

The majority of cases (65%) of hemolytic disease of the newborn have relatively minor consequences and are caused by ABO blood-group incompatibility between the mother and fetus. Type A or B fetuses carried by type O mothers most commonly develop these reactions. A type O mother is most likely to develop IgG antibody to the A or B blood-group antigens either through natural exposure or through exposure to fetal blood-group A or B antigens in successive pregnancies. Usually the fetal anemia resulting from this incompatibility is mild; the major clinical manifestation is a slight elevation of bilirubin, with jaundice. Depending on the severity of the anemia and jaundice, a blood-exchange transfusion may be required in these infants. In general the reaction is mild, however, and exposure of the infant to low levels of UV light is enough to break down the bilirubin and avoid any cerebral damage.

Drug-Induced Hemolytic Anemia

Certain antibiotics (e.g., penicillin, cephalosporin, and streptomycin) can adsorb nonspecifically to proteins on RBC membranes, forming a complex similar to a hapten-carrier complex. In some patients, such drug-protein complexes induce formation of antibodies, which then bind to the adsorbed drug on red blood cells, inducing complement-mediated lysis and thus progressive anemia. When the drug is withdrawn, the hemolytic anemia disappears. Penicillin is notable in that it can induce all four types of hypersensitivity with various clinical manifestations (Table 18-8).

TABLE 18-8 PENICILLIN-INDUCED HYPERSENSITIVE REACTIONS

Type of hypersensitive reaction	Antibody or lymphocytes induced	Clinical manifestations
I	IgE	Urticaria, systemic anaphylaxis
II	IgM, IgG	Hemolytic anemia
III	IgG	Serum sickness, glomerulonephritis
IV	T_{DTH} cells	Contact dermatitis

Autoimmune Type II Reactions

Individuals with certain autoimmune diseases produce autoantibodies against a variety of cellular antigens. These antibodies can mediate cellular destruction by way of a type II mechanism involving complement-mediated lysis. These diseases, which are discussed in Chapter 19, include autoimmune hemolytic anemia, idiopathic thrombocytopenia purpura, Hashimoto's thyroiditis, Goodpasture's syndrome, and myasthenia gravis.

Immune Complex–Mediated (Type III) Hypersensitivity

The reaction of antibody with antigen generates immune complexes. Generally this complexing of antigen with antibody facilitates the clearance of antigen by phagocytic cells. In some cases, however, large amounts of immune complexes can lead to tissue-damaging type III hypersensitive reactions. The magnitude of the reaction depends on the quantity of immune complexes as well as their distribution within the body. Depending on where these complexes are carried, different tissue-damaging reactions can be observed. When the complexes are deposited in tissue very near the site of antigen entry, a localized *Arthus reaction* develops. When the complexes are formed in the blood, a reaction can develop wherever the complexes are deposited (e.g., on blood-vessel walls, in the synovial membrane of joints, on the glomerular basement membrane of the kidney, on the choroid plexus of the brain). In any case, tissue is damaged at the site of deposition.

Type III hypersensitive reactions develop when immune complexes activate the complement system's array of immune effector molecules. The C3a, C4a, and C5a complement split products are anaphylatoxins that cause localized mast-cell degranulation and consequent increase in local vascular permeability. C3a, C5a, and C5b67 are also chemotactic factors for neutrophils, which can accumulate in large numbers at the site of immune-complex deposition. Larger immune complexes are deposited on the basement membrane of blood-vessel walls or kidney glomeruli, whereas smaller complexes may pass through the basement membrane and be deposited in the subepithelium. The type of lesion that results depends on the site of deposition of the complexes.

Much of the tissue damage in type III reactions stems from release of lytic enzymes by neutrophils as they attempt to phagocytose immune complexes. A neutrophil binds to an immune complex by means of the type I complement receptor, which is specific for the C3b complement component. Because the complex is attached to the basement-membrane surface, phagocytosis is impeded, allowing lytic enzymes to be released during the unsuccessful attempts of the neutrophil to ingest the adhering immune complex. Further activation of the membrane-attack mechanism of the complement system can also contribute to the tissue destruction. In addition, the activation of complement can induce aggregation of platelets, and the resulting release of clotting factors can lead to formation of microthrombi.

Localized Type III Reactions

Injection of an antigen intradermally or subcutaneously into an animal that has high levels of circulating antibody specific for that antigen leads to formation of localized immune complexes, which mediate an acute Arthus reaction within 4–8 h (Figure 18-14). Microscopic examination of the tissue reveals neutrophils adhering to the vascular endothelium and then migrating into the tissues at the site of immune-complex deposition. As the reaction develops, localized tissue and vascular damage results in an accumulation of fluid (edema) and red blood cells (erythema) at the site. The severity of the reaction can vary from mild swelling and redness to tissue necrosis.

Following an insect bite, a sensitive individual may have a rapid, localized type I reaction at the site. Often, some 4–8 h later, a typical Arthus reaction also develops at the site with pronounced erythema and edema. Intrapulmonary Arthus-type reactions induced by bacterial spores, fungi, or dried fecal proteins can also cause pneumonitis or alveolitis. These reactions are known by a variety of common names reflecting the source of the antigen. For example, "farmer's lung" develops after inhalation of thermophilic actinomycetes from moldy hay, and "pigeon fancier's disease" results from inhalation of a serum protein in dust derived from dried pigeon feces.

Generalized Type III Reactions

When large amounts of antigen enter the bloodstream and bind to antibody, circulating immune complexes can form. If antigen is in excess, small complexes form; because these are not easily cleared by the phagocytic cells, they can cause tissue-damaging type III reactions at various sites. Historically, generalized type III reactions were often observed after the administration of antitoxins containing foreign serum, such as horse antitetanus or antidiphtheria serum. In such cases, the recipient of a foreign antiserum develops antibodies specific for the foreign serum proteins; these antibodies then form circulating immune complexes with the foreign serum antigens. Typically within days or weeks after exposure to foreign serum antigens, an individual begins to manifest a combination of symptoms that are called *serum sickness* (Figure 18-15). These symptoms include fever, weakness, generalized vasculitis (rashes) with edema and erythema, lymphadenopathy, arthritis, and sometimes glomerulonephritis. The precise manifestations of

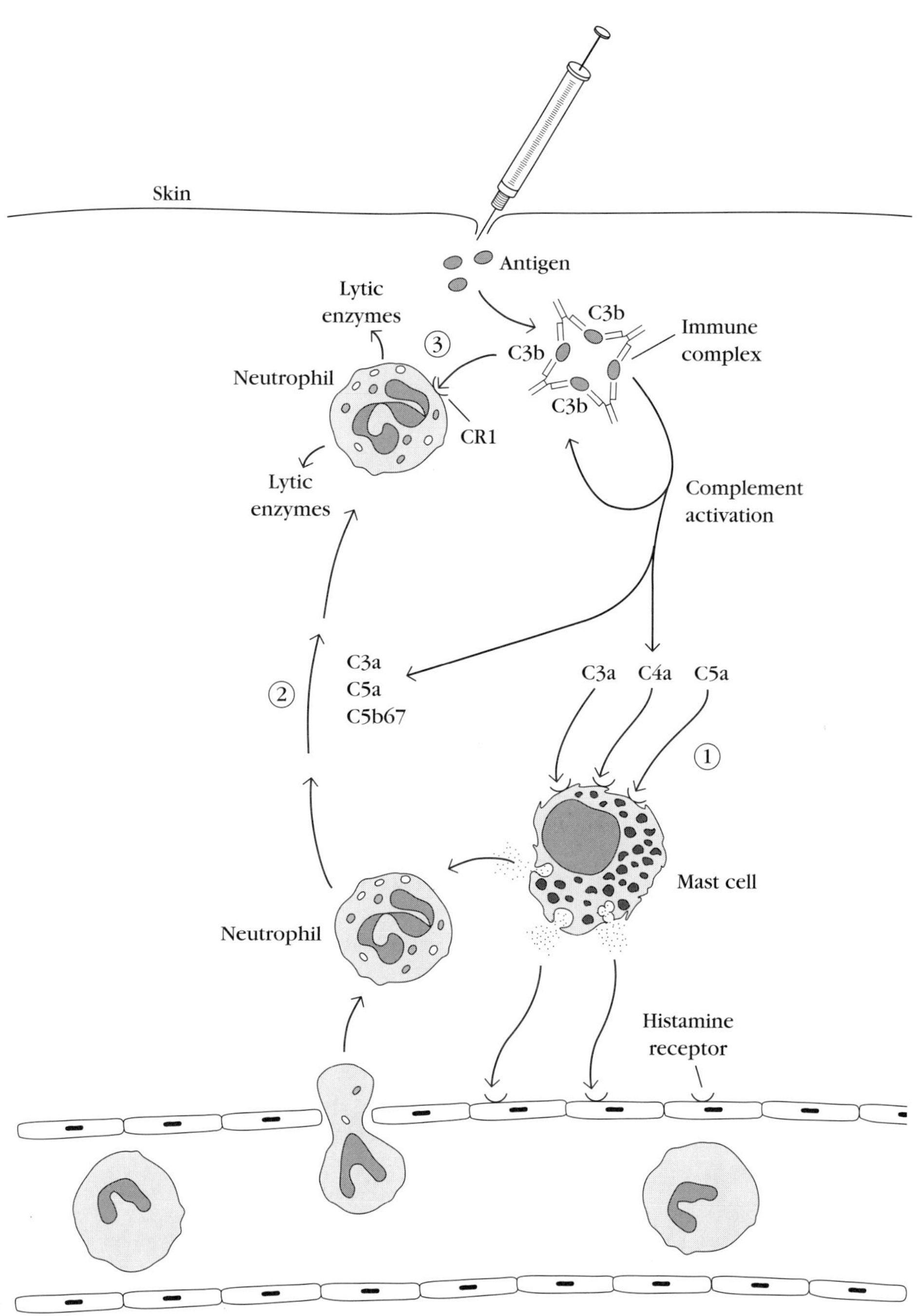

FIGURE 18-14 Development of a localized Arthus reaction (type III hypersensitive reaction). Complement activation initiated by immune complexes (classical pathway) produces complement intermediates that (1) mediate mast-cell degranulation, (2) chemotactically attract neutrophils, and (3) stimulate release of lytic enzymes from neutrophils trying to phagocytose C3b-coated immune complexes. See text for further discussion.

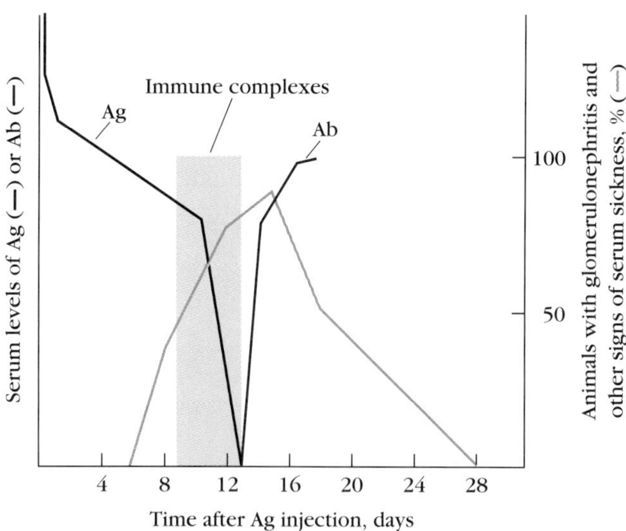

FIGURE 18-15 Correlation between immune-complex formation and development of symptoms of serum sickness. A large dose of antigen (BSA) was injected into a rabbit at day 0. As antibody formed, it complexed with the antigen and was deposited in the kidneys, joints, and capillaries. The symptoms of serum sickness corresponded to the peak in immune-complex formation. As the immune complexes were cleared, free circulating antibody was detected and the symptoms of serum sickness subsided. [Based on F. G. Germuth, Jr., 1953, *J. Exp. Med.* **97**:257.]

serum sickness depend on the quantity of immune complexes formed as well as the overall size of the complexes, which determine the site of tissue deposition.

Formation of circulating immune complexes contributes to the pathogenesis of a number of conditions other than serum sickness. These include the following:

Autoimmune Diseases
- Systemic lupus erythematosus
- Rheumatoid arthritis
- Goodpasture's syndrome

Drug Reactions
- Allergies to penicillin and sulphonamides

Tumors

Infectious Diseases
- Poststreptococcal glomerulonephritis
- Meningitis
- Hepatitis
- Mononucleosis
- Malaria
- Trypanosomiasis

Complexes of antibody with various bacterial, viral, and parasitic antigens have been shown to induce a variety of type III hypersensitive reactions including skin rashes, arthritic symptoms, and glomerulonephritis. Poststreptococcal glomerulonephritis, for example, develops when circulating complexes of antibody and streptococcal antigens are deposited in the kidney and damage the glomeruli. A number of autoimmune diseases stem from circulating complexes of antibody and self-proteins, glycoproteins, or even DNA. In systemic lupus erythematosus, complexes of DNA and anti-DNA antibodies accumulate in synovial membranes, causing arthritic symptoms, or accumulate on the basement membrane of the kidney, causing progressive kidney damage. Type III reactions are also common in cancer patients, in whom complexes of antibody with shed tumor antigens can build up in the circulation, leading to skin rashes, arthritic symptoms, and/or kidney damage.

T_{DTH}-Mediated (Type IV) Hypersensitivity

Type IV hypersensitive reactions develop when antigen activates sensitized T_{DTH} cells; these cells generally appear to be a T_H1 subpopulation although sometimes T_C cells are involved. As illustrated in Figure 15-13, activation of T_{DTH} cells by antigen on appropriate antigen-presenting cells results in the secretion of various cytokines including interleukin 2 (IL-2), interferon gamma (IFN-γ), macrophage migration-inhibition factor (MIF), and tumor necrosis factor β (TNF-β). The overall effect of these cytokines is to draw macrophages into the area and activate them, promoting increased phagocytotic activity and increased concentrations of lytic enzymes for more effective killing. As lytic enzymes leak out of the activated macrophages into the surrounding tissue, localized tissue destruction can ensue. These reactions typically take 48–72 h to develop, the time required for initial T_{DTH}-cell activation and lymphokine secretion to mediate accumulation of macrophages and the subsequent release of their lytic enzymes.

As discussed in Chapter 15, several lines of evidence suggest that the type IV (or DTH) reaction is important in host defense against parasites and bacteria that can live intracellularly. Antibodies cannot reach these organisms (because they are inside the host's cells), but the heightened phagocytotic activity and the buildup of lytic enzymes from macrophages in the area leads to nonspecific destruction of cells, and thus of the intracellular pathogen. When this defense process is not entirely effective, however, the continued presence of the pathogen's antigens can provoke a chronic DTH reaction, which is characterized by excessive numbers of macrophages, continual release of lytic enzymes, and consequent tissue destruction. The granulomatous skin lesions seen with *Mycobacterium leprae* and the lung cavitation seen with *Mycobacterium tuberculosis* are both examples of the tissue damage that can result when chronic delayed-type hypersensitive reactions develop (see Figure 21-8).

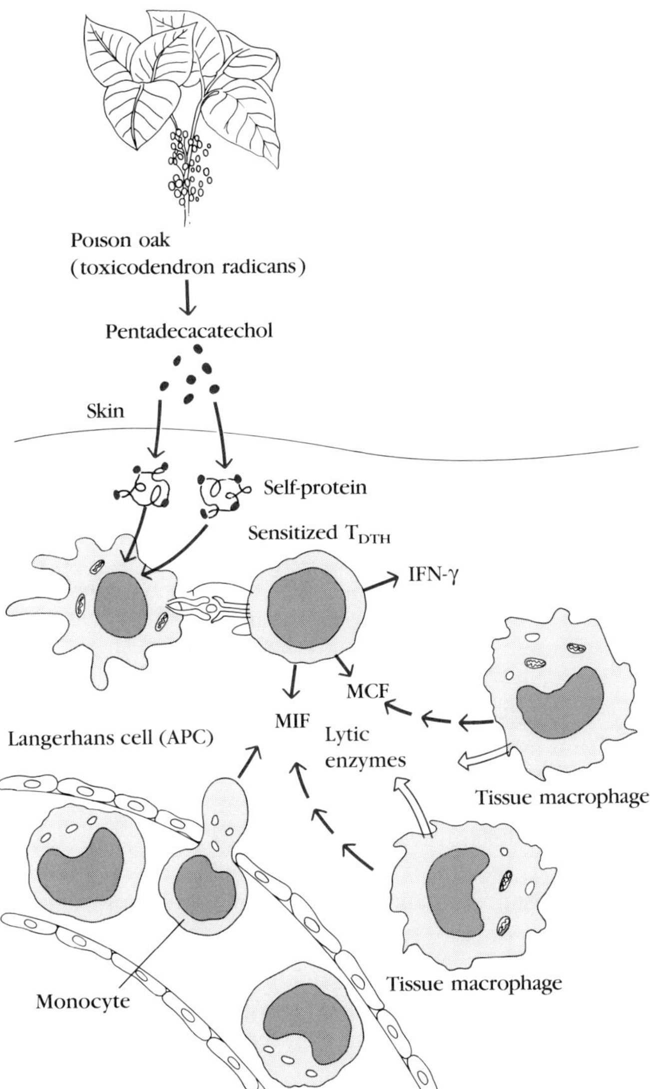

FIGURE 18-16 Development of delayed-type hypersensitivity reaction following second exposure to poison oak. Cytokines such as IFN-γ, MCF, and MIF released from sensitized T_{DTH} cells mediate this reaction. Tissue damage results from lytic enzymes released from activated macrophages. MCF = macrophage-chemotactic factor; MIF = migration-inhibition factor. See also Figures 15-13 and 15-14.

The reaction to an intradermal injection of an antigen can serve as a test for the presence of T_{DTH} cells previously sensitized by that antigen. The use of the PPD antigen to detect previous exposure to *M. tuberculosis* was described in Chapter 15. Similar skin tests to detect previous exposure to the bacterium causing leprosy and the fungus causing coccidiomycosis utilize lepromin and coccidiodin, respectively, as test antigens. In these tests, the appearance of swelling and redness at the injection site within 48–72 h constitutes a positive reaction. The depletion in $CD4^+$ T cells associated with AIDS can be monitored by repeated skin testing with any of the various antigens that induce a type IV DTH response in most normal individuals. As AIDS progresses, the decline in T_{DTH} cells is reflected in decreased skin reactivity to such antigens.

Many contact-dermatitis reactions, including the response to formaldehyde, trinitrophenol, nickel, turpentine, various cosmetics and hair dyes, poison oak, and poison ivy, are mediated by T_{DTH} cells. Most of these substances are small molecules that can complex with skin proteins. This complex is internalized by antigen-presenting cells in the skin (such as Langerhans cells), then processed and presented together with class II MHC molecules, causing activation of sensitized T_{DTH} cells. In the reaction to poison oak, for example, a pentadecacatechol compound from the leaves of the plant complexes with skin proteins. T_H cells react with this compound appropriately expressed by local antigen-presenting cells and differentiate into sensitized T_{DTH} cells. A subsequent exposure to pentadecacatechol will elicit activation of T_{DTH} cells and induce cytokine production. Approximately 48–72 h after exposure, the secreted cytokines cause macrophages to accumulate at the site. Activation of these macrophages and release of their lytic enzymes results in the redness and pustules that characterize a reaction to poison oak (Figure 18-16).

Summary

1. Hypersensitive reactions are inflammatory reactions within the humoral or cell-mediated branches of the immune system that lead to extensive tissue damage or even death. These reactions are classified into four main types based on the mechanism that induces them. Each type generates characteristic effector molecules and clinical manifestations.

2. A type I hypersensitive reaction is mediated by IgE antibodies, whose Fc region binds to receptors on mast cells or blood basophils. Cross-linkage by allergen of the fixed IgE initiates a sequence of intracellular events leading to mast-cell or basophil degranulation with release of pharmacologically active mediators. The mediators are the immune effector molecules in this reaction. The principal effects of these mediators are smooth-muscle contraction and vasodilation.

3. A type II hypersensitive reaction occurs when antibody reacts with antigenic determinants present on the surface of cells, leading to cell damage or death through complement-mediated lysis or antibody-dependent cell-mediated cytotoxicity (ADCC).

4. A type III hypersensitive reaction is mediated by the formation of immune complexes and the ensuing activation of complement. Complement split products serve as immune effector molecules that cause localized vasodilation and chemotactically attract neutrophils. Deposition of immune complexes near the site of antigen entry can induce an Arthus reaction in which lytic enzymes released by the accumulated neutrophils and the complement membrane-attack complex cause localized tissue damage. Generalized type III reactions occur when circulating immune complexes are deposited at various sites; the manifestations of these reactions vary depending on the site of tissue deposition.

5. A type IV hypersensitive reaction involves the cell-mediated branch of the immune system. Antigen activation of sensitized T_{DTH} cells induces release of various cytokines, which serve as the immune effector molecules in this reaction. The net effect of these cytokines is to cause an accumulation and activation of macrophages, which release lytic enzymes that cause localized tissue damage.

References

ANSARI, A. A., L. R. FRIEDHOFF, D. A. MEYERS et al. 1989. Human immune responsiveness to Lolium perenne pollen allergen Lol p III (rye III) is associated with HLA-DR3 and DR5. *Hum. Immunol.* **25**:59.

AUBRY, J. P., S. POCHON, P. GRABER, K. U. JANSEN, and J. Y. BONNEFOY. 1992. CD21 is a ligand for CD23 and regulates IgE production. *Nature* **358**:505.

BONNEFOY, J. Y., S. PPCHON, J. P. AUBRY et al. 1993. A new pair of surface molecules involved in human IgE regulation. *Immunol. Today* **14**:1.

FINKELMAN, F. D., I. M. KATONA, J. URBAN et al. 1988. IL-4 is required to generate and sustain in vivo IgE response. *J. Immunol.* **141**:2335.

GORDON, J. R., P. R. BURD, and S. J. GALI. 1990. Mast cells as a source of multifunctional cytokines. *Immunol. Today* **11**:457.

ISHIZAKA, K. 1989. Regulation of immunoglobulin E biosynthesis. *Adv. Immunol* **47**:1.

ISHIZAKA, K. 1988. IgE-binding factors and regulation of the IgE antibody response. *Annu. Rev. Immunol.* **6**:513.

KAWAKAMI, T., N. INAGAKI, M. TAKEI et al. 1992. Tyrosine phosphorylation is required for mast cell activation by FcεRI cross-linking. *J. Immunol.* **148**:3513.

KUHN, R., K. RAJEWSKI, and W. MULLER. 1991. Generation and analysis of interleukin-4 deficient mice. *Science* **254**:707.

PAUL-EUGENE, N., J. P. KOLB, A. CALENDA et al. 1993. Functional interaction between β_2-adrenoceptor agonists and interleukin-4 in the regulation of CD23 expression and release and IgE production in human. *Molec. Immunol.* **30**:157.

THOMAS, P., H. GOMI, T. TAKEUCHI et al. 1992. Glycosylation-inhibiting factor from human T cell hybridomas constructed from peripheral blood lymphocytes of a bee venom-sensitive allergic patient. *J. Immunol.* **148**:729.

WILLIAMS, J., S. JOHNSON, J. J. MASCALI et al. 1992. Regulation of low affinity IgE receptor (CD23) expression on mononuclear phagocytes in normal and asthmatic subjects. *J. Immunol.* **149**:2823.

Study Questions

1. Indicate whether each of the following statements is true or false. If you think a statement is false, explain why.
   a. Mice infected with *Nippostrongylus brasiliensis* show decreased production of IgE.
   b. IL-4 decreases IgE production by B cells.
   c. Babies can acquire IgE-mediated allergies by passive transfer of maternal antibody.
   d. Antihistamines are effective for the treatment of type III hypersensitivity.
   e. Most pollen allergens contain a single allergenic component.

2. In an immunology laboratory exercise, you are studying the response of mice injected intradermally with complete antibodies to the IgE Fc receptors (FcεRI) or with Fab fragments of such antibodies.
   a. Predict the response expected with each type of antibody.
   b. Would the responses observed depend on whether or not the mice were allergic? Explain.

3. Serum sickness can result when an individual is given a large dose of antiserum such as an antitoxin to snake venom. How could you take advantage of recent technological advances to produce an antitoxin that

would not produce serum sickness in patients who receive it?

4. What immunologic mechanisms most likely account for a person developing each of the following reactions following an insect bite?
   a. Within 1–2 min after being bitten, swelling and redness appear at the site and then disappear by 1 h.
   b. 6–8 h later swelling and redness again appear and persist for 24 h.
   c. 72 h later the tissue becomes inflamed, and tissue necrosis follows.

5. In the table below, indicate whether each immunologic event listed does (+) or does not (−) occur in each type of hypersensitive response.

For use with Question 5.

Immunologic event	Type I hypersensitivity	Type II hypersensitivity	Type III hypersensitivity	Type IV hypersensitivity
IgE-mediated degranulation of mast cells				
Lysis of antibody-coated blood cells by complement				
Tissue destruction in response to poison oak				
C3a- and C5a-mediated mast-cell degranulation				
Chemotaxis of neutrophils				
Chemotaxis of eosinophils				
Activation of macrophages by IFN-γ				
Deposition of antigen-antibody complexes on basement membranes of capillaries				
Sudden death due to vascular collapse (shock) shortly after injection or ingestion of antigen				

AUTOIMMUNITY

The response of the immune system against self-components is termed *autoimmunity.* Normally the mechanisms of self-tolerance protect an individual from potentially self-reactive lymphocytes. In the 1960s, it was believed that all self-reactive lymphocytes were eliminated during their development and that a failure to eliminate these lymphocytes led to autoimmune consequences. Since the late 1970s a broad body of experimental evidence has countered that belief, revealing that not all self-reactive lymphocytes are deleted during T-cell and B-cell maturation. Instead normal healthy individuals have been shown to possess mature, recirculating self-reactive lymphocytes. Since the presence of these self-reactive lymphocytes does not inevitably result in autoimmune reactions, their activity must be regulated in normal individuals through clonal anergy or clonal suppression. A breakdown in this regulation can lead to activation of self-reactive clones of T or B cells, generating humoral or cell-mediated responses against self-antigens. These reactions can cause serious damage to cells or organs, sometimes with fatal consequences. This chapter describes some common autoimmune diseases in humans and experimental animal models used to study autoimmunity. In addition various mechanisms that may contribute to induction of autoimmune reactions are discussed, as well as current and experimental therapies for treating them.

Autoimmune Diseases in Humans

Autoimmune diseases affect 5–7% of the population, often causing chronic debilitating illnesses. In general, autoimmune diseases can be divided into two categories: organ-specific and systemic autoimmune disease (Table 19-1). In organ-specific autoimmune disease, the immune response is directed to a target antigen unique to a single organ or gland, so that the manifestations are largely limited to that organ. In systemic autoimmune disease, the response is directed toward a broad range of target antigens and involves a number of organs and tissues.

Table 19-1 Some autoimmune diseases in humans

Disease	Self-antigen	Immune response
	Organ-specific autoimmune diseases	
Addison's disease	Adrenal cells	Autoantibodies
Autoimmune hemolytic anemia	RBC membrane proteins	Autoantibodies
Goodpasture's syndrome	Renal and lung basement membranes	Autoantibodies
Graves' disease	Thyroid-stimulating hormone receptor	Autoantibody (stimulating)
Hashimoto's thyroiditis	Thyroid proteins and cells	T_{DTH} cells, autoantibodies
Idiopathic thrombocytopenia purpura	Platelet membrane proteins	Autoantibodies
Insulin-dependent diabetes mellitus	Pancreatic beta cells	T_{DTH} cells, autoantibodies
Myasthenia gravis	Acetylcholine receptors	Autoantibody (blocking)
Myocardial infarction	Heart	Autoantibodies
Pernicious anemia	Gastric parietal cells: (intrinsic factor)	Autoantibody
Poststreptococcal glomerulonephritis	Kidney	Antigen-antibody complexes
Spontaneous infertility	Sperm	Autoantibodies
	Systemic autoimmune disease	
Ankylosing spondylitis	Vertebrae	Immune complexes
Multiple sclerosis	Brain or white matter	T_{DTH} and T_C cells, autoantibodies
Rheumatoid arthritis	Connective tissue, IgG	Autoantibodies, immune complexes
Scleroderma	Nuclei, heart, lungs, gastrointestinal tract, kidney	Autoantibodies
Sjögren's syndrome	Salivary gland, liver, kidney, thyroid	Autoantibodies
Systemic lupus erythematosus (SLE)	DNA, nuclear protein, RBC and platelet membranes	Autoantibodies, immune complexes

Organ-Specific Autoimmune Diseases

In organ-specific autoimmune diseases, target organs may be subjected to direct cellular damage by humoral or cell-mediated mechanisms; alternatively, the function of a target organ may be stimulated or blocked by autoantibodies.

Diseases Mediated by Direct Cellular Damage

Autoimmune diseases involving direct cellular damage occur when lymphocytes or antibodies bind to cell-membrane antigens, causing cellular lysis and/or an inflammatory response in the affected organ. Gradually the cellular structure of an affected organ is replaced by connective tissue and the function of the organ declines. A few examples of this type of autoimmune disease are briefly discussed in this section.

HASHIMOTO'S THYROIDITIS. In this autoimmune disease, most frequently seen in middle-aged women, an individual produces autoantibodies and sensitized T_{DTH} cells specific for thyroid antigens. The DTH response is characterized by an intense infiltration of the thyroid gland by lymphocytes, macrophages, and plasma cells, which form lymphocytic follicles and germinal centers (Figure 19-1). The ensuing inflammatory response causes a goiter, or visible enlargement of the thyroid gland. Antibodies are formed to a number of thyroid proteins, including thyroglobulin and thyroid peroxidase, both of which are involved in the uptake of iodine. Binding of the autoantibodies to these proteins interferes with iodine uptake and leads to decreased production of thyroid hormones (hypothyroidism).

AUTOIMMUNE ANEMIAS. Autoimmune anemias include pernicious anemia, autoimmune hemolytic anemia, and drug-induced hemolytic anemia. Pernicious anemia is caused by autoantibodies to a membrane-bound intestinal protein, called intrinsic factor. Binding of intrinsic factor to vitamin B_{12} in the small intestine facilitates uptake of the vitamin. Binding of the autoantibody to intrinsic factor prevents this process, thus blocking intrinsic factor–mediated absorption of

(a)

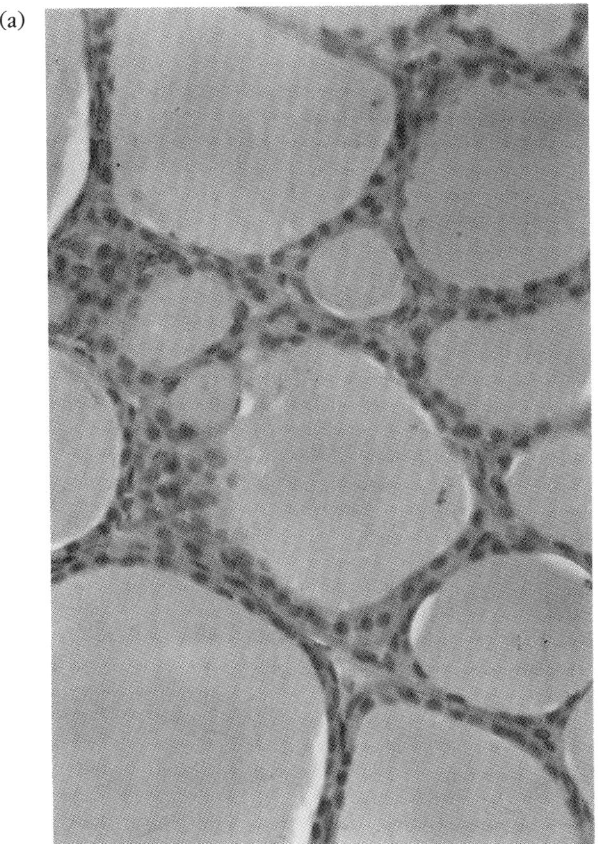

(b)

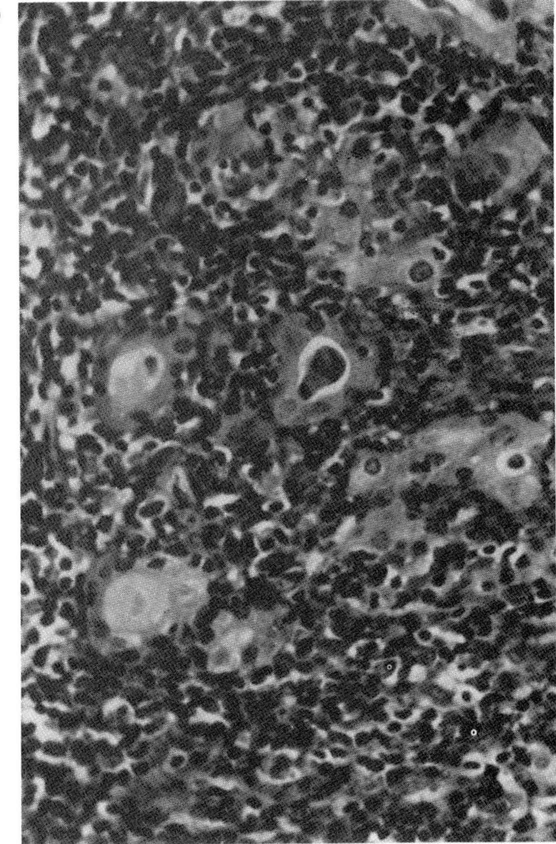

FIGURE 19-1 Photomicrographs of (a) normal thyroid gland and (b) gland in Hashimoto's thyroiditis showing intense lymphocyte infiltration. [From L. V. Crowley, 1983, *Introduction to Human Disease,* Wadsworth Health Sciences.]

vitamin B_{12}. In the absence of vitamin B_{12}, which is necessary for proper hematopoiesis, the number of functional mature red blood cells is decreased. Pernicious anemia is treated with injections of vitamin B_{12}, thus circumventing the defect in absorption.

An individual with autoimmune hemolytic anemia makes autoantibody to RBC antigens, triggering complement-mediated lysis or antibody-mediated opsonization and phagocytosis of the red blood cells. The majority of autoimmune hemolytic anemias can be divided into warm and cold types. In warm hemolytic anemias the autoantibodies have optimal serologic activity at 37° C, and in cold hemolytic anemias the autoantibodies have optimal activity at 4° C but also react at 25° C and 31° C. Warm hemolytic anemias generally involve IgG autoantibodies, which often are specific for the Rh antigens. Cold hemolytic anemias generally involve IgM autoantibodies specific for the I and H RBC antigens. Clinical manifestation of cold hemolytic anemia occurs when blood vessels, such as those in the skin of the hands of face, are exposed to the cold. The condition is reversed by warming the affected areas. The immunodiagnostic test for autoimmune hemolytic anemias generally involves a Coombs test in which the red cells are incubated with an anti-human IgG antiserum. If IgG autoantibodies are present on the red cells, the cells are agglutinated by the antiserum.

GOODPASTURE'S SYNDROME. In Goodpasture's syndrome, autoantibodies specific for certain basement-membrane antigens bind to the basement membranes of the kidney glomeruli and the alveoli of the lungs. Subsequent complement activation leads to direct cellular damage and an ensuing inflammatory response mediated by a buildup of complement split products. Damage to the glomerular and aveolar basement membranes leads to progressive kidney damage and pulmonary hemorrhage with death often within several months of the onset of symptoms. Staining of biopsies, from patients with Goodpasture's syndrome, with fluorescent-labeled anti-IgG and anti-C3b reveals linear deposits of IgG and C3b along the basement membranes (Figure 19-2).

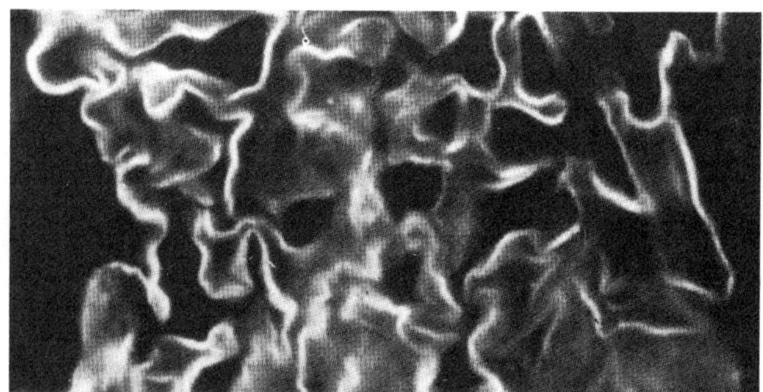

FIGURE 19-2 Fluorescent anti-IgG staining of a kidney biopsy from a patient with Goodpasture's syndrome reveals linear deposits of autoantibody along the basement membrane. [From J. A. Charlesworth and B. A. Pussell, 1986, in *Clinical Immunology Illustrated,* J. V. Wells and D. S. Nelson (eds.), Williams & Wilkins, p. 191.]

INSULIN-DEPENDENT DIABETES MELLITUS. A disease afflicting 0.2% of the population, insulin-dependent diabetes mellitus (IDDM) is caused by an autoimmune attack on the pancreas. The attack is directed against specialized insulin-producing cells (beta cells) that are located in spherical clusters (the islets of Langerhans) scattered throughout the pancreas. The autoimmune attack destroys the beta cells resulting in decreased production of insulin and consequently increased levels of blood glucose.

This disease is characterized by a condition called insulitis in which a large numbers T_{DTH} cells infiltrate the islets of Langerhans (Figure 19-3). A cell-mediated DTH response develops with the infiltration and activation of large numbers of macrophages. The subsequent beta-cell destruction is thought to be mediated by cytokines released during the DTH response and by lytic enzymes released from the activated macrophages. IFN-γ, TNF-α, and IL-1 have each been implicated in destruction of the beta cells. Autoantibodies to beta cells may contribute to cell destruction by facilitating either antibody-plus-complement lysis or antibody-dependent cell-mediated cytotoxicity (ADCC).

Diseases Mediated by Stimulating Autoantibodies

In some autoimmune diseases antibodies act as agonists, binding to hormone receptors in lieu of the normal ligand and stimulating inappropriate activity. This usually leads to an overproduction of mediators or an increase in cell growth. This type of autoimmunity is exemplified by *Graves' disease,* which involves the thyroid gland.

The production of thyroid hormones is carefully regulated by thyroid-stimulating hormone (TSH), which is produced by the pituitary gland. Binding of TSH to a receptor on thyroid cells activates adenylate cyclase and stimulates the synthesis of two thyroid hormones, thyroxine and triiodothyronine. A patient with Graves' disease produces autoantibody to the receptor for TSH. Binding of these autoantibodies to the receptor mimics the normal action of TSH, activating adenylate cyclase and resulting in production of the thyroid hormones. Unlike TSH, however, the autoantibodies are not regulated, and consequently they overstimulate the thyroid. For this reason these autoantibodies are called *long-acting thyroid-stimulating (LATS)* antibodies (Figure 19-4a).

(a)

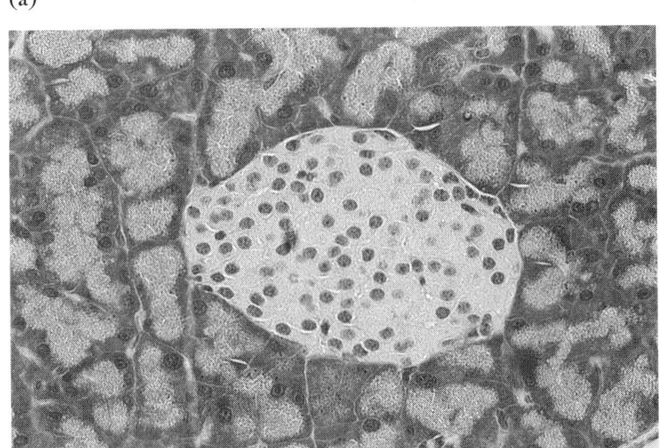

(b)

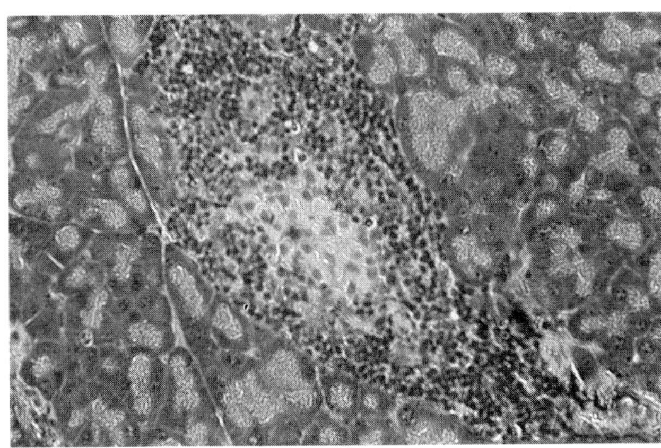

FIGURE 19-3 Photomicrographs of islet of Langerhans (a) in pancreas from a normal mouse and (b) in pancreas from a mouse with a disease resembling insulin-dependent diabetes mellitus. Note the lymphocyte infiltration into the islet (insulitis) in (b). [From M. A. Atkinson and N. K. Maclaren, 1990, *Sci. Am.* **263**(1):62.]

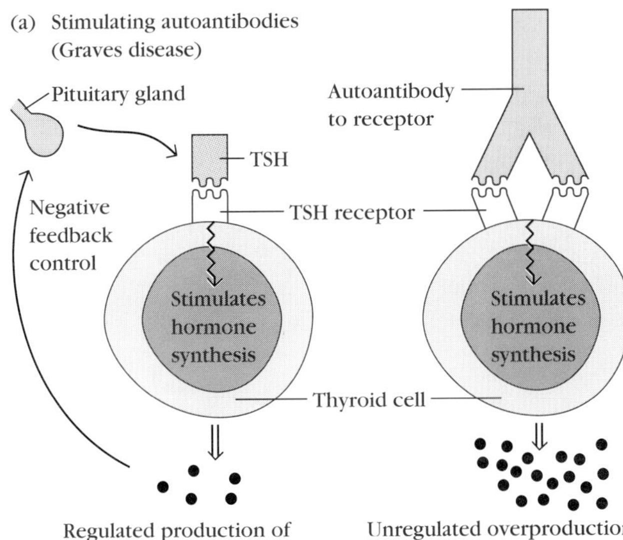

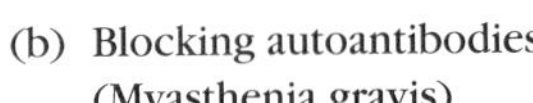

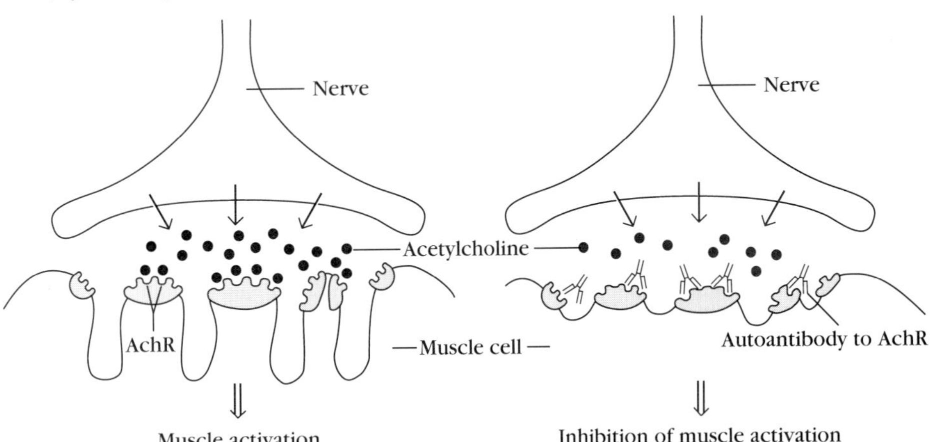

FIGURE 19-4 Autoantibodies to cell-membrane receptors can either enhance or block receptor activity. (a) In Graves' disease, autoantibody to the receptor for thyroid-stimulating hormone (TSH) induces unregulated activation of the thyroid, leading to overproduction of the thyroid hormones (purple circles). (b) In myasthenia gravis, autoantibody to the acetylcholine receptor (AChR) binds to the receptor and blocks binding of acetylcholine (purple circles) and subsequent muscle activation. In addition, the autoantibody induces complement activation resulting in damage to the muscle end-plate with a reduction in acetylcholine receptors as the disease progresses.

Diseases Mediated by Blocking Autoantibodies

In some cases of autoimmunity, autoantibodies bind to hormone receptors but act as antagonists, inhibiting receptor function. These diseases generally involve impaired secretion of mediators and gradual atrophy of the affected organ. In *myasthenia gravis,* the prototype disease of this type, autoantibodies are produced to the acetylcholine receptors on the motor end-plates of muscles. Binding of these autoantibodies to the receptors prevents binding by acetylcholine thereby inhibiting muscle activation. The antibodies also induce complement-mediated degradation of the receptor, resulting in progressive weakening of the skeletal muscles (Figure 19-4b).

Systemic Autoimmune Diseases

Autoimmune diseases with systemic manifestations reflect a generalized defect in immune regulation that results in hyperactive T cells and B cells. Tissue damage is widespread, both from cell-mediated immune responses and from direct cellular damage caused by autoantibodies or by accumulation of immune complexes.

SYSTEMIC LUPUS ERYTHEMATOSUS (SLE). One of the best examples of a systemic autoimmune disease, SLE usually appears in women between 20 and 40 years of age and is characterized by fever, weakness, joint pain, erythematous lesions, pleurisy, and kidney dysfunction. Affected individuals may produce autoantibodies to a vast array of tissue antigens such as DNA, histones, RBCs, platelets, leukocytes, and clotting factors; interaction of these autoantibodies with their specific antigens produces various symptoms. Autoantibody specific for RBCs and platelets, for example, can lead to complement-mediated lysis, resulting in hemolytic anemia and thrombocytopenia, respectively. When immune complexes of autoantibodies with various nuclear antigens are deposited along the walls of small blood vessels, these complexes activate the complement system and generate membrane-attack complexes, which damage the blood-vessel wall, resulting in vasculitis and glomerulonephritis.

Complement activation also generates such complement split products as C3a and C5a; serum levels of C3a and C5a may be three to four times higher in patients with severe SLE than in normal individuals (Figure 19-5). C5a induces increased expression of the type 3 complement receptor (CR3) on neutrophils, facilitating neutrophil aggregation and attachment to the vascular endothelium. As neutrophils attach to small blood vessels, the number of circulating neutrophils declines (neutropenia) and various occlusions of the small blood vessels develop (vasculitis). These occlusions can lead to widespread tissue damage.

Laboratory diagnosis of SLE focuses on the characteristic antinuclear antibodies, which are directed against double-stranded or single-stranded DNA,

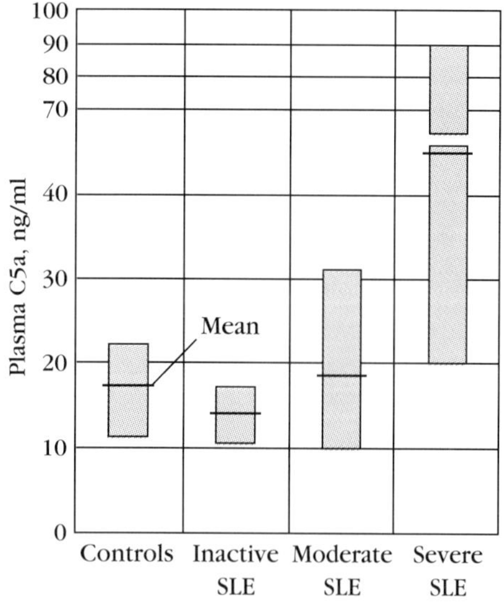

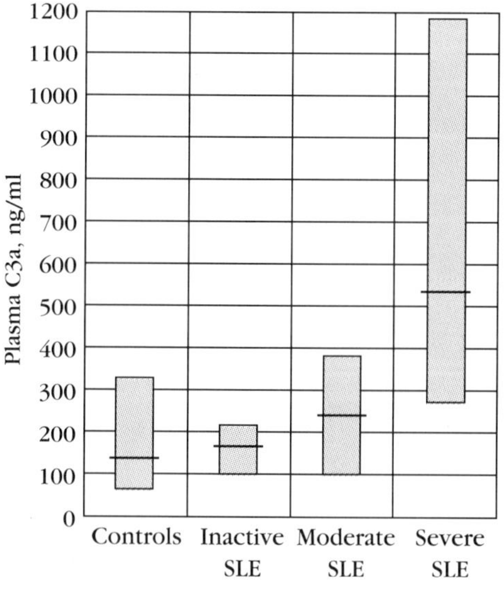

FIGURE 19-5 Antigen-antibody complexes produced in SLE induce complement activation with production of complement split products. Among patients with severe SLE the levels of complement split products C3a and C5a are significantly higher than in controls. [Modified from S. B. Abramson and G. Weissmann, 1988, *Hosp. Prac.* **15**(Dec.):45.]

nucleoprotein, histones, and nucleolar RNA. Indirect immunofluorescent staining of serum from SLE patients produces various characteristic nuclei-staining patterns. Another diagnostic test for SLE is the LE test. When peripheral blood from SLE patients is incubated at 37° C, the lymphocytes release their nuclei. Antibodies to nuclear antigens then react with the nuclei, and neutrophils in the blood sample phagocytose the antibody-coated nuclei, forming a characteristic cell called the LE cell. Because the LE test is difficult to perform and also relatively insensitive, it is seldom used anymore to diagnose SLE.

MULTIPLE SCLEROSIS (MS). Multiple sclerosis, an autoimmune disease affecting the central nervous system, is the most common cause of neurologic disability associated with disease in Western countries. Individuals with this disease produce autoreactive T cells that participate in the formation of inflammatory lesions along the myelin sheath of nerve fibers. Patients with active disease have activated T lymphocytes in their cerebrospinal fluid, which infiltrate the brain tissue and cause characteristic inflammatory lesions, destroying the myelin. Since myelin functions as an insulation of the nerve fibers, a breakdown in the myelin sheath leads to numerous neurologic dysfunctions.

RHEUMATOID ARTHRITIS. Rheumatoid arthritis is a common autoimmune disorder, most often affecting women from 40 to 60 years old. The major symptom is chronic inflammation of the joints, although the hematologic, cardiovascular, and respiratory systems are often affected as well. In many cases of rheumatoid arthritis a group of autoantibodies is produced that are reactive with determinants in the Fc region of IgG. These autoantibodies are call *rheumatoid factors*. The classical rheumatoid factor is an IgM antibody reactive to the Fc of IgG. Such autoantibodies bind to normal circulating IgG, forming IgM-IgG complexes that are then deposited in the joints. The immune complexes can then activate the complement cascade, resulting in a chronic inflammation of the joints.

ANIMAL MODELS FOR AUTOIMMUNE DISEASE

Animal models for autoimmune diseases have contributed to our understanding of autoimmunity in humans. Autoimmunity develops spontaneously in certain inbred strains of animals; autoimmunity also can be induced by certain experimental manipulations (Table 19-2). Both types of autoimmune diseases have provided valuable insights into the mechanism of autoimmunity and into potential treatments.

Spontaneous Autoimmunity in Animals

A number of autoimmune diseases that develop spontaneously in animals exhibit important clinical and pathologic similarities with certain autoimmune diseases in humans. Certain inbred mouse strains in particular have been valuable models for increasing understanding of the immunologic defects involved in the development of autoimmunity.

New Zealand Black (NZB) mice and F_1 hybrids of NZB and New Zealand White (NZW) mice spontaneously develop autoimmune diseases closely paralleling systemic lupus erythematosus. The NZB mice spontaneously develop autoimmune hemolytic anemia between 2 and 4 months of age and die prematurely by 18 months. Various autoantibodies can be detected, including antibodies to erythrocytes, nuclear proteins, DNA, and T lymphocytes. The autoimmune manifestations are even more severe when NZB mice are crossed with NZW mice. These F_1 (NZB $\times$ NZW) hybrids produce increased levels of anti-DNA and antinuclear antibodies and develop glomerulonephritis from immune-complex deposits in the kidney. As is true of SLE, the incidence of autoimmunity in these F_1 hybrids is greater in females, a phenomenon apparently related to estrogen levels. The effect of androgens and estrogens on development of autoimmune symptoms in these mice was studied by N. Talal. In his study, male and female F_1 (NZB $\times$ NZW) mice were castrated before puberty and then given hormone replacements. In both male and female mice that received androgens, there was a delay in the onset of autoimmunity and a reduction in its severity. Estrogens had the opposite effect, promoting early onset of autoimmunity with increased severity.

Another important animal model is the nonobese diabetic (NOD) mouse, which spontaneously develops a form of diabetes that resembles human insulin-dependent diabetes mellitus (IDDM). Like the human disease, the NOD mouse disease begins with lymphocytic infiltration into the islets of the pancreas. Also, as in IDDM, there is a strong association between certain MHC alleles and development of diabetes in these mice. Experiments with these mice have shown that T cells from diabetic mice can transfer diabetes to nondiabetic recipients. For example, when the immune system of normal mice is destroyed by lethal x-irradiation and then the mouse is reconstituted with an injection of bone marrow cells from NOD mice, the reconstituted mice develop diabetes; conversely, when the immune system of still healthy NOD mice is destroyed by x-irradiation and then reconstituted with normal bone marrow cells, the NOD mice do not develop diabetes. The role of $CD4^+$ and $CD8^+$ T cells in the development of diabetes has been studied in these

TABLE 19-2 EXPERIMENTAL ANIMAL MODELS OF AUTOIMMUNE DISEASES

Animal model	Possible human disease counterpart	Inducing antigen	Disease transferred by T cells
	Spontaneous autoimmune disease		
Nonobese diabetic (NOD) mouse	Insulin-dependent diabetes mellitus (IDDM)	Unknown	Yes
F_1 (NZB × NZW) mouse	Systemic lupus erythematosus (SLE)	Unknown	Yes
Obese-strain chicken	Hashimoto's thyroiditis	Thyroglobulin	Yes
	Experimentally induced autoimmune disease*		
Experimental autoimmune myasthenia gravis (EAMG)	Myasthenia gravis	Acetylcholine receptor	Yes
Experimental autoimmune encephalomyelitis (EAE)	Multiple sclerosis (MS)	Myelin basic protein (MBP); proteolipid protein (PLP)	Yes
Autoimmune arthritis (AA)	Rheumatoid arthritis	*M. tuberculosis* (proteoglycans)	Yes
Experimental autoimmune thyroiditis (EAT)	Hashimoto's thyroiditis	Thyroglobulin	Yes

* These diseases can be induced by injecting appropriate animals with the indicated antigen in complete Freund's adjuvant. Except for autoimmune arthritis, the antigens used correspond to the self-antigens associated with the human-disease counterpart. Rheumatoid arthritis involves reaction to proteoglycans, which are self-antigens associated with connective tissue.

mice. Since spleen cells from NOD mice can transfer diabetes into normal recipients, it is possible to selectively deplete either $CD4^+$ or $CD8^+$ T cells from the NOD spleen-cell suspension and then determine whether the depleted spleen cells can still transfer diabetes to normal mice. Such experiments have revealed that removal of either the $CD4^+$ or $CD8^+$ cells inhibits the transfer of diabetes, suggesting that both populations are necessary for the development of diabetes.

Several other spontaneously occurring autoimmune diseases have been discovered in animals and have served as models for similar human diseases. Among these are Obese-strain chickens, which develop both humoral and cell-mediated reactivity to thyroglobulin resembling that seen in Hashimoto's thyroiditis.

Experimentally Induced Autoimmunity in Animals

A number of experimental animal models have autoimmune dysfunctions similar to certain human autoimmune diseases (see Table 19-2). One of the first such animal models was discovered serendipitously in 1973 when rabbits were immunized with acetylcholine receptors purified from electric eels. The animals soon developed muscular weakness similar to that seen in myasthenia gravis. Soon this experimental autoimmune myasthenia gravis (EAMG) was shown to be caused when antibody to the acetylcholine receptor blocked muscle stimulation by acetylcholine in the synapse. Within a year this animal model had proved its value with the discovery that autoantibodies to the acetylcholine receptor were the cause of myasthenia gravis in humans.

Experimental autoimmune encephalomyelitis (EAE) is another animal model that has greatly improved understanding of autoimmunity. EAE can be induced in a variety of species by immunization with myelin basic protein (MBP) in complete Freund's adjuvant. Within 2–3 weeks the animals develop cellular infiltration of the myelin sheaths of the central nervous system, resulting in demyelination and development of paralysis. Most of the animals die, but some recover and are now resistant to the development of disease after a subsequent injection of MBP and adjuvant. EAE is considered to be a good laboratory model for multiple sclerosis.

Experimental autoimmune thyroiditis (EAT) can be induced in a number of animals by immunization with thyroglobulin in complete Freund's adjuvant. Both humoral antibodies and T_{DTH} cells directed against the thyroglobulin develop, resulting in thyroid inflammation. EAT appears to best mimic Hashimoto's thyroiditis. In contrast to both EAE and EAT, which are induced by immunization with self-antigens, autoimmune arthritis (AA) is induced by immunization of rats with *Mycobacterium tuberculosis* in complete Freund's adjuvant. These animals develop an arthritis whose features are similar to those of rheumatoid arthritis in humans.

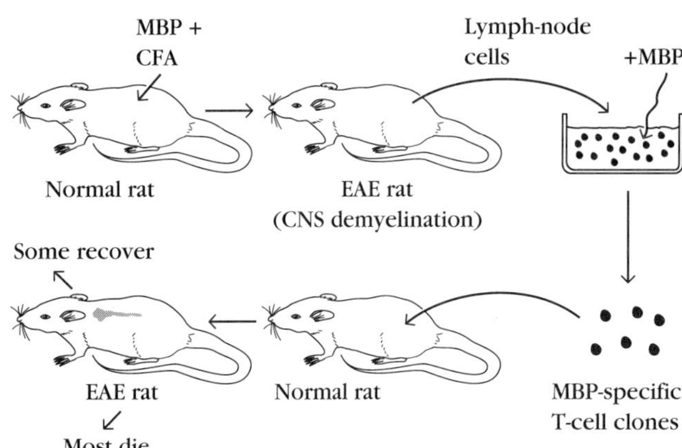

FIGURE 19-6 Experimental autoimmune encephalomyelitis (EAE) can be induced by injecting rats with myelin basic protein (MBP) in complete Freund's adjuvant (CFA). MBP-specific T-cell clones can be generated by culturing lymph-node cells from EAE rats with MBP. These T cells can then transfer the disease to normal animals.

Role of the $CD4^+$ T Cell, MHC, and T-Cell Receptor in Autoimmunity

The inappropriate response to self-antigens that characterizes all autoimmune diseases can involve either the humoral or the cell-mediated branch. Identifying the underlying defect in human autoimmune diseases has been difficult. Characterization of the immune defect in the various animal models has been more successful. Surprisingly, each of the animal models has implicated the $CD4^+$ T cell as the primary mediator of autoimmune disease. T-cell recognition of antigen, of course, involves a trimolecular complex of the T-cell receptor, an MHC molecule, and antigenic peptide (see Figure 11-13). Thus an individual susceptible to autoimmunity must possess MHC molecules and T-cell receptors capable of binding self-antigens.

Evidence for $CD4^+$ T-Cell Role

Autoimmune T-cell clones have been obtained from all of the animal models listed in Table 19-2 by culturing lymphocytes from the autoimmune animals in the presence of various T-cell growth factors and then inducing proliferation of specific autoimmune clones with the various autoantigens. For example, when lymph-node cells from EAE rats are cultured in vitro with myelin basic protein, clones of activated T cells emerge. When these MBP-specific T-cell clones are injected intravenously in sufficient numbers into normal syngeneic animals, the cells penetrate the blood-brain barrier and induce demyelination; EAE develops within 5 days (Figure 19-6). With a similar experimental protocol, T-cell clones specific for thyroglobulin and for *M. tuberculosis* can be isolated from EAT and AA animals, respectively. In each case the T-cell clone induces the experimental autoimmune disease in normal animals. Examination of these T cells has revealed that they bear the CD4 membrane marker. In a number of animal models for autoimmune diseases it has been possible to reverse the autoimmunity by depleting the T-cell population with antibody directed against CD4. For example, weekly injections of anti-CD4 monoclonal antibody abolished the autoimmune symptoms in NZB × NZW mice and in mice with EAE.

Evidence for Association with the MHC

Several types of studies have supported an association between expression of a particular MHC allele and susceptibility to autoimmunity. Some of these studies have used the EAE animal model, whose inducing antigen—myelin basic protein (MBP)—has been well characterized and sequenced. Various MBP peptides have been assessed for their ability to activate T_H cells and elicit autoimmune encephalomyelitis reactions. The results of such experiments show that inbred mice expressing different MHC haplotypes develop EAE in response to different MBP peptides (Figure 19-7). Moreover, the same peptides that induce EAE in a given strain also induce maximal T_H-cell proliferation.

By using antibodies to type the HLA alleles expressed by individuals with various autoimmune diseases (see Figure 24-7), it has been shown that some HLA alleles occur at a much higher frequency among autoimmune individuals than in the general population. The association between the expression of a

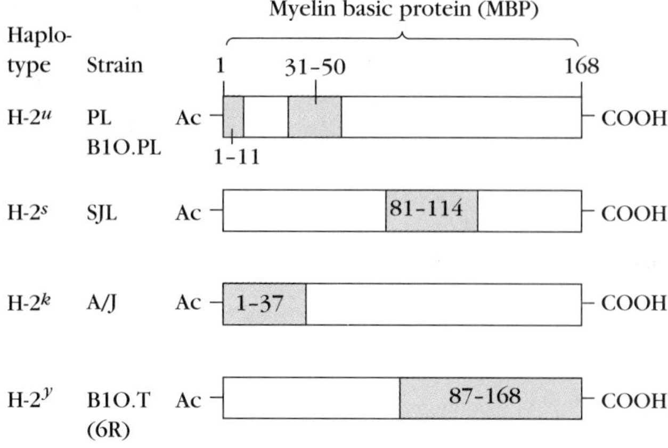

FIGURE 19-7 MBP peptides (purple) that induce EAE and maximal T-cell proliferation in various inbred mouse strains. The haplotype of the mouse strain appears to determine which peptides are encephalitogenic.

given HLA allele and an autoimmune disease is expressed as the relative risk:

$$\text{Relative risk} = \frac{(\text{patient with HLA allele}) \times (\text{controls without HLA allele})}{(\text{patients without HLA allele}) \times (\text{controls with HLA allele})}$$

A relative risk value of 1 means that the HLA allele is expressed with the same frequency in the autoimmune and control subpopulations whereas a relative risk value substantially above 1 indicates an association between the HLA allele and the autoimmune disease. However, the existence of such an association should not be interpreted to imply that the expression of a particular MHC allele has caused the disease because the relationship between MHC alleles and development of autoimmune disease is complex. That these diseases are not inherited via simple mendelian segregation of MHC alleles can be seen in identical twins when both inherit the MHC risk factor but only one develops autoimmunity. This finding suggests that multiple genetic factors and environmental factors have roles in the development of autoimmunity, with the MHC playing an important but not exclusive role. As the antigens inducing human autoimmune diseases are identified and sequenced, it will be possible to analyze the linkage between the MHC and various diseases more fully.

Table 19-3 lists a number of autoimmune diseases for which an association between a particular MHC allele and disease susceptibility have been demonstrated. One difficulty in associating a particular MHC allele with autoimmunity is the genetic phenomenon of *linkage disequilibrium* in which two alleles are inherited together with a higher frequency than normally expected. Initially class I MHC alleles were shown to be associated with autoimmunity. But later most autoimmune diseases were shown to be much more strongly associated with class II MHC alleles. The fact that some of the class I MHC alleles were in linkage disequilibrium with the class II MHC alleles made their contribution to autoimmune susceptibility appear more pronounced than it actually was.

By using the polymerase chain reaction, H. McDevitt and his co-workers analyzed the nucleotide sequences of class II MHC genes from patients with different autoimmune diseases. They found that certain short sequences within the α_1 and β_1 domains of class II MHC molecules appear to play a major role in susceptibility and resistance to autoimmunity. These sequences are thought to be located within the peptide-binding groove of the class II MHC molecule. In patients with insulin-dependent diabetes mellitus (IDDM) and in the mouse model for diabetes (the NOD mouse), a single amino acid change at residue 57 in the HLA-DQ

TABLE 19-3 HLA ALLELES ASSOCIATED WITH INCREASED RISK FOR VARIOUS AUTOIMMUNE DISEASES

Disease	HLA allele	Relative risk*
Ankylosing spondylitis	B27	90
Goodpasture's syndrome	DR2	16
Graves' disease	B8/DR3	3–4
Insulin-dependent diabetes mellitus	DR4/DR3 DR3/DQW8	20 100
Juvenile rheumatoid arthritis	B27/DR5	4
Multiple sclerosis	DR2	5
Myasthenia gravis	DR3	10
Pernicious anemia	DR5	5
Psoriatic arthritis (central)	B27	11
Reiter's syndrome	B27	37
Rheumatoid arthritis	Dw4/DR4	10
Sjögren's syndrome	Dw3	6
Systemic lupus erythematosus	DR3	5
Ulcerative colitis	B5	4

* Likelihood of developing disease compared to the general population, which is assigned a risk value of 1.

β chain was found to correlate with resistance or susceptibility to diabetes. An aspartic residue at position 57 of the DQ β chain correlated with resistance to IDDM, whereas a valine, serine, or alanine at this position correlated with susceptibility to IDDM. Presumably the differences in amino acids at this position influence the binding of different self-peptides to the DQ molecule.

Evidence for Association with the T-Cell Receptor

The presence of T-cell receptors containing particular V_α and V_β domains also has been linked to a number of autoimmune diseases including experimental EAE and its human counterpart, multiple sclerosis. In one approach, T cells specific for various encephalitogenic peptides of MBP were cloned and their T-cell receptors analyzed. In PL/J mice, for example, T-cell clones were obtained by culturing T cells with the acetylated amino-terminal nonapeptide of MBP presented in association with a class II IA^u MHC molecule. Analysis of the T-cell receptors on these clones revealed a restricted repertoire of V_α and V_β domains: 100% of the T-cell clones expressed $V_\alpha4.3$, and 80% of the T-cell clones expressed $V_\beta8.2$. In human autoimmune diseases, evidence for restricted TCR expression has been obtained in both multiple sclerosis and myasthenia gravis. The preferential expression of TCR variable-region genes in these autoimmune T-cell clones suggests that a single epitope might induce the clonal expansion of a small number of pathogenic T cells.

Proposed Mechanisms for Induction of Autoimmunity

A variety of mechanisms have been proposed to account for the T-cell–mediated generation of autoimmune diseases (Figure 19-8). Evidence exists for each of these mechanisms, and it is likely that autoimmunity does not develop from a single event but rather from a number of different events.

Release of Sequestered Antigens

As discussed in Chapter 16, the induction of tolerance in self-reactive T cells is thought to occur through exposure of immature lymphocytes to self-antigens during development. Any tissue antigens that are sequestered from the circulation, and therefore are not seen

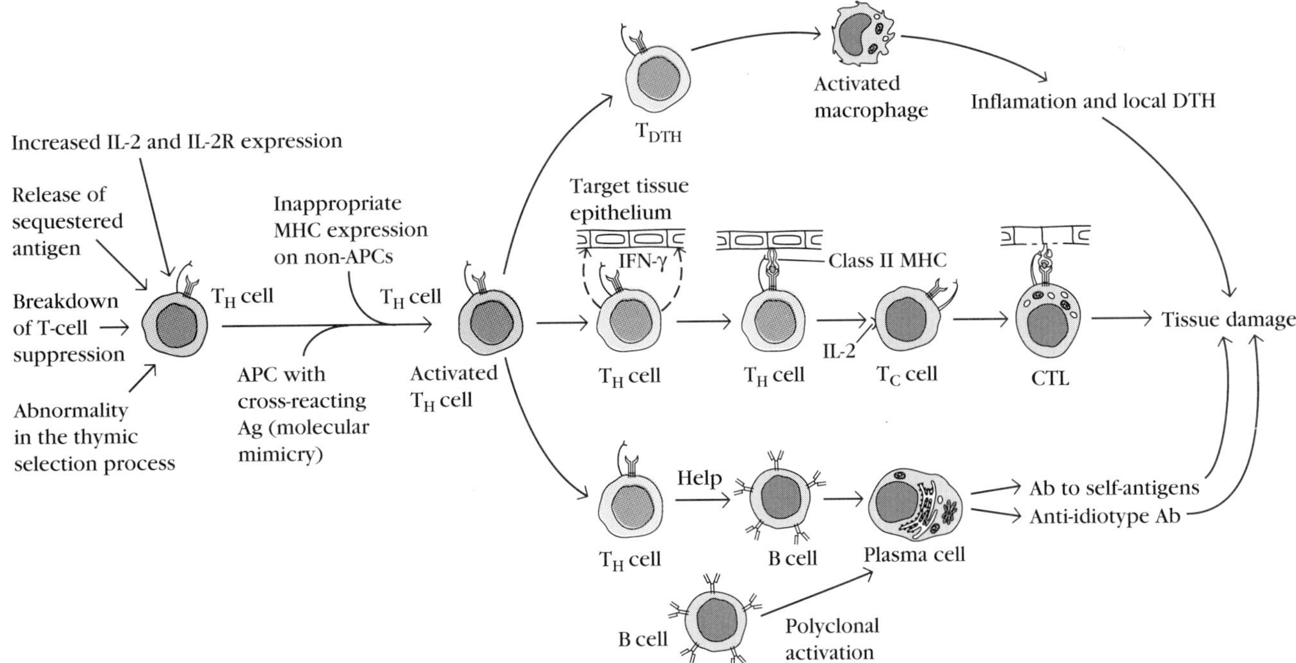

FIGURE 19-8 Proposed mechanisms leading to autoimmunity. Once activated self-reactive T_H cells (purple) are generated, they act in various ways to mediate an autoimmune response, in this case involving tissue damage. In all likelihood, several mechanisms are involved in each autoimmune disease. See text for details. [Adapted from V. Kumar et al., 1989, *Annu. Rev. Immunol.* **7**:657.]

by the developing immune system, will not induce self-tolerance. Exposure of mature T cells to such normally sequestered antigens at a later date might result in their activation.

Myelin basic protein is an example of an antigen normally sequestered from the immune system, in this case by the blood-brain barrier. In the EAE model, animals are injected directly with MBP, together with adjuvant, under conditions that maximize immune exposure. In this type of animal model, the immune system is exposed to sequestered self-antigens under nonphysiologic conditions, but trauma to tissues following either an accident or a viral or bacterial infection might also release sequestered antigens into the circulation. A few tissue antigens are known to fall into this category. For example, sperm arise late in development and are sequestered from the circulation, but after a vasectomy, some sperm antigens are released into the circulation and can induce autoantibody formation in some men. Similarly the release of lens protein after eye damage or of heart-muscle antigens after myocardial infarction has been shown to lead to autoantibody formation on occasion.

Molecular Mimicry

A number of viruses and bacteria have been shown to possess antigenic determinants that are identical to or similar to normal host-cell components. This *molecular mimicry* appears to occur in a wide variety of organisms (Table 19-4). In one study 600 different monoclonal antibodies, specific for 11 different viruses, were tested to evaluate their reactivity with normal tissue antigens. More than 3% of the virus-specific antibodies tested also bound to normal tissue, suggesting

TABLE 19-4 MOLECULAR MIMICRY BETWEEN PROTEINS OF INFECTIOUS ORGANISMS AND HUMAN HOST PROTEINS

Protein*	Residue†	Sequence‡
Human cytomegalovirus IE2	79	PDPLGRPDED
HLA-DR molecule	60	VTELGRPDAE
Poliovirus VP2	70	STTKESRGTT
Acetylcholine receptor	176	TVIKESRGTK
Papilloma virus E2	76	SLHLESLKDS
Insulin receptor	66	VYGLESLKDL
Rabies virus glycoprotein	147	TKESLVIIS
Insulin receptor	764	NKESLVISE
Klebsiella pneumoniae nitrogenase	186	SRQTDREDE
HLA-B27 molecule	70	KAQTDREDL
Adenovirus 12 E1B	384	LRRGMFRPSQCN
α-Gliadin	206	LGQGSFRPSQQN
Human immunodeficiency virus p24	160	GVETTTPS
Human IgG constant region	466	GVETTTPS
Measles virus P3	13	LECIRALK
Corticotropin	18	LECIRACK
Measles virus P3	31	EISDNLGQE
Myelin basic protein	61	EISFKLGQE

* In each pair, the human protein is listed second. The proteins in each pair have been shown to exhibit immunologic cross-reactivity.

† Each number indicates the position in the intact protein of the amino-terminal amino acid in the indicated peptide.

‡ Amino acid residues are indicated by single-letter code.

SOURCE: Adapted from M. B. A. Oldstone, 1987, *Cell* **50**:819.

that molecular mimicry is a fairly common phenomenon.

Molecular mimicry has been suggested as one mechanism leading to autoimmunity. One of the best examples of this type of autoimmune reaction is post-rabies encephalitis, which used to develop in some individuals who had received the rabies vaccine. In the past, the rabies virus was grown in rabbit brain-cell cultures, and preparations of the vaccine included antigens derived from the rabbit brain cells. In a vaccinated person these rabbit brain-cell antigens could induce formation of antibodies and activated T cells, which could cross-react with the recipient's own brain cells and lead to encephalitis. Cross-reacting antibodies are also thought to be the cause of heart damage in rheumatic fever, which usually develops after a *Streptococcus* infection. In this case the antibodies are to streptococcal antigens, but they cross-react with the heart muscle.

Since the encephalitogenic MBP peptides are known, the extent to which they are molecularly mimicked by proteins from other organisms can be assessed. In one study, the sequence of one encephalitogenic MBP peptide (66–75) was compared with the known sequences of a large number of viral proteins. This computer analysis revealed sequence homologies between this MBP peptide and a number of animal viruses, including influenza, polyoma, adenovirus, Rous sarcoma, Abelson leukemia, poliomyelitis, Epstein-Barr, and hepatitis B. One peptide from the polymerase enzyme of the hepatitis B virus was particularly striking: a sequence of six of its 10 amino acids was homologous with a sequence in the encephalitogenic MBP peptide. To test the hypothesis that molecular mimicry can generate autoimmunity, rabbits were immunized with this hepatitis B virus peptide. The peptide was shown to induce both the formation of antibody and the proliferation of T cells that cross-reacted with MBP; in addition, central nervous system tissue from the immunized rabbits showed cellular infiltration characteristic of that seen in EAE. These findings suggest that infection with certain viruses expressing epitopes that mimic sequestered self-components may induce autoimmunity to those components. Susceptibility to this type of autoimmunity may also be influenced by the MHC haplotype of the individual, since certain class I and class II MHC molecules may be more effective than others in presenting the homologous peptide for T-cell activation.

Another group of proteins implicated in autoimmunity through molecular mimicry are the heat-shock proteins, which are produced by mammalian cells in response to elevated temperatures or other cellular stresses. These proteins, however, are not unique to mammalian cells and are found in a wide variety of bacterial and parasitic pathogens. These proteins exhibit remarkable evolutionary conservation: Mammalian and microbial heat-shock proteins share more than 50% sequence identity. Despite their sequence homology, these proteins have been shown to serve as major immunodominant antigens in a variety of bacterial and parasitic infections. In human mycobacterial infection, for example, nearly 40% of the T-cell response is specific for microbial heat-shock protein (hsp65). This has led to the suggestion that the high degree of sequence homology between microbial heat-shock protein (hsp65) and the human heat-shock protein (hsp60) may result in autoimmune consequences through molecular mimicry.

Several types of evidence support the role of heat-shock proteins in autoimmunity. For example, individuals with rheumatoid arthritis have been shown to have T cells responsive to hsp65, and antibodies to hsp65 have been detected in NOD mice about 2 months before the onset of autoimmune destruction of pancreatic beta cells. In addition, T-cell clones reactive with hsp65 have been isolated from prediabetic NOD mice. When these T-cell clones were injected into mice of an H-2 compatible, nondiabetic strain, the nondiabetic mice developed diabetes.

Perhaps the most compelling evidence that molecular mimicry between heat-shock proteins and tissue-specific proteins plays a role in autoimmunity comes from work by D. Jones, A. Coulson, and G. Duff on insulin-dependent diabetes mellitus (IDDM). These researchers found that individuals with IDDM have antibody specific for hsp65; moreover, this anti-hsp65 antibody was shown to cross-react with glutamic acid decarboxylase (GAD), a pancreatic enzyme localized in the insulin-producing beta cells of the islets of Langerhans. Sequence analyses revealed that hsp65, human hsp60, and GAD exhibit striking sequence homology. Based on these results, Jones, Coulson, and Duff hypothesized that heat-shock proteins are homologous with a number of tissue-specific proteins. To test this hypothesis, they compared by computer analysis the sequences of known human proteins with the overlapping sequences, each containing about 25 amino acid residues, that constitute the entire sequence of human hsp60. As a control, computer analysis was performed with the overlapping 25-residue sequences of human albumin. The results of this study revealed that hsp60 exhibited sequence homology with 86 human peptides of which 19 were known autoantigens that had already been implicated in autoimmune pathogenesis (Table 19-5). Among the autoantigens that exhibited sequence homology with human hsp60 were those implicated in IDDM, Hashimoto's thyroiditis, scleroderma, rheumatoid arthritis, multiple sclerosis, and Addison's disease. In contrast, the

TABLE 19-5 MOLECULAR MIMICRY BETWEEN HUMAN HEAT-SHOCK PROTEIN HSP60 AND OTHER CELLULAR PROTEINS

Antigen	Amino acid region	Sequence*
Thyroglobulin	393–403	E K R W A S P R V A R
hsp60	65–75	E Q S W G S P K V T K
DNA-binding protein	73–82	E A G E A T T T T T
hsp60	108–117	E A G D G T T T A T
Cytokeratin	545–555	G G M G G G L G G G
hsp60	562–571	G G M G G G M G G G
Neurofilament triplet protein	727–749	V P E K K K A E S P V K E - E A V A E V V T I T
hsp60	152–175	I A E L K K Q S K P V T T P E E I A Q V A T I S

* Amino acid residues are indicated by single-letter code. Identical residues are in purple; conserved substitutions are underlined in purple.

SOURCE: D. B. Jones et al., 1993, *Immunol. Today* **14**:115.

albumin control showed sequence homology with 138 human peptides, but of these, only 4 were known autoantigens.

Despite the evidence linking autoimmunity to responses to heat-shock proteins, such responses cannot be the whole story in the pathogenesis of autoimmunity. This conclusion is easily demonstrated by immunizing normal individuals with killed mycobacteria. Although most produce T cells reactive with hsp65, they do not develop an autoimmunity. Several proposals have been suggested to account for this finding. One hypothesis is that an immune response to heat-shock proteins occurs naturally but that it is normally kept in check by a population of regulatory T cells specific for anti-hsp T cells. Another hypothesis is that some MHC alleles bind to and present heat-shock peptides that do not mimic self-proteins, whereas other MHC alleles present heat-shock peptides that do mimic self-proteins, thus inducing autoimmune responses.

Inappropriate Expression of Class II MHC Molecules

The pancreatic beta cells of individuals with insulin-dependent diabetes mellitus (IDDM) express high levels of both class I and class II MHC molecules, whereas healthy beta cells express lower levels of class I and do not express class II at all. Similarly, in Graves' disease thyroid acinar cells have been shown to express class II MHC molecules on their membranes. This inappropriate expression of class II MHC molecules, which are normally expressed only on antigen-presenting cells, may serve to sensitize T_H cells to peptides derived from the beta cells or thyroid cells, allowing activation of B cells or T_C cells or sensitization of T_{DTH} cells against self-antigens.

Other evidence suggests that certain agents can induce some cells that should not express class II MHC molecules to express them. For example, the T-cell mitogen phytohemagglutinin (PHA) has been shown to induce thyroid cells to express class II molecules. In vitro studies reveal that interferon gamma (IFN-γ) also induces increases in class II MHC molecules on a wide variety of cells, including pancreatic beta cells, intestinal epithelial cells, melanoma cells, and thyroid acinar cells. M. Feldman and G. F. Bottazzo hypothesized that trauma or viral infection in an organ may induce a localized inflammatory response, and thus increased concentrations of IFN-γ, in the affected organ. If IFN-γ induces class II MHC expression on non-antigen-presenting cells, inappropriate T_H-cell activation might follow, with autoimmune consequences. It is noteworthy that SLE patients with active disease have higher serum titers of IFN-γ than patients with inactive disease. Feldman and Bottazzo suggested that the increase in IFN-γ in these patients may lead to inappropriate expression of class II MHC molecules and thus to T-cell activation against a variety of autoantigens.

The role of inappropriate class II MHC expression has been studied in transgenic mice in which the injected DNA included class II MHC genes linked to the insulin promoter, which is activated only in pancreatic beta cells. In these transgenic mice, class II MHC molecules were expressed at high levels in pancreatic beta cells but not in other tissues. The mice became diabetic and suffered degeneration of their beta cells, suggesting a link between inappropriate class II MHC expression and diabetes in these mice. One puzzling aspect of this experiment, however, was that lymphocytes and inflammatory cells were not observed to penetrate the pancreas in these mice, as occurs in insulin-dependent diabetes mellitus. Might, then, the diabetes observed in these mice be due to some other component of the transgenic system and not to autoimmunity? For example, the abnormally high levels of class II MHC molecules in these transgenic mice may in itself inhibit the normal secretory functions of the pancreatic beta cell and decrease insulin secretion. Or class II MHC molecules may actually bind to insulin and reduce its activity, giving rise to diabetes without autoimmunity. Although the actual mechanism of diabetes in these class II MHC transgenic mice has not been established, the association between inappropriate class II MHC expression and autoimmunity is intriguing.

Cytokine Imbalance

There is now considerable evidence to suggest that preferential activation of T_H1 cells plays a central role in the pathogenesis of a number of autoimmune diseases. The cytokines that set the T_H1 subset apart are IFN-γ, TNF-β, and IL-2. The ability to transfer autoimmunity in EAE with cloned T cells specific for myelin basic protein has enabled researchers to characterize the pathogenic T-cell subpopulation. The results of these studies have revealed that animals manifesting EAE have large numbers of T_H1-like cells, whereas those animals that spontaneously recover have higher numbers of the T_H2 subset. There is also evidence for T_H1 involvement in insulin-dependent diabetes mellitus (IDDM) and in its animal model, the NOD mouse.

Since the T_H1 subset is the principal producer of IL-2, it is not surprising that higher levels of IL-2 have been observed in a number of autoimmune diseases. Elevated IL-2 serum levels have been observed in active SLE patients, in patients with multiple sclerosis, and in an animal model for Hashimoto's thyroiditis, the Obese chicken. Abnormalities in the IL-2 receptor have also been observed. Normal resting T cells do not express the α subunit of the IL-2 receptor until they have been activated. In a number of autoimmune diseases, including rheumatoid arthritis, SLE, and IDDM, there appears to be abnormal expression of the IL-2R α subunit. G. Kroemer and G. Wick have suggested that perturbations in the regulation of expression of IL-2 and the high-affinity IL-2 receptor may have several possible consequences that could lead to autoimmune manifestations (Figure 19-9). Increased expression of IL-2 and IL-2R, for example, could promote T-cell activation, resulting in production of other cytokines and possibly leading to various effector functions that might cause tissue damage. Overproduction of IL-2 or other cytokines from activated T_H cells also could result in excessive B-cell activation and autoantibody production. Finally, increased expression of IL-2 and IL-2R on thymocytes might allow some thymocytes to escape clonal deletion within the thymus.

An interesting transgenic mouse system that implicates T_H1-derived cytokines in autoimmunity was developed by N. Sarvetnick. In this system an IFN-γ transgene was genetically engineered with the insulin promoter, so that the transgenic mice secreted IFN-γ from their pancreatic beta cells (Figure 19-10a). Since IFN-γ up-regulates class II MHC expression, these mice also expressed class II MHC molecules on their pancreatic beta cells. The mice developed diabetes, which (in contrast to the class II transgenic system previously described) was associated with cellular infiltration of lymphocytes and inflammatory cells similar to the infiltration seen in autoimmune NOD mice and in patients with insulin-dependent diabetes mellitus (Figure 19-10b). Although inappropriate class II MHC expression on the beta cells may be involved in the autoimmune reaction, other factors also may play a

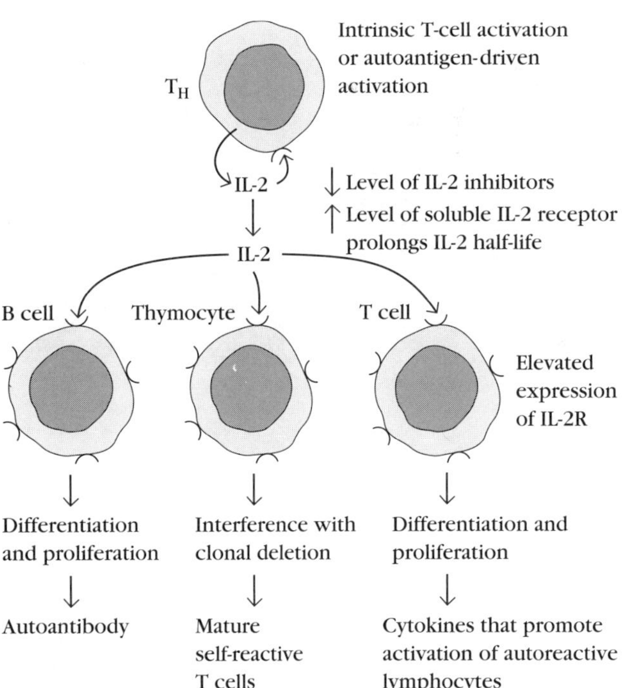

FIGURE 19-9 Perturbations in the regulation of IL-2 and IL-2R expression have been postulated to lead to autoimmune consequences. [Adapted from G. Kroemer and G. Wick, 1989, *Immunol. Today* **10**:246.]

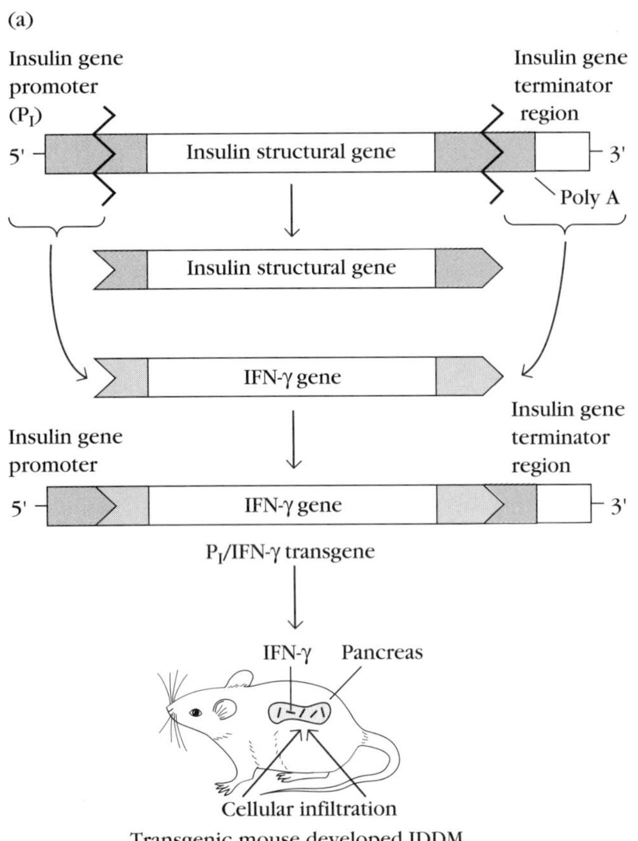

(b)

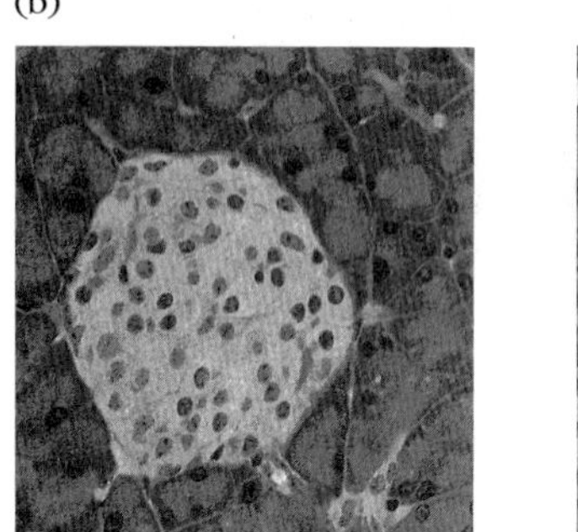

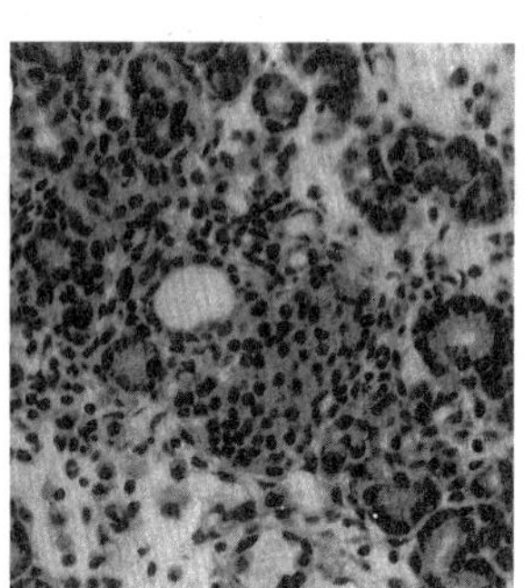

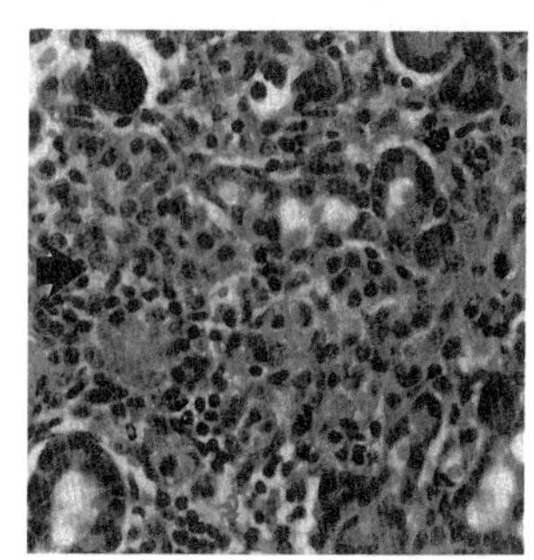

FIGURE 19-10 Insulin-dependent diabetes mellitus (IDDM) in transgenic mice. (a) Production of transgenic mice containing an IFN-γ transgene linked to the insulin promoter (P_I). The transgenics, which expressed the P_I/IFN-γ transgene only in the pancreas, developed symptoms characteristic of IDDM. (b) Pancreatic islets of Langerhans from a normal BALB/c mouse *(left)* and from P_I/IFN-γ transgenics at 3 weeks *(center)* and 6 weeks *(right)* showing infiltration of inflammatory cells. [Part (b) from N. Sarvetnick, 1988, *Cell* **52**:773.]

role in development of autoimmunity in this system. For example, IFN-γ is known to induce production of several other cytokines, including IL-1 and TNF. Therefore, the development of autoimmunity in this transgenic system may involve antigen presentation by class II MHC molecules on the pancreatic beta cells, together with a costimulatory signal, such as IL-1, that may activate self-reactive T cells. There is also some evidence to suggest that IL-1, IFN-γ and TNF may directly impair the secretory function of human beta cells.

Dysfunction of the Idiotype Network Regulatory Pathways

As discussed in Chapter 16, production of anti-idiotype antibody that presents an internal image of a foreign antigen is thought to enhance the immune response and thus contribute to host defense (see Figure 16-3). However, production of anti-idiotype antibodies to self-proteins may contribute to autoimmune reactions in some cases.

The first evidence linking anti-idiotype antibody and autoimmunity was discovered serendipitiously. B. F. Erlanger and colleagues were studying the acetylcholine analog Bis Q, a potent agonist of the acetylcholine receptor (AChR); the molecular structure of Bis Q is complementary to the combining site of the AChR. They immunized rabbits with Bis Q to make anti-Bis Q. When other rabbits were immunized with anti-Bis Q, they developed signs of myasthenia gravis (Figure 19-11). In later experiments hybridomas secreting monoclonal anti-idiotype antibodies (anti-anti-Bis Q) were produced. When these hybridomas were injected into the peritoneal cavity of three female and three male mice, all the female mice developed myasthenia gravis.

In Graves' disease antibodies are produced to the receptor for thyroid-stimulating hormone (TSH). These antibodies bind to the receptor and stimulate the thyroid inappropriately (see Figure 19-4a). Experimentally it is possible to make antibody specific for TSH and then make antibody to this antibody (anti-idiotype). This anti-idiotype antibody has been shown to stimulate the TSH receptor. So far, one patient with Graves' diseases has been shown to have developed an idiotype–anti-idiotype network of antibodies that participate in the autoimmune response.

Dysfunction of T-Cell–Mediated Immune Regulation

Studies of immune dysfunction in NZB mice have revealed a loss of T-cell–mediated suppression activity that parallels the development of autoimmunity. As noted earlier, these mice exhibit hyperactive B-cell and T-cell responses to numerous self-proteins, mimicking SLE. When thymocytes from NZB mice 1–3 months old were injected into older NZB mice, there was a delay in the onset of the usual spontaneous autoimmune disease, suggesting that the young thymocytes had restored the immune imbalance in the NZB mouse. The Obese chicken also shows less T-cell–mediated suppression activity than control populations. When thymocytes from normal chickens were added to an in vitro culture of CTLs specific for thyroglobulin-coated chicken RBCs, the thymocytes suppressed the cytotoxic response. However, when thymocytes from 3-week-old Obese chickens were added to the in vitro culture, there was no such suppression of cytotoxicity. The development of autoimmune thyroiditis in these young chickens may therefore reflect a decrease in their T-cell suppression activity. Patients with a systemic autoimmune disease (e.g., systemic

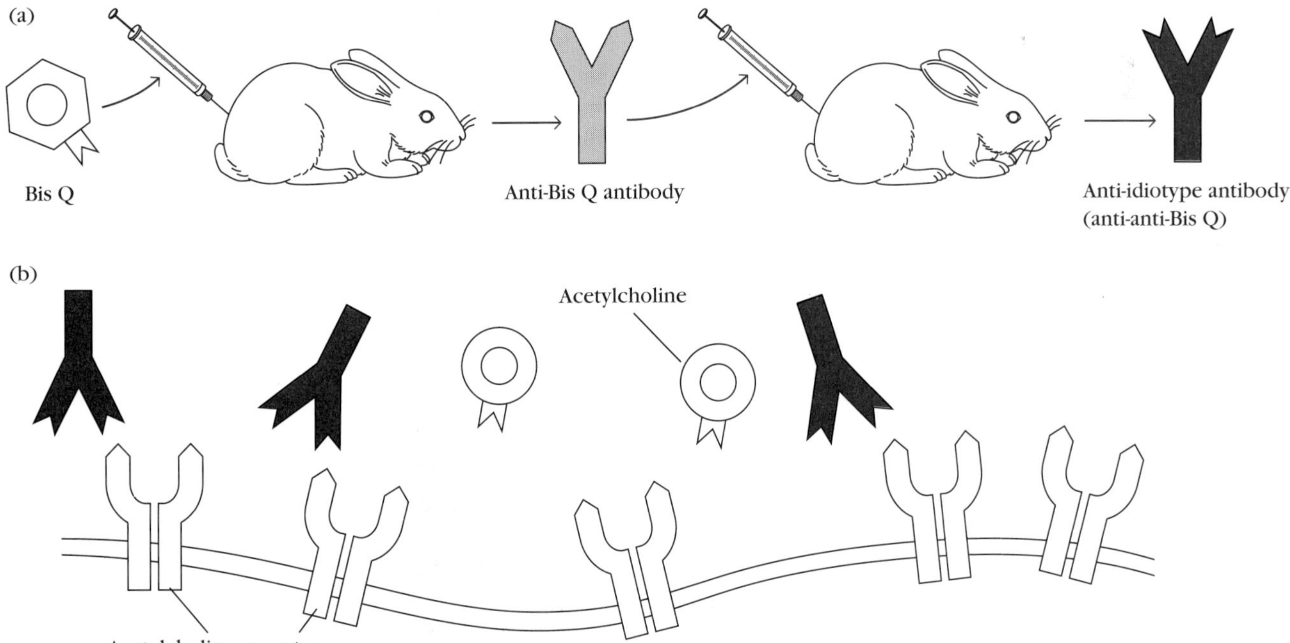

FIGURE 19-11 (a) Induction of experimental myasthenia gravis in rabbits by immunization with antibodies to Bis Q, an acetylcholine analog. The antibodies to Bis Q induce production of anti-idiotype antibodies (purple) in these rabbits. (b) Some of the anti-idiotype antibody binds to the acetylcholine receptor, blocking binding of acetylcholine and causing symptoms of myasthenia gravis.

lupus erythematosus, rheumatoid arthritis, multiple sclerosis) also appear to have a general regulatory T-cell defect that causes hyperactivity of both B cells and T cells.

Work with experimental autoimmune encephalomyelitis (EAE) has suggested that restoration of the regulatory T-cell subpopulation can reverse autoimmunity. As outlined in Figure 19-6, EAE can be induced in rats by injection of myelin basic protein (MBP) in adjuvant or of T-cell lines activated in vitro with MBP. Some rats, however, recover spontaneously and are resistant to further attempts to induce EAE by injection of MBP in adjuvant. There is a great deal of interest in understanding the immune state of these resistant rats. In one study female rats were injected with a male MBP-reactive T-cell line activated in vitro with MBP. As expected, these rats developed EAE and some of them recovered and became resistant to EAE induction by MBP. Months later two populations of thymocytes were isolated from the thymus of these resistant rats. One population bore the male karyotype of the original MBP-reactive T-cell line, which must have survived in the thymus of the resistant female rats. The other population of thymocytes was derived from the resistant female rats and was shown to specifically suppress the MBP-reactive T cells in vitro. This finding suggests that the presence of a low number of autoimmune MBP-specific T cells within the thymus had induced a population of T cells capable of specifically suppressing the autoimmune T cells and thus inducing resistance to EAE. Analysis of these T cells revealed that they were T_H1 cells, suggesting that restoration of the balance of T_H1 cells had reversed the autoimmunity.

Polyclonal B-Cell Activation

A number of viruses and bacteria can induce nonspecific polyclonal B-cell activation. Gram-negative bacteria, cytomegalovirus, and Epstein-Barr virus (EBV) are all known to be such activators, inducing the proliferation of numerous clones of B cells that express IgM in the absence of T_H cells. If B cells reactive to self-antigens are activated by this mechanism, autoantibodies can appear. During infectious mononucleosis, which is caused by EBV, a variety of autoantibodies are produced, including autoantibodies reactive to T and B cells, rheumatoid factors, and antinuclear antibodies. Similarly, lymphocytes from patients with SLE produce large quantities of IgM in culture, suggesting that they have been polyclonally activated. Many AIDS patients also show high levels of nonspecific antibody and autoantibodies to RBCs and platelets. These patients are often coinfected with other viruses such as EBV and cytomegalovirus, which may induce the polyclonal B-cell activation that results in autoantibody production.

Treatment of Autoimmune Diseases

Ideally, treatment for autoimmune diseases should be aimed at reducing only the autoimmune response while leaving the rest of the immune system intact. To date, this ideal has not been reached.

Current Therapies

Current therapies for autoimmune diseases are not cures by merely palliatives, aimed at reducing symptoms to provide the patient with an acceptable quality of life. For the most part these treatments provide nonspecific suppression of the immune system and thus do not distinguish between a pathologic autoimmune response and a protective immune response. Immunosuppressive drugs (e.g., corticosteroids, azathioprine, and cyclophosphamide) are often given with the intent of slowing proliferation of lymphocytes. By depressing the immune response in general, such drugs can reduce the severity of autoimmune symptoms. The general reduction in immune responsiveness, however, puts the patient at greater risk for infection or the development of cancer. A somewhat more selective approach employs cyclosporin A to treat autoimmunity. Since this agent blocks signal transduction mediated by the T-cell receptor, it should only inhibit antigen-activated T cells while sparing nonactivated ones.

Another therapeutic approach that has had some success with some autoimmune diseases (e.g., myasthenia gravis) is removal of the thymus. Because patients with this disease often have thymic abnormalities (e.g., thymic hyperplasia or thymomas), adult thymectomy often increases the likelihood of remission of symptoms.

Patients with Graves' disease, myasthenia gravis, rheumatoid arthritis, and systemic lupus erythematosus may experience short-term benefit from plasmapheresis. In this process plasma is removed from a patient's blood by continuous-flow centrifugation. The red blood cells are then resuspended in a suitable medium and returned to the patient. Plasmapheresis has been beneficial to patients with autoimmune diseases involving antigen-antibody complexes, which are removed with the plasma. Removal of the complexes, although only temporary, can result in a short-term reduction in symptoms.

Experimental Therapeutic Approaches

Studies with experimental autoimmune animal models have provided evidence that it is indeed possible to induce specific immunity to the development of autoimmunity. Several of these approaches are described in this section and outlined in Figure 19-12.

T-Cell Vaccination

I. R. Cohen and his co-workers have been pioneers in T-cell vaccination. The basis for this approach came from experiments with the EAE animal model. When rats were injected with low doses ($<10^4$) of cloned T cells specific for MBP, they did not develop symptoms of EAE and instead became resistant to the development of EAE when later challenged with a lethal dose of activated MBP-specific T cells or MBP in adjuvant. Later findings revealed that the efficacy of these autoimmune T-cell clones as a vaccine could be enhanced by cross-linking the cell-membrane components with formaldehyde or glutaraldehyde. When such cross-linked T cells were injected into animals with active EAE, permanent remission of symptoms was observed. The cross-linked T cells apparently elicit regulatory T cells specific for TCR variable-region determinants of the autoimmune clones. Presumably these regulatory T cells act to suppress the autoimmune T cells that mediate EAE.

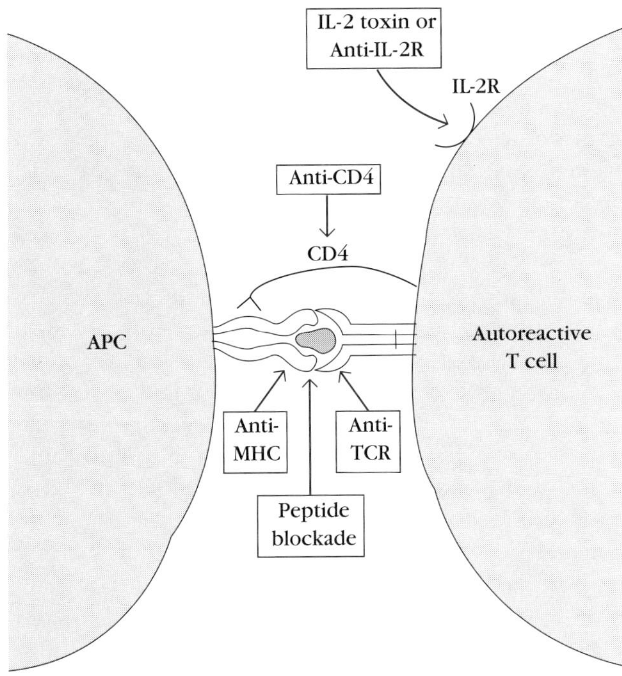

FIGURE 19-12 Some experimental agents for immunointervention in autoimmune disease. See text for discussion.

Because of the effectiveness of T-cell vaccination in animal models, this approach has been tried with a few human patients. For example, a 42-year-old woman with severe progressive multiple sclerosis was injected subcutaneously with T cells that had been isolated from her own cerebrosprinal fluid, cloned in vitro, and cross-linked with formaldehyde. The progression of her disease is currently being monitored. If this approach works, it represents a specific therapy that reduces only a specific autoimmune response without affecting overall immune responsiveness.

The finding that encephalitogenic T cells specific for MBP express T-cell receptors with a limited repertoire of V_α and V_β domains has led some researchers to use the restricted TCR V-region peptides as a possible vaccine. In the Lewis rat, for example, the encephalitogenic T-cell clones use $V_\beta 8.2$ almost exclusively. A synthetic peptide vaccine spanning the CDR2 region of the $V_\beta 8.2$ chain was shown to protect Lewis rats from developing EAE following an injection of MBP and adjuvant. When this same V-region peptide was injected into rats exhibiting severe EAE (characterized by hind limb paralysis), disease progression was arrested and the animals clinically recovered within 3 days. Thus the synthetic TCR V-region peptide not only functioned as a vaccine to prevent clinical signs of EAE from developing, it also was an effective treatment for animals with established disease. As noted earlier, both multiple sclerosis and myasthenia gravis appear to be associated with restricted expression of TCR V-region genes, suggesting that a similar approach might be effective in patients with these diseases.

Peptide Blockade of MHC Molecules

Identification and sequencing of various autoantigens has led to the development of new approaches to modulate autoimmune T-cell activity. In EAE, for example, the encephalitogenic peptides of MBP have been well characterized. Synthetic peptides differing by only one amino acid from their MBP counterpart have been shown to bind to the appropriate MHC molecule. Moreover, when sufficient amounts of such a peptide were administered along with the corresponding encephalitogenic MBP peptide, the clinical development of EAE was blocked. Presumably, the synthetic peptide acts as a competitor, occupying the antigen-binding cleft on MHC molecules and thus preventing binding of the MBP peptide.

In other studies blocking peptides complexed to soluble class II MHC molecules reversed the clinical progression of EAE in mice, presumably by inducing a state of clonal anergy in the autoimmune T cells. In a somewhat similar approach, a complex was formed between the blocking peptide, a class II MHC molecule, and the toxin adriamycin. This complex was shown to kill autoimmune EAE T cells in vitro.

Monoclonal-Antibody Treatment

Monoclonal antibodies have been used successfully to treat autoimmune disease in several animal models. For example, a high percentage of F_1 (NZB × NZW) mice given weekly injections of high doses of monoclonal antibody specific for the CD4 membrane molecule recovered from their autoimmune lupus-like symptoms (Figure 19-13). Similar positive results were observed in NOD mice, in which treatment with an anti-CD4 monoclonal led to disappearance of the lymphocytic infiltration and diabetic symptoms. Because anti-CD4 monoclonals block or deplete all T_H cells, regardless of their specificity, they can threaten the overall immune responsiveness of the recipient. One remedy for this disadvantage is to try to block antigen-activated T_H cells, since these cells are involved in the autoimmune state. To do this, researchers have used monoclonal antibody directed against the α subunit of the high-affinity IL-2 receptor. Since only antigen-activated T_H cells express the high-affinity IL-2R α subunit, monoclonal antibody to the α subunit (anti-TAC) might specifically block autoreactive T_H cells. Because the IL-2R α subunit is expressed at higher levels on autoimmune T cells, monoclonal antibody to the α subunit (anti-TAC) might block autoreactive T cells. This approach was tested in adult rats injected with activated MBP-specific T cells in the presence or absence of monoclonal antibody specific for the IL-2 receptor. All the control rats died of EAE, whereas six of the nine treated with the monoclonal antibody had no symptoms, and the symptoms in the other three were mild.

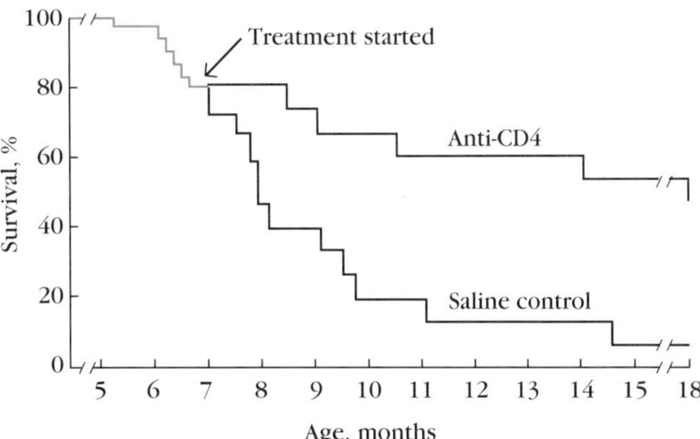

FIGURE 19-13 Effect of weekly injections of anti-CD4 monoclonal antibody on survival of F_1 (NZB × NZW) mice exhibiting autoimmune lupus-like symptoms. [From D. Wofsy, 1988, in *Monoclonal Antibody Therapy,* Prog. Allergy, H. Waldmann (ed.).]

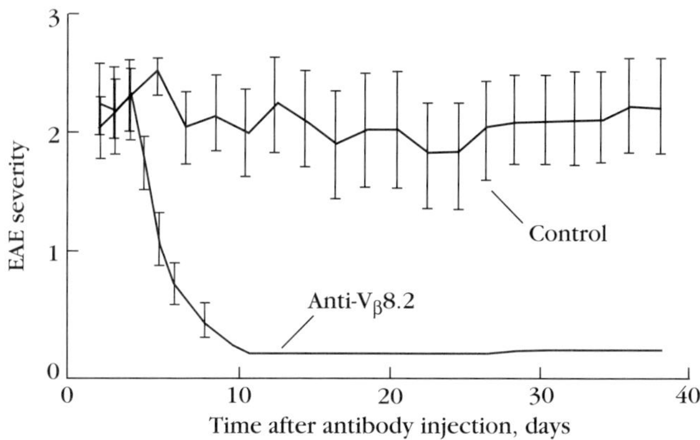

FIGURE 19-14 Effect of injection of monoclonal antibody to the $V_\beta 8.2$ T-cell receptor on PL/J mice exhibiting EAE symptoms. EAE was induced by injecting mice with MBP-specific T-cell clones. EAE severity scale: 3 = total paralysis of lower limbs; 2 = partial paralysis of lower limbs; 1 = limp tail; 0 = normal (no symptoms). [Adapted from H. Acha-Orbea et al., 1989, *Ann. Rev. Immunol.* **7**:371.]

The association of autoimmune disease with restricted TCR expression in a number of animal models has prompted researchers to see if blockage of the preferred receptors with monoclonal antibody might be therapeutic. Injection of PL/J mice with monoclonal antibody specific for the $V_\beta 8.2$ T-cell receptor prevented EAE induction with MBP in adjuvant. Even more exciting was the finding that the anti-$V_\beta 8.2$ monoclonal antibody could also reverse the symptoms of autoimmunity in mice manifesting induced EAE (Figure 19-14) and that these mice manifested long-term remission. Clearly, the use of monoclonal antibodies as a treatment for human autoimmune diseases presents exciting possibilities.

Similarly, the association of various MHC alleles with autoimmunity (see Table 19-3), as well as the evidence for increased or inappropriate MHC expression in some autoimmune disease, offers the possibility that monoclonal antibodies against appropriate MHC molecules might retard development of autoimmunity. Moreover, since antigen-presenting cells express many class II MHC molecules, it should theoretically be possible to selectively block an MHC molecule that is associated with autoimmunity, while sparing the other class II MHC molecules. In one study, injection of mice with monoclonal antibodies to class II MHC molecules prior to injection of myelin basic protein blocked the development of EAE. If, instead, the antibody was given after the injection of myelin basic protein, development of EAE was delayed but not prevented. In nonhuman primates, monoclonal antibodies to HLA-DR and HLA-DQ have been shown to reverse EAE.

Tolerance Induction by Oral Antigen

When antigens are administered orally, they tend to induce a state of immunologic unresponsiveness (tolerance). For example, mice fed MBP do not develop EAE following subsequent injection of MBP. This finding led H. Weiner, D. Hafler, and their colleagues to design a double-blind pilot trial in which 30 individuals with multiple sclerosis were fed either a placebo or 300 mg of bovine myelin every day for a year. The results of this study revealed that T cells specific for MBP were reduced in the myelin-fed group; there also was some suggestion that MS symptoms were reduced in the male recipients (although the reduction fell shy of statistical significance) but not in the female recipients. The difference in response between males and females may reflect differences in the HLA-DR phenotype: Most of the males were HLA-DR2$^-$ and most of the females were HLA-DR2$^+$. Further investigation is needed to determine whether individuals with different HLA-DR phenotypes respond differently to the oral myelin. If further trials of this sort demonstrate the efficacy of this type of treatment, it will certainly prove to be a simple and risk-free treatment for patients with autoimmune disease.

Summary

1. Human autoimmune diseases can be divided into organ-specific and systemic diseases. The organ-specific diseases involve an autoimmune response directed primarily against a single organ or gland. In contrast, the systemic diseases are directed against a broad spectrum of tissues and have manifestations in a variety of organs.

2. There are both spontaneous and experimental animal models for autoimmune diseases. Spontaneous models include a disease in NZB and (NZB $\times$ NZW) F_1 mice that parallels systemic lupus erythematosus, a thyroiditis seen in Obese-strain chickens that parallels Hashimoto's thyroiditis, and a diabetes in NOD mice that resembles human insulin-dependent diabetes mellitus. Several experimental animal models have been developed by immunizing animals with self-antigens in the presence of adjuvant. In experimental autoimmune myasthenia gravis (EAMG), the antigen is the acetylcholine receptor; in experimental autoimmune encephalomyelitis (EAE), the antigen is myelin basic protein; in experimental autoimmune thyroiditis (EAT), the antigen is thyroglobulin.

3. The experimental autoimmune animal models have revealed a central role for the CD4$^+$ T_H cell in the development of autoimmunity. In each of the experimentally induced autoimmune diseases, autoimmune T-cell clones can be isolated that induce the autoimmune disease in normal animals. The MHC haplotype of the experimental animal determines the ability to present various autoantigens to T_H cells. In addition, some autoimmune animals utilize a restricted repertoire of TCR genes, which may predispose the animal toward T-cell activity in response to a given self-antigen.

4. A variety of mechanisms have been proposed for autoimmunity, including release of sequestered antigens, molecular mimicry, inappropriate class II MHC expression on cells, a cytokine imbalance, a dysfunction of the idiotype network, a dysfunction of T-cell–mediated suppression, and polyclonal activation of lymphocytes. Evidence exists for each of these mechanisms, reflecting the many different pathways leading to autoimmune reactions.

5. Current therapies for autoimmune diseases include treatment with immunosuppressive drugs, thymectomy, and plasmapheresis for diseases involving immune complexes. These therapies, which are relatively nonspecific, may have significant side effects. Several more specific approaches have shown some success in various animal models for autoimmune diseases. These include vaccination with T cells specific for a given autoantigen, administration of synthetic blocking peptides that compete with autoantigen for binding to MHC molecules, treatment with monoclonal antibodies that react with some component specifically involved in an autoimmune reaction, and induction of tolerance to autoantigens by administering them orally.

References

ADORINI, L., J. C. GUERY, G. RODRIGUEZ-TARDUCHY, and S. TREMBLEAU. 1993. Selective immunosuppression. *Immunol. Today* **14**:285.

COHEN, I. R. 1989. T cell vaccination against autoimmune disease. *Hosp. Prac.* (Feb. 15):57.

COHEN, I. R. 1991. Autoimmunity to chaperonins in the pathogenesis of arthritis and diabetes. *Annu. Rev. Immunol.* **9**:567.

FAUSTMAN, D., L. XIANGPING, H. Y. LIN et al. 1991. Linkage of faulty major histocompatibility complex class I to autoimmune diabetes. *Science* **254**:1756.

FELDMANN, M., C. H. JUNE, A. MCMICHAEL et al. 1992. T-cell-targeted immunotherapy. *Immunol. Today* **13:**84.

HASKINS, K., and M. MCDUFFIE. 1990. Acceleration of diabetes in young NOD mice with a CD4+ islet-specific T cell clone. *Science* **249**:1433.

JONES, D. B., A. F. W. COULSON, AND G. W. DUFF. 1993. Sequence homologies between hsp60 and autoantigens. *Immunol. Today* **14**:115.

KRONENBERG, M. 1991. Self-tolerance and autoimmunity. *Cell* **65**:537.

KUMAR, V., D. H. KONO, J. L. URBAN, and L. HOOD. 1989. The T cell receptor repertoire and autoimmune diseases. *Annu. Rev. Immunol.* **7**:657.

MARTIN, R., H. F. MCFARLAND, and D. E. MCFARLIN. 1992. Immunological aspects of demyelinating disease. *Annu. Rev. Immunol.* **10**:153.

NAPARSTEK, Y., and P. H. PLOTZ. 1993. The role of autoantibodies in autoimmune disease. *Annu. Rev. Immunol.* **11**:79.

OFFNER, H., G. A. HASHIM, and A. A. VANDENBARK. 1991. T cell receptor peptide therapy triggers autoregulation of experimental encephalomyelitis. *Science* **251**:430.

OKSENBERG, J. R., et al. 1989. T cell receptor V_α and C_α alleles associated with multiple sclerosis and myasthenia gravis. *Proc. Nat'l. Acad. Sci. USA.* **86**:988.

SEBOUN, E., et al. 1989. A susceptibility locus for multiple sclerosis is linked to the T cell receptor β- chain complex. *Cell* **57**:1095.

SHIZURU, J. A., and N. SARVETNICK. 1991. Transgenic mice for the study of diabetes mellitus. *Trends Endocrinol. Metab.* **2**:97.

SINHA, A. A., M. T. LOPEZ, and H. O. MCDEVITT. 1990. Autoimmune diseases: the failure of self-tolerance. *Science* **248**:1380.

STEINMAN, L. 1991. The development of rational strategies for selective immunotherapy against autoimmune demyelinating disease. *Adv. Immunol.* **49**:357.

STEINMAN, L., J. R. OSKENBERG, and C. C. A. BERNARD. 1992. Association of susceptibility to multiple sclerosis with TCR genes. *Immunol. Today* **13**:49.

WALDMAN, H. 1989. Manipulation of T cell responses with monoclonal antibodies. *Annu. Rev. Immunol.* **7**:407.

WALDMANN, T. A. 1993. The IL-2/IL-2 receptor system: a target for rational immune intervention. *Immunol. Today* **14**:264.

WEINER, H. L., G. A. MACKIN, M. MATSUI et al. 1993. Double-blind pilot trial of oral tolerization with myelin antigens in multiple sclerosis. *Science* **259**:1321.

WOFSY, D. 1988. Treatment of autoimmune diseases with monoclonal antibodies. *Prog. Allergy* **45**:106.

ZAMVIL, S. S., and L. STEINMAN. 1990. The T lymphocyte in experimental allergic encephalomyelitis. *Annu. Rev. Immunol.* **8**:579.

Study Questions

1. Match each of the following autoimmune diseases (a–l) with the most appropriate characteristic (1–12) listed below.

a. ______ Experimental autoimmune encephalitis (EAE)
b. ______ Goodpasture's syndrome
c. ______ Graves' disease
d. ______ Systemic lupus erythematosus (SLE)
e. ______ Insulin-dependent diabetes mellitus (IDDM)
f. ______ Rheumatoid arthritis
g. ______ Hashimoto's thyroiditis
h. ______ Experimental autoimmune myasthenia gravis (EAMG)
i. ______ Myasthenia gravis
j. ______ Pernicious anemia
k. ______ Multiple sclerosis
l. ______ utoimmune hemolytic anemia

1. Autoantibodies to intrinsic factor block vitamin B_{12} absorption
2. Autoantibodies to acetylcholine receptor
3. T_{DTH}-cell reaction to thyroid antigens
4. Autoantibodies to RBC antigens
5. T-cell response to myelin
6. Induced by injection of myelin basic protein + complete Freund's adjuvant
7. Autoantibody to IgG
8. Autoantibodies to receptor for thyroid-stimulating hormone
9. Autoantibodies to basement membrane
10. Autoantibodies to DNA and DNA-associated protein
11. Induced by injection of acetylcholine receptors
12. T_{DTH}-cell response to pancreatic beta cells

2. Experimental autoimmune encephalitis (EAE) has proved to be a useful animal model of autoimmune disorders.

a. Discuss how this animal model is generated.
b. What is unusual about the animals that recover from EAE?
c. How has this animal model indicated a role for T cells in the development of autoimmunity?

3. Molecular mimicry is one mechanism proposed to account for the development of autoimmunity. How has induction of EAE with myelin basic protein contributed to understanding of molecular mimicry in autoimmune disease?

4. Describe at least three different mechanisms by which a localized viral infection might contribute to

the development of an organ-specific autoimmune disease.

5. In a system developed by Sarvetnik, transgenic mice expressing the IFN-γ transgene linked to the insulin promoter developed diabetes.
   a. Why was the insulin promoter used?
   b. What is the evidence that the diabetes in these mice is due to autoimmune damage?
   c. What is unusual about MHC expression in this system?
   d. How might this system mimic events that might be caused by a localized viral infection in the pancreas?

6. In patients with multiple sclerosis, elevated expression of IL-2 and the IL-2 receptor is often observed. How might this contribute to development of this autoimmune disease?

7. Monoclonal antibodies have been administered for therapy in various autoimmune animal models. What monoclonal antibodies have been used and what is the rationale for these approaches?

VACCINES

The discipline of immunology has its roots in the early vaccination trials of Edward Jenner and Louis Pasteur. Since these early efforts, vaccines have been developed for many diseases that were once major afflictions of mankind. The incidence of diseases such as diphtheria, measles, mumps, pertussis (whooping cough), rubella (German measles), poliomyelitis, and tetanus has declined dramatically as vaccination has become more common. According to the World Health Organization, immunization of children in Third World countries increased from 5% to 60% between 1974 and the late 1980s. Despite this progress, more than 5 million infants worldwide continue to die every year from diseases that could be avoided by existing vaccines. Among them are 2 million deaths from measles and 800,000 from neonatal tetanus, both of which can be completely avoided by immunization. Clearly, vaccination is a cost-effective weapon for disease prevention. Perhaps in no case have its benefits been as dramatically evident as in the eradication by the smallpox vaccine of one of mankind's long-standing and most terrible scourges. Since October of 1977 there has not been a single naturally acquired case of smallpox anywhere in the world.

Unfortunately, because of economic or scientific obstacles, vaccines are either nonexistent or not readily available for several diseases associated with significant morbidity or mortality rates. For example, more than 250 million people are chronically infected with hepatitis B virus (HBV); malaria causes 1–2 million deaths each year; diarrheal diseases (e.g., infections caused by rotavirus, *Shigella* sp., *Vibrio cholerae,* and toxin-producing *Escherichia coli*) annually kill an estimated 4–5 million people; the common cold and influenza continue to inflict untold millions yearly. And despite unprecedented efforts, no effective vaccine has been developed against human immunodeficiency virus (HIV), which had infected an estimated 10–20 million people by 1993.

Recent advances in immunology have led to the development of new and promising vaccine strategies. Knowledge of the differences in epitopes recognized by T cells and B cells has enabled immunologists to begin to design vaccines to maximize activation of the humoral or cell-mediated branch of the immune system. As differences in antigen-processing pathways became evident, scientists began to design vaccines to maximize antigen presentation with class I or class II MHC molecules. Genetic engineering techniques can be used to develop vaccines to maximize the immune response to selected epitopes. This chapter focuses on some of the existing vaccine strategies as well as on some experimental designs that may become the vaccines of the future.

Active and Passive Immunization

Immunity to infectious microorganisms can be achieved by active or passive immunization. In each case, immunity can be acquired by natural processes or by artificial means involving injection of antibodies or vaccines (Table 20-1).

Passive Immunization

Passive immunization, in which preformed antibodies are transferred to a recipient, can occur naturally by transplacental transfer of maternal antibodies to the developing fetus. Maternal antibodies to diphtheria, tetanus, streptococci, rubeola, rubella, mumps, and poliovirus all afford passively acquired protection to the developing fetus. Maternal antibodies present in colostrum also provide passive immunity to the infant.

Passive immunization also can be achieved by injecting a recipient with preformed antibodies. Passive immunization is used to provide immediate protection to individuals who have been exposed to an infectious organism and are suspected of lacking active immunity to that organism. As an example, individuals with wounds who have not received up-to-date active immunization against tetanus are given an injection of horse antiserum to tetanus toxin. The preformed horse antibody neutralizes any tetanus toxin produced by *Clostridium tetani* in the wound. Passive immunization is routinely administered to individuals exposed to botulism, tetanus, diphtheria, hepatitis, measles, and rabies (Table 20-2). Passively administered antiserum is also administered to provide protection from snake bites and black widow spider bites. Because

Table 20-1 Acquisition of immunity through passive and active immunization

Type	Acquired through
Passive immunization	Natural maternal antibody Artificial immune serum
Active immunization	Natural infection Artificial infection: Attenuated organisms Inactivated organisms Purified microbial macromolecules Cloned microbial antigens (alone or in vectors) Synthetic peptides Anti-idiotype antibodies Multivalent complexes

Table 20-2 Common agents used for passive immunization

Disease	Agent
Black widow spider bite	Horse antivenin
Botulism	Horse antitoxin
Diphtheria	Horse antitoxin
Hepatitis A and B	Pooled human immune gamma globulin
Measles	Pooled human immune gamma globulin
Rabies	Pooled human immune gamma globulin
Snake bite	Horse antivenin
Tetanus	Pooled human immune gamma globulin or horse antitoxin

passive immunization does not activate the immune system, there is no memory response.

Passive immunization should only be given when necessary because certain risks are associated with the injection of preformed antibody. If the antibody was produced in another species, such as a horse, the recipient can mount a strong response to the isotypic determinants of the foreign antibody. This anti-isotype response can lead to certain complications. Some individuals, for example, produce IgE antibody specific for a passive antibody. Immune complexes of this IgE bound to the passively administered antibody can mediate systemic mast-cell degranulation, leading to systemic anaphylaxis. Other individuals produce IgG or IgM antibodies specific for the foreign antibody, which form complement-activating immune complexes. The deposition of these complexes in the tissues can lead to type III hypersensitive reactions. Even when human gamma globulin is administered passively, the recipient can generate an anti-allotype response to the human immunoglobulin, although its level is usually much lower than that of an anti-isotype response.

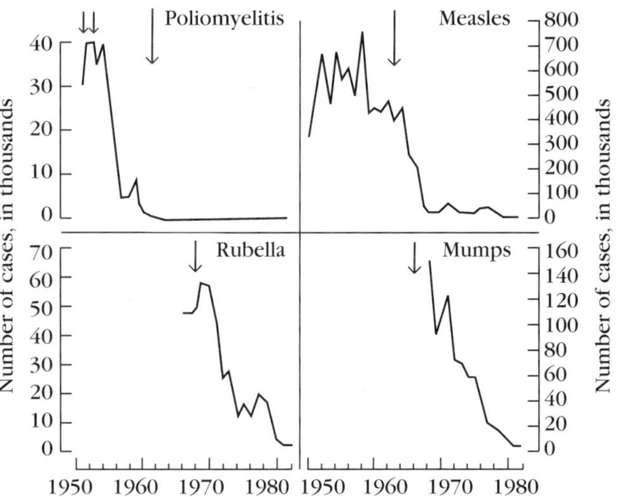

FIGURE 20-1 Reported annual number of cases of poliomyelitis, measles, rubella (German measles), and mumps in the United States (1950–1980) as reported by the Centers for Disease Control. The effect of introduction of vaccines (indicated by purple arrows) on the incidence of these diseases is obvious. [Data from Centers for Disease Control, adapted from C. A. Mims and D. O. White, 1984, *Viral Pathogenesis and Immunology,* Blackwell Scientific.]

Active Immunization

The goal of active immunization is to elicit protective immunity and immunologic memory so that a subsequent exposure to the pathogenic agent will elicit a heightened immune response with successful elimination of the pathogen. Active immunization can be achieved through natural infection with a microorganism, or it can be acquired artificially through vaccination. In active immunization, as the name implies, the immune system plays an active role, with proliferation of antigen-reactive T and B cells resulting in memory-cell formation. Active immunization with various types of vaccines has played an important role in the reduction of deaths from infectious diseases, especially among children.

TABLE 20-3 ROUTINE IMMUNIZATION SCHEDULE FOR INFANTS AND CHILDREN

Age	Vaccine
2 months	Diphtheria-pertussis-tetanus (DPT) Poliomyelitis (OPV)
4 months	Diphtheria-pertussis-tetanus Poliomyelitis
6 months	Diphtheria-pertussis-tetanus
15 months	Measles-mumps-rubella (MMR)
15–24 months	Diphtheria-pertussis-tetanus Poliomyelitis
18 months– 5 years	*Hemophilus influenzae* type b conjugate (Hib)
4–6 years	Diphtheria-pertussis-tetanus Poliomyelitis Measles-mumps-rubella
14–16 years	Diphtheria-tetanus

Active immunization of children is begun at about 2 months of age. A prescribed program of childhood immunizations, outlined in Table 20-3, includes the diphtheria-pertussis-tetanus (DPT) combined vaccine, trivalent oral polio vaccine (OPV), measles-mumps-rubella (MMR) combined vaccine, and the recently developed *Hemophilus influenzae* (Hib) vaccine. Childhood immunization has brought about a marked reduction in various childhood diseases in the United States (Figure 20-1). As long as widespread, effective immunization programs are maintained, the incidence of these childhood diseases should remain low.

As indicated in Table 20-3, childhood immunization often requires multiple boosters at appropriately timed intervals to achieve effective immunity. One reason for this is the persistence of maternal antibodies in the young infant. For example, passively acquired maternal antibodies bind to epitopes on the DPT vaccine and block adequate immune-system activation; therefore, this vaccine must be given several times after the maternal antibody has been catabolized to achieve adequate immunity. Passively acquired maternal antibody also interferes with the effectiveness of the measles vaccine; for this reason, the MMR vaccine is not given before 15 months of age. In Third World countries, however, the measles vaccine is administered at 9 months, even though maternal antibodies are still present, because 30–50% of young children in these countries contract the disease before 15 months of age. Multiple immunizations with the oral polio vaccine are required to ensure that an adequate immune response is generated to each of the three strains of poliovirus that make up the vaccine.

Adult immunization policies vary depending on the risk group. Vaccines for meningitis, pneumonia, and influenza are often given to groups living in close quarters (e.g., military recruits) or to individuals with reduced immunity (e.g., the elderly). International travelers are also routinely immunized against such endemic diseases as cholera, yellow fever, plague, typhoid, hepatitis, typhus, and polio. Some of the commonly administered active immunization agents are listed in Table 20-4.

Vaccination is not 100% effective. Instead, with any vaccine a small percentage of recipients will respond poorly and therefore will not be adequately protected. This is not a serious problem if the majority of the population is immune to an infectious agent. In this case the probability of a susceptible individual contacting an infected individual is so low that the susceptible individual is not likely to become infected. This phenomenon is known as ***herd immunity***. The appearance of measles epidemics among college students and unvaccinated preschool-age children in the United States during the mid- to late-1980s resulted partly from an overall decrease in vaccinations among the population that had lowered the herd immunity of the population (Figure 20-2). Among preschool-age children, 88% of those who developed measles were unvaccinated. Most of the college students who contracted measles had been vaccinated as children; the failure of the vaccine to protect them may have resulted from the presence of passively acquired maternal antibodies that reduced their overall response to the vaccine. This increase in the incidence of measles prompted the Immunization Practices Advisory Committee of the Centers for Disease Control to recommend that children receive two immunizations with the combined measles-mumps-rubella vaccine, one at 15 months of age and one at entry to kindergarten.

TABLE 20-4 CLASSIFICATION OF COMMON VACCINES FOR HUMANS

Disease or pathogen	Type of vaccine
Whole bacterial cells	
Cholera	Inactivated
Pertussis	Inactivated
Plague	Inactivated
Tuberculosis	Attenuated BCG*
Capsular polysaccharide	
Meningitis	Polysaccharide
Pneumococcal pneumonia	14 antigenically distinct polysaccharides
Hemophilus influenzae type b	Polysaccharide-protein carrier
Toxoids	
Diphtheria	Recombinant inactivated exotoxin
Tetanus	Recombinant inactivated exotoxin
Whole viral particles	
Influenza	Inactivated
Measles	Attenuated
Mumps	Attenuated
Rubella	Attenuated
Polio (Salk)	Inactivated
Polio (Sabin)	Attenuated
Rabies	Inactivated
Yellow fever	Attenuated
Viral antigens	
Hepatitis B	Recombinant surface antigen (HbsAg)

* Bacillus Calmette-Guerin is an avirulent strain of *Mycobacterium bovis.*

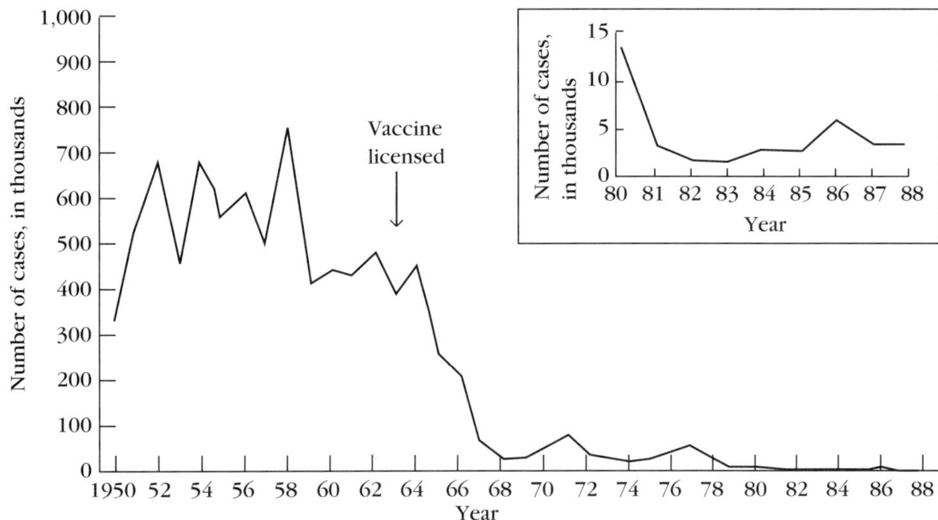

FIGURE 20-2 Introduction of the measles vaccine in 1962 led to a dramatic decrease in the annual incidence of this disease in the United States. Occasional outbreaks of measles in the 1980s *(inset)* occurred mainly among unvaccinated young children and among college students; most of the latter had been vaccinated, but only once, when they were young. [Data from Centers for Disease Control.]

Designing Vaccines for Active Immunization

Several factors must be kept in mind in developing a successful vaccine. First and foremost, the development of an immune response does not necessarily mean that a state of immunity has been achieved. Often the branch of the immune system that is activated is critical, and therefore vaccine design must recognize the important differences between activation of the humoral and cell-mediated branches. A second factor is the development of immunologic memory. For example, a vaccine may induce a primary response that is protective but may fail to induce memory-cell formation, leaving the host unprotected after the primary response to the vaccine subsides.

The role of memory cells in immunity depends, in part, on the incubation period of the pathogen. In the case of influenza virus, which has a very short incubation period of less than 3 days, disease symptoms are already under way by the time memory cells are activated. Effective protection against influenza therefore depends on maintaining high levels of neutralizing antibody by repeated reimmunizations. For pathogens with a longer incubation period, demonstrable neutralizing antibody at the time of infection is not necessary. The poliovirus, for example, has a long incubation period, requiring more than 3 days to begin to infect the central nervous system. An incubation period of this length provides the necessary time for memory B cells to respond with production of high levels of serum antibody. The vaccine for polio is therefore designed to induce high levels of immunologic memory. Following immunization with the Salk vaccine, serum antibody levels peak within 2 weeks and then decline, but the memory response continues to climb, reaching maximal levels at 6 months and persisting for years (Figure 20-3). If an immunized

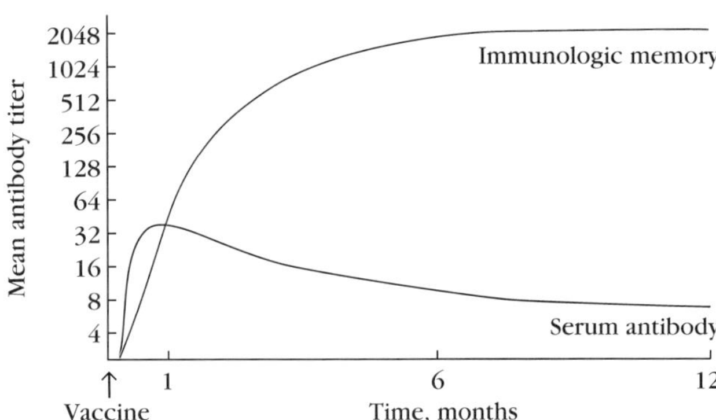

FIGURE 20-3 Immunization with a single dose of the Salk polio vaccine induces a rapid increase in serum antibody levels, which peak by 2 weeks and then decline. Induction of immunologic memory follows a slower time course, reaching maximal levels 6 months after vaccination. The persistence of the memory response for years following primary vaccination is responsible for immunity to poliomyelitis. [From M. Zanetti et al., 1987, *Immunol. Today* **8**:18.]

individual is later exposed to the poliovirus, these memory cells will respond by differentiating into plasma cells that produce high levels of serum antibody, which protect the individual from infection.

Vaccines designed to induce humoral antibody production must display epitopes that are accessible to the immunoglobulin receptor on B cells. As discussed in Chapter 4, B cells generally recognize epitopes that are hydrophilic and that display segmental mobility on x-ray crystallographic analysis. Many of these epitopes are not sequential and thus require the native structure of the protein to generate their conformation (see Figure 4-6). Inactivated or attenuated bacterial or viral vaccines often display native epitopes and thus induce humoral antibody production. Purified proteins and polysaccharides are also effective inducers of humoral immunity. Vaccination intended to produce humoral immunity also must take into account the location of the potential pathogen and the ability of different antibody isotypes to get to that location and neutralize the pathogen. In designing a vaccine for gonorrhea, for example, one of the major stumbling blocks has been the need to induce production of secretory IgA antibodies, which can block bacterial attachment to host mucous membrane cells. When vaccines are administered by injection, they tend to induce production of IgM and IgG but not secretory IgA. What is needed is a means of administering the vaccine at mucous membrane sites and keeping the vaccine at these sites long enough to induce a secretory IgA response.

For some infectious agents—notably viruses, bacteria, protozoa, and fungi that are intracellular pathogens—a cell-mediated immune response is necessary to confer immunity. A vaccine designed to induce this type of response must activate T cells as strongly as possible. Unlike B cells, which recognize epitopes on native antigen, T cells recognize antigen that has been processed and is presented along with MHC molecules. T-cell epitopes tend to be internal, hydrophobic, and linear peptides that are not revealed until the protein is denatured and unfolded in the course of antigen processing. These requirements place certain constraints on potential vaccines: To activate $CD4^+$ T cells, a vaccine must be processed by antigen-presenting cells and presented in association with class II MHC molecules; to activate $CD8^+$ T cells, a vaccine must be capable of replicating in host cells where its peptides can associate with class I MHC molecules. For this reason attenuated vaccines that permit some limited viral replication or bacterial growth within host cells are most effective for the induction of cytotoxic activity. In addition to the differences in processing routes for class I and for class II MHC presentation (see Figure 10-8), potential vaccines for inducing a cell-mediated response are limited by constraints arising from the preferential interaction of MHC molecules with different peptides (see Table 9-6). Therefore, an immunodominant T-cell epitope for one individual may not serve as an immunodominant T-cell epitope for another individual who expresses a different set of MHC antigen-presenting molecules.

In the remainder of this chapter, various approaches to the design of vaccines—both currently used vaccines and experimental ones—are described and examined in terms of their ability to induce humoral and cell-mediated immunity and memory-cell production.

Whole-Organism Vaccines

As Table 20-4 indicates, many of the common vaccines currently in use consist of inactivated (killed) or live but attenuated (avirulent) bacterial cells or viral particles. The primary characteristics of these two types of vaccines are compared in Table 20-5.

Attenuated Viral or Bacterial Vaccines

In some cases microorganisms can be *attenuated* so that they lose their pathogenicity while retaining their capacity for transient growth within an inoculated host. Attenuation can often be achieved by growing a pathogenic bacterium or virus for prolonged periods under abnormal culture conditions. This procedure selects mutants that are better suited to growth in the abnormal culture conditions and are therefore less capable of growth in the original host. For example, an attenuated strain of *Mycobacterium bovis* called Bacillus Calmette-Guerin (BCG) was developed by growing *M. bovis* on a medium containing increased concentrations of bile. After 13 years this strain had adapted to growth with increased bile and had become sufficiently attenuated that it was suitable as a vaccine for tuberculosis. The Sabin polio vaccine and the measles vaccine consist of viral strains that have been successfully attenuated and now serve as successful vaccines. The poliovirus used in the Sabin vaccine was attenuated by growth in monkey kidney epithelial cells. The measles vaccine contains a strain of rubella virus that was grown in duck embryo cells and later in human cell lines.

Attenuated vaccines have some advantages and some disadvantages. Because of their capacity for transient growth, such vaccines provide prolonged immune-system exposure to the individual epitopes on the attenuated organisms, resulting in increased immunogenicity and memory-cell production. As a consequence, these vaccines often require only a single

TABLE 20-5 COMPARISON OF ATTENUATED (LIVE) AND INACTIVATED (KILLED) VACCINES

Characteristic	Attenuated vaccine	Inactivated vaccine
Production	Virulent pathogen is grown under abnormal culture conditions to select for avirulent organisms	Virulent pathogen is inactivated by chemicals or irradiation with γ-rays
Booster requirement	Generally requires only a single booster	Requires multiple boosters
Relative stability	Less stable	More stable (advantageous for Third World countries where refrigeration is limited)
Type of immunity induced	Produces humoral and cell-mediated immunity	Produces mainly humoral immunity
Reversion tendency	May revert to virulent form	Cannot revert to virulent form

immunization, eliminating the need for repeated boosters. This property is a major advantage in Third World countries where epidemiologic studies have shown that roughly 20% of individuals fail to return for each subsequent booster. The ability of many attenuated vaccines to replicate within host cells makes them particularly suitable to induce a cell-mediated response.

The Sabin polio vaccine, consisting of three attenuated strains of poliovirus, is administered orally to children on a sugar cube or in sugar liquid. The attenuated viruses colonize the intestine and induce protective immunity to all three strains of virulent poliovirus. The ability of the attenuated Sabin vaccine to colonize the intestines enables it to induce production of secretory IgA, which serves as an important defense against naturally acquired poliovirus. Unlike most attenuated vaccines that require a single immunizing dose, the Sabin polio vaccine requires boosters because the three strains of attenuated poliovirus in the vaccine interfere with one another's replication in the intestine. With the first immunization, one strain will predominate in its growth, inducing immunity to that strain. With the second immunization, the immunity generated by the previous immunization will limit the growth of the previously predominant strain, enabling one of the two remaining strains to predominate and induce immunity. Finally with the third immunization, immunity to all three strains is achieved.

The major disadvantage of attenuated vaccines is the possibility of their reversion to a virulent form. The rate of reversion of the Sabin polio vaccine leading to subsequent paralytic disease is about one case in four million doses of vaccine. Another concern with attenuated vaccines is the presence of other viruses as contaminants. In 1960 it was discovered that the oncogenic virus SV40 had contaminated some monkey kidney cultures used in production of the Sabin vaccine; as a result more stringent vaccine testing was required to eliminate this contaminant. Attenuated vaccines may also be associated with complications similar to those seen in the natural disease. A small percentage of recipients of the measles vaccine, for example, develop postvaccine encephalitis. Although these complications are undesirable, the risk of such complications is far less than that observed in a naturally acquired measles infection.

In some cases, however, postvaccine complications may render a potential vaccine unacceptable. This situation is illustrated by recent trials with a new experimental measles vaccine. This vaccine—a new attenuated strain of the virus called the Edmonston-Zagreb strain—is immunogenic in infants as young as 4–6 months old. As noted earlier, maternal antibodies render the standard measles vaccine ineffective when it is given before 9 months of age. The new vaccine was developed for use in Third World countries where many infants are infected with the measles virus at a very early age. Unfortunately, trials of the Edmonston-Zagreb vaccine in Guinea-Bissau, Senegal, and Haiti had to be halted when many vaccinated children began dying from common endemic disorders such as diarrhea, pneumonia, and parasitic diseases. Mortality rates were higher in girls than boys, an unexplained finding. The high rate of postvaccine complications with the Edmonston-Zagreb strain may result from vaccine-mediated immunosuppression, since the measles virus is known to cause transient immunosuppression. Some have speculated that the potent immunogenicity of the Edmonston-Zagreb strain, even in the presence of maternal antibodies, may be associated with potent immunosuppressive effects, placing vaccinated infants at risk for infections with other endemic pathogens that unvaccinated infants can resist.

Genetic engineering techniques provide a way to attenuate a virus irreversibly by selectively removing genes that are necessary for virulence. This has been done with a herpes virus vaccine for pigs, in which the thymidine kinase gene was removed. Because thymidine kinase is required for the virus to grow in certain types of cells (e.g., neurons), removal of this gene rendered the virus incapable of causing disease. It is possible that similar genetic engineering techniques could eliminate the risk of reversion of the attenuated polio vaccine. One strategy for developing an AIDS vaccine involves research on HIV variants in the hope of developing an irreversibly attenuated strain.

Inactivated Viral or Bacterial Vaccines

Another common approach in vaccine production is to inactivate the pathogen by heat or chemical means so that the pathogen is no longer capable of replication in the host. It is critically important to maintain the structure of epitopes on surface antigens during inactivation. Heat inactivation generally is unsatisfactory because it causes extensive protein denaturation; thus any epitopes that depend on higher orders of protein structure are likely to be altered. Chemical inactivation with formaldehyde or various alkylating agents has had success. The Salk polio vaccine and the pertussis (whooping cough) vaccine both depend on formaldehyde inactivation. In contrast with attenuated vaccines, whose immunogenicity is increased by their transient growth, killed vaccines tend to require repeated boosters to maintain the immune status of the host. In addition, killed vaccines induce a predominantly humoral antibody response; they are less effective than attenuated vaccines in inducing cell-mediated immunity and in eliciting an IgA response.

Even though they contain killed pathogens, inactivated whole-organism vaccines still are associated with certain risks. A serious complication with the first Salk vaccines was inadequate formaldehyde killing of the virus in two vaccine lots, which caused paralytic polio in a high percentage of recipients. The pertussis vaccine highlights another problem that can arise with a complex whole-organism vaccine. Encephalitis-type reactions occur in a small percentage of infants receiving this vaccine (Table 20-6), and it has not been possible to establish just what components of the organism are responsible for these reactions.

TABLE 20-6 RISKS VERSUS BENEFITS OF THE PERTUSSIS VACCINE FOR WHOOPING COUGH

	Risk of occurrence after	
Problem	Vaccination	Disease
Seizures	1:1750	1:25–1:50
Encephalitis	1:110,000	1:1000–1:4000
Severe brain damage	1:310,000	1:2000–1:8000
Death	1:1,000,000	1:200–1:1000

SOURCE: I. Tizard, *Immunology: An introduction,* 2d ed., Saunders.

Purified Macromolecules as Vaccines

Some of the risks of vaccines based on attenuated or killed microorganisms can be avoided with vaccines that consist of specific, purified macromolecules. The vaccines for meningococcal meningitis and pneumococcal pneumonia use a mixture of purified capsular polysaccharides as the immunogen. One of the limitations with polysaccharide vaccines is their inability to activate T_H cells. They activate B cells in a thymus-independent manner, resulting in IgM but no IgG production and little, if any, development of memory cells. One method that has been utilized to bypass this limitation is to conjugate the polysaccharide antigen to some sort of protein carrier. For example, the vaccine for *Haemophilus influenzae* type b (Hib), the major cause of bacterial meningitis in children under 5 years of age, consists of type b capsular polysaccharide covalently linked to a protein carrier, tetanus toxoid. The polysaccharide-protein conjugate is considerably more immunogenic than the polysaccharide alone, and because it activates T_H cells, it enables class switching from IgM to IgG. Although this type of vaccine can induce memory B cells, it cannot induce memory T cells specific for the pathogen. In the case of the Hib vaccine, it appears that the memory B cells can be activated to some degree in the absence of a memory T_H-cell population, thus accounting for the efficacy of this vaccine.

One of the problems encountered with vaccines containing purified surface macromolecules is the difficulty of obtaining sufficient quantities of the purified component. This limitation can be overcome with recombinant DNA techniques whereby a gene encoding an immunogenic protein is expressed in bacterial, yeast, or insect cells. Diphtheria and tetanus vaccines, for example, can be made by purifying the recombinant bacterial exotoxin and then inactivating the toxin with formaldehyde to form a *toxoid*. Vaccination with the toxoid induces antitoxoid antibodies, which are also capable of binding to the toxin and neutralizing its toxic effect. In production of toxoid vaccines the conditions must be closely controlled to achieve detoxification without excessive modification of the epitope structure.

Recombinant Antigen Vaccines

DNA encoding antigenic determinants can be isolated and cloned in bacteria, yeast, or mammalian cells. A number of genes from viral, bacterial, and protozoan pathogens have been successfully cloned and are presently being developed as vaccines. The DNA encoding the relevant antigen can be cloned in bacterial, yeast, insect, or mammalian expression systems. The first successful recombinant vaccine was developed for the major antigen (VP1) of the foot-and-mouth disease virus. In this case, viral RNA encoding the VP1 surface antigen was transcribed into cDNA using reverse transcriptase. The VP1 cDNA was then inserted into an *Escherichia coli* plasmid and cloned in *E. coli* (see Figure 2-5). This procedure allowed production of large quantities of the VP1 antigen, which was then purified and used as a vaccine in animals.

The first recombinant antigen vaccine approved for human use was the hepatitis B vaccine. This vaccine was developed by cloning the gene for the major surface antigen of hepatitis B virus (HBsAg) in yeast cells. The recombinant yeast cells are grown in large fermenters and HBsAg accumulates intracellularly in the cells. The yeast cells are harvested and disrupted by high pressure, releasing the recombinant HBsAg, which is then purified by conventional biochemical techniques. The recombinant hepatitis B vaccine has been administered to over 8000 individuals and has been shown to induce the production of protective antibodies. This vaccine holds much promise for the 250 million carriers of chronic hepatitis B worldwide!

Several recombinant vaccines for human immunodeficiency virus are presently being assessed in volunteers as potential vaccines for AIDS (see Chapter 23). Other recombinant vaccines that are being developed in animal models include the β subunit of cholera toxin, the enterotoxin of *E. coli,* the circumsporozoite protein of the malaria parasite, and a glycoprotein membrane antigen from Epstein-Barr virus. Animals immunized with these recombinant vaccines have in some cases mounted a protective immune response to a subsequent challenge with the live pathogen. One disadvantage of recombinant protein or glycoprotein vaccines is that they are processed as exogenous antigens and therefore do not tend to induce much activation of class I MHC–restricted T_C cells.

Recombinant Vector Vaccines

It is possible to introduce genes encoding major antigens of especially virulent pathogens into attenuated viruses or bacteria. The attenuated organism serves as a vector, replicating within the host and expressing the gene product of the pathogen. A number of organisms have been used for vector vaccines including vaccinia virus, attenuated poliovirus, adenoviruses, attenuated strains of *Salmonella,* and the BCG strain of *Myobacterium bovis.*

Vaccinia virus, the attenuated vaccine used to eradicate smallpox, has been widely employed as a vector vaccine. This large, complex virus, with a genome of about 200 genes, can be engineered to carry several dozen foreign genes without impairing its capacity to infect host cells and replicate. The gene encoding the desired antigen is inserted into a plasmid vector adjacent to a vaccinia promoter and flanked on either side by vaccinia thymidine kinase sequences. Tissue culture cells are then simultaneously infected with vaccinia virus and transfected with the recombinant plasmid. The desired gene and promoter are inserted into the vaccinia virus genome by homologous recombination at the site of the nonessential vaccinia thymidine kinase gene, resulting in a thymidine kinase–negative recombinant virus. Tissue culture cells infected with recombinant (thymidine kinase–negative) vaccinia viruses are then selected by adding bromodeoxyuridine (BUdr), a thymidine analog, which will kill all thymidine kinase–positive cells (Figure 20-4).

The genetically engineered vaccinia expresses high levels of the inserted gene product, which can then serve as a potent immunogen in an inoculated host. E. Paoletti has inserted genes from hepatitis B virus, herpes simplex, and influenza into vaccinia virus. Vaccine trials in the laboratory have shown that this engineered vaccinia induces antibodies to all three engineered gene products. Like the smallpox vaccine, genetically engineered vaccinia can be administered simply by dermal scratching, causing a limited localized, infection in host cells. If the foreign gene product expressed by the vaccinia is a viral envelope protein, it is inserted into the membrane of the infected host cell, inducing development of T-cell–mediated immunity as well as antibody-mediated immunity. Vaccinia virus engineered with the envelope glycoproteins of the human immunodeficiency virus (HIV) is currently being assessed both in chimpanzees and in human volunteers as a potential vaccine for AIDS. There are

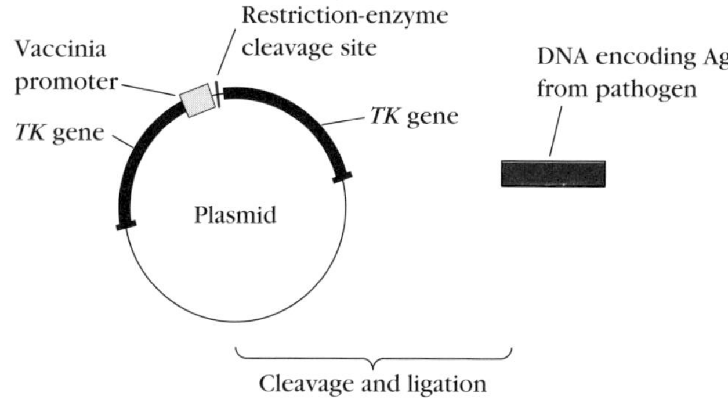

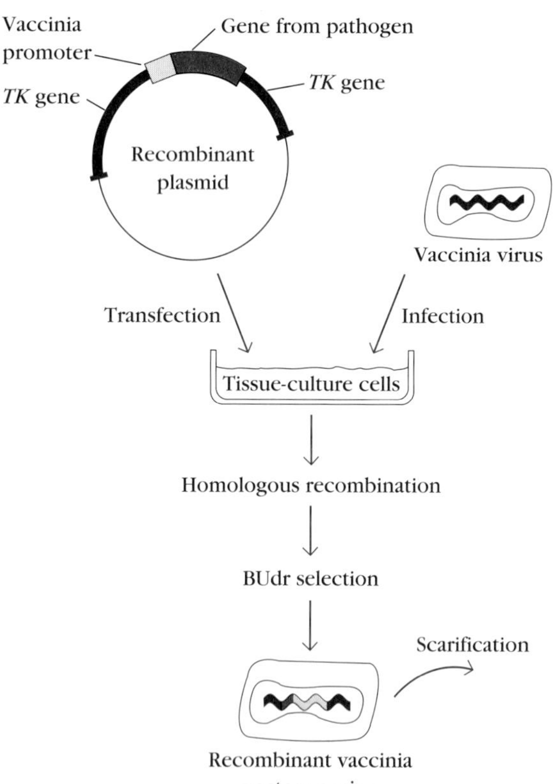

FIGURE 20-4 Production of vaccinia vector vaccine containing a gene encoding an antigen from a pathogen (purple). When tissue-culture cells are incubated with the recombinant plasmid and vaccinia virus, homologous recombination occurs at the site of the vaccinia thymidine kinase *(TK)* gene. Cells containing the recombinant vaccinia virus are selected by addition of bromodeoxyuridine (BUdr), which kills TK^{+} cells. [Adapted from B. Moss, 1985, *Immunol. Today* **6**:243.]

questions, however, about the suitability of a vaccinia vector vaccine for individuals with AIDS. In the early 1980s, an individual infected with HIV developed disseminated vaccinia after being vaccinated for smallpox with vaccinia. In healthy individuals an attenuated vaccine has only limited growth, but in individuals with immune deficiency even an attenuated vaccine can be potentially fatal.

Other attenuated vector vaccines may prove to be safer than the vaccinia vaccine. An attenuated strain of *Salmonella typhimurium* has been engineered with genes from the bacterium that causes cholera. The advantage of this vector vaccine is that *Salmonella* infects cells of the mucosal lining of the gut and therefore will induce secretory IgA production. For a number of diseases, including cholera and gonorrhea, increased levels of secretory IgA at mucous membrane surfaces is necessary for immunity. The Sabin vaccine strain of poliovirus is another candidate for a safe and effective vector vaccine. In this case the poliovirus vector is genetically engineered so that a portion of the gene encoding the outer capsid protein of poliovirus is replaced by DNA encoding the epitope of choice. The resulting poliovirus chimera will express the desired epitope in a highly accessible presentation protruding from the poliovirus nucleocapsid. A chimeric poliovirus vector vaccine expressing epitopes from the envelope glycoproteins of HIV has been shown to induce high levels of neutralizing antibodies specific for HIV in animal models.

Synthetic Peptide Vaccines

Construction of synthetic peptides for use as vaccines to induce either humoral or cell-mediated immunity requires an understanding of the nature of T-cell and B-cell epitopes. Potential B-cell epitopes of a protein antigen can be identified by examining its structure for peptide sequences representing sites that are accessible, hydrophilic, and mobile. Because x-ray crystallographic analysis has not been performed on most proteins, B-cell epitopes are generally chosen by identifying strongly hydrophilic sequences. The assumption is that strongly hydrophilic sequences are most likely to represent accessible surface regions that constitute B-cell epitopes. Ideally, vaccines for inducing humoral immunity should include peptides composing immunodominant B-cell epitopes. Such epitopes can be identified by determining the dominant antibody in the sera of individuals who are recovering from a disease and then testing peptides for their ability to react with that antibody with a high affinity. In one such experiment, two linear synthetic peptides representing potential B-cell epitopes of HBsAg were tested for their binding affinity to pooled antisera from individuals who had recovered from hepatitis B. It was found that a synthetic peptide consisting of cyclical repeats of amino acids 139–147 had a 10-fold higher affinity than cyclical repeats of amino acids 124–137.

The cyclical peptide 139–147 was therefore chosen as a potential candidate for a synthetic hepatitis B vaccine.

An effective memory response for both humoral and cell-mediated immunity requires generation of a population of memory T_H cells. A successful vaccine must therefore include immunodominant T-cell epitopes. With synthetic peptide vaccines it is difficult to identify those epitopes owing to the role, unpredictable as yet, of the MHC in influencing immunodominance for the T-cell system. T cells recognize processed peptides that, in the majority of cases, appear to represent internal amphipathic peptides. As illustrated in Figure 4-8, these peptides must have a site (the agretope) that enables them to interact with MHC molecules as well as a site (the epitope) that enables them to interact with the T-cell receptor. MHC molecules differ in their ability to present peptides to T cells. In one experiment congenic and recombinant congenic strains of mice were tested for their ability to recognize synthetic peptides of an internal core protein (nucleoprotein) of the influenza virus. As the data in Table 20-7 show, mouse strains with different MHC haplotypes recognized and responded to different peptides. To determine whether the K or D class I MHC molecules were responsible for peptide recognition in these strains, the class I MHC genes from each strain were transfected individually into L cells. The transfected fibroblasts were incubated with the various peptides and tested for their ability to activate a CTL response with influenza-primed T_C cells from the corresponding strain. The D^b molecule was the restriction element in the C57BL/6 strain, the K^k molecule was the restriction element in the CBA strain, and the K^d molecule was the restriction element in the BALB/c strain (see Table 20-7). These results highlight the important differences among MHC molecules in peptide presentation. The MHC polymorphism within a species will therefore influence the level of T-cell responsiveness by different individuals to different peptides.

Moreover, different subpopulations of T cells probably recognize different epitopes. Experiments by E. Sercarz have identified some peptides that induce a strong helper response and other peptides that induce immunologic suppression. These helper and suppressor peptides generally represent different, nonoverlapping amino acid sequences. For example, immunization with the amino-terminal residues (1–17) of hen egg-white lysozyme suppressed the response to native lysozyme. By identifying suppressing peptides and eliminating them from synthetic vaccines, it might be possible to generate enhanced immunity. These suppressing peptides may also be valuable in situations where it is desirable to decrease the immune response, as in treating autoimmune diseases.

In designing synthetic peptide vaccines against viruses, the current approach is to look for invariant regions, whose amino acid sequence is highly conserved. Some regions of the hemagglutinin (HA) molecule of influenza virus, for example, display high levels of amino acid variation, which generate the type and subtype differences enabling the virus to escape the immune system. But invariant regions, which mediate essential biological functions, also are present in the HA molecule. For example, the sialic acid–binding site on HA allows the virus to bind to sialic acid residues on cell surfaces. Although this region on the intact viral particle does not normally induce antibody formation, synthetic peptide vaccines of this conserved region were found to neutralize viral infectivity

TABLE 20-7 EFFECT OF MHC HAPLOTYPE ON RECOGNITION OF INFLUENZA NUCLEOPROTEIN PEPTIDES BY INBRED MOUSE STRAINS

			CML response in vitro with transfected class I MHC alleles†	
Strain	MHC haplotype	Peptide producing response in vivo*	*D*	*K*
C57BL/6	H-2^b	365–380	+	–
CBA	H-2^k	50–63	–	+
BALB/c	H-2^d	147–161	–	+

* Mice from each strain were injected with the various peptides conjugated to a carrier protein. Only the indicated peptides induced a T-cell response as measured by a CML assay.

† The *D* and *K* alleles from each strain were transfected individually into fibroblast L cells. The transfected cells were then incubated with the appropriate peptide and antigen-primed T_c cells from the corresponding strain and the CML response was measured.

SOURCE: Based on D. C. Wraith, 1987, *Immunol. Today* **8**:239.

against a number of different influenza types and subtypes. These studies provide optimism for a long-awaited influenza vaccine, which is discussed in Chapter 21. Synthetic peptide vaccines are being evaluated for hepatitis B virus, the malaria parasite, diphtheria toxin, and various proteins and glycoproteins of HIV.

Multivalent Subunit Vaccines

One of the limitations with synthetic peptide vaccines and recombinant protein vaccines is that these vaccines tend to be poorly immunogenic; in addition, they tend to induce humoral antibody production but are less able to induce a cell-mediated response. What is needed is some method of structuring a vaccine to contain immunodominant B-cell *and* T-cell epitopes. Furthermore, if a CTL response is desired, it is also necessary to be able to deliver the vaccine intracellularly so that the peptides can be processed and presented together with class I MHC molecules. A number of innovative techniques are currently being employed to develop multivalent vaccines that can present multiple copies of a given peptide or a mixture of peptides to the immune system.

One approach is to prepare solid matrix-antibody-antigen (SMAA) complexes by attaching monoclonal antibodies to particulate solid matrices and then saturating the antibody with the desired antigen. The resulting complexes are then used as vaccines. By attaching different monoclonal antibodies to the solid matrix, it is possible to bind a mixture of peptides or proteins, composing immunodominant epitopes for both T cells and B cells, to the solid matrix (Figure 20-5a). These multivalent complexes have been shown to induce vigorous humoral and cell-mediated responses. Their particulate nature contributes to their increased immunogenicity by facilitating phagocytosis by phagocytic cells.

Another means of obtaining a multivalent vaccine is to utilize detergent to incorporate protein or peptide antigens into lipid vesicles (called liposomes), into immunostimulating complexes (called ISCOMs), or into protein micelles (Figure 20-5b). Micelles are formed by mixing proteins in detergent and then removing the detergent. The individual proteins will orient themselves with the hydrophilic residues oriented toward the aqueous environment and the hydrophobic residues at the center so as to exclude their interaction with the aqueous environment. Liposomes containing protein antigens are prepared by mixing the proteins with a suspension of phospholipids under conditions that form vesicles bounded by a bilayer. The proteins are incorporated into the bilayer with the hydrophilic

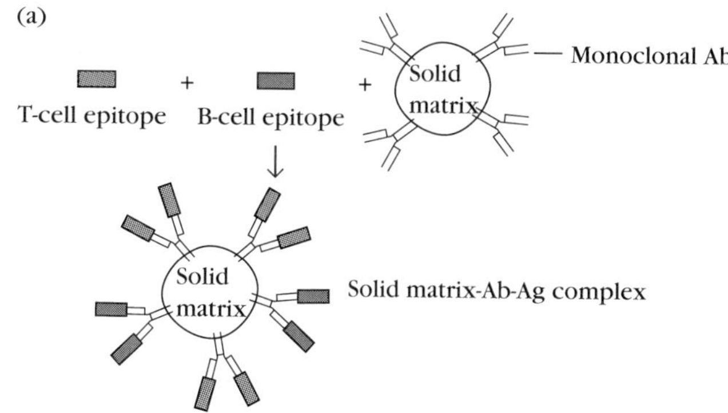

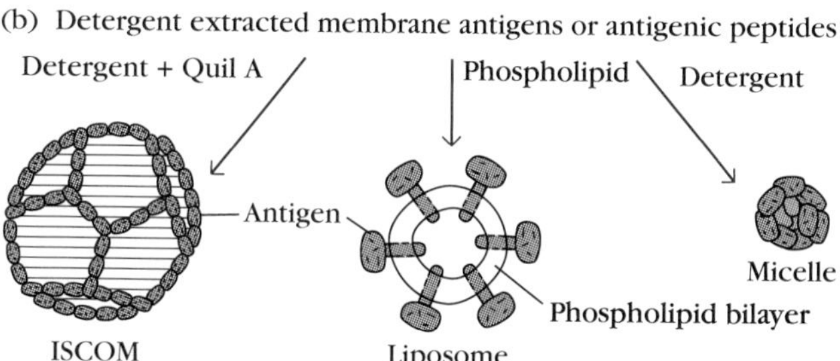

FIGURE 20-5 Multivalent subunit vaccines. (a) Solid matrix-antibody-antigen complexes can be designed to contain synthetic peptides representing both T-cell epitopes (purple) and B-cell epitopes (gray). (b) Protein micelles, liposomes, and immunostimulating complexes (ISCOMs) can all be prepared with extracted antigens or antigenic peptides (purple). In each case, the hydrophilic residues of the antigen are oriented outward.

residues exposed. ISCOMs are prepared by mixing protein or peptide antigens with detergent and a glycoside called Quil A, which forms micelles that interact with the antigen. The peptide or protein is expressed as a multivalent complex on the surface of the micelle. Membrane proteins from different pathogens including influenza virus, measles virus, hepatitis B virus, and HIV have been incorporated into micelles, liposomes, and ISCOMs and are currently being assessed as potential vaccines. In addition to their increased immunogenicity, liposomes and ISCOMs appear to deliver the antigen into cells and therefore are able to induce cell-mediated immunity.

Anti-Idiotype Vaccines

The discovery that an anti-idiotype antibody can in effect serve as the internal image of an antigen (see Figure 16-5) opened the door to the potential introduction of anti-idiotype antibodies as vaccines. What they promise, of course, is the generation of an effective immune response to a dangerous pathogen

TABLE 20-8 EVALUATION OF SOME ANTI-IDIOTYPE VACCINES

Infectious agents	Nature of anti-idiotype vaccine	Species tested	Adjuvant	Protection
		Viruses		
Hepatitis	P/M	Mice	+	+
Rabies	P	Mice	+	ND
Tobacco mosaic	P	Mice	+	ND
Polio type II	M	Mice	−	−
Reovirus	M	Mice	−	ND
Sendai	M	Mice	−	+
		Bacteria		
Streptococcus pneumoniae	M	Mice	−	+
Escherichia coli	M	Mice	+	+
Listeria monocytogenes	M	Mice	+	+
		Parasites		
Trypanosoma rhodesiense	M	Mice	−	+
Schistosoma mansoni	M	Rats	−	+
Trypanosoma cruzi	P	Mice	+	ND

KEY: P = polyclonal antibody; M = monoclonal antibody; ND = not determined.

SOURCE: M. Zanetti et al., 1987, *Immunol Today* **8**:18.

without exposure of the vaccinated individual to any form of the pathogen. One anti-idiotype vaccine currently being developed for protection against HIV is designed to bind to a conserved region on the gp120 envelope glycoprotein that is required for binding to the CD4 membrane molecule on host cells. Table 20-8 lists some of the anti-idiotype vaccines that have been evaluated. For a more complete discussion of these vaccines see Chapter 16.

SUMMARY

1. A state of immunity can be induced by passive or active immunization. Passive immunization involves transfer of preformed antibodies and provides short-term protection without the requirement for an active immune response. Active immunization induces clonal selection and results in memory-cell formation.

2. The current vaccines for humans are attenuated (avirulent) microorganisms, inactivated (killed) microorganisms, or purified macromolecules. Attenuated vaccines have the advantage of transient growth and therefore stimulate a more pronounced immune response and memory-cell production without the requirement for additional boosters. Inactivated vaccines require repeated boosters but pose no risk of reversion to a pathogenic state. The use of purified macromolecules, which are less complex than whole-organism vaccines, avoids certain complications due to unknown side effects. By applying recombinant DNA techniques, it is possible to produce large quantities of a defined antigen for immunization.

3. In developing a vaccine, the branch of the immune system to be activated must be considered. To induce humoral immunity, epitopes must be accessible to B-cell immunoglobulin receptors and should represent immunodominant epitopes of the infectious agent. To induce cell-mediated immunity, a vaccine capable of transient intracellular growth is desirable to maximize the presentation of antigens with MHC molecules.

4. Vaccinia virus can be engineered to carry multiple genes from infectious microorganisms. An advantage of this vector approach is that there is some replication of the engineered vaccinia virus in host cells, which serves to maximize cell-mediated immunity to the expressed antigens.

5. Peptides can be synthesized that represent immunodominant T- or B-cell epitopes. This approach has enabled immunologists to produce defined vaccines that may make possible the selective activation of the humoral or cell-mediated branches of the immune system.

6. Anti-idiotype vaccines offer the possibility of achieving a state of immunity without having to expose the recipient to the uncertainties of vaccines derived from whole organisms or purified macromolecules.

References

BLOOM, B. 1989. Vaccines for the third world. *Nature* **342**:115.

ETLINGER, H. M. 1992. Carrier sequence selection—one key to successful vaccines. *Immunol. Today* **13**:52.

EVANS, D. J., J. MCKEATING, J. M. MEREDITH et al. 1989. An engineered poliovirus chimera elicits broadly reactive HIV-1 neutralizing antibodies. *Nature* **339**:385.

HENDERSON, D. A. 1976. The eradication of smallpox. *Sci. Am.* **235**:25.

MILCH, D. R. 1989. Synthetic T and B cell recognition sites: implications for vaccine development. *Adv. Immunol.* **45**:195.

RANDALL, R. E. 1989. Solid matrix-antibody-antigen (SMAA) complexes for constructing multivalent subunit vaccines. *Immunol. Today* **10**:336.

ROBBINS, A., and P. FREEMAN. 1988. Obstacles to developing vaccines for the third world. *Sci. Am.* **259**(Nov.):126.

STEWARD, M. W., and C. R. HOWARD. 1987. Synthetic peptides: a next generation of vaccines? *Immunol. Today* **8**:51.

STOVER, C. K., V. FDELA CRUG, and T. R. FUERSTETAL. 1991. New use of BCG for recombinant vaccines. *Nature* **351**:456.

TAKAHSHI, H., T. TAKESHITA, B. MOREINA et al. 1990. Induction of $CD8^+$ cytotoxic T cells by immunization with purified HIV-1 envelope protein in Iscoms. *Nature* **344**:873.

WEISS, R. 1992. Measles battle loses potent weapon. *Science* **258**:546.

ZANETTI, M., E. SERCARZ, and J. SALK. 1987. The immunology of new generation vaccines. *Immunol. Today* **8**:18.

ZUCKERMAN, A. J. (ed.). 1989. *Recent Developments in Prophylactic Immunization.* Immunology and Medicine Series Vol. 12. Kluwer Academic Publishers.

Study Questions

1. Indicate whether each of the following statements is true or false. If you think a statement is false, explain why.
   a. Transplacental transfer of maternal IgG antibodies against measles confers short-term immunity on the fetus.
   b. Attenuated vaccines are more likely to induce cell-mediated immunity than killed vaccines are.
   c. Hydrophilic peptides are more likely to represent immunodominant B-cell epitopes than hydrophobic peptides.
   d. Macromolecules generally contain a large number of potential epitopes.

2. What are the advantages and disadvantages of using attenuated organisms as vaccines?

3. A child who had never been immunized to tetanus stepped on a rusty nail and got a deep puncture wound. The doctor cleaned out the wound and gave the child an injection of tetanus antitoxin. Why was antitoxin given instead of a booster shot of tetanus toxoid? If the child receives no further treatment and steps on a rusty nail again 3 years later, will he be immune to tetanus?

4. What are the advantages of the Sabin polio vaccine compared with the Salk vaccine?

5. In an attempt to prepare a synthetic peptide vaccine you have analyzed a protein antigen for (a) amphipathic peptides and (b) mobile peptides. How might each of these peptides be used as a vaccine to induce different immune responses?

6. You have developed a synthetic peptide vaccine representing an immunodominant T-cell epitope for strain A mice. When the vaccine is tested in strain B mice, no T-cell response occurs. What is the most likely explanation for this finding? How could you test this hypothesis?

7. Explain the relationship between the incubation period of an antigen and the approach needed to achieve effective active immunization.

8. The Salk polio vaccine has been recommended for use by HIV-infected children instead of the Sabin polio vaccine. Why do you think this recommendation was made?

IMMUNE RESPONSE TO INFECTIOUS DISEASES

In order for a pathogen to establish an infection in a susceptible host, a series of coordinated events is required to circumvent the specific and nonspecific host defenses. Generally, pathogens use a variety of strategies to escape immune destruction. Many pathogens reduce their own antigenicity either by growing within host cells, where they are sequestered from immune attack, or by shedding their membrane antigens. Other pathogens mimic host-cell membrane molecules, either by expressing molecules with similar sequences or by acquiring a covering of host membrane molecules. In some cases pathogens are able to selectively suppress the immune response or regulate the response to generate a branch of immune activation that is ineffective. Continual variation in surface antigens is another strategy that enables a pathogen to elude the immune system. This antigenic variation may occur by the gradual accumulation of mutations (antigenic drift), or it may involve an abrupt change in surface antigens (antigenic shift).

Infectious diseases, which have plagued human populations throughout history, still cause the death of millions each year. Although widespread use of vaccines and drug therapy has dramatically reduced mortality due to infectious diseases in developed countries, infectious diseases continue to be the leading cause of death in the Third World. It is estimated that over 600 million people are infected with tropical diseases (Table 21-1), resulting in some 20 million deaths each

TABLE 21-1 INFECTIOUS DISEASES: THE LEADING KILLERS IN 1990

Cause of death	Estimated number
Acute respiratory infections	6,900,000
Diarrheal diseases	4,200,000
Tuberculosis	3,300,000
Malaria	1,000,000–2,000,000
Hepatitis	1,000,000–2,000,000
Measles alone	220,000
Meningitis, bacterial	200,000
Schistosomiasis (parasitic tropical disease)	200,000
Pertussis alone (whooping cough)	100,000
Amoebiasis (parasitic infection)	40,000–60,000
Hookworm (parasitic infection)	50,000–60,000
Rabies	35,000
Yellow fever (epidemic)	30,000
African trypanosomiasis (sleeping sickness)	20,000 or more

SOURCE: World Health Organization, 1992, *Global Health Situation and Projections;* cited in A. Gibbons, 1992, *Science* **256**:1135.

year. Despite these alarming numbers, estimated expenditures for research on infectious diseases prevalent in the Third World are less than 5% of total health-research expenditures worldwide. Not only is this a tragedy for these countries, but some of these diseases are beginning to emerge or re-emerge in developed countries. For example, some U. S. troops returned from the Persian Gulf with schistosomiasis; cholera cases have recently increased worldwide with more than 30 cases reported in the United States in 1992; and a new drug-resistant strain of *Mycobacterium tuberculosis* is spreading at an alarming rate within the United States.

In this chapter the concepts discussed in earlier chapters, such as antigenicity (Chapter 4), immune effector mechanisms (Chapters 6, 14, 15, 17, and 18), immune regulation (Chapter 16), and vaccine development (Chapter 20), are applied to selected infectious diseases caused by viruses, bacteria, protozoa, and helminths—the four major types of pathogens.

VIRAL INFECTIONS

A number of specific immune effector mechanisms, together with nonspecific defense mechanisms, are called into play to eliminate an infecting virus (Table 21-2). At the same time the virus acts to subvert one or more of these mechanisms in order to prolong its own survival. The outcome of the infection will depend on how effectively the host's defensive mechanisms resist the offensive tactics of the virus.

TABLE 21-2 MECHANISMS OF HUMORAL AND CELL-MEDIATED IMMUNE RESPONSES TO VIRUSES

Response type	Effector molecule or cell	Activity
Humoral	Antibody (especially secretory IgA)	Blocks binding of virus to host cells, thus preventing infection or reinfection
	IgG, IgM, and IgA antibody	Blocks fusion of viral envelope with host-cell plasma membrane
	IgG and IgM antibody	Enhances phagocytosis of viral particles (opsonization)
	IgM antibody	Agglutinates viral particles
	Complement activated by IgG or IgM antibody	Mediates opsonization by C3b and lysis of enveloped viral particles by membrane-attack complex
Cell-mediated	IFN-γ secreted by T_H or T_C cells	Has direct antiviral activity
	Cytotoxic T lymphocytes (CTLs)	Kill virus-infected self-cells
	NK cells and macrophages	Kill virus-infected cells by ADCC

Viral Neutralization by Humoral Antibody

Antibodies specific for viral surface antigens are often crucial in containing the spread of a virus during acute infection and in protecting against reinfection. Most viruses express surface receptor molecules that enable them to initiate infection by binding specifically to host-cell membrane molecules. For example, influenza virus binds to sialic acid residues in cell-membrane glycoproteins and glycolipids; rhinovirus binds to intercellular adhesion molecules (ICAMs); and Epstein-Barr virus binds to type 2 complement receptors on B cells. If antibody is produced to the viral receptor, it can block infection altogether by preventing binding of viral particles to host cells. Secretory IgA in mucous secretions plays an important role in host defense against viruses by blocking viral attachment to mucosal epithelial cells. The advantage of the attenuated oral polio vaccine, discussed in Chapter 20, is that it induces production of secretory IgA, which effectively blocks attachment of poliovirus along the gastrointestinal tract.

Viral neutralization by antibody sometimes involves other mechanisms, which operate following viral attachment to host cells. In some cases antibodies may block viral penetration by binding to epitopes that are necessary to mediate fusion of the viral envelope with the plasma membrane. If the induced antibody is of a complement-activating isotype, lysis of enveloped virions can ensue. Antibody or complement can also agglutinate viral particles and function as an opsonizing agent to facilitate Fc or C3b receptor-mediated phagocytosis of the viral particles.

Cell-Mediated Antiviral Mechanisms

Although antibodies have an important role in containing the spread of a virus in the acute phases of infection, they are not usually able to eliminate the virus once infection has occurred—particularly if the virus is capable of entering a latent state in which its DNA is integrated into host chromosomal DNA. Once an infection is established, cell-mediated immune mechanisms are most important in host defense. In general $CD8^+$ cytotoxic T cells and $CD4^+$ T_H1 cells are the main components of cell-mediated antiviral defense, although in some cases $CD4^+$ cytotoxic T cells have also been implicated. Activated T_H1 cells produce a number of cytokines, including IL-2, IFN-γ, and TNF, that serve, either directly or indirectly, to defend against viruses. IFN-γ acts directly by inducing an antiviral state in cells. IL-2 acts indirectly by assisting in the activation of CTL precursors into an effector population. Both IL-2 and IFN-γ activate NK cells, which play an important role in host defense during the first days of many viral infections until a specific CTL response develops.

In most viral infections specific CTL activity arises within 3–4 days after infection, peaks by 7–10 days, and then declines. Within 7–10 days of primary infection most virions are eliminated, paralleling the development of CTLs. CTLs specific for the virus eliminate virus-infected self-cells and thus eliminate potential sources of new viral production. The role of CTLs in defense against viruses is demonstrated by the ability of virus-specific CTLs to confer protection on nonimmune recipients. The viral specificity of the CTL can be demonstrated using adoptive transfer of specific CTL clones. Adoptive transfer of a CTL clone specific for influenza virus X will protect mice against influenza virus X but not against influenza virus Y.

Viral Evasion of Host-Defense Mechanisms

Despite their restricted genome size, a number of viruses have been found to encode proteins that interfere at various levels with specific or nonspecific host defenses. Presumably the advantage of such proteins is that they enable viruses to replicate more effectively amidst antiviral host defenses. A major nonspecific defense against viruses are the interferons α and β, which are produced by various cells in response to a viral infection. These cytokines induce an antiviral protein called DAI in nearby uninfected cells. Recently, a number of viruses, including adenoviruses and Epstein-Barr virus, have been shown to overcome the antiviral effect of the interferons by blocking or inhibiting the action of DAI.

Antibody-mediated destruction of viruses requires complement activation resulting either in direct lysis of the viral particle or opsonization and elimination of the virus via phagocytic cells. A number of viruses have strategies to evade complement-mediated destruction. Vaccinia virus, for example, secretes a protein that binds to the C4b complement component, inhibiting the classical complement pathway; and herpes simplex viruses have a glycoprotein component that binds to the C3b complement component inhibiting both the classical and alternative pathways.

A number of viruses escape immune attack by constantly changing their antigens. In the case of the influenza virus, which is discussed more fully later, continual antigenic variation results in the frequent emergence of new infectious strains of the virus. The absence of protective immunity to these newly emerging strains leads to repeated epidemics of influenza. Antigenic variation among rhinoviruses, the causative agent of the common cold, is responsible for the inability to produce an effective vaccine for colds. Nowhere is antigenic variation greater than in the human immunodeficiency virus (HIV), the causative agent of AIDS. Estimates suggest that HIV accumulates mutations at a rate 65-times faster than influenza virus. Because of the importance of AIDS, Chapter 23 is devoted in its entirety to this disease.

A large number of viruses evade the immune response by causing generalized immunosuppression. Among these are the paramyxoviruses causing mumps, the measles virus, Epstein-Barr virus (EBV), cytomegalovirus, and HIV. In some cases immunosuppression is caused by direct viral infection of lymphocytes or macrophages. The virus can then directly destroy the immune cells by cytolytic mechanisms or alter the function of these cells. In other cases immunosuppression occurs as a result of a cytokine imbalance. A recent study, for example, has shown that EBV produces a protein, called BCRF1, that is homologous to IL-10 and, like IL-10, suppresses cytokine production by the T_H1 subset, resulting in decreased levels of IL-2, TNF, and IFN-γ. Other viruses suppress the immune response by suppressing class I MHC expression: cytomegaloviruses produce a protein that binds to β_2-microglobulin, blocking class I MHC expression on the membrane; and adenoviruses synthesize an integral membrane protein that binds to class I MHC molecules within the endoplasmic reticulum preventing their translocation to the cell membrane. Recent evidence suggests that the immunosuppression that is often observed in retrovirus infections may be due to a retroviral envelope protein, called p15E, that inhibits signal transduction by protein kinase C during T-cell activation (see Figure 12-13).

Influenza

The influenza virus infects the upper respiratory tract and major central airways in humans, horses, birds, pigs, and even seals. It has been responsible for some of the worst pandemics (worldwide epidemics) in human history, one of which killed more than 20 million people in 1918–1919, a toll surpassing the number of casualties in World War I. Some areas, such as Alaska and the Pacific Islands, lost more than half of their population during that pandemic.

Properties of the Influenza Virus

Influenza viral particles, or virions, are roughly spherical or ovoid in shape, with an average diameter of 90–100 nm. The virions are surrounded by an outer envelope—a lipid bilayer acquired from the plasma membrane of the infected host cell during the process of budding. Inserted into the envelope are two glycoproteins, *hemagglutinin* (HA) and *neuraminidase* (NA), which form radiating projections that are visible in electron micrographs (Figure 21-1). The hemagglutinin projections, in the form of trimers, are responsible for the attachment of the virus to host cells. There are approximately 1000 hemagglutinin projections per influenza virion. The hemagglutinin trimer binds to sialic acid groups on host-cell glycoproteins and glycolipids by way of a conserved amino acid sequence that forms a small groove in the hemagglutinin molecule. Neuraminidase, as its name indicates, cleaves *N*-acetylneuramic (sialic) acid from nascent viral glycoproteins and host-cell membrane glycoproteins, an activity that presumably facilitates viral budding from the infected host cell. Within the envelope an inner layer of matrix protein surrounds the nucleocapsid, which consists of eight different strands of ssRNA associated with protein and RNA polymerase (Figure 21-2). Each RNA strand encodes a different influenza protein.

Three basic types of influenza (A, B, and C) can be distinguished by differences in their nucleoprotein and matrix proteins. Type A is the most common and is responsible for the major human pandemics. Antigenic variation in hemagglutinin and neuraminidase has allowed type A influenza virus to be subtyped. According to the nomenclature of the World Health Organization, each virus strain is defined by its animal

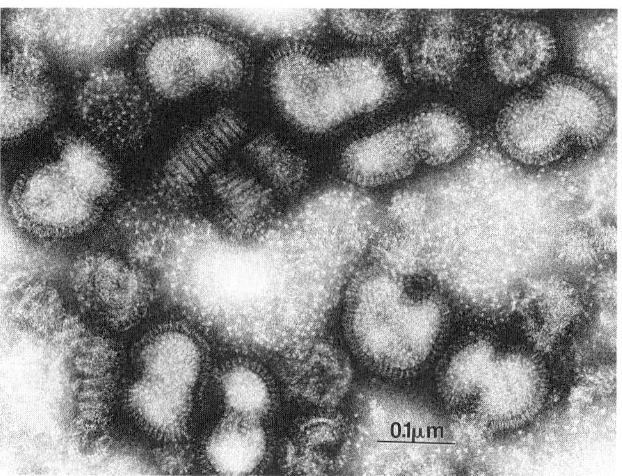

FIGURE 21-1 Electron micrograph of influenza virus reveals roughly spherical viral particles enclosed in a lipid bilayer with protruding hemagglutinin (HA) and neuraminadase (NA) glycoprotein spikes. [Courtesy of G. Murti, Department of Virology, St. Jude Children's Research Hospital, Memphis, TN.]

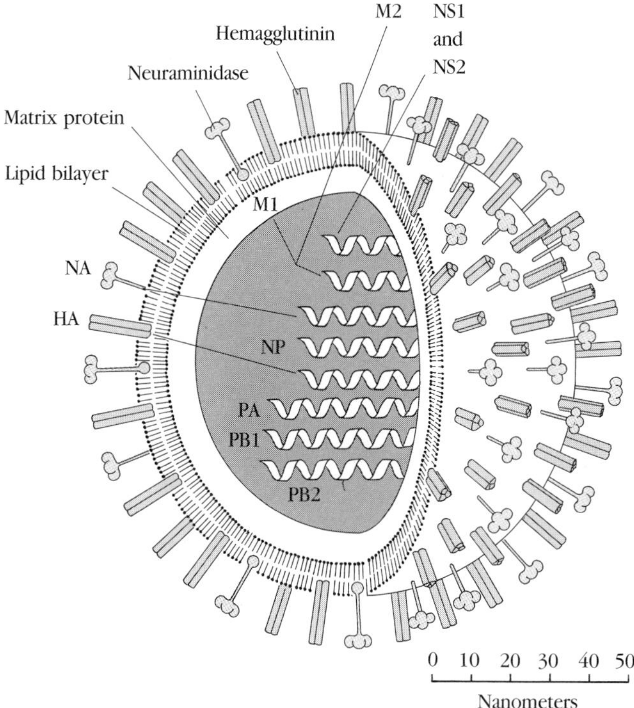

FIGURE 21-2 Representative structure of influenza. The envelope is covered with neuraminadase and hemagglutinin spikes. Inside is an inner layer of matrix protein surrounding the nucleocapsid, which consists of eight ssRNA strands associated with nucleoprotein. The eight RNA strands encode ten proteins: PB1, PB2, PA, HA (hemagglutinin), NP (nucleoprotein), NA (neuraminadase), M1, M2, NS1, and NS2.

host of origin (specified, if other than human), geographical origin, strain number, year of isolation, and antigenic description of HA and NA (Table 21-3). For example, A/SW/Iowa/15/30 (H1N1) designates strain-A isolate 15 that arose in swine in Iowa in 1930, and A/Hong Kong/1/68 (H3N2) denotes strain-A isolate 1 that arose in humans in Hong Kong in 1968; the H and N spikes are antigenically distinct in these two strains.

The distinguishing feature of influenza virus is its variability. The virus can change its surface antigens so completely that the immune response to one viral epidemic gives little or no protection against a subsequent epidemic. The antigenic variation results primarily from changes in the hemagglutinin and neuraminidase spikes protruding from the viral envelope (Figure 21-3). Two different mechanisms generate antigenic variation in HA and NA: *antigenic drift* and *antigenic shift.* Antigenic drift involves a series of spontaneous point mutations that occur gradually, resulting in minor changes in HA and NA. Antigenic shift results in the sudden emergence of a new subtype of influenza bearing an HA and possibly NA dramatically different from that of the preceding virus.

The first human influenza virus was isolated in 1934 and was given the subtype designation H0N1. This subtype persisted until 1947 when a major antigenic shift generated a new subtype, H1N1. This subtype supplanted the previous subtype and became prevalent worldwide until 1957 when H2N2 emerged. The H2N2 subtype prevailed for the next decade and was replaced in 1968 by H3N2. The last antigenic shift in 1977 saw the re-emergence of H1N1. With each antigenic shift, hemagglutinin and neuraminidase undergo major sequence changes, resulting in major antigenic variations for which the immune system displays an absence of memory. Thus each antigenic shift finds the population immunologically unprepared, resulting in a major pandemic of influenza.

Between pandemics the influenza virus undergoes antigenic drift, generating minor antigenic variations, which account for strain differences. The immune response contributes to the emergence of these different influenza strains. As an individual infected with a given influenza strain mounts an effective immune response, the strain is eliminated. However, the accumulation of point mutations alters the antigenicity of some variants sufficiently so that they are able to escape immune elimination. These variants become a new strain of influenza, causing another local epidemic cycle. The role of antibody in such immunologic selection can be

TABLE 21-3 SOME INFLUENZA A STRAINS AND THEIR HEMAGGLUTININ (H) AND NEURAMINIDASE (N) SUBTYPE

Species	Virus strain designation	Antigenic subtype
Human	A/Puerto Rico/8/34	H0N1
	A/Fort Monmouth/1/47	H1N1
	A/Singapore/1/57	H2N2
	A/Hong Kong/1/68	H3N2
	A/USSR/80/77	H1N1
	A/Brazil/11/78	H1N1
	A/Bangkok/1/79	H3N2
	A/Taiwan/1/86	H1N1
Swine	A/Sw/Iowa/15/30	H1N1
	A/Sw/Taiwan/70	H3N2
Horse (Equine)	A/Eq/Prague/1/56	H7N7
	A/Eq/Miami/1/63	H3N8
Birds	A/Fowl/Dutch/27	H7N7
	A/Tern/South America/61	H5N3
	A/Turkey/Ontario/68	H8N4

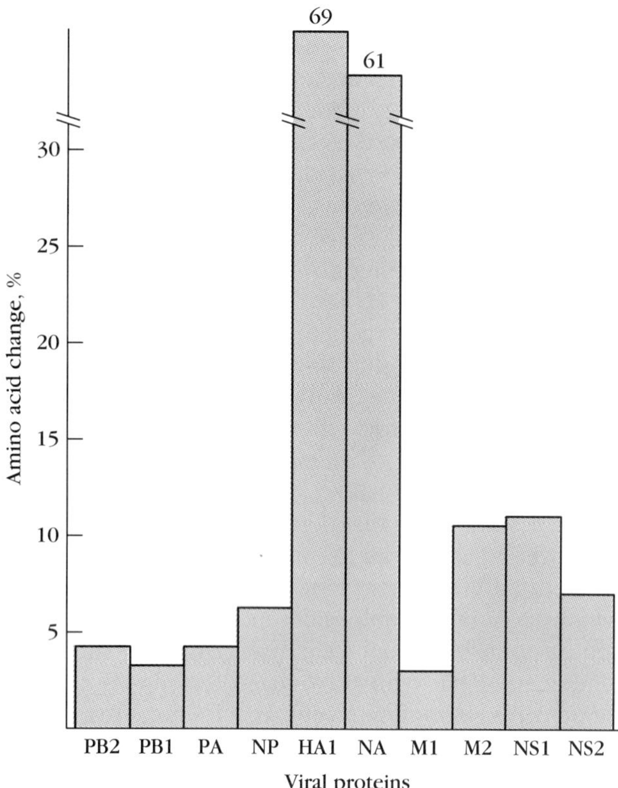

FIGURE 21-3 Amino acid sequence variation in 10 influenza viral proteins from two H3N2 strains and one H1N1 strain. The surface glycoproteins hemagglutinin (HA) and neuraminidase (NA) showed significant sequence variation; in contrast, the sequences of internal viral proteins, such as matrix proteins (M1 and M2) and nucleoprotein (NP), were largely conserved. [From G. G. Brownlee, 1986, in *Options for the Control of Influenza,* Alan R. Liss.]

demonstrated in the laboratory by mixing an influenza strain with monoclonal antibody specific for that strain and then culturing the virus in cells. The antibody will neutralize all unaltered viral particles and only those viral particles with mutations resulting in altered antigenicity will escape. Within a short period in culture, a new influenza strain can be shown to emerge.

Antigenic shift is thought to occur through genetic reassortment between influenza virions from humans and from various animals, including horses, pigs, and ducks. The fact that influenza contains eight separate strands of ssRNA makes possible the reassortment of the RNA strands of human and animal virions within a single cell coinfected with both viruses. Evidence for in vivo genetic reassortment between influenza A viruses from human and domestic pigs was obtained by R. G. Webster and C. H. Campbell in 1971. After infecting a pig simultaneously with human Hong Kong influenza (H3N2) and with swine influenza (H1N1), they were able to recover virions expressing H3N1. In some cases, an apparent antigenic shift may represent the re-emergence of a previous strain that has remained hidden for several decades. For example, in May of 1977 a strain of influenza, A/USSR/77 (H1N1), appeared that proved to be identical to a strain that had caused an epidemic 27 years earlier. The virus could have been preserved over the years in a frozen state or in an animal reservoir. When such a re-emergence occurs, the HA and NA antigens expressed are not really new; however, they will be seen by the immune system as if they were new because no memory cells specific for these antigenic subtypes will exist in the

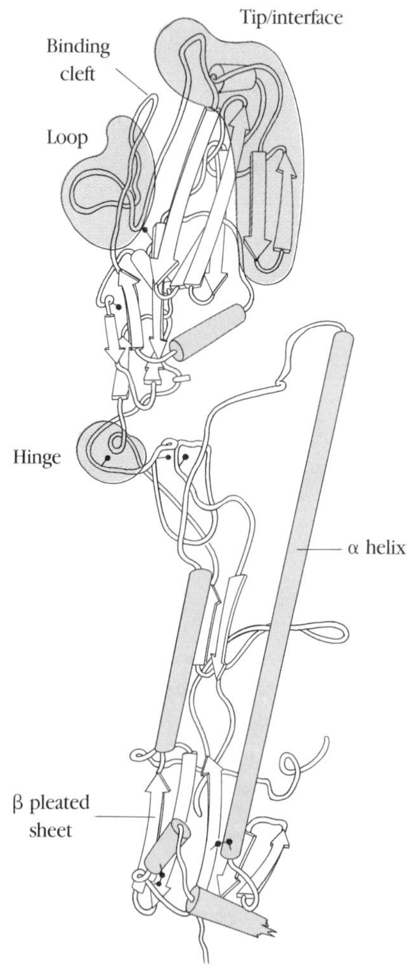

FIGURE 21-4 Structure of hemagglutinin molecule showing cleft that binds to sialic acid on host cells and regions where antigenic drift is prevalent (purple areas). Antibodies to two of these regions—designated the loop and tip/interface—are important in blocking viral infections. Continual changes in amino acid residues in these regions allow the influenza virus to evade the antibody response. Small black dots represent residues that exhibit a high degree of variation among virus strains. [From D. C. Wiley et al., 1981, *Nature* **289**:373.]

population. Thus from an immunologic point of view, the re-emergence of a previous influenza A strain can have the same effect as an antigenic shift that generates a new subtype.

Host Response to Influenza Infection

Humoral antibody specific for the HA molecule is produced during an influenza infection. This antibody protects against influenza infection, but its specificity is strain-specific and is readily bypassed by antigenic drift in the HA and NA glycoproteins. Antigenic drift in the HA molecule results in amino acid substitutions in several antigenic domains at the molecule's distal end (Figure 21-4). Two of these domains are on either side of the conserved sialic acid-binding cleft, which is necessary for binding of virions to target cells. Serum antibodies to these regions, which are important in blocking initial viral infectivity, peak within a few days of infection and then decrease over the next 6 months; the titers then plateau and remain relatively stable for the next several years. This antibody does not appear to be required for recovery from influenza, as patients with agammaglobulinemia recover from the disease. Instead the serum antibody appears to play a significant role in resistance to reinfection by the same strain. When serum antibody levels are high for a particular HA molecule, both mice and humans are resistant to infection by virions expressing that particular HA molecule. If mice are infected with influenza virus and antibody production is experimentally suppressed, the mice recover from the infection only to become reinfected with the same viral strain.

Cell-mediated immunity involving CTLs specific for influenza-infected host cells develops 3–4 days after infection, reaches a peak by day 8 and then disappears by about day 20. In mice, transfer of influenza-specific T_C clones has been shown to confer immunity to a lethal dose of influenza virus on syngeneic adoptive-transfer recipients. Unlike the humoral response, which is specific for each influenza subtype, CTL activity can be cross-reactive; that is, CTLs sometimes recognize and kill syngeneic cells infected with any type A influenza subtype (Table 21-4). This cross-reactivity is important for the development of a better vaccine for influenza, since current vaccines—which are designed to induce antibodies to HA and NA—yield poor protection owing to the continual changes in these glycoproteins. If a vaccine could induce CTL memory that is cross-reactive for all three human pandemic viral subtypes (H1N1, H2N2, and H3N2), then the vaccine might be more protective. It is therefore important to determine which influenza antigens induce cross-reactive CTLs and to characterize the cross-reactive epitopes on these antigens. As discussed in Chapter 20, a vaccine intended to maximize CTL activity must be infectious and capable of replicating within host cells to some extent. Thus, inactivated influenza preparations, which cannot replicate in host cells, are relatively ineffective at inducing CTL activity.

One of the cross-reactive influenza antigens, an internal viral protein called *nucleoprotein,* is recognized by a subset of CTLs that are indeed cross-reactive for all three human pandemic influenza A subtypes. Different inbred strains of mice show individual variation in their ability to respond to influenza nucleoprotein. In some strains 40% of the cross-reactive CTL clones respond to influenza nucleoprotein, but in other strains none of the cross-reactive CTL clones respond to the nucleoprotein. Among strains that respond to nucleoprotein, however, there are differences in the ability to recognize various peptides

TABLE 21-4 CROSS-REACTIVITY OF CTL RESPONSE TO INFLUENZA TYPE A VIRUS*

	^{51}Cr release from infected target cells (%)				
Subtype used to challenge primed lymphocytes in vitro	H2N1	H2N2	H3N2	H0N1	Control (uninfected)
H2N1	48	50	52	35	1
H2N2	45	53	53	40	2
H3N2	46	52	52	37	3
H0N1	34	52	45	42	1

* Mice were primed with an H2N1 subtype of influenza. The mouse splenic lymphocytes were isolated and challenged in vitro with macrophages infected with the influenza subtypes indicated. The CTL activity generated was then measured by monitoring ^{51}Cr release from syngeneic ^{51}Cr-labeled target cells infected with the indicated influenza subtypes.

SOURCE: Adapted from H. J. Zweerink et al., 1977, *Eur. J. Immunol.* **7**:630.

derived from nucleoprotein. Experiments described in Chapter 20 indicate that these differences are related to the MHC haplotype of the mouse strains. Furthermore, generation of CTL activity in response to a particular nucleoprotein peptide depends on expression of a particular class I MHC molecule on the target cells (see Table 20-7).

These results with influenza nucleoprotein peptides highlight the important role of the MHC in determining the immunodominant T-cell epitopes. In the design of a vaccine for influenza, the results from these mouse studies must be considered. A vaccine consisting only of nucleoprotein might not be immunogenic in all individuals, because (as suggested by the mouse data) some MHC haplotypes appear unable to respond to nucleoprotein. And if a synthetic peptide vaccine is chosen, it should consist of a "cocktail" of several peptides, because the mouse data reveal differences among class I MHC molecules in their ability to present different influenza nucleoprotein peptides.

Bacterial Infections

Immunity to bacterial infections is achieved by means of antibody unless the bacterium is capable of intracellular growth, in which case delayed-type hypersensitivity has an important role. Bacteria enter the body either through a number of natural entry routes (e.g., the respiratory tract, the gastrointestinal tract, and the genitourinary tract) or through unnatural routes opened up by breaks in mucous membranes or skin. Depending on the number of organisms entering and the virulence of the organism, different levels of host defense are enlisted. If the inoculum size and the virulence are both low, then localized tissue phagocytes may be able to mount a nonspecific defense and eliminate the bacteria. Larger inoculums or organisms with increased virulence tend to induce an immune response.

Immune Response to Extracellular and Intracellular Bacteria

Infection by extracellular bacteria induces production of humoral antibodies, which are ordinarily secreted by plasma cells in regional lymph nodes and the submucosa of the respiratory and gastrointestinal tracts. The antibodies act at several levels to bring about destruction of the invading organisms (Figure 21-5). Antibody that binds to accessible antigens on the surface of a bacterium can, together with the C3b component of complement, act as an opsonin that increases phagocytosis and thus clearance of the bacterium (see Figure 17-11). Antibody-mediated activation of the complement system can also induce localized production of immune effector molecules that help to develop an amplified and more effective inflammatory response. For example, the complement split products C3a, C4a, and C5a act as anaphylatoxins, inducing local mast-cell degranulation and thus vasodilation and the extravasation of lymphocytes and neutrophils from the blood into tissue space. Other complement split products serve as chemotactic factors for neutrophils, thereby contributing to the buildup of phagocytic cells at the site of infection. In the case of some bacteria—notably the gram-negative organisms—complement activation can lead to lysis of the organism. If the bacterium secretes an exotoxin or endotoxin, antibody may bind to the toxin and neutralize it. The antibody-toxin complexes are then cleared by phagocytic cells in the same manner as any antigen-antibody complex.

Infections caused by bacteria that are capable of intracellular growth within phagocytic cells tend to induce a cell-mediated immune response, specifically, delayed-type hypersensitivity. In this response cytokines secreted by T_{DTH} cells are important—notably IFN-γ, which activates macrophages to achieve more effective killing of intracellular pathogens (see Figure 15-15).

Bacterial Evasion of Host-Defense Mechanisms

Bacteria have evolved various mechanisms for enhancing their ability to colonize host mucous membranes and for circumventing host immune responses (Table 21-5). A number of gram-negative bacteria have pili (long hair-like projections), which enable them to attach to the membrane of the intestinal or genitourinary tracts, the first step in infection (Figure 21-6). Other bacteria, such as *Bordetella pertussis,* secrete adhesion molecules that attach to both the bacterium and the ciliated epithelial cells of the upper respiratory tract. Secretory IgA antibodies can block bacterial attachment to mucosal epithelial cells. However, some bacteria (e.g., *Neisseria gonorrhoeae, Hemophilus influenzae,* and *Neisseria meningitidis*) secrete proteases that cleave secretory IgA at the hinge region; the resulting Fab and Fc fragments have a shortened half-life in mucous secretions and are not able to agglutinate microorganisms.

Another way that bacteria evade the IgA response of the host and increase their ability to attach to epithelial cells is by changing their surface antigens. An example of this is provided by *N. gonorrhoeae,* which attaches to epithelial cells of the urethra or cervix by means of

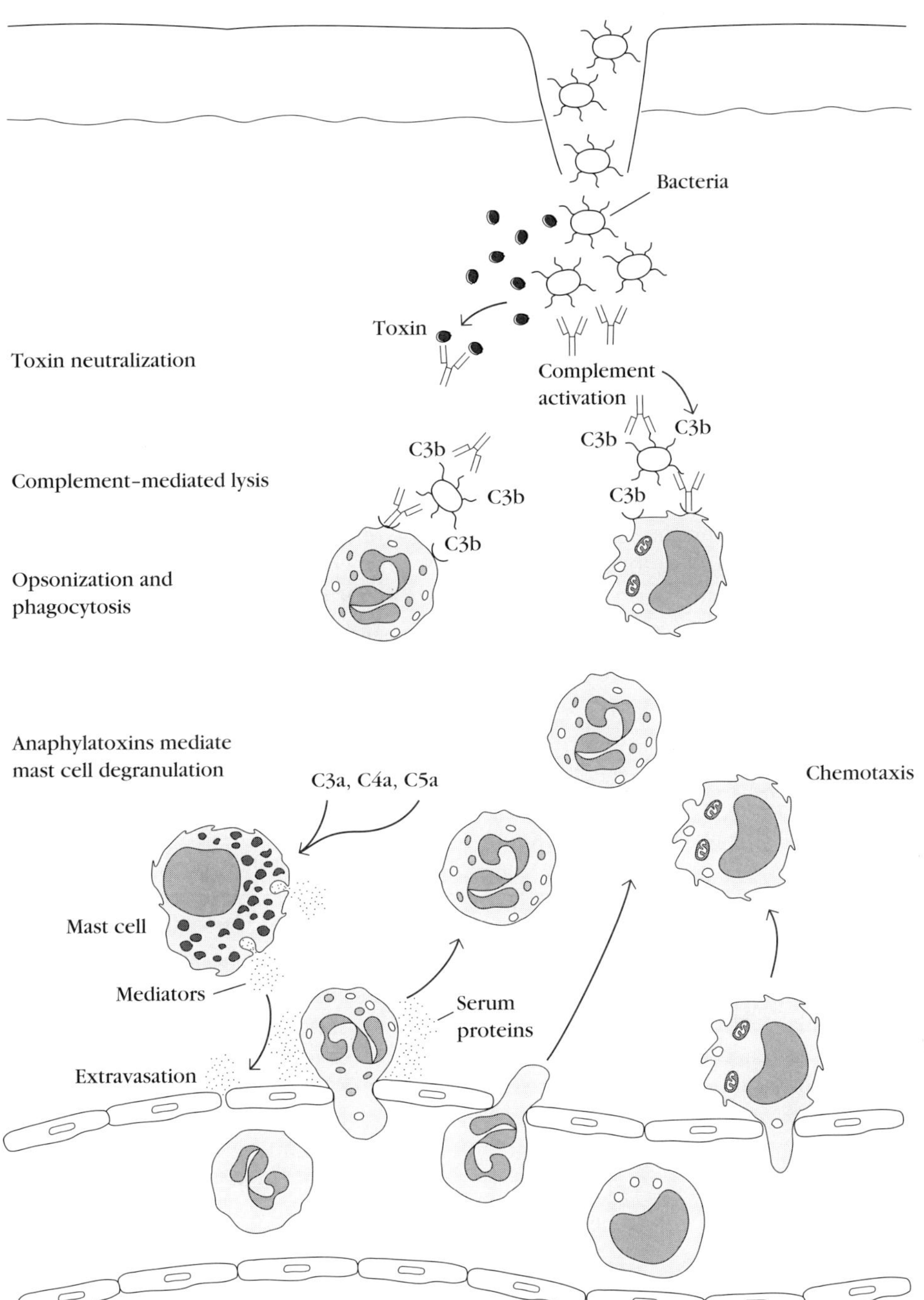

FIGURE 21-5 Antibody-mediated mechanisms for combating infection by extracellular bacteria. (1) Antibody neutralizes bacterial toxins (purple circles). (2) Complement activation on bacterial surfaces leads to complement-mediated lysis of bacteria. (3) Antibody and the complement split product C3b bind to bacteria, serving as opsonins to increase phagocytosis. (4) C3a and C5a, generated by antibody-initiated complement activation, induce local mast-cell degranulation, releasing substances that mediate vasodilation and extravasation of lymphocytes and neutrophils. (5) Other complement split products are chemotactic for neutrophils.

pili. In this organism, pilin, the protein component of the pili, has been shown to consist of constant, variable, and hypervariable amino acids. Variation in the pilin amino acid sequence is generated by gene rearrangements of the coding sequences. The pilin locus consists of one or two expression genes and 10–20 silent genes. Each gene is arranged into six regions called "minicassettes." Pilin variation is generated by a process of gene conversion in which one or more minicassettes from the silent genes replace a

TABLE 21-5 HOST IMMUNE RESPONSES TO BACTERIAL INFECTION AND BACTERIAL EVASION MECHANISMS

Infection process	Host defense	Bacterial evasion mechanisms
Attachment to host cells	Blockage of attachment by secretory IgA antibodies	Secretion of proteases that cleave secretory IgA dimers *(Neisseria meningitidis, N. gonorrhoeae, Hemophilus influenzae)* Antigenic variation in attachment structures (pili of *N. gonorrhoeae*)
Proliferation	Phagocytosis (Ab- and C3b-mediated opsonization)	Production of surface structures (polysaccharide capsule, M protein, fibrin coat) that inhibit phagocytic cells Intracellular mechanisms for surviving within phagocytic cells Induction of apoptosis in macrophages *(Shigella flexneri)*
	Complement-mediated lysis and localized inflammatory response	Generalized resistance to complement-mediated lysis by gram-positive bacteria Insertion of membrane-attack complex prevented by long side chain in cell-wall LPS (some gram-negative bacteria) Secretion of elastase that inactivates C3a and C5a *(Pseudomonas)*
Invasion of host tissues	Ab-mediated agglutination	Secretion of hyaluronidase, which enhances bacterial invasiveness
Toxin-induced damage to host cells	Neutralization of toxin by antibody	

minicassette of the expression gene (Figure 21-7). This process generates enormous antigenic diversity of the pilin proteins, similar to that achieved by immunoglobulin-gene rearrangements. The continual changes in the structure of pilin may contribute to the pathogenicity of *N. gonorrhoeae,* by increasing the likelihood of expression of pili that bind more firmly to epithelial cells. In addition, the continual changes in the pilin sequence allows the organism to evade neutralization by humoral antibody.

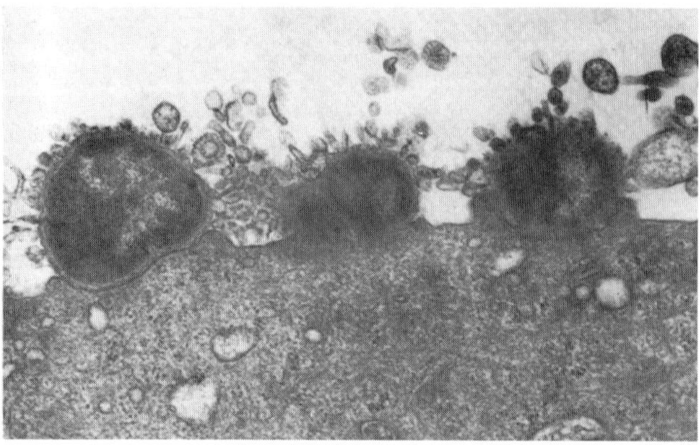

FIGURE 21-6 Electron micrograph of *Neisseria gonorrhoeae* attaching to urethral epithelial cells. Pili (P) extend from the gonococcal surface and mediate the attachment. [From M. E. Ward and P. J. Watt, 1972, *J. Inf. Dis.* **126**:601.]

Numerous bacteria have developed ways to resist phagocytosis or to counteract various complement-mediated immune responses. A number of bacteria, for example, possess surface structures that serve to inhibit phagocytosis. A classic example is *Streptococcus pneumoniae,* whose polysaccharide capsule is very effective in preventing phagocytosis. On other bacteria, such as *Streptococcus pyogenes,* a surface protein projection, called the M protein, inhibits phagocytosis. And some pathogenic staphylococci secrete a coagulase enzyme that produces a fibrin coat around the organism, shielding it from phagocytic cells. Some bacteria are able to interfere with the complement system. In some gram-negative bacteria, for example, long side chains on the lipid A moiety of the cell-wall core polysaccharide help to resist complement-mediated lysis. *Pseudomonas* secretes an enzyme, elastase, that inactivates both the C3a and C5a anaphylatoxins, thereby diminishing the localized inflammatory reaction.

A number of bacteria escape host-defense mechanisms by their ability to survive intracellularly within

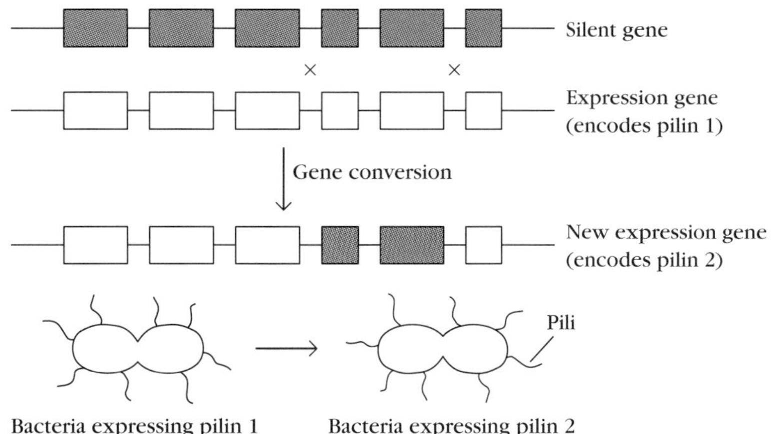

FIGURE 21-7 Variation of pilin sequences is generated by DNA rearrangements. The pilin locus consists of one or two expression genes and a series of 10–20 silent genes. Each gene contains a series of "minicassettes." One or more minicassettes of the expression gene can be replaced by a minicassette of one of the silent genes. [Modified from T. F. Meyer, 1990, *Annu. Rev. Microbiol.* **44**:460.]

phagocytic cells. Some, such as *Mycobacterium tuberculosis* and *Mycobacterium leprae,* do this by escaping the phagolysosome and growing within the more favorable environment of the cytoplasm. Other bacteria, such as *Mycobacterium avium* and *Chlamydia,* block lysosomal fusion with the phagolysosome; and some Mycobacteria are resistant to the oxidative attack that takes place within the phagolysosome.

Contribution of the Immune Response to Bacterial Pathogenesis

In some cases disease is caused not by the bacterial pathogen but by the immune response to the pathogen. As discussed in Chapter 13, pathogen-stimulated overproduction of cytokines leads to the symptoms of bacterial septic shock, food poisoning, and toxic-shock syndrome. In the case of bacterial septic shock, cell-wall endotoxins of some gram-negative bacteria activate macrophages, resulting in release of high levels of IL-1 and TNF-α, which can cause septic shock. In the case of staphylococcal food poisoning and toxic-shock syndrome, exotoxins produced by the pathogens function as superantigens, which can activate all T cells expressing T-cell receptors with a particular V_β domain (see Table 12-2). The resulting overproduction of cytokines by activated T_H cells causes many of the symptoms associated with these diseases.

The ability of some bacteria to survive intracellularly within pathogenic cells can result in chronic antigenic activation of T_{DTH} cells, leading to tissue destruction by a delayed-type hypersensitivity reaction (see Chapter 15). Cytokines secreted by these activated T cells can lead to extensive macrophage accumulation and activation (called a granuloma). The localized concentrations of lysosomal enzymes in these granulomas can cause extensive tissue necrosis. Much of the tissue damage seen with *Mycobacterium tuberculosis* is due to a delayed-type hypersensitivity response.

Diphtheria *(Corynebacterium diphtheriae)*

Diphtheria is the prototype of a bacterial disease caused by a secreted exotoxin for which immunity can be induced by immunization with a toxoid. The causative agent, a gram-positive, rodlike organism called *Corynebacterium diphtheriae,* was first described by Klebs in 1883 and was shown a year later by Loeffler to cause diphtheria in guinea pigs and rabbits. Autopsies on the infected animals revealed that while bacterial growth was limited to the site of inoculation, there was widespread damage to a variety of organs including the heart, liver, and kidneys. This led Loeffler to speculate that the neurologic and cardiologic manifestations of the disease were caused by a toxic substance elaborated by the organism. Loeffler's hypothesis was validated in 1888 when Roux and Yersin produced the disease in animals by injection of a sterile filtrate from a culture of *C. diphtheriae.* Two years later, von Behring showed that an antiserum to the toxin was able to prevent death in infected animals. He prepared a toxoid by treating the toxin with iodine trichloride and demonstrated that the toxoid could induce protective antibodies in animals. However the toxoid was still quite toxic and therefore unsuitable for use in humans. In 1923 Ramon found that exposure of the toxin to heat and formalin rendered it nontoxic but did not destroy its antigenicity. Clinical trials with the formalin-treated toxoid revealed that it was able to confer a high level of protection to diphtheria upon recipients. As widespread use of the toxoid increased, the number of cases of diphtheria decreased dramatically. In the 1920s there were approximately 200 cases of diphtheria per 100,000 population in the United States. In 1989 the Centers for Disease Control reported only three cases of diphtheria in the United States.

Natural infection with *C. diphtheriae* occurs only in humans. The disease is spread from one individual to another by airborne respiratory droplets. The organism colonizes the nasopharyngeal tract, remaining in the superficial layers of the respiratory mucosa. Growth of the organism itself causes little tissue damage, and only a mild inflammatory reaction develops. The virulence of the organism is completely dependent on its potent exotoxin. The toxin causes destruction of the underlying tissue resulting in the formation of a tough fibrinous membrane ("pseudomembrane") composed of fibrin, white blood cells, and dead respiratory epithelial cells. The membrane itself can lead to suffocation. The exotoxin also is responsible for widespread systemic manifestations. Often there is pronounced myocardial damage (often leading to congestive heart failure) and neurologic damage (ranging from mild weakness to complete paralysis).

The toxin that causes diphtheria symptoms is encoded by the *tox* gene carried by phage β. Only strains of *C. diphtheriae* that carry phage β in a state of lysogeny (in which the β-prophage DNA persists within the bacterial cell) are able to produce the exotoxin. The exotoxin, which is synthesized as a single polypeptide precursor, can be dissociated into two fragments (A and B) by mild trypsin digestion. Fragment B binds to ganglioside receptors on susceptible cells, facilitating the transport of fragment A across the plasma membrane. Toxicity results from the inhibitory effect of fragment A on protein synthesis. This fragment catalyzes the covalent modification of elongation factor 2 (EF-2), which is present in mammalian cells but not in bacteria. Loss of EF-2 inhibits interaction of mRNA and tRNA on ribosomes, thus preventing further addition of amino acids to a growing polypeptide chain. Fragment A is extremely potent; a single molecule has been shown to kill a cell. Removal of fragment B from the exotoxin prevents fragment A from entering the cell, thus rendering the exotoxin nontoxic. As discussed in Chapter 7, an immunotoxin can be prepared by replacing fragment B with a monoclonal antibody specific for a tumor-cell surface antigen; in this way the toxin A fragment can be targeted to tumor cells (see Figure 7-10).

Today, diphtheria toxoid is prepared by treating diphtheria toxin with formaldehyde. The reaction with formaldehyde cross-links the toxin, resulting in an irreversible loss in its toxicity while enhancing its antigenicity. The toxoid is administered together with tetanus toxoid and inactivated *Bordetella pertussis* in a combined vaccine that is given to children beginning at 6–8 weeks of age. Immunization with the toxoid induces the production of antibodies (antitoxin), which can bind to the toxin and neutralize its activity. Because antitoxin levels decline slowly over time, booster doses are recommended at 10-year intervals to maintain antitoxin levels within the protective range. Interestingly, antibodies specific for epitopes on fragment B of the diphtheria toxin are critical for toxin neutralization because these antibodies block binding of the toxin to cellular receptors and the subsequent translocation of fragment A into cells.

Tuberculosis *(Mycobacterium tuberculosis)*

Tuberculosis is the leading cause of death in the world from a single infectious agent, killing about 3 million individuals every year and accounting for 18.5% of all deaths in adults between the ages of 15 and 59. About 2 billion people, roughly one-third to one-half of the world's population, are infected with the causative agent *Mycobacterium tuberculosis* and are at risk of developing the disease. Long thought to have been eliminated as a public health problem in the United States, tuberculosis reemerged in the early 1990s, particularly in the inner cities and in areas where HIV-infection levels are high. In 1991, 26,000 Americans were diagnosed with tuberculosis; this figure is the proverbial tip of the iceberg, because for every diagnosed case of tuberculosis, experts estimate that there are more than 600 infected individuals who have not yet developed symptoms. The situation is especially frightening because of the rapid emergence of *M. tuberculosis* strains that are resistant to antibiotics; some strains exhibit resistance to nine of the 11 antibiotics presently used in treating tuberculosis.

Although several *Mycobacterium* species can cause tuberculosis, *M. tuberculosis* is the principal causative agent. This organism is spread easily, and pulmonary infection usually results from inhalation of small droplets of respiratory secretions containing a few bacilli. The inhaled bacilli are ingested by alveolar macrophages and are able to survive and multiply intracellularly by inhibiting formation of phagolysosomes. When the infected macrophages lyse, as they eventually do, large numbers of bacilli are released. A cell-mediated response involving T_{DTH} cells, which is required for immunity to tuberculosis, may be responsible for much of the tissue damage in the disease. T_{DTH} activity is the basis for the tuberculin skin test to the purified protein derivative (PPD) from *M. tuberculosis* (see Chapter 15).

One of two basic clinical patterns follows infection with *M. tuberculosis.* In the most common clinical pattern, which occurs in about 90% of those infected, T_{DTH} cells are activated within 2–6 weeks after infection, inducing the infiltration of large numbers of activated macrophages. These cells wall-off the organism inside a granulomatous lesion called a *tubercle.* A tubercle consists of a few small lymphocytes and a compact collection of activated macrophages, which sometimes differentiate into epitheloid cells or multinucleated giant cells. Because the activated macrophages suppress proliferation of the phagocytosed bacilli, infection is contained. Cytokines produced by T_{DTH} cells play an important role in the response by activating macrophages, so that they are able to kill or inhibit growth of the organism. The role of IFN-γ in the immune response to mycobacteria has been demonstrated with knock-out mice lacking IFN-γ. These mice died when they were infected with an attenuated strain of mycobacteria (BCG), whereas IFN-γ^{+} normal mice survived (see Figure 15-16).

Although the intracellular bacilli are contained within tubercles, not all of them are killed. Moreover, massive activation of macrophages within tubercles by T_{DTH}-cell cytokines often results in the concentrated release of lytic enzymes. These enzymes destroy nearby healthy cells, resulting in circular regions of necrotic tissue, which eventually form a lesion with a cheeselike consistency Figure 21-8. As these caseous lesions heal, they become calcified and are readily visible on x-rays, where they are called *Ghon complexes.*

In about 10% of individuals infected with *M. tuberculosis,* the disease progresses to chronic pulmonary tuberculosis or extrapulmonary tuberculosis. This progression may occur years after the primary infection. In this clinical pattern accumulation of large concentrations of mycobacterial antigens within tubercles leads to extensive T_{DTH}-cell activation and ensuing macrophage activation. The resulting high concentrations of lytic enzymes cause the necrotic caseous lesions to liquify, creating a rich medium that allows the tubercle bacilli to proliferate extracellularly. Eventually the lesions rupture, and the bacilli disseminate in the lung and/or are spread through the blood and lymphatic vessels to the pleural cavity, bone, urogenital system, meninges, peritoneum, or skin.

Tuberculosis is treated with several drugs, used in combination, including isoniazid, rifampin, streptomycin, pyrazinamide, and ethambutol. Of these, a combination therapy of isoniazid and rifampin has

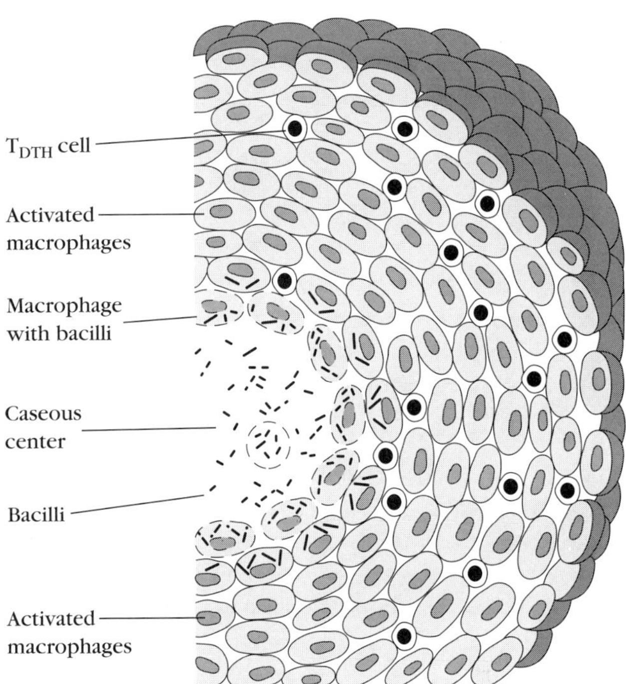

FIGURE 21-8 A tubercle formed in pulmonary tuberculosis. [From: A. M. Dannenberg, 1993, *Hospital Practice* Jan. **15**:51.]

been particularly effective. The intracellular growth of *M. tuberculosis* makes it difficult for drugs to reach the bacilli. For this reason drug therapy must be continued for at least 9 months. Some patients with tuberculosis do not exhibit any clinical symptoms at all, and other patients with symptoms often begin to feel better within 2–4 weeks after treatment begins. Because the combined antibiotics have undesirable side effects, patients often stop taking the medications, and it is difficult to get patients to comply with medication regimes. Because such brief treatment does not eradicate the organism, a multidrug-resistant strain can emerge. Noncompliance with required treatment regimes, one of the most troubling aspects of the recent surge in tuberculosis cases, clearly compromises efforts to contain spread of the disease.

Presently, the only vaccine for *M. tuberculosis* is an attenuated strain of *M. bovis* called BCG. The vaccine appears to provide fairly effective protection against extrapulmonary tuberculosis but has been inconsistent against pulmonary tuberculosis. In different studies, BCG has provided protection in anywhere from 0 to 80% of vaccinated individuals; in some cases, BCG vaccination has even increased the risk of infection. Moreover, following BCG vaccination, the skin test cannot be used as an effective monitor of exposure to *M. tuberculosis.* Because of the variable effectiveness of the BCG vaccine and the inability to monitor for exposure with the skin test following BCG vaccination, this vaccine is not used in the United States. However, the alarming increase in multidrug-resistant strains has stimulated renewed efforts to develop a more effective tuberculosis vaccine.

Lyme Disease *(Borrelia burgdorferi)*

In 1975 about 60 cases of a new and mysterious disease were reported in Lyme, Connecticut. The disease symptoms included unexplained "bull's-eye" rashes, headaches, and arthritis; in some cases severe neurologic complications developed, including excruciating headaches, meningitis, loss of memory, and mood swings. An epidemiologic study was initiated in hope of identifying the causative agent. The disease was shown to have a higher incidence in individuals living in heavily wooded areas, and a close geographic clustering of infected individuals was found. In addition, the disease was shown to be contracted during the summer months between June and September. Finally in 1977, nine patients with the disease remembered having been bitten by a tick at the site of the characteristic rash. Fortuitously, the tick had been saved by one patient and was examined by Willy Burgdorfer, a noted authority on tickborne diseases. He found the tick (an *Ixodes* species) to be teaming with a new species of gram-negative spirochete, which was subsequently named *Borrelia burgdorferi* after its discoverer.

As an infected tick takes a blood meal, *B. burgdorferi* enters the bloodstream. Experiments with fluorescent antibodies to *B. burgdorferi* have revealed the presence of low numbers of the spirochete at the site of the bite and in various organs including kidney, spleen, liver, cerebrospinal fluid, and brain tissue. The clinical symptoms of Lyme disease generally begin with a characteristic rash, beginning as a red papule and spreading to form what appears as a bull's eye 10–50 cm in diameter. Following the rash, arthritic symptoms and neurologic symptoms often develop. Roughly 80% of individuals with Lyme disease develop some arthritic symptoms ranging from joint pain to chronic joint destruction. Neurologic symptoms develop in about 60% of Lyme patients. Most report headaches, but about 15% develop meningitis and encephalitis. The disease can be successfully treated with broad-spectrum antibiotics such as penicillin and tetracycline. Interestingly, though, soon after the antibiotic is administered, there is a temporary exacerbation of symptoms (called the Jarish-Herxheimer reaction).

Antibodies to a protein associated with the flagella of *B. burgdorferi* can often be detected after infection. However, these antibodies do not appear to confer protection against the spirochete and may even contribute to the pathogenesis of Lyme disease. Immune complexes, consisting of spirochete antigens and antibody, are thought to result in a type III hypersensitive reaction. Deposition of complexes near the original bite results in the characteristic rash; deposition of complexes in the joints is thought to induce an inflammatory response resulting in arthritic symptoms; deposition of the complexes in the vasculature and along the meninges leads to neurologic symptoms. As was discussed in Chapter 17, antigen-antibody complexes activate the complement system. Complement activation can result in direct lytic damage to the joints or vasculature. Alternatively, complement split products, such as C3a and C5a, will induce neutrophil chemotaxis and activation. Some of the tissue damage may then result from lytic enzymes released by the activated neutrophils.

G. Habicht, G. Beck, and J. Benach have suggested that interleukin 1 (IL-1) is involved in the pathogenesis of Lyme disease. Like other gram-negative bacteria, *Borrelia* has a cell wall containing lipopolysaccharide (LPS). These researchers observed that when macrophages are cultured together with *B. burgdorferi,* the macrophages secrete high levels of IL-1. They suggested that high levels of IL-1 released by macrophages in Lyme disease may be responsible for many of the symptoms of the disease. For example, when IL-1 is injected into rabbit skin, a characteristic rash appears. Furthermore, when IL-1 is added to cultured synovial cells, the cells begin to secrete collagenase and prostaglandins. The release of collagenase in a joint could lead to the degradation of collagen and destruction of the joint. They have suggested that the exacerbation of symptoms seen with antibiotic treatment may result from massive killing of *B. burgdorferi,* releasing large quantities of LPS from the gram-negative cell wall. The LPS in turn is hypothesized to induce excessive release of IL-1, resulting in increased severity of symptoms, until the LPS levels subside.

In order to understand the role of the immune response in Lyme disease, some researchers have studied the infection in mice, which are a major reservoir of *B. burgdorferi.* Ticks acquire the spirochetes from infected mice and transmit them to humans. Unlike humans, however, normal mice infected with *B. burgdorferi* do not develop Lyme disease, although mutant *scid* mice, which lack functional T and B cells, are susceptible to the disease. This finding has led to the speculation that the immune response in normal mice protects the animals from the disease. Comparison of the immune response to *B. burgdorferi* in normal mice and humans has shown that mice produce high levels of antibodies to two envelope outer-surface proteins, whereas humans fail to do so; instead, most infected humans produce antibodies to a flagellar antigen. The ability of these antibodies to protect against Lyme disease was studied using *scid* mice. Monoclonal antibodies to the outer-surface proteins protected *scid* mice from disease, whereas monoclonal antibodies to the flagellar antigen did not. These results offer the possibility that a vaccine for Lyme disease consisting of the outer-surface proteins might induce protective antibodies in humans.

Protozoan Diseases

Protozoans are unicellular eukaryotic organisms. They are responsible for several serious diseases in humans, including amebiasis, Chagas' disease, African sleeping sickness, malaria, leishmaniasis, and toxoplasmosis. The type of immune response that develops and the effectiveness of the response depends in part on the location of the parasite within the host. Many protozoans have stages in which they are free within the bloodstream, and it is during these stages that humoral antibody is most effective. Many of these same pathogens are also capable of intracellular growth, and during these stages cell-mediated immune reactions are effective in host defense. In the development of vaccines for protozoan diseases, the branch of the immune system that is most likely to confer protection must be carefully considered.

Malaria (*Plasmodium* Species)

Malaria, one of the most important diseases in the world today, is estimated to infect 600 million people worldwide and to cause 1–2 million deaths every year. Malaria is caused by various species of the genus *Plasmodium,* of which *P. falciparum* is the most virulent and prevalent. The alarming development of multiple drug resistance in *Plasmodium* and the increased resistance of its vector, the *Anopheles* mosquito, to DDT underscore the importance of developing new strategies to hinder the spread of malaria.

Plasmodium *Life Cycle and Pathogenesis of Malaria*

Plasmodium progresses through a remarkable series of developmental and maturational stages in its extremely complex life cycle. Female *Anopheles* mosquitos, which feed on blood meals, serve as the vector for *Plasmodium,* and part of the parasite's life cycle takes place within the mosquito. (Because male *Anopheles* mosquitos feed on plant juices, they do not transmit *Plasmodium.*)

Human infection begins when *sporozoites,* one of the *Plasmodium* stages, are introduced into an individual's bloodstream as an infected mosquito takes a blood meal (Figure 21-9). Within 30 min the sporozoites disappear from the blood as they migrate to the liver, where they infect hepatocytes. Sporozoites are long, slender cells that are covered by a 45-kDa protein

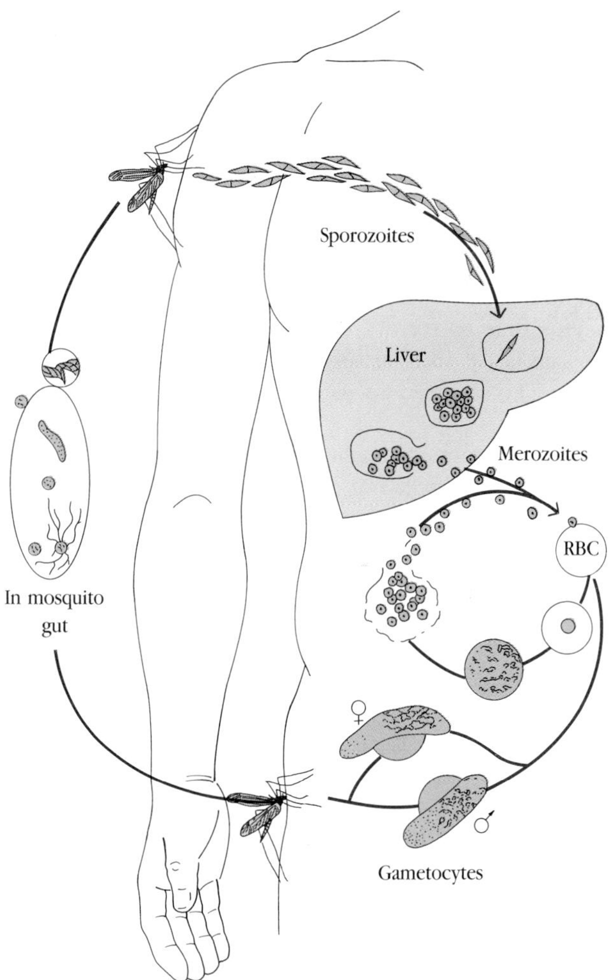

FIGURE 21-9 The life cycle of *Plasmodium.* Sporozoites enter the bloodstream when an infected mosquito takes a blood meal. The sporozoites migrate to the liver where they multiply, transforming liver hepatocytes into giant multinucleate schizonts, which release thousands of merozoites into the bloodstream. The merozoites infect red blood cells, which eventually rupture, releasing more merozoites. Eventually some of the merozoites differentiate into male and female gametocytes, which are ingested by a mosquito and differentiate into the sporozoite stage within the salivary gland of the mosquito.

called circumsporozoite (CS) antigen, which probably mediates adhesion of sporozoites to hepatocytes. Such adhesion has been demonstrated in vitro, and recombinant CS antigens have been shown to bind to hepatocytes in vitro. The binding site on the CS antigen is a conserved region in the carboxy-terminal end (called region II) that has a high degree of sequence homology with cell-adhesion molecules.

Within the liver, the sporozoites multiply extensively and undergo a complex series of transformations that culminate in the formation and release of *merozoites* in about a week. It has been estimated that a liver hepatocyte infected with a single sporozoite can release 5,000–10,000 merozoites. The released merozoites infect red blood cells, initiating the symptoms and pathology of malaria. Within a red blood cell, merozoites replicate and undergo successive differentiations; eventually the cell ruptures and releases new merozoites, which go on to infect more red blood cells. Eventually some of the merozoites differentiate into male and female *gametocytes,* which are ingested by a female *Anopheles* mosquito during a blood meal. Within the mosquito's gut, the male and female gametocytes fuse to form a zygote, which multiplies and differentiates into sporozoites within the salivary gland. The infected mosquito is now set to initiate the cycle once again.

The symptoms of malaria are recurrent chills, fever, and sweating. The symptoms peak roughly every 48 h, when successive generations of merozoites are released from infected red blood cells. An infected individual eventually becomes weak and anemic and shows splenomegaly. The large numbers of merozoites formed can block capillaries, causing intense headaches, renal failure, heart failure, or cerebral damage—often with fatal consequences. There is speculation that some of the symptoms of malaria may be caused not by *Plasmodium* itself but instead by excessive production of cytokines. This hypothesis stemmed from the observation that cancer patients treated in clinical trials with recombinant tumor necrosis factor (TNF) developed symptoms that mimicked malaria. The relation between TNF and malaria symptoms was studied by infecting mice with a mouse-specific strain of *Plasmodium,* which causes rapid death by cerebral malaria. Injection of these mice with antibodies to TNF was shown to prevent the rapid death.

Host Response to Plasmodium *Infection*

In regions where malaria is endemic, the immune response to *Plasmodium* infection is poor. Children less than 14 years old mount the lowest immune response and consequently are most likely to develop malaria. In some regions the childhood mortality rate for malaria reaches 50%, and worldwide the disease kills about a million children a year. The low immune response to *Plasmodium* among children can be demonstrated by measuring serum antibody levels to the sporozoite stage. Only 22% of the children living in endemic areas have detectable antibodies to the sporozoite stage, whereas 84% of the adults have such antibodies. Even in adults the degree of immunity is far from complete, however, and most people living in endemic regions have lifelong low-level *Plasmodium* infections.

A number of factors may contribute to the low levels of immune responsiveness to *Plasmodium.* The maturational changes from sporozoite to merozoite to gametocyte allow the organism to keep changing its surface molecules, resulting in continual changes in the antigens seen by the immune system. The intracellular phases of the life cycle in liver cells and erythrocytes also reduce the degree of immune activation generated by the pathogen and allow the organism to multiply while it is shielded from the attacking immune system. Furthermore, the most accessible stage, the sporozoite, circulates in the blood for only about 30 min before it infects liver hepatocytes; it is unlikely that much immune activation can occur in such a short period of time. And even when an antibody response does develop to sporozoites, *Plasmodium* has evolved a way of overcoming that response by sloughing off the surface CS-antigen coat, thus rendering the antibodies ineffective.

Design of Malaria Vaccines

Clearly an effective vaccine for malaria should be designed to maximize the most effective immune defense mechanisms. Unfortunately, little is known of the roles that humoral and cell-mediated responses play in the development of protective immunity to this disease. Current approaches to design of malaria vaccines largely focus on the sporozoite stage. One experimental vaccine, for example, consists of *Plasmodium* sporozoites attenuated by x-irradiation. In a recent study 9 volunteers were repeatedly immunized by the bite of *P. falciparum*–infected, irradiated mosquitos. Later challenge by the bites of mosquitos infected with virulent *P. falciparum* revealed that 6 of the 9 recipients were completely protected. As encouraging as these results are, the need to breed mosquitos to obtain *Plasmodium* sporozoites makes this approach impracticable for immunizing the millions of people living in endemic malaria regions. For example, an enormous insectory would be required to breed mosquitos in which to prepare enough irradiated sporozoites to vaccinate just one small village in such regions.

Another approach focuses on identification of immunodominant B- and T-cell epitopes on the various *Plasmodium* stages. Once these epitopes are identified, synthetic peptide vaccines containing these epitopes could be prepared or monoclonal antibodies could be developed that are specific for these epitopes. Both of these approaches are currently being explored. The target antigen recognized by humoral antibodies induced by the irradiated-sporozoite vaccine is CS antigen. In *P. falciparum* the CS antigen contains 412 amino acids with a central region consisting of approximately 40 repeats of an Asn-Ala-Asn-Pro (NANP) sequence (Figure 21-10). On either side of the repeat are two regions of conserved amino acid sequences designated regions I and II. As noted previously, region II enables the sporozoites to bind to hepatocytes. Both the repeat region and the conserved sequence in region II are potential vaccine components. Sera from *P. falciparum*–infected individuals living in endemic areas contain antibodies to the repeat region, but the levels of these antibodies are insufficient to prevent infection. However, when people are immunized with x-irradiated sporozoites, the repeat region is the immunodominant B-cell epitope and high titers of antibody are produced to this region. In addition, monoclonal antibodies specific for these repeats on the CS antigen were found to protect mice against a challenge of live plasmodia, suggesting that synthetic peptide vaccines based on the repeat might induce protective antibody. The first step in designing such a synthetic peptide vaccine was to determine the number of repeats that function as the immunodominant B-cell epitope. Experiments with synthetic peptides incorporating from one to five repeats of NANP demonstrated that $(NANP)_3$ represented the entire immunodominant B-cell epitope; that is, it could completely block antibody binding to sporozoites.

In one trial the $(NANP)_3$ synthetic peptide was conjugated to tetanus toxoid in alum and administered intramuscularly to 35 healthy male volunteers. Of

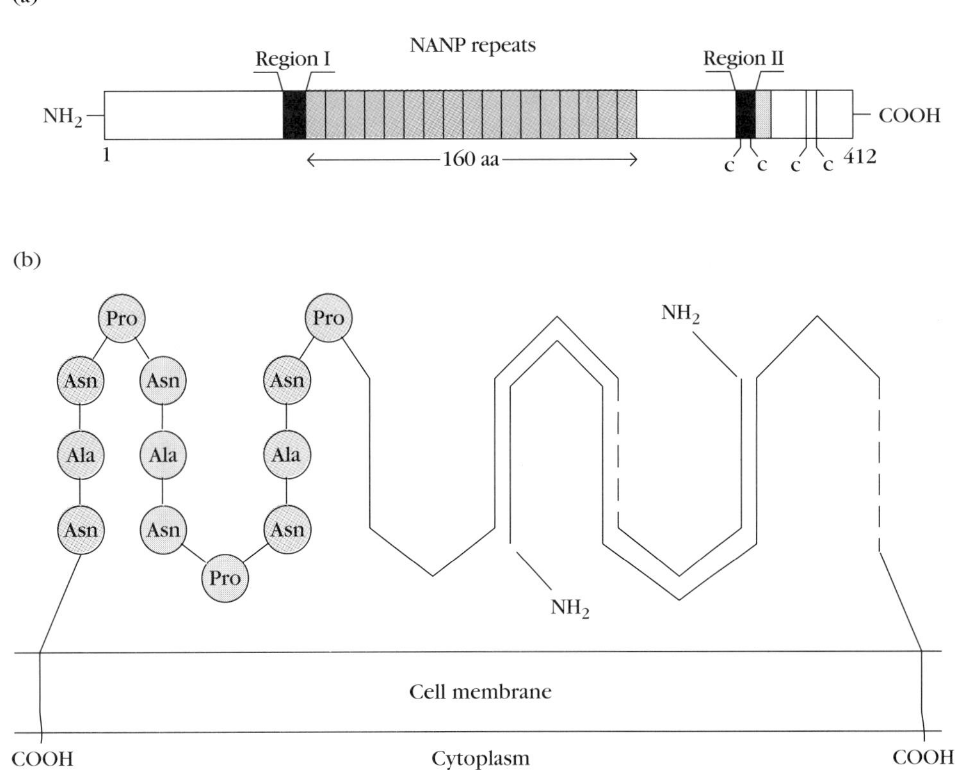

FIGURE 21-10 Schematic diagrams of circumsporozoite (CS) antigen on surface of *P. falciparum.* (a) The entire molecule of 412 amino acids contains a central region (purple), consisting of about 40 repeats of the NANP tetrapeptide, and two flanking conserved regions (black). Region II is involved in binding sporozoites to hepatocytes. (b) NANP repeat region (not to scale) bends sharply at each proline and hydrogen bonds to itself or to an adjacent molecule. A sequence of three repeats—that is, $(NANP)_3$—serves as the immunodominant B-cell epitope on CS antigen. [Part (a) adapted from E. H. Nardin and R. S. Nussenzweig, 1993, *Annu. Rev. Immunol.* **11**:687.]

these volunteers, 71% developed antibody to a 160-μg dose of the vaccine. Three of the volunteers with high serum antibody levels were subsequently infected with live *P. falciparum* by infected *Anopheles* mosquitos; four unimmunized volunteers were also infected. All four unimmunized volunteers developed merozoites in an average of 8.5 days. In contrast, one recipient of the vaccine appeared to be immune and never developed merozoites or any symptoms of malaria; the other two recipients developed merozoites, but they did not appear until day 11, considerably later than usual. Similar degrees of protection have been reported by other researchers. Such results show promise, but a success rate of one in three is not what one would hope for.

The $(NANP)_3$-tetanus toxoid trials illustrate one common problem with vaccines in which a synthetic peptide representing only the immunodominant B-cell epitope is coupled to an unrelated carrier protein. Although a humoral antibody response is generated to $(NANP)_3$, the T-cell response induced by this vaccine is directed to the tetanus toxoid carrier; therefore, the vaccine fails to generate a T-memory response specific for *Plasmodium*. What is needed is a vaccine incorporating both B- and T-cell immunodominant epitopes. In an attempt to identify T-cell epitopes on CS antigen, different inbred mouse strains were immunized with a recombinant vaccinia virus expressing the CS antigen. Of the different mice strains tested, only mice possessing IA^b or IA^k class II MHC alleles were able to produce a high antibody response to the CS antigen. This would suggest that only IA^b and IA^k class II molecules can present peptides from CS antigen to T_H cells and thereby achieve B-cell activation.

In order to identify the T-cell epitope on CS antigen that is recognized by IA^k-bearing mice, linear peptide sequences of CS antigen were analyzed by a computer program to identify peptides having significant amphipathic α helices. Such peptides present both hydrophobic and hydrophilic surfaces and are thought to bind effectively to MHC molecules and the T-cell receptor. The peptide sequence designated Th2R had the highest amphipathic index (Figure 21-11). When IA^k-bearing mice were immunized with a synthetic peptide containing the B-cell epitope NANP conjugated to the Th2R peptide, the mice responded with a high level of antibody production. By analyzing peptide sequences for those properties known to be important for T-cell epitopes (such as amphipathic helices), then, it was possible to design a successful synthetic vaccine for the IA^k-bearing mice. It is hoped that additional studies of this type will identify other T-cell epitopes that can be presented by other MHC alleles. Presumably an effective vaccine would include a mixture of these peptides.

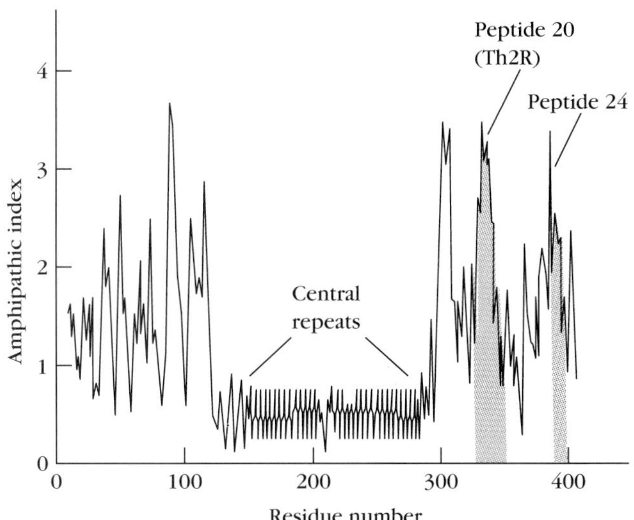

FIGURE 21-11 Identification of amphipathic peptides in circumsporozoite (CS) antigen of *P. falciparum*. Overlapping blocks of 11 residues were analyzed by computer and assigned an amphipathic index, which was plotted at the center position of each block. The area under each peak corresponds to the amphipathic score. The peaks with the highest amphipathic scores correspond to peptides 20 (Th2R) and 24. Th2R is the major T-cell epitope on CS antigen recognized by IA^k-bearing mice. In humans, both Th2R and peptide 24 function as T-cell epitopes. [Adapted from M. F. Good et al., 1987, *Science* **235**:1059.]

CS antigen also appears to be poorly immunogenic for T cells in humans. For example, when peripheral-blood lymphocytes from individuals living in malarial endemic areas were incubated with overlapping synthetic peptides spanning the entire length of CS antigen, the cells from 40% of the individuals did not proliferate (were not activated) in response to any of the peptides. Interestingly, among the 60% of cell samples that did respond to the synthetic peptides, the two peptides that were most recognized, peptides 20 (Th2R) and 24, were also the peptides having the highest amphipathic indices. Comparison of the sequence variation of CS peptides from one plasmodium to the next revealed that these two peptides (Th2R and 24) exhibited more variation than other peptide sequences. This variability might contribute to the ability of *Plasmodium* to escape the immune response. Some researchers speculate that the immune response may actually select for such variants, which would be more likely to escape an effective cell-mediated response. Because of this possibility, it might be fruitful to screen other sporozoite proteins for amphipathic sequences showing less variation.

The variation in the major T-cell epitopes of CS antigen may place a fundamental limit on the effectiveness of the cell-mediated immune response to *Plasmodium*. Yet a number of findings have suggested that cell-mediated immunity—acting in concert with humoral antibody or acting independently—is important in malaria. For example, when mice are immunized with x-irradiated sporozoites, they are immune to a subsequent challenge with live sporozoites, as mentioned above. However, if immunized mice are treated with anti-CD8 to deplete their $CD8^+$ T cells, that immunity is abolished (Table 21-6). In addition, T cells from mice rendered immune with irradiated-sporozoite vaccine are able to confer immunity on adoptive-transfer recipients. T cells could contribute to immunity to malaria either through a delayed-type hypersensitive response or by cell-mediated lysis by CTLs. $CD4^+$ cells may recognize sporozoite antigens associated with class II MHC molecules on liver Kupffer cells (a type of macrophage). The target for $CD8^+$ CTLs is thought to be sporozoite antigens presented by class I MHC molecules on infected liver hepatocytes. The ability of sporozoites to escape an effective cell-mediated immune response may allow such large numbers of merozoites to become established that successful elimination of *Plasmodium* by the immune system is reduced.

African Sleeping Sickness (*Trypanosoma* Species)

Two species of African trypanosomes, which are flagellated protozoans, can cause sleeping sickness, a chronic, debilitating disease transmitted to humans and cattle by the bite of the tsetse fly. In the bloodstream a trypanosome differentiates into a long, slender form that continues to divide every 4–6 h. The disease progresses through several stages, beginning with an early (systemic) stage in which trypanosomes multiply in the blood and progressing to a neurologic stage in which the parasite infects the central nervous system, causing meningoencephalitis and eventually the loss of consciousness.

Following infection, the number of trypanosomes within the bloodstream increases and decreases rapidly in successive waves of parasitemia, which continue indefinitely. As parasite numbers increase, an effective humoral antibody response to trypanosomal surface antigens develops; these antibodies eliminate most of the parasites from the bloodstream, both by complement-mediated lysis and by opsonization and subsequent phagocytosis. Although most of the trypanosomes are successfully eliminated from the blood, about 1% of the organisms, which bear an antigenically different surface glycoprotein, escape the initial antibody response. These surviving organisms now begin to proliferate in the bloodstream, and a new wave of parasitemia is observed. The successive waves of parasitemia reflect a unique mechanism of *antigenic shift* by which the trypanosomes can evade the immune response to their glycoprotein antigens. This process is so effective that each new variant that arises in the course of a single infection is able to escape the humoral antibodies generated in response to the preceding variant, so that waves of parasitemia occur (Figure 21-12b).

Trypanosomes are covered by a glycoprotein coat, called *variant surface glycoprotein* (VSG), and antigenic shift of this surface glycoprotein enables the organism to escape immunologic clearance and so generate successive waves of parasitemia. Several unusual genetic processes generate the extensive variation in

TABLE 21-6 EFFECT OF REMOVAL OF $CD4^+$ OR $CD8^+$ T CELLS ON IMMUNITY TO *PLASMODIUM* INFECTION IN MICE IMMUNIZED WITH X-IRRADIATED–SPOROZOITE VACCINE*

Immunization	In vivo treatment	Infected/total mice	Median days to detectable parasitemia
No (control)	None	15/15	5
Yes	None	0/10	Not detected
Yes	Anti-CD8	9/9	5
Yes	Anti-CD4	0/5	Not detected

* After immunization and in vivo treatment as indicated, mice were challenged with a mouse-specific strain of *Plasmodium*. The number that became infected and the development of parasitemia were monitored.

SOURCE: Data from W. R. Weiss, 1988, *Proc. Nat'l Acad. Sci. USA* **85**:573; cited in M. F. Good et al., 1988, *Annu. Rev. Immunol.* **6**:663.

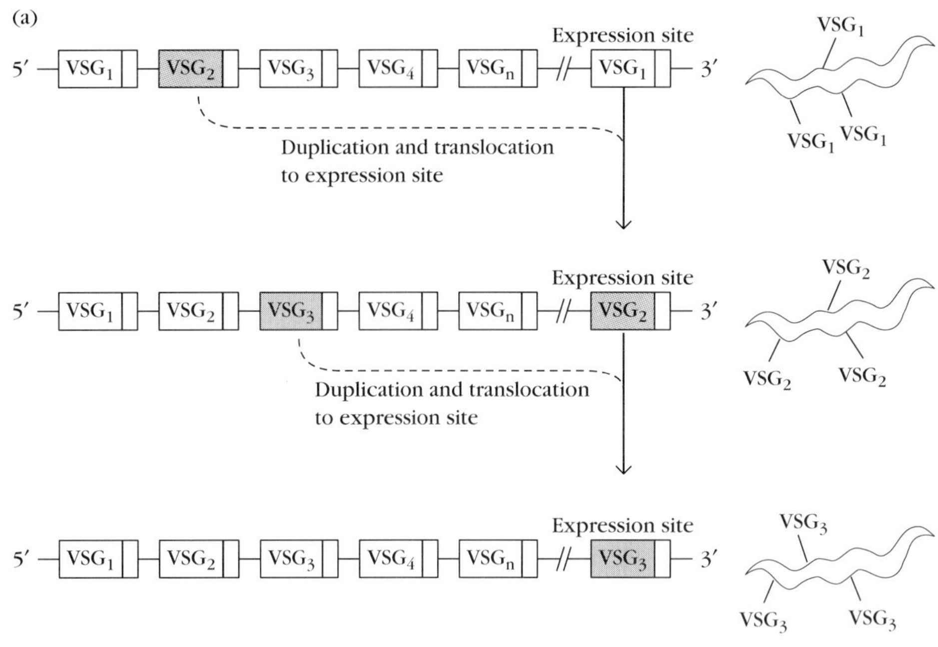

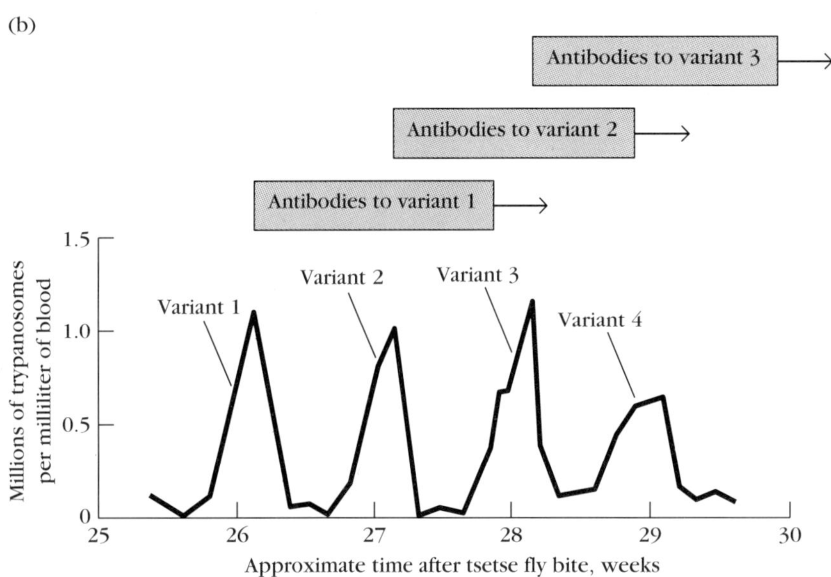

FIGURE 21-12 (a) Antigenic shifts in trypanosomes occur by the duplication of gene segments encoding variant VSG molecules and their translocation to an expression site located close to the telomere. (b) Successive waves of parasitemia following infection with *Trypanosoma* result from antigenic shifts in the parasite's variable surface glycoprotein (VSG). Each variant that arises is unaffected by the humoral antibodies induced by the previous variant. [Part (b) adapted from John Donelson, 1988, *The Biology of Parasitism,* Alan R. Liss.]

the VSG. An individual trypanosome carries a large repertoire of VSG genes, each encoding a different VSG primary sequence. *Trypanosoma brucei,* for example, contains more than 1000 VSG genes in its genome, clustered at multiple chromosomal sites. A trypanosome expresses only a single VSG gene at a single time. Activation of a VSG gene results in duplication of the gene and its transposition to a transcriptionally active expression site (ES) at the telomeric end of specific chromosomes (Figure 21-11a). Activation of a new VSG gene displaces the previous gene from the telomeric expression site. A number of chromosomes in the trypanosome have transcriptionally active expression sites at the telomeric ends, so that a number of VSG genes can potentially be expressed, but unknown control mechanisms limit expression to a single VSG expression site at a time.

One interesting observation is that there appears to be some order to the VSG variation during infection. Each new variant arises not by clonal outgrowth from a single variant cell but instead from the growth of multiple cells that have activated the same VSG gene in the current wave of parasite growth. It is not known how this process is regulated among individual trypanosomes. Clearly the continual shifts in epitopes displayed by the VSG makes the development of a vaccine for African sleeping sickness extremely difficult.

Diseases Caused by Parasitic Worms (Helminths)

Unlike protozoans, which are unicellular and often grow within human cells, helminths are large multicellular organisms that do not ordinarily multiply within humans and are not intracellular pathogens. Although helminths are more accessible to the immune system than protozoans, most infected individuals carry relatively few of these parasites; for this reason the immune system is not strongly engaged and the level of immunity generated to helminths is often very poor. Parasitic worms are responsible for a wide variety of diseases in both humans and animals. More than a billion people are infected with *Ascaris,* a parasitic roundworm that infects the small intestine, and more than 300 million people are infected with *Schistosoma,* a trematode worm that causes a chronic debilitating infection. Several helminths are important pathogens of domestic animals and invade humans who ingest contaminated food. These helminths include *Taenia,* a tapeworm of cattle and pigs, and *Trichinella,* the roundworm of pigs that causes trichinosis.

Schistosomiasis (*Schistosoma* Species)

Several *Schistosoma* species are responsible for the chronic, debilitating, and sometimes fatal disease schistosomiasis (formerly known as bilharzia). Three species, *S. mansoni, S. japonicum,* and *S. haematobium,* are the major pathogens in humans, infecting individuals in Africa, the Middle East, South America, the Caribbean, China, Southeast Asia, and the Philippines. A rise in the incidence of schistosomiasis in recent years has paralleled the increasing worldwide use of irrigation, which has expanded the habitat of the fresh water snail that serves as the intermediate host for schistosomes.

Infection occurs through contact with free-swimming infectious larvae, called cercariae, which are released from an infected snail at the rate of 300–3000 per day. When cercariae contact human skin, they secrete digestive enzymes that help them to bore into the skin, where they shed their tail and are transformed into schistosomules. The schistosomules enter the capillaries and migrate to the lungs, then to the liver, and finally to the primary site of infection, which varies with the species. *S. mansoni* and *S. japonicum* infect the intestinal mesenteric veins; *S. haematobium* infects the veins of the urinary bladder. Once established in their final tissue site, schistosomules mature into male and female adult worms. The worms mate and the females produce at least 300 spiny eggs a day. Unlike protozoan parasites, schistosomes and other helminths do not multiply within their hosts. The eggs produced by the female worm do not mature into adult worms in humans; instead, some of them pass into the feces or urine and are excreted to infect more snails. The number of worms in an infected individual increases only through repeated exposure to the free-swimming cercariae, and so most infected individuals carry rather low numbers of worms.

Most of the symptoms of schistosomiasis are initiated by the egg stage. Not all the eggs are eliminated through the feces or urine; as many as half of them remain in the host, where they invade the intestinal wall, liver, or bladder and cause hemorrhage. A chronic state can then develop lasting for 20 years or more in which the adult worms persist and the unexcreted eggs induce cell-mediated delayed-type hypersensitive reactions, resulting in large granulomas that are gradually walled off by fibrous tissue. Although the eggs are contained by the formation of the granuloma, often the granuloma itself obstructs the venous blood flow to the liver or bladder.

Although an immune response does develop to the schistosomes, it is not sufficient to eliminate the adult worms in most individuals, even though the intravascular sites of schistosome infestation should make the worm an easy target for immune elimination. Instead the worms survive for up to 20 years. The schistosomules would appear to be the forms most susceptible to immune attack, but because they are motile, they can evade the localized cellular buildup of immune and inflammatory cells. Adult schistosome worms also possess several unique protective mechanisms that help them to escape the immune defenses. The adult worm has been shown to decrease the expression of antigens on its outer membrane and also to enclose

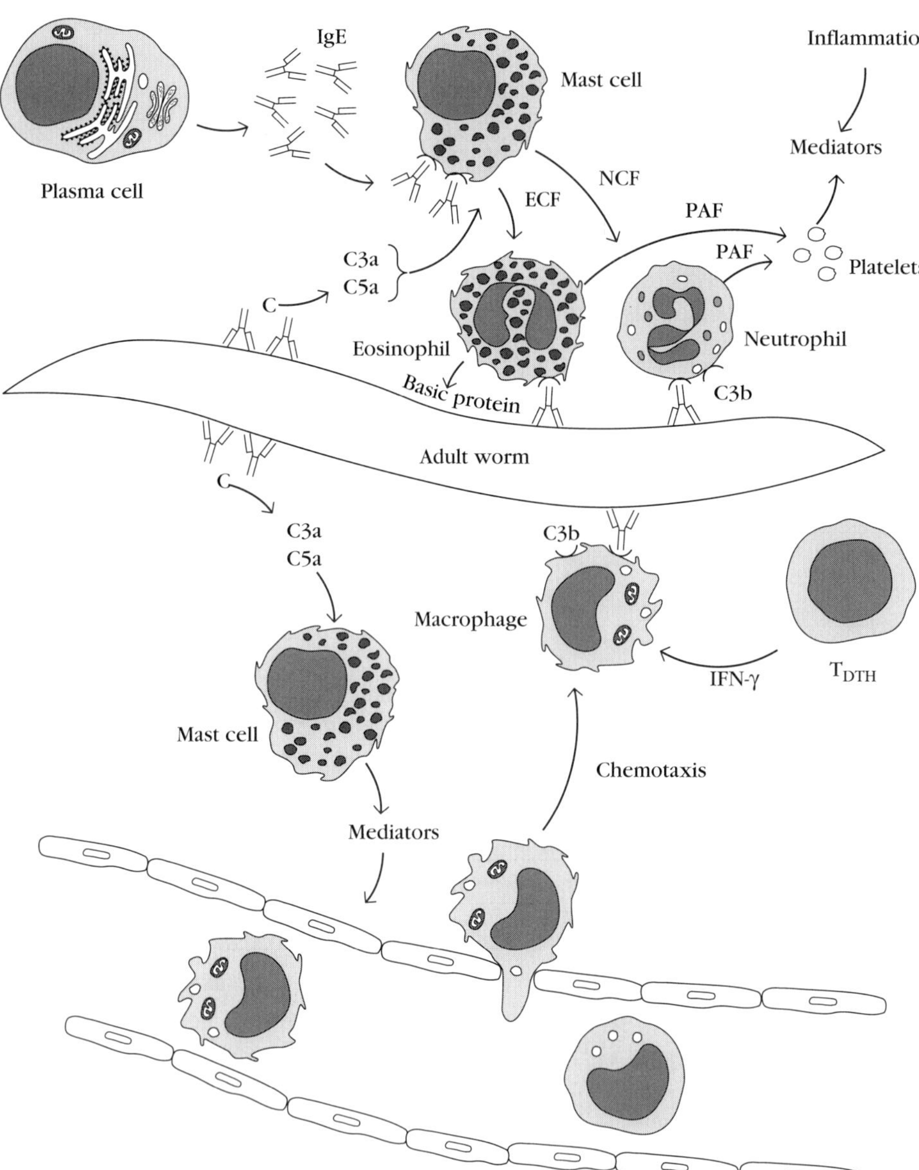

FIGURE 21-13 Overview of the immune response generated against *Schistosoma mansoni.* The response includes both humoral and cell-mediated components. C = complement; ECF = eosinophil chemotactic factor; NCF = neutrophil chemotactic factor; PAF = platelet-activating factor.

itself in a glycolipid and glycoprotein coat derived from the host, masking the presence of its own antigens. Among the antigens observed on the adult worm are the host's own ABO blood-group antigens and histocompatibility antigens! The immune response is of course diminished by this covering of the host's self-antigens, which probably contributes to the lifelong persistence of these organisms.

The role of humoral and cell-mediated responses in protective immunity to schistosomiasis is controversial. Following infection with *S. mansoni,* a humoral response develops that is characterized by high titers of antischistosome antibodies of the IgE isotype, localized increases in mast cells and their subsequent degranulation, and increased numbers of eosinophils (Figure 21-13). These manifestations suggest that cytokines produced by a T_H2-like subset are important: IL-4, which induces B cells to class-switch to IgE production; IL-5, which induces bone marrow precursors to differentiate into eosinophils; and IL-3 (along with IL-4), which stimulates mast-cell growth. Degranulation of mast cells releases mediators that increase the infiltration of such inflammatory cells as macrophages and eosinophils. The eosinophils express Fc receptors for IgE and IgG and bind to the antibody-coated parasite. Once bound to the parasite, an eosinophil can participate in antibody-dependent cell-mediated cytotoxicity (ADCC), releasing mediators from its granules that damage the parasite (see Figure 15-11). One eosinophil mediator, called basic protein, has been shown to be particularly toxic to helminths.

Immunization studies with mice, however, suggest that this humoral IgE response may not provide protective immunity. When mice are immunized with *S. mansoni* vaccine, the protective immune response that develops is not an IgE response, but rather is a cell-mediated T_{DTH} response characterized by IFN-γ production and macrophage accumulation (see Figure 21-12). Furthermore, inbred strains of mice with deficiencies in mast cells or IgE develop protective immunity following vaccination, whereas inbred strains with deficiencies in cell-mediated T_{DTH} responses fail to develop protective immunity in response to the vaccine. These studies suggest that the T_{DTH} response may be important in immunity to schistosomiasis. This led A. Sher and his colleagues to speculate that schistosomes may have evolved a clever defense mechanism by their ability to induce an ineffective T_H2-like response. This response would ensure that sufficient levels of IL-10 are produced to inhibit the effective response generated by the T_H1-like subset.

Antigens present on the membrane of cercariae and young schistosomules look promising as possible vaccine components because these stages appear to be most susceptible to immune attack. Some monoclonal antibodies to cercariae and young schistosomules have been shown to passively transfer resistance to mice and rats challenged with live cercariae. These protective monoclonal antibodies were then used to identify surface antigens on cercariae and schistosomules as possible candidates for vaccine development. With monoclonal-antibody affinity columns the schistosome membrane antigens were purified from crude membrane extracts. When mice were immunized and boosted with these purified antigens, they exhibited increased resistance to a later challenge with live cercariae. Schistosome cDNA libraries were then established and screened with the monoclonal antibodies to identify those encoding the surface antigens. Experiments using cloned cercariae or schistosomule antigens are presently under way to assess their ability to induce protective immunity in animal models. In developing an effective vaccine for schistosomiasis, however, a fine line separates a beneficial immune response, which at best limits the parasite load, from a detrimental response, which in itself may become pathologic.

Summary

1. The immune response to viral infections involves both humoral and cell-mediated components. Antibody to the viral receptor can block viral infections of host cells. However, a number of viruses, including influenza, are able to mutate their receptor molecules and thus evade the humoral antibody response. Once a viral infection has been established, cell-mediated immunity appears to be more important. The cell-mediated response may develop in response to such internal viral proteins as the nucleoprotein of the viral core. These internal proteins are expressed together with class I MHC molecules on the membrane of infected host cells and serve to activate CTL activity.

2. Immunity to bacterial infections is generally mediated by antibody unless the bacterium is capable of intracellular growth, in which case delayed-type hypersensitivity is important for host defense. Antibody can induce localized production of immune effector molecules of the complement system, thus facilitating development of an inflammatory response. Antibody can also activate complement-mediated lysis of the bacterium, neutralize toxins, and serve as an opsonin to increase phagocytosis. Bacteria can evade the humoral antibody response by several mechanisms. Some bacteria secrete protease enzymes that cleave IgA dimers, thus reducing the effectiveness of IgA in the mucous secretions. Other bacteria escape phagocytosis by producing surface capsules or protein that inhibit adherence to phagocytes, by secreting toxins that kill phagocytes, or through their ability to survive within phagocytes.

3. Both humoral and cell-mediated immune responses have been implicated in immunity to protozoan infections. The effectiveness of the response depends in part on the site of the parasite. In general, humoral antibody is effective against blood-borne stages, but once protozoans infect host cells, cell-mediated immunity is necessary. Protozoans escape the immune response through several mechanisms. Some —notably *Trypanosoma brucei*—are covered by a glycoprotein coat that is constantly changed by a genetic-switch mechanism. Others (including *Plasmodium*) slough off their glycoprotein coat after antibody has bound. In addition, the glycoprotein coat of *Plasmodium* contains few T-cell epitopes, and those that are present are in regions of the glycoprotein exhibiting the most variation among organisms.

4. Because of their size, the helminths are extracellular parasites and are generally attacked by antibody-mediated defenses. Because relatively few of these organisms are carried in an affected individual and because they do not multiply within the host, immune system exposure to helminths is limited and consequently only a low level of immunity is induced.

References

BLOOM, B. R., and C. J. L. MURRAY. 1992. Tuberculosis: commentary on a reemergent killer. *Science* **257**:1055.

BODMER, H. C., R. M. PEMBERTON, J. ROTHBARD, and B. A. ASKONAS. 1988. Enhanced recognition of a modified antigen by cytotoxic T cells specific for influenza nucleoprotein. *Cell* **52**:253.

BORST, P. 1991. Molecular genetics of antigenic variation. *Immunoparasit. Today* (March):A29.

BRAUN, R. 1988. Molecular and cellular biology of malaria. *Bioessays.* **8**:194.

BRETSCHER, P. A. 1992. A strategy to improve the efficacy of vaccination against tuberculosis and leprosy. *Immunol. Today* **13**:342.

CAPRON, A., and J. P. DESSAINT. 1992. Immunologic aspects of schistosomiasis. *Annu. Rev. Med.* **43**:209.

DOHERTY, P. C., W. ALLEN, M. EICHELBERGER, and S. R. CARDING. 1992. Roles of $\alpha\beta$ and $\gamma\delta$ T cell subsets in viral immunity. *Annu. Rev. Immunol.* **10**:123.

GOOD, M. F. 1992. A malaria vaccine strategy based on the induction of cellular immunity. *Immunol. Today* **13**:126.

GOOD, M. F., J. A. BERZOFSKY, and L. H. MILLER. 1988. The T cell response to the malaria circumsporozoite protein: an immunological approach to vaccine design. *Annu. Rev. Immunol.* **6**:663.

GOODING, L. R. 1992. Virus proteins that counteract host immune defenses. *Cell* **71**:5.

GREVE, J. M., G. DAVIS, A. M. MEYER et al. 1989. The major human rhinovirus receptor is ICAM-1. *Cell* **56**:839.

HABICHT, G. S., G. BECK, and J. L. BENACH. 1987. Lyme disease. *Sci. Am.* **257** (July):

HALL, B. F., and K. A. JOINER. 1991. Strategies of obligate intracellular parasites for evading host defences. *Immunoparasit. Today* (March):A22.

KAUFMANN, S. H. E. 1993. Immunity to intracellular bacteria. *Annu. Rev. Immunol.* **11**:129.

LOCKSLEY, R. M., and P. SCOTT. 1991. Helper T-cell subsets in mouse leishmaniasis: induction, expansion, and effector. *Immunoparasit. Today* (March):A58.

MAHMOUD, A. A. F. 1989. Parasitic protozoa and helminths: biological and immunological challenges. *Science* **246**:1015.

MCCONKEY, G. A., A. P. WATERS, T. F. MCCUTCHAN et al. 1990. The generation of genetic diversity in malarial parasites. *Annu. Rev. Microbiol.* **44**:479.

MEYER, T. F., C. P. GIBBS, and R. HASS. 1990. Variation and control of protein expression in Neisseria. *Annu. Rev. Microbiol.* **44**:451.

MIMS, C. A. 1987. *Pathogenesis of Infectious Disease.* Academic Press.

MITCHELL, G. F. 1987. Cellular and molecular aspects of host-parasite relationships. In *Progress in Immunology VI.* B. Cinander and R. G. Miller (eds.). Academic Press.

NARDIN, E. H., and R. S. NUSSENZWEIG. 1993. T cell responses to pre-erythrocytic stages of malaria: role in protection and vaccine development against pre-erythrocyte stages. *Annu. Rev. Immunol.* **11**:687.

PALA, P., and B. A. ASKONAS. 1986. Low responder MHC alleles for Tc recognition of influenza nucleoprotein. *Immunogenetics* **23**:379.

PLAYFAIR, H. L., J. TAVERNE, C. A. W. BATE, and J. B. DE SOUZA. 1990. The malaria vaccine: anti-parasite or anti-disease? *Immunol. Today* **11**:25.

ROBERTSON, B. D., and T. F. MEYER. 1992. Genetic variation in pathogenic bacteria. *Trends Genet.* **8**:422.

ROTH, J. A. (ed.). 1988. *Virulence Mechanisms of Bacterial Pathogens.* American Society for Microbiology.

SHER, A., and R. L. COFFMAN. 1992. Regulation of immunity to parasites by T cells and T-cell derived cytokines. *Annu. Rev. Immunol.* **10**:385.

SIMON, M. M., U. E. SCHAIBLE, R. WALLICH, and M. D. KRAMER. 1991. A mouse model for *Borrelia burgdorferi* infection: approach to a vaccine against Lyme disease. *Immunol. Today* **12**:11.

STAUNTON, D. E., V. J. MERLUZZI, R. ROTHLEIN et al. 1989. A cell adhesion molecule, ICAM-1, is the major surface receptor for rhinoviruses. *Cell* **56**:849.

TAYLOR, P. M., J. DAVEY, K. HOWLAND et al. 1987. Class I MHC molecules rather than other mouse genes dictate influenza epitope recognition by cytotoxic T cells. *Immunogenetics* **26**:267.

TOWNSEND, A. R. M., J. ROTHBARD, F. M. GOTCH et al. 1986. The epitopes of influenza nucleoprotein recognized by cytotoxic T lymphocytes can be defined with short synthetic peptides. *Cell* **44**:959.

VIGNALI, D. A. A., Q. D. BICKLE, M. G. TAYLOR et al. 1989. Immunity to *Schistosoma mansoni* in vivo: contradiction or clarification? *Immunol. Today* **10**:410.

WEISS, R. 1992. On the track of "killer" TB. *Science* **255**:148.

Study Questions

1. The effect of the MHC on the immune response to peptides of the influenza virus nucleoprotein was studied in H-2^b mice that had been previously immunized with live influenza virions. The CTL activity of primed lymphocytes was determined by in vitro CML assays using H-2^k fibroblasts as target cells. The target cells had been transfected with different H-2^b class I MHC genes and were infected either with live influ-

For use with Question 1.

Target cell (H-2^k fibroblast)	Test antigen	CTL activity of influenza-primed H-2^b lymphocytes (% lysis)
(A) Untransfected	Live influenza	0
(B) Transfected with class I D^b	Live influenza	60
(C) Transfected with class I D^b	Nucleoprotein peptide 365–380	50
(D) Transfected with class I D^b	Nucleoprotein peptide 50–63	2
(E) Transfected with class I K^b	Nucleoprotein peptide 365–380	0.5
(F) Transfected with class I K^b	Nucleoprotein peptide 50–63	1

enza or incubated with nucleoprotein synthetic peptides. The results of these assays are shown in the table above:

a. Why was there no killing of the target cells in system A even though the target cells were infected with live influenza?
b. Why was a CTL response generated to the nucleoprotein in system C, even though it is an internal viral protein?
c. Why was there a good CTL response in system C to peptide 365–380, whereas there was no response in system D to peptide 50–63?
d. If you were going to develop a synthetic peptide vaccine for influenza in humans, how would these results obtained in mice influence your design of a vaccine?

2. a. Describe the nonspecific defenses that operate when a disease-producing microorganism enters the body.
b. What additional defense mechanisms does the immune system contribute?

3. Discuss the role of humoral and the cell-mediated responses in immunity to influenza.

4. The humoral response to influenza is subtype specific, whereas the cell-mediated response has been shown to cross-react with all influenza A subtypes.
a. Discuss the significance of this observation in terms of vaccine development for influenza.
b. Why might an internal viral protein, such as nucleoprotein, serve as a potential vaccine?

5. M. F. Good and co-workers analyzed the effect of MHC haplotype on the antibody response to a malarial circumsporozoite (CS) peptide antigen in several recombinant congenic mouse strains. Their results are shown in the table below.
a. Based on the results of this study, which MHC molecule(s) serve(s) as restriction element(s) for this peptide antigen?
b. Since antigen recognition by B cells is not MHC restricted, why is the humoral antibody response influenced by the MHC haplotype?

For use with Question 5.

Strain	H-2 alleles					Antibody response to CS peptide
	K	*IA*	*IE*	*S*	*D*	
B10.BR	*k*	*k*	*k*	*k*	*k*	<1
B10.A (4R)	*k*	*k*	*b*	*b*	*b*	<1
B10.HTT	*s*	*s*	*k*	*k*	*d*	<1
B10.A (5R)	*b*	*b*	*k*	*d*	*d*	67
B10	*b*	*b*	*b*	*b*	*b*	73
B10.MBR	*b*	*k*	*k*	*k*	*a*	<1

SOURCE: Adapted from M. F. Good et al., 1988, *Annu. Rev. Immunol.* **6**:633.

6. Discuss the unique mechanisms each of the following pathogens has for escaping the immune response: (a) African trypanosomes, (b) plasmodium species, and (c) influenza virus.

IMMUNODEFICIENCY DISEASES

The immunodeficiency diseases include a diverse spectrum of illnesses that stem from various abnormalities of the immune system. The basic clinical manifestations are frequent, prolonged, severe infections, which are often caused by organisms of normally low pathogenicity. An immunodeficiency disease may result from a primary congenital defect or may be acquired from a secondary cause, such as a viral or bacterial infection, malnutrition, or a drug treatment. Acquired immune deficiency syndrome (AIDS) is the most significant immunodeficiency arising from secondary causes, in this case a retrovirus named human immunodeficiency virus (HIV). Because of its worldwide impact and scientific importance, AIDS is covered separately in the next chapter. This chapter focuses on selected primary immunodeficiency diseases affecting the various branches of the immune system.

Classification of Immunodeficiencies

Immunodeficiency diseases can result from congenital or acquired defects in hematopoietic stem cells, T cells, B cells, phagocytic cells, and the complement system. The diseases discussed in this chapter are summarized in Table 22-1, classified according to the branch of the immune system that is primarily involved. Figure 22-1

TABLE 22-1 SOME IMMUNODEFICIENCY DISEASES

Disease	Immune-system deficiency	Possible mechanism
	Phagocytic deficiencies	
Congenital agranulocytosis	Decreased neutrophil count	Decreased production of G-CSF
Leukocyte-adhesion deficiency (LAD)	Failure of neutrophils and monocytes to extravasate Defective CTL killing Defective T-cell help in B-cell activation	Defective synthesis of β chain of integrin adhesion molecules
Lazy-leukocyte syndrome	Decreased neutrophil chemotaxis	Not known
Chronic granulomatous disease (CGD)	Defective killing by neutrophils of phagocytosed bacteria	Decreased H_2O_2 production due to defective NADPH oxidase (cytochrome *b*)
	Humoral deficiencies	
X-linked agammaglobulinemia (XLA)	Reduction in B-cell count Absence of immunoglobulins	Block in maturation of pre-B cells due to defective V-D-J gene rearrangement
X-linked hyper-IgM (XHM) syndrome	Low levels of IgG and IgA Very high levels of IgM	Defect in class switching
Common variable hypogammaglobulinemia (CVH)	Decreased plasma-cell levels but usually normal B-cell levels Variable reduction in secreted Ig of all isotypes	Defective differentiation of B cells to plasma cells due to defective processing of Ig transcripts, lack of cytokine receptors on B cells, or abnormal T-cell response
Selective immunoglobulin deficiencies	Decreased levels of one or more Ig isotypes	Defect in maturation of plasma cells or necessary T-cell–derived cytokines
	Cell-mediated deficiencies	
DiGeorge syndrome	Decreased T-cell counts	Lack of T-cell maturation due to absence of thymus
Nude mice	Decreased T-cell counts	Lack of T-cell maturation due to absence of thymus

(Continued)

shows the stages in hematopoiesis and development of leukocytes in which congenital defects result in various immunodeficiency diseases. The prevalence of several of these diseases is given in Table 22-2.

PHAGOCYTIC DEFICIENCIES

Defects in phagocytic defense can result either from a reduction in the numbers of phagocytic cells or from a reduction in their function. Decreases in phagocyte production, extravasation, chemotaxis, and killing have each been implicated in immunodeficiencies. In each case the hallmarks are recurrent bacterial or fungal infections. The clinical manifestations, which generally are related to the magnitude of the defect, range from mild skin infections to life-threatening systemic infections. The most common infectious organisms include *Staphylococcus aureus, Streptococcus pneumoniae, Escherichia coli,* and various species of *Pseudomonas, Candida,* and *Aspergillus.*

Table 22-1 (continued) Some immunodeficiency diseases

Disease	Immune-system deficiency	Possible mechanism
	Combined immunodeficiencies	
Reticular dysgenesis	Decreased numbers of all cells of lymphoid and myeloid lineages	Defective maturation of hematopoietic stem cells
Bare-lymphocyte syndrome	Some reduction in $CD4^+$ T-cell counts Reduced B-cell and T_C-cell activation Decreased T_{DTH}-cell activity	Failure to express class I and/or class II MHC molecules on cells
Severe combined immunodeficiency disease (SCID)	Marked reduction in T- and B-cell counts in all forms	Various mechanisms
X-linked SCID		Defective T- and B-cell maturation
Autosomal recessive SCID		Defective T- and B-cell maturation
ADA-deficiency SCID		Selective killing of lymphocytes by metabolites that accumulate in absence of adenosine deaminase (ADA)
PNP-deficiency SCID		Selective killing of lymphocytes by metabolites that accumulate in the absence of purine nucleoside phosphorylase (PNP)
CB-17 *scid* mouse		Aberrant D-J joining of Ig heavy-chain and TCR β- and δ-chain gene segments
Wiskott-Aldrich syndrome (WAS)	Low levels of IgM Elevated levels of IgA and IgE Abnormal T-cell function with progressive dysfunction	Defective glycosylation of membrane glycoproteins (CD43) on lymphocytes
	Complement deficiencies	
(See Table 17-9)		

Reduction in Neutrophil Count (Neutropenia)

Quantitative deficiencies in neutrophils can range from an almost complete absence of cells, called *agranulocytosis,* to a reduction in peripheral blood neutrophils below 1500/mm^3, called *granulocytopenia* or *neutropenia.* These quantitative deficiencies may result from congenital defects or may be acquired through extrinsic factors. Acquired neutropenias are much more common than congenital ones.

Congenital neutropenias often involve a genetic defect affecting the myeloid progenitor stem cell that results in reduced production of neutrophils during hematopoiesis (see Figure 22-1). In *congenital agranulocytosis* myeloid stem cells are present in the bone marrow but rarely differentiate beyond the pro-

Table 22-2 Prevalence of selected immunodeficiency diseases

Disease	Worldwide prevalence
IgA immunodeficiency	1 : 700
Hereditary angioedema (deficiency in C1 inhibitor)*	1 : 1000
Common variable hypogammaglobulinemia	1 : 70,000
Severe combined immunodeficiency disease (SCID)—all forms	1 : 100,000
X-linked agammaglobulinemia	1 : 200,000

* Complement deficiencies are discussed in Chapter 17.

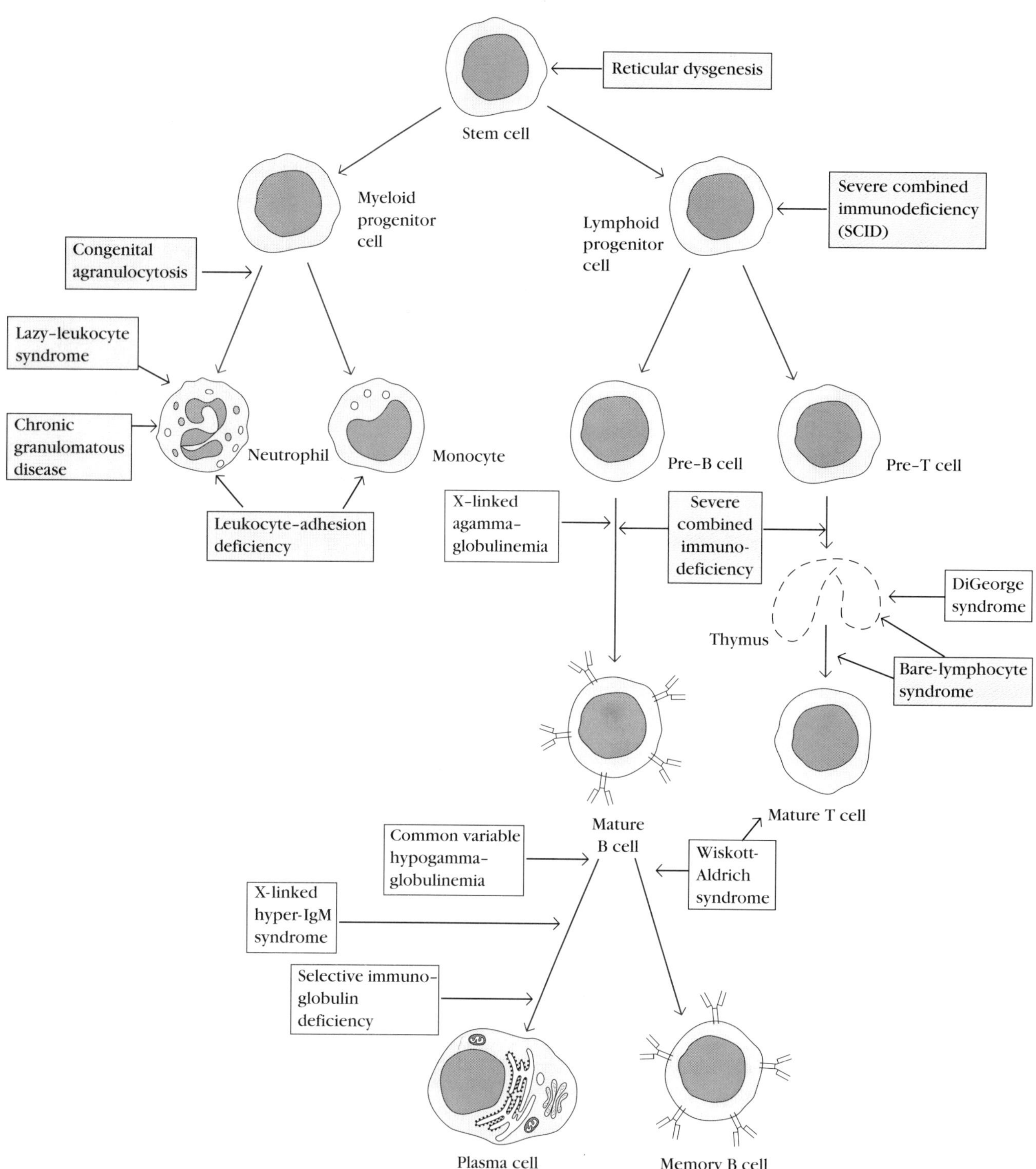

FIGURE 22-1 Stages in hematopoiesis in which common congenital defects result in various immunodeficiency diseases. Gray screen indicates phagocytic deficiencies; purple outline, humoral deficiencies; black outline, cell-mediated deficiencies; purple screen, combined immunodeficiencies.

myelocyte stage. As a result, children born with this condition show severe neutropenia with counts of less than 200 cells/mm³. These children frequently manifest bacterial infections as early as the first month of life. Experimental evidence suggests that this genetic defect results in decreased production of granulocyte colony-stimulating factor (G-CSF) and thus in a failure of the myeloid stem cell to differentiate along the granulocytic lineage (see Figure 3-2).

Because neutrophils have a short life span, their precursors divide rapidly in the bone marrow to maintain homeostatic levels of these cells. For this reason agents, such as radiation and certain drugs (e.g., chemotherapeutic drugs), that specifically damage rapidly dividing cells are likely to cause neutropenia. Occasionally neutropenia develops in such autoimmune diseases as Sjögren's syndrome or systemic lupus erythematosus; in these conditions, autoantibodies cause neutrophil destruction. Transient neutropenia often develops after certain bacterial or viral infections. It is not uncommon for children to manifest neutropenia after certain viral infections, but this neutropenia is transient, and neutrophil counts return to normal as the infection is cleared.

Defective Phagocytic Function

An effective phagocytic defense system involves a series of processes that interact in sequence to ingest and kill microorganisms. These processes include the adherence of phagocytes to vascular endothelial cells, emigration across the vascular endothelium, chemotaxis through subendothelial connective tissue to the site of immune reaction, attachment to the microorganism, phagocytosis, and subsequent killing and digestion. A dysfunction in any one of these processes may severely limit the effectiveness of the phagocytic defense system (see Table 22-1).

Adherence Defect

The development of an effective inflammatory response involves the adherence of neutrophils and monocytes to capillary endothelial cells near the site of the immune reaction. These adherent neutrophils and monocytes migrate through the capillary wall into extravascular sites, where an effective inflammatory response develops. A recently described autosomal recessive defect, called *leukocyte-adhesion deficiency (LAD),* involves an impairment of a variety of functions involving leukocyte adhesion. Included among the deficiencies is the inability of neutrophils, monocytes, and lymphocytes to adhere to vascular endothelial cells, thus preventing extravasation of these cells into the extravascular tissue spaces. Also impaired is the ability of CTLs and NK cells to adhere to their target cells and of T_H-cells and B cells to form conjugates. Individuals with this defect manifest recurrent bacterial infections and impaired wound healing.

The molecular basis of LAD has been shown to be defective biosynthesis of the β-chain component (CD18) of one subfamily of integrin adhesion molecules. The integrin molecules affected by this defect include the type 3 and type 4 complement receptors (CR3 and CR4), which bind the complement degradation product C3bi, and LFA-1, which binds the intercellular adhesion molecule ICAM-1. CR3, CR4, and LFA-1 are all heterodimeric glycoproteins in which a unique α chain is noncovalently associated in the cell membrane with a common β chain. The β-chain defect in LAD results in a loss of all three membrane glycoproteins (Table 22-3).

Each of the three integrin receptors has its own role in leukocyte adhesion (Table 22-4). Monoclonal antibody to the β chain strongly inhibits adhesion of phagocytes to endothelial cells, random locomotion, and chemotaxis, suggesting that the β chain takes part in all these processes. Phagocytes from individuals with LAD show diminished in vitro adherence to cultured human endothelial cells. Activation of normal neutrophils with agents such as phorbol myristate acetate produces an increase in adherence from a baseline of 5–10% to 50–80% after activation; unactivated neutrophils from individuals with LAD exhibit 2–5% adherence, and there is no appreciable increase in adherence after activation.

Chemotactic Defect

A large number of clinical disorders reflect defects in neutrophil chemotaxis. These disorders may be caused by an intrinsic defect in the neutrophil itself or by an extrinsic defect such as a complement deficiency and a corresponding reduction in the chemotactic factors of the complement cascade (C3a, C5a, C5b67). One syndrome, called *lazy-leukocyte syndrome,* involves a congenital defect in which neutrophil migration is severely impaired.

Killing Defect

Chronic granulomatous disease (CGD) is the most prevalent defect associated with defective intracellular killing of ingested bacteria. The disease is inherited as an X-linked recessive disorder that is manifested in boys during the first 2 years of life. (A milder autosomal recessive form of this disease has been observed; this form can also occur in girls and often is not

TABLE 22-3 PERCENTAGE OF GRANULOCYTES BEARING CR3, CR4, AND LFA-1 IN PATIENTS WITH LEUKOCYTE-ADHESION DEFICIENCY (LAD) AND IN NORMAL CONTROLS*

	Percentage of cells bearing				
LAD status	CR3 M α chain	LFA-1 L α chain	CR4 X α chain	Common β chain	Unrelated molecule (CR1)
Severe					
Patient 1	0.1	0.15	0.1	0.15	94
Patient 2	0.0	0.0	0.3	0.1	100
Moderate					
Patient 3	6.0	11.0	7.0	4.4	92
Patient 4	4.0	31	3.5	2.5	99
Patient 5	4.0	26	4.0	6.0	87
Patient 6	3.0	24	2.0	4.0	109
Normal control	57.0	66.5	42.1	54.5	101

* Granulocytes were incubated with fluorochrome-labeled monoclonal antibody specific for the indicated receptor chains and then analyzed with a fluorescence-activated cell sorter (FACS) to determine the percentage of cells binding antibody.

SOURCE: D. C. Anderson et al., 1986, *J. Infect. Dis.* **152**:668.

TABLE 22-4 PROPERTIES OF INTEGRIN MOLECULES THAT ARE ABSENT IN LEUKOCYTE-ADHESION DEFICIENCY

	Integrin molecule*		
Property	LFA-1	CR3	CR4
CD designation	CD11a/CD18	CD11b/CD18	CD11c/CD18
Subunit composition	αLβ2	αMβ2	αXβ2
Subunit molecular mass M_r (kDa)			
α chain	175,000	165,000	150,000
β chain	95,000	95,000	95,000
Cellular expression	Lymphocytes Monocytes Macrophages Granulocytes Natural killer cells	Monocytes Macrophages Granulocytes Natural killer cells	Monocytes Macrophages Granulocytes
Ligand	ICAM-1 ICAM-2	C3bi	C3bi
Functions inhibited with monoclonal antibody	Extravasation CTL killing T-B conjugate formation ADCC	Opsonization Granulocyte adherence, aggregation, and chemotaxis ADCC	Granulocyte adherence and aggregation

* CR3 = type 3 complement receptor, also known as Mac-1; CR4 = type 4 complement receptor, also known as p 150,90. LFA-1, CR3, and CR4 are heterodimers containing a common β chain but different α chains designated L, M, and X, respectively.

recognized until young adulthood.) Clinically, CGD is characterized by disseminated granulomatous lesions in various organs. Children with this disease often die of septicemia by 7 years of age.

The deficiency in CGD is in the bactericidal activity of neutrophils. Neutrophils from affected individuals can phagocytose bacteria but are unable to kill bacteria that contain the enzyme catalase. (Catalase-negative bacteria are not a problem because bacteria form H_2O_2 during their own metabolism, and in the absence of catalase these bacteria cannot detoxify their own H_2O_2 and are unable to survive even in the defective phagocytes.) During normal phagocytosis there is a burst of respiratory oxidative activity, increased oxygen consumption, and a shift of glucose metabolism to the hexose monophosphate shunt. As glucose is metabolized, reduced pyridine nucleotides (NADH and NADPH) accumulate and convert O_2 into the bactericidal H_2O_2 and potent superoxides (see Table 3-4). The levels of H_2O_2 and superoxides are normally high enough to kill even catalase-positive bacteria. Neutrophils from CGD patients, however, show no increase in O_2 consumption, no increase in utilization of the hexose monophosphate shunt, and no H_2O_2 production during phagocytosis. The underlying defect appears to be in one of the genes encoding a subunit of cytochrome *b*, which is necessary for NADP recycling. The resulting decrease in the levels of reduced pyridine nucleotides leads to decreased H_2O_2 production; in this environment ingested catalase-positive bacteria can survive in neutrophils. The bacteria are carried by the cells into various organs, where they give rise to the characteristic disseminated granulomatous lesions.

Humoral Deficiencies

B-cell immunodeficiency disorders include a diverse spectrum of diseases ranging from the complete absence of mature recirculating B cells, plasma cells, and immunoglobulin to the selective absence of only certain classes of immunoglobulins (see Table 22-1). Patients with these disorders usually are subject to recurrent bacterial infections but display normal immunity to most viral and fungal infections because the T-cell branch of the immune system is largely unaffected. The most common infections in patients with humoral immunodeficiencies involve such encapsulated bacteria as staphylococci, streptococci, and pneumococci because antibody is critical for the opsonization and clearance of these organisms. The severity of the disorder parallels the degree of antibody deficiency.

X-Linked Agammaglobulinemia

A severe *X-linked agammaglobulinemia (XLA),* described by Bruton in 1952, was the first immunodeficiency disorder to be recognized. Male infants with this disorder begin to manifest severe recurrent bacterial infections, especially of *Streptococcus pneumoniae, Staphylococcus aureus,* and *Hemophilus influenzae,* at about 6 months as the level of passively acquired maternal antibody declines and they are left unprotected.

The defect responsible for XLA, which has been mapped to the long arm of the X chromosome, is one of several X-chromosome defects that result in immunodeficiency diseases (Figure 22-2). In addition to XLA, this group of diseases includes X-linked severe combined immunodeficiency (XSCID), Wiskott-Aldrich syndrome, X-linked chronic granulomatous disease, and X-linked hyper-IgM syndrome (XHM). These X-linked disorders exhibit several features in common: They each are recessive, occur with a frequency of 1 in $10^3 - 10^6$ males, affect cells of the hematopoietic system, and occur in atypical forms in some patients; also, carriers of each disorder are normal by all immunologic criteria. Because of these similarities, some researchers have suggested that the defective genes responsible for these disorders are members of a gene family arising from a common ancestral gene.

The defect causing XLA involves the maturation of pre-B cells to mature B cells in the bone marrow (see Figure 8-22). Patients have normal numbers of pre-B cells in their bone marrow but lack (or have severely reduced levels of) mature B cells and plasma cells. In

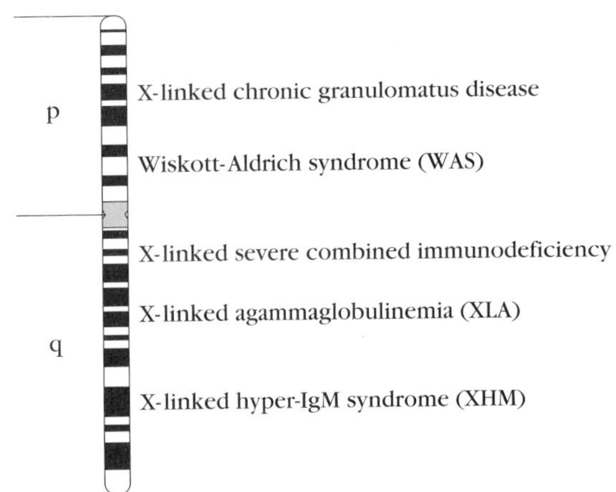

FIGURE 22-2 Several X-linked immunodeficiency diseases result from defects in loci in the long arm of the X chromosome. [From M. E. Conley, 1992, *Annu. Rev. Immunol.* **10**:215.]

normal individuals, for example, 5–15% of peripheral-blood lymphocytes are B cells, whereas in XLA patients less than 0.1% of the peripheral lymphocytes are B cells. Fluorescent antibody staining has revealed a complete absence of recirculating mature B cells and lack of cells in the B-cell–dependent areas of the peripheral lymphoid tissues in affected individuals. The lymph nodes are unusually small and lack germinal centers. In one study, pre-B cells from the bone marrow of XLA patients were shown to contain cytoplasmic μ heavy chains but no κ or λ light chains. The cytoplasmic μ heavy chains were found to be unusual in that they lacked the V_H sequence and therefore were shorter than normal. The defect in these cases is in the V-D-J rearrangement process, which occurs during B-cell maturation, and appears to result in defective heavy-chain production in the affected individuals. In other studies, however, analyses of B cells from XLA patients revealed normal VDJ rearrangement, but these patients expressed high levels of membrane IgM and other membrane markers of an immature B-cell phenotype.

X-linked agammaglobulinemia can be diagnosed relatively easily by serum electrophoresis. IgG levels of affected individuals are usually 10–20% of normal levels, and other isotypes are often not detectable. Treatment of patients with XLA requires periodic gamma-globulin injections to passively protect them against common bacterial infections. Treated patients are still susceptible to sinopulmonary infections because secretory IgA is not transferred by gamma-globulin injections.

X-Linked Hyper-IgM Syndrome

A peculiar immunoglobulin deficiency, known as *X-linked hyper-IgM (XHM) syndrome,* is characterized by a deficiency of IgG and IgA but markedly elevated levels of IgM as high as 10 mg/ml (normal IgM is 1.5 mg/ml). Although XHM syndrome is primarily an X-linked recessive disorder, some forms appear to be acquired and affect both men and women. Affected individuals have high counts of IgM-secreting plasma cells in their peripheral blood and lymphoid tissue. In addition, XHM patients often have high levels of autoantibodies to neutrophils, platelets, and red blood cells.

Although affected individuals exhibit normal counts of B cells expressing membrane-bound IgM or IgD, they appear to lack B cells expressing membrane-bound IgG or IgA. This finding suggests that XHM syndrome may involve a defect in class switching. This defect might be in the B-cell switch mechanism itself (see Figure 8-18) or in the T cells that produce cytokines necessary for class switching. The latter possibility is supported by one study in which B cells from an XHM patient class-switched from IgM to IgG or IgA when incubated with T-lymphoma cells. However, other studies have shown that when T cells from an XHM patient are mixed with normal B cells expressing IgM, the B cells class-switch to IgG or IgA. These contradictory results may indicate that more than one defect can lead to XHM syndrome.

Common Variable Hypogammaglobulinemia

Common variable hypogammaglobulinemia (CVH) refers to a heterogeneous group of disorders that cause late-onset hypogammaglobulinemia. No definitive genetic basis has been demonstrated for CVH, although familial inheritance patterns have been reported. Patients with this disorder typically develop recurrent bacterial infections beginning between 15 and 35 years of age because their serum immunoglobulin levels are severely reduced.

A variety of immune deficiencies have been observed in affected individuals. In some cases the number of mature B cells is reduced; usually, however, B-cell levels are normal and the intrinsic defect appears to be in the differentiation of mature B cells into functional antibody-secreting plasma cells. A variety of defects could render plasma cells unable to synthesize the secreted form of the antibody molecule. For example, a defect in polyadenylation of the primary Ig transcript might prevent the loss of the M1 and M2 exons, which is necessary for the expression of secreted antibody (see Figure 8-21). In other cases defective heavy-chain glycosylation may prevent secretion of antibodies by plasma cells. Another possibility is that B cells in CVH patients lack receptors for the cytokines that trigger the activation and differentiation of B cells into antibody-secreting cells (see Figure 14-12). Alternatively, the defect may be in the T cells that play a role in the humoral response. Some CVH patients, for example, have been shown to have defective T_H cells that cannot mediate B-cell activation and differentiation. In contrast, other patients have an excess of T cells that may act as suppressors and prevent plasma cells from secreting immunoglobulin.

Selective Immunoglobulin Deficiencies

Some immunodeficiency disorders involve a deficiency in a single immunoglobulin class or subclass. Most common is a selective IgA deficiency, which occurs in 1 in 600–800 people. Although some affected individuals are completely asymptomatic, many develop recurrent respiratory infections and gastrointestinal symptoms of malabsorption and infection. This is not surprising in view of the important role of secretory IgA in the mucous secretions of the respiratory and gastrointestinal tracts. Affected individuals also have an increased incidence of severe allergic reactions, presumably due to increased penetration of allergens through mucosal surfaces and subsequent stimulation of IgE production. The B cells of patients with IgA deficiency generally bear membrane IgA; the defect appears to be in the maturation of these cells into IgA-secreting plasma cells. It is not known whether the defect is in the B cell itself or whether the defect is at the level of T-cell help. It has been suggested that there may be a decrease in IL-5 or TGF-β, which are known to mediate a class switch to IgA. In some cases the defect has been shown in vitro to be caused by T-cell–mediated suppression of IgA production by B cells.

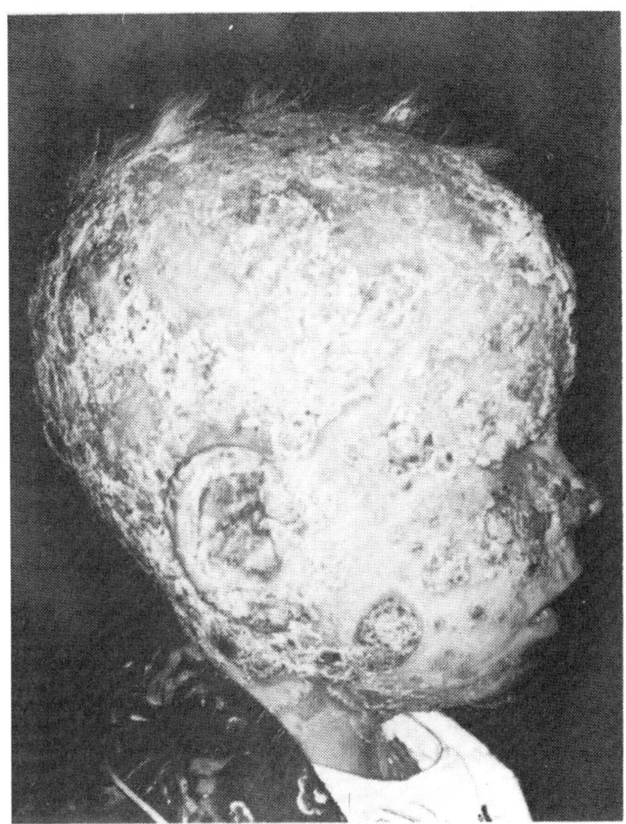

FIGURE 22-3 Chronic cutaneous candidiasis in a boy with defective cell-mediated immunity. [From R. J. Schlegel et al., 1970, *Pediatrics* **45**:926.]

Cell-Mediated Deficiencies

Because of the central role of T cells in the immune system, a T-cell deficiency can affect both the humoral and the cell-mediated responses. The impact on the cell-mediated system can be severe, with a reduction in both delayed-type hypersensitive responses and cell-mediated cytotoxicity. Whereas defects in the humoral system are associated primarily with infections by encapsulated bacteria, defects in the cell-mediated system are associated with increased susceptibility to viral, protozoan, and fungal infections. Intracellular pathogens such as *Candida albicans* (Figure 22-3), *Pneumocystis carinii,* and *Mycobacteria* are often implicated, reflecting the importance of T cells in eliminating intracellular pathogens. Infections with viruses that are rarely pathogenic for the normal individual (such as cytomegalovirus or even an attenuated measles vaccine) may be life-threatening for those with impaired cell-mediated immunity. T-cell defects generally affect the humoral system, too, because of the requirement for T_H cells in B-cell activation. Generally there is some decrease in antibody levels, particularly in the production of specific antibody following immunization.

DiGeorge Syndrome (Congenital Thymic Aplasia)

In 1965 DiGeorge first described a syndrome characterized by the absence of a thymus; hypoparathyroidism, cardiovascular anomalies, characteristic facial features (Figure 22-4), and increased incidence of infections. The syndrome reflects a failure of the third and fourth pharyngeal pouches to develop between 10 and 12 weeks of gestation, a time when several organs, including the aortic arch of the heart, are developing. Children born with this defect often have seizures on the first day of life due to low calcium in the blood, a result of the hypoparathyroid condition. Cardiac defects are the most common cause of death. If the child survives the neonatal period, increased susceptibility to various opportunistic infections is observed. Generally these children have effective humoral immunity against common bacterial infections but are extremely susceptible to viral, protozoan, and fungal infections; even the common attenuated measles vaccine may be life-threatening to affected children.

Evaluation of children with complete DiGeorge syndrome reveals a severe decrease in the total number of T cells, which can be demonstrated by flow cytometry. Functionally, there is an absence of T_{DTH} skin-test reactivity to common antigens, a decreased response to T-cell mitogens such as PHA, and decreased responsiveness to allogeneic cells in the

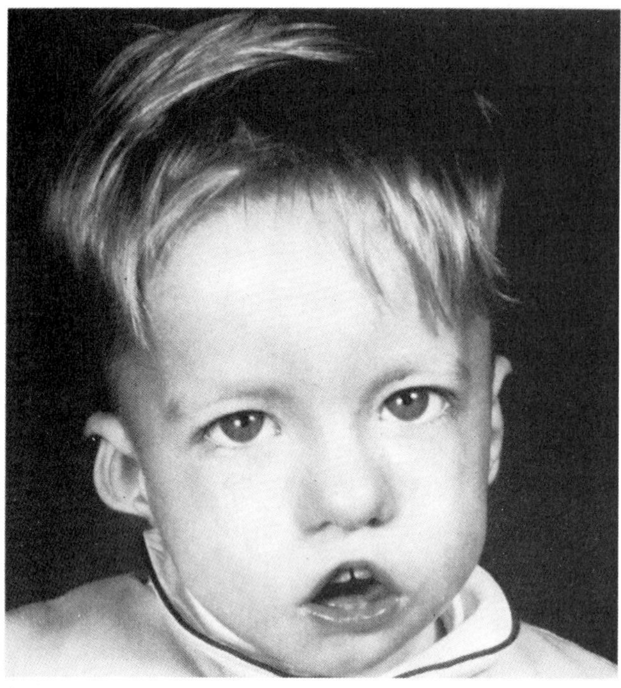

FIGURE 22-4 A child with DiGeorge syndrome showing characteristic dysplasia of ears and mouth and abnormally long distance between the eyes. [From F. S. Rosen, in R. Kretschmer et al., 1968, *New Engl. J. Med.* **279**:1295.]

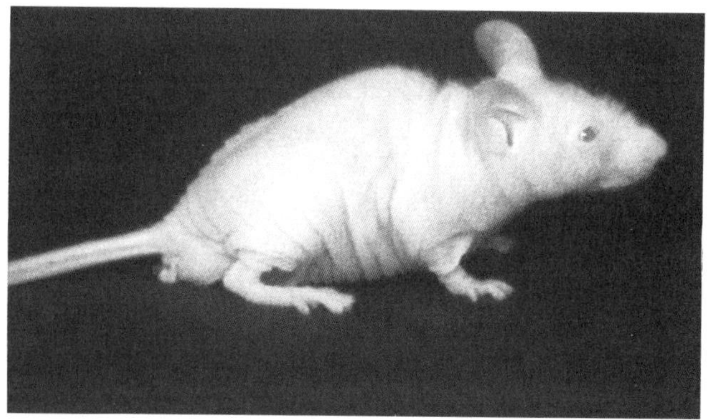

FIGURE 22-5 A nude mouse *(nu/nu)*. [Courtesy of Jackson Laboratories.]

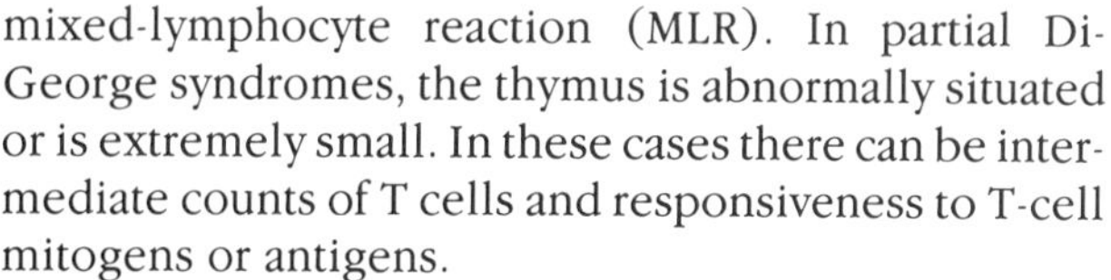

mixed-lymphocyte reaction (MLR). In partial DiGeorge syndromes, the thymus is abnormally situated or is extremely small. In these cases there can be intermediate counts of T cells and responsiveness to T-cell mitogens or antigens.

Treatment for DiGeorge syndrome involves the grafting of fetal thymus tissue. The age of the thymus tissue is important: fetal thymuses older than 14 weeks of gestation should not be used because they have T cells that can cause graft-versus-host disease in the immune-suppressed recipient. The grafted thymic tissue provides a source of thymic hormones and a cellular environment in which T-cell stem cells can mature and differentiate. Once mature T cells are formed, unfortunately, the grafted thymus can sometimes be rejected by the very cells it helped to mature.

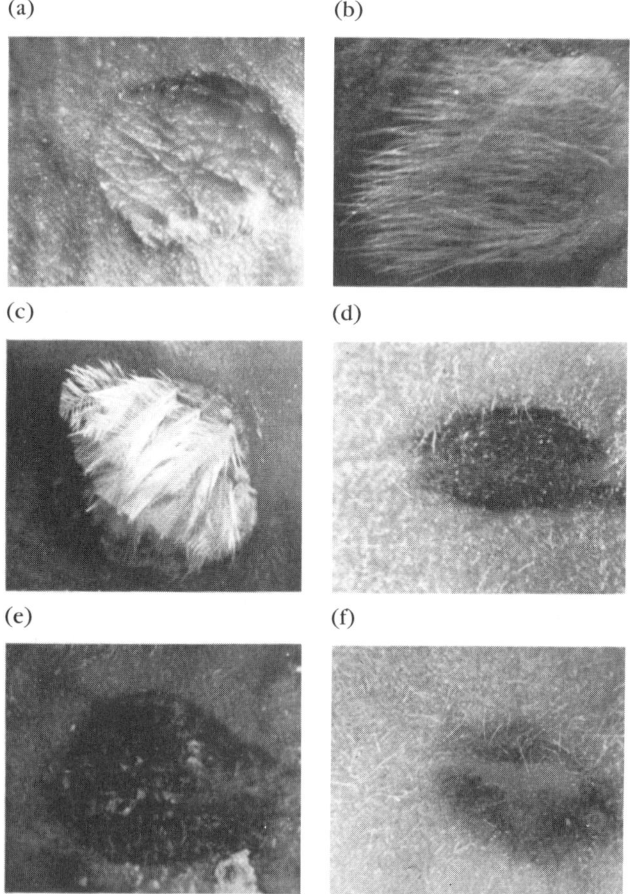

FIGURE 22-6 Grafts from other species (xenogeneic grafts) accepted by nude mice. The figure shows mice with the following grafts: (a) human skin after 60 days; (b) cat skin after 51 days; (c) chicken skin with feathers at 32 days; (d) chameleon skin at 41 days; (e) lizard skin at 28 days; and (f) tree frog skin at 40 days. [From D. D. Manning et al., 1973, *J. Exp. Med.* **138**:488.]

Nude Mice

An autosomal recessive thymic defect in mice resembles DiGeorge syndrome. Among the many defects exhibited by these mice is an absence of hair follicles, and they are called *nude* mice because of their strange hairless state (Figure 22-5). What makes these mice interesting from an immunologic perspective is that they lack a thymus or have a vestigial thymus and show varying degrees of cell-mediated immunodeficiency. The defect is inherited and controlled by a recessive gene on chromosome 11; *nu/nu* homozygotes are hairless and lack a thymus, whereas *nu/+* heterozygotes are normal. This homozygous recessive gene has been bred into several inbred mouse strains, and these animals have served as important model systems. Because these mice lack a thymus, the pre-T cells fail to mature and there is a marked absence of cell-mediated immunity. This lack of a functioning cell-mediated response is best demonstrated in these mice by their ability to accept foreign skin grafts. Even xenogeneic grafts of human skin or chicken skin, feathers and all, are accepted by nude mice (Figure 22-6).

Combined Humoral and Cell-Mediated Deficiencies

As one might expect, combined deficiencies of the humoral and cell-mediated branches are the most serious of the immunodeficiency disorders (see Table 22-1). The onset of infections begins early in infancy and the prognosis for these infants is early death unless some therapeutic intervention reconstitutes the defective immune system. Considerable success has been achieved with bone marrow transplantation from HLA-matched donors.

Reticular Dysgenesis

Reticular dysgenesis is a rare, fatal congenital disease in which the lymphoid and myeloid stem cells fail to differentiate during hematopoiesis. Children born with this defect lack phagocytic cells of the monocyte and granulocyte series and also T and B lymphocytes. The developmental failure must therefore be at a very early stage in hematopoiesis, before the stem cell differentiates into separate lymphoid and myeloid lineages (see Figure 22-1). Children born with this disorder die shortly after birth.

Bare-Lymphocyte Syndrome

Several severe combined immunodeficiency diseases caused by a deficiency in expression of MHC molecules are collectively referred to as *bare-lymphocyte syndrome*. These disorders are classified into three types: Type I bare-lymphocyte syndrome involves defective class I MHC expression; type II syndrome, defective class II MHC expression; and type III syndrome, defective class I and class II MHC expression. The absence or reduced levels of MHC molecules impairs antigen presentation to T cells. Consequently, individuals born with bare-lymphocyte syndrome suffer recurrent bacterial and viral infections and often die by 5 years of age.

The defect causing type II bare-lymphocyte syndrome has begun to be unraveled at the molecular level. Antigen-presenting cells (e.g., B cells, macrophages, dendritic cells), which normally express class II MHC molecules, do not do so in patients with the type II syndrome. Moreover, IFN-γ, which induces increased class II MHC expression in normal individuals, does not induce class II expression in patients with this syndrome. The observation that none of the three class II MHC molecules (DP, DQ, and DR) is expressed in affected individuals suggests that the genes encoding these molecules are regulated coordinately. As discussed in Chapter 9, regulation of MHC expression depends in part on DNA-binding proteins (transcription factors) that bind to the promoters associated with each MHC gene. The finding that the *DP, DQ,* and *DR* promoters contain several conserved motifs suggests that each of these class II genes is activated by binding of the same transcription factor(s). A defect in binding of this factor to the conserved class II MHC promoter motif would lead to the coordinated loss of all three class II molecules observed in bare-lymphocyte syndrome. A study by C. J. Kara and L. H. Glimcher provides some support for this hypothesis. These researchers showed that some cases of bare-lymphocyte syndrome were caused by a defect in the class II MHC promoter region, causing the chromatin structure to be less accessible to DNA-binding proteins. They speculated that the loss of a common DNA-binding factor in bare-lymphocyte syndrome may render the DNA less accessible to other transcriptional activating factors.

Severe Combined Immunodeficiency Disease

A group of diseases characterized by markedly depressed counts of T cells and B cells is referred to as *severe combined immunodeficiency disease (SCID)*. This disorder is associated with increased susceptibility to viral, bacterial, fungal, and protozoan diseases; a failure to thrive and reduced weight gain are also usually observed. The degree of immune compromise is so severe that organisms that are nonpathogenic for the normal individual can cause serious or even life-threatening infections in the SCID patient. Infants born with SCID generally develop recurrent infections at 3–6 months of age. The most common manifestations are pneumonia due to *Pneumocystis carinii,* prolonged diarrhea due to rotavirus or bacterial infections of the gastrointestinal tract, and moniliasis caused by the common yeast, *Candida albicans.* These children are so severely compromised that even attenuated vaccines such as the oral Sabin polio vaccine or the measles vaccine can cause progressive infection and death. The disease received national attention in the 1970s when the plight of a boy named David, who lived inside a sterile plastic bubble, was much publicized.

Individuals with SCID exhibit structural and functional abnormalities in both the humoral and cell-mediated branches of the immune system. Recirculating lymphocyte counts generally are dramatically reduced; the tonsils usually are absent; peripheral lymph nodes are absent or extremely small; and the usual thymic shadow does not show on an x-ray. Functional abnormalities in SCID patients generally include quite low antibody levels, negative skin test for delayed-type hypersensitivity, little if any proliferation in mitogen-stimulation assays, and markedly reduced cytokine production.

Over half of all SCID cases result from an X-linked recessive defect; the remaining cases are caused by an autosomal recessive defect (see Table 22-1). The basic defect in most forms of human SCID has not been established. Possible causes include a defect in stem-cell differentiation or a defect in thymic and bone marrow processing. Bone marrow transplantation from HLA-identical siblings has successfully reconstituted the immune system in some SCID children. Because 60% of SCID patients do not have HLA-identical siblings, marrow from haploidentical parental donors often is administered. The problem with HLA-mismatched bone marrow is that fatal graft-versus-host disease can develop. This fatal reaction can be avoided by treating the donor bone marrow with monoclonal anti-T-cell antibody plus complement to deplete T cells prior to transplantation.

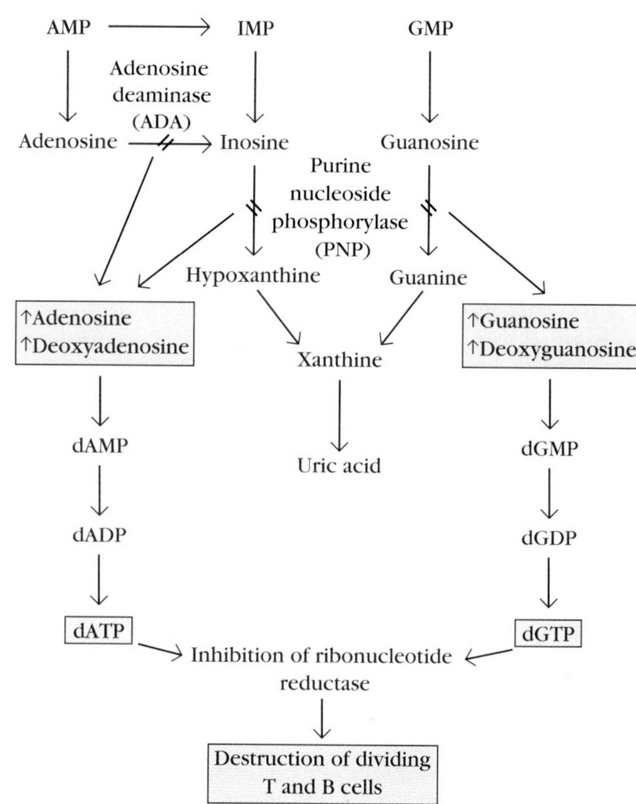

FIGURE 22-7 Molecular basis of severe combined immunodeficiency disease resulting from genetic defect in adenosine deaminase (ADA) or purine nucleoside phosphorylase (PNP). The normal pathway of AMP and GMP degradation, which yields uric acid, involves steps catalyzed by ADA and PNP; the latter enzyme acts on both inosine and guanosine. The accumulation of dGTP and/or dATP in the absence of PNP or ADA, respectively, leads to inhibition of ribonucleotide reductase and the selective killing of dividing T and B cells.

ADA Deficiency and PNP Deficiency

The defects causing two autosomal recessive forms of SCID have been established. In both cases the disease results from an inherited deficiency of an enzyme—either adenosine deaminase (ADA) or purine nucleoside phosphorylase (PNP). A deficiency of PNP or ADA results in accumulation of dGTP and/or dATP, respectively; both of these metabolites are selectively toxic to dividing B and T cells (Figure 22-7). Thus individuals with either ADA or PNP deficiency have markedly reduced counts of mature B and T cells.

Patients with ADA deficiency have been treated successfully with infusions of the purified enzyme, and in 1990 the first gene therapy in humans was performed in two young girls suffering from ADA-deficiency SCID. The gene therapy was accomplished with a retrovirus in which key retroviral genes had been replaced with the *ADA* gene. The patients' bone marrow cells were removed and infected in vitro with the engineered retrovirus; the genetically altered bone marrow cells then were reinfused back into the little girls. A major limitation with this technique has been the inability to identify and isolate the pluripotent stem cell in humans (see Chapter 3). Because the hematopoietic cells carrying the engineered ADA gene are not pluripotent, they are not capable of self-renewal; for this reason this therapy has short-term effects only and must be repeated every few months. A report in *Science,* dated October 1992, indicated that both girls were doing well with fully functioning immune systems. A similar gene therapy was used more recently to treat a newborn baby boy born with ADA-deficiency SCID. In this case, however, cord blood was used since it contains a rich supply of stem cells. The 4-day-old infant was injected with cord blood cells containing the engineered ADA gene. If the gene was inserted into pluripotent stem cells, then a long-term cure may be achieved.

Scid *Mice and* Scid*-Human Mice*

An autosomal recessive mutation resulting in severe combined immunodeficiency disease developed spontaneously in CB-17 mice. Like humans with this disease, CB-17 *scid* mice fail to develop mature T and B cells; these mice can be kept alive by housing them in a sterile environment. When normal mouse bone marrow cells are injected into *scid* mice, normal T and B cells develop. These mice have proven to be a valuable model system for the study of immunodeficiency and hematopoiesis. The defect in CB-17 *scid* mice is in the recombinase enzyme machinery that normally catalyzes functional rearrangements of variable-region gene segments in immunoglobulin and T-cell receptor DNA. As illustrated in Figure 8-9, *scid* mice have a defect in joining of the D and J coding sequences resulting in the deletion of one or both of the coding sequences. Interest in *scid* mice has mushroomed recently with the development of *scid*-human mice (see Figure 2-1).

Wiskott-Aldrich Syndrome

Wiskott-Aldrich syndrome (WAS), an X-linked recessive disease affecting boys, is characterized by a spectrum of abnormalities including eczema, thrombocytopenia, increased susceptibility to bacterial infections, and bloody diarrhea. Patients with this syndrome have normal levels of IgG, low levels of IgM, and elevated levels of IgA and IgE. They generally exhibit an absence of isohemagglutinins and fail to produce antibodies to polysaccharide antigens in general. The absence of antibodies to polysaccharide antigens leaves these patients at risk for infections with encapsulated pyogenic bacteria. T-cell function is variable and tends to get progressively worse as WAS patients grow older; most patients do not exhibit cutaneous delayed-type hypersensitivity. Lymphocytes from WAS patients are smaller and have fewer microvilli than normal lymphocytes. These morphologic abnormalities result from an alteration in or complete absence of a cell-membrane glycoprotein called sialophorin (CD43). WAS patients have been treated successfully with bone marrow transplantation.

Complement Deficiencies

Immunodeficiency diseases resulting from defects in the complement system are discussed in Chapter 17. Many complement deficiencies are associated with increased susceptibility to bacterial infections and/or immune-complex diseases (see Table 17-9).

Summary

1. Immunodeficiency diseases can affect any component of the immune system. Disorders involving the phagocytic system, complement system, humoral system, or cell-mediated system have all been reported.

2. Phagocytic disorders can result from quantitative deficiencies (agranulocytosis or neutropenia) or from a functional defect in one of the steps of phagocytosis (leukocyte adhesion, chemotaxis, phagocytosis, or killing). Examples include congenital agranulocytosis, leukocyte-adhesion deficiency, lazy-leukocyte syndrome, and chronic granulomatous disease.

3. Humoral immunodeficiencies can result from defects in B-cell maturation, intrinsic defects of mature B cells, ineffective T_H-cell activation, or inappropriate suppression by T cells. Examples of humoral deficiencies include X-linked agammaglobulinemia, X-linked hyper-IgM syndrome, common variable immunodeficiency, and selective IgA deficiency.

4. Cell-mediated immunodeficiencies can result from defective T-cell maturation due to thymic aplasia. DiGeorge syndrome is an example of a cell-mediated immune defect.

5. Combined humoral and cell-mediated immunodeficiencies can result from defects in stem-cell differentiation (reticular dysgenesis), from failure to express MHC molecules (bare-lymphocyte syndrome), from defective T- and B-cell maturation (severe combined immunodeficiency disease), or from deficiencies in adenosine deaminase or purine nucleoside phosphorylase, which result in selective killing of T and B cells (ADA-deficiency SCID and PNP-deficiency SCID).

References

ANDERSON, D. C., and T. A. SPRINGER. 1987. Leukocyte adhesion deficiency: an inherited defect in the Mac-1, LFA-1 and p150,95 glycoproteins. *Annu. Rev. Med.* **38**:175.

BOSMA, M. J., and A. M. CARROLL. 1991. The scid mouse mutant: definition, characterization, and potential uses. *Annu. Rev. Immunol.* **9**:323.

CONLEY, M. E. 1992. Molecular approaches to analysis of X-linked immunodeficiencies. *Annu. Rev. Immunol.* **10**:215.

COURNOYER, D., and C. T. CASKEY. 1993. Gene therapy of the immune system. *Annu. Rev. Immunol.* **11**:297.

HOLZMANN, B., and I. L. WEISSMAN. 1989. Integrin molecules involved in lymphocyte homing to Peyer's patches. *Immunol. Rev.* **108**:45.

KANTOFF, P. W., S. M. FREEMAN, and W. F. ANDERSON. 1988. Prospects for gene therapy for immunodeficiency diseases. *Annu. Rev. Immunol.* **6**:581.

KARA, C. J., and L. H. GLIMCHER. 1991. In vivo footprinting of MHC class II genes: bare promoters in the bare lymphocyte syndrome. *Science* **252**:709.

MALYNN, B. A., J. K. BLACKWELL, G. M. FULOP, et al. 1988. The *scid* defect affects the final step of the immunoglobulin VDJ recombinase mechanism. *Cell* **54**:453.

MCCUNE, J. M., R. NAMIKAWA, H. KANESHIMA, et al. 1988. The SCID-Hu mouse: murine model for the analysis of human hematolymphoid differentiation and function. *Science* **241**:1632.

ROSEN, F. S., M. D. COOPER, and R. J. WEDGWOOD. 1984. The primary immunodeficiencies. *New Eng. J. Med.* **311**:235 and 300.

SPICKETT, G. P., and J. FARRANT. 1989. The role of lymphokines in common variable hypogammaglobulinemia. *Immunol. Today* **10**(6):192.

THOMPSON, L. 1992. At age 2, gene therapy enters a growth phase. *Science* **258**:744.

VERMA, I. M. 1990. Gene therapy. *Sci. Am.* **263**(5):68.

YANCOPOULOS, G. D., and F. W. ALT. 1988. Reconstruction of an immune system. *Science* **241**:1581.

YEDNOCK, T. A., and S. R. ROSEN. 1989. Lymphocyte homing. *Adv. Immunol.* **44**:313.

Study Questions

1. Indicate whether each of the following statements is true or false. If you think a statement is false, explain why.
   a. DiGeorge syndrome is a congenital birth defect resulting in absence of the thymus.
   b. X-linked agammaglobulinemia (XLA) is a combined B-cell and T-cell immunodeficiency disease.
   c. The hallmark of a phagocytic deficiency is increased susceptibility to viral infections.
   d. In chronic granulomatous disease, H_2O_2 produced by catalase-negative bacteria results in bacterial killing in the defective granulocytes.
   e. Gamma-globulin injections are given to treat individuals with X-linked agammaglobulinemia.
   f. D_H-J_H joining is defective in CB-17 *scid* mice.
   g. Mice with the *scid* defect lack functional B and T lymphocytes.
   h. A thymic transplant can restore the immune defect in CB-17 *scid* mice.
   i. Children born with DiGeorge syndrome often manifest increased infections with encapsulated bacteria.
   j. Failure to express class II MHC molecules in bare-lymphocyte syndrome affects cell-mediated immunity only.

2. Granulocytes from patients with leukocyte-adhesion deficiency (LAD) express greatly reduced amounts of three integrin molecules designated CR3, CR4, and LFA-1.
   a. What is the nature of the defect that results in decreased or in no expression of these receptors in LAD patients?
   b. What is the normal function of the integrin molecule LFA-1? Give specific examples.
   c. Would you expect LAD patients to exhibit normal levels of specific antibody following antigenic challenge? Explain your answer.

3. a. Do rearranged Ig heavy-chain genes in *scid* mice differ from those in normal mice?
   b. In *scid* mice, rearrangement of κ light-chain DNA is not attempted. Explain why.
   c. If you introduced a functional μ heavy-chain gene into *scid* progenitor B cells by a gene-transfer method, would the κ light-chain DNA undergo a normal rearrangement? Explain your answer.
   d. If you compared gene rearrangements in TCR α- and β-chain DNA in T-cell thymomas derived from *scid* mice and normal CB-17 mice, what differences would you detect?

4. As indicated in several chapters, *scid*-human mice are a valuable experimental system for studying human lymphoid cells within an animal model.
   a. Describe the procedure for preparing *scid*-human mice.
   b. Why are human fetal liver cells used in this procedure?
   c. Why are the human cells not rejected by the recipient mouse?
   d. Why does graft-versus-host disease not develop in the recipient mouse?

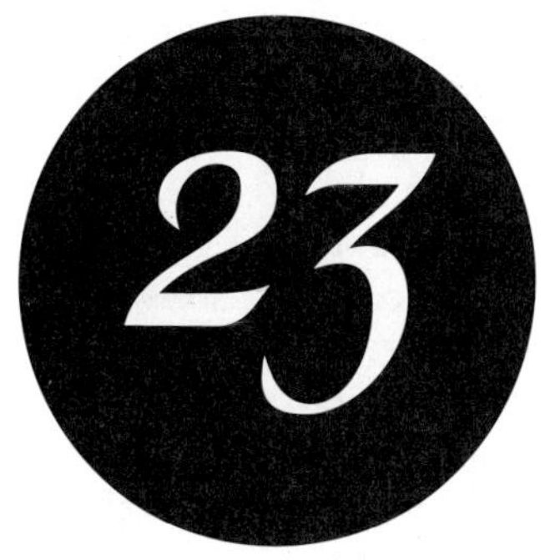

THE IMMUNE SYSTEM IN AIDS

Since the early 1980s, the spread of the disease now known as acquired immunodeficiency syndrome (AIDS) has been dramatic. Many predict that AIDS eventually will cause millions of deaths and sorely stress health care systems worldwide in the next decade or two. AIDS —the epitome of an acquired immunodeficiency disease—renders its victims susceptible to various opportunistic infections and rare forms of cancer, which are the immediate cause of death. As the number of reported AIDS cases escalated, the acquisition of scientific information about AIDS exhibited a comparable surge, with reports in the scientific literature increasing logarithmically from 1982 to the present. Never has so much been learned about a disease and its causative agent in such a short time. This explosion of information about AIDS has expanded our understanding about the immune system to such an extent that this entire chapter is devoted to AIDS, the immunodeficiences associated with it, and efforts to develop AIDS vaccines.

Discovery of AIDS and Its Causative Agent

In the summer of 1981, five cases of *Pneumocystis carinii* pneumonia, all in young homosexual men from the same area of Los Angeles, were reported to the Centers for Disease Control (CDC), the agency of the U.S. Public Health Service responsible for monitoring infectious diseases in the United States. Soon after, the CDC began to get reports of *Pneumocystis carinii* pneumonia, Kaposi's sarcoma, and various opportunistic infections clustered in young homosexual men living in New York City, San Francisco, and Los Angeles. *Pneumocystis carinii* had been known as a widespread, generally harmless protozoan rarely associated with pneumonia; Kaposi's sarcoma had been recognized as a rare tumor of blood-vessel tissue associated with aging. What caught the attention of the CDC was that these diseases had previously been limited to individuals with impaired cell-mediated immunity. Such diseases might be expected in individuals born with immune deficiencies, in transplant recipients receiving immunosuppressive drugs, or in cancer patients receiving chemotherapy, but their presence in young and previously healthy men with no obvious condition that would impair immunity was alarming. In December 1981, reports in the *New England Journal of Medicine* confirmed the linkage to immune-system compromise by demonstrating that the original victims of the still-unnamed disorder had decreased counts of $CD4^+$ T cells. In early 1982 the CDC suggested that this distinct new disorder be called *acquired immunodeficiency syndrome,* now commonly known as AIDS. The syndrome appeared to be a collection of symptoms associated with an immune-system deficiency that was not inborn or imposed but somehow acquired.

Incidence of AIDS

Although AIDS was first identified in homosexual men in the United States, it was soon observed in other groups, including users of intravenous (IV) drugs, hemophiliacs, recipients of blood transfusions, sexual partners of AIDS patients, and eventually in infants of mothers with the disease. Such findings suggested that AIDS was transmissible; in order to monitor the disease, the CDC asked in 1982 that all AIDS cases be reported. Since that time the spectrum of clinical disease has broadened as the number of reported cases has increased exponentially. What began as five cases reported in a CDC newsletter in 1981 mushroomed to staggering proportions within a few years. Between 1980 and 1985 there were an estimated 70,000 cases of AIDS worldwide; by 1986 to 1988 the number of AIDS cases had risen to 300,000; and by 1992 there were 612,000 cases. In the United States, a total of 242,146 AIDS cases had been reported as of December 1992, and projected estimates forecast 500,000 cases by 1995. The CDC estimated that, by the early 1990s, 1–2 million Americans had been infected with the virus that causes AIDS. In 1993, conservative estimates by the World Health Organization suggested that 12 million people are infected worldwide. As shown in Figure 23-1, the greatest number of infected individuals live in Africa, but the incidence of infection is predicted to increase most dramatically in Asia during the remainder of this decade. The estimated rate of infection among women is substantially lower than that in men in the Americas and Western Europe, but not in sub-Saharan Africa (Table 23-1). The high rates of infection among men and the likely increase in infection rates among women and children portend widespread economic and social disaster unless effective interventions are developed.

Identification of Human Immunodeficiency Virus (HIV)

Initial attempts to identify the cause of AIDS in homosexual men focused on a number of hypotheses. Sperm was known to be immunosuppressive, and some investigators suggested that the entry of sperm antigens into the blood through rectal tearing might account for the immunosuppression seen in AIDS. Others thought that antigen overload might in itself suppress the immune system. In addition, amyl nitrite, a sexual stimulant used by some homosexuals, was known to have immunosuppressive capabilities. However, the development of AIDS in hemophiliacs who had received injections of factor VIII from pooled and concentrated human plasma began to point to a viral agent. Several known viruses such as Epstein-Barr virus and cytomegalovirus were considered. It was not long, however, before a new retrovirus was identified as being associated with AIDS by several independent groups.

Luc Montagnier's group at the Pasteur Institute isolated a retrovirus from a patient manifesting persistent generalized lymphadenopathy in 1983 and called it *LAV* for lymphadenopathy-associated virus. In 1984 Robert Gallo's group at the National Cancer Institute identified a retrovirus that was called *HTLV-III* for human T-cell lymphotrophic virus type III. The virus was independently identified by Jay Levy's group at the University of California at San Francisco and called *ARV* (AIDS-related virus). Subsequent studies revealed that the three viral isolates were the same virus. For a while all three names were used in the literature, leading to some confusion. Then, in 1986, an international committee renamed the virus *human immunodeficiency virus,* or *HIV.* Following the discovery of an antigenic variant in 1986, the original virus was designated HIV-1 and the variant was designated HIV-2. Both HIV-1 and HIV-2 are genetically related to the simian immunodeficiency viruses (SIVs), which are found in African primates.

Evolutionary Relationships of HIV

The retroviruses can be divided into two groups: transforming and cytopathic. The *transforming retroviruses* induce changes in cell growth that lead to

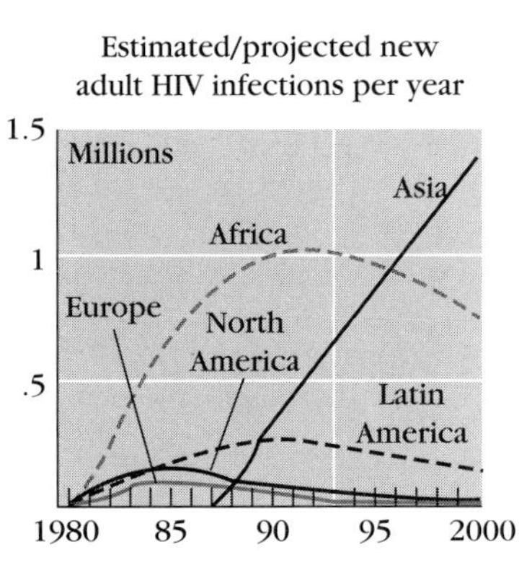

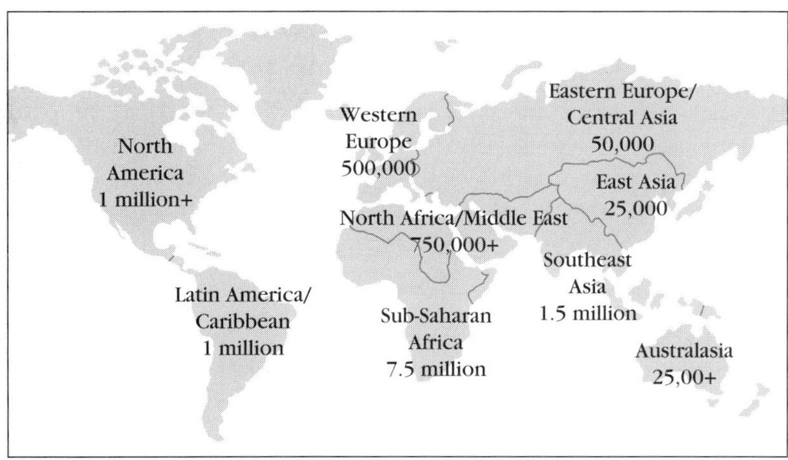

FIGURE 23-1 Estimated incidence and distribution of infection with HIV, the virus causing AIDS. [Data from World Health Organization, 1993; adapted from *Newsweek,* March 22, 1993.]

cancer. These viruses often carry genes, called *oncogenes,* that influence cellular growth. Included in this group are bovine leukemia virus, avian type C virus, mammalian type C virus, and human T-cell lymphotrophic virus type 1 and 2 (HTLV-1 and HTLV-2). The best studied of this group is HTLV-1 which causes T-cell leukemia. This retrovirus does not carry an oncogene, but it induces cancer nevertheless. Infection of T lymphocytes with HTLV-1 causes the cells to begin to express the high-affinity receptor for IL-2; as the cell secretes IL-2, it autostimulates its own division in an unregulated way, causing T-cell leukemia (see Figure 25-4).

The *cytopathic retroviruses* are members of the lentivirus family. One branch of this group includes visna virus, caprine arthritis encephalitis virus, equine infectious anemia virus, and feline immunodeficiency virus. The other branch of this group includes human immunodeficiency virus (HIV-1 and HIV-2) and simian immunodeficiency virus (SIV). HIV-1 infection is epidemic in Central Africa, the Americas, Western Europe, North Africa, the Middle East, Haiti, and Southeast Asia (see Figure 23-1). This virus infects humans, chimpanzees, and the pigtailed macaque but causes immune suppression only in humans and the pigtailed macaque. How infected chimpanzees escape immune suppression is unknown. HIV-2 was originally isolated from samples that originated in Senegal in West Africa. Infection with HIV-2 is endemic in many countries of West Africa; it generally is much rarer in other parts of the world, although a small number of cases of HIV-2 infection have been reported in Europe and the Americas. Most HIV-2 strains appear to spread more slowly and to be less pathogenic that HIV-1. HIV-2, which infects humans, chimpanzees, macaque monkeys, and baboons, also has a broader host range than HIV-1. Infection of macaque monkeys with some strains of HIV-2 results in symptoms of immune suppression and holds promise as an animal model for AIDS.

Various strains of simian immunodeficiency viruses have been isolated from different African primates: SIV_{AGM} from African green monkeys, SIV_{MND} from mandrills, SIV_{MAC} from captive macaque (rhesus) monkeys, SIV_{SM} from captive sooty mangabeys, and SIV_{CPZ} from wild chimpanzees. SIV_{AGM} is present in an estimated 40% of the African green monkey population in some parts of Africa. Although SIV_{AGM} infection of African green monkeys does not cause immune suppression, injection of SIV_{AGM} into macaques leads to a fatal AIDS-like disease (called *simian AIDS,* or *SAIDS*) and to death within 3–36 months. Comparisons of the DNA sequences of various HIV-1, HIV-2, and SIV isolates have revealed that both HIV-1 and HIV-2 are more closely related to SIV than to each other. For example, HIV-1 and HIV-2 exhibit only 40–50% DNA sequence homology, whereas HIV-2 has 75% homology with strains of SIV_{SM}, SIV_{MAC}, and SIV_{AGM}.

TABLE 23-1 ESTIMATED PROPORTION OF MEN AND WOMEN INFECTED WITH HIV*

	Men	Women
North America	1 in 75	1 in 700
South America	1 in 125	1 in 500
Western Europe	1 in 200	1 in 1400
Sub-Saharan Africa	1 in 40	1 in 40

* Incidence by sex is for adults aged 15 to 49.
SOURCE: WHO Communicable Disease Scotland Weekly Report 25/8/90 and *Science,* 1991, **252**:372.

Origin of HIV and Initial Appearance of AIDS

The presence of SIV in several African primate species and the discovery of the sequence homology between SIV and HIV led to speculation that HIV arose from SIV. According to this hypothesis, SIV arose first as a nonpathogenic lentivirus in African nonhuman primates, was transmitted to humans, and then gave rise to HIV. Some evidence in support of cross-species transfer of SIV has been reported. For example, four technicians working in primate research laboratories have been shown to be infected with SIV. No one knows whether these individuals will develop AIDS, but their SIV infection demonstrates the possibility of cross-species transmission.

One hypothesis concerning the introduction of SIV into humans was proposed by an anthropologist who studied the Idjiwi tribe of eastern Zaire. Members of this tribe apply monkey blood to the pubic area as a part of an initiation ritual. If the monkey blood contained SIV, human infection may have occurred during initiation rituals. Some believe that SIV may have begun to spread in Africa after the Second World War when antibiotics began to be given by syringes. Because syringes were often in limited supply, they were generally reused and may have served as a means to transmit the virus from a rural population, such as the Idjiwi tribe, to an urban population where the virus could continue to spread by sexual contact.

A second hypothesis that provides a reasonable mechanism for the cross-species transfer of SIV from monkeys to humans appeared in the *Journal of the Royal Society of Medicine* in 1989. The authors suggested that the early polio vaccines may have been contaminated with SIV and administration of infected vaccine to humans may have provided a vehicle for massive cross-species transfer of SIV into humans. Since the first polio vaccine administered in Africa was grown in cultures of kidney cells from African green monkeys, which are known to have a high incidence of SIV infection, the possibility of vaccine contamination appears plausible. Indeed, when two frozen stocks of the early African polio vaccine were tested in 1992, one of the stocks tested positive for SIV.

Many scientists now believe that SIV was introduced into humans in Africa, perhaps on numerous occasions. Following this cross-species transfer, SIV may have mutated into a retrovirus (now known as HIV) not only capable of replicating in humans but also far more pathogenic in humans than SIV. Although the time and place of the initial appearance of AIDS is likely to remain unknown, two findings date HIV as far back as 1959. After the HIV antibody test was developed, a frozen human blood sample collected in 1959 in Zaire was shown to contain antibodies to HIV. Also in 1959 a merchant seaman from Manchester, England, died from pneumonia after an apparent immunologic collapse. Fortunately, some tissue from the dead seaman was preserved in paraffin wax, and in 1990 the PCR technique was used to prove that DNA from HIV was in his bone marrow, spleen, kidney, and pharyngeal mucosa. The seaman's wife and youngest child also died of a similar syndrome, suggesting that the man had infected his wife and that the wife had infected the youngest child during pregnancy. It is unlikely that these two isolated cases in 1959 mark the beginning of AIDS, and one is left wondering how many cases went unnoticed in 1958, 1957. . . . ?

HIV: Structure and Infectious Process

All members of the lentivirus family of retroviruses, including HIV-1, HIV-2, and SIV, share numerous structural and molecular features. These viruses have an RNA genome and two associated molecules of *reverse transcriptase,* which catalyzes the "reverse transcription" of viral RNA into DNA. Surrounding the viral genome are two layers of protein forming a cylindrical protein core. In HIV these core proteins are designated p17 and p24 (Figure 23-2). Surrounding the core is an envelope that the virus acquires from the infected host cell by a process called budding. The host-cell membrane is modified by the insertion of two HIV glycoproteins, gp120 and gp41. The gp41 glycoprotein spans the membrane; gp120 is associated with gp41 but extends beyond the membrane. Both gp120 and gp41 have important roles in the binding of HIV to cells in the infection process.

For quite some time it has been known that the envelope of HIV is studded with human proteins (including class I and class II MHC molecules) acquired by the virus as it buds from the human cell membrane. More recent research has revealed that the level of these human proteins is far greater than had been previously thought. In fact, more human proteins were found on the envelope of HIV than molecules of gp120! This startling finding is discussed later in the chapter.

HIV Infection of Target Cells

Entry of HIV into target cells involves two steps: binding of virions to receptors on target cells followed by fusion of the viral envelope with the plasma membrane of the target cells. The two envelope glycoproteins—

(a)

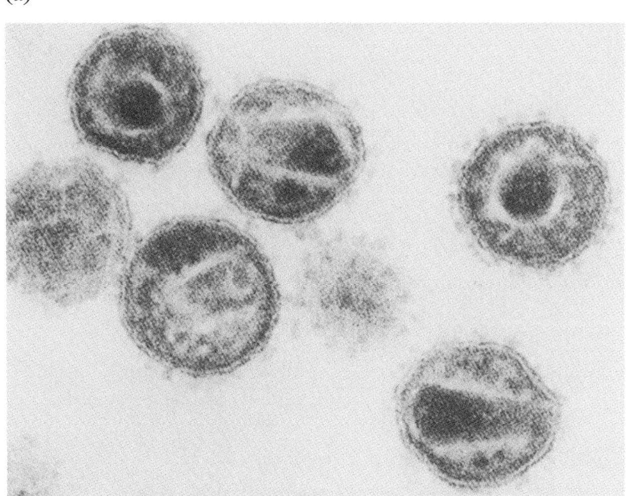

(b)

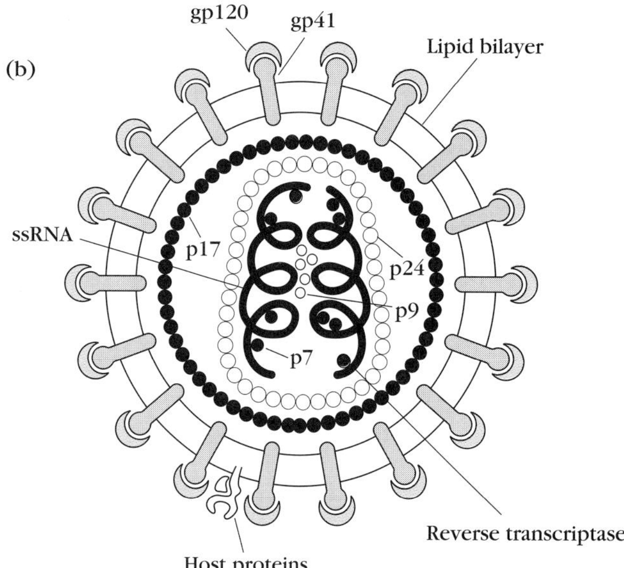

FIGURE 23-2 (a) Electron micrograph of HIV virions magnified 200,000 times. The glycoprotein projections are faintly visible as "knobs" extending from the periphery of each virion. (b) Cross-sectional diagram of HIV virion. Each virion expresses 72 glycoprotein projections composed of gp120 (light purple) and gp41 (gray). Gp 41 is a transmembrane molecule that crosses the lipid bilayer of the envelope. Gp120 is noncovalently associated with gp41 and serves as the viral receptor for CD4 on host cells. The viral envelope also contains some host-cell membrane proteins such as class I and class II MHC molecules. Within the envelope is the viral core, or nucleocapsid, which includes a layer of a protein called p17 and an inner layer of a protein called p24. The HIV genome consists of two copies of ssRNA, which are associated with two molecules of reverse transcriptase (dark purple) and nucleoid proteins p7 and p9. [Part (a) from micrograph by Hans Geldenblom of the Robert Koch Institute (Berlin) in R. C. Gallo and L. Montagnier, 1988, *Sci. Am.* **259**:40; part (b) adapted from B. M. Peterlin and P. A. Luciw, 1988, *AIDS* **2**:S29.]

gp120 and gp41—that make up the surface projections on HIV play vital roles in these initial steps in HIV infection. Once inside a target cell, the viral RNA is copied into DNA. The viral DNA is then integrated into the host-cell DNA, forming a *provirus,* which may remain in a latent state or be activated and transcribed into viral proteins.

Entry of HIV into Cells

The first step in HIV infection is binding of viral gp120 to receptors on target cells. The major cellular receptor for HIV is CD4. Because the T_H cell expresses the highest levels of CD4, HIV is said to be *lymphotrophic.* Other cells that bind HIV include macrophages, monocytes, dendritic cells, Langerhans cells, hematopoietic stem cells, certain rectal-lining cells, and microglial cells. These cells express low levels of CD4 and thus can bind less HIV than T_H cells. HIV-1 has a 25-fold higher affinity for CD4 than does HIV-2. The lower binding affinity of HIV-2 for CD4 may account, in part, for its lower pathogenicity compared with HIV-1. The importance of CD4 in HIV binding can be demonstrated by transfecting the gene encoding CD4 into certain cells in tissue culture that lack CD4; such cells, formerly resistant to HIV, become susceptible to HIV after the CD4 gene is transfected into them.

Although CD4 is the high-affinity receptor for HIV, studies have shown that expression of CD4 by a cell is not sufficient for HIV infection. For example, when the gene for human CD4 was transfected into mouse cells, the transfected cells still cannot be infected with HIV even though these cells express CD4 on their membrane. This led to the speculation that some other membrane molecule must participate in the process of HIV entry. At the time that this book went to press an additional membrane receptor for HIV, called CD26, was identified by Ara Hovanessian and his colleagues at the Pasteur Institute. The CD26 receptor has protease activity and binds to another site on gp120. Both CD4 and CD26 binding to gp120 appear to be required for HIV infection. The role of CD26 was demonstrated by showing that mouse cells could be infected by HIV after they were transfected with both CD4 and CD26 genes.

After binding of HIV to its receptors, the viral envelope fuses with the target-cell plasma membrane. The fusion event appears to be induced by a hydrophobic region—called the *fusogenic domain*—near the amino-terminal end of gp41. Following fusion, the HIV nucleocapsid is internalized, and the viral RNA is uncoated, establishing a productive infection (Figure 23-3a, steps 1-4). A model has been proposed for the combined roles of CD4 and CD26 in this process: HIV first binds to CD4 via a conserved *CD4 binding site* on gp120. CD26 then binds to another region on gp120, called the *V-3 loop.* Presumably proteolytic cleavage within the V-3 loop of gp120 induces a conformational change that exposes the fusogenic domain of gp41. The exposed fusogenic domain then mediates fusion of the viral envelope with the target-cell membrane (Figure 23-3b). There is currently a great deal of interest in the role of CD26 in the HIV entry process. Hovanessian reported that when the protease activity of CD26 was blocked that HIV entry was also blocked. This finding raises hope that a new therapeutic approach may soon be developed to block HIV infection.

Integration of HIV into Host Genome

Once the HIV RNA has been introduced into a target cell and uncoated, it is transcribed into DNA by the viral reverse transcriptase enzyme. The viral DNA then integrates into the host-cell genome, forming a *provirus,* which can remain in a *latent state* (see Figure 23-3a, steps 5-7). Integration of the HIV DNA into the host-cell chromosomal DNA is mediated by a viral enzyme called *integrase,* which is packaged together with the reverse transcriptase enzyme in the virion. Once integrated, the viral DNA is permanently associated with the host-cell DNA and is passed on to daughter cells as the cell divides. In the latent state the viral genes are not expressed, and therefore the virus is able to remain hidden from the host immune system.

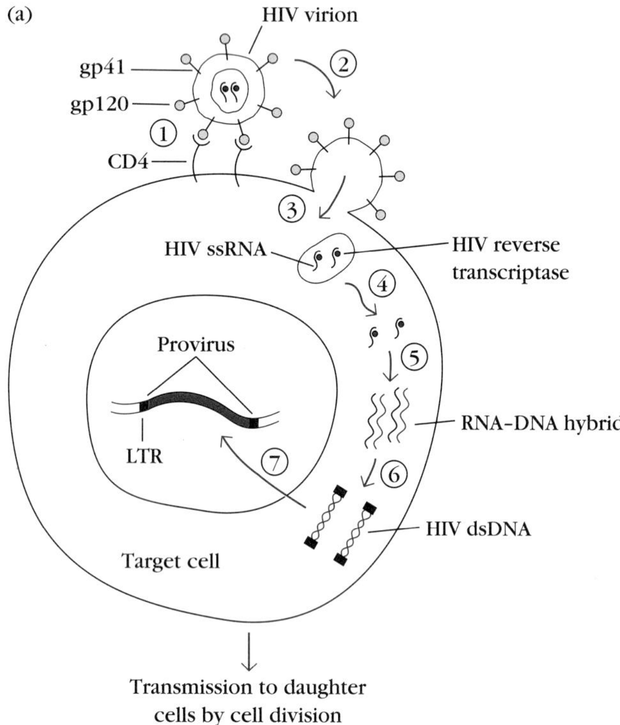

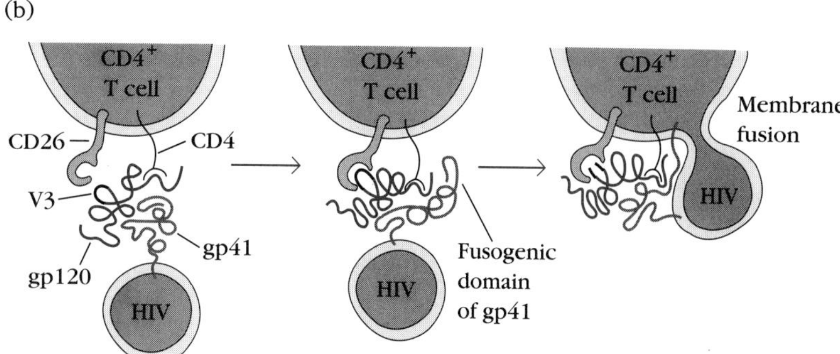

FIGURE 23-3 Entry of HIV into cells and integration of viral DNA. (a) Binding of gp120 to CD4 on the target cell's plasma membrane (1) is followed by fusion (2), allowing entry of the HIV nucleocapsid containing the viral genome (3). The core proteins are removed (4), releasing ssRNA and reverse transcriptase, which copies the ssRNA forming RNA-DNA hybrids (5). After the original RNA template is partially degraded by ribonuclease H, synthesis of the second DNA strand proceeds (6). The viral dsDNA is then translocated to the nucleus and integrated into the host chromosomal DNA by the viral integrase enzyme (7). (b) Proposed model of HIV fusion with a target cell. After viral gp120 (light purple) binds to CD4, the V3-loop (black) binds to CD26 (gray). Proteolytic cleavage of the V3 loop by CD26 induces a conformational change in gp120 and gp41 exposing the fusogenic domain in gp41 (purple). The fusogenic domain then mediates fusion between the viral envelope and target-cell plasma membrane.

Activation of HIV Provirus

The HIV provirus remains in the latent state until events within a virus-infected cell trigger activation of the provirus. Proviral activation initiates transcription of the structural genes into mRNA, which is then translated into viral proteins. As the viral proteins begin to assemble within the host cell, the host-cell plasma membrane is modified by insertion of gp41 and associated gp120. The viral RNA and core proteins then assemble beneath the modified membrane, acquiring the modified host plasma membrane as its envelope in a process called *budding* (Figure 23-4a).

In some cases activation of the HIV provirus and budding of newly assembled viral particles lead to lysis of an infected cell, whereas in other cases an infected cell may survive these events. The level of CD4 expressed on a cell influences the consequences of HIV budding; as viral gp120 is expressed on the cell membrane, it binds to CD4 on the membrane (Figure 23-4b). If the CD4 level is high, this membrane autofusion destroys the membrane's integrity, resulting in lysis and cell death. However, if the CD4 level is low (e.g., in macrophages, monocytes, and dendritic cells), the budding of HIV and subsequent autofusion does not lead to extensive membrane damage, and the cell continues to live producing low levels of HIV.

Role of Infected Cells in HIV Transmission

It is now known that HIV not only binds to but also can infect a rather wide variety of cell types (Table 23-2). HIV can exist as a provirus and replicate in any of these cells; however, as indicated in the previous section, cells that express only low levels of CD4 tend to survive HIV infection. Even though other cells are infected by HIV, T lymphocytes are the major cell type to be depleted as a result of HIV infection. What this means is that other cells, notably macrophages and dendritic cells, can harbor the virus, protecting it from the immune system and serving as a reservoir from which the virus can be transmitted throughout the body or from one individual to another. Examination of lymph nodes from AIDS patients, for example, has shown that most of the HIV particles are in or near dendritic cells, not in T cells, suggesting that dendritic cells are a major site of HIV replication. The ability of HIV to infect microglial cells, which are macrophage-like cells located in the central nervous system, may lead to some of the neurologic manifestations in AIDS.

(a)

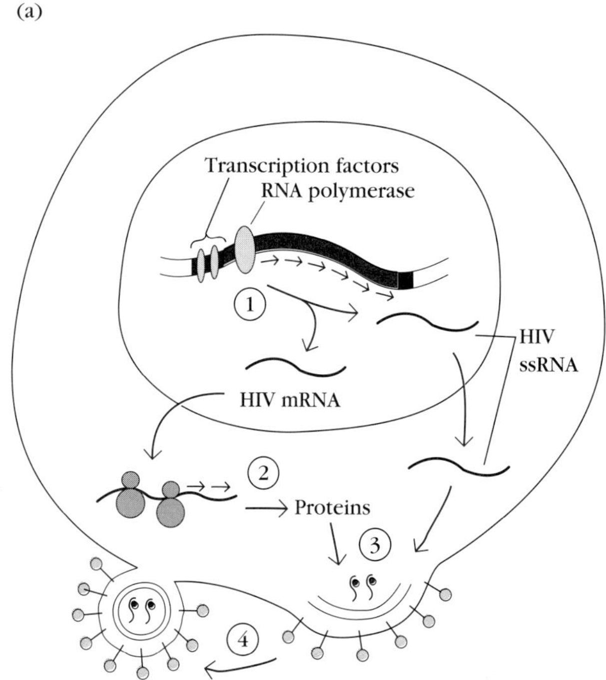

(b)

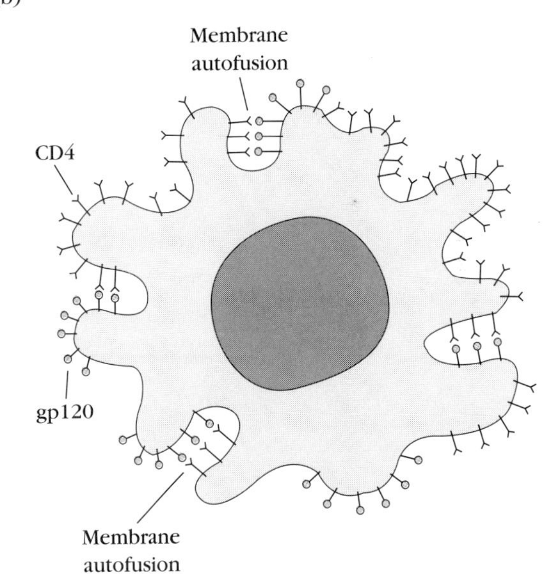

FIGURE 23-4 Activation of HIV provirus and conversion to lytic cycle. (a) Binding of various transcription factors can activate the HIV provirus leading to transcription of the proviral DNA (1) and synthesis of viral structural proteins (2). After the HIV ssRNA and proteins assemble beneath the host-cell membrane (3), the membrane buds out forming the viral envelope (4). (b) Viral gp120 expressed on the host-cell plasma membrane binds to membrane CD4 as budding occurs. In cells expressing high levels of CD4, this autofusion disrupts the membrane integrity and leads to cell lysis.

TABLE 23-2 CELL TYPES THAT CAN BE INFECTED BY HIV

Hematopoietic/immune cells	Brain/glial cells	Others
T lymphocytes	Astrocytes and oligodentrocytes	Fibroblasts
B lymphocytes	Microglia	Sperm
Primary monocytes/macrophages	Glial cell lines	Liver sinusoid epithelium
Kuppfer cells (liver macrophages)	Fetal neural cells	Bowel epithelium
Monocyte cell lines	Brain capillary endothelium	Colon carcinoma cells
Bone marrow precursor cells		Osteosarcoma cells
Dendritic cells		Rhabdomyosarcoma cells
Langerhans cells		Fetal chorionic villi
		Rabbit macrophages

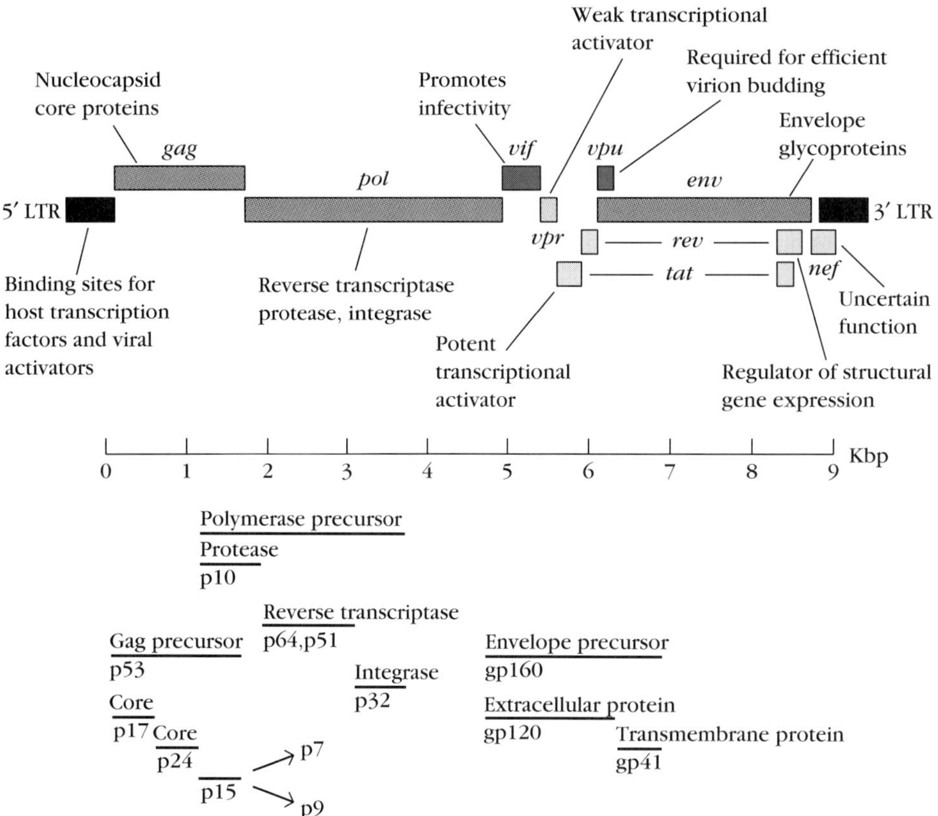

FIGURE 23-5 Genetic organization of HIV-1 *(top)*. The three major genes (purple)—*gag, pol,* and *env*—encode polyproteins, which are cleaved to yield the nucleocapsid core proteins, enzymes required for replication, and envelope core proteins *(bottom)*. Of the remaining six genes, three (light gray) encode regulatory proteins that play a major role in controlling expression; two (dark gray) encode proteins required for virion maturation; and one (light purple) encodes a weak transcriptional activator. As indicated, the coding sequences of several genes overlap. Differential RNA processing of the single primary transcript and translation of the resulting mRNAs in different reading frames yields the various gene products. Both *tat* and *rev* are split genes; the exons are spliced together during RNA processing, and depending on the reading frame during translation, either Tat or Rev is synthesized. The 5′ long terminal repeat (LTR) contains sequences to which various regulatory proteins bind. The organization of the HIV-2 genome is very similar, except the *vpu* gene is replaced by *vpx* in HIV-2. See Table 23-3 for a summary of the functions of the viral proteins.

Normally the HIV level is quite low in semen and vaginal fluid, and the level of free virus is lower still in other body fluids, such as urine, saliva, and tears. The major transmission routes are by sexual intercourse, transfusion of blood or blood products, IV drug use involving shared needles, and transplacental transfer from an infected mother to the fetus; each of these routes are likely to involve cell-associated virus. These findings and the results of other studies strongly suggest that the most important mode of HIV transmission from an infected individual to an uninfected one probably is HIV-infected cells, in particular macrophages, dendritic cells, and lymphocytes.

HIV Genome

The HIV genome is more complex than that of other known retroviruses. The organization of the HIV-1 genome is diagrammed in Figure 23-5, and the functions of the corresponding proteins are summarized in Table 23-3. All retroviral proviruses are flanked by repetitive sequences called long-terminal repeats (LTRs). The 5′ LTR contains enhancer and promoter sequences essential for proviral transcription; the 3′ LTR is required for polyadenylation of the RNA transcripts. Like all other retroviruses, the HIV provirus contains the *gag, env,* and *pol* genes, which encode, respectively, the viral core proteins, the surface envelope glycoproteins, and the nonstructural proteins required for replication. Each of these genes encodes a large polyprotein precursor that is cleaved to render the final gene products. The polyprotein encoded by *pol* is cleaved to generate three enzymes: reverse transcriptase, protease, and integrase. The *gag* gene encodes a precursor polyprotein that is cleaved by the *pol*-encoded protease to yield p24, p7, p9, and p17. Both p17 and p24 make up the protein core of the viral particle. The *env* gene encodes a glycosylated precursor polyprotein (gp160) that is cleaved by a host-cell protease to yield gp120 and gp41.

In addition to *gag, env,* and *pol,* the HIV genome contains six additional genes: virion infectivity factor *(vif),* viral protein R *(vpr),* transactivator *(tat),* regulator of expression of virion proteins *(rev),* negative

TABLE 23-3 PROTEINS ENCODED BY HIV-1 GENES AND THEIR FUNCTIONS

Gene	Protein products	Functions of final products
gag	53-kDa precursor (p53) ↓ p17, p24, p9, & p7	*Nucleocapsid core proteins* p17 is associated with inner surface of envelope p24 forms inner protein layer of nucleocapsid p9 is a component of nucleoid core p7 binds directly to genomic RNA
env	160-kDa precursor (gp160) ↓ gp120 & gp41	*Envelope glycoproteins* gp120 protrudes from envelope and binds CD4 gp41 is a transmembrane protein that contains an external domain required for fusion with target cells
pol	Precursor ↓ p64, p51, p10, & p32	*Enzymes* p64 and p51 have reverse transcriptase activity; p64 also has RNase activity p10 has protease activity p32 has integrase activity
vif	p23	Promotes infectivity of cell-free virions
vpr	p15	Activates transcription weakly
tat	p14	Activates transcription strongly
rev	p19	Controls proportions of mRNAs for structural and regulatory proteins
nef	p27	Has uncertain regulatory functions*
vpu	p16	Is required for efficient viral assembly and budding from host cells

* Early studies suggested that the protein encoded by this gene inhibited HIV transcription; hence the gene was named *nef* for "negative factor." More recent studies, however, have called this function into question.

regulatory factor *(nef)*, and either viral protein U *(vpu)* found in HIV-1 or viral protein X *(vpx)* found in HIV-2. Three of these genes—*tat, rev,* and *nef*—encode regulatory proteins that control the expression of the structural genes *gag, pol,* and *env.* Two of these genes—*tat* and *rev*—are split genes, which are read in different reading frames on the polyribosome to yield the *tat* gene product or the *rev* gene product.

The product of the *tat* gene, a small 86-aa protein called Tat, is conserved in HIV-1, HIV-2, and SIV. Tat activates proviral expression by interacting with a short sequence of RNA located at the 5′ end of all transcripts just downstream of the start site. The RNA sequence, known as the TAR element (for trans-acting responsive), forms a 59-nucleotide RNA stem-loop structure. The binding of Tat to the RNA stem-loop structure has two effects: It increases the initiation of transcription and it stabilizes the RNA polymerase complex as it moves along the proviral DNA, so that RNA transcription does not terminate prematurely. Thus, in the presence of Tat, transcription of the proviral genome increases by several thousandfold.

Following transcription of the HIV proviral DNA, the first viral proteins to appear are the regulatory proteins Tat, Rev, and Nef (Figure 23-6). Later, there is a shift in expression from the regulatory proteins to the viral structural and enzymatic proteins encoded by *gag, env,* and *pol.* Once transcription of the integrated provirus begins, the first RNAs to appear are multiply spliced transcripts (~2 kb) encoding the regulatory proteins Tat, Rev, and Nef. Later, singly spliced transcripts (~4 kb) encoding the viral structural proteins and full-length unspliced genomic RNA (~9 kb) are produced. This shift from multiply spliced transcripts to larger singly spliced and unspliced transcripts is regulated by the level of Rev.

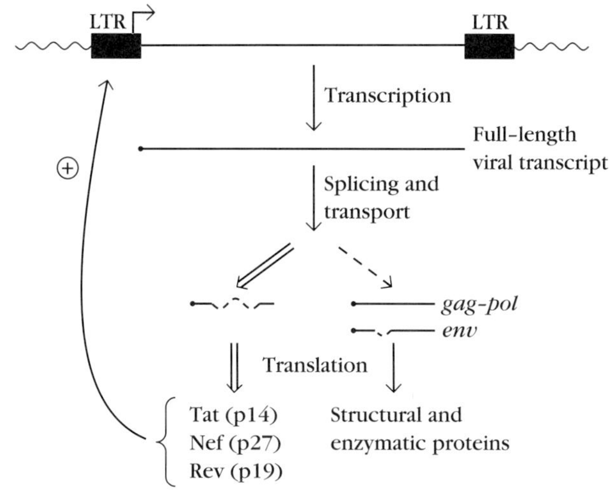

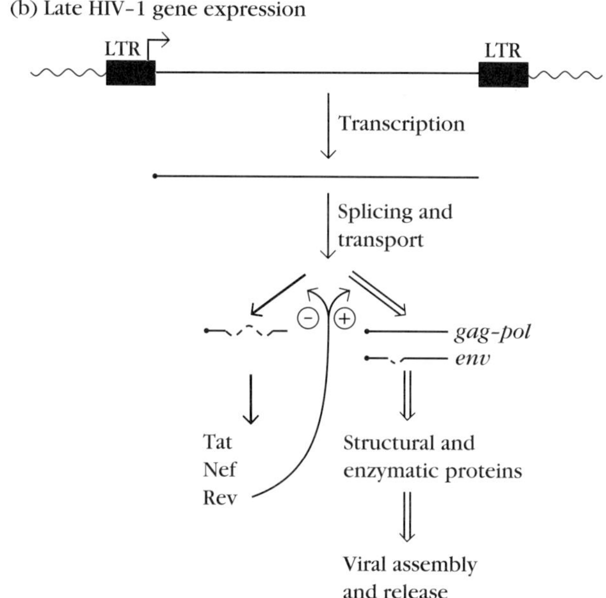

FIGURE 23-6 Stages in the expression of HIV-1 proviral DNA. (a) Early in expression the predominant products formed are the HIV regulatory proteins, including Tat, Rev, and Nef. Tat and Nef act on the 5′ LTR to regulate HIV transcription. (b) Late in HIV expression there is a shift from production of regulatory proteins to production of the structural and enzymatic proteins encoded by *gag, env,* and *pol.* This shift appears to depend upon the levels of Rev, which can increase the transport and translation of the mRNAs encoding the structural and enzymatic proteins necessary for viral assembly. [Adapted from W. C. Greene, 1991, *New Engl. J. Med.* **324**:308.]

Mechanism of HIV Activation: Latency to Lytic Cycle

Transcription of HIV proviral DNA into RNA and mRNA is catalyzed by RNA polymerase, which initially binds to the promoter in the 5′ LTR. The HIV promoter is relatively weak and has a low affinity for RNA polymerase. For this reason, once RNA polymerase has bound to the HIV promoter and begins to transcribe the proviral DNA, it tends to dissociate and thus generates only short, truncated RNA transcripts (Figure 23-7a). Synthesis of full-length HIV-1 transcripts can occur only after the weak promoter is converted into a strong, fully active promoter. Thus, activation of the HIV provirus and its progression from latency to the

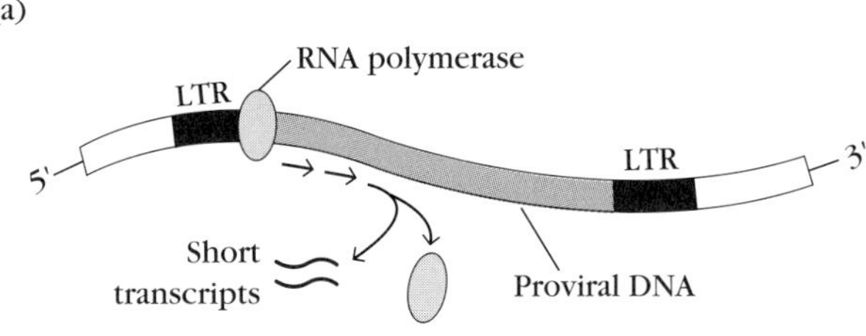

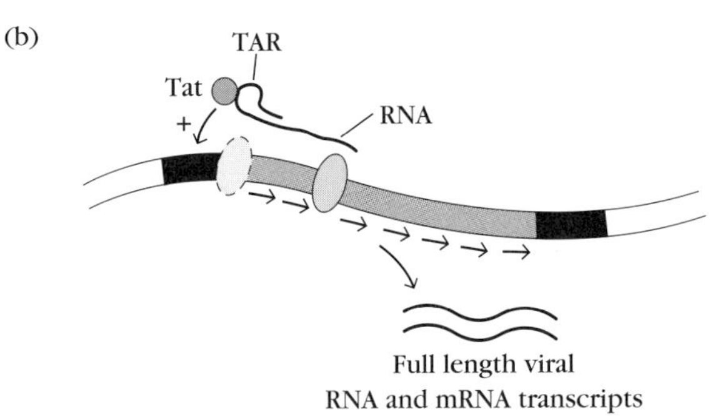

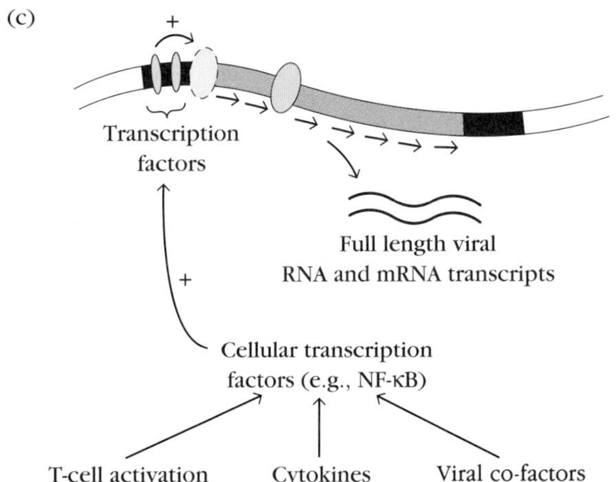

FIGURE 23-7 Activation of HIV provirus. (a) In the absence of activation, the HIV promoter binds RNA polymerase weakly. As a result, the enzyme dissociates before the entire proviral genome is transcribed, thus maintaining the latent state. (b) Conversion of the promoter to one that binds RNA polymerase strongly can be mediated by the HIV regulatory protein Tat, which binds to the TAR element in the nascent RNA transcript. (c) Promoter conversion also is induced by binding of certain transcription factors whose production is stimulated by antigen activation of HIV-infected T cells or by infection with other viruses. Promoter conversion leads to production of full-length viral transcripts and initiates the lytic cycle.

lytic state depends on this conversion in promoter activity.

Several factors have been shown to influence conversion of the weak HIV promoter into a strong one (Figure 23-7b,c). For example, binding of the HIV regulatory protein Tat to the TAR element in the emerging RNA transcript mediates this promoter conversion. In addition, certain host-cell transcription factors, such as NFκB, can bind to the HIV promoter, converting it from a weak to a strong promoter. When T lymphocytes are activated by antigen, they produce various transcription factors including NFκB, which promotes transcription of the gene encoding interleukin 2 (see Figure 12-13). Thus, when an HIV-infected T lymphocyte is activated by antigen, synthesis of NFκB increases; this factor then stimulates expression of the HIV proteins as well as IL-2 and its receptor, which are encoded by host-cell genes.

In addition to Tat and NFκB, several viruses have been shown to enhance transcription of the HIV proviral DNA, thus accelerating the progression of AIDS. These viruses include HTLV-1, cytomegalovirus, herpes simplex virus, Epstein-Barr virus, adenovirus, papovaviruses, and hepatitis B virus. Many of these viruses can infect an HIV-infected cell and induce production of transcription factors (e.g., NFκB) that bind to the proviral promoter, converting it from a weak to an active promoter. These findings explain why many HIV-infected intravenous drug users progress to full-blown AIDS much more rapidly than HIV-infected individuals who do not use IV drugs. If an infected drug user continues to use IV drugs, then antigen introduced into the bloodstream may result in T-cell activation and consequently transcription of HIV. In addition, IV drug users often are coinfected with other viruses such as hepatitis B virus or cytomegalovirus, which would have a similar effect.

Genetic Variation in HIV

HIV is capable of tremendous genetic variation, with mutations in the viral genome occurring at rates millions of times faster than what is observed in human DNA. The influenza virus causing the common flu also has a high mutation rate, which has hampered development of a flu vaccine. Yet the rate of mutation in HIV is 65 times that observed for influenza! Sequencing studies reveal that no two AIDS patients carry the identical virus; furthermore, HIV isolates taken from the same individual at different times also can differ substantially. The DNA sequence diversity seen in HIV is generated by its reverse transcriptase enzyme, which has been shown to be extremely error-prone and thus gives rise to numerous base substitutions, additions, and deletions. An estimated 5–10 errors are introduced into the HIV genome during each round of replication. As discussed in a later section, these changes make development of an HIV vaccine extremely difficult, because antibodies or cell-mediated immunity directed against one isolate may not recognize another isolate.

Role of Immune System in Selecting HIV Variants

In one study HIV was isolated from peripheral-blood lymphocytes from an infected individual on two different occasions separated by 16 months. The viral isolates recovered at these different times showed an average of 13% variation in their DNA sequences. The variation was enough to change the viral isolates' biological activity, as evidenced by differences in their ability to grow in T lymphocytes and in macrophages.

The emergence of distinct HIV isolates in infected individuals results partly from immune-system selection of HIV variants. After an individual is infected with HIV, specific neutralizing antibodies are made to viral protein or glycoprotein components. These antibodies bind to HIV and have been shown to block its ability to infect T cells in vitro. Furthermore, when HIV is grown in T-cell lines in the presence of human serum containing neutralizing antibody, a viral population resistant to the neutralizing antibody emerges after 4–5 weeks in culture. What this means is that although an individual may initially produce antibody that can inactivate HIV, the high mutation rate, coupled with the high rate of viral replication, enables some viral progeny to become resistant to the effects of the antibody. These resistant viruses survive and continue to infect additional cells and replicate, so that eventually a population of resistant viral particles emerges.

Variation in the Envelope Glycoproteins

The external presentation of gp120 and gp41 on the envelope of HIV makes these two glycoproteins potential targets for antibody-mediated neutralization of viral infectivity. For this reason considerable research has focused on the structure and antigenicity of these two envelope glycoproteins. Gp120 and gp41 are synthesized from a glycosylated precursor protein (gp160) in the rough endoplasmic reticulum of the infected cell. The precursor is cleaved, generating a small carboxyl-terminal fragment (gp41), which spans the membrane, and a larger amino-terminal fragment (gp120), which remains noncovalently associated with gp41 on the membrane (see Figure 23-2b).

Both gp120 and gp41 show a great deal of sequence variation. Of all the protein products of HIV, gp120 shows the most sequence variation with gp41 ranking second. When the gp120 and gp41 sequences of different isolates are compared, some regions are constant from one isolate to another and other regions are hypervariable (Figure 23-8). The constant regions are thought to be conserved for some necessary viral function. For example, both the CD4-binding site in gp120 and the fusogenic domain in gp41 are conserved regions.

A number of laboratories have focused their research on producing neutralizing antibodies to accessible, conserved regions of gp120 or gp41. Antibodies to the conserved region of gp120 that is the putative CD4-binding site have been shown to block binding of soluble gp120 to CD4. Unfortunately, these antibodies are not effective at blocking HIV infection. This may be because there are so many gp120-CD4 interactions at the interface of the virus and cell that they act cooperatively, increasing the likelihood of HIV binding to the target cell and rendering the neutralizing antibody ineffective. Antibodies to this conserved region on gp120 are present in HIV-infected individuals, but the titer is low.

Another conserved region that appears promising as a potential target for neutralizing antibody is a subregion within the third hypervariable region of gp120 known as the *V3 loop,* which spans residues 307 to 330 (see Figure 23-8). This region extends as a loop formed by two disulfide-linked cysteine residues at position 303 and 337. The two cysteines are highly conserved and are present in all HIV-1 isolates studied to date. As noted earlier, the V3 loop of gp120 may play a role in exposing the fusogenic domain in gp41 (see Figure 23-3b), and antibodies to the V3 loop have been shown to be quite effective at neutralizing viral infectivity. Unfortunately, the V3 loop is the most variable sequence in gp120, differing by as much as 50% between HIV-1 isolates. Thus most neutralizing antibodies to the V3 loop are strain specific.

There is, however, a small subregion within the V3 loop that is largely conserved. This subregion, which was identified by sequencing the V3 loop of over 200 HIV isolates, is located at the crown of the loop. HIV isolates can be grouped into a small number of classes based on the crown sequence. For example, 30% of HIV isolates in North America have a crown sequence designated MN (Figure 23-9). Antibodies to the MN crown sequence of the V3 loop have been shown to block infectivity of all MN viral isolates. There is a great deal of interest in producing antibodies to the different crown sequences of the V3 loop as a possible vaccine approach. This approach is discussed in the section on vaccines.

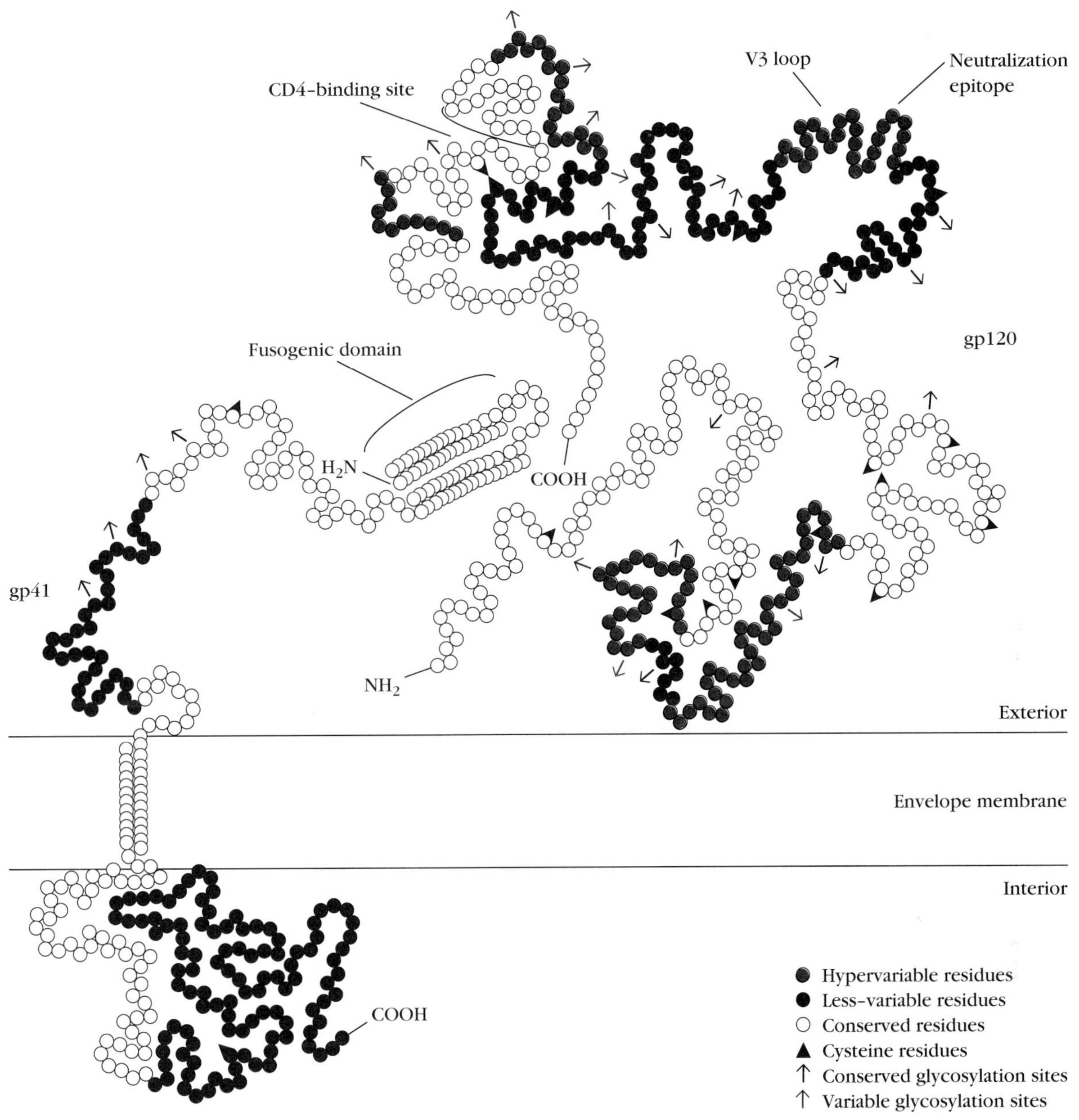

FIGURE 23-8 Schematic diagram of HIV-1 envelope glycoproteins showing hypervariable amino acid residues (purple), less variable residues (black), and conserved residues (white). Neutralizing antibodies are produced predominantly to an epitope that overlaps with one of the hypervariable regions in gp120, designated the V3 loop. For this reason, neutralizing antibodies to HIV generally are strain specific. Note that the CD4-binding site on gp120 and the fusogenic domain in gp41, both of which mediate essential viral functions, have conserved amino acid sequences. [Adapted from R. C. Gallo, 1988, *J. Acquired Immune Deficiency Syndromes* **1**:521.]

Clinical Diagnosis of AIDS

The disease manifestations initially recognized by the CDC as being indicative of AIDS were limited to a few opportunistic infections or Kaposi's sarcoma. It soon became apparent, however, that a much broader range of indicator diseases should be included in the diagnosis of AIDS. In an effort to reflect the diversity of disease symptoms in AIDS, the CDC has classified the indicator diseases into various categories. The CDC classification initially was published in 1986 and was revised in 1993 (Table 23-4). The revised classification consists of three clinical categories (A, B, and C), each of which is subdivided into three ranges of $CD4^+$ T-cell counts ($\geq 500/\mu l$, $200–499/\mu l$, and $<200/\mu l$), as shown in Table 23-5.

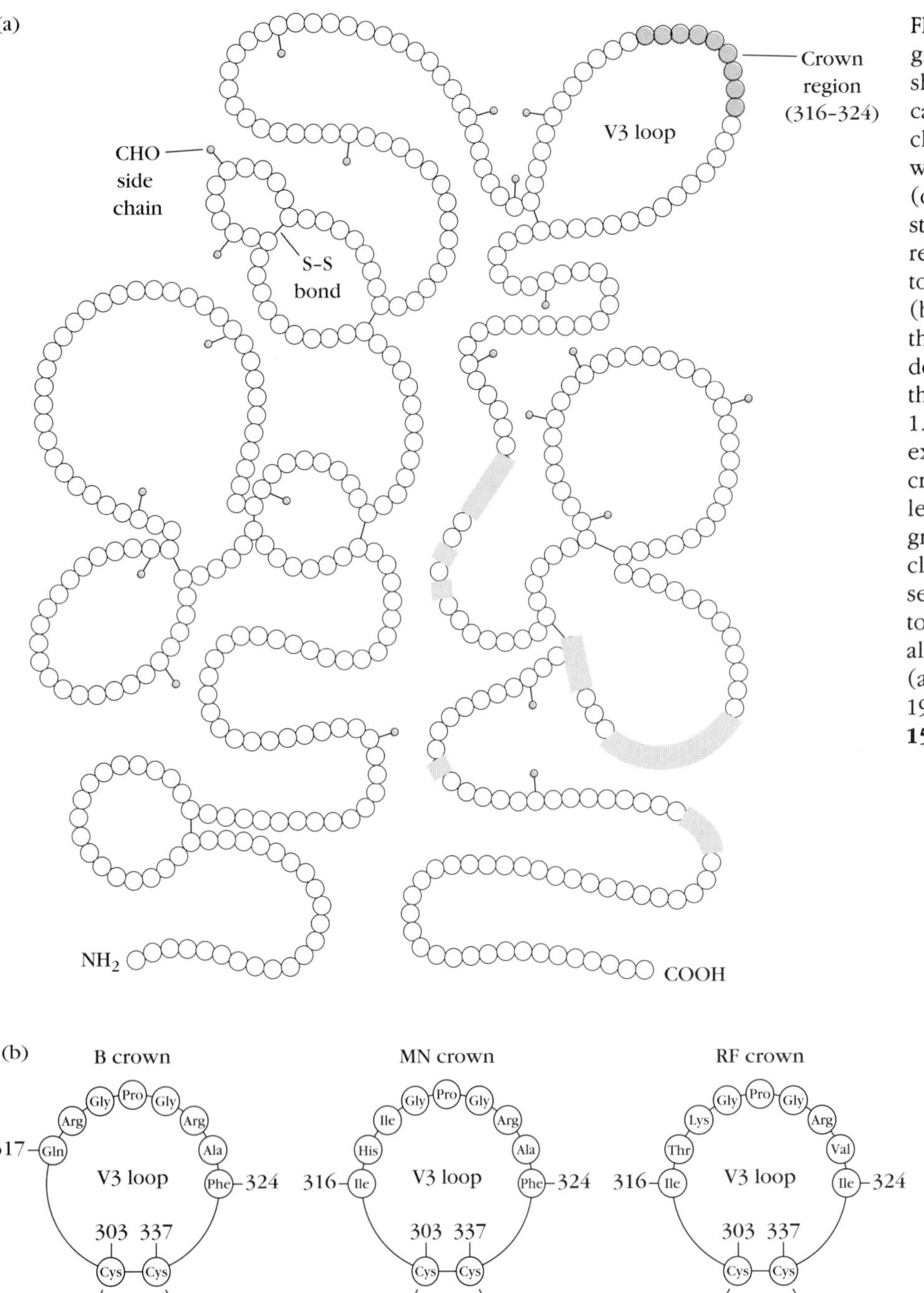

FIGURE 23-9 (a) Schematic diagram of gp120 from HIV-1 showing disulfide bonds and carbohydrate (CHO) side chains. The crown region, which extends from residue 316 (or 317) to 324 in various strains, is shaded light purple; residues important in binding to CD4 are shaded gray. (b) Amino acid sequences of three crown regions—designated B, MN, and RF—in the V3 loop of gp120 from HIV-1. Although the entire V3 loop exhibits extensive variation, the crown region exhibits much less. Thus HIV isolates can be grouped into a small number of classes based on their crown sequence. Small numbers refer to residue positions in the overall gp120 sequence. [Part (a) adapted from S. Putney, 1992, *Trends Biochem. Sci.* **15**(5):191.]

Category A includes three general presentations of HIV infection. Initial HIV infection sometimes causes an acute mononucleosis-like illness, which is generally followed by an asymptomatic latency period. Often, however, individuals manifest no apparent symptoms at all upon initial HIV infection and pass without any indications into an asymptomatic latency period. Finally, a significant number of individuals infected with HIV have a persistent generalized lymphadenopathy, characterized by enlargement of multiple lymph nodes, but no concurrent illness. In all three cases, the individual is infected with HIV and is usually antibody positive in an ELISA or Western-blot test but is not diagnosed as having AIDS unless the $CD4^+$ T-cell count drops below 200/μl.

Category B includes various symptomatic conditions attributable to HIV infection that are not included in category C. These conditions are attributed to di-

Table 23-4 CDC classification of AIDS indicator diseases (1993 revision)

Clinical categories in individuals with documented HIV infection:

*Category A**
- Asymptomatic: no symptoms at the time of HIV infection
- Acute infection: glandular fever-like illness lasting a few weeks at the time of infection
- Persistent generalized lymphadenopathy (PGL): lymph node enlargement persisting for 3 or more months with no evidence of infection

Category B†
- Bacillary angiomatosis
- Candidiasis, oropharyngeal (thrush)
- Candidiasis, vulvovaginal: persistent, frequent, or poorly responsive to therapy
- Cervical dysplasia (moderate or severe)/cervical carcinoma in situ
- Constitutional symptoms such as fever or diarrhea lasting ≥1 month
- Hairy leukoplakia, oral
- Herpes zoster (shingles) involving at least two distinct episodes or more than one dermatome
- Idiopathic thrombocytopenic purpura
- Listeriosis
- Pelvic inflammatory disease, particularly by tubo-ovarian abscess
- Peripheral neuropathy

Category C
- Candidiasis of bronchi, trachae, or lungs
- Candidiasis, esophageal
- Cervical cancer (invasive)
- Coccidioidomycosis, disseminated or extrapulmonary
- Cryptococcosis, extrapulmonary
- Cryptosporidiosis, chronic intestinal (>1 month's duration)
- Cytomegalovirus disease (other than liver, spleen, or nodes)
- Cytomegalovirus retinitis (with loss of vision)
- Encephalopathy, HIV-related
- Herpes simplex: chronic ulcer(s) (>1 month's duration) or bronchitis, pneumonitis, or esophagitis
- Histoplasmosis, disseminated or extrapulmonary
- Isosporiasis, chronic intestinal (>1 months duration)
- Kaposi's sarcoma
- Lymphoma, Burkitt's
- Lymphoma, immunoblastic
- *Mycobacterium avium* complex or *M. kansasii,* disseminated or extrapulmonary
- *Mycobacterium,* other species, disseminated or extrapulmonary
- *Pneumocystis carinii* pneumonia
- Progressive multifocal leukoencephalopathy
- *Salmonella* septicemia (recurrent)
- Toxoplasmosis of brain
- Wasting syndrome due to HIV

* Conditions listed in categories B and C must not have occurred.
† Conditions listed in category C must not have occurred.

Table 23-5 CDC classification system for HIV infection (1993 revision)

	Clinical categories*		
CD4+ T-cell count	(A)	(B)	(C)
(1) ≥500/μl	A1	B1	**C1**
(2) 200–499/μl	A2	B2	**C2**
(3) <200/μl	**A3**	**B3**	**C3**

* See Table 23-4 for listing of indicator diseases in each clinical category. Categories in boldface are now reported as an AIDS diagnosis.

minished cell-mediated immunity and require clinical management that is complicated by HIV infection. Included in this category are several diseases seen in women with AIDS such as vulvovaginal candidiasis, cervical dysplasia, cervical carcinoma, and pelvic inflammatory disease. Also included in this category are various constitutional symptoms such as persistent fever and diarrhea, oral candidiasis, hairy leukoplakia, and peripheral neuropathy. Individuals manifesting category B symptoms and a $CD4^+$ T-cell count below 200/μl are diagnosed as having AIDS.

Category C includes a variety of conditions: HIV wasting syndrome, esophageal candidiasis, invasive cervical cancer, Kaposi's sarcoma, lymphoma (immunoblastic or Burkitt's), *Pneumocystis carinii* pneumonia, HIV-related encephalopathy, infections with various *Mycobacterium* species, histoplasmosis, cryptococcosis, toxoplasmosis of the brain, and diseases caused by cytomegalovirus. HIV-infected individuals who manifest category C symptoms are diagnosed as having AIDS regardless of what their $CD4^+$ T-cell count is.

HIV Destruction of $CD4^+$ T Cells

One of the early observations of immune-system impairment in HIV infection was a reduction in the number of $CD4^+$ T cells. Uninfected individuals have approximately 1100 $CD4^+$ T cells/μl of whole blood; in AIDS patients the numbers drop dramatically, often reaching levels below 200/μl. Normally the ratio of $CD4^+$ to $CD8^+$ T cells in the peripheral blood is about 2.0, but in AIDS patients the ratio is reversed, becoming less than 1.0 and sometimes reaching values below 0.2. When lymphocytes are stained with fluorescent anti-CD4 monoclonal antibody and passed through a fluorescence-activated cell sorter, the $CD4^+$ T cells appear as a distinct peak; in AIDS patients this peak is markedly reduced.

The number of $CD4^+$ lymphocytes in the peripheral blood also has been shown to vary among clinical subgroups of AIDS patients (Figure 23-10). Although there is considerable variation in the counts among individuals in each group, the average count for the control group differs significantly from those of all the HIV-infected groups exhibiting symptoms. Once the $CD4^+$ T-cell count falls below 200/μl, an individual is quite susceptible to opportunistic infections and neoplasms. About 40% of AIDS patients manifesting opportunistic infections have no detectable $CD4^+$ T cells at all. The very low number or complete absence of $CD4^+$ T cells in these patients probably explains their susceptibility to opportunistic infections, and also the finding that such patients have the shortest life expectancy of all AIDS patients.

The average $CD8^+$ T-cell count is actually higher in some subgroups of AIDS patients than in uninfected controls. Early in the disease, CTL activity against HIV-infected cells can be detected, but as the disease progresses, the CTL activity appears to decline. There is some evidence that at least some of the $CD8^+$ T cells in HIV-infected individuals may act to suppress the immune response.

Depletion of HIV-Infected $CD4^+$ T Cells

As explained previously, as long as the HIV provirus in an infected $CD4^+$ T cell remains in the latent state, no damage to the cell is evident. However, once the provirus is activated and new HIV virions begin to assemble and bud from the infected cell, extensive damage to the cell membrane can occur, leading to death of the cell (Figure 23-11a). In addition, the humoral or cell-mediated response generated against HIV may lead to destruction of HIV-infected $CD4^+$ T cells. Those infected $CD4^+$ T cells expressing gp120 and gp41 on their membrane can be killed by antibody-plus-com-

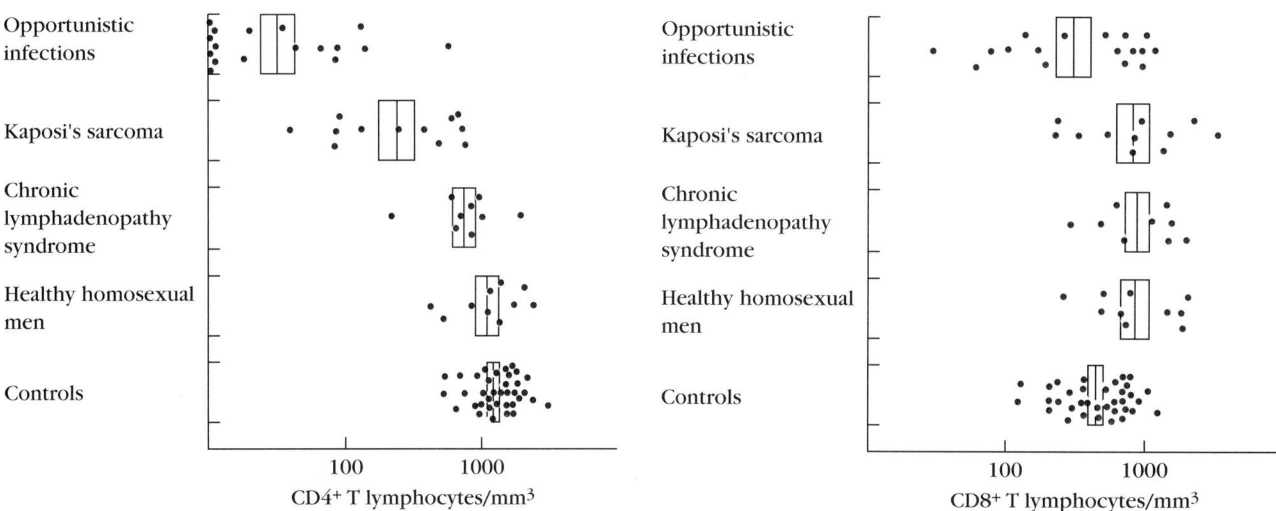

FIGURE 23-10 Quantitation of $CD4^+$ and $CD8^+$ T lymphocytes in normal controls and in clinical subpopulations of AIDS patients. [From H. C. Lane and A. S. Fauci, 1985, *Annu. Rev. Immunol.* **3**:477.]

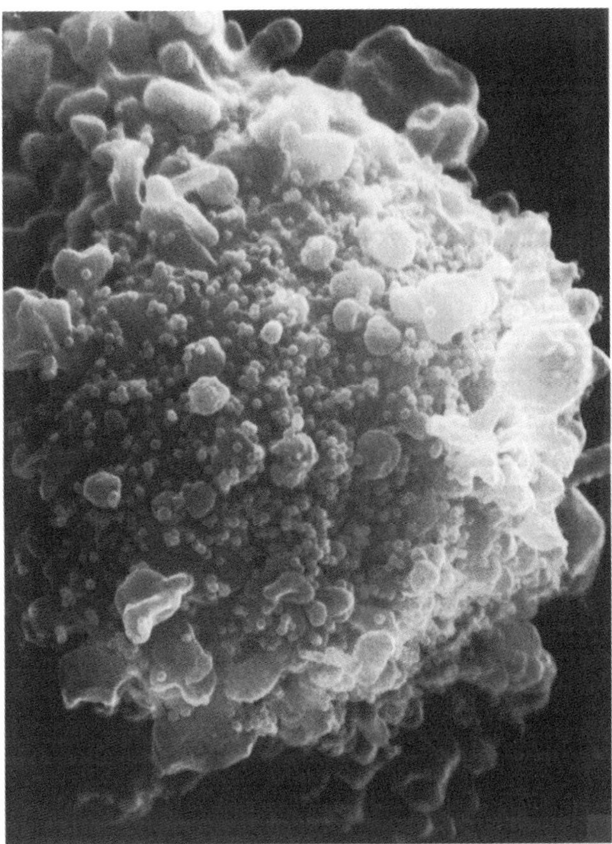

(a)

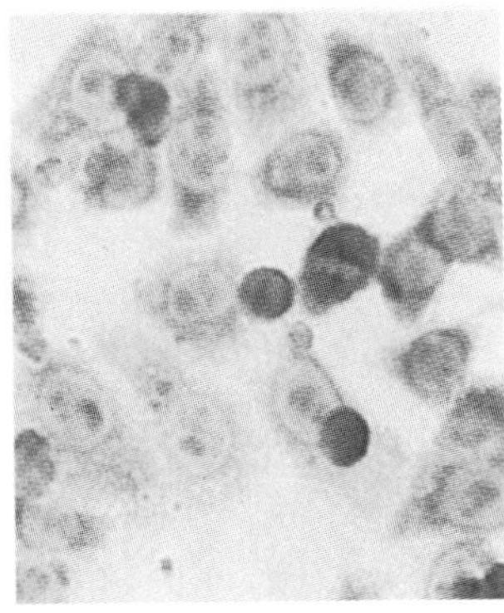

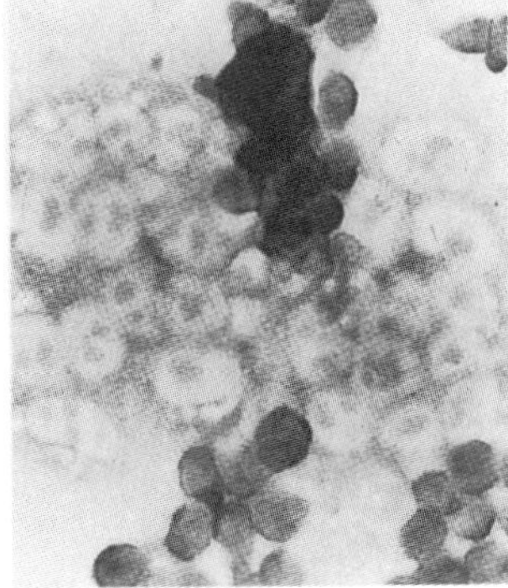

(b)

FIGURE 23-11 (a) Destruction of HIV-infected T cells can occur as HIV buds from the infected T cell. (b) Destruction of uninfected T cells can occur through syncytia formation caused by HIV. On the left HeLa cells lacking CD4 are exposed to HIV in culture. These cells cannot be infected and do not show syncytia formation. At right, CD4-transfected HeLa cells expressing CD4 are infected by HIV. Giant multinucleated syncytia are formed following HIV infection. [Part (a) photo courtesy of R. C. Gallo, 1988, *J. Acquired Immune Deficiency Syndromes* **1**:521–535; part (b) from J. N. Weber and R. A. Weiss, 1988, *Sci. Am.* **259**(October):101.]

plement lysis; those that express viral peptides associated with class I MHC molecules can be killed by a CTL response against the altered self-cells. Both processes represent a normal immune response against a virus, a process that should serve to eliminate virus-infected cells and thus prevent further spread of the virus. The irony in the case of HIV is that the immune response to eliminate the virus kills off the central cells of the immune system itself.

The actual number of HIV-infected $CD4^+$ T cells present in AIDS patients is somewhat controversial. Analyses of peripheral blood from infected but asymptomatic individuals indicate that only 0.01–1.0% of $CD4^+$ cells is infected. As AIDS progresses, the proportion of infected $CD4^+$ T cells increases, reaching levels of 1% or greater. Recent evidence, however, suggests that the level of HIV infection in recirculating $CD4^+$ cells may be substantially less than that in noncirculating T cells. For example, analyses of lymph node biopsies from HIV-infected individuals reveal that lymph node tissue contains 10–100 times as many HIV particles as do circulating $CD4^+$ T cells. Because antigen-activated T cells loose their homing receptors and cease recirculating, such activated T cells are preferentially located in peripheral lymphoid tissue. Furthermore, as noted earlier, antigen activation of HIV-infected T cells stimulates the lytic cycle. For these reasons, the higher levels of HIV infection in lymph node T cells compared with recirculating T cells is not surprising.

While upper estimates of HIV infection approach 1% of $CD4^+$ T cells, this still cannot account for the dramatic decline in T-cell counts, which often reaches levels of 90%. Thus the decline in $CD4^+$ T-cell numbers and function cannot result entirely from HIV-mediated damage to infected cells.

Depletion of Uninfected $CD4^+$ T Cells

In asymptomatic HIV-infected individuals, $CD4^+$ T cells begin to lose their capacity to respond to foreign antigen long before their numbers plummet. Various mechanisms other than direct virus-mediated damage have been proposed to account for the decline of $CD4^+$ T-cell function and the dramatic depletion of $CD4^+$ T cells seen in AIDS patients. Several of the hypotheses that have been put forth to account for this depletion of uninfected T cells are described in this section.

Syncytia Formation

In vitro experiments reveal that an HIV-infected $CD4^+$ T cell can form a giant multinucleated cell, called a *syncytium,* by fusing with as many as 500 uninfected

$CD4^+$ T cells (Figure 23-11b). These giant multinucleated cells produce large quantities of the virus for a short period of time and then die within 48 h of their formation. Some evidence suggests that soluble gp120 alone may interact with CD4 membrane molecules to induce cell fusion leading to syncytia formation. In one study a recombinant vaccinia virus containing the gp120 gene was able to cause syncytia formation and subsequent cell death in a $CD4^+$ T-cell line in vitro. Taken together, these findings suggest that the fusion of activated virus-infected $CD4^+$ T cells expressing gp120 with other, uninfected $CD4^+$ T cells may lead to the progressive depletion of $CD4^+$ T cells that is seen in AIDS patients.

These findings also raise some concern about the use of gp120 (or a recombinant vaccinia virus carrying the gp120 gene) as a vaccine because the vaccine itself might induce syncytia formation. Not all researchers, however, think that syncytia formation is a primary cause of $CD4^+$ T-cell depletion in AIDS. Syncytia formation has been observed in the brain and lymph nodes of some AIDS patients, but the inability to detect widespread formation of syncytia in vivo has led some to suggest that the formation of these giant cells may be an in vitro phenomenon and bear little relevance to the disease process.

Destruction Mediated by Soluble gp120

The finding that the blood and lymph of AIDS patients contains large quantities of soluble gp120 is the basis for several other hypotheses to account for the depletion of uninfected $CD4^+$ T cells (Figure 23-12). The noncovalent interaction of gp120 and gp41 is unstable, allowing large quantities of free gp120 to be shed into the surrounding fluid. Because gp120 has a high affinity for $CD4^+$, it can bind to CD4 molecules on normal, uninfected $CD4^+$ T cells. Such binding may block in-

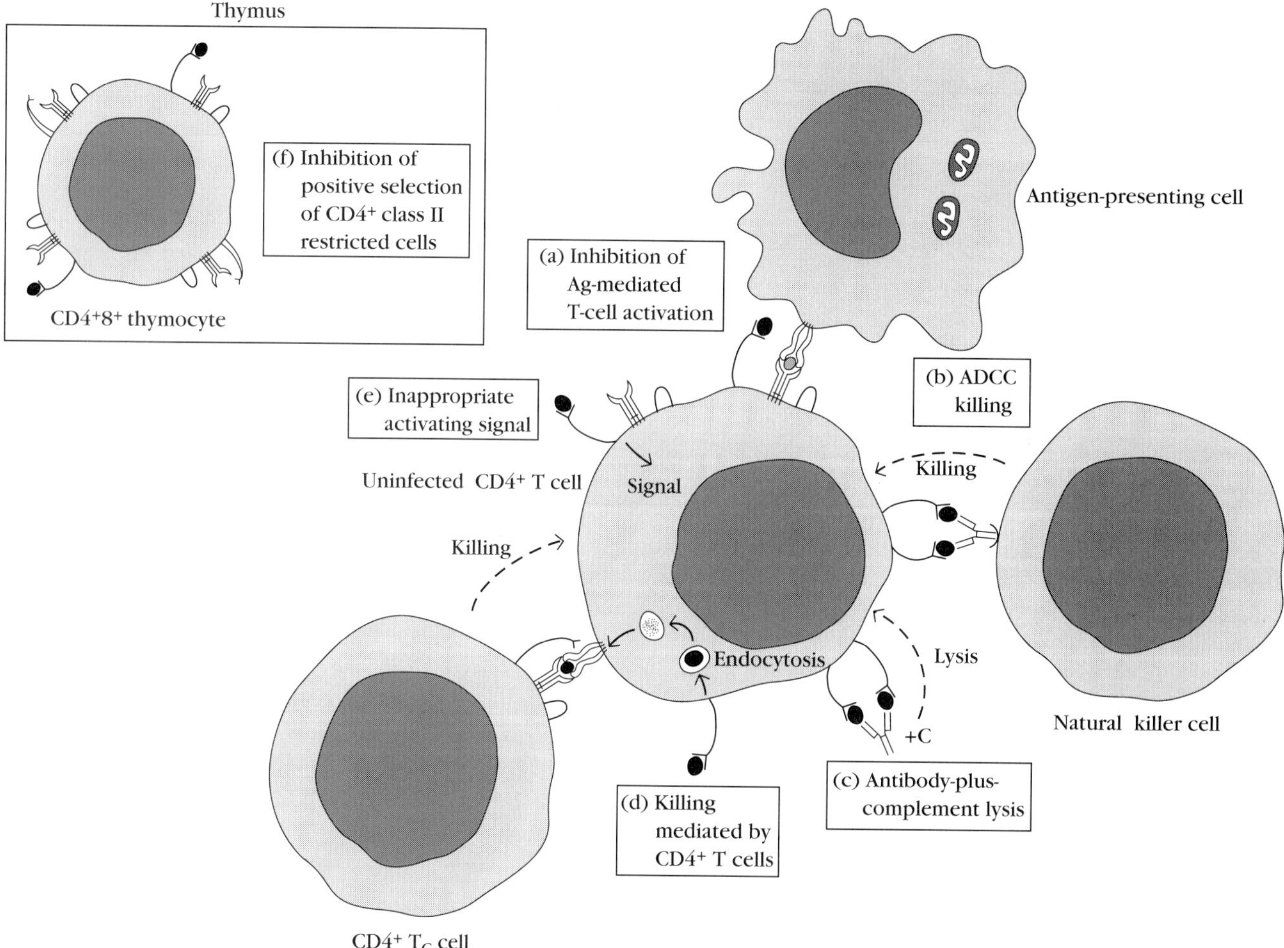

FIGURE 23-12 Possible mechanisms by which soluble gp120 (purple) may induce depletion of uninfected $CD4^+$ T cells. See text for discussion. C = complement.

teraction of CD4 with class II MHC molecules on antigen-presenting cells, thus preventing the subsequent transduction of part of the activating signal.

Another possibility is that binding of soluble gp120 to CD4 membrane molecules may induce destruction of uninfected T cells by antibody-plus-complement lysis or by antibody-dependent cell-mediated cytotoxicity (ADCC). Since numerous other cell types express CD4 (see Table 23-2), these mechanisms might be expected to cause their destruction as well. In fact, however, only $CD4^+$ T cells are extensively depleted in AIDS patients, and depletion of other CD4-bearing cells is much lower. The probable explanation of this difference lies in the density of CD4 molecules, which is considerably higher on $CD4^+$ T cells than on macrophages and other CD4-bearing cells. Except for $CD4^+$ T cells, the density of CD4 molecules most likely is too low to induce ADCC or antibody-plus-complement lysis of other $CD4^+$ cells.

Another hypothesis is that antigen-activated but uninfected $CD4^+$ T cells are destroyed by $CD4^+$, class II–restricted T cytotoxic cells. Although T cells that are $CD4^+$ and class II restricted generally function as helper cells, small numbers exhibit cytotoxic activity instead. In one study such atypical T_C cells specific for gp120 were isolated from a normal individual and cloned. When these cloned T cells were added to normal $CD4^+$ T cells in the presence of soluble gp120, the cloned cells began to kill the normal cells. Since antigen-activated human T cells express class II MHC molecules, these results led to speculation that binding of soluble gp120 to CD4 molecules on an uninfected, activated T cell might result in receptor-mediated endocytosis of gp120. The internalized gp120 might then be processed and presented together with class II MHC molecules on the cell membrane of the uninfected $CD4^+$ T cell. Cytotoxic $CD4^+$ T cells specific for gp120 associated with class II MHC molecules could then selectively deplete these uninfected $CD4^+$ T cells (see Figure 23-12d).

Interference with T-Cell Maturation

Depletion of T cells normally induces T-cell maturation within the thymus to restore the peripheral T-cell numbers. Some researchers have suggested that soluble gp120 in AIDS patients binds to CD4 on thymocytes, thus interfering with the positive selection of class II MHC–restricted cells that occurs during T-cell maturation (see Figure 12-4). In the experiments outlined in Figure 12-5, antibody to class II MHC molecules selectively interfered with maturation of $CD4^+$ T cells. By analogy, binding of soluble gp120 to CD4 also might interfere with the maturation process (see Figure 23-12f). Destruction of mature $CD4^+$ T cells in the periphery, coupled with a lack of replacement by developing thymocytes, could explain the progressive $CD4^+$ T-cell depletion in AIDS patients.

Inappropriate Programmed Cell Death

Another possible explanation for $CD4^+$ T-cell depletion in AIDS patients is that binding of soluble gp120 to CD4 on uninfected cells results in an inappropriate signal leading to programmed cell death, or apoptosis. As discussed in Chapter 12, CD4 is involved in transmitting an activating signal to the interior of a T cell after it interacts with an antigen–class II MHC complex. In normal T-cell activation the T-cell receptor first transmits a signal after recognizing a peptide–class II MHC complex on an antigen-presenting cell; then the CD4 molecule on the T cell binds to the class II MHC molecule and transmits a subsequent signal (Figure 23-13a).

The order of the two signals appears to be crucial. For example, when T cells are first incubated with anti-CD4 antibody, which stimulates the second signal, and then are activated with antigen, they exhibit programmed cell death (Figure 23-13b). Similar results are obtained when normal $CD4^+$ T cells are incubated with gp120 and anti-gp120; when these T cells are later activated with anti-CD3, they undergo programmed cell death (Figure 23-13c). Based on these findings, some have proposed that binding of gp120 to CD4 on uninfected T cells in AIDS patients primes these cells for programmed cell death when they are later activated by antigen. This hypothesis predicts that the rate of $CD4^+$ T-cell depletion depends on the level of T-cell activation.

A study reported in 1992 indicates that depletion of $CD4^+$ T cells in AIDS patients shows similarities to the T-cell depletion that occurs following superantigen activation. Superantigens can bind simultaneously to the V_β region of the T-cell receptor and to a class II MHC molecule on an antigen-presenting cell (see Figure 4-15). A given superantigen is able to activate all T cells expressing a particular V_β gene sequence. Since there are about 20 different V_β gene segments, a superantigen is able to activate 1 in 20 T cells, whereas a normal antigenic peptide can activate on the order of only 1 in 100,000 T cells. If uninfected T cells are poised to undergo programmed cell death as the result of binding soluble gp120, a superantigen may provide the necessary activation signal to initiate programmed cell death. One characteristic of superantigen deletion is a characteristic "hole" in the T-cell repertoire. For example, if a superantigen binds to T cells expressing the $V_\beta3$ gene segment, then all T cells expressing $V_\beta3$ will be deleted, but all other T cells will remain. Several retroviruses have been shown to encode superan-

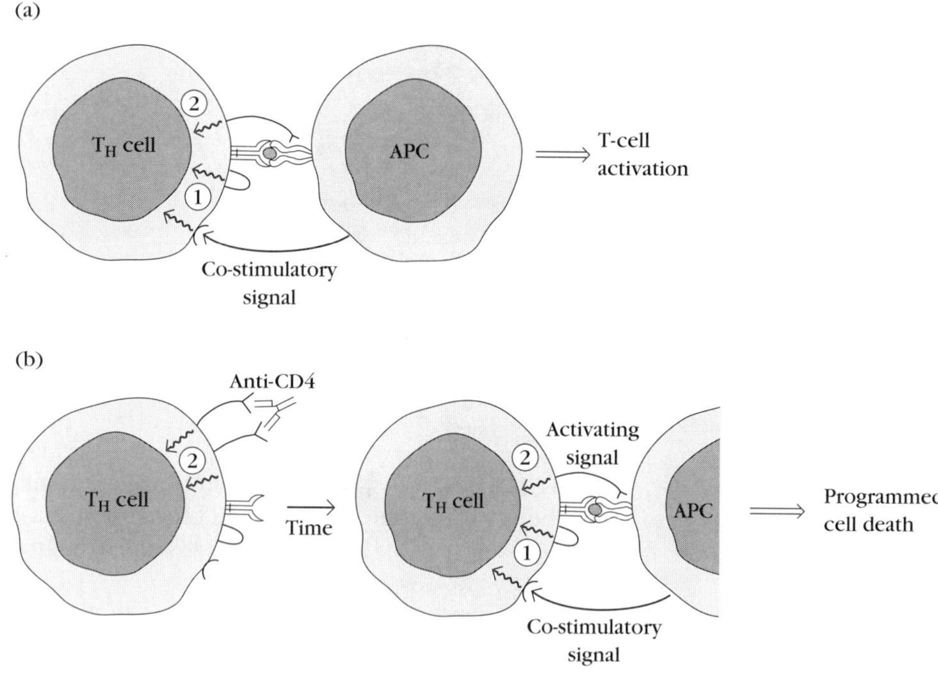

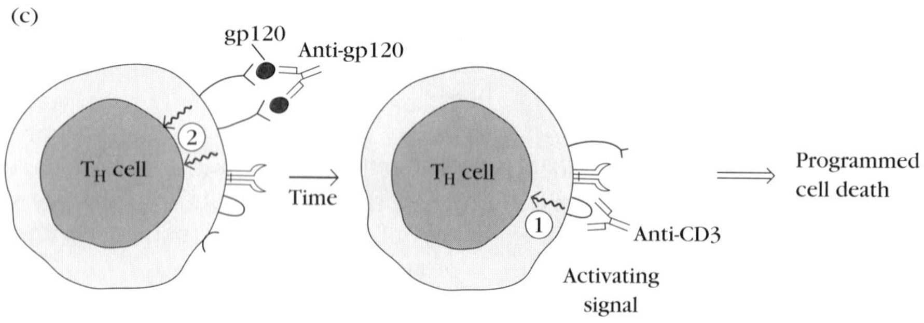

FIGURE 23-13 Experimental demonstration that inappropriate signal can prime T_H cells for programmed cell death. (a) Normal T-cell activation requires two signals, as well as a co-stimulatory signal. Signal 1 is transmitted when a T-cell receptor and associated CD3 molecule recognize a peptide–class II MHC complex; signal 2 is transmitted when CD4 on the T cell interacts with the class II molecule. (b, c) When normal T_H cells are treated experimentally so as to induce signal 2 and then activated by antigen or anti-CD3 to induce signal 1 (activating signal), the cells undergo programmed cell death (apoptosis).

tigens that induce this type of characteristic deletion of subsets of T cells expressing particular V_β gene segments. This finding has led to speculation that a gene product of HIV may act as a superantigen, inducing programmed cell death in all T cells expressing T-cell receptors with a V_β that binds this product. Support for this hypothesis came from comparisons of the T-cell repertoires of six AIDS patients with those of six uninfected controls. The α-chain repertoires were the same in both groups, but the β-chain repertoires of the AIDS group showed a loss of T cells expressing certain V_β sequences.

Immunologic Abnormalities in AIDS

The total collapse of the immune system in AIDS reflects the central role of $CD4^+$ T cells in both humoral and cell-mediated responses. Not surprisingly, AIDS patients manifest a variety of immunologic abnormalities (Table 23-6). HIV infection initially leads to viremia in which viral particles can be readily detected in circulating lymphocytes. Shortly thereafter the virus largely disappears from the circulating lymphocytes; in most individuals, nearly a decade passes before large numbers of virus-infected cells are detected again in circulating lymphocytes. This observation led to the belief that following initial infection, HIV entered a long latency lasting nearly a decade. Recently this belief has been challenged. As mentioned previously, peripheral lymphoid tissue such as lymph nodes, spleen, tonsils, and adenoids reveal active viral replication and levels of HIV that are 10–100 times higher than that observed in circulating lymphocytes. Thus, although the $CD4^+$ T-cell count may remain high in the early years following infection, this count may not accurately reflect the impact of HIV on lymphocytes residing in peripheral lymphoid tissue.

TABLE 23-6 IMMUNOLOGIC ABNORMALITIES ASSOCIATED WITH HIV INFECTION

Stage of infection	Typical abnormalities observed
	Lymph node structure
Early	Infection and destruction of dendritic cells; some structural disruption
Late	Extensive damage and tissue necrosis; loss of follicular dendritic cells and germinal centers; inability to trap antigens or support activation of T and B cells
	T helper (T_H) cells
Early	Lack of in vitro proliferative response to specific antigen
Late	Marked decrease in T_H-cell numbers and corresponding helper activities
	Antibody production
Early	Enhanced nonspecific IgG and IgA production but reduced IgM synthesis
Late	Lack of proliferation of HIV-specific B cells; absence of detectable anti-HIV antibodies in some patients
	Cytokine production
Early	Increased levels of some cytokines
Late	Shift in cytokine production from T_H1 subset to T_H2 subset
	Delayed-type hypersensitivity
Early	Highly significant reduction in proliferative capacity of T_{DTH} cells and reduction in skin-test reactivity
Late	Elimination of DTH response; complete absence of skin-test reactivity
	T cytotoxic (T_C) cells
Early	Comparatively normal reactivity
Late	Reduction but not elimination of CTL activity due to impaired ability to generate CTLs from T_C cells

Pathologic Changes in Lymph Nodes

Soon after an individual is infected with HIV, circulating antibodies are thought to form complexes with viral particles, and the virus appears to disappear from the bloodstream. Although some virions are eliminated by phagocytosis, others infect cells of the regional lymph nodes establishing a massive covert infection. The infection appears to occur as antibody-HIV complexes carried into a node are trapped by Fc receptors along the long cytoplasmic processes of follicular dendritic cells within the germinal center. Biopsies from patients with early HIV infection (those with $CD4^+$ T-cell counts $\geq 500/\mu l$) reveal millions of HIV viral particles along the long processes of the follicular dendritic cells. As $CD4^+$ T cells traffic through the lymph nodes, some probably become infected by the HIV particles associated with the follicular dendritic cells.

The peripheral lymph nodes of HIV-infected individuals undergo striking changes in structure as AIDS progresses. These changes begin with the HIV infection and subsequent death of the follicular dendritic cells; eventually the germinal center becomes involuted due to the loss of these cells. Lymph node biopsies of HIV-infected patients reveal a progression of structural changes. In patients with intermediate HIV infection (i.e., those with $CD4^+$ T-cell counts of 200–499/μl), the lymph nodes begin to show signs of disruption. Interdigitating dendritic cells also are infected and killed by HIV. Because these cells play a vital role in $CD4^+$ T-cell activation, a reduction in dendritic cell numbers may result in a corresponding reduction in T-cell activity. Finally, in patients with advanced disease (those with $CD4^+$ T-cell counts $<200/\mu l$), lymph nodes show extensive damage and tissue necrosis, with loss of follicular dendritic cells and consequently the loss of germinal centers. As the lymph node architecture is destroyed, the nodes are less able to trap HIV particles or provide a suitable environment for T-cell and B-cell activation. At this point there is a significant increase in detectable virus in the peripheral blood and a corresponding increase in manifestations of AIDS.

Reduced Antigen-Specific Responses by T_H Cells

One of the earliest immunologic abnormalities associated with AIDS is the reduced ability of T lymphocytes to proliferate in vitro in response to mitogens or soluble antigens. This is illustrated by the data in Table 23-7, which compares the in vitro proliferative response to pokeweed mitogen and tetanus toxoid by T

TABLE 23-7 COMPARISON OF IN VITRO PROLIFERATIVE RESPONSE OF PERIPHERAL-BLOOD LYMPHOCYTES FROM AIDS PATIENTS AND NORMAL CONTROLS*

	[^{3}H]thymidine incorporated (cpm)			
	Pokeweed mitogen		Tetanus toxoid	
Cell sample†	AIDS	Control	AIDS	Control
Unfractionated	1,400 ± 800	10,800 ± 1,900	<100	20,300 ± 6,400
CD4$^+$ T cells	17,800 ± 2,600	19,600 ± 2,200	<100	16,900 ± 1,200
CD8$^+$ T cells	3,100 ± 515	4,400 ± 680	<100	45,300 ± 600

* Lymphocytes were cultured in the presence of [^{3}H]thymidine and either pokeweed mitogen or tetanus toxoid. At the end of a 5-day culture period, the amount of radioactivity (cpm) incorporated into cells was determined.

† Cell numbers in the unfractionated sample were not equalized and represent the cell counts in peripheral blood. After separation of CD4$^+$ and CD8$^+$ T cells, cell numbers in the AIDS and control samples were equalized.

SOURCE: Data from H. C. Lane and A. S. Fauci, 1985, *Annu. Rev. Immunol.* **3**:477.

lymphocytes from AIDS patients and normal controls. The researchers in this study wanted to know if the decrease observed with unfractionated T cells from AIDS patients reflected reduced numbers of T cells compared with controls or some inherent defect in the T cells. They therefore separated CD4$^+$ and CD8$^+$ T cells with a fluorescence-activated cell sorter, adjusted cell numbers so that comparable numbers of cells were present in the AIDS and control samples, and repeated the proliferation assays. The results with these adjusted samples showed that CD4$^+$ T cells from AIDS patients responded at near-normal levels to pokeweed mitogen; the low response to mitogen with the unfractionated cell sample thus reflected the smaller number of T cells in this sample compared with that of controls. On the other hand, the CD4$^+$ cells from AIDS patients, even when cell numbers were equalized, remained unable to respond to tetanus toxoid antigen. This study demonstrates one of the earliest abnormalities seen in AIDS patients: the inability of CD4$^+$ T cells to proliferate in response to a specific antigen. The absence of antigen-specific T-cell proliferation lends support for various hypotheses suggesting that the CD4$^+$ T cells in AIDS patients may have received an inappropriate activating signal, inducing these cells to become anergic or programming the cells for death by apoptosis.

Ineffective Antibody Response

Many HIV-infected individuals can produce antibodies to various HIV gene products, including both envelope glycoproteins (gp160, gp41, and gp120) and core proteins (p55, p17, and p24). Unfortunately the presence of high titers of circulating antibody to HIV proteins in no way indicates protective immunity. One reason the antibody has so little effect seems to be frequent antigenic drift in HIV. Furthermore, the decline of CD4$^+$ T_H cells in AIDS patients eventually affects the functioning of B cells in the humoral response. As AIDS progresses, patients are increasingly unable, for lack of T_H cells, to mount a humoral antibody response to new antigens. The decline in antibody levels as AIDS progresses can be so pronounced that some patients screen as antibody negative in the HIV ELISA test during advanced stages of the disease. Some studies have indicated that anti-HIV antibody may actually be detrimental because binding of antibody-HIV immune complexes to Fc receptors on macrophages and subsequent receptor-mediated endocytosis may lead to increased HIV infection of macrophages.

Cytokine Imbalance

Several findings suggest that an imbalance in expression of cytokines or cytokine receptors may contribute to the pathogenesis of AIDS. Elevated levels of IL-1, IL-6, GM-CSF, OSM, TNF-α, and TNF-β have been reported in both serum and cerebrospinal fluid of AIDS patients. The higher levels of cytokines may also contribute to some of the symptoms seen in AIDS patients (Figure 23-14). For example, IL-1 is known to cause fever and may be responsible for the persistent fevers seen in AIDS patients. High levels of IL-1 have also been reported in patients with Alzheimer's disease; it

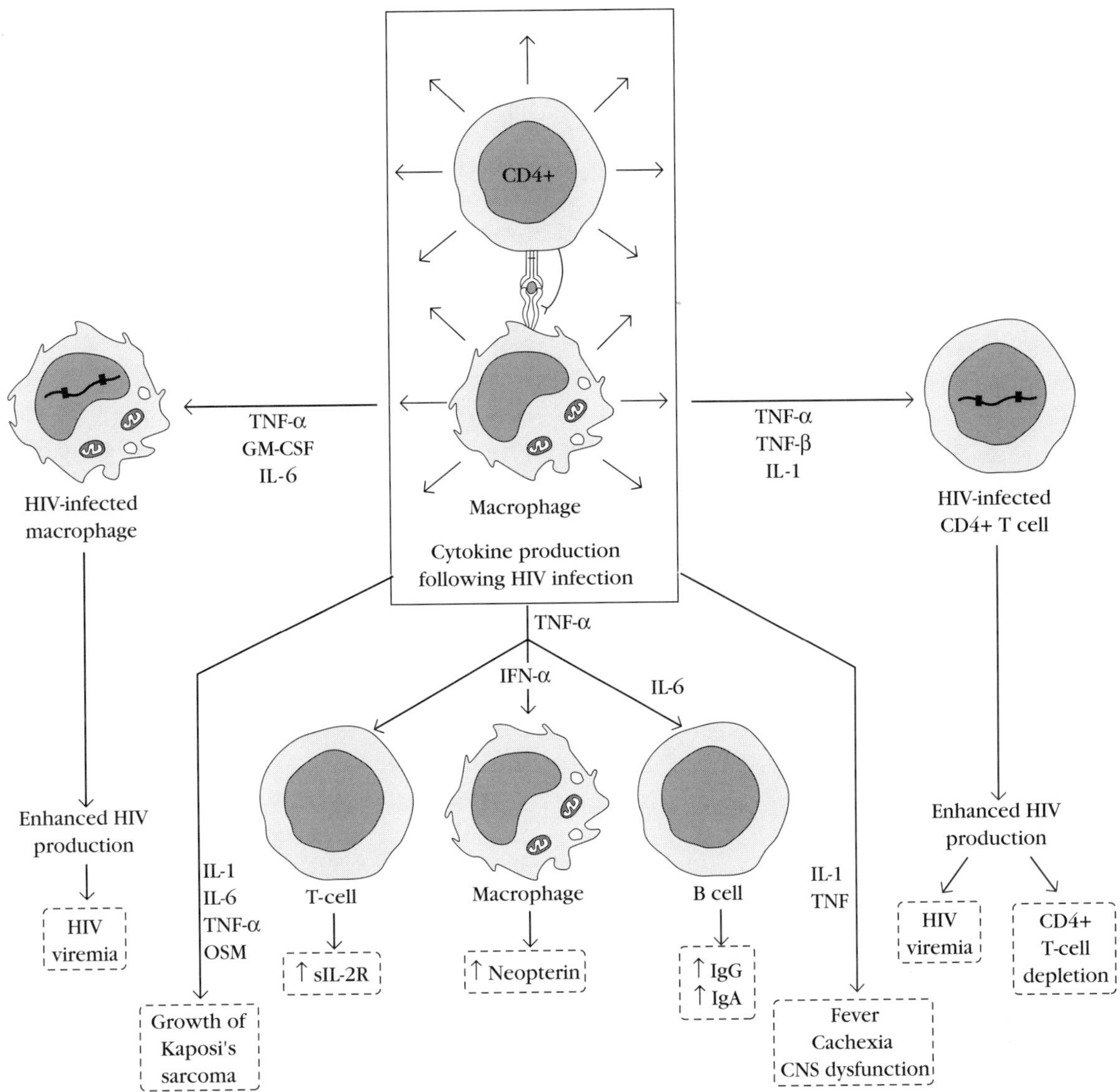

FIGURE 23-14 Effects of increased levels of various cytokines following HIV infection. IL = interleukin; IFN = interferon; OSM = oncostatin M; sIL-2R = soluble receptor for IL-2; TNF = tumor necrosis factor; GM-CSF = granulocyte-monocyte colony-stimulating factor. [Adapted from T. Matsuyama, N. Kobayashi, and N. Yamamoto, 1991, *AIDS* **5**:1405.]

is possible that some of the symptoms of dementia in AIDS patients may be due to similar effects caused by IL-1. Another cytokine, TNF, has been shown to cause weight loss and may play a role in AIDS wasting syndrome. Additionally, IL-1, IL-6, TNF-α, and OSM have been reported to induce proliferation of Kaposi's sarcoma cells. In vitro studies also suggest that elevated levels of cytokines may contribute to the progression of HIV from latency to lytic infection. For example, TNF-α, IL-6, and GM-CSF induce expression of HIV reverse transcriptase in infected monocytes (Table 23-8), and TNF-α, TNF-β, and IL-1 induce HIV expression in infected $CD4^+$ T cells.

M. Clerici and G. M. Shearer noted that as AIDS progresses IL-2 and IFN-γ levels decrease, whereas IL-4 and IL-10 levels increase (Figure 23-15). This observation suggests that the activity of the T_H1 subset decreases and that of the T_H2 subset increases during AIDS progression. The T_H1 response would be expected to generate activity of T_{DTH} cells or CTLs. A T_H2 response, on the other hand, would lead to antibody production. Thus this shift from T_H1 to T_H2 activity may contribute to the progression of AIDS.

Decreased DTH Response

As just noted, both IL-2 and IFN-γ have been shown to decrease with time following HIV infection. The decline in IFN-γ most likely reflects a decrease in T_{DTH}-

TABLE 23-8 CYTOKINE INDUCTION OF HIV REVERSE TRANSCRIPTASE IN HIV-INFECTED MONOCYTES

Cytokine	Reverse transcriptase activity (cpm/μl)
M-CSF	200
GM-CSF	950
IFN-γ	300
TGF-β	200
TNF-α	1200
IL-6	1250
IL-4	200
IL-3	200
IL-2	200
IL-1	200
Unstimulated	200

SOURCE: Data from A. S. Fauci, 1989, Cytokine induction of HIV expression, *Colloque Des Cent Gardes,* Marnes La Coquette, Paris, France.

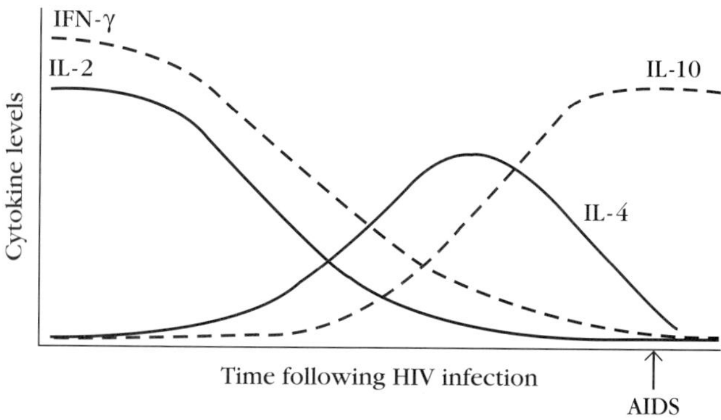

FIGURE 23-15 Following HIV infection there is a shift in cytokines that indicates progression into AIDS. IL-2 and IFN-γ levels are initially quite high but begin to drop with time following HIV infection. In contrast the levels of IL-4 and IL-10 begin to increase. This shift in cytokines suggests a shift from initial T_H1 activity following HIV infection to T_H2 activity as the disease progresses into full-blown AIDS. (Based on data from M. Clerici and G. M. Shearer, 1993, *Immunology Today* **14**(3): 107.)

TABLE 23-9 SKIN-TEST REACTIVITY TO VARIOUS TEST ANTIGENS IN AIDS PATIENTS AND NORMAL CONTROLS

	No. responding/No. tested (%)	
Antigen	AIDS patients ($n = 20$)	Controls ($n = 10$)
Control	0	0
Tetanus	10	90
Diphtheria	5	80
Streptococcus	15	70
Tuberculosis	0	60
Candida	10	90
Trichophyton	0	80
Proteus	40	50

SOURCE: DATA FROM H. C. LANE AND A. S. FAUCI, 1985, *Annu. Rev. Immunol.* 3:477.

cell function and is responsible for the significant reduction in skin-test reactivity in AIDS patients (Table 23-9). As discussed in Chapter 15, the delayed-type hypersensitive response is an important host-defense mechanism against intracellular pathogens such as *Pneumocystis carinii, Mycobacterium tuberculosis, Mycobacterium avium, Candida albicans, Histoplasma,* and *Cryptococcus.* Given the limited ability of AIDS patients to mount a DTH response, it is not surprising that they exhibit increased susceptibility to intracellular pathogens.

Impaired CTL Activity

Although the level of $CD8^+$ T_C cells is near normal in AIDS patients, their ability to generate CTLs from T_C cells, which requires IL-2 (see Figure 15-1), is impaired because of their reduced IL-2 levels. Therefore, despite the presence of adequate numbers of T_C cells, AIDS patients have limited abilities to eliminate virus-infected cells and tumor cells. In one study, the cytolytic activity of $CD8^+$ T cells from AIDS patients infected with cytomegalovirus (CMV) and from CMV-infected controls was compared. In CML assays (see Figure 9-11b) with CMV-infected target cells, the T cells from the AIDS patients showed lower ability to kill CMV-infected target cells than did T cells from the controls.

Moreover, because HIV antigens are not expressed on latently infected host cells, these cells are safe from CTL-mediated killing until activation of the provirus initiates expression of the viral antigens. IL-2 also stimulates the activation and proliferation of natural killer (NK) cells, which are important in nonspecific killing of tumor cells. Because of their reduced IL-2 levels, AIDS patients have diminished NK-cell activity; not surprisingly they commonly develop various types of tumors.

Disturbances in Immune Regulation

Several observations indicate that regulation of the immune system is disturbed in AIDS patients, although the mechanisms underlying these disturbances are not entirely clear. For example, many AIDS patients exhibit various autoimmune manifestations including the presence of autoantibodies and immune complexes, disease symptoms similar to systemic lupus erythematosus, glomerulonephritis, autoimmune thrombocytopenia purpura, and various skin disorders. These autoimmune symptoms may reflect a decline in T-cell–mediated immune suppression (see Chapter 19). In addition, a generalized loss of regulation in the humoral branch results in a nonspecific increase in immunoglobulins of the IgG and IgA classes, presumably because B cells are being activated in a nonspecific, unregulated way; the loss of specific T-cell–mediated suppression may be partly responsible. It is also possible that the presence of cytomegalovirus and Epstein-Barr virus in AIDS patients may be partly responsible, since these viruses are known to activate B cells nonspecifically.

Serologic Profile of HIV Infection

Most HIV-infected individuals develop symptoms of AIDS between 8 and 10 years after infection, but approximately 25% of infected individuals have remained symptom-free for some 10–12 years. Whether all HIV-infected individuals eventually will develop AIDS is not known; nor is it possible to predict how quickly any given infected individual will develop symptoms. By compiling detailed information about the various serologic events associated with HIV infection, clinicians hope to develop ways to predict, with some degree of accuracy, the likelihood of progression into AIDS. The $CD4^+$ T-cell count, although widely used clinically, is only a crude predictor of progression. In order to increase the accuracy of AIDS progression, several other serologic events are also being monitored.

Following HIV infection a sequence of serologic events occurs that can be used to diagnose HIV infection and to predict the progression from latency to lytic infection, culminating in an AIDS diagnosis (Figure 23-16). Soon after infection, the virus appears to replicate actively and the viral core protein p24 can be detected in the serum by ELISA or RIA. The p24 antigen is detectable in the serum for only a few weeks following infection and then disappears as the antibody response *(seroconversion)* develops. In most cases the time between infection and seroconversion is 6 weeks, but in some individuals the lag period has lasted for more than 3 years.

At seroconversion IgM antibody to HIV antigens can be detected; within a few weeks of seroconversion these IgM antibodies decline and anti-HIV IgG antibodies appear. The IgG antibodies are specific for many of the HIV structural proteins (e.g., gp160, gp120, gp41, p24, and p17). The appearance of antibody to the p24 core protein is particularly useful as its presence correlates with viral latency. As long as the antibody to p24 remains high, an individual remains asymptomatic. When the antibody to p24 begins to decline, there is a corresponding increase in the p24 antigen in the serum. This decline in antibody to p24 and increase in p24 antigen are associated with the progression of HIV from latency to lytic infection and have been used clinically to predict the onset of overt disease. Progression from latent HIV infection to AIDS can be predicted more reliably by use of $CD4^+$ T-cell counts and p24 levels than by T-cell counts alone. For example, of HIV-infected individuals who have $CD4^+$ T-cell counts greater than 400/μl and also are positive for p24, about 45% will progress to AIDS within 3 years.

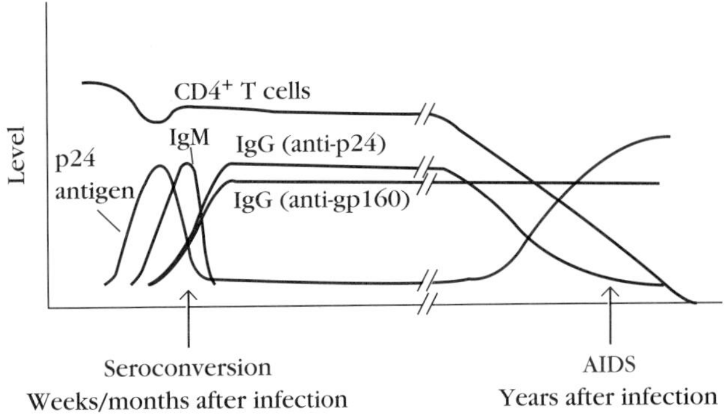

FIGURE 23-16 Serologic profile of HIV infection.

However, of infected individuals who are p24 positive and have $CD4^+$ T-cell counts less than 400/μl, 80% will progress to AIDS within 3 years.

In addition to p24 levels, serum levels of several other cellular products of activated lymphocytes or macrophages have been shown to serve as prognostic indicators of AIDS progression. Among these immune activation markers are β_2-microglobulin, neopterin, soluble CD8, and soluble IL-2 receptor. Elevated levels of β_2-microglobulin may reflect CTL- or virus-mediated destruction of cells resulting in the release of class I MHC molecules and the associated β_2-microglobulin. Neopterin is a metabolite produced following activation of macrophages by IFN-γ. Soluble CD8 and soluble IL-2 receptor are both cell-membrane molecules released from activated T cells. In one study 185 asymptomatic HIV-infected individuals were monitored for 36 months to correlate progression to AIDS with the presence of p24 antigen and one or more immune activation markers. Of those individuals who at the beginning of the study had $CD4^+$ T-cell counts between 200 and 499/μl and were negative for p24 and the immune activation markers, only 3–6% progressed to AIDS. In striking contrast, 60–90% of those individuals with similar T-cell counts but positive for p24 and two of the immune activation markers progressed to AIDS during the study period.

Screening Tests for HIV Infection

The standard screening test for HIV infection is an ELISA for serum antibody to HIV in which viral antigens are absorbed onto a solid phase. The patient's serum is added, unbound antibody is washed away, and then an enzyme-conjugated goat antihuman immunoglobulin reagent is added. After excess reagent is washed away, the substrate for the enzyme is added. A colored reaction product indicates that the patient has antibody to the HIV antigens and must therefore have been exposed to the virus. There is a lag period between the time of HIV infection and the appearance of enough antibody to be detected in the ELISA assay. Because of the lag period, potentially infectious individuals may screen negative for HIV infection. The importance of the lag period between HIV infection and seroconversion was demonstrated in 1991 by a news report of the transmission of HIV from an infected organ donor to a number of transplant recipients. In this case, the organ donor had been infected with HIV but had not yet seroconverted. Thus when an ELISA test was performed prior to organ transplantation, the donor screened negative for HIV infection. The lag period is often referred to as a "window of opportunity" and is a time when a HIV-infected individual will screen negative using an ELISA test for HIV-specific antibody. Also, as mentioned previously, AIDS patients often test negative for antibody in the late stages of the disease, when serum antibody levels drop as a result of depleted levels of T_H cells.

More sensitive and expensive tests, such as the Western blot and the polymerase chain reaction (PCR), are used to confirm HIV infection or to detect low-level infection. In a Western-blot assay, HIV proteins and glycoproteins are separated by electrophoresis and then transferred to a nitrocellulose membrane. The patient's serum is added to the nitrocellulose and allowed to react, and then a radiolabeled goat antihuman immunoglobulin reagent is added (see Figure 6-15). The presence of radioactive bands corresponding to the molecular weight of HIV antigens indicates the presence in the patient of antibody to HIV. In 1987 the CDC recommended that a positive HIV ELISA test should be confirmed by another ELISA and then by a positive Western blot. The polymerase chain reaction can be used to amplify a small number of proviral DNA copies isolated from a large amount of cellular DNA (see Figure 2-9). The PCR technique has made it possible to demonstrate HIV infection in a number of individuals who had tested negative by the ELISA and Western-blot assays.

Development of an AIDS Vaccine

The development of a vaccine requires knowledge of the infectious agent, characterization of the immune response to the agent, and determination of what type of immune response is protective. There are no shortcuts, and the development of most vaccines has been a long and arduous process. For example, development and testing of the most recent hepatitis B vaccine took 17 years. Human clinical trials of a vaccine must be conducted according to guidelines set by the Food and Drug Administration (FDA). A vaccine is first tested in appropriate animals to determine whether it is safe. Three phases of human clinical trials are then conducted. Phase I and phase II human trials are intended to evaluate the safety, dosage, and immunogenicity of a vaccine preparation. Phase III trials are designed to determine the effectiveness of a vaccine.

The first human phase I clinical trial of an AIDS vaccine began in September 1987 when 81 volunteers were immunized with genetically engineered gp160.

Phase II trials, with larger numbers of volunteers, attempt to extend the phase I findings on safety, dosage, and immunogenicity. Phase III trials require much larger numbers of volunteers so that the degree of vaccine protection afforded by the vaccine can be assessed by statistical measures. Because of the high mortality of HIV infection, the FDA has tried to shorten some aspects of the review process. All AIDS-related drug and vaccine treatments, for instance, have been given a special designation, 1-AA, that automatically moves them ahead in the review process.

Obstacles to Development of an AIDS Vaccine

Despite the extensive efforts to develop an AIDS vaccine and the actions of the FDA to hasten testing and review, several properties of HIV itself hamper vaccine development. For any vaccine to be successful it must be able to induce an immune response that renders the host protected against the pathogen. Unfortunately, the type of immune response that is protective against HIV is not yet known. Moreover, as was seen in the development of a vaccine for measles, some types of immune response actually may increase the likelihood of infection. J. Levy has shown that certain subclasses of antibody to HIV mediate uptake of the virus into macrophages via Fc receptors and thus enhance infection. Therefore, until the mechanisms of protective immunity to HIV are more fully understood, researchers will not be able to focus their energy on one type of immune response and may develop vaccines that do not elicit protective immunity.

As discussed earlier, HIV constantly mutates and changes its surface glycoproteins, allowing it to evade the immune response. Such antigenic shift, which occurs in a variety of other viruses, has been a major obstacle to development of an AIDS vaccine. The challenge facing researchers is to develop a single vaccine (or mixture of a small number of vaccines) that is effective against myriad antigenically diverse HIV strains. A number of published reports of experimental vaccine trials appear hopeful, but the implications of these trials may be limited. In these studies a state of immunity that protects the animal against a later challenge with live SIV or HIV has been induced; however, to date the strain of the virus used for the subsequent challenge has been the same as the strain used for immunization. Knowing that HIV has such a high mutation rate, one must continually ask whether the animal will be protected against other strains of the virus that differ antigenically from the immunizing strain.

Before his death in 1993, Albert Sabin, the developer of the oral polio vaccine, raised another caution in regard to interpreting the effectiveness of the initial AIDS vaccine trials. Sabin pointed out that all animal vaccine trials to date have challenged the animal with the live virus, not with virus-infected cells. Since the HIV-infected cell has been shown to be the major vehicle of transmission, Sabin suggested that test animals should be challenged with virus-infected cells rather than with the free virus. He believed that it will be much more difficult to generate immunity to HIV-infected cells than to the free virus and therefore cautioned against unwarranted optimism about the positive results of the early vaccine trials.

Another major hindrance to developing an AIDS vaccine has been the lack of a suitable animal model. The chimpanzee and the pigtailed macaque monkey are the only natural animal models for HIV-1 infection. Although HIV can produce a persistent infection in the chimpanzee, the infection does not lead to an immune deficiency (Table 23-10). Testing of a potential vaccine in chimpanzees must therefore focus on inhibition of viral replication rather than on the immunodeficiency manifestations. Moreover, use of

TABLE 23-10 INFECTIVITY AND PATHOGENICITY OF HIV-1, HIV-2, AND SIV_{AGM} IN VARIOUS ANIMALS

Virus	Animal	Infection	AIDS
HIV-1	Human	+	+
	Chimpanzee	+	−
	Scid-human mouse	+	?
	Pigtailed macaque	+	?
HIV-2	Human	+	+
	Chimpanzee	+	−
	Macaque (rhesus) monkey	+	+
	Baboon	+	−
SIV_{AGM}	African green monkey	+	−
	Macaque (rhesus) monkey	+	+ (SAIDS)

chimpanzees for AIDS-vaccine testing poses an increasing threat to the already dwindling chimpanzee population. The pharmaceutical industry has been pushing vigorously for the World Health Organization to relax restrictions on the importation of chimpanzees from Africa. The contention is that a shortage of captive chimpanzees (fewer than 600 in the United States) is impeding the development of vaccines for AIDS. Yet a 1988 paper in *Nature* from scientists in the United States, the Netherlands, Germany, and France highlights the threat of extinction to wild chimpanzees. The authors maintain that many chimpanzees of breeding age will be killed as attempts are made to capture infants for export; they estimate that 10 chimpanzees die for every infant that eventually reaches its overseas destination. Certainly these issues point to the need for proper management, sharing of research information among competing groups, and attention to priorities as vaccine trials go forward in chimpanzees in research laboratories around the world.

Development of *scid*-human mice has given AIDS researchers some optimism in their search for a practical animal model. Two distinct approaches to developing the *scid*-human mouse have proved useful. In the approach developed by M. McCune, the immune system of CB-17 *scid* mice is reconstituted with human fetal liver, mesenteric lymph node, and thymus (see Figure 2-1). In the other approach, developed by D. Mosier, *scid* mice are reconstituted with human peripheral-blood mononuclear cells. In both systems the mice become populated with human T and B lymphocytes and with other white blood cells. When *scid*-human mice are challenged with HIV, the human CD4$^+$ T cells and myeloid cells have been shown to become infected. Mosier, for example, found a significant depletion in the CD4$^+$ T cells of *scid*-human mice within 8 weeks of HIV infection (Figure 23-17). These mice may prove to be a workable animal model for studying the mechanism of immune suppression in AIDS and for evaluating potential drug and vaccine therapies.

Indeed, *scid*-human mice have already proved useful for in vivo evaluation of antiviral agents and AIDS vaccines. McCune, for example, demonstrated that azido-3′-deoxythymidine (AZT), the first therapeutic drug approved for AIDS patients, inhibits HIV infection in *scid*-human mice developed by his method. Studies with these mice helped to define therapeutic levels of AZT and dideoxyinosine (ddI) for use in humans. Mosier also showed that *scid*-human mice were protected from a later challenge with HIV when they were produced with peripheral-blood cells from human volunteers who had been immunized with a recombinant vaccinia virus vaccine expressing gp160.

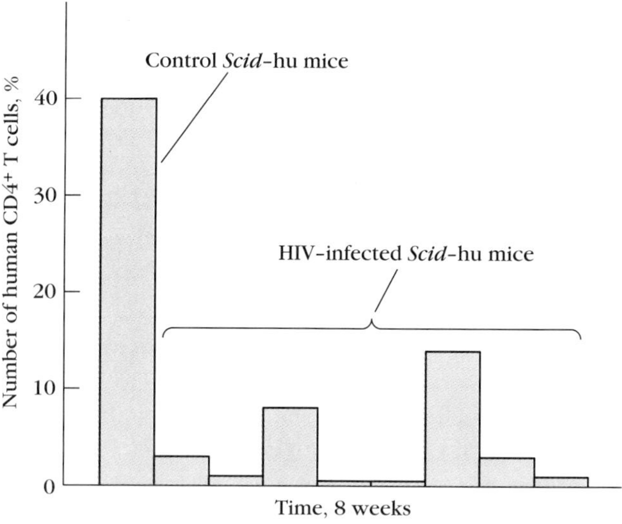

FIGURE 23-17 Depletion of CD4$^+$ T cells in HIV-infected *scid*-human mice 8 weeks after infection. [Data from D. E. Mosier et al., 1991, *Science* **251**:791.]

Experimental AIDS Vaccines

Ever since HIV was identified as the causative agent of AIDS, tremendous effort has been directed toward the development of a safe and effective vaccine. Several types of vaccines have been designed, including inactivated whole virus, live recombinant viruses, attenuated virus, recombinant DNA products, synthetic peptides, and anti-idiotype antibodies. A summary of human trials of AIDS vaccines under way as of mid-1993 is presented in Table 23-11.

Inactivated Whole Viruses

Inactivated preparations of HIV-1 and SIV have been produced by irradiating the virus and treating it with formaldehyde. This procedure, similar to that used to develop the Salk polio vaccine, inactivates the retroviral genome and releases much of the gp120 from the envelope. The noninfectious SIV or HIV preparation is then used as a vaccine. The results of trials with such vaccines are summarized in Table 23-12.

In the two trials of inactivated SIV, macaque monkeys were immunized with the vaccine and then challenged with doses of live SIV considerably higher than the established minimum infectious dose. All the unvaccinated controls became infected and all developed SAIDS, whereas none of the vaccinated monkeys developed SAIDS during the trial period, although some of them became infected.

TABLE 23-11 SURVEY OF AIDS VACCINE TRIALS IN HUMANS IN PROGRESS IN MID-1993

Type of vaccine	Company	Recipients	Status
Inactivated HIV	Immunization Products Ltd.	HIV-infected asymptomatic patients	Phase II/III
gp160	Immuno AG National Institutes of Health	AIDS patients	Phase I
gp160	MicroGeneSys	HIV-infected asymptomatic patients HIV-negative volunteers HIV-infected pregnant women, newborns, and children	Phase II Phase I/II Phase I*
gp120 (MN crown)	Genentech	HIV-infected adults, pregnant women, newborns and children	Phase I*
gp 120 (SF-2 crown)	Chiron, Ciba-Geigy	AIDS patients; HIV-infected pregnant woman, newborns, and children	Phase I*
p24	MicroGeneSys	AIDS patients	Phase I
p24 synthetic peptide	Viral technologies	Uninfected volunteers	Phase I
Vector vaccine (gp 120 in canary pox)	Pasteur Merieux	Uninfected volunteers	Phase I
Anti-idiotype antibody	IDEC Pharmaceuticals	HIV-infected asymptomatic patients	Phase I

* Trials begun in early 1993.

TABLE 23-12 TRIALS WITH INACTIVATED SIV_{AGM} AND HIV-1 VACCINES

Date	Recipient (no.)	Inactivated vaccine	Challenge	Observations
June 1989	Macaques (6)	SIV	Live SIV	2/6 no detectable SIV 4/6 detectable SIV 6/6 no SAIDS/no deaths
	Macaques (4): controls	None	Live SIV	4/4 SAIDS 3/4 died
Dec. 1989	Macaques (9)	SIV	Live SIV	8/9 no detectable SIV 8/9 no SAIDS
	Macaques (7): controls	None	Live SIV	7/7 detectable SIV 7/7 SAIDS
June 1989	Chimpanzee (3)	HIV	Live HIV	3/3 no detectable HIV
1988–1989	HIV-infected humans (19)	HIV	None	7/19 increased $CD4^+$ T cells; of these, 6/7 increased skin-test response 4/19 decreased $CD4^+$ T cells; of these, 4/4 decreased skin-test response

Inactivated HIV-1 has been tested in chimpanzees that were subsequently challenged with live HIV and in HIV-infected humans. In one trial, the vaccine was given to three chimpanzees, two of which were already infected with HIV. Following two booster injections with the vaccine, all three chimpanzees were given a large injection of live HIV. All three vaccinated chimps were shown to clear the HIV, and all three have remained free of virus. Although these animal trials with inactivated SIV and HIV are hopeful, it is important to keep in mind that the animals were vaccinated and subsequently challenged with the same strain of SIV or HIV. As discussed previously, these trials offer no evidence that such vaccines will offer widespread protection against unrelated strains of the virus.

An additional problem with interpreting the results of animal trials with SIV vaccines arises because these vaccines are prepared by growing SIV in human T cells. Thus, as SIV buds out of the human cells, it acquires human cell-membrane antigens (e.g., class I MHC molecules) on its envelope. In fact, the level of human MHC molecules on the SIV envelope is actually higher than the level of viral gp120! In an article published in *Science* (December 1992), L. O. Arthur and co-workers suggested that the immunity induced by inactivated SIV vaccine actually may represent an immune response by the macaque to the human antigens in the vaccine rather than the SIV antigens. They uncovered this possibility quite by accident when they immunized some control macaques with uninfected human cells for comparison with animals immunized with inactivated SIV. Much to their surprise both groups of macaques were protected against a later challenge with live SIV, even though the control group had been immunized only with human cells. These results indicate that the immune response mounted by the controls against human cell-membrane antigens allowed the animals to subsequently eliminate live SIV virus. This finding clearly raises serious questions about the interpretation of results with inactivated SIV vaccine.

An inactivated-HIV vaccine was tested in 1988–1989 in clinical phase I trials on 19 HIV-infected humans who manifested early symptoms of AIDS; the objective was to boost their immune response to viral antigens. Of these 19 individuals, 7 showed an increase in their $CD4^+$ T-cell count following vaccination, and 6 of these 7 also showed an increase in cell-mediated immunity, demonstrated by skin testing. However, in 4 of the 19 vaccine recipients the level of $CD4^+$ T cells decreased following vaccination, as did the skin-test response. It is not known why some individuals responded positively to the vaccine and others did not. In any case, the inactivated-vaccine approach is not without potential risks, as work with feline leukemia virus (FeLV), a retrovirus that causes leukemia in cats, has demonstrated. When cats were vaccinated with an irradiated and formaldehyde-treated preparation of FeLV, some of them actually developed enhanced susceptibility to infection compared with unvaccinated controls.

Cloned Envelope Glycoproteins

Several groups have applied gene-engineering techniques to clone the gp120 gene or the entire gp160 gene in order to produce large quantities of gp120 or gp160 for immunization. The first of the cloned gp160 vaccines, which was produced by MicroGeneSys Inc., was administered in September 1987 to 140 healthy seronegative volunteers. The vaccine induced largely-humoral immunity to HIV. The antibodies elicited in the volunteers were shown to inhibit viral replication in vitro, but the inhibition was always strain specific—a result of the antigenic variation of gp160. Presently phase II clinical trials are under way in patients with early HIV infection; phase I and II clinical trials are under way in uninfected volunteers. Phase I trials also were started in 1993 in HIV-infected pregnant women, newborns, and children.

Phase I clinical trials of two genetically engineered gp120 vaccines began in the spring of 1993. One vaccine, produced by Genentech, consists of gp120 from the MN strain of HIV-1. The MN sequence is a conserved crown sequence present in a high proportion of HIV isolates in North America (see Figure 23-9). The other vaccine, produced by Chiron, contains gp120 from the SF-2 strain, which has another conserved crown sequence. Earlier animal trials of Genentech's recombinant gp120 vaccine were promising. In these animal trials four chimpanzees were immunized, two with recombinant gp160 and two with recombinant gp120, and then challenged with live HIV-1. The control unimmunized group and both chimpanzees immunized with gp160 became infected with HIV-1 within 7 weeks of challenge. However, the two chimpanzees that were immunized with the recombinant gp120 were reported to show no sign of HIV infection, even by the very sensitive PCR technique, for more than 6 months.

One limitation with vaccines of this sort is that they are soluble glycoproteins and therefore are processed as exogenous antigen; thus, they are not very likely to induce a significant $CD8^+$ CTL response. In order to induce $CD8^+$ CTLs specific for gp120 or gp160, the antigen must be introduced by a route that will favor antigen processing and presentation together with class I MHC molecules. Two types of vaccines discussed in Chapter 20 are being developed to accomplish this end (see Figure 20-5b). Gp120-containing liposomes have been constructed; these can fuse with cells, enabling the gp120 to be processed by an endogenous pathway. Gp120 also has been incorporated into immunostimulating complexes (ISCOMs), which are particles with a mean diameter of 35 nm that hold protein antigens in an adjuvant-containing micelle. ISCOMs can penetrate the plasma membrane and deliver the antigen to the cytoplasm where it would likely be processed as an endogenous antigen and presented together with class I MHC molecules. Gp120-containing ISCOMs have been reported to induce $CD8^+$ CTLs specific for gp120.

Several possible concerns about vaccines employing gp120 or gp160 have yet to be evaluated. One concern, mentioned already, is whether gp120 itself might induce syncytia formation and thus increase T-cell depletion. Another concern is that a strong humoral-antibody response might increase the cellular spread of HIV infection through binding of antibody-HIV complexes to Fc receptors on macrophages. A third concern stems from the observation that gp160 shares amino acid sequences in common with certain class II MHC molecules. It is not known whether individuals possessing these class II MHC molecules might be at risk for developing some type of autoimmune reaction when immunized with gp160. Finally the tremendous genetic variation in gp120 and gp160 among different HIV strains makes it unlikely that any one vaccine would provide protection against an unrelated HIV strain.

Attenuated Viruses

In general, attenuated viral vaccines are produced by growing live viruses under unusual culture conditions that force the virus to mutate to survive in the new conditions. The Sabin polio vaccine, for example, was produced by growing the live polio virus in monkey kidney cell cultures. The majority of viral vaccines used today are attenuated vaccines; these include the measles, mumps, rubella, and polio vaccines. Because the vaccine is live, it is able to infect cells and grow for a limited amount of time before the immune response eliminates the virus. During this time, the attenuated virus is able to induce a potent immune response, often with cell-mediated CTLs produced to the endogenously produced viral antigens. In addition, attenuated viral vaccines tend to produce a good memory cell response, which accounts for the life-long immunity generated by these vaccines. The limitation of these vaccines is the risk that the attenuated virus may be able to mutate back to a virulent strain.

Because of the high rate of mutation in HIV and its virulence, attenuated HIV strains were long considered too dangerous for use as vaccines. This prevailing opinion has been called into question by the work of R. Desrosiers and his colleagues. These researchers eliminated the regulatory gene *nef* from a highly virulent strain of SIV. When the *nef*-deleted strain of SIV was injected into six macaques, the animals did not develop symptoms of SAIDS. The macaques were then challenged with a small dose of infectious live SIV and remained healthy. Finally, the researchers challenged the animals with a huge dose of infectious SIV and found that the animals still continued to remain healthy. The beauty of this system is that removal of the *nef* gene makes it impossible for the virus to mutate back to a virulent form.

Recombinant Viruses Carrying HIV Genes

Recombinant vector vaccines are another approach that may prove useful in the search for an effective AIDS vaccine. Vaccinia virus and the Sabin polio virus are both live attenuated viruses that have proved to be safe and successful vaccines for smallpox and polio, respectively. Both of these viruses can be engineered to carry genes from HIV-1, and the recombinant virus can then be used as an HIV vaccine. Because the recombinant virus is attenuated (not inactivated), it is able to infect host cells and would therefore be expected to induce CTL activity. As with any attenuated vaccine, the prolonged exposure to the viral antigens tends to induce a very good immune response without the need of additional boosters.

Vaccinia virus, which is a large virus, can be engineered to carry several dozen foreign genes without impairing its capacity to infect host cells and to replicate in them. A genetically engineered vaccinia virus can be administered simply by dermal scratching; the virus causes a limited localized infection in host cells (see Figure 20-4). The foreign genes are expressed by the vaccinia, and if the foreign gene product is a viral envelope protein, it is inserted into the membrane of the infected host cell and there stimulates the development of T-cell–mediated immunity. Vaccinia virus carrying gp160 has been shown to infect host cells at the site of scarification; the gp160 is glycosylated, cleaved into gp120 and gp41, and inserted into the plasma membrane of the infected host cells. A number of HIV genes have been engineered into vaccinia virus, including *env, tat, pol,* and *gag.*

In experiments conducted by researchers at the Oncogen Corporation, chimpanzees were immunized with vaccinia virus carrying the gp120 gene. The vaccine induced production of protective antibodies to gp120 and sensitization of T_C cells. When the sensitized T_C cells from the immunized chimpanzees were tested in an in vitro CML reaction, they killed target cells infected with the recombinant vaccinia virus. These initial findings appeared hopeful, but unfortunately later clinical trials revealed that the immunized chimpanzees were not protected from infection with live HIV-1.

Trials of this same type of vaccine were conducted by Daniel Zagury and co-workers of the Pasteur Institute. Healthy human volunteers (including Zagury himself) were immunized by scarification with recombinant vaccinia virus expressing the gp160 envelope glycoprotein. The primary response was weak, and the volunteers were subsequently boosted intramuscularly with their own cells, which had first been infected in vitro with the recombinant vaccinia virus. These individuals showed enhanced in vitro cell-mediated immunity to HIV following each booster immunization. Such an approach to large-scale clinical trials is limited logistically by the difficulty of immunization with autologous cells infected in vitro with recombinant vaccinia virus. Zagury's vaccinia-based HIV vaccine trials were criticized because of questions about the degree of informed consent in the test trials on human subjects in Zaire, which were conducted without the prior approval of a Zairian or French human subjects ethics committee. Consequently, the French minister of health, Bruno Durieux, eventually imposed a ban on these vaccine trials, and the National Institutes of Health in the United States rescinded permission for Robert Gallo at the National Cancer Institute to collaborate with Zagury. Adding to the controversy was the finding that three recipients of the vaccine died from disseminated vaccinia infection. Although, vaccinia is a safe vaccine in healthy individuals, the attenuated virus can cause disseminated lesions in individuals with immune-system compromise. At the VII International Conference on AIDS in Florence, Zagury announced that he would discontinue the vaccinia vaccine trials. This case demonstrates the importance of ethical awareness in scientific research, particularly where the welfare of human subjects is involved.

Synthetic Crown-Sequence Peptides

The principal neutralizing epitope of HIV overlaps with the V3 loop of gp120 (see Figure 23-8), and antibodies to the V3 loop have been shown to protect chimpanzees from HIV infection. Because of the high level of variation in the V3 loop, antibody neutralization is always strain specific. However, the so-called crown sequence in the V3 loop is conserved to a considerable degree (see Figure 23-9). Approximately 30% of North American HIV isolates have the crown sequence designated MN. Synthetic peptides of different HIV crown sequences, including the MN sequence, have been prepared and tested for their ability to activate T-cell proliferation and cytotoxicity in vitro. These synthetic peptides appear to activate a population of T_H cells and to induce some cytotoxic activity; however, because these peptides are processed as exogenous antigens, the T cytotoxic cells induced were all $CD4^+$, class II restricted. These studies suggest that cocktails of synthetic peptides, representing the crown sequences of the predominant HIV isolates, might induce protective antibody or $CD4^+$ T cytotoxic cells.

Cloned CD4

A number of laboratories have cloned CD4 and used it as a vaccine in an effort to block HIV infection. Because gp120 binds to CD4 with such high affinity, the hope is that soluble CD4 may bind effectively to gp120 on HIV and thus block viral binding to host cells (Figure 23-18a). In vitro studies have revealed that soluble cloned CD4 can indeed inhibit HIV binding and infection of T cells and can also inhibit syncytia formation. In one study four SIV-infected macaques were given daily intramuscular injections of 2 mg of soluble cloned CD4 for 50 days. Before the CD4 treatment, SIV could be isolated from peripheral-blood cultures or bone marrow cultures from all the infected monkeys. Within 2 weeks of the first CD4 injection, the virus could not be recovered from either peripheral-blood or bone marrow cultures in three of the four monkeys. Cell cultures from these three monkeys remained free of SIV for 18–43 days after the CD4 injections were stopped. The one monkey that failed to show this effect had already shown severe T-cell depletion at the beginning of the study and died 3 days after the end of treatment; autopsy suggested that death was due to simian AIDS rather than to the CD4 treatment. Results with soluble cloned CD4 look hopeful, and phase 1 clinical trials in AIDS patients are now in progress.

One of the problems with a soluble CD4 vaccine in humans is that CD4 has a half-life of only 30–120 min in serum, which necessitates frequent injections. D. J. Capon and colleagues reported overcoming this limitation in an ingenious way by linking the CD4 gene to the constant-region gene of human IgG1. The CD4-immunoglobulin hybrid encoded by this recombinant gene, called an *immunoadhesin,* exhibits the

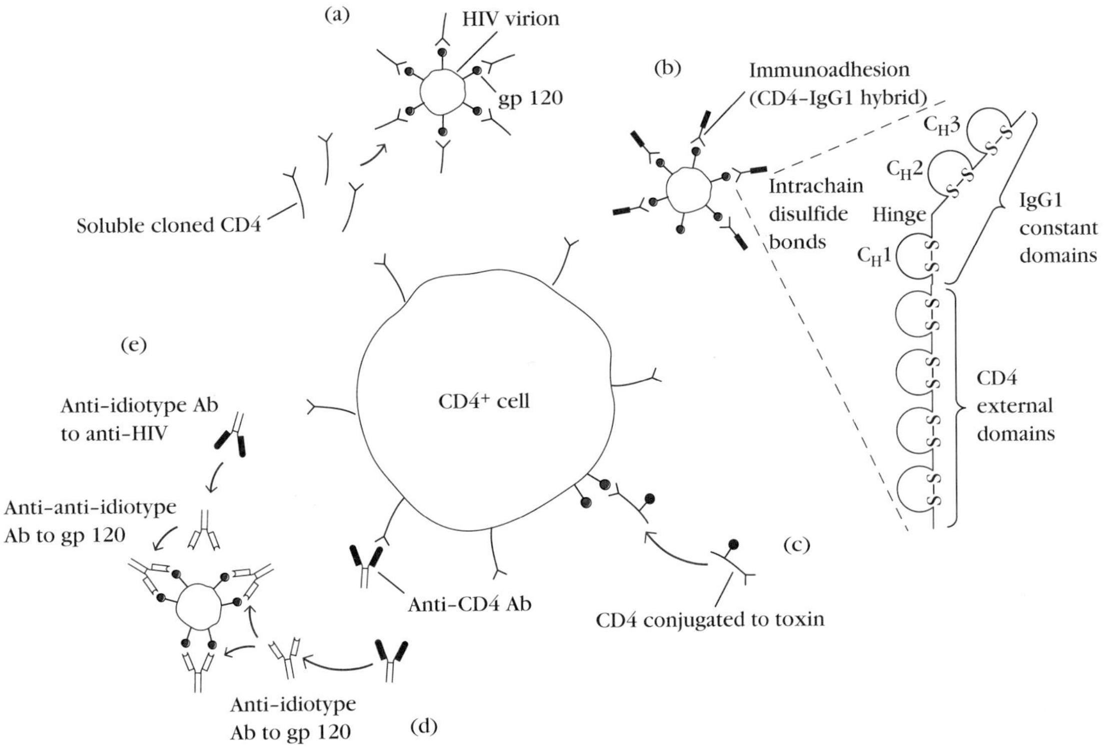

FIGURE 23-18 Mechanisms by which various reagents can interfere with the gp120-CD4 interaction, which is necessary for HIV to infect T cells. (a) Soluble cloned CD4 binds to gp120 on HIV virions. (b) An immunoadhesin formed from the external domains of CD4 and the constant region of IgG1 also binds to gp120 on virions. The half-life of this immunoadhesin in the blood is considerably longer than that of soluble CD4. (c) Binding of CD4 linked to a toxin to viral gp120 on HIV-infected cells leads to death of the cell. (d,e) Both anti-CD4 antibody (d) and anti-idiotype antibody specific for the paratope on anti-HIV antibody (e) can induce production of antibodies that bind to gp120 without exposing the individual to HIV or to HIV components.

high-affinity binding of gp120 characteristic of CD4 but has the longer serum half-life characteristic of IgG1 (Figure 23-18b). Initial animal studies with this immunoadhesin revealed that its half-life is 200-fold longer than that of soluble CD4; in humans the half-life of this immunoadhesin is expected to approach 21 days. It is also possible to engineer immunoadhesins with different immunoglobulin Fc regions to induce different effector functions such as opsonization or complement activation.

Another approach utilizing soluble CD4 that has been tried is to conjugate a toxin chemically to CD4. Any HIV-infected cell expressing gp120 on its membrane should bind the soluble CD4 toxin and be killed (Figure 23-18c). It is hoped that alternating administration of soluble CD4, to bind the free virus and inhibit infection of additional T cells, followed by CD4-toxin, to kill HIV-infected cells, might prove effective.

Anti-Idiotype Antibodies

Anti-idiotype antibody specific for the antigen-binding site (the paratope) on anti-HIV antibody is an attractive vaccine approach, especially when undesirable or uncontrollable side effects might be induced with an attenuated or killed whole-pathogen vaccine. When anti-idiotype antibody specific for the paratope is administered, an animal makes antibody to the binding site on the anti-idiotype antibody, and this antibody (called anti-anti-idiotype antibody) will also bind to the original antigen (see Figure 16-5). In this way an animal can become immune to an antigen without having to see the antigen; it is exposed instead to anti-idiotype antibody. Kaprowski has produced anti-idiotype antibody to HIV antigens and then injected it into animals to produce anti-anti-idiotype antibody, which also binds to HIV antigens. The beauty of this scheme is that it avoids immunizing with the virus or viral components. Following the same principle, researchers have immunized animals with anti-CD4 monoclonals to generate an anti-idiotype response to the antibody. This induced anti-idiotype antibody blocks the CD4-binding site on HIV (Figure 23-18d,e).

Summary

1. HIV—an enveloped retrovirus containing ssRNA as its genome—is the causative agent for AIDS. The virus infects host cells when its envelope glycoprotein gp120 binds to CD4 molecules on cell membranes. Upon entry into a cell, the virus copies its RNA into DNA with a viral reverse transcriptase. The DNA can then integrate into the host chromosomal DNA forming a provirus, which can remain in a latent state for varying periods of time.

2. Activation of an HIV-infected $CD4^+$ T cell also triggers activation of the provirus, resulting in transcription of the viral structural proteins and assembly of viral particles at the host cell's plasma membrane. Viral particles are released from the host cell by a process called budding, in which portions of the host-cell plasma membrane modified with viral glycoproteins become the viral envelope. Destruction of the host-cell plasma membrane in this process can lead to cell death.

3. Destruction of $CD4^+$ T_H cells following HIV infection leads to severe immune-system depression, reflecting the necessary role of T_H cells in activation of B cells and T_C cells, delayed-type hypersensitivity, and IL-2–mediated activation of NK cells.

4. Since less than 0.01% of the $CD4^+$ T cells in an HIV-infected individual are actually infected with the virus, the extensive depletion of T_H cells that is observed means that uninfected $CD4^+$ T_H cells also are destroyed. Several mechanisms have been proposed to account for destruction of uninfected T_H cells. One theory is that binding of soluble gp120 to CD4 on uninfected cells may lead to their destruction by antibody-plus-complement lysis or antibody-dependent cell-mediated cytotoxicity. Another hypothesis speculates that soluble gp120 may induce an unusual population of $CD4^+$ T_C cells specific for gp120 peptides presented by class II MHC molecules on activated T_H cells. Still other hypotheses suggest that soluble gp120 may bind to CD4 and either block T_H-cell activation or induce an inappropriate signal resulting in programmed cell death.

5. Several approaches are being tried in the extensive effort to develop an effective AIDS vaccine. Experimental vaccines that have been developed and tested to some extent include the following: inactivated HIV, cloned envelope glycoproteins, recombinant vaccinia virus carrying HIV envelope-protein genes, synthetic peptides of the gp120 crown sequence, soluble CD4 and CD4-IgG1 hybrids (immunoadhesins), and anti-idiotype antibody specific for gp120 epitopes or the CD4-binding site on gp120. Development of an effective AIDS vaccine has been hampered by the extensive antigenic variation exhibited by HIV; the ability of HIV to exist as a provirus in host cells, where it is unaccessible to the immune system; and the lack of a good animal model for AIDS.

References

ARTHUR, L. O., J. W. BESS JR., R. C. SOWDER II et al. 1992. Cellular proteins bound to immunodeficiency viruses: implications for pathogenesis and vaccines. *Science* **258**:1935.

ASCHER, M. S., and H. W. SHEPPARD. 1990. AIDS as immune system activation. *J. Acquired Immune Deficiency Syndromes* **3**:177.

BERZOFSKY, J. A. 1991. Approaches and issues in the development of vaccines against HIV. *J. Acquired Immune Deficiency Syndrome* **4**:451.

BOLOGNESI, D. P. 1990. Progress in vaccine development against SIV and HIV. *J. Acquired Immune Deficiency Syndromes* **3**:390.

CAPON, D. J., S. M. CHAMOW, J. MORDENTI et al. 1989. Designing CD4 immunoadhesins for AIDS therapy. *Nature* **337**:525.

CAPON, D. J., and R. H. R. WARD. 1991. The CD4-gp120 interaction and AIDS pathogenesis. *Annu. Rev. Immunol.* **9**:649.

CENTERS FOR DISEASE CONTROL. 1990. HIV/AIDS surveillance report. April:**1**.

COHEN, J. 1992. AIDS vaccines: is older better? *Science* **258**:1880.

CONSTANTINE, N. T. 1993. Serologic tests for the retroviruses: approaching a decade of evolution. *AIDS* **7**:1.

DANIEL, M., F. KIRCHOFF, S. C. CZAJAK et al. 1992. Protective effects of a live attenuated SIV vaccine with a deletion in the nef gene. *Science* **258**:1938.

EIDEN, L. E., and J. D. LIFSON. 1992. HIV interactions with CD4: a continuum of conformations and consequences. *Immunol. Today* **13**:201.

FAUCI, A. S. 1988. The human immunodeficiency virus: infectivity and mechanisms of pathogenesis. *Science* **239**:617.

FOX, C. H., and M. COTTLER-FOX. 1992. The pathobiology of HIV infection. *Immunol. Today* **13**:353.

GALLO, R. C. 1990. Mechanism of disease induction by HIV. *J. Acquired Immune Deficiency Syndromes* **3**:380.

GERMAINE, R. N. 1988. Antigen processing and $CD4^+$ T cell depletion in AIDS. *Cell* **54**:441.

GREENE, W. C. 1991. The molecular biology of human immunodeficiency virus type I infection. *New Engl. J. Med.* **324**:308.

HABESHAW, J., E. HOUNSELL, and A. DALGLEISH. 1992. Does the HIV envelope induce a chronic graft-versus-host-like disease? *Immunol. Today* **13**:207.

HASELTINE, W. A. 1991. Molecular biology of the human immunodeficiency virus type I. *FASEB* **5**:2349.

IMBERTI, L., A. SOTTINI, A. BETTINARDI et al. 1991. Selective depletion in HIV infection of T cells that bear specific T cell receptor V_β sequences. *Science* **254**:860.

KARON, J. M., T. J. DONDERO, and J. W. CURRAN. 1988. The projected incidence of AIDS and estimated prevalence of HIV infection in the United States. *J. Acquired Immune Deficiency Syndromes* **1**:542.

LAURENCE, J. 1988. Vaccines and immunology overview. *AIDS* **2** (Suppl. 1):91.

MCCUNE, J. M., R. NAMIKAWA, C. C. SHIH et al. 1990. Suppression of HIV infection in AZT-treated SCID-hu mice. *Science* **247**:564.

MCCUNE, J. M., H. KANESHIMA, J. KROWKA et al. 1991. The SCID-hu mouse: a small animal model for HIV infection and pathogenesis. *Annu. Rev. Immunol.* **9**:399.

MATSUYAMA, T., N. KOBAYASHI, and N. YAMAMOTO. 1991. Cytokines and HIV infection: is AIDS a tumor necrosis factor disease? *AIDS* **5**:1405.

MOSIER, D. E., R. J. GULIZIA, S. M. BAIRD et al. 1991. Human immunodeficiency virus infection of human-PBL-SCID mice. *Science* **251**:791.

MURPHEY-CORB, M., L. N. MARTIN, B. DAVISON-FAIRBURN, et al. 1989. A formalin inactivated whole SIV vaccine confers protection in macaques. *Science* **246**:1293.

NAMIKAWA, R., H. KANESHIMA, M. LIEBERMAN et al. 1988. Infection of the SCID-hu mouse by HIV-1. *Science* **242**:1684.

PETERLIN, B. M., and P. A. LUCIW. 1988. Molecular biology of HIV. *AIDS 1988* **2**(Suppl. 1):29.

PUTNEY, S. 1992. How antibodies block HIV infection: paths to an AIDS vaccine. *TIBS* **17**:191.

ROSENBERG, Z. F., and A. S. FAUCI. 1990. Immunopathogenic mechanisms of HIV infection: cytokine induction of HIV expression. *Immunol. Today* **11**:176.

ROSENBERG, Z. F., and A. S. FAUCI. 1991. Immunopathogenesis of HIV infection. *FASEB* **5**:2382.

TILL, M. A., V. GHETIE, T. GREGORY et al. 1990. Immunoconjugates containing ricin A chain and either human anti-gp41 or CD4 kill H9 cells infected with different isolates of HIV but do not inhibit normal T or B cell function. *J. Acquired Immune Deficiency Syndromes* **3**:609.

WEISS, R. A., P. R. CLAPHAM, M. O. MCCLURE et al. 1988. Human immunodeficiency viruses: neutralization and receptors. *J. Acquired Immune Deficiency Syndromes* **1**:536.

WIGZELL, H. 1988. Immunopathogenesis of HIV infection. *J. Acquired Immune Deficiency Syndromes* **1**:559.

WIGZELL, H. 1991. Prospects for an HIV-vaccine. *FASEB* **5**:2406.

Study Questions

1. Indicate whether each of the following statements is true or false. If you think a statement is false, explain why.
   a. HIV-1 and HIV-2 are more closely related to each other than to SIV.
   b. HIV-1 causes immune suppression in both humans and chimpanzees.
   c. SIV is endemic in the African green monkey.
   d. The Tat protein of HIV appears to increase proviral transcription.
   e. T-cell activation increases transcription of the HIV proviral genome.
   f. HIV can only infect cells expressing CD4.
   g. Patients with advanced stages of AIDS always have detectable antibody to HIV.
   h. The polymerase chain reaction is a sensitive test that can be used to detect antibodies to HIV.
   i. Production of antibody to HIV sometimes increases the likelihood of HIV infection.

2. What is the rationale for administering soluble CD4 to AIDS patients? What is a major limitation of this approach and what experimental procedures are being developed to overcome this limitation?

3. Would you expect to see much p17 and p24 in the blood of HIV-infected individuals in the asymptomatic latency period?

4. If p24 levels begin to increase dramatically in the blood of an HIV-infected individual, what would this indicate about HIV infection?

5. Why do clinicians monitor the level of skin-test reactivity in HIV-infected individuals? What change might you expect to see in skin-test reactivity with progression into AIDS?

6. What type of immune response would probably be induced by immunization with a recombinant vaccinia virus carrying the HIV gene encoding gp120?

TRANSPLANTATION IMMUNOLOGY

Transplantation, as the term is used in immunology, refers to the act of transferring cells, tissues, or organs from one site to another. The surgical procedures for many kinds of transplantation were developed by the turn of the century. With the surgical technology in place, scientists began to ask whether organs or tissues might be transplanted from one individual to another. In the early 1900s a Viennese surgeon observed that he could surgically remove a kidney from an animal and then transplant it back into the same animal and restore kidney function. When the kidney was transplanted to a different animal, however, it soon ceased to function. Experimental transplantation between animals continued through the 1920s and 1930s, but every attempt was a dismal failure. Autopsies revealed massive infiltrations of white blood cells into the donated organ or tissue.

Several observations by P. B. Medawar in the early 1940s convinced him that graft rejection was due to an immunologic response. While working with burn patients during World War II, he noticed that grafts of skin from one site to another on the same patient were readily accepted, whereas grafts from relatives were rejected. In one patient a skin graft from a brother had been rejected; when a second graft from the same donor was attempted, the rejection occurred much faster and with much greater intensity. This observation led Medawar to experiment with animals and to discover that prior sensitization with donor cells led to heightened rejection of a subsequent graft. In 1945 he published a paper suggesting that graft rejection resulted from an immunologic response to the donor organ.

Medawar's suggestion proved to be correct. No matter how skilled the surgeon is, a surgically successful transplant can be thwarted by an immunologic attack. The very system that had evolved to recognize and destroy altered self-cells was simply performing its function by recognizing and destroying the foreign cells of the graft. The subdiscipline of transplantation immunology sought to understand the immunologic basis of graft rejection. Active experimentation sought techniques for reducing immune-system activation and thus promoting graft acceptance. Various immunosuppressive agents soon were developed to diminish the immunologic attack. Within just 10 years of Medawar's 1945 paper, the first kidney transplantation in humans was successfully performed. Today transplantations that once were widely publicized have become commonplace events. Transplantations of kidney, heart, lung, liver, bone marrow, and cornea are performed with ever-increasing frequency and success. This chapter describes the mechanisms underlying graft rejection and various procedures that are used to prolong graft survival.

The Immunologic Basis of Graft Rejection

The degree of immune response to a graft varies with the type of graft. Various terms are used to denote different types of transplants. *Autograft* refers to self-tissue transferred from one body site to another in the same individual. These grafts are often performed on patients with burns by transferring healthy skin to the burned area. *Isografts* are grafts between genetically identical individuals. In inbred strains of mice an isograft can be performed from one mouse to another syngeneic mouse. In humans an isograft can be performed between genetically identical (monozygotic) twins. Neither autografts nor isografts are usually rejected, owing to the genetic identity between graft and host. *Allografts* are grafts between genetically different members of the same species. In mice an allograft is performed by transferring tissue or an organ from one inbred strain to another. In humans most organ grafts from one individual to another are allografts, unless an identical twin is available as a donor. Because an allograft is genetically dissimilar to the host, it is often recognized as foreign by the immune system and is rejected in an allograft reaction. *Xenografts* are grafts between different species such as the graft of a baboon heart to a human. Obviously, xenografts exhibit the greatest genetic disparity and therefore engender the most vigorous graft rejection.

Specificity and Memory of Rejection Response

The time sequence of allograft rejection varies according to the tissue involved. In general, skin grafts are rejected faster than more vascularized tissues such as kidney or heart. Despite these time differences, the immune response culminating in graft rejection always displays the attributes of specificity and memory. If an inbred mouse of strain A is grafted with skin from strain B, primary graft rejection—known as *first-set rejection*—takes place (Figure 24-1). As the reaction develops, the vascularized transplant becomes infiltrated with lymphocytes, monocytes, and other inflammatory cells; there is decreased vascularization of the transplanted tissue by 6–9 days, visible necrosis by 10 days, and complete rejection by 14 days. Immunologic memory is demonstrated when another strain-B graft is transferred to the original strain-A mouse. A graft-rejection reaction develops more quickly than after the first graft with complete rejection occurring within 5–6 days; this secondary response is designated *second-set rejection.* The specificity of second-set rejection can be demonstrated by grafting an unrelated strain-C graft at the same time as the second strain-B graft. Rejection of the strain-C graft proceeds according to first-set rejection kinetics, whereas the strain-B graft is rejected in an accelerated second-set fashion.

Role of Cell-Mediated Responses

In the early 1950s A. Mitchison showed in adoptive-transfer experiments that lymphocytes, but not serum antibody, could transfer allograft immunity. Later studies began to implicate T cells in allograft rejection. For example, nude mice, which lack a thymus and consequently lack functional T cells, were found to be incapable of allograft rejection; indeed these mice even accept xenografts (see Figure 22-6). In other studies, T cells derived from an allograft-primed mouse were shown to transfer second-set graft rejection to unprimed syngeneic recipients, as long as that recipient was grafted with the same allogeneic tissue (Figure 24-2).

Analysis of the T-cell subpopulations involved in allograft rejection has implicated both $CD4^+$ and $CD8^+$

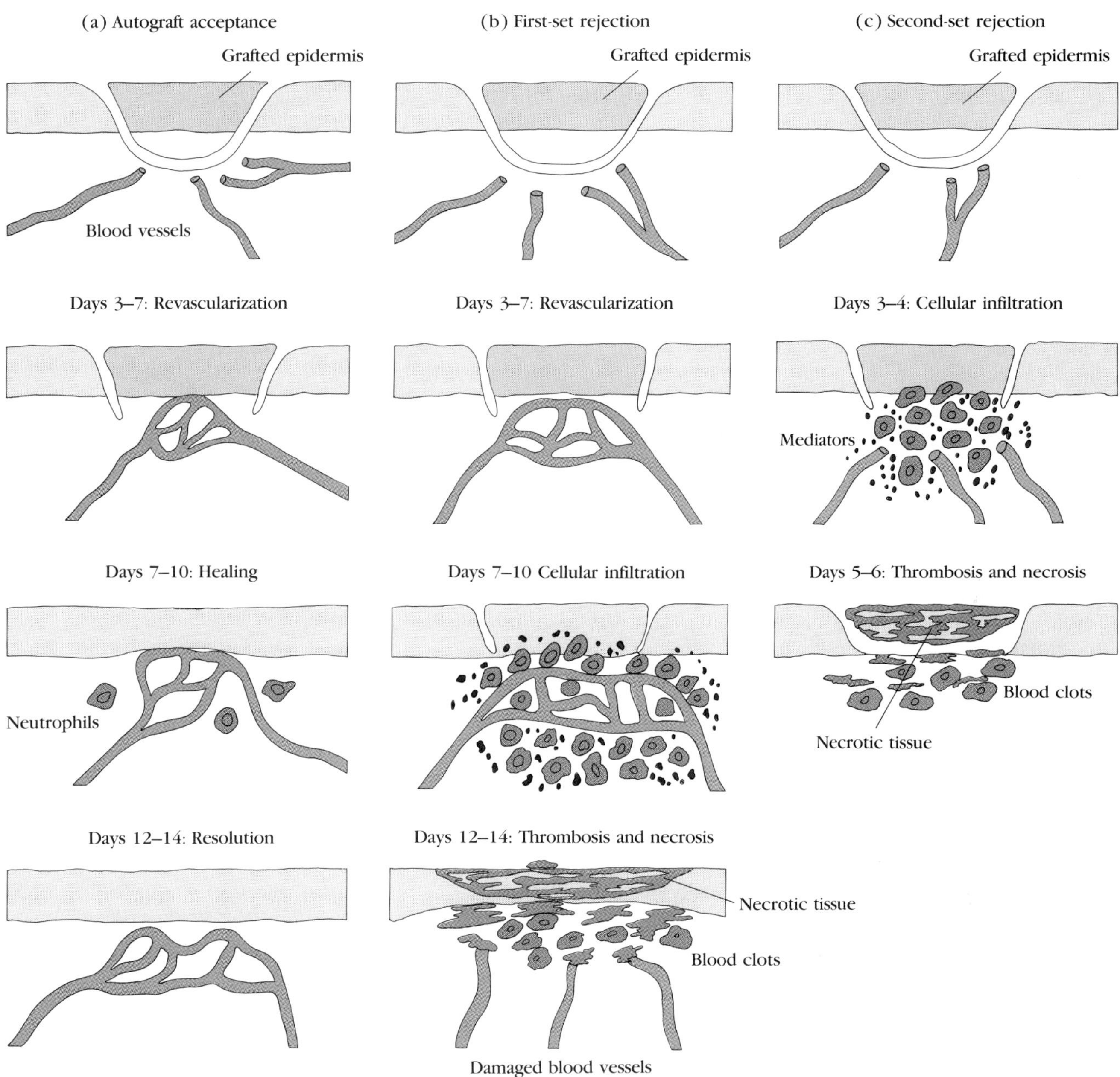

FIGURE 24-1 Schematic diagrams of the process of graft acceptance and rejection. (a) Acceptance of an autograft is completed within 12–14 days. (b) First-set rejection of an allograft begins 7–10 days after grafting, with full rejection occurring by 12–14 days. (c) Second-set rejection of an allograft begins within 3–4 days, with full rejection by 5–6 days. The cellular infiltrate that invades an allograft contains lymphocytes, phagocytes, and other inflammatory cells.

populations. In one study the role of $CD4^+$ and $CD8^+$ T-cell subpopulations in rejection of skin allografts was analyzed by injecting the recipient mice with monoclonal antibodies to deplete one or both types of T cells and then measuring the rate of graft rejection. As shown in Figure 24-3, removal of the $CD8^+$ population alone had no effect on graft survival, and the graft was rejected at the same rate as in control mice (15 days). Removal of the $CD4^+$ T-cell population alone prolonged graft survival from 15 days to 30 days. However, removal of both the $CD4^+$ and the $CD8^+$ T cells resulted in long-term survival (up to 60 days) of the allografts. This study indicates that both $CD4^+$ and $CD8^+$ T-cells participate in rejection and that the collaboration of both subpopulations results in more pronounced graft rejection.

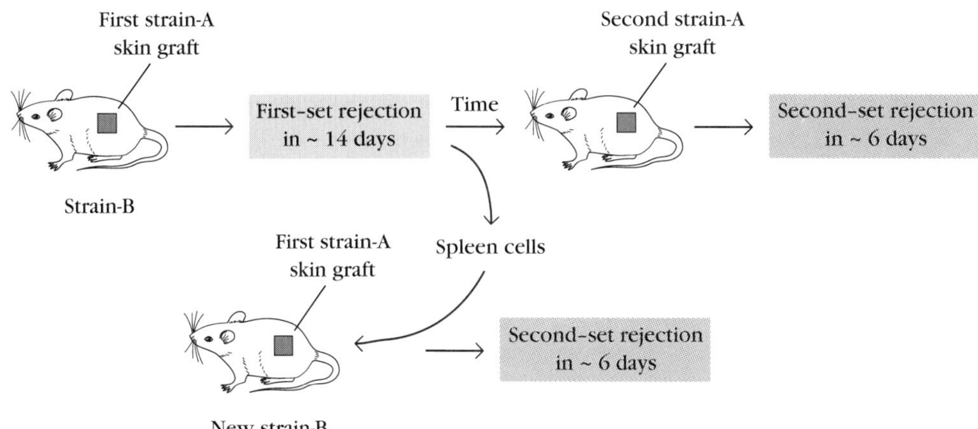

FIGURE 24-2 T cells derived from an allograft-primed mouse mediate second-set rejection of an allograft (from the same allogeneic strain) in an unprimed mouse.

Transplantation Antigens

Tissues that are antigenically similar are said to be *histocompatible;* such tissues do not induce an immunologic response that leads to tissue rejection. Tissues displaying significant antigenic differences are *histoincompatible;* such tissues induce an immune response leading to tissue rejection. The various antigens that determine histocompatibility are encoded by more than 40 different loci, but the loci responsible for the most vigorous allograft-rejection reactions are located within the major histocompatibility complex (MHC). The organization of the MHC—called the H-2 complex in mice and the HLA complex in humans—was described in Chapter 9 (see Figure 9-1). Because the MHC loci are closely linked, they are usually inherited as a complete set, called the haplotype, from each parent. Within an inbred strain of mice, all animals are homozygous at each MHC locus. When mice from two different inbred strains are mated, all the F_1 progeny inherit one haplotype from each parent (see Figure 9-2b); these F_1 offspring can accept grafts from either parent. MHC inheritance in outbred populations is very different because the high polymorphism exhibited at each MHC locus gives a high probability of heterozygosity at most loci. In matings between outbred mice, there is only a 25% chance that any two offspring will inherit identical MHC haplotypes (see Figure 9-2c), unless the parents share one or more haplotypes in common. Therefore, for purposes of organ or bone marrow grafts, there is a 25% chance of identity within the MHC between siblings. With parent-to-child grafts, the donor and host will always have one haplotype in common but will be mismatched for the other haplotype.

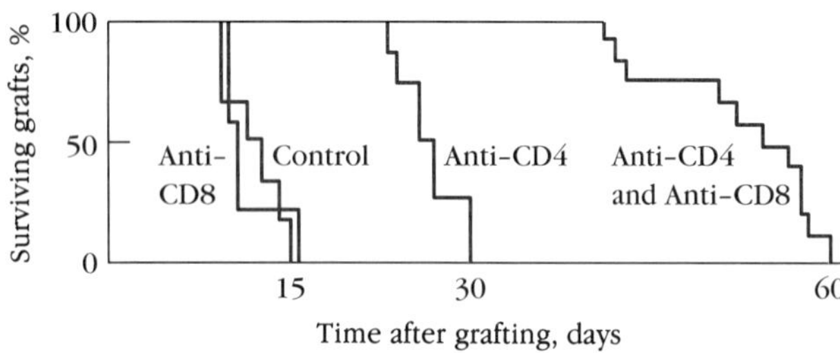

FIGURE 24-3 Experimental demonstration of the role of $CD4^+$ and $CD8^+$ T cells in allograft rejection in mice. Animals were treated with either anti-CD4 or anti-CD8 monoclonal antibody and then grafted with allogeneic skin; the rate of graft rejection was monitored and compared with that in untreated grafted controls. Removal of $CD8^+$ T cells alone had no effect on graft survival, whereas removal of $CD4^+$ T cells prolonged graft survival by about 15 days. However, removal of both T-cell populations resulted in much longer graft survival. [Adapted from S. P. Cobbold et al., 1986, *Nature* **323**:165.]

Identity at the MHC of donor and host is not the sole factor determining tissue acceptance. When tissue is transplanted between genetically different individuals, even if their MHC antigens are identical, the transplanted tissue is likely to be rejected because of differences at various minor histocompatibility loci. Unlike the major histocompatibility antigens, which are recognized directly by T_H and T_C cells (see Chapter 11), minor histocompatibility antigens are recognized only when they are presented in the context of self-MHC molecules. In addition, the tissue rejection induced by minor histocompatibility differences is usually less vigorous than that induced by major histocompatibility differences. Still, reaction to these minor tissue differences often results in graft rejection. For this reason, transplantation even between HLA-identical individuals requires some degree of immune suppression.

Mechanisms Involved in Graft Rejection

Graft rejection is caused principally by a cell-mediated immune response to *alloantigens* (primarily MHC molecules) expressed on cells of the graft. Both delayed-type hypersensitive and cell-mediated cytotoxicity reactions have been implicated. The process of graft rejection can be divided into two stages: (1) a sensitization phase in which antigen-reactive lymphocytes of the recipient proliferate in response to alloantigens on the graft and (2) an effector stage in which immune destruction of the graft takes place.

Sensitization Stage

During the sensitization phase $CD4^+$ and $CD8^+$ T cells recognize alloantigens expressed on cells of the foreign graft and proliferate in response. Both major and minor histocompatibility alloantigens can be recognized. In general the response to the minor histocompatibility antigens is weak, although the combined response to several minor differences can sometimes be quite vigorous. The response to the major histocompatibility antigens involves recognition of both the MHC molecule and an associated peptide ligand in the cleft of the MHC molecule. The peptides present in the groove of allogeneic class I MHC molecules are derived from proteins synthesized within the allogeneic cell. The peptides present in the groove of allogeneic class II MHC molecules are generally proteins taken up and processed through the endocytic pathway of the allogeneic antigen-presenting cell. In some cases peptide fragments of allogeneic class I MHC molecules can be presented within the groove of a class II molecule.

Activation of host T_H cells requires the interaction with an antigen-presenting cell (APC) expressing an appropriate antigenic ligand–MHC complex and providing the requisite co-stimulatory signal. Depending upon the tissue, different populations of cells within a graft may function as APCs. Because dendritic cells are found in most tissues and because they constitutively express high levels of class II MHC molecules, they generally serve as the major APC in grafts. APCs of host origin can also migrate into a graft and endocytose the foreign alloantigens (both major and minor histocompatibility molecules) and present them as processed peptides together with self-MHC molecules.

In some organ and tissue grafts (e.g., grafts of kidney, thymus, and pancreatic islets), a population of donor APCs called *passenger leukocytes* has been shown to migrate from the graft to the regional lymph nodes (Figure 24-4). These passenger leukocytes have been shown to be dendritic cells, which express high levels of class II MHC molecules (together with normal levels of class I MHC molecules) and are widespread in most mammalian tissues with the exception of the brain. Because passenger leukocytes express the allogeneic MHC antigens of the donor graft, they are recognized as foreign and therefore stimulate immune activation of T lymphocytes in the lymph node.

Passenger leukocytes are not the only cells in a graft that can present alloantigens to the immune system. In fact, in skin grafts and some other grafts, passenger leukocytes do not seem to play any role at all. Other cell types that have been implicated in alloantigen presentation to the immune system include Langerhans cells and endothelial cells lining the blood vessels. Both of these cell types express class I and class II MHC antigens.

Immunologic involvement varies with different types of transplants. When skin is grafted, for example, the graft at first does not contain functional blood vessels. Host lymphocytes, carried to the tissue by capillaries or lymphatics, encounter the foreign antigens of the skin graft and are carried by the afferent lymphatics to regional lymph nodes. Effector lymphocytes are generated in the regional nodes and are carried by the lymphatics back to the graft to mount an immunologic attack. In kidney or heart transplants the blood vasculature is immediately restored by suturing major blood vessels of the graft together with those of the host. Blood-borne lymphocytes encounter the alloantigens of the graft and are carried by blood vessels to the spleen or by the lymphatics to regional lymph nodes. Here, within the spleen or lymph nodes effector cells are generated and are then transported back to the graft by blood or lymph vessels.

Recognition of the foreign alloantigens expressed on the cells of a graft induces vigorous T-cell proliferation in the host. This proliferation can be demonstrated in vitro in a mixed-lymphocyte reaction. Both dendritic cells and vascular endothelial cells from an allogeneic graft induce vigorous proliferation of host T cells in an MLR. The major proliferating cell is the $CD4^+$ T cell, which recognizes class II alloantigens directly or alloantigen peptides presented by host antigen-presenting cells. This amplified population of activated T_H cells is thought to play a central role in inducing the various effector mechanisms of allograft rejection.

Effector Stage

A variety of effector mechanisms participate in allograft rejection. The most common are cell-mediated reactions involving delayed-typed hypersensitivity

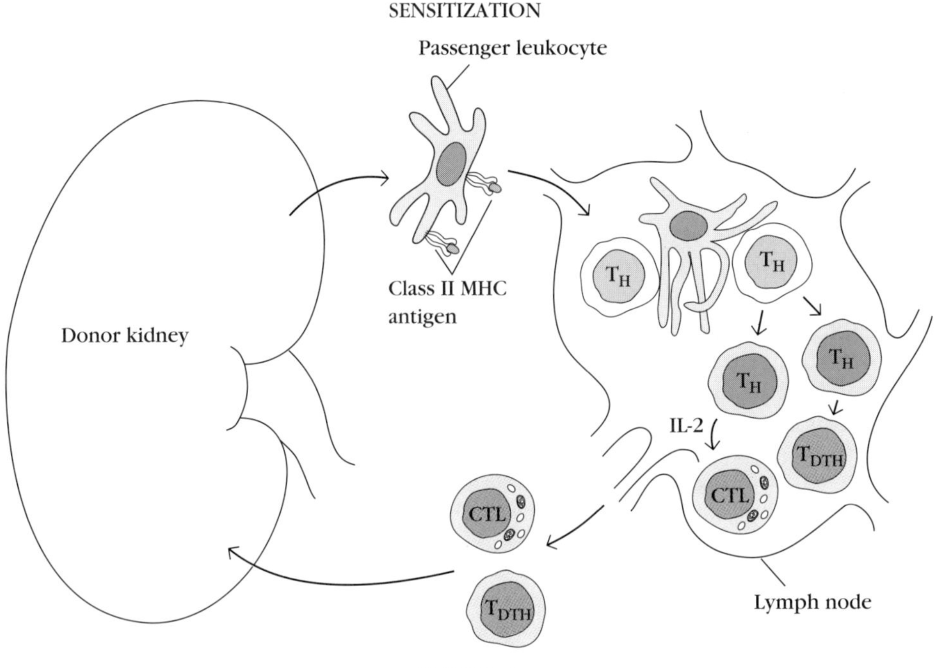

FIGURE 24-4 Migration of passenger leukocytes from a donor graft to regional lymph nodes of the recipient results in the activation of T_H cells in response to different class II MHC antigens expressed by the passenger leukocytes. These activated T_H cells (gray) then induce generation of T_{DTH} cells and/or CTLs (purple), both of which mediate graft rejection.

and CTL-mediated cytotoxicity; less common mechanisms are antibody plus complement lysis and destruction by antibody-dependent cell-mediated cytotoxicity (ADCC). The hallmark of graft rejection involving cell-mediated reactions is an influx of T lymphocytes and macrophages into the graft. Histologically, the infiltration in many cases resembles that seen during a delayed-type hypersensitive response in which cytokines produced by T_{DTH} cells promote macrophage infiltration (see Figure 15-14). Recognition of foreign class I alloantigens on the graft by host $CD8^+$ cells can lead to CTL-mediated killing (see Figure 15-5). In some cases graft rejection is mediated by $CD4^+$ T cells that function as class II MHC–restricted cytotoxic cells.

In each of these effector mechanisms, cytokines secreted by T_H cells play a central role (Figure 24-5). For example, IL-2, IFN-γ, and TNF-β have each been shown to be important mediators of graft rejection. IL-2 promotes T-cell proliferation and is necessary for the generation of effector CTLs (see Figure 15-1). IFN-γ is central to the development of a DTH response, promoting the influx of macrophages into the graft and their subsequent activation into more destructive cells. TNF-β has been shown to have direct cytotoxic activity on the cells of a graft. A number of cytokines promote graft rejection by inducing expression of class I or class II MHC molecules on graft cells. The interferons (α, β, and γ), TNF-β, and TNF-α all increase class I MHC expression, and IFN-γ increases class II MHC expression as well. During a graft rejection episode, these cytokines will increase, inducing a variety of cell types within the graft to express class I or class II MHC molecules. In rat cardiac allografts, for example, dendritic cells are initially the only cells that express class II MHC molecules, but as an allograft reaction begins, localized production of IFN-γ in the graft induces vascular endothelial cells and myocytes to begin to express class II MHC molecules as well.

Clinical Manifestations of Graft Rejection

Graft rejection reactions have various time courses depending upon the type of tissue or organ grafted and the immune response involved. *Hyperacute* rejection reactions occur within the first 24 h after transplantation; *acute* rejection reactions usually begin in the first few weeks after transplantation; and *chronic* rejection reactions can occur from months to years after transplantation.

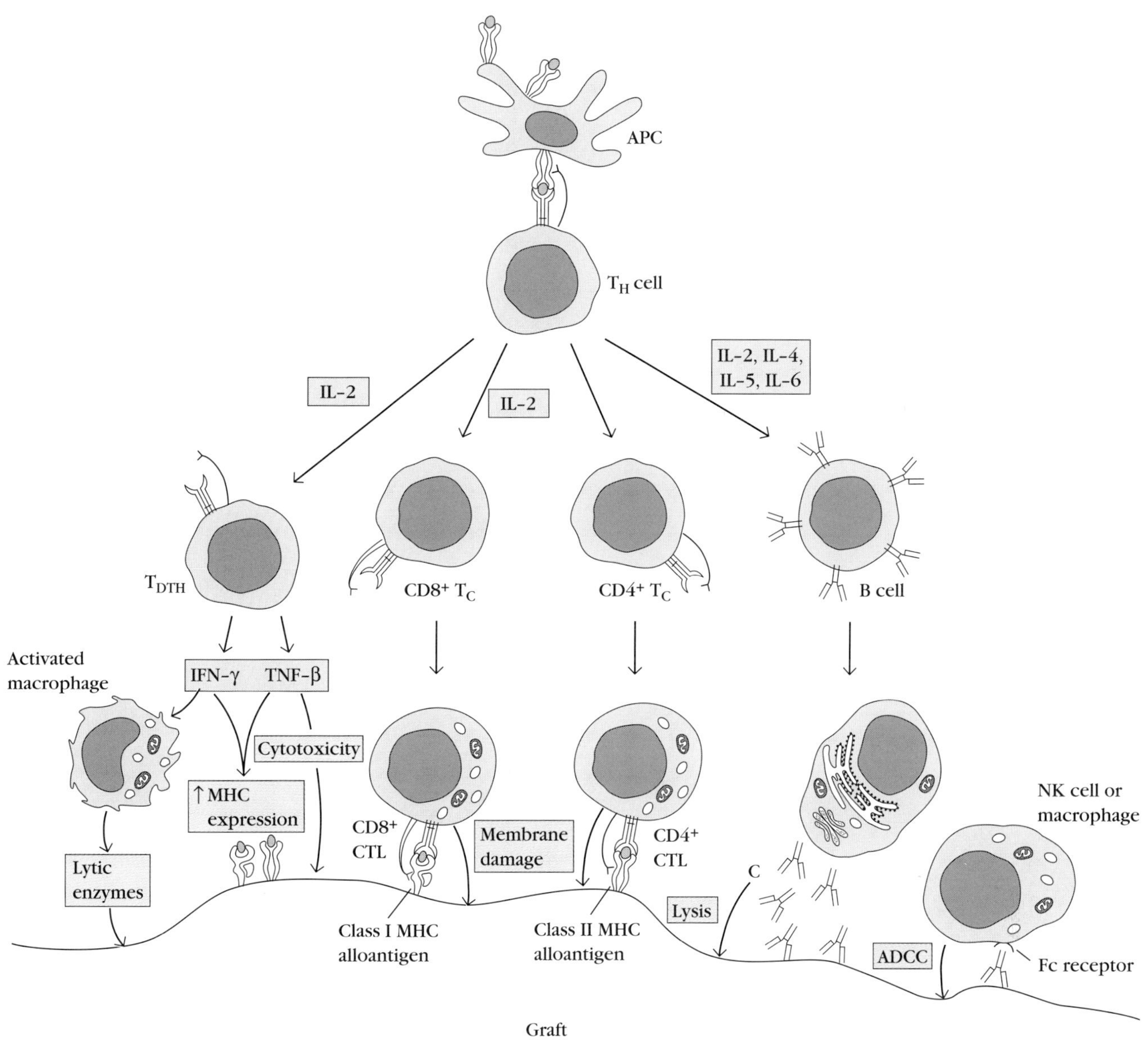

FIGURE 24-5 Effector mechanisms (purple blocks) involved in allograft rejection. The generation or activity of various effector cells depends directly or indirectly on cytokines (gray blocks) secreted by activated T_H cells. C = complement; ADCC = antibody-dependent cell-mediated cytotoxicity.

Hyperacute Rejection

In rare instances a transplant is rejected almost immediately—so quickly in fact that the grafted tissue never becomes vascularized. These hyperacute reactions are caused by pre-existing host serum antibodies specific for antigens of the graft. The antigen-antibody complexes that form activate the complement system, resulting in an intense infiltration of neutrophils into the grafted tissue. The ensuing inflammatory reaction causes massive blood clots within the capillaries, preventing vascularization of the graft (Figure 24-6).

Several mechanisms can account for the presence of pre-existing antibodies specific for allogeneic MHC antigens. Recipients of repeated blood transfusions sometimes develop significant levels of antibodies to MHC antigens expressed on white blood cells present in the transfused blood. If some of these MHC antigens are the same as those on a subsequent graft, then the antibodies can react with the graft, inducing a hyperacute rejection reaction. With repeated pregnancies women are exposed to the paternal alloantigens of the fetus and may develop antibodies to these antigens. If a woman receives a graft expressing any of these same

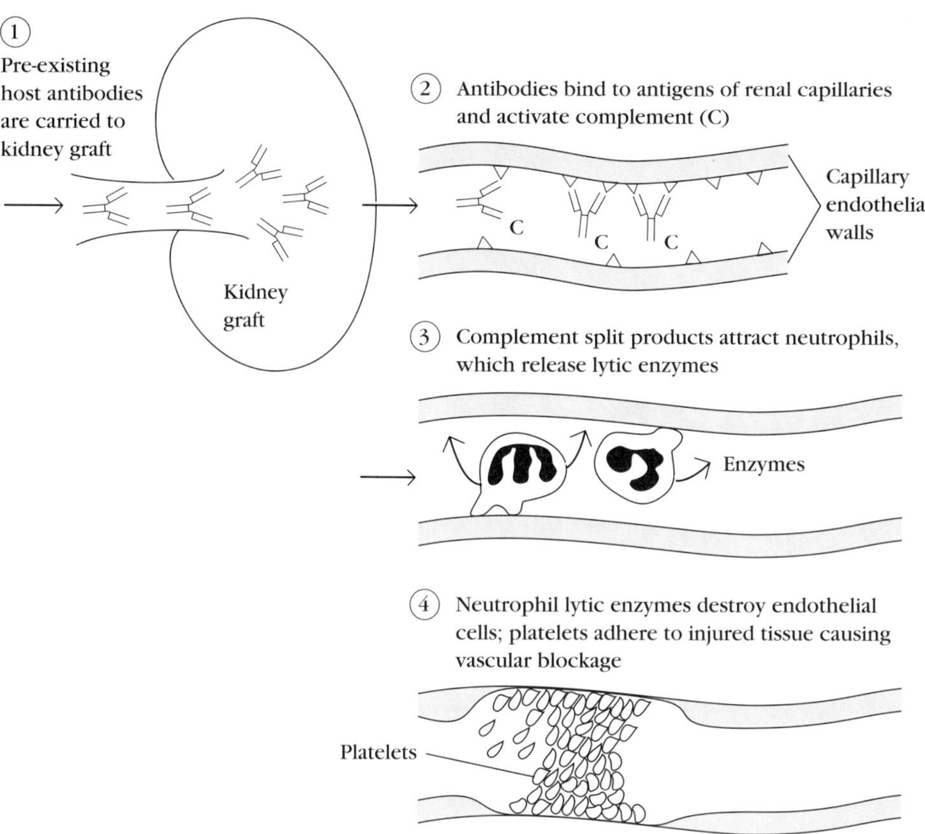

FIGURE 24-6 Steps in the hyperacute rejection of a kidney graft. In this type of rejection reaction, the graft never becomes vascularized.

MHC antigens, it is subject to a hyperacute rejection reaction. Finally, individuals who have had previous grafts sometimes have high levels of antibodies to the allogeneic MHC antigens of this graft; these antibodies will mediate hyperacute rejection of any subsequent graft that expresses some of the same allogeneic antigens. In some cases the pre-existing antibodies participating in hyperacute graft rejection may be specific for blood-group antigens in the graft. If tissue typing and ABO blood-group typing are performed prior to transplantation, these pre-existing antibodies can be detected and grafts that would result in hyperacute rejection can be avoided.

Acute Rejection

Allograft rejection that is cell-mediated manifests as an acute rejection of the graft beginning about 10 days after transplantation (see Figure 24-1b). Histopathologic examination reveals a massive infiltration of macrophages and lymphocytes at the site of tissue destruction, suggestive of T_H-cell activation and proliferation. Acute graft rejection is effected by the mechanisms described previously (see Figure 24-5).

Chronic Rejection

Chronic rejection reactions develop months or years after acute rejection reactions have subsided. The mechanisms of chronic rejection include both humoral and cell-mediated responses. Chronic rejection reactions are often difficult to manage with immunosuppressive drugs and may necessitate another transplantation.

Tissue Typing

Since differences in blood-group and major histocompatibility antigens are responsible for the most intense graft rejection reactions, various tissue-typing procedures have been developed to screen potential donor and recipient cells and assess the likelihood of tissue compatibility. Initially, donor and recipient are screened for ABO blood-group compatibility by typing their RBC antigens (see Figure 18-12). The A, B, and O antigens are expressed on donor RBCs, epithelial cells, and endothelial cells. Antibodies produced in

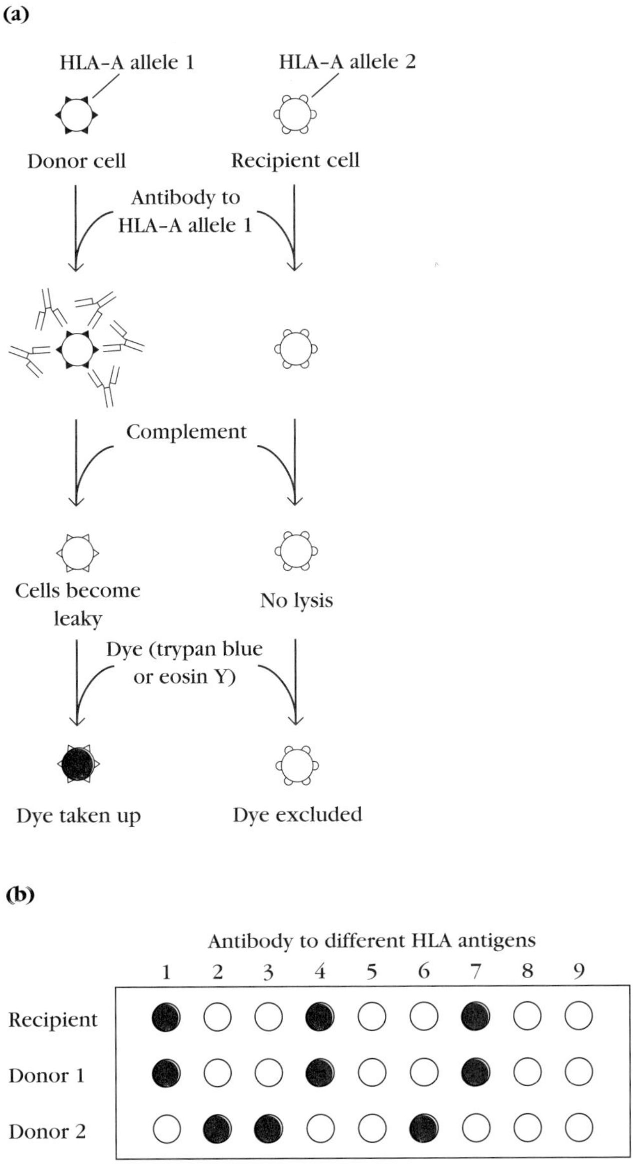

FIGURE 24-7 Microcytotoxicity HLA typing. (a) White blood cells from potential donors and the recipient are added to separate wells of a microtiter plate. The example depicts only one HLA antigen on donor and recipient cells and shows the reaction sequence on addition of antibody to one of these antigens. (b) Because cells express numerous HLA antigens, they are separately tested with a battery of monoclonal antibodies specific for various HLA antigens. Here, donor 1 shares antigens 1, 4, and 7 with the recipient, whereas donor 2 has no antigens in common with the recipient.

the recipient to any of these antigens that are present on transplanted tissue will induce antibody plus complement lysis of the incompatible cells.

HLA typing of potential donors and a recipient can be accomplished with a microcytotoxicity test (Figure 24-7). In this test white blood cells from the potential donors and recipient are distributed into a separate series of wells on a microtiter plate, and then monoclonal antibodies specific for various class I and class II MHC alleles are added to different wells. After incubation, complement is added to the wells, and cytotoxicity is assessed by the uptake or exclusion of various dyes (e.g., trypan blue or eosin Y) by the cells. If the white blood cells express the MHC allele for which a particular monoclonal antibody is specific, then the cells will be lysed on addition of complement, and these dead cells will take up a dye such as trypan blue. HLA typing based on antibody-mediated microcytotoxicity can indicate the presence or absence of various MHC alleles. The results of such typing of a hypothetical family are shown in Table 24-1. In this example, only siblings 1 and 4 are fully HLA compatible.

Even when a fully HLA-compatible donor is not available, transplantation may be successful. For example, in Table 24-1, sibling 1 shares some HLA antigens with sibling 2 and with the father. In this situation, a one-way MLR can be used to assess quantitatively the degree of class II MHC compatibility between potential donors and a recipient (see Figure 9-12). Lymphocytes from a potential donor that have been treated with mitomycin C or x-irradiated serve as the stimulator cells, and lymphocytes from the recipient serve as responder cells. Proliferation is indicated by the uptake of [^{3}H]thymidine. The greater the class II MHC differences between the donor and recipient cells, the more [^{3}H]thymidine uptake will be observed in an MLR assay. Intense proliferation of the donor lymphocytes indicates a poor prognosis for graft survival. The advantage of the MLR over microcytotoxicity typing is that it gives a better indication of the degree of T_H-cell activation generated in response to the class II MHC antigens of the potential graft. The disadvantage of the MLR is that it takes about 6 days to run the assay. If the potential donor is a cadaver, for example, it is not possible to wait 6 days for the results of the MLR, and in that case the microcytotoxicity test must be relied on.

General Immunosuppressive Therapy

Allogeneic transplantation requires some degree of immunosuppression if the transplant is to survive. Most of the immunosuppressive treatments that have been developed have the disadvantage of being non-

TABLE 24-1 HLA TISSUE TYPING OF A HYPOTHETICAL FAMILY BASED ON MICROCYTOTOXICITY TESTING WITH MONOCLONAL ANTIBODIES TO VARIOUS HLA-A, -B, -C, AND -DR ALLELIC ANTIGENS

	Allelic antigens at each locus														
	A				*B*				*C*			*DR*			
Family member	1	2	3	9	5	7	8	12	1	2	4	1	2	3	7
Father	+	−	+	−	−	+	+	−	+	−	−	−	+	+	−
Mother	−	+	−	+	+	−	−	+	−	+	+	+	−	−	+
Sib 1	+	−	−	+	−	−	+	+	+	−	+	−	−	+	+
Sib 2	+	+	−	−	+	−	+	−	+	+	−	+	−	+	−
Sib 3	−	+	+	−	+	+	−	−	−	+	−	+	+	−	−
Sib 4	+	−	−	+	−	−	+	+	+	−	+	−	−	+	+

	Inferred genotype								
Family member	*A,*	*B,*	*C,*	*DR*	*A,*	*B,*	*C,*	*DR*	Haplotype designation
Father	*A1,*	*B8,*	*C1,*	*D3*	*A3,*	*B7,*	*—,*	*D2*	*a/b*
Mother	*A2,*	*B5,*	*C2,*	*D1*	*A9,*	*B12,*	*C4,*	*D7*	*c/d*
Sib 1	*A1,*	*B8,*	*C1,*	*D3*	*A9,*	*B12,*	*C4,*	*D7*	*a/d*
Sib 2	*A1,*	*B8,*	*C1,*	*D3*	*A2,*	*B5,*	*C2,*	*D1*	*a/c*
Sib 3	*A3,*	*B7,*	*—,*	*D2*	*A2,*	*B5,*	*C2,*	*D1*	*b/c*
Sib 4	*A1,*	*B8,*	*C1,*	*D3*	*A9,*	*B12,*	*C4,*	*D7*	*a/d*

SOURCE: Adapted from A. Svejgaard et al., 1979, *The HLA System: An Introductory Survey,* S. Karger, Basel, cited in W. E. Paul, 1984, *Fundamental Immunology,* Raven, Press.

specific; that is, they result in generalized immunosuppression, which places the recipient at increased risk for infection. In addition, many immunosuppressive measures are aimed at slowing the proliferation of activated lymphocytes. However, because any rapidly dividing nonimmune cells (e.g., epithelial cells of the gut or bone marrow hematopoietic stem cells) are also affected, serious or even life-threatening complications can occur.

Mitotic Inhibitors

Azathioprine (Imuran), a potent mitotic inhibitor, is often given just before and after transplantation to diminish T-cell proliferation in response to the alloantigens of the graft. Azathioprine acts on cells in the S phase of the cell cycle to block synthesis of inosinic acid, which is a precursor of the purines adenylic and guanylic acid. Both B-cell and T-cell proliferation is diminished in the presence of azathioprine. Functional immune assays such as the MLR, CML, and skin test show a significant decline following azathioprine treatment, indicating an overall decrease in T-cell numbers.

Two other mitotic inhibitors that are sometimes used in conjunction with other immunosuppressive agents are cyclophosphamide and methotrexate. Cyclophosphamide is an alkylating agent that inserts into the DNA helix and becomes cross-linked, leading to disruption of the DNA chain. It is especially effective against rapidly dividing cells and therefore is sometimes given at the time of grafting to block T-cell proliferation. Methotrexate acts as a folic acid antagonist to block purine biosynthesis.

Corticosteroids

The corticosteroids, which are cholesterol derivatives, include prednisone, prednisolone, and methylprednisolone. The lipophilic nature of these hormones enables them to cross the plasma membrane and bind to receptors in the cytosol; the receptor-corticosteroid complexes are subsequently transported to the nucleus where they bind to specific regulatory DNA sequences, either up-regulating or down-regulating transcription.

Corticosteroids are potent anti-inflammatory agents that exert their effects at many levels of the immune response. Corticosteroid treatment causes a decrease in the number of circulating lymphocytes as the result either of steroid-induced lysis of lymphocytes (lympholysis) or of alterations in lymphocyte-circulation patterns. Some species (e.g., hamster, mouse, rat, and rabbit) are particularly sensitive to corticosteroid-induced lympholysis. In these animals corticosteroid treatment at dosages as low as 10^{-7} *M* causes such widespread lympholysis that the weight of the thymus is reduced by 90%; the spleen and lymph nodes also shrink visibly (see Figure 3-17). Immature thymocytes in these species appear to be particularly sensitive to corticosteroid-mediated killing. Corticosteroids display markedly different effects on immature and mature thymocytes in rodents. Corticosteroids induce programmed cell death by apoptosis in immature thymocytes, whereas mature thymocytes are resistant to this activity. Within 2 h following in vitro incubation with corticosteroids, immature thymocytes begin to show the characteristic morphology of apoptosis, and by 24 h 90% of the chromatin is degraded into the characteristic nucleosome ladder. The steps involved in the induction of apoptosis by corticosteroids remain to be determined. In humans, guinea pigs, and monkeys, corticosteroids do not induce apoptosis but instead affect lymphocyte-circulation patterns, causing a decrease in thymic weight and a marked decrease in the number of circulating lymphocytes.

Corticosteroids also reduce both the phagocytic and killing ability of macrophages and neutrophils, and this effect may contribute to their anti-inflammatory action. In addition, chemotaxis is reduced, so that fewer inflammatory cells are attracted to the site of T_H-cell activation. In the presence of corticosteroids class II MHC expression and IL-1 production by macrophages is dramatically reduced; such reductions would be expected to lead to corresponding reductions in T_H-cell activation. Corticosteroids also stabilize the lysosomal membrane, so that decreased levels of lysosomal enzymes are released at the site of inflammation.

Cyclosporin A

FK506

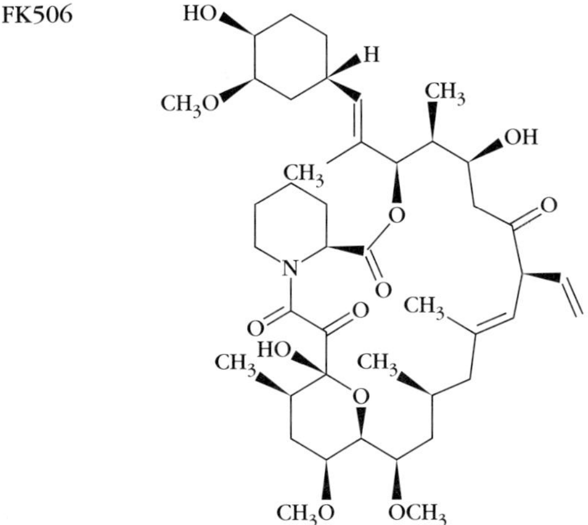

Rapamycin

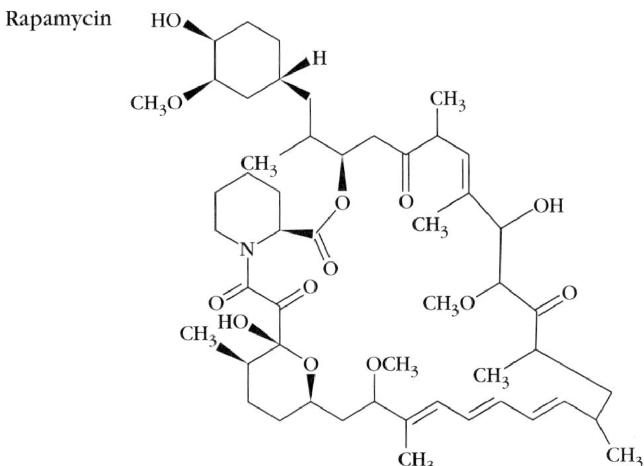

FIGURE 24-8 Chemical structures of three immunosuppressive fungal metabolites. Cyclosporin A and FK506 inhibit activation of T_H cells, and rapamycin inhibits proliferation and differentiation of activated T_H cells. [From: N. H. Sigal and F. J. Dumont. 1992. *Annu. Rev. Immunol.* **10**:519.]

Cyclosporin A, FK506, and Rapamycin

Cyclosporin A (CsA), FK506, and rapamycin are fungal metabolites with potent immunosuppressive properties (Figure 24-8). Although chemically unrelated, CsA and FK506 have similar actions. Both drugs block activation of resting T cells by inhibiting the transcription of genes encoding IL-2 and the high-affinity IL-2 receptor (IL-2R), which are essential for activation. As shown in Figure 12-14, CsA and FK506 exert this effect by binding to cytoplasmic proteins called immunophilins, forming a complex that blocks the phosphatase activity of calcineurin. This prevents the formation and nuclear translocation of the cytoplasmic subunit NF-ATc and its subsequent assembly into NF-AT, a DNA-binding protein necessary for transcription of the genes encoding IL-2 and IL-2R. Rapamycin is structurally similar to FK506 and also binds to an immunophilin. However, the rapamycin-immunophilin complex does not inhibit calcineurin activity; instead it blocks the proliferation and differentiation of activated T_H cells in the G_1 phase of the cell cycle. All three drugs, by inhibiting T_H-cell proliferation and thus T_H-cell cytokine expression, reduce the subsequent activation of various effector populations involved in graft rejection, including T_{DTH} cells, T_C cells, NK cells, macrophages, and B cells.

The profound immunosuppressive properties of these three agents has made them a mainstay in heart, liver, kidney, and bone marrow transplantation. Cyclosporin A has been shown to prolong graft survival in kidney, liver, heart, and heart-lung transplants. In one study of 209 kidney transplants from cadaver donors, the 1-year survival rate was 64% among recipients receiving other immunosuppressive treatments and 80% among those receiving cyclosporin A. Similar results have been obtained with liver transplants (Figure 24-9). Despite these impressive results, cyclosporin A does have some negative side effects, the most notable of which is its toxicity to the kidneys. Acute nephrotoxicity is quite common, in some cases progressing to chronic nephrotoxicity and drug-induced kidney failure. FK506 and rapamycin are newer drugs and require longer experience in clinical trials before a fuller assessment of their merits can be made. They are 10 – 100 times more potent as immune suppressants than CsA and therefore can be administered at lower doses and consequently have fewer side effects than CsA.

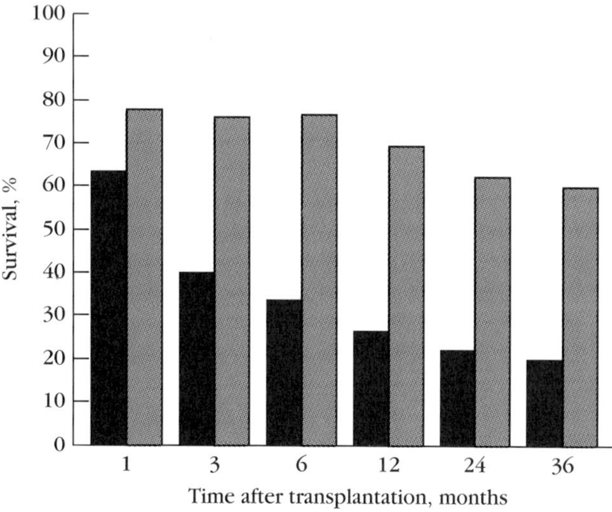

FIGURE 24-9 Comparison of survival rates of liver transplants in 84 patients who were immunosuppressed with azathioprine and corticosteroids (black) and in 55 patients who were immunosuppressed with cyclosporin A and corticosteroids (purple). [Adapted from S. M. Sabesin and J. W. Williams, 1987, *Hosp. Pract.* (July 15):p.75.]

Total Lymphoid Irradiation

Because lymphocytes are extremely sensitive to x-rays, x-irradiation can be used to eliminate recipient lymphocytes before grafting. In total lymphoid x-irradiation the recipient receives multiple x-ray exposures to the thymus, spleen, and lymph nodes and then receives the transplant. The typical protocol involves daily x-irradiation treatments of about 200 rads per day for several weeks until a total of 3400 rads has been administered. The recipient is grafted in this immune-suppressed state. Because the bone marrow is not x-irradiated, lymphoid stem cells proliferate and renew the population of recirculating lymphocytes. These newly formed lymphocytes appear to be more tolerant to the antigens of the graft.

Antilymphocyte Serum

Antilymphocyte serum can be prepared by immunizing an animal with allogeneic or xenogeneic thymocytes, spleen cells, lymph-node cells, or thoracic-duct lymphocytes. For transplantation in humans, antilymphocyte serum is often prepared by immunizing a horse or a rabbit with human lymphocytes. The injection of antilymphocyte serum at the time of grafting results in decreased levels of circulating lymphocytes (lymphocytopenia) and in decreased cell-mediated immunity; it has variable effects on humoral immunity. The lymphocyte depletion does not appear to be caused by antibody plus complement lysis; it may be that antibody coats the lymphocytes and acts as an opsonin, promoting phagocytosis of antibody-coated cells mediated by Fc receptors on phagocytes (see Figure 17-11a).

In experimental animals antilymphocyte serum has been shown to prolong kidney, liver, and cardiac allografts. In human transplantation the serum is always given along with other immunosuppressive drugs, and so it has been difficult to determine its individual effectiveness. Further, it is difficult to predict the effectiveness of a particular serum batch, perhaps because of variation in the concentrations of antibodies specific for one or another lymphocyte membrane molecule or variation in the major antibody isotypes. Some antilymphocyte sera may be quite effective at lymphocyte depletion, and others may be quite poor. Finally, a major drawback to the use of horse or rabbit antilymphocyte serum in humans is that it may induce a potent antibody response in the recipient to the antigenic determinants of the foreign antiserum that can result in serum sickness or anaphylactic shock.

Specific Immunosuppressive Therapy

The major limitation with each of the immunosuppressive treatments discussed thus far is that they lack specificity and therefore result in more-or-less generalized immunosuppression and increase the recipient's risk for infection. Ideally what is needed is an antigen-specific immunosuppressant that will reduce the immune response to the alloantigens of the graft while preserving the response to unrelated antigens. Although this goal has not yet been achieved, steps are being made toward increasing the specificity of immunosuppression.

Monoclonal Antibodies to T-Cell Components or Cytokines

Thus far, monoclonal antibodies have been used successfully to suppress T-cell activity in general or to suppress the activity of broad subpopulations of T cells. The technology has not yet advanced to the point of using monoclonal antibodies to suppress only alloantigen-activated T cells, but animal models suggest that monoclonal antibodies are the immune suppressors of the future.

Monoclonal antibody to the CD3 molecule of the TCR complex has been shown in some cases to block T-cell activation. Injection of such monoclonal antibodies results in a rapid depletion of T cells from the circulation. This depletion appears to be caused by binding of antibody-coated T cells to Fc receptors on phagocytic cells, which then phagocytose and clear the T cells from the circulation. The success of anti-CD3 monoclonal antibody in reversing rejection episodes in animal models has led to its approval by the Food and Drug Administration for clinical trials. In some cases, anti-CD3 has reversed acute rejection in human patients.

Monoclonal antibodies specific for the high-affinity IL-2 receptor (anti-TAC) have been used successfully to increase graft survival. Since the high-affinity IL-2 receptor is expressed only on activated T cells, exposure to anti-TAC following grafting should specifically block proliferation of T cells activated in response to the alloantigens of the graft. In one experiment, treatment of mice and rats with anti-TAC monoclonal antibody markedly increased the acceptance of cardiac and kidney transplants from allogeneic donors (Table 24-2).

Both CD3 and the high-affinity IL-2 receptor are expressed on all activated T cells. Monoclonal antibodies specific for membrane molecules that are present only on particular T-cell subpopulations also have been developed. For example, monoclonal antibody to CD4 has been shown to prolong graft survival. In one study, monkeys were given a single large dose of anti-CD4 just before they received a kidney transplant. Graft survival in the anti-CD4–treated animals was markedly increased compared with that in untreated control animals. Interestingly, the anti-CD4 did not reduce the $CD4^+$ T-cell count but instead appeared to induce the T cells to enter an immunosuppressed state.

Monoclonal antibodies to the adhesion molecules ICAM-1 and LFA-1 permitted indefinite survival of cardiac grafts between allogeneic mice in experiments by M. Isobe and co-workers. The two monoclonal antibodies (anti-ICAM-1 and anti-LFA-1) were administered simultaneously for 6 days following transplantation. However, when either monoclonal antibody was administered alone, the cardiac transplant was rejected. The requirement that both monoclonal antibodies be given at the same time is thought to reflect the redundancy of adhesion molecules: LFA-1 is known to bind to ICAM-2 in addition to ICAM-1; and ICAM-1 is known to bind to Mac-1 and CD43 in addition to LFA-1. Only when both pairs are blocked at the same time will adhesion and signal transduction through this ligand pair be blocked.

Table 24-2 Effect of treatment with anti-TAC monoclonal antibody* on survival of cardiac allografts in rats

Anti-TAC dose (μg/kg/day)	Treatment period (days after grafting)	Mean graft survival in days (range)
—	—	8 (4–9)
25	0–9	13 (12–14)
100	0–9	14 (13–16)
300	0–9	20 (20–21)
300	5–9	17 (15–26)
300	5–9/15–19	27 (26–28)

* Anti-TAC binds to the IL-2 receptor.

SOURCE: Data from J. W. Kupiec-Weglinski et al., 1986, *Proc. Nat'l. Acad. Sci. USA* **83**:2624.

Monoclonal antibody therapy, which usually is employed to deplete or inactivate T cells in graft recipients, also has been used to treat bone marrow before it is transplanted. Such treatment is designed to deplete the immunocompetent T cells in the bone marrow transplant, which can cause graft-versus-host disease, as discussed in the next section. The effectiveness of an anti-T-cell monoclonal antibody in reducing T-cell populations can be maximized by selecting monoclonal antibody isotypes that are good activators of the complement system.

One difficulty with monoclonal antibody intervention for prolonging graft survival is that the antibodies are generally of mouse origin. The recipient often develops an antibody response to the mouse monoclonal antibody, rapidly clearing it from the body. To avoid this limitation, human monoclonal antibodies and mouse-human chimeric antibodies (see Figure 7-12) are being evaluated in experimental trials.

Because cytokines appear to play an important role in allograft rejection, another strategy to prolong graft survival is to inject animals with monoclonal antibodies specific for the implicated cytokines, particularly TNF-α, IFN-γ, and IL-2. Monoclonal antibodies to TNF-α have been shown to prolong bone marrow transplants in mice and to reduce the incidence of graft-versus-host disease. Monoclonal antibodies to IFN-γ and to IL-2 have each been reported in some cases to prolong cardiac transplants in rats. Anticytokine antibodies have not yet been used in human transplantations.

Agents That Block the Co-stimulatory Signal

The requirement for a co-stimulatory signal in T_H-cell activation makes it a potential target in immunosuppression. As discussed in Chapter 12, T_H-cell activation requires a co-stimulatory signal in addition to the signal mediated by the T-cell receptor. One such co-stimulatory signal is mediated by interaction of the B7 molecule on the membrane of antigen-presenting cells and the CD28 or CTLA-4 molecule on T cells (see Figure 12-12). In the absence of a co-stimulatory signal, antigen-activated T cells become anergic (see Figure 12-15). CD28 is expressed on both resting and activated T cells and binds B7 with a moderate affinity; CTLA-4 is expressed at much lower levels only on activated T cells but binds B7 with a 20-fold higher affinity.

Demonstration of the B7-mediated co-stimulatory signal suggests that blocking the co-stimulatory signal following transplantation would cause the host's T cells to become anergic, thus enabling the grafted tissue to survive. D. J. Lenschow, J. A. Bluestone, and colleagues tested this approach by transplanting human pancreatic islets into mice that were injected with CTLA-4Ig, a soluble fusion protein consisting of the extracellular domains of CTLA-4 and the constant region of the IgG1 heavy chain. (Inclusion of the IgG1 heavy-chain constant region increases the half-life of the soluble fusion protein.) The xenogeneic graft exhibited long-term survival in treated mice but was quickly rejected in untreated controls. Presumably, the soluble CTLA-4Ig binds to B7 on antigen-presenting cells, so the co-stimulatory signal is not generated when host T cells recognize the graft antigens.

Donor-Cell Microchimerism

Recent studies suggest that immunosuppressive drugs act not only by blocking T-cell activation but also by inducing host tolerance to the allogeneic cells. As a result of this tolerance, donor leukocytes can migrate from a graft and survive within the recipient, producing a state of long-term microchimerism in the recipient. Several studies have demonstrated that long-term transplant survivors exhibit donor-cell microchimerism, prompting the suggestion that graft acceptance depends upon establishment of a microchimeric state.

Evidence that microchimerism plays an important role in graft acceptance first came from studies of long-term survivors of kidney transplants. Five individuals who were among the original kidney transplant patients in the 1960s were examined in 1992. Biopsies on the still functioning kidney grafts revealed that the interstitial cells of the allograft were from the recipient, whereas the nephrons were from the donor. In addition, this study revealed the presence of dendritic cells from the donor in the skin and lymph nodes of the recipient. Another study conducted in 1992 involved 25 individuals who had received liver transplants 2–22 years previously and had been immunosuppressed with azathioprine or cyclosporin A. Examination of these individuals revealed donor-cell microchimerism in the skin, lymph nodes, heart, lungs, spleen, intestine, kidneys, bone marrow, and thymus. Although there were relatively few donor cells at each site, the widespread distribution of these donor cells suggests that substantial numbers of them survive within the recipient.

The growing awareness of the importance of microchimerism in graft acceptance suggests that administration of immunosuppressive drugs may be discontinued once a stable chimera is achieved. A 1993 report of 44 human liver transplant recipients who had survived 11–23 years revealed that 6 had stopped taking all immunosuppressive drugs and yet remained clinically stable. These findings led to initiation of clinical trials, which are currently under way, to determine if immunosuppressive drugs can be slowly eliminated in liver transplant recipients after chimerism is established without inducing graft rejection.

The mechanism by which microchimerism leads to immune suppression and graft acceptance remains to be determined. T. E. Starzl and co-workers believe that graft success depends upon both the migration of recipient leukocytes into the graft and the migration of donor leukocytes out from the graft. The net effect would be a two-directional immune reaction leading to immunologic tolerance to the alloantigens of the graft. Because dendritic cells are the major cell type in the chimeras, it has been suggested that they may function as APCs inducing a state of tolerance in the alloreactive T_H cells.

Clinical Transplantation

The clinical results of transplantation of various cells, tissues, and organs in humans have improved considerably in the past few years, largely because of the use of immunosuppressive agents such as cyclosporin A. Nowadays, kidney and corneal transplantations are performed with high success rates; heart, lung, and liver transplantations are accomplished with somewhat lower, but still promising, success rates. In contrast, transplantations of bone marrow and pancreas exhibit even lower rates of success and are performed as a last resort only after other treatment possibilities have been exhausted.

Bone Marrow Transplants

In the past decade bone marrow transplantation has been increasingly adopted as a therapy for a number of malignant and nonmalignant hematologic diseases, including leukemia, lymphoma, aplastic anemia, thalassemia major, and immunodeficiency diseases in general. In 1990, over 4000 allogeneic bone marrow transplantations were performed. The bone marrow, which is obtained from a donor by multiple needle aspirations, consists of erythroid, myeloid, monocytoid, megakaryocytic, and lymphocytic lineages. The graft, which usually consists of about 10^9 cells per kilogram of host body weight, is injected intravenously into the recipient. The first successful bone marrow transplantations were performed between identical twins. However, development of the tissue-typing procedures described earlier now makes it possible to identify allogeneic donors with identical or near-identical HLA antigens as the recipients.

In the usual procedure, the recipient of a bone marrow transplant is immunologically suppressed before grafting. Leukemia patients, for example, are often treated with cyclophosphamide and total-body irradiation to kill all cancerous cells. The immune-suppressed state of the recipient makes graft rejection rare; however, because the donor bone marrow contains immunocompetent cells, the graft may reject the host, causing *graft-versus-host disease (GVHD).* This is quite common in bone marrow transplantation, affecting between 50 and 70% of transplant patients. Graft-versus-host disease develops as donor T cells recognize alloantigens on the host cells. The activation and proliferation of these T cells and the subsequent production of cytokines generate inflammatory reactions in the skin, gastrointestinal tract, and liver. If it is severe, GVHD can result in generalized erythroderma of the skin, gastrointestinal hemorrhage, and liver failure.

GVHD involves both an afferent phase and an efferent phase. In the afferent phase, T_H cells from the donor bone marrow recognize recipient peptide-MHC complexes displayed on antigen-presenting cells. Antigen presentation, together with a co-stimulatory signal, induces T_H-cell activation, production of IL-2, and proliferation. Cytokines elaborated by the T_H cell induce the effector phase of GVHD by activating a variety of secondary effector cells including NK cells, CTLs, and macrophages. Although CTLs can act directly to cause tissue damage, cytokines such as TNF may play a more important role in the effector phase of GVDH. TNF, which is released by a variety of cells (e.g., T_H cells, CTLs, NK cells, and macrophages), has been shown to mediate direct cytolytic damage to cells. The role that TNF plays in GVHD in mice is demonstrated by the ability of monoclonal antibody to TNF to block the development of GVHD following bone marrow transplantation in mice.

Various treatments are administered to prevent GVHD in bone marrow transplantation. The transplant recipient is usually placed on a regimen of immunosuppressive drugs, which often include cyclosporin and methotrexate. Another approach has been to deplete T cells from the donor bone marrow before transplantation with anti-T-cell antisera or monoclonal antibodies specific for T cells. Complete T-cell depletion from donor bone marrow, however, makes it more likely that the marrow will be rejected, and so the usual procedure is now a partial T-cell depletion. Apparently a low level of donor T-cell activity, which results in a low-level GVHD, is actually beneficial because it prevents any residual host T cells from becoming sensitized to the graft. In leukemia patients low-level GVHD also seems to result in destruction of leukemic cells, thus making it less likely for the leukemia to recur.

Organ Transplants

The impact of basic scientific research on clinical medicine is highlighted by the success rates for organ transplantation. In the case of kidney transplants, the survival rate in 1967 was 45%; by the early 1990s, the rate had been improved to about 90%. Currently more than 10,000 kidney transplantations are performed every year in the United States. Heart, heart-lung, and liver transplantations are also being done with remarkable success (Table 24-3). A number of other experimental transplantations (e.g., of the pancreas and parts of the intestine) have been performed but have not yet attained a level of success that warrants widespread application.

Several factors have contributed to the increase in successful organ transplants, most notably HLA typing and immunosuppressive treatments. Comparisons of HLA antigen differences and graft survival have shown that matching of the class II D antigens is most important for success. The data in Figure 24-10, for example, reveal that survival of kidney grafts depends primarily on donor-recipient matching of the HLA-D antigens; matching or mismatching of the class I HLA-A and HLA-B antigens has little effect on graft survival unless there is mismatching of the D antigens. In heart transplants, due to a shortage of transplantable organs and insufficient time, it is not possible to match HLA antigens prior to grafting. In order to assess the effect that differences in HLA antigens have on heart-transplant success, a number of studies have compared HLA antigen differences to graft-recipient survival rates. In one study of heart-transplant recipients, the 1000-day survival rate of the recipients was 90% when there was a single mismatch in HLA-DR antigens between the donor and recipient; the survival rate dropped to 65% when two HLA-DR antigens were mismatched.

TABLE 24-3 SURVIVAL RATES FOR ORGAN ALLOGRAFTS IN HUMANS

Organ allograft	1-year survival rate (%)
Kidney (sibling)	90
Kidney (cadaver)	80
Heart	80
Heart-lung	74
Liver	70
Pancreas	40

SOURCE: J. R. Batchelor and Y. L. Chai, 1986, *Prog. Immunol.* **6**:1002.

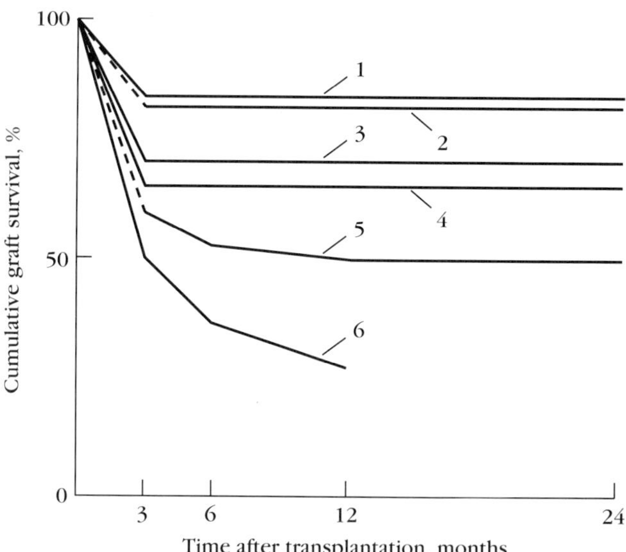

Curve no.	HLA mismatches (no.) A,B	HLA mismatches (no.) D
1	0	0
2	1 or 2	0
3	3 or 4	0
4	0	1 or 2
5	1 or 2	1 or 2
6	3 or 4	1 or 2

FIGURE 24-10 The effect of HLA-A, -B and -D antigen matching on survival of kidney grafts. Mismatching of HLA-A or HLA-B antigens has little effect on graft survival unless HLA-D is also mismatched. [Adapted from T. Moen et al., 1980, *N. Eng. J. Med.* **303**:850.]

An important finding that has emerged from experimental transplant models is that the critical period for graft rejection is from 2 to 4 weeks after grafting. If immunosuppressive drugs or monoclonal antibody therapy can prevent graft rejection during this critical period, when acute graft rejection would normally occur, then the prognosis for long-term graft survival improves dramatically. A number of reasons have been suggested for the decrease in immunogenicity shown by grafts that survive the critical period. One suggestion is that passenger leukocytes leave the graft, home to draining lymph nodes, and induce immune activation soon after grafting. If immune activation is decreased with immunosuppressive drugs or monoclonal antibodies until these allogeneic leukocytes die off, the potential for immune activation will dramatically decrease. There is also some speculation that, with time, continual alloantigen expression by the graft may induce a state of immunologic tolerance.

Transplantation of human pancreatic islet cells has been shown to reverse insulin-dependent diabetes mellitus, which is caused by degeneration of the insulin-producing islet cells of the pancreas. In the past, however, islet-cell allografts have often been rejected, even when the recipient is given potent immunosuppressive therapy. In an attempt to find a way to reduce rejection of islet-cell grafts, A. M. Posselt, A. Naji, and their colleagues injected rat pancreatic islet cells directly into the thymus of an allogeneic diabetic recipient rat. They found that the allogeneic islet cells survived indefinitely in the recipient, suggesting that the presence of alloantigens in the thymus induced the host's developing thymocytes to become tolerant to the alloantigens on the islet cells. This novel approach, reported in 1990, may well be applicable to other types of transplants and offers the promise of significantly improving graft survival rates without compromising the recipient's immune system.

Transplants to Immunologically Privileged Sites

There are certain sites in the body, called *immunologically privileged sites,* where an allograft can be placed without engendering a rejection reaction. These sites include the anterior chamber of the eye, the cornea, the cheek pouch of the Syrian hamster, the uterus, the testes, and the brain. Each of these sites is characterized by an absence of lymphatic vessels and sometimes an absence of blood vessels as well. Consequently, the alloantigens of the graft are not generally able to sensitize the recipient's lymphocytes, and the graft shows an increased likelihood of acceptance, even when HLA antigens are not matched.

The privileged location of the cornea has allowed cornea transplants to be highly successful. The brain is another immunologically privileged site because the blood-brain barrier prevents the entry and exit of many molecules into or out of the brain. Transplantations of fetal brain-stem neurons into primates has been shown to reduce the symptoms of Parkinson's disease, and recently human fetal neurons have been transplanted into several patients with Parkinson's disease. The successful transplantation of allogeneic pancreatic islet cells into the thymus, discussed in the preceding section, has led to the speculation that the thymus may also be an immunologically privileged site.

Immunologically privileged sites fail to induce an immune response because they are effectively sequestered from the cells of the immune system. A recent publication suggests that it is possible to achieve this goal experimentally. Pancreatic islet cells were encapsulated in semipermeable membranes (fabricated from an acrylic copolymer) and then transplanted into diabetic mice. The islet cells survived and produced insulin but were not rejected because immune cells could not contact the transplanted islet cells. This novel transplant method enabled the diabetic mice to produce normal levels of insulin.

Summary

1. Graft rejection is an immunologic response displaying the attributes of specificity, memory, and self/nonself recognition. The reaction generally involves the cell-mediated branch of the immune system with tissue damage mediated by T_{DTH} cells and/or CTLs.

2. The immune response is generated to tissue antigens on the transplanted tissue that differ from those of the host. Although more than 40 different loci encode such antigens, the loci responsible for the most vigorous graft-rejection reactions are contained within the major histocompatibility complex (MHC), called the HLA complex in humans. Even when a donor and recipient have identical HLA antigens, differences in minor histocompatibility loci outside the MHC can also contribute to graft rejection.

3. The process of graft rejection can be divided into a sensitization stage and an effector stage. During the sensitization stage, passenger leukocytes, derived from the donor graft, migrate from the graft to the regional lymph nodes, where they are recognized as foreign by immune T_H cells, stimulating T_H-cell proliferation. Following T_H-cell proliferation, a population of effector cells is generated, which migrates to the graft and mediates graft rejection.

4. The degree to which a recipient and potential graft donors are matched for MHC antigens can be assessed by tissue typing. In the microcytotoxicity test, monoclonal antibodies are used to detect the presence of various class I and class II MHC antigens on donor and recipient cells. The more MHC antigens that a donor and recipient have in common, the more likely is a graft to survive. The mixed-lymphocyte reaction (MLR) can be used to quantitatively assess the class II MHC compatibility of a recipient and potential donors. In an MLR assay, donor and recipient lymphocytes are incubated together in the presence of [^{3}H]thymidine; the uptake of the labeled thymidine is directly related to T_H-cell proliferation. The closer the MHC match, the less proliferation occurs.

5. Graft rejection can be suppressed by specific and nonspecific immunosuppressive agents. Nonspecific agents include purine analogs, corticosteroids, cyclosporin A, total lymphoid x-irradiation, and antilymphocyte serum. Experimental approaches using monoclonal antibodies offer the possibility of specific immunosuppression. These approaches include blocking proliferation of antigen-activated T cells with monoclonal antibodies to the IL-2 receptor or depletion of T-cell populations with monoclonal antibodies to CD3 or CD4. Another new approach that offers considerable promise is blocking of the co-stimulatory signal by binding inhibitors that interfere with the interaction of B7 and CD28 or CTLA-4. In the absence of this co-stimulatory signal, antigen-activated T_H cells become anergic.

6. A major complication in bone marrow transplantation is a graft-versus-host reaction mediated by the lymphocytes contained within the donor marrow. T-cell depletion from the donor marrow with antibody specific for T-cell populations reduces the risk of graft-versus-host disease. Transplantations of a variety of organs are being performed with remarkable success. HLA typing together with immunosuppressive therapy have contributed to the high success rate for organ transplants.

References

BRADLEY, J. A., A. McI. MOWAT, and E. M. BOLTON. 1992. Processed MHC class I alloantigen as the stimulus for CD4+ T-cell dependent antibody-mediated graft rejection. *Immunol. Today.*

COLVIN, R. B. 1990. Cellular and molecular mechanisms of allograft rejection. *Annu. Rev. Med.* **41**:361.

FERRARA, J. L. M., and H. J. DEEG. 1991. Graft-versus-host disease. *N. Engl. J. Med.* **324**:667.

ISOBE, M., H. YAGITA, K. OKUMURA, and A. IHARA. 1992. Specific acceptance of cardiac allograft after treatment with antibodies to ICAM-1 and LFA-1. *Science* **255**:1125.

LACY, P. E., O. D. HEGRE, A. GERASIMIDI-VAZEOU et al. 1991. Maintenance of normoglycemia in diabetic mice by subcutaneous xenografts of encapsulated islets. *Science* **254**:1972.

LENSCHOW, D. J., Y. ZENG, J. R. THISTLEWAITE et al. 1992. Long-term survival of xenogeneic pancreatic islets induced by CTLA-4Ig. *Science* **257**:789.

PARKMAN, R. 1991. The biology of bone marrow transplantation for severe combined immune deficiency. *Adv. Immunol.* **49**:381.

POSSELT, A. M., et al. 1990. Induction of donor-specific unresponsiveness by intrathymic islet transplantation. *Science* **249**:1293.

ROSENBERG, A. S., and A. SINGER. 1992. Cellular basis of skin allograft rejection: an in vivo model of immune-mediated tissue destruction. *Annu. Rev. Immunol.* **10**:333.

SHERMAN, L. A., and S. CHATTOPADHYAY. 1993. The molecular basis of allorecognition. *Annu. Rev. Immunol.* **11**:385.

SIGAL, N. H., and F. J. DUMONT. 1992. Cyclosporin A, FK-506, and rapamycin: pharmacologic probes of lymphocyte signal transduction. *Annu. Rev. Immunol.* **10**:519.

STARZL, T. E., A. J. DEMETRIS, N. MURASE et al. 1993. Donor-cell chimerism permitted by immunosuppressive drugs: a new view of organ transplantation. *Immunol. Today* **14**:326.

Study Questions

1. You are a pediatrician treating a child who needs a kidney transplant. The child does not have an identical twin, but both parents and several siblings will donate a kidney if the MHC match with the patient is good.
   a. What is the best possible MHC match that could be achieved in this situation?
   b. In which relative(s) might you find it? Why?
   c. What test(s) would you perform in order to find the best-matched kidney?

2. Indicate in the Response column in the accompanying table whether a skin graft from each donor to each recipient listed would result in a rejection (R) or an acceptance (A) response. If you believe a rejection reaction would occur, then indicate in the right-hand column whether it would be a first-set rejection (FSR), occurring in 12–14 days, or a second-set rejection (SSR), occurring in 5–6 days. All the mouse strains listed in the table have different H-2 haplotypes.

3. Graft-versus-host (GVHD) frequently develops after certain types of transplantations.
   a. Briefly outline the mechanisms involved in GVDH.
   b. Under what conditions is GVHD likely to occur?
   c. Some researchers have found that GVHD can be diminished by prior treatment of the graft with monoclonal antibody and complement or monoclonal antibody conjugated to toxins. List at least two cell-surface antigens to which monoclonal antibodies could be prepared and used for this purpose, and give the rationale for your choices.

4. A child who requires a kidney transplant has been offered a kidney from both parents and from five siblings.
   a. Cells from the potential donors are screened with monoclonal antibodies to the HLA-A, -B, and -C antigens in a microcytotoxicity assay. In addition, ABO blood-group typing is performed. Based on the results in the accompanying table, a kidney graft from which donor(s) is most likely to survive?

For use with Question 2.

Donor	Recipient	Response	Type of rejection
BALB/c	C3H		
BALB/c	Rat		
BALB/c	Nude mouse		
BALB/c	C3H, had previous BALB/c graft		
BALB/c	C3H, had previous C57BL/6 graft		
BALB/c	BALB/c		
BALB/c	F_1 (BALB/c × C3H)		
BALB/c	F_1 (C3H × C57BL/6)		
F_1 (BALB/c × C3H)	BALB/c		
F_1 (BALB/c × C3H)	BALB/c, had previous F_1 graft		

b. Now a one-way MLR is performed using various combinations of mitomycin-treated lymphocytes. The results, expressed as counts per minute of [^{3}H]thymidine incorporated, are shown in the accompanying table; the stimulation index is listed below in parentheses. Based on these data, a graft from which donor(s) is most likely to be accepted?

For use with Question 4a.

	ABO type	HLA-A type	HLA-B type	HLA-C type
Recipient	O	*A1/A2*	*B8/B12*	*Cw3*
Potential donors:				
Mother	A	*A1/A2*	*B8/B12*	*Cw1/Cw3*
Father	O	*A2*	*B12/B15*	*Cw3*
Sibling A	O	*A1/A2*	*B8/B15*	*Cw3*
Sibling B	O	*A2*	*B12*	*Cw1/Cw3*
Sibling C	O	*A1/A2*	*B8/B12*	*Cw3*
Sibling D	A	*A1/A2*	*B8/B12*	*Cw3*
Sibling E	O	*A1/A2*	*B8/B15*	*Cw3*

For use with Question 4b.

Responder cells	Mitomycin C–treated stimulator cells					
	Patient	Sib A	Sib B	Sib C	Sib D	Sib E
Patient	1,672 (1.0)	1,800 (1.1)	13,479 (8.1)	5,210 (3.1)	13,927 (8.3)	13,808 (8.3)
Sib A	1,495 (1.6)	933 (1.0)	11,606 (12.4)	8,443 (9.1)	11,708 (12.6)	13,430 (14.4)
Sib B	25,418 (9.9)	26,209 (10.2)	2,570 (1.0)	13,170 (5.1)	19,722 (7.7)	4,510 (1.8)
Sib C	10,722 (6.2)	10,714 (5.9)	13,032 (7.5)	1,731 (1.0)	1,740 (1.0)	14,365 (8.3)
Sib D	15,988 (5.1)	13,492 (4.2)	18,519 (5.9)	3,300 (1.1)	3,151 (1.0)	18,334 (5.9)
Sib E	5,777 (6.5)	8,053 (9.1)	2,024 (2.3)	6,895 (7.8)	10,720 (12.1)	888 (1.0)

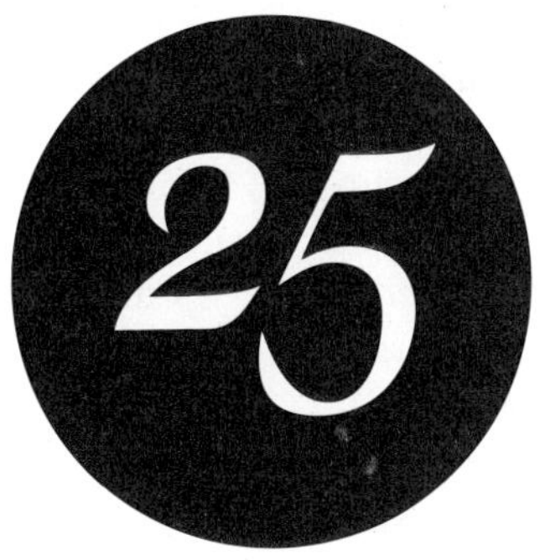

CANCER AND THE IMMUNE SYSTEM

As the death toll from infectious disease has declined in the Western world, cancer has become the second-ranking cause of death, led only by heart disease. Current estimates project that one person in three in the United States will develop cancer, and that one person in five will die from cancer. From an immunologic perspective, cancer cells can be viewed as altered self-cells that have escaped normal growth-regulating mechanisms. This chapter examines the unique properties of cancer cells, paying particular attention to those properties that can be recognized by the immune system. The immune responses that develop to cancer cells, as well as the methods by which cancers manage to evade those responses, are then described. Finally, current clinical and experimental immunotherapies for cancer are discussed.

Cancer: Origin and Terminology

In a mature animal, a balance usually is maintained between cell renewal and cell death in most organs and tissues. The various types of mature cells in the body have a given life span; as these cells die, new cells are generated by the proliferation and differentiation of various types of stem cells. Under normal circumstances, the production of new cells is so regulated that the numbers of any particular type of cell remain constant. Occasionally, though, cells arise that are no longer responsive to normal growth-control mechanisms. These cells give rise to clones of cells that can expand to a considerable size, producing a *tumor,* or *neoplasm.* A tumor that is not capable of indefinite growth and does not invade the healthy surrounding tissue extensively is *benign.* A tumor that continues to grow and becomes progressively invasive is *malignant;* the term *cancer* refers specifically to a malignant tumor. In addition to uncontrolled growth, malignant tumors exhibit *metastasis;* in this process, small clusters of cancerous cells dislodge from a tumor, invade the blood or lymphatic vessels, and are carried to other tissues, where they continue to proliferate. In this way a primary tumor at one site can give rise to a secondary tumor at another site (Figure 25-1).

Malignant tumors are classified according to the embryonic origin of the tissue from which the tumor is derived. *Carcinomas* are tumors arising from endodermal or ectodermal tissues such as skin or the epithelial lining of internal organs and glands. *Sarcomas,* which arise less frequently, are derived from mesodermal connective tissues such as bone, fat, and cartilage. The *leukemias* and *lymphomas* are malignant tumors of hematopoietic cells of the bone marrow. Leukemias proliferate as single cells, whereas lymphomas tend to grow as tumor masses.

Cancer cells exhibit a number of properties that distinguish them from normal cells. The most important of these properties are as follows:

- *Clonal origin:* Most cancer cells are derived from a single neoplastic cell possessing a regulatory defect, which is inherited by the clonal progeny.
- *Unregulated growth in vivo:* Because cancer cells do not respond to normal regulatory mechanisms, they can proliferate indefinitely (unlike normal cells).
- *Altered tissue-specific affinity:* The loss of the normal tissue-specific affinity enables some cancer cells

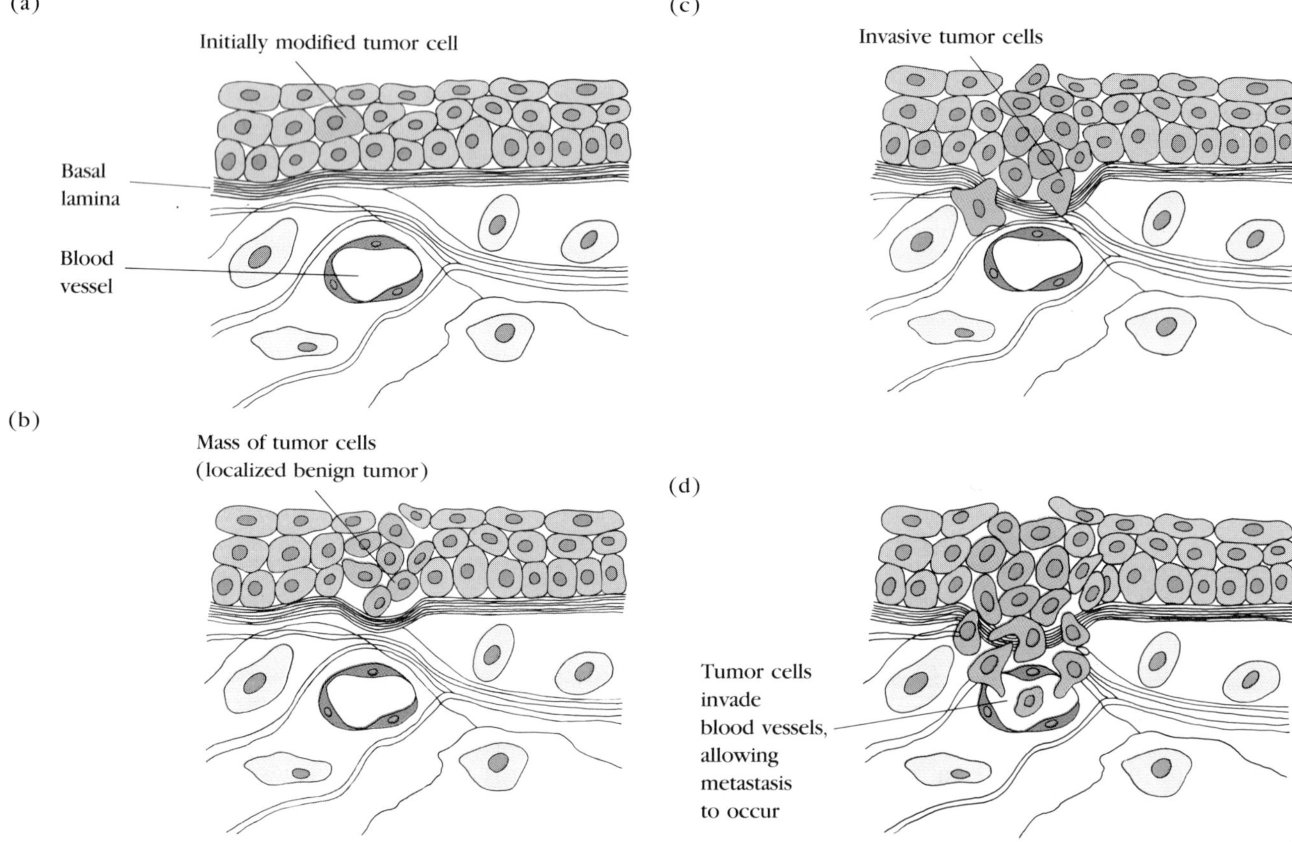

FIGURE 25-1 Tumor growth and metastasis. (a) A single cell develops altered growth properties at a tissue site. (b) The altered cell proliferates, forming a mass of localized tumor cells, or benign tumor. (c) The tumor cells become progressively more invasive, invading the underlying basal lamina. The tumor is now classified as malignant. (d) The malignant tumor metastasizes by generating small clusters of cancer cells that dislodge from the tumor and are carried by the blood or lymph to other sites in the body. [Adapted from J. Darnell et al., 1990, *Molecular Cell Biology,* 2d ed., Scientific American Books.]

to grow beyond the boundaries of their tissue of origin; that is, they can metastasize and grow in diverse tissue sites. Other cancer cells appear to acquire affinity for specific but "wrong" tissues; this property may account for the tendency of certain cancers to metastasize preferentially to particular tissue sites.

- *Altered biochemical activities:* Cancer cells acquire several biochemical activities that may contribute to their invasiveness and ability to metastasize. These include increased glycolytic activity, which may allow tumors to grow at decreased oxygen levels; secretion of several enzymes that degrade the basement membrane and underlying stroma surrounding a tissue; and production of angiogenesis factors, which induce formation of blood vessels within a tumor to supply the oxygen and nutrients necessary for sustained tumor growth.

- *Abnormal cytoskeleton:* Cancer cells possess a disorganized cytoskeleton, whereas normal cells possess an organized network of microtubules and microfilaments. One result of the cytoskeletal changes is an overall change in the morphology of cancer cells compared with normal cells.

- *Chromosomal abnormalities:* Instead of the usual diploid complement of chromosomes, cancer cells generally exhibit *aneuploidy;* that is, they contain either more or less than the normal number of chromosomes. In addition, chromosomal deletions, translocations, and gene duplications are associated with various types of cancer cells (Figure 25-2).

- *Immortal in vitro growth:* Whereas normal cells can be subcultured only a limited number of times, cancer cells can be subcultured indefinitely; that is, they exhibit immortal growth.

(a) Chronic myelogenous leukemia

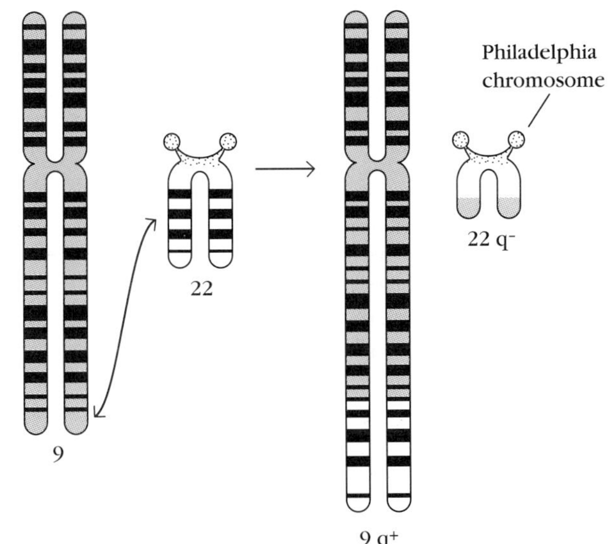

(b) Burkitt's lymphoma

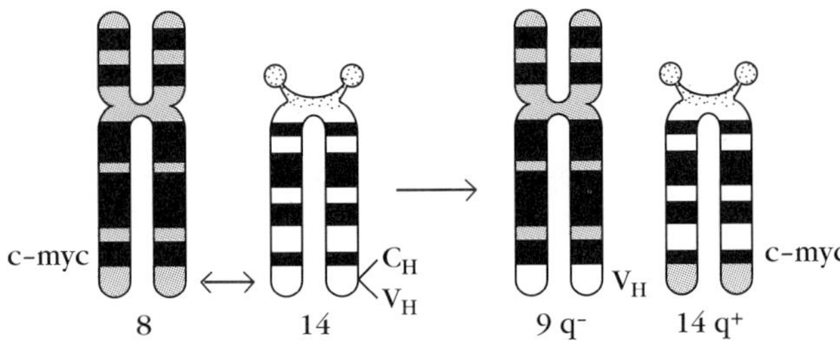

FIGURE 25-2 Chromosomal translocations in (a) chronic myelogenous leukemia (CML) and (b) Burkitt's lymphoma. Leukemic cells from all patients with CML contain the so-called Philadelphia chromosome, which results from a translocation between chromosomes 9 and 22. Cancer cells from some patients with Burkitt's lymphoma exhibit a translocation that moves part of chromosome 8 to chromosome 14. It is now known that this translocation involves c-*myc,* a cellular oncogene. Abnormalities such as these are detected by banding analysis of metaphase chromosomes. Normal chromosomes are shown on the left, and translocated chromosomes on the right.

Malignant Transformation of Cells

Treatment of normal cultured cells with chemical carcinogens, irradiation, and certain viruses can alter the morphology and growth properties of the cells. In some cases this process, referred to as *transformation,* makes the cells able to induce tumors when they are injected into animals; such cells are said to have undergone *malignant transformation,* and they often exhibit in vitro culture properties similar to those of cancer cells. They have decreased requirements for growth factors and serum, are no longer anchorage-dependent, grow in a density-independent fashion—and they are immortal. The process of malignant transformation has been studied extensively as a model of cancer induction.

Transformation Induced by Chemical or Physical Carcinogens

In the early 1900s two Japanese researchers applied coal tar to the ears of rabbits repeatedly over a period of a year and found that tumors appeared. Since this initial demonstration of chemically induced malignant transformation in animals, various chemical and physical agents have been shown to induce transformation by mutagenesis. Some chemical carcinogens, such as alkylating agents, are directly mutagenic; others are not mutagenic in vitro but are converted into potent mutagens in vivo, usually by enzymes of the liver. Physical carcinogens, such as ultraviolet light and ionizing radiation, are also potent mutagens. Ultraviolet light induces the formation of thymine dimers, and x-irradiation induces a range of mutations including chromosome breakage. The importance of these mutations in the induction of cancer is illustrated in certain diseases such as xeroderma pigmentosum. This rare disease in humans is caused by a defect in the gene encoding a DNA-repair enzyme called UV-specific endonuclease. Individuals with this disease are unable to repair UV-induced thymine dimers and consequently develop skin cancers.

Induction of malignant transformation with chemical or physical carcinogens appears to involve multiple steps and at least two distinct phases: *initiation* and *promotion*. Initiation involves changes in the genome but does not, in itself, lead to malignant transformation. Following initiation, promoters stimulate cell division and lead to malignant transformation.

Virus-Induced Transformation

The first evidence that a virus could induce malignant transformation came from the experiments of Peyton Rous in 1910. Rous prepared cell-free filtrates of chicken sarcomas and injected them into healthy chickens; he found that these filtrates alone could induce the formation of sarcomas. When Rous characterized the filtrate, he discovered that an RNA virus (which came to be called the Rous sarcoma virus) was the agent responsible for malignant transformation. In 1966, at the age of 85, Rous received a Nobel prize for this work. Since Rous' initial discovery, a number of DNA and RNA viruses have been shown to induce malignant transformation.

Two of the best-studied DNA viruses known to cause malignant transformation are SV40 and polyoma. In both cases the viral genomes, which integrate randomly into the host chromosomal DNA, include several genes that are expressed early in the course of viral replication. SV40 encodes two early proteins called T and t, and polyoma encodes three early proteins called T, mid-T, and t. Each of these proteins plays a role in malignant transformation of virus-infected cells.

Most RNA viruses replicate in the cytoplasm and do not induce malignant transformation. The exceptions are retroviruses, which transcribe their RNA into DNA by means of a reverse transcriptase enzyme and then integrate the DNA transcript into the host's chromosomal DNA. This process is similar in the cytopathic retroviruses such as HIV-1 and HIV-2 and in the transforming retroviruses, which induce changes in the host cell that lead to malignant transformation. In some cases, retrovirus-induced transformation is related to the presence of *oncogenes,* or "cancer genes," carried by the retrovirus. One of the best-studied transforming retroviruses is the Rous sarcoma virus. This virus carries an oncogene called v-*src,* which encodes a 60-kDa phosphoprotein (v-Src) that catalyzes the addition of phosphate to tyrosine residues on proteins. The first evidence that oncogenes alone could induce malignant transformation came from studies on the v-*src* oncogene from Rous sarcoma virus. When the v-*src* oncogene from Rous sarcoma virus was cloned and transfected into normal cells in culture, the cells underwent malignant transformation.

Oncogenes and Cancer Induction

In 1971 Howard Temin suggested that oncogenes might not be unique to transforming viruses but might also be found in normal cells; indeed, he proposed that oncogenes might be acquired by a virus from the genome of an infected cell. He called these cellular genes *proto-oncogenes,* or *cellular oncogenes* (c-*onc*), to distinguish them from their viral counterpart (v-*onc*). In the mid-1970s J. M. Bishop and H. E. Varmus set out to determine whether these putative proto-oncogenes exist in normal cells. Using a radioactive v-*src* DNA probe, they identified a homologous DNA sequence in normal chicken cells, which was designated c-*src.* Since these early discoveries, numerous cellular oncogenes have been identified.

Sequence comparisons of viral and cellular oncogenes reveal that they are highly conserved in evolution. For example, sequences related to *src* have been detected in species as distant as humans, *Drosophila,* and even yeast, implying that the proteins encoded by these genes may have fundamental functions related to regulation of cellular growth or differentiation. Although most proto-oncogenes consist of a series of exons and introns, their viral counterparts consist of uninterrupted coding sequences, suggesting that the virus might have acquired the oncogene sequence via an intermediate RNA transcript from which the intron sequences were removed during RNA processing. The actual coding sequences of viral oncogenes and cellular proto-oncogenes exhibit a high degree of homology; in some cases a single point mutation is all that distinguishes a viral oncogene from the corresponding proto-oncogene. It is now believed that most, if not all, oncogenes (both viral and cellular) are derived from cellular genes that encode various growth-controlling proteins. In addition, the proteins encoded by a particular oncogene and its corresponding proto-oncogene appear to have very similar functions. As discussed below, the conversion of a proto-oncogene into an oncogene appears in many cases to involve a change in the level of expression of a normal growth-controlling protein.

Function of Oncogenes

In normal cells, oncogenes generally are expressed at relatively low levels, and their expression is often limited to certain stages of the cell cycle and cellular differentiation. A number of oncogenes are activated as cells enter the cell cycle, moving from G_0 into G_1 or from G_1 into the S phase of DNA synthesis. For example, as discussed in Chapter 12, within 45 min following T_H-cell activation, three oncogene products—c-Fos, c-Myc, and c-Abl—can be detected (see Table 12-6). In this situation, these products serve a normal function in T-cell proliferation and/or differentiation.

Homeostasis in normal tissue is maintained by a highly regulated process of cellular proliferation balanced by cell death. If there is an imbalance, either at the level of cellular proliferation or at the level of cell death then a cancerous state will develop. Oncogenes have been shown to play an important role in this process, either by regulating cellular proliferation or by regulating cell death. Oncogenes can be divided into three categories reflecting these different activities (Table 25-1).

Induction of Cellular Proliferation

One category of oncogenes encode proteins that induce cellular proliferation. Some of these proteins function as growth factors, growth-factor receptors, or transcription factors; others function in signal-transduction pathways. Included in this category is *sis,* which encodes a form of platelet-derived growth factor, and *fms, erbB,* and *neu,* which encode growth-factor receptors. In normal cells the expression of growth factors and their receptors is carefully regulated. Usually, one population of cells secretes a growth factor that acts on another population of cells carrying the receptor for that factor, thus stimulating proliferation of the second population. Inappropriate expression of either a growth factor or its receptor can result in uncontrolled proliferation. Other oncogenes in this category encode products that function in signal-transduction pathways or as transcription factors. The *src* and *abl* oncogenes encode tyrosine kinases; the *ras* oncogene encodes a GTP-binding protein; the

TABLE 25-1 FUNCTIONAL CLASSIFICATION OF ONCOGENES

Type/name	Nature of gene product
	Category I: oncogenes that induce cellular proliferation
Growth factors	
sis	A form of platelet-derived growth factor (PDGF)
Growth-factor receptors	
fms	Receptor for colony-stimulating factor 1 (CSF-1)
erbB	Receptor for epidermal growth factor (EGF)
neu	Protein related to EGF receptor
erbA	Receptor for thyroid hormone
Signal transducers	
src	Tyrosine kinase
abl	Tyrosine kinase
Ha-*ras*	GTP-binding protein with GTPase activity
N-*ras*	GTP-binding protein with GTPase activity
K-*ras*	GTP-binding protein with GTPase activity
Transcription factors	
jun	Component of transcription factor AP1
fos	Component of transcription factor AP1
myc	DNA-binding protein
	Category II: oncogenes that inhibit cellular proliferation*
Rb	Suppressor of retinoblastoma
p53	Nuclear phosphoprotein that inhibits formation of small-cell lung cancer and colon cancers
DCC	Suppressor of colon carcinoma
APC	Suppressor of adenomatous polyposis
NF1	Suppressor of neurofibromatosis
WT1	Suppressor of Wilm's tumor
	Category III: oncogenes that regulate programmed cell death
bcl-2	Suppressor of apoptosis

* The activity of the category II oncogene products is not well understood. However, loss or mutation in these oncogenes is associated with development of the indicated cancers.

myc, jun, and *fos* oncogenes encode transcription factors. Overactivity of any of these oncogenes may result in unregulated proliferation.

Inhibition of Cellular Proliferation

A second category of oncogenes—called tumor-suppressor genes, or anti-oncogenes—function to inhibit excessive cell proliferation. Inactivation of these oncogenes abolishes their inhibitory activity, resulting in unregulated proliferation. To date, somatic inactivation of six suppressor genes have been identified in different human cancers (see Table 25-1). The prototype of this category of oncogenes is *Rb*, the retinoblastoma gene. Hereditary retinoblastoma is a rare childhood cancer in which tumors develop from neural precursor cells in the immature retina. The affected child inherits a mutated *Rb* allele; somatic inactivation of the remaining *Rb* allele leads to tumor growth. Probably the single most frequent abnormality in human cancer is mutations in *p53*, which encodes a nuclear phosphoprotein. Over 90% of small-cell lung cancer and over 50% of breast and colon cancers have been shown to be associated with mutations in *p53*.

Regulation of Programmed Cell Death

A third category of oncogenes regulates programmed cell death. These genes encode proteins that either block or induce apoptosis. Included in this category of oncogenes is *bcl-2,* an anti-apoptosis gene. This oncogene was originally discovered from a chromosomal translocation associated with B-cell follicular lymphoma. Since its discovery, *bcl-2* has been shown to play an important role in regulating cell survival during hematopoiesis and in survival of selected B cells and T cells during maturation (see Chapters 12 and 14). Interestingly, the Epstein-Barr virus contains a gene that has sequence homology to *bcl-2* and may act in a similar manner to suppress apoptosis.

Conversion of Proto-oncogenes to Oncogenes

In 1972 R. J. Huebner and G. J. Todaro suggested that mutations or genetic rearrangements of proto-oncogenes by carcinogens or viruses might alter the normal regulated function of these genes, converting them into potent cancer-causing oncogenes (Figure 25-3). Considerable evidence supporting this hypothesis has accumulated. For example, some malignantly transformed cells contain multiple copies of cellular oncogenes, resulting in increased production of oncogene products (Table 25-2). Several groups have identified c-*myc* oncogenes in homogeneously staining regions (HSRs) of chromosomes from cancer cells; these HSRs represent long tandem arrays of amplified genes.

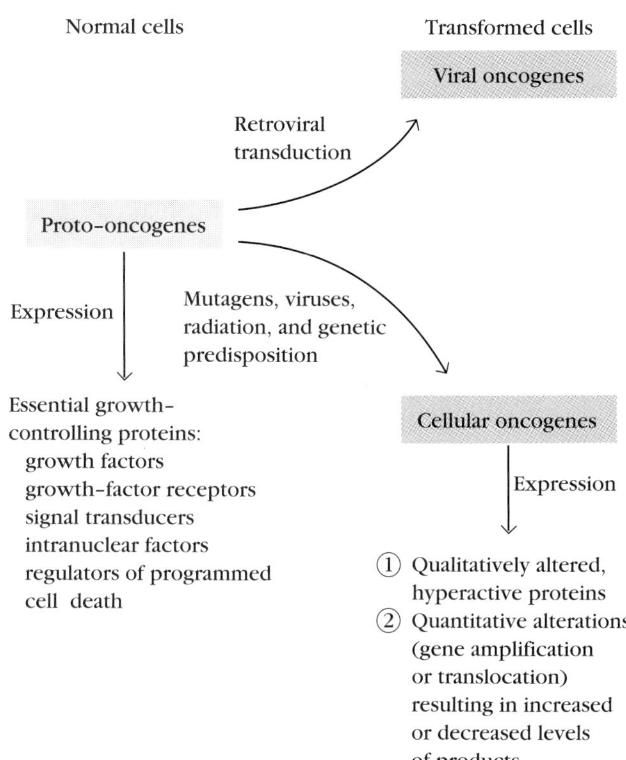

FIGURE 25-3 Conversion of proto-oncogenes into oncogenes can involve mutation, resulting in production of qualitatively different gene products, or DNA amplification or translocation, resulting in increased or decreased expression of gene products.

As noted earlier, some cancer cells exhibit chromosomal translocations. It turns out that these translocations usually involve movement of a proto-oncogene from one chromosomal site to another. In many cases of Burkitt's lymphoma, for example, c-*myc* is moved from its usual position on chromosome 8 to a position near the immunoglobulin heavy-chain enhancer on chromosome 14 (see Figure 25-2b). As a result of this translocation, synthesis of the c-Myc protein, which functions as a transcription factor, increases.

Mutation in proto-oncogenes has also been associated with cellular transformation and may be a major mechanism by which chemical carcinogens or x-irradiation convert a proto-oncogene into a cancer-inducing oncogene. A single-point mutation in c-*ras* has been detected in human lung carcinoma, prostate carcinoma, bladder carcinoma, and neuroblastoma. This single mutation appears to reduce the GTPase activity of the Ras protein and may alter its function in the

TABLE 25-2 AMPLIFICATION OF ONCOGENES IN HUMAN TUMORS

Amplified gene	Tumor	Degree of amplification
c-*myc*	Promyelocytic leukemia cell line, HL60	20 ×
	Small-cell lung carcinoma cell lines	5–30 ×
N-*myc*	Primary neuroblastomas (stages III and IV) and neuroblastoma cell lines	5–1000 ×
	Retinoblastoma cell line and primary tumors	10–200 ×
	Small-cell lung carcinoma cell lines and tumors	50 ×
L-*myc*	Small-cell lung carcinoma cell lines and tumors	10–20 ×
c-*myb*	Acute myeloid leukemia	5–10 ×
	Colon carcinoma cell lines	10 ×
c-*erbB*	Epidermoid carcinoma cell line	30 ×
	Primary gliomas*	—
c-K-*ras-2*	Primary carcinomas of lung, colon, bladder, and rectum	4–20 ×
N-*ras*	Mammary carcinoma cell line	5–10 ×

* No amplification given.

SOURCE: Modified from H. E. Varmus, 1984, *Annu. Rev. Genet.* **18**:553.

regulation of cellular growth. Finally, viral integration into the host-cell genome may in itself serve to convert a proto-oncogene into a transforming oncogene. For example, avian leukosis virus (ALV) is a retrovirus that does not carry any viral oncogenes and yet is able to transform B cells into lymphomas. This particular retrovirus has been shown to integrate within the c-*myc* proto-oncogene between exon 1 and exons 2 and 3. Exon 1 of c-*myc* has an unknown function; exons 2 and 3 encode the Myc protein. Insertion of the virus at this position has been shown in some cases to allow the provirus promoter to increase transcription of exons 2 and 3, resulting in increased synthesis of c-Myc.

A variety of tumors have been shown to express significantly increased levels of growth factors or growth-factor receptors. In adult T-cell leukemia, discussed in Chapter 13, T cells infected with the HTLV-1 retrovirus show constitutive expression of IL-2 and the IL-2 receptor, enabling the cells to autostimulate their own proliferation in the absence of antigen activation (Figure 25-4). Expression of the receptor for epidermal growth factor, which is encoded by c-*erbB,* has also been shown to be amplified in many cancer cells. And in breast cancer, increased synthesis of the growth-factor receptor encoded by c-*neu* has been linked with a poor prognosis.

One of the best examples of the association between increased expression of growth factors and cancer induction involves transforming growth factor (TGF-α). TGF-α, which is secreted by a variety of transformed cells, is similar in both structure and function to epidermal growth factor (EGF), and like EGF it is also able to bind to the EGF receptor on cells. Increased expression of both TGF-α and the EGF receptor have been observed in many cancer cells and in cells that

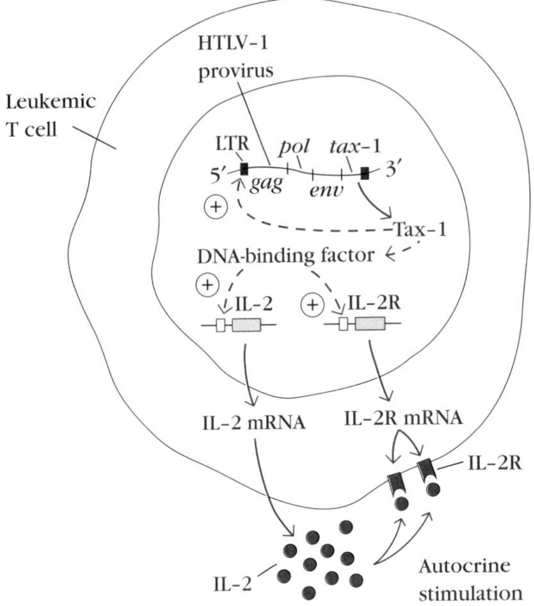

FIGURE 25-4 In adult T-cell leukemia, infection of T cells with HTLV-1 leads to constitutive expression of IL-2 and the IL-2 receptor (IL-2R), resulting in antigen-independent autostimulation of T-cell proliferation. Tax-1, encoded by the HTLV-1 genome, binds to the 5′ LTR, promoting transcription of the provirus. Tax-1 also stimulates expression of an unknown DNA-binding factor (or factors) that binds to the promoters (open boxes) of the IL-2 and IL-2R genes. As a result, IL-2 and IL-2R are expressed in the absence of antigen activation, leading to proliferation of infected T cells.

have been transformed with retroviruses, viral oncogenes, and carcinogens. TGF-α is thought to act as an autocrine activator of the EGF receptor. The effects of TGF-α overproduction have been studied by producing transgenic mice containing a TGF-α transgene linked to a metallothionine promoter. In these mice, the level of TGF-α expression could be controlled by adjusting their zinc intake. Experiments with these mice revealed that when TGF-α expression was high, they developed carcinomas of the liver and breast and also exhibited enlargement of the pancreas; however, when TGF-α expression was low, none of these changes was observed. Thus overexpression of the gene encoding TGF-α enables it to function as an oncogene in this system.

Induction of Cancer: A Multistep Process

The development from a normal cell to a cancerous cell is thought to be a multistep process of clonal evolution driven by a series of somatic mutations that progressively convert the cell from normal growth to a precancerous state and finally into a cancerous state.

The presence of a myriad of chromosomal abnormalities in precancerous and cancerous cells lends support to the role of multiple mutations in the development of cancer. In human colon cancer the progression to a more malignant phenotype correlates with an increase in the number of genetic alterations (Figure 25-5). Colon cancer begins as small, benign tumors in the colorectal epithelium, called adenomas. These precancerous tumors grow, gradually becoming increasingly disorganized in their intracellular organization until they acquire the malignant phenotype. These well-defined morphologic stages of colon cancer have allowed researchers to establish the sequence of mutations in the progression to a more malignant phenotype. The progression involves inactivation or loss of three anti-oncogenes (*APC, DCC,* and *p53*) and activation of one cellular proliferation oncogene (K-*ras*).

Studies with transgenic mice also support the role of multiple steps in the induction of cancer. Transgenic mice expressing high levels of Bcl-2 develop a population of small resting B cells, derived from secondary lymphoid follicles, that have greatly extended life spans. Gradually these transgenic mice develop lymphomas. Analysis of lymphomas in these transgenic mice have shown that approximately half have a c-*myc* translocation to the immunoglobulin H-chain locus. The synergism of Myc and Bcl-2 is highlighted in double-transgenic mice (produced by mating the *bcl-2*$^+$ transgenic mice with *myc*$^+$ transgenic mice). In this case the mice develop a very rapid onset leukemia.

Tumors of the Immune System

Tumors of the immune system are classified as lymphomas or leukemias. Lymphomas proliferate as solid tumors within a lymphoid tissue such as the bone marrow, lymph nodes, or thymus; they include Hodgkin's and non-Hodgkin's lymphomas. Leukemias tend to proliferate as single cells and are detected by increased cell numbers in the blood or lymph. Leukemia can develop in lymphoid or myeloid lineages. Historically the leukemias were classified as acute or chronic

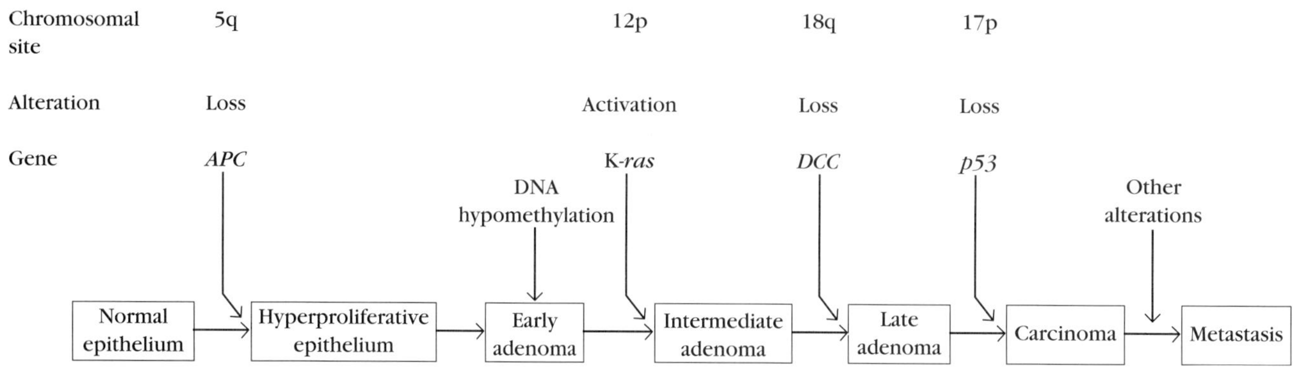

FIGURE 25-5 Model of sequential genetic alterations leading to metastatic colon cancer. Each of the stages indicated at the bottom are morphologically distinct, allowing researchers to determine the sequence of genetic alterations. [Adapted from B. Vogelstein and K. W. Kinzler, 1993, *Trends Genet.* **9**:138.]

according to the clinical progression of the disease. The acute leukemias appeared suddenly and progressed rapidly, whereas the chronic leukemias were much less aggressive and developed slowly as mild, barely symptomatic diseases. These clinical distinctions apply to untreated leukemias; with current treatments the acute leukemias often have a good prognosis, and permanent remission can often be achieved. Now the major distinction between acute and chronic leukemias is the maturity of the cell involved. Acute leukemias tend to arise in less mature cells, whereas chronic leukemias arise in mature cells. The acute leukemias include acute lymphocytic leukemia (ALL) and acute myelogenous leukemia (AML); these diseases can develop at any age and have a rapid onset. The chronic leukemias include chronic lymphocytic leukemia (CLL) and chronic myelogenous leukemia (CML); these diseases develop slowly and are seen in adults.

A number of B- and T-cell leukemias and lymphomas have been shown to involve chromosomal translocations in which a proto-oncogene is translocated into the immunoglobulin genes or T-cell-receptor genes. One of the best-characterized involves the translocation of c-*myc* in Burkitt's lymphoma and in mouse plasmacytomas. In 75% of Burkitt's lymphoma patients, c-*myc* is translocated from chromosome 8 to the Ig heavy-chain gene cluster on chromosome 14 (see Figure 25-2b). In the remaining patients, c-*myc* remains on chromosome 8 and the κ or λ light-chain genes are translocated to a region 3′ of c-*myc*. Kappa-gene translocations from chromosome 2 to chromosome 8 occur 9% of the time, and λ-gene translocations from chromosome 22 to chromosome 8 occur 16% of the time.

Translocations of c-*myc* to the Ig heavy-chain gene cluster on chromosome 14 have been analyzed in some detail. In some cases the entire c-*myc* gene is translocated head-to-head to a region near the heavy-chain enhancer. In other cases exons 1, 2, and 3 or exons 2 and 3 of c-*myc* are translocated head-to-head to the S_μ or S_α switch site (Figure 25-6). In each case the translocation removes the *myc* coding exons from the regulatory mechanisms operating in chromosome 8 and places them in the immunoglobulin-gene region, which is a very active region that is expressed constitutively in these cells. Transgenic mice have been used to study the consequences of constitutive *myc* expression in lymphoid cells. In one study mice containing a transgene consisting of all three c-*myc* exons and the immunoglobulin heavy-chain enhancer were produced. Of 15 transgenic pups born, 13 developed lymphomas of the B-cell lineage within just a few months of birth.

Various hypotheses have been suggested to account for *myc*-related oncogenesis. Some researchers have suggested that the presence of the immunoglobulin enhancer may result in overproduction of the *myc*

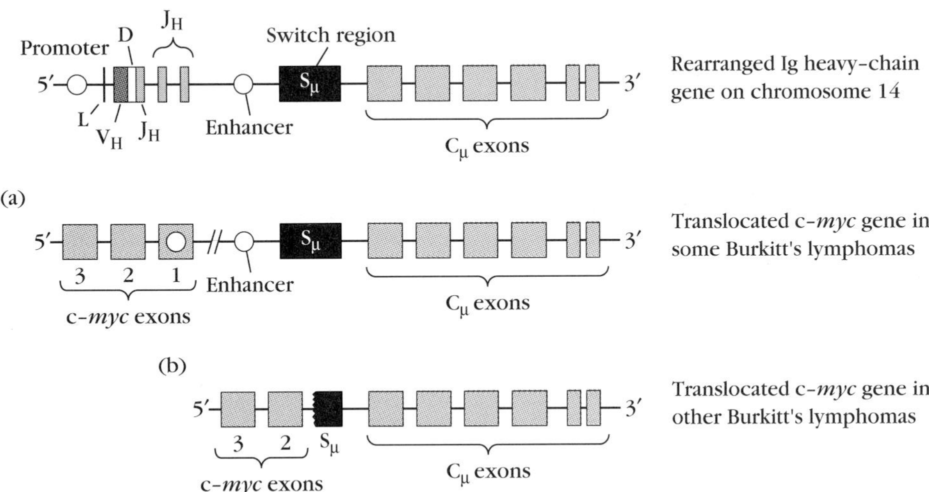

FIGURE 25-6 Analysis of the c-*myc* gene translocation to the immunoglobulin heavy-chain gene cluster on chromosome 14 in Burkitt's lymphoma has revealed several insertion sites. (a) Insertion of the entire c-*myc* gene near the heavy-chain enhancer. (b) Insertion of exons 2 and 3 of c-*myc* at the S_μ switch site. Only exons 2 and 3 of c-*myc* are coding exons.

gene product. Another hypothesis, based on the unusual level of mutations observed in exon 1 of c-*myc* after translocation, is that somatic mutation within the immunoglobulin V-region genes may induce mutations in the oncogene that lead to faulty regulation through its exon 1 or to changes in the function of its protein product.

Tumor Antigens

The subdiscipline of tumor immunology involves the study of cell-membrane antigens on tumor cells and the immunologic response to these antigens. Two types of tumor antigens have been identified on tumor cells: *tumor-specific antigens (TSAs)* and *tumor-associated antigens (TAAs).* Tumor-specific antigens are unique to tumor cells and do not occur on other cells in the body. Tumor-associated antigens are not unique to the tumor cells and instead are also expressed on normal cells under conditions that fail to induce a state of immunologic tolerance to the antigen. The expression of the antigen on the tumor may occur under conditions that enable the immune system to respond to the antigen. Tumor-associated antigens may be antigens that are expressed on normal cells during fetal development when the immune system is immature and unable to respond or they may be antigens that are normally present at extremely low levels on normal cells but which are expressed at much higher levels on tumor cells.

Tumor antigens, whether tumor-specific or tumor-associated, must be capable of inducing either a humoral or cell-mediated immune response. Although a few tumor antigens have been shown to induce the production of humoral antibodies, most tumor antigens fail to induce humoral antibodies and instead induce a cell-mediated response. The presence of tumor antigens that elicit a cell-mediated response has been demonstrated by the rejection of tumors transplanted into syngeneic recipients; because of this phenomenon, these tumor antigens are referred to as *tumor-specific transplantation antigens (TSTAs)* or *tumor-associated transplantation antigens (TATAs).* It has been difficult to characterize tumor transplantation antigens because they do not generally elicit an antibody response and therefore they cannot be isolated by immunoprecipitation. Many are peptides that are presented together with MHC molecules on the surface of tumor cells and have been characterized by their ability to induce antigen-specific CTLs.

Tumor-Specific Antigens

Tumor-specific antigens have been demonstrated on tumors induced with chemical or physical carcinogens and on some virally induced tumors. It has been much more difficult to demonstrate the presence of tumor-specific antigens on spontaneously occurring tumors. This may be because the immune response to such tumors has eliminated all of the tumor cells bearing recognizable antigens and in this way has selected for cells bearing lower levels of tumor-specific antigens.

Chemically or Physically Induced Tumor Antigens

A variety of chemical and physical carcinogens have been used to induce tumors in animals. Methylcholanthrene and ultraviolet light are two carcinogens that have been used extensively to generate tumorigenic

Table 25-3 Immune response to methylcholanthrene (MCA) or polyoma virus (PV)*

Transplanted killed tumor cells	Source of live tumor cells for challenge	Tumor growth
	Chemically induced	
MCA-induced sarcoma A	MCA-induced sarcoma A	−
MCA-induced sarcoma A	MCA-induced sarcoma B	+
	Virally induced	
PV-induced sarcoma A	PV-induced sarcoma A	−
PV-induced sarcoma A	PV-induced sarcoma B	−
PV-induced sarcoma A	SV40-induced sarcoma C	+

* Tumors were induced either with MCA or PV, and killed cells from the induced tumors were injected into syngeneic animals, which were then challenged with live cells from the indicated tumor-cell lines. The absence of tumor growth after live challenge indicates that the immune response induced by tumor antigens on the killed cells provided protection against the live cells.

cell lines. When syngeneic animals are injected with killed cells from a carcinogen-induced tumor-cell line, the animals develop a specific immunologic response that is unique for the specific tumor-cell line and does not recognize other tumor-cell lines induced in syngeneic animals by the same chemical or physical carcinogen (Table 25-3). Even when the same chemical carcinogen induces two separate tumors at different sites in the same animal, the tumor antigens are distinct and the immune response to one tumor does not protect against the other tumor.

The tumor-specific transplantation antigens of chemically induced tumors have been difficult to characterize because they cannot be identified by induced antibodies but only by their T-cell–mediated rejection. One experimental approach that has allowed identification of genes encoding some TSTAs is outlined in Figure 25-7. When a mouse tumor-cell line is treated in vitro with a chemical mutagen, it is possible to convert the cell line from a tumorigenic line, designated tum$^+$, that forms progressive tumor growth to a mutant cell line that is no longer capable of inducing a tumor in syngeneic mice. These mutant tumor-cell lines are designated as tum$^-$ variants. Most tum$^-$ variants have been shown to express TSTAs that are not expressed by the original tum$^+$ tumor-cell line. When

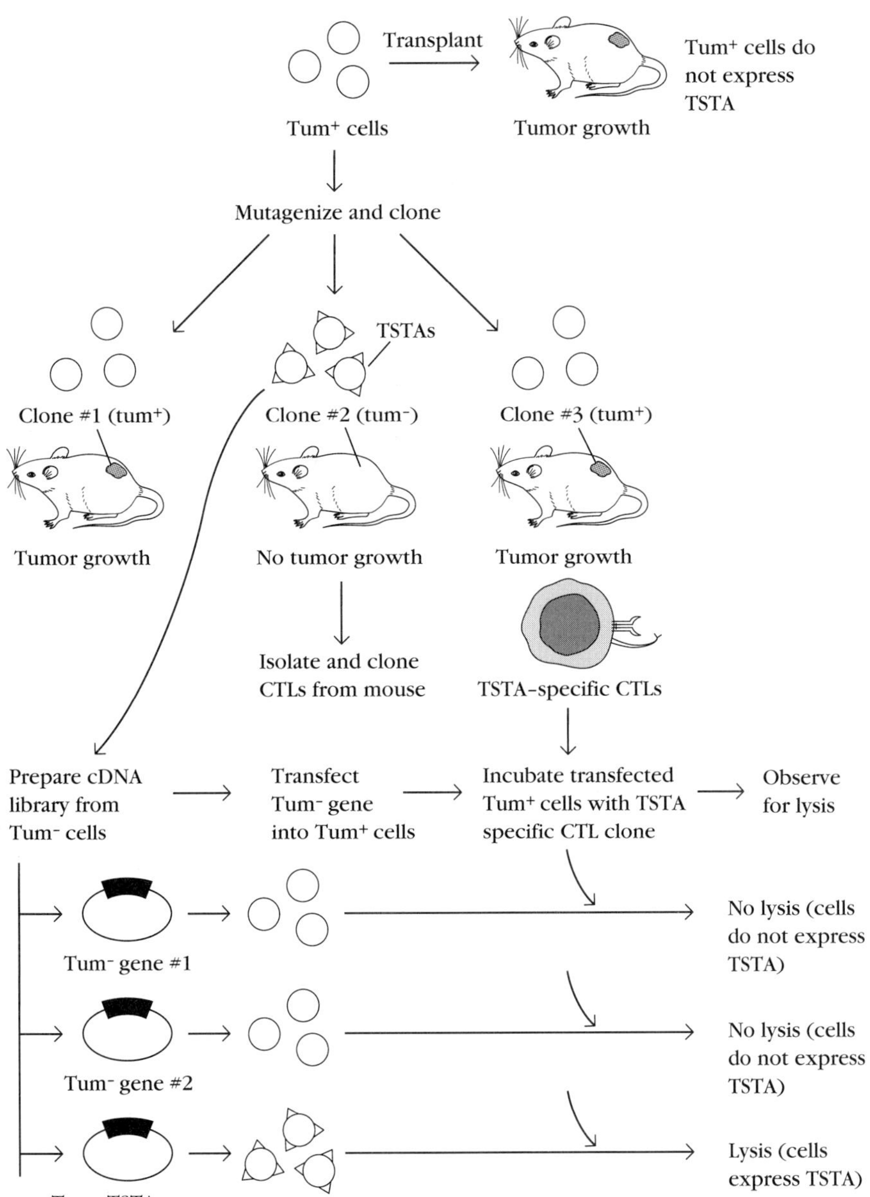

FIGURE 25-7 General procedure for identification of genes encoding tumor-specific transplantation antigens (TSTAs). Most TSTAs can be detected only by the cell-mediated rejection they elicit. In the first part of this procedure, a nontumorigenic (tum$^-$) cell line is generated; this cell line expresses a TSTA that is recognized by syngeneic mice, which mount a cell-mediated response against it. To isolate the gene encoding the TSTA, a cosmid gene library is prepared from the tum$^-$ cell line, the genes are transfected into tum$^+$ cells, and the transfected cells are incubated with TSTA-specific CTLs.

tum$^-$ cells are injected into syngeneic mice, these unique TSTAs are recognized by specific CTLs, which destroy the tumor cells, thus preventing tumor growth.

To identify the genes encoding the TSTAs of a tum$^-$ cell line, a cosmid DNA library is prepared from the tum$^-$ cells. Genes from the tum$^-$ cells then are transfected back into the original tum$^+$ cells, and the transfected tum$^+$ cells are tested for their ability to activate cloned CTLs specific for the tum$^-$ TSTA. A number of diverse TSTAs have been identified by this method. The genes encoding these TSTAs have in some cases been shown to differ from normal cellular genes by a single-point mutation. In one case the mutated protein encoded by a particular tum$^-$ gene was shown to be presented as a short peptide in association with a class I MHC molecule on the tum$^-$ cells or on the transfected tum$^+$ cells. This experimental system has shown that at least some TSTAs may represent mutated forms of normal cellular proteins. In addition, these TSTAs are not always cell-membrane molecules of the tumor but sometimes are cytoplasmic proteins that are processed and presented as short peptides together with class I MHC molecules on the surface of the tumor cells where they can be recognized by CTLs as altered self-cells.

Virally Induced Tumor Antigens

In contrast to chemically induced tumors, virally induced tumors express tumor antigens shared by all tumors induced by the same virus. For example, when syngeneic mice are injected with killed cells from a particular polyoma-induced tumor, the recipients are protected against subsequent challenge with live cells from any polyoma-induced tumors (see Table 25-3). Likewise, when lymphocytes are transferred from mice with a virus-induced tumor into normal syngeneic recipients, the recipients reject subsequent transplants of all syngeneic tumors induced by the same virus. In the case of both SV40- and polyoma-induced tumors, the presence of tumor antigens is related to the neoplastic state of the cell. Although viral antigens have not yet been established in human cancers, Burkitt's lymphoma cells have been shown to express a nuclear antigen of the Epstein-Barr virus that may indeed be a tumor-specific antigen for this type of tumor.

The nature of virally induced tumor antigens has been studied extensively in mice bearing polyoma- and SV40-induced tumors. In both cases the tumor antigens are encoded by viral genes shown to play a role in malignant transformation. For SV40 the early viral protein designated *large T* (where "T" stands for tumor) serves as a tumor-specific antigen. In the case of polyoma virus the tumor-specific antigen is the early viral protein called *middle T* (or mid-T). In both cases the tumor antigens are not part of the envelope proteins of the virion but instead are proteins expressed primarily in the nucleus of the tumor cell. At first the nuclear location of these tumor antigens was a surprise to researchers, but as data began to accumulate on antigen-processing pathways, it became clear that these nuclear proteins might be processed in tumor cells and presented with class I or class II MHC molecules on the tumor-cell membrane, thus serving to activate T_H and T_C cells.

The potential value of these virally induced tumor antigens can be seen in animal models. In one experiment mice immunized with a preparation of genetically engineered polyoma virus tumor antigen were shown to be immune to subsequent injections of live polyoma-induced tumor cells. In another experiment mice were immunized with a vaccinia virus vaccine engineered with the gene encoding the polyoma middle-T antigen. These mice also developed immunity, rejecting later injections of live polyoma-induced tumor cells (Figure 25-8). Clearly if virally induced tumor antigens can be demonstrated on some human tumors, immunotherapeutic approaches to the treatment of these human tumors might be possible.

Tumor-Associated Antigens

The majority of tumor antigens are not unique to tumor cells but also are present on normal cells and are called tumor-associated antigens. These antigens may be expressed only on fetal cells but not on adult cells, or they may be antigens expressed at low levels on normal cells but at much higher levels by tumor cells. Several growth-factor receptors are expressed at significantly increased levels on tumor cells and can serve as tumor-associated antigens. Among these growth-factor receptors is the EGF receptor. A variety of tumor cells have been shown to express the EGF receptor at levels 100 times greater than that in normal cells. Another example of a tumor-associated antigen is a protein, designated p97, on melanoma cells. This protein functions as a transferrin growth factor by aiding in the transport of iron into cells. Whereas normal cells express less than 8,000 molecules of p97 per cell, melanoma cells express 50,000–500,000 molecules of p97 per cell. The gene encoding p97 has been cloned, and a recombinant vaccinia virus vaccine has been prepared carrying the cloned gene. When this vaccine was injected into mice, it induced both humoral and cell-mediated immune responses, which protected the mice against live melanoma cells expressing the p97 antigen. Results such as this highlight the importance of identifying tumor antigens as potential targets of tumor immunotherapy.

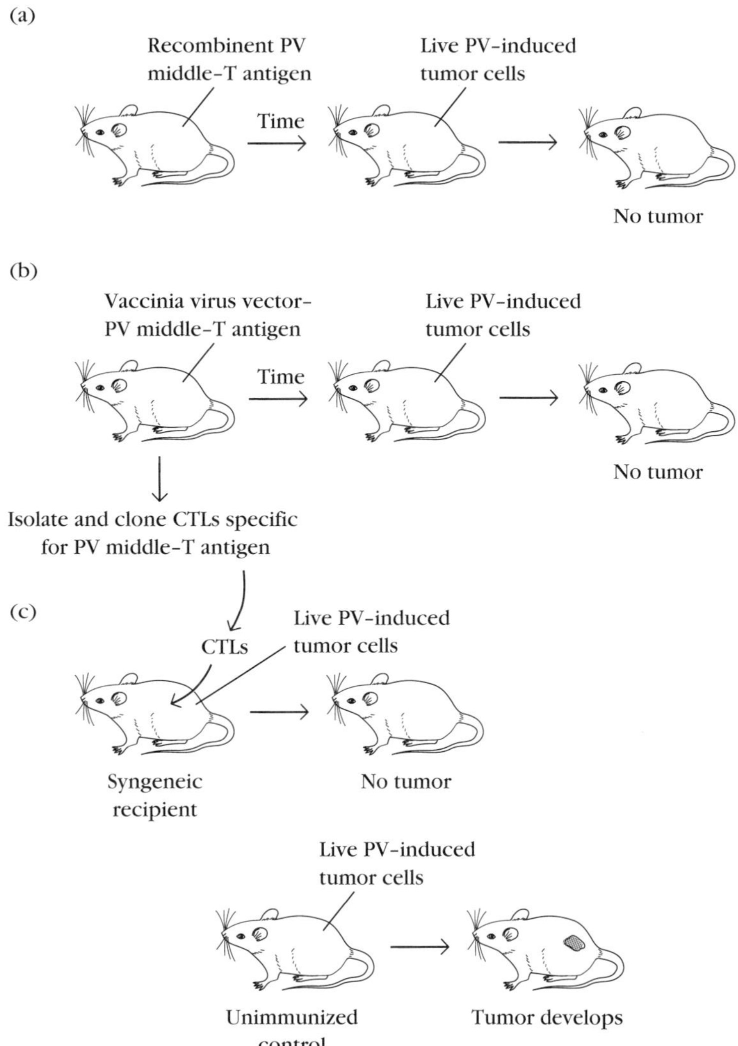

FIGURE 25-8 Experimental induction of immunity against tumor cells induced by polyoma virus (PV) has been achieved by immunizing mice with recombinant polyoma middle-T antigen (a), with a vaccinia vector vaccine containing the gene encoding middle-T antigen (b), or with CTLs specific for middle-T antigen (c). Unimmunized mice *(bottom)* develop tumors when injected with live polyoma-induced tumor cells, whereas the immunized mice do not.

Oncofetal Tumor Antigens

Oncofetal antigens, as the name implies, are found not only on cancerous cells but also on normal fetal cells. These antigens appear early in embryonic development, before the immune system acquires immunocompetence; if these antigens later appear on cancer cells, they are recognized as nonself and induce an immunologic response. Two examples of oncofetal antigens are alpha-fetoprotein (AFP) and carcinoembryonic antigen (CEA). Although the serum concentration of AFP drops from milligram levels in fetal serum to nanogram levels in normal adult serum, elevated AFP levels are found in a majority of patients with liver cancer (Table 25-4). CEA is a membrane glycoprotein found on gastrointestinal and liver cells of 2- to 6-month-old fetuses. Approximately 90% of patients with advanced colorectal cancer, and 50% of patients with early colorectal cancer have increased levels of CEA in their serum; some patients with other types of cancer also exhibit increased CEA levels. However, because AFP and CEA can be found in trace amounts in some normal adults and in some noncancerous disease states, the presence of these oncofetal antigens is not diagnostic of tumors but rather serves to monitor tumor growth. If, for example, a patient has had

TABLE 25-4 ELEVATION OF ALPHA-FETOPROTEIN (AFP) AND CARCINOEMBRYONIC ANTIGEN (CEA) IN SERUM OF PATIENTS WITH VARIOUS DISEASES

Disease	No. of patients tested	% of patients with high AFP or CEA levels*
AFP > 400 μg/ml		
Alcoholic cirrhosis	NA	0
Hepatitis	NA	1
Hepatocellular carcinoma	NA	69
Other carcinoma	NA	0
CEA > 10 ng/ml		
Cancerous		
Breast carcinoma	125	14
Colorectal carcinoma	544	35
Gastric carcinoma	79	19
Noncarcinoma malignancy	228	2
Pancreatic carcinoma	55	35
Pulmonary carcinoma	181	26
Noncancerous		
Alcoholic cirrhosis	120	2
Cholecystitis	39	1
Nonmalignant disease	115	0
Pulmonary emphysema	49	4
Rectal polyps	90	1
Ulcerative colitis	146	5

* Although trace amounts of both AFP and CEA can be found in some healthy adults, none would have levels greater than those indicated in the table.

surgery to remove a colorectal carcinoma, CEA levels are monitored following surgery. An increase in the CEA level is an indication of resumed tumor growth.

Oncogene Proteins as Tumor Antigens

A number of tumors have been shown to express tumor-associated antigens encoded by cellular oncogenes. These antigens are also present in normal cells encoded by the corresponding proto-oncogene. In many cases there is no qualitative difference between the oncogene and proto-oncogene products; instead, the increased levels of the oncogene product can be recognized by the immune system. For example, as noted earlier, human breast-cancer cells exhibit elevated expression of oncogene-encoded Neu protein, a growth-factor receptor, whereas normal adult cells express only trace amounts of Neu protein. Because of this difference in the Neu level, anti-Neu monoclonal antibodies can recognize and selectively eliminate breast-cancer cells without damaging normal cells.

A few tumors have been shown to express a proto-oncogene product that is qualitatively different from the normal protein. For example, single-point mutations in the *ras* proto-oncogene have been detected in a number of tumors including 17 out of 17 cases of malignant prostate cancer. If these qualitative changes can be recognized effectively by the immune system as tumor-specific antigens, they will lend themselves to various cancer immunotherapy approaches.

IMMUNE RESPONSE TO TUMORS

In experimental animals tumor antigens can be shown to induce humoral and cell-mediated immune responses, which in some cases result in tumor elimination. Generally the tumor antigens on UV-induced tumors or tumors induced by oncogenic viruses tend to induce a strong immune response, the tumor antigens on chemically induced tumors tend to induce less immune reactivity, and tumors that arise spontaneously in animals tend to be poorly immunogenic. It is not known why spontaneous tumors lack tumor antigens capable of inducing strong immune reactivity. One theory is that the immune response eliminates any tumor cells bearing strong tumor antigens and that only weakly immunogenic tumor cells survive. The various humoral and cell-mediated responses that have been shown to play a role in tumor immunity are discussed in this section.

Role of CTLs

Tumor-bearing mice generate T_C cells and effector CTLs with specificity for the tumor cells. The activity of these T_C cells can be measured in an in vitro CML assay with ^{51}Cr-labeled tumor cells (see Figure 9-11). In this reaction the CTLs can be shown to recognize tumor antigens associated with class I MHC molecules, so that there is a direct membrane interaction between CTLs and the tumor cells. After a CTL forms a conjugate with a target cancer cell, the CTL releases perforin monomers, which polymerize and insert into the cancer-cell membrane, forming a 5- to 20-nm pore (see Figure 15-8). Another constituent of the perforin-containing granules in CTLs is the soluble toxin TNF-β (lymphotoxin). It has been hypothesized that formation of the perforin pore on the membrane of a cancer cell may facilitate entry of TNF-β.

The protective effect of CTLs against tumor cells can be demonstrated in vivo with the Winn assay (Figure 25-9). In this assay lymphocytes are isolated from the spleen or lymph nodes of mice undergoing successful tumor regression. The lymphocytes are then mixed with live tumor cells from the same animals and injected into syngeneic recipients. As a control, lymphocytes isolated from normal mice are mixed with the live tumor cells and injected into syngeneic recipients. After an appropriate time, the tumors are removed from the recipients and weighed. One of the problems in extrapolating these results to real-life tumor immunity is that the ratio of the cytotoxic cells mixed with the tumor cells must be quite high to ensure direct contact between the two cell types. In reality such high ratios of CTLs to tumor cells may be achieved only at the periphery of a tumor, where CTLs can contact it. This has led some to question the importance of CTLs in tumor immunity.

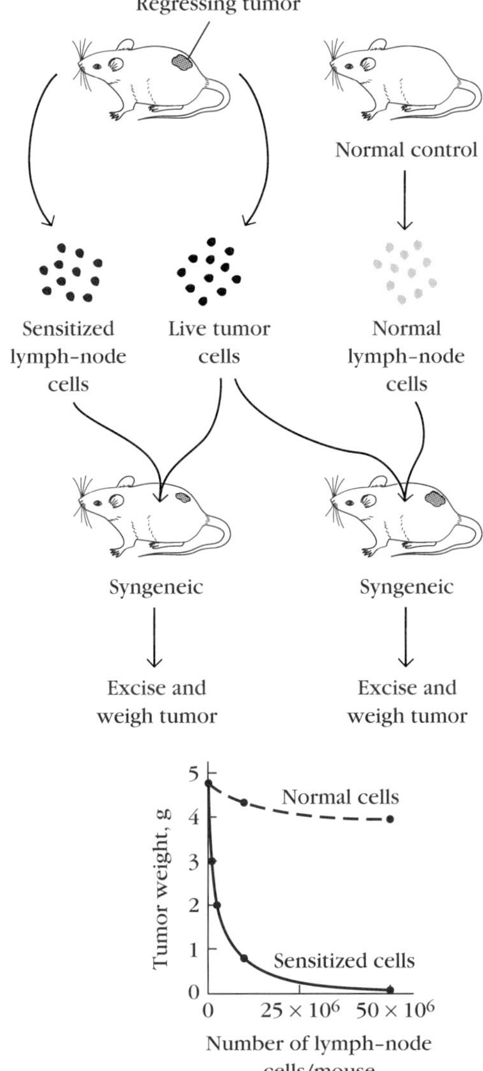

FIGURE 25-9 Winn assay for assessing CTL-mediated immunity to tumor cells in vivo. Constant numbers of live tumor cells are mixed with varying numbers of lymph-node cells from mice showing tumor regression or from normal control mice and then injected into syngeneic recipients. After 3 weeks, the resulting tumors are removed and weighed. Typical results are shown in the graph at the bottom.

Role of Natural Killer Cells

Natural killer (NK) cells acquired their name from the observation that normal animals have high levels of lymphocytes capable of lysing a wide variety of tumor cells. Unlike B and T cells, these lymphocytes do not exhibit immunologic memory; that is, prior priming with a given tumor does not heighten NK-cell reactivity to a later challenge with the same tumor. NK cells are a heterogeneous group of large granular lymphocytes that constitute 0.6–2.4% of the total lymphocyte population. As noted in Chapter 15, NK cells do not express membrane-bound immunoglobulin, the T-cell receptor, or CD3. Although it is not known how NK cells recognize tumor cells, it is known that the recognition is not MHC-restricted. In some cases Fc receptors on NK cells can bind to antibody-coated tumor cells, bringing the NK cell into contact with the tumor and facilitating tumor-cell killing. In this type of killing, referred to as antibody-dependent cell-mediated cytotoxicity (ADCC), the antibody provides the antitumor specificity but the killing is done by the nonspecific NK cell (see Figure 15-11). NK cells are thought to exocytose granules containing perforin, which mediates pore formation in tumor cells (much like CTLs do). In addition, a soluble NK cytotoxic factor (NKCF) found to be secreted by NK cells appears to be cytotoxic only for tumor cells. The importance of NK cells in tumor immunity can be seen in a genetic defect in the mouse strain called beige and in Chédiak-Higashi syndrome in humans. In both cases there is marked impairment of NK cells and an increased incidence of certain types of cancer.

In addition to NK cells there are some T_C cells that express either the $\alpha\beta$ or $\gamma\delta$ T-cell receptor and CD3 but are not MHC-restricted and appear to resemble NK cells in their nonspecific tumor recognition and killing. This cell population is sometimes grouped among the NK cells, but they should actually be referred to as natural cytotoxic cells (NC cells) or as T_C

cells with NK-like function rather than as NK cells. The cytotoxic activity of both NK and NC cells can be enhanced by in vitro treatment with IFN-γ or IL-2. This finding is being exploited in one type of experimental immunotherapy described later in this chapter.

Role of Macrophages

Numerous observations indicate that macrophages play a significant role in the immune response to tumors. For example, macrophages are often observed to cluster around tumors, and their presence is often correlated with tumor regression. Also, macrophages isolated from tumor-bearing animals have been shown to inhibit tumor growth in vitro.

The antitumor activity of macrophages probably is mediated by several macrophage products. Activation of macrophages with IFN-γ and macrophage-activating factor (MAF) not only increases their secretion of various products but also increases their cytotoxicity to tumor cells. Activated macrophages secrete increased levels of lytic enzymes. These enzymes can reach high levels around a tumor, especially if antitumor antibodies bind to Fc receptors on macrophages and serve to bridge the macrophages to the tumor. Macrophages also secrete a cytokine called tumor necrosis factor α (TNF-α) that has potent antitumor activity. The gene for TNF-α has been isolated; when cloned TNF-α is injected into tumor-bearing animals, it has been found to induce hemorrhage and necrosis of the tumor (see Figure 13-14a).

Role of Humoral Antibody

Tumor-cell antigens often elicit the production of specific serum antibodies. These antibodies can play a protective role in eliminating the tumor through several mechanisms. In some cases the antibody can activate the complement system, leading to assembly of the membrane-attack complex (MAC), pore formation, and complement-mediated lysis. Some tumors, however, have been shown to endocytose the MAC pore and repair the membrane before the cell is lysed. In these cases complement split products such as C3a, C4a, C5a, and C5b67 can still play a significant role by inducing localized mast-cell degranulation and the release of mediators that facilitate the influx of inflammatory cells, especially neutrophils and macrophages. Antibodies bound to tumor cells may also facilitate antibody-dependent cell-mediated cytotoxicity (ADCC). Both macrophages and NK cells have receptors for the Fc region of certain antibody classes. The antibody thus serves to bring these nonspecific immune cells into contact with the tumor.

Paradoxically, in some cases antibodies have been shown to interfere with the immune response to a tumor. A number of experiments have demonstrated that tumor-specific antibody can block in vitro CML reactions to tumor cells, perhaps by binding to the tumor antigens and masking them from CTLs or NK cells. The role of antibody in enhancing tumor growth is discussed more fully later in this chapter.

Immune Surveillance Theory

The immune surveillance theory was first conceptualized in the early 1900s by Paul Ehrlich. He suggested that cancer cells frequently arise in the body but are recognized as foreign and eliminated by the immune system. Some 50 years later Lewis Thomas suggested that the cell-mediated branch of the immune system had evolved to patrol the body and eliminate cancer cells. According to these concepts, tumors arise only if cancer cells are able to escape immune surveillance, either by reducing their expression of tumor antigens or by an impairment in the immune response to these cells.

Among the early observations that seemed to support the immune surveillance theory was the increased incidence of cancer in transplantation patients on immunosuppressive drugs. Other findings, however, were difficult to reconcile with this theory. Nude mice, for example, lack a thymus and consequently lack functional T cells. According to the immune surveillance theory these mice should show an increase in cancer, but instead nude mice are no more susceptible to cancer than other mice. Furthermore, although individuals on immunosuppressive drugs do show an increased incidence of cancer, the cancers are largely restricted to cancers of the immune system. Contrary to what the immune surveillance theory would have predicted, other common cancers, such as lung, breast, and colon cancer are not increased in these individuals. One possible explanation for the selective increase in immune-system cancers is that the immunosuppressive agents themselves may exert a direct carcinogenic effect on immune cells.

Experimental data concerning the effect of tumor-cell dosage on the ability of the immune system to respond also are incompatible with the immune surveillance theory. For example, animals injected with very low or very high doses of tumor cells develop tumors, whereas those injected with intermediate doses do not. The mechanism by which a low dose of tumor cells "sneaks through" is difficult to reconcile with the immune surveillance theory. Finally, this theory assumes that cancer cells and normal cells exhibit qualitative antigen differences. In fact, as discussed in previous sections, many types of tumors do not express tumor-specific antigens, and any immune response that develops must be induced by quantitative differences in antigen expression by normal cells and tumor cells.

The basic concept of the immune surveillance theory—that malignant tumors arise only if the immune system is somehow impaired or if the tumor cells lose their immunogenicity, enabling them to escape immune surveillance—at this time remains unproven. Nevertheless, it is clear that an immune response can be generated to tumor cells and therapeutic approaches aimed at increasing that response may serve as a defense against malignant cells.

Tumor Evasion of the Immune System

Although the immune system clearly can respond to tumor cells, the fact that so many individuals die each year from cancer suggests that the immune response to tumor cells often is ineffective. This section describes several mechanisms by which tumor cells appear to evade the immune system.

Immunologic Enhancement of Tumor Growth

Following the discovery that antibodies could be produced to tumor-specific antigens, attempts were made to protect animals against tumor growth by active immunization with tumor antigens or by passive immunization with antitumor antibodies. Much to the surprise of the researchers, these immunizations did not protect against tumor growth; in many cases they actually enhanced growth of the tumor. The tumor-enhancing ability of immune sera subsequently was studied in in vitro CML reactions. Serum taken from animals with progressive tumor growth was found to block the CML reaction, whereas serum taken from animals with regressing tumors had little or no blocking activity. K. E. and I. Hellstrom extended these findings by showing that children with progressive neuroblastoma had high levels of some kind of blocking factor in their sera and that children with regressive neuroblastoma did not have such factors. Since these first reports, blocking factors have been found to be associated with a number of human tumors.

In some cases, antitumor antibody itself acts as a blocking factor. Presumably the antibody binds to tumor-specific antigens and masks the antigens from cytotoxic T cells. In many cases the blocking factors are not antibodies alone but rather antibodies complexed to tumor antigens. These immune complexes have been shown to block the in vitro CML reaction to tumor cells and may inhibit T_C-cell activity either by blocking tumor antigens or by binding to Fc receptors on the T_C cells. The complexes also may inhibit ADCC by binding to Fc receptors on NK cells or macrophages and blocking their activity.

Modulation of Tumor Antigens

Certain tumor-specific antigens have been observed to disappear from the surface of tumor cells in the presence of serum antibody and then to reappear after the antibody is no longer present. This phenomenon, called *antigenic modulation,* is readily observed when leukemic T cells are injected into mice previously immunized with a leukemic T-cell antigen (TL antigen). These mice develop high titers of anti-TL antibody, which binds to the TL antigen on the leukemic cells and induces capping, endocytosis, and/or shedding of the antigen-antibody complex. As long as antibody is present, these leukemic T cells fail to display the TL antigen and thus cannot be eliminated.

Reduction in Class I MHC Molecules on Tumor Cells

Since $CD8^+$ CTLs recognize only antigen associated with class I MHC molecules, any alteration in the expression of class I MHC molecules on tumor cells may exert a profound effect on the CTL-mediated immune response. Malignant transformation of cells is often associated with a reduction (or even a complete loss) of class I MHC molecules, and a number of tumors have been shown to express decreased levels of class I MHC molecules (Table 25-5). Class I MHC expression can be quantitated with radiolabeled monoclonal antibody to β_2-microglobulin, which is invariant and is always expressed together with the α chain of class I molecules on the cell membrane. In many cases the decrease in class I MHC expression is accompanied by progressive tumor growth, and so the absence of MHC molecules on a tumor is generally an indication of a poor prognosis. For example, malignant porocarcinoma cells have been found to stain poorly with radiolabeled antibody to β_2-microglobulin, indicating weak class I MHC expression, whereas benign porocarcinoma cells stain well with the radiolabeled antibody, owing to their strong class I MHC expression.

The correlation between weak class I MHC expression and tumor progression has been studied

TABLE 25-5 SOME TUMORS WITH ALTERED MHC EXPRESSION AND THE BIOLOGICAL CONSEQUENCES

Experimental tumor systems	Altered MHC expression	Biological consequences
AKR mouse leukemia	Absence of H-2K	Increased tumorigenicity
Murine D122 Lewis lung carcinoma	Reduced H-2K/H-2D ratio	Increased metastasis
Methylcholanthrene-induced murine T10 sarcoma	Absence of H-2K and increased H-2D	Increased metastasis
SV40-transformed mouse cells	Absence of H-2K	Increased tumorigenicity
Radiation leukemia virus (RadLV)–transformed mouse cells	Absence of class I	Lethal leukemogenesis
Herpes simplex virus type 2 (HSV-2)–infected cells	Reduced class I molecules	Resistance to lysis by CTLs
Human Burkitt's lymphoma	Absence of class I	Resistance to lysis by CTLs
Human urothelial cell line TGr III	Reduced class I	Increased tumorigenicity and invasiveness
Human small-cell lung cancer	Deficient class I	Increased tumorigenicity and early metastasis
Human neuroblastoma	Deficient class I	Increased N-*myc* expression
Human mucinous colorectal carcinoma	Reduced class I	Poor prognosis
Human melanomas	Reduced class I	Increased invasiveness and thicker primary form

SOURCE: From K. M. Hui, 1989, *BioEssays* **11**:23.

extensively in AKR-strain mice, which have a high incidence of spontaneously occurring leukemias. Leukemic cells from these mice often have normal levels of class I H-2D molecules but significantly reduced levels of class I H-2K molecules. On the other hand, in vitro CML assays of lymphocytes from AKR mice, using leukemic cells as the target cells, reveal that only tumor antigens associated with H-2K molecules are recognized. The relationship between expression of H-2K molecules and tumor progression was studied in AKR mice by inoculating groups of mice with one of two leukemic cell lines: one with no detectable H-2K molecules and one with a high level of H-2K molecules. With the cell line lacking H-2K, only 3×10^3 cells were enough to produce a tumor, whereas with the line expressing high H-2K nearly a thousand-fold greater inoculum (2×10^6 cells) was required to induce a tumor. However, when a cloned gene encoding H-2K was transfected into the class I-deficient leukemic cell line, even substantial inoculum sizes failed to induce a tumor, presumably because class IK-restricted CTLs were able to kill the transfected leukemic cells. As illustrated in Figure 25-10, the immune response itself may play a role in selecting tumor cells with decreased class I MHC expression.

CANCER IMMUNOTHERAPY

The discussion in this and previous chapters indicates that various immune mechanisms exist for responding to tumor cells, although the response frequently is not sufficient to prevent tumor growth. One approach to cancer treatment is to augment or supplement these natural defense mechanisms. Several types of cancer immunotherapy in current use or under development are described in this concluding section.

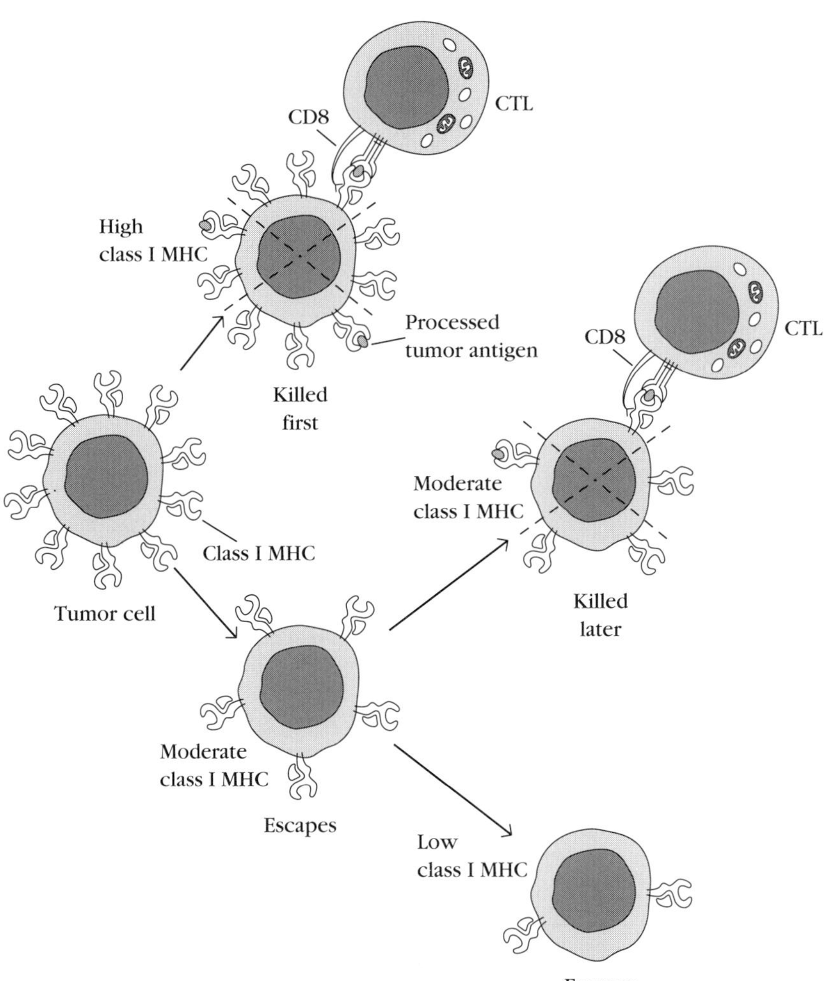

FIGURE 25-10 Down-regulation of class I MHC expression on tumor cells may allow a tumor to escape CTL-mediated recognition. The immune response may play a role in selecting for tumor cells expressing lower levels of class I MHC molecules by preferentially eliminating those cells expressing high levels of class I molecules. With time, malignant tumor cells may express progressively fewer MHC molecules and thus escape CTL-mediated destruction.

Immune Adjuvants

A number of immunotherapeutic approaches involve nonspecific activation of the immune system to boost the response to tumor cells. Several adjuvants previously shown to enhance immune responses to various microorganisms have also been shown to enhance antitumor responses. The most widely used adjuvant in tumor immunotherapy is the attenuated strain of *Mycobacterium bovis* called bacillus Calmette-Guérin (BCG). This adjuvant activates macrophages and thus increases their production of interleukin 1 and the membrane molecule B7. Both of these molecules can mediate a co-stimulatory signal necessary for T_H-cell activation, resulting in generalized increases in both humoral and cell-mediated responses. The effects of BCG as a tumor immunoagent are clearest when it is injected directly into a tumor, thereby stimulating localized immune activation within the tumor. A number of clinical studies have reported beneficial effects of BCG in slowing the growth of metastatic breast tumors, basal-cell tumors, and malignant melanoma. At first these reports were hailed as a "cancer cure," but continuing studies have shown that although the immune response to such tumors is definitely heightened by BCG treatment, the increase is not usually enough to eliminate the tumors. Other adjuvants that have been tried usually have shown less antitumor activity than BCG. These agents include *Corynebacterium parvum,* an antihelminth drug called levamisole, and azimezone and isoprinosine. The two latter compounds are mitogens that can activate lymphocytes in the absence of antigen.

Dinitrochlorobenezene (DNCB) is an allergen that induces delayed-type hypersensitive reactions when painted on the skin of test animals. Painting DNCB directly on skin cancers generates a localized DTH response that leads in some cases to complete regression of the cancers. DNCB has been shown to be particularly effective when painted on basal-cell carcinomas, causing complete regression in a third of the tumors and partial regression in another third of them.

Cytokine Therapy

Cloning of the various cytokine genes has facilitated their large-scale production. A variety of experimental and clinical approaches have been developed to use recombinant cytokines, either singly or in combination, to augment the immune response against cancer. Among the cytokines that have been evaluated in cancer immunotherapy are interferons α, β, and γ; IL-1, IL-2, IL-4, and IL-5; GM-CSF and TNF. There are scattered hopeful results from these trials but many obstacles remain. The most notable obstacle is the complexity of the cytokine network itself. This complexity makes it very difficult to know precisely how intervention with a given recombinant cytokine will affect the production of other cytokines. And since some cytokines act antagonistically, it is possible that intervention with a recombinant cytokine, designed to enhance a particular branch of the immune response, may actually lead to suppression. In addition, cytokine immunotherapy is plagued by difficulties with administering the cytokines in a localized fashion. In some cases systemic administration of high levels of a given cytokine has been shown to lead to serious and even life-threatening consequences. Although the results of several experimental and clinical trials of cytokine therapy for cancer are discussed here, it is important to keep in mind that this therapeutic approach is still in its infancy.

Interferons

Large quantities of purified recombinant preparations of the interferons, IFN-α, IFN-β, and IFN-γ, are now available, each of which has shown some promise in the treatment of human cancer. To date, most of the clinical trials have involved IFN-α. Daily injections of recombinant IFN-α have been shown to induce partial or complete tumor regression in some patients with hematologic malignancies such as leukemias, lymphomas, and myelomas and with solid tumors such as melanoma, Kaposi's sarcoma, renal cancer, and breast cancer. The effectiveness of IFN-α in inducing tumor regression depends in part on the degree of tumor malignancy. For example, when patients with relapsing non-Hodgkin's lymphoma were treated with daily injections of recombinant IFN-α, 15 out of 30 patients with low-level or intermediate-level malignancies exhibited complete or partial remission, whereas 6 of 7 patients with highly malignant lymphomas were completely unresponsive to the interferon treatment.

Interferon-mediated antitumor activity may involve several mechanisms. All three types of interferon have been shown to increase class I MHC expression on tumor cells; IFN-γ has also been shown to increase class II MHC expression on macrophages. Given the evidence for decreased levels of class I MHC molecules on malignant tumors, the interferons may act by restoring MHC expression, thereby increasing CTL activity against tumors. In addition, the interferons have been shown to inhibit cell division of both normal and malignantly transformed cells in vitro. It is possible that some of the antitumor effects of the interferons are related to this ability to directly inhibit tumor-cell proliferation. Finally, IFN-γ increases the activity of T_C cells, macrophages, and NK cells, all of which play a role in the immune response to tumor cells, as described in an earlier section.

Tumor Necrosis Factors

The tumor necrosis factors, TNF-α and TNF-β, have been shown to exhibit direct antitumor activity, killing some tumor cells and reducing the rate of proliferation of others while sparing normal cells (Figure 25-11). In the presence of TNF-α or TNF-β a tumor undergoes visible hemorrhagic necrosis and tumor regression. TNF-α has also been shown to inhibit tumor-induced vascularization (angiogenesis) by damaging the vascular endothelial cells in the vicinity of a tumor, thereby decreasing the flow of blood and oxygen that is necessary for progressive tumor growth.

Progress in understanding the functional activity of TNF-α and TNF-β has been facilitated by the recent cloning of their genes and the production of large amounts of both factors by recombinant DNA technology. Phase I clinical trials of recombinant TNF-α in cancer patients appeared quite promising, and again early news stories hailed TNF-α as the "cure for cancer." Later reports showed that although TNF-α holds some promise, it is far from being an antitumor wonder drug. Some patients treated with TNF-α have had complete tumor regression, but only if TNF-α was injected directly into the tumor. For other patients direct tumor injection elicited some effects, but tumor regression was not complete. TNF-α therapy has several limitations: its short half-life necessitates frequent injections; and its adverse side effects include fever, chills, blood-pressure changes, and decreased counts of white blood cells.

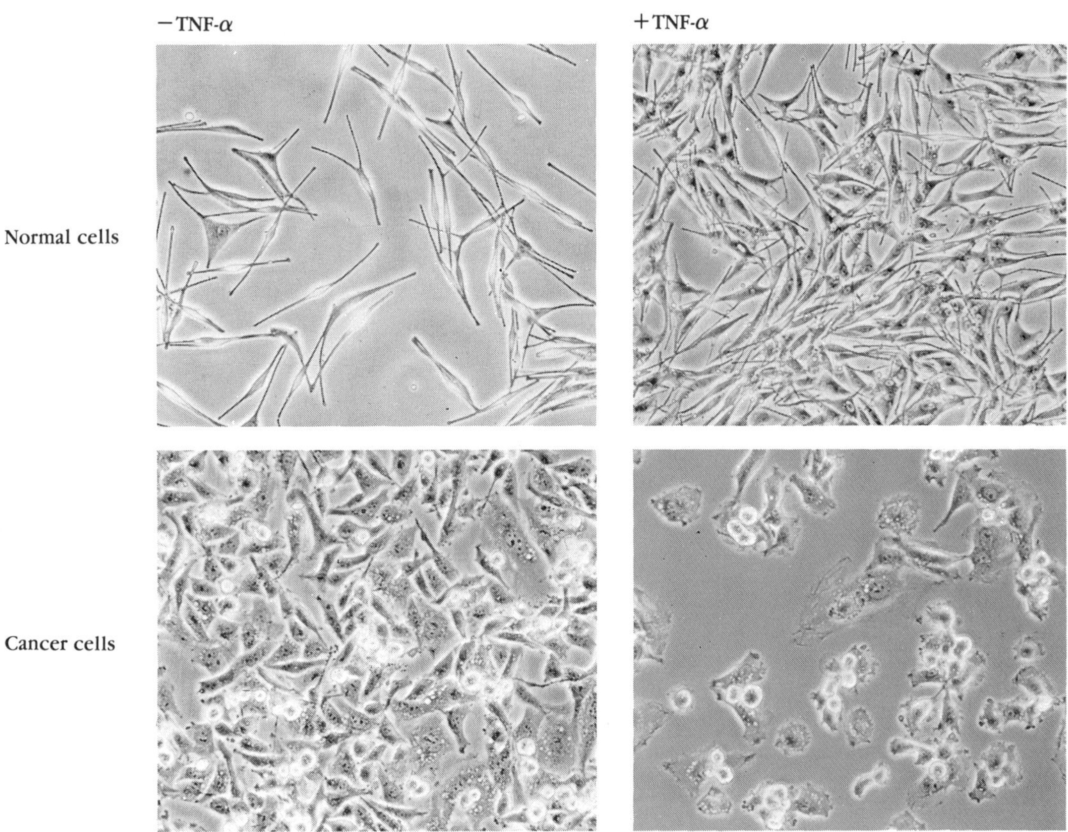

FIGURE 25-11 Photomicrographs of cultured normal melanocytes *(top)* and of cultured cancerous melanoma cells *(bottom)* in the presence and absence of tumor necrosis factor α (TNF-α). Note that in the presence of TNF-α, the cancer cells stop proliferating, whereas TNF-α has no inhibitory effect on proliferation of the normal cells. [From L. J. Old, 1988, *Sci. Am.* **258**(May):59.]

In Vitro–Activated LAK and TIL Cells

Animal studies have shown that lymphocytes can be activated against tumor antigens in vitro by culturing the lymphocytes with x-irradiated tumor cells in the presence of IL-2. These activated lymphocytes mediate more effective tumor destruction than untreated lymphocytes when they are reinjected into the original tumor-bearing animal. It is difficult, however, to activate in vitro enough lymphocytes with antitumor specificity to be useful in cancer therapy. In 1980 S. Rosenberg, who was sensitizing lymphocytes to tumor antigens by this method, found that in the presence of high concentrations of cloned IL-2 and without the addition of tumor antigens, large numbers of activated lymphoid cells were generated that could kill fresh tumor cells but not normal cells. He called these cells *lymphokine-activated killer (LAK) cells.* In one study, for example, Rosenberg found that infusion of LAK cells plus recombinant IL-2 into tumor-bearing animals mediated effective tumor-cell destruction (Figure 25-12). LAK cells appear to be a heterogeneous population of lymphoid cells that includes natural killer (NK) cells and natural cytotoxic (NC) cells; the relative numbers of the two cell types depend on the source of the lymphocytes and the conditions of IL-2 activation.

Because large numbers of LAK cells can be generated in vitro and because these cells are active against a wide variety of tumors, their effectiveness in human tumor immunotherapy has been evaluated in several clinical trials. In these trials, peripheral-blood lymphocytes were removed from patients with various advanced metastatic cancers and were activated in vitro to generate LAK cells. Patients were then infused with their autologous LAK cells together with IL-2. A trial with 25 patients in 1985 resulted in cancer regression in some patients. A more extensive trial with 222 patients in 1987 resulted in complete regression in 16 patients. However, a number of undesirable side

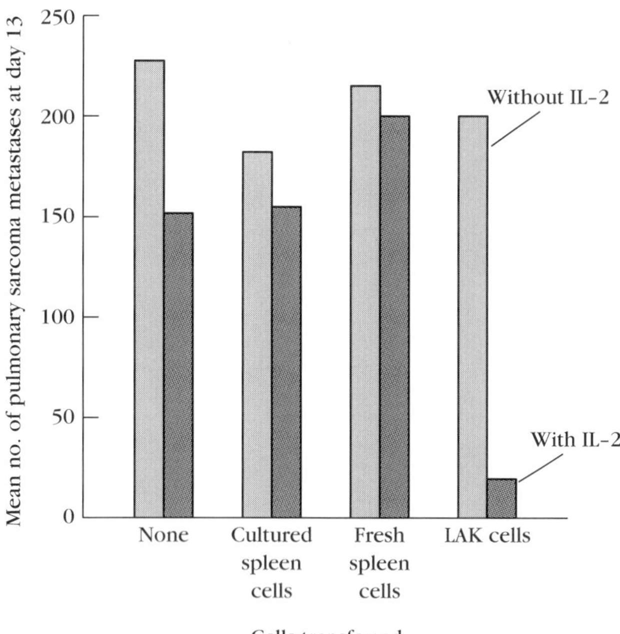

FIGURE 25-12 Experimental demonstration of tumor-destroying activity of LAK cells plus IL-2. Spleen cells or LAK cells, in the presence or absence of recombinant IL-2, were infused into mice with pulmonary sarcoma. The animals were evaluated 13 days later for the number of pulmonary sarcoma metastases. The LAK cells were prepared by isolating lymphocytes from tumor-bearing animals and incubating them in vitro with high concentrations of IL-2. Note that tumor regression occurred only when LAK cells and IL-2 were infused. [Data from S. Rosenberg et al., 1988, *Ann. Int. Med.*, **108**:853.]

effects are associated with the high levels of IL-2 required for LAK-cell activity. The most noteworthy is vascular leak syndrome, which involves emigration of lymphoid cells and plasma from the peripheral blood into the tissues, leading to shock.

Tumors contain lymphocytes that have infiltrated the tumor and presumably are taking part in an antitumor response. By taking small biopsy samples of tumors, one can obtain a population of these lymphocytes and expand it in vitro with IL-2. These activated *tumor-infiltrating lymphocytes* are called *TIL cells.* Many TIL cells have a wide range of antitumor activity and appear to be indistinguishable from LAK cells. However, some TIL cells have specific cytolytic activity against their autologous tumor. These tumor-specific TIL cells are of interest because they have increased antitumor activity and require 100-fold lower levels of IL-2 for their activity than do LAK cells. In one study TIL cells were expanded in vitro from biopsy samples taken from patients with malignant melanoma, renal-cell carcinoma, and small-cell lung cancer. The expanded TIL cells were reinjected into autologous patients together with continuous infusions of recombinant IL-2. Renal-cell carcinomas and malignant melanomas showed partial regression in 29% and 23% of the patients, respectively.

Gene Therapy

The early 1990s saw remarkable progress in efforts to apply somatic gene therapy in human patients. As of June 1992, 18 gene-therapy trials approved by the Recombinant DNA Advisory Committee were under way or planned, and 11 of these trials involved transfer of genes into human patients (Table 25-6). The first approved human gene-transfer experiment, which was performed in 1990, used a retrovirus to deliver a neomycin gene into TIL cells. The neomycin-marked TIL cells were then injected back into patients with advanced melanoma, and the distribution and survival of the neomycin-marked TIL cells was monitored. The genetically engineered TIL cells were shown to survive from 3 weeks to 2 months in these patients and to produce no detrimental effects. Once safety was established, a gene-therapy experiment was initiated in January 1991. TIL cells from 50 patients with advanced malignant melanoma were engineered with the gene for TNF-α, and these engineered TIL cells were then infused into the autologous patients. The rationale of this approach is that the TIL cells will attack the tumor, releasing high localized concentrations of TNF-α, which then will mediate tumor destruction. As of June 1992, no negative side effects had been observed, even in patients receiving 10^{11} TNF-modified TIL cells. These patients are still being monitored.

In October 1991, S. Rosenberg began a gene-therapy trial in which cancer patients were vaccinated with genetically engineered cancer cells. In this study, which is still in progress, melanoma cells were surgically removed from patients with advanced malignant melanoma and genetically engineered with the gene for IL-2 or TNF. The modified melanoma cells then were injected back into the autologous patients. The hope is that the patient's immune cells will recognize the engineered tumor cells and become activated by the cytokine.

In a somewhat similar approach to gene therapy, the gene encoding HLA-B7 has been introduced into melanoma cells. It is hoped that increased expression of this class I MHC molecule may enable these engineered cells to serve as a vaccine. Another vaccine approach is to engineer the cancer cells so that they will provide the requisite co-stimulatory signal for CTL activation. As discussed in Chapter 15, melanoma cells lack the co-stimulatory ligand B7 and thus are unable

TABLE 25-6 APPROVED GENE-THERAPY TRIALS WITH HUMAN CANCER PATIENTS

Disease	Gene inserted	Principal investigator
Advanced cancers	Tumor necrosis factor	Steven Rosenberg, NCI
Advanced cancers	Tumor necrosis factor	Steven Rosenberg, NCI
Advanced cancers	Interleukin-2	Steven Rosenberg, NCI
Ovarian cancer	Thymidine kinase	Scott Freeman, U. Rochester
Malignant melanoma	HLA-B7	Gary Nabel, U. Michigan
Neuroblastoma	Interleukin-2	Malcolm Brenner, St. Jude's, Memphis
Brain tumor	Thymidine kinase	Kenneth Culver, NCI
Malignant melanoma	Interleukin-2	Eli Gilboa, Sloan-Kettering
Kidney cancer	Interleukin-2	Eli Gilboa, Sloan-Kettering
Cancer	Interleukin-4	Michael Lotze, U. Pittsburg
Lung cancer	Antisense *ras/p53*	Jack Roth, M.D. Anderson

SOURCE: Adapted from L. Thompson, 1992, *Science* **258**:744.

to activate CTL precursors. However, when melanoma cells are genetically engineered with the gene encoding B7, then they can induce CTL activation (see Figure 15-2).

Because of the demonstrated involvement of oncogenes in many types of cancer, another possible gene-therapy approach is to inhibit the function of activated oncogenes or to replace the function of defective tumor-suppressor genes (anti-oncogenes). Lung cancer cells, for example, have mutations in two oncogenes that contribute to the cancerous state: a mutation in K-*ras* that causes the cells to proliferate and deletion of *p53,* an anti-oncogene that normally suppresses cell growth. In a trial with lung cancer patients to be conducted by K. Roth, gene therapy will be used to introduce an active *p53* to suppress cell growth and an antisense gene to block the effects of the mutated K-*ras.*

Monoclonal Antibodies

Various monoclonal antibodies have been tested experimentally as immunotherapeutic agents for cancer. The preparation and potential uses of immunotoxins specific for tumor cells was discussed in Chapter 7. These agents consist of the inhibitor chain of a toxin (e.g., diphtheria toxin) linked to an antibody against a tumor-specific or tumor-associated antigen (see Figure 7-10). In vitro studies have demonstrated that these "magic bullets" can kill tumor cells without harming normal cells.

In another approach, monoclonal antibody to CD3, which is known to activate T cells in vitro, has been administered to mice in an effort to induce nonspecific T-cell activation in vivo. In one study, T cells from C3H-strain mice that had previously been activated by injections of anti-CD3 monoclonal antibody were isolated and analyzed. In comparison with control mice, the T cells from treated mice exhibited increased expression of IL-2 and increased functional activity in both MLR and CML assays. To determine whether such nonspecific T-cell activation might increase tumor immunity, C3H mice were injected with live fibrosarcoma cells with or without anti-CD3 and the tumor volume was measured over time. The fibrosarcoma tumor was chosen because it grows progressively in most C3H mice and kills the mice by developing into a large tumor mass. In one experiment, only 35% of mice injected with 4 μg of anti-CD3 had tumors 4 weeks after being injected with live fibrosarcoma cells, whereas 95% of the untreated mice had tumors. In the treated mice that did develop tumors, the tumor volume was significantly less than in the untreated controls. When the treated mice were later given a secondary challenge with live fibrosarcoma cells, they were immune and did not develop tumors. Interestingly, the $F(ab')_2$ fragment of anti-CD3 was ineffective in reducing tumor development.

Although these findings with anti-CD3 are hopeful for tumor immunotherapy, the experiments also demonstrated the fine line between immune enhancement and immune suppression. The concentration of the anti-CD3 monoclonal was shown to be critical: a 4-μg dose enhanced tumor immunity, but a 40-μg dose appeared to be immunosuppressive, causing enhanced tumor growth and earlier death (Figure 25-13). Until the steps leading to immune activation and immune suppression are more clearly understood, approaches such as this one are clearly too risky for clinical human trials.

Monoclonal antibodies can also be used to bridge activated T cells directly to a tumor. In this approach two different monoclonal antibodies are produced; one specific for a tumor-cell membrane molecule and one specific for the CD3 membrane molecule of the TCR complex. A hybrid monoclonal antibody, or heteroconjugate, is then prepared with specificity for the tumor antigen and for CD3 (see Figure 7-12d). In vitro experiments with these heteroconjugates have revealed that they are able to cross-link and activate T cells directly on the surface of the tumor cell.

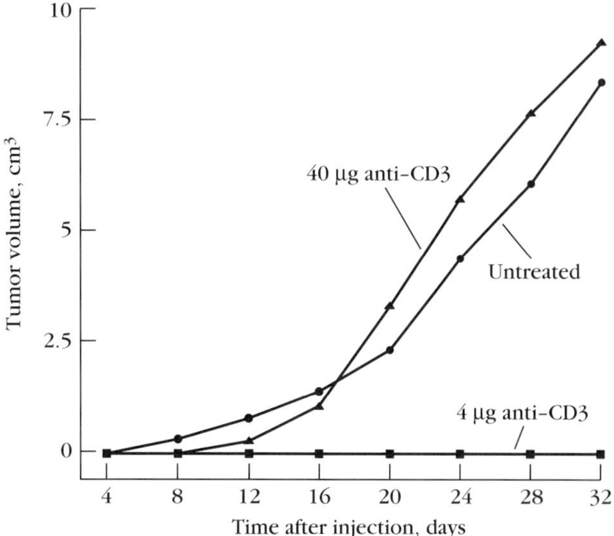

FIGURE 25-13 Effect of anti-CD3 monoclonal antibody on tumor growth in C3H mice. Animals were injected with live fibrosarcoma cells and simultaneously with 4 μg or 40 μg of anti-CD3 or with saline buffer; tumor volume was then determined at various times after the injections. The low dose of anti-CD3 inhibited tumor growth effectively, whereas the high dose did not do so and even appeared to enhance tumor growth somewhat in comparison with untreated controls. [Adapted from J. D. Ellenhorn et al., 1988, *Science*, **242**:569.]

The finding that a variety of tumors express significantly increased levels of growth-factor receptors suggests that treatment with monoclonal antibodies against these receptors might inhibit tumor-cell activity. Monoclonal antibodies to the EGF receptor, to the p97 (transferrin) receptor, and to the IL-2 receptor have each been produced. In one study hundreds of mice with a lethal tumor were treated with chemotherapy alone or with chemotherapy plus monoclonal antibody to the EGF receptor. Chemotherapy alone failed to slow tumor growth in these mice, but every mouse that received the combined therapy recovered fully and the tumor did not recur following treatment. In a phase I clinical trial at Memorial Sloan-Kettering Cancer Center, patients with squamous-cell lung carcinoma are being treated with monoclonal antibody to EGF receptor. The results of this trial have not been published yet.

Tumor-Cell Vaccines

In a novel approach to developing tumor vaccines, a patient's own tumor cells are killed by x-irradiation, mixed with BCG, and reinjected into the patient. One woman treated in this way had been diagnosed in 1986 with advanced malignant melanoma with literally hundreds of tumors on her right leg. Within 7 weeks after receiving this experimental vaccine, the tumors in her leg had disappeared, and the woman was still alive more than 3 years after treatment. Recent reports indicate that about 25% of patients with malignant melanoma have shown complete or partial remission after treatment with killed autologous tumor cells plus BCG.

Summary

1. Tumor cells differ from normal cells in numerous ways. Among these differences are changes in growth regulation, various biochemical changes, cytoskeletal changes, chromosomal abnormalities, and the ability to grow indefinitely in in vitro culture.

2. Normal cells can be transformed by chemical and physical carcinogens and by transforming viruses. Transformed cells exhibit altered growth properties and are sometimes capable of inducing cancer when they are injected into animals. A study of transformed cells has revealed the important role of cellular and viral oncogenes in the transformation process.

3. In a number of B- and T-cell leukemias and lymphomas, proto-oncogenes have been translocated to the immunoglobulin or T-cell-receptor genes. In its

new site the translocated gene may come under the influence of an enhancer and be transcribed at higher levels or may undergo an unusually high level of mutation owing to somatic mutation mechanisms at work in the B-cell immunoglobulin genes.

4. Tumor cells display a number of surface structures that can be recognized as antigenic by the immune system. Among these antigens are oncofetal antigens, virally encoded antigens, and increased levels of oncogene products. The immune response to tumors includes CTL-mediated lysis, NK-cell activity, macrophage-mediated tumor destruction, and destruction mediated by ADCC. Several cytotoxic factors, including TNF-α and TNF-β, help to mediate tumor-cell killing. Tumors may evade the immune response by modulating their tumor antigens, by reducing their expression of class I MHC molecules, and by antibody-mediated or immune-complex–mediated inhibition of CTL activity.

5. Experimental cancer immunotherapy has taken a variety of approaches. In some cases, injections of cytokines such as IFN-α and TNF-α have been shown to have beneficial effects. In another approach lymphocytes are activated in vitro with high concentrations of IL-2, thereby inducing LAK cells or TIL cells with antitumor activity. Infusions of LAK cells plus IL-2 have reduced tumor development in experimental animals. Monoclonal antibodies specific for tumor antigens have also been used to produce immunotoxins. Monoclonal antibodies to CD3 and to various growth-factor receptors are being evaluated. Vaccines of killed autologous tumor cells mixed with BCG have shown some success in treatment of malignant melanomas. Gene therapy, the most recent experimental approach, currently is being evaluated in a number of approved human trials. The general technique involves removing tumor cells from a patient, genetically altering them in some way that will increase the immune response to them, and then reinjecting the altered cells into the patient.

References

AISENBERG, A. C. 1993. Utility of gene rearrangements in lymphoid malignancies. *Annu. Rev. Med.* **44**:75.

CARBONE, D. P., and J. D. MINNA. 1993. Antioncogenes and human cancer. *Annu. Rev. Med.* **44**:451.

COHEN, J. J. 1993. Apoptosis. *Immunol. Today* **14**:136.

CORY, S., and J. M. ADAMS. 1988. Transgenic mice and oncogenesis. *Annu. Rev. Immunol.* **6**:25.

COURNOYER, D., and C. T. CASKEY. 1993. Gene therapy of the immune system. *Annu. Rev. Immunol.* **11**:297.

GREENBERG, P. D. 1991. Adoptive T cell therapy of tumors: mechanisms operative in the recognition and elimination of tumor cells. *Adv. Immunol.* **49**:281.

HELLSTROM, K. E., and I. HELLSTROM. 1989. Oncogene-associated tumor antigens as targets for immunotherapy. *FASEB* **3**:1715.

HUBER, B. E. 1989. Therapeutic opportunities involving cellular oncogenes: novel approaches fostered by biotechnology. *FASEB* **3**:5.

HUI, K. M. 1989. Re-expression of major histocompatibility complex (MHC) class I molecules on malignant tumor cells and its effect on host-tumor interaction. *BioEssays* **11**:22.

JHAPPAN, C., et al. 1990. TGF-α overexpression in transgenic mice induces liver neoplasia and abnormal development of the mammary gland and pancreas. *Cell* **61**:1137.

KRADIN, R. L., et al. 1989. Tumor infiltrating lymphocytes and interleukin-2 treatment of advanced cancer. *Lancet* (March 18):577.

LANG, R. A., and A. W. BURGESS. 1990. Autocrine growth factors and tumourigenic transformation. *Immunol. Today* **11**:244.

LIVINGSTONE, L. R., A. WHITE, J. SPROUSE et al. 1992. Altered cell cycle arrest and gene amplification potential accompany loss of wild type p53. *Cell* **70**:923.

LURQUIN, C., A. V. PEL, B. MARIAME et al. 1989. Structure of the gene of Tum$^-$ transplantation antigen P91A: the mutated exon encodes a peptide recognized with L^d by cytolytic T cells. *Cell* **58**:293.

MARX, J. 1990. Oncogenes evoke new cancer therapies. *Science* **249**:1376.

RUSSEL, S. J. 1990. Lymphokine gene therapy for cancer. *Immunol. Today* **11**:196.

SANDGREN, E. P., N. C. LUETTEKE, R. D. PALMITER et al. 1990. Overexpression of TGF-α in transgenic mice: induction of epithelial hyperplasia, pancreatic metaplasia, and carcinoma of the breast. *Cell* **61**:1121.

SCHREIBER, H., P. L. WARD, D. A. ROWLEY, and H. J. STAUSS. 1988. Unique tumor-specific antigens. *Annu. Rev. Immunol.* **6**:465.

SHOWE, L. C., and C. M. CROCE. 1987. The role of chromosomal translocations in B and T cell neoplasia. *Annu. Rev. Immunol.* **5**:253.

SUGIMURA, T. 1992. Multistep carcinogenesis: a 1992 perspective. *Science* **258**:603.

TOPALIAN, S. L., D. SOLOMON, and S. A. ROSENBERG. 1989. Tumor-specific cytolysis by lymphocytes infiltrating human melanomas. *J. Immunol.* **142**:3714.

VOGELSTEIN, B., and K. W. KINZLER. 1993. The multistep nature of cancer. *Trends Genet.* **9**:138.

WILLIAMS, G. T., C. A. SMITH, N. J. MCCARTHY, and E. A. GRIMES. 1992. Apoptosis: final control point in cell biology. *Trends Cell Biol.* **2**:263.

Study Questions

1. Indicate whether each of the following statements is true or false. If you think a statement is false, explain why.
   a. Cancer cells divide much more rapidly than normal cells.
   b. The c-*myc* gene is expressed in activated T_H cells.
   c. Multiple copies of cellular oncogenes are sometimes observed in cancer cells.
   d. Viral integration into the cellular genome may convert a proto-oncogene into a transforming oncogene.
   e. All oncogenic retroviruses carry viral oncogenes.
   f. The immune response against a virus-induced tumor protects against another tumor induced by the same virus.
   g. LAK cells are tumor specific.

2. You are a clinical immunologist studying acute lymphoblastic leukemia (ALL). Leukemic cells from most patients with ALL have the morphology of lymphocytes but do not express cell-surface markers characteristic of mature B or T cells. You have isolated cells from ALL patients that do not express membrane Ig but do react with monoclonal antibody against a normal pre-B cell marker (B-200). You therefore suspect that these leukemic cells are pre-B cells. How would you confirm this commitment to the B-cell lineage by means of genetic analysis?

3. In a recent experiment melanoma cells were isolated from patients with early or advanced stages of malignant melanoma. At the same time T cells specific for tetanus toxoid antigen were isolated and cloned from each patient.
   a. When early-stage melanoma cells were cultured together with tetanus toxoid antigen and the tetanus toxoid–specific T-cell clones, the T-cell clones were observed to proliferate. This proliferation was blocked by addition of chloroquine or by addition of monoclonal antibody to HLA-DR. Proliferation was not blocked by addition of monoclonal antibody to HLA-A, -B, -DQ, or -DP. What might these findings indicate about the early-stage melanoma cells in this experimental system?
   b. When the same experiment was repeated with advanced-stage melanoma cells, the tetanus toxoid T-cell clones failed to proliferate in response to the tetanus toxoid antigen. What might this indicate about advanced-stage melanoma cells?
   c. When early and advanced malignant melanoma cells were fixed with paraformaldehyde and incubated with processed tetanus toxoid, only the early-stage melanoma cells could induce proliferation of the tetanus toxoid T-cell clones. What might this indicate about early-stage melanoma cells?
   d. How might you confirm your hypothesis experimentally?

4. What is the rationale behind the use of anti-CD3 as an antitumor immunoagent? What is a critical consideration with this approach?

5. Various cytokines have been evaluated for use in tumor immunotherapy. Describe four mechanisms by which cytokines mediate antitumor effects and the cytokines that induce each type of effect.

GLOSSARY

Acquired immunity host defenses that are mediated by B and T cells following exposure to antigen and that exhibit specificity, diversity, memory, and self/nonself recognition.

Acquired immunodeficiency syndrome (AIDS) a disease caused by human immunodeficiency virus (HIV) that is marked by significant depletion of $CD4^+$ T cells resulting in increased susceptibility to a variety of infections and cancers.

Activity immunity acquired immunity that is induced by natural exposure to a pathogen or by **vaccination.**

Acute-phase proteins hepatocyte-derived serum proteins that are produced during the early stages of an inflammatory response.

Adherent cells cells of the monocyte-macrophage lineage and other stromal cells that in culture normally adhere to glass or plastic forming a layer.

Adjuvant a substance (e.g., Freund's adjuvant, alum, bacterial **LPS**) that nonspecifically enhances or potentiates the immune response to an antigen.

Adoptive transfer an experimental technique in which lymphocytes from an antigen-primed donor are transferred to an x-irradiated recipient that lacks a functional immune system.

Affinity the binding strength between a single receptor site (e.g., one binding site on an antibody) and a ligand (e.g., an antigenic determinant). The association constant is a quantitative measure of affinity.

Affinity maturation the increase in average antibody affinity for an antigen that occurs during the course of immune response.

Agretope the region of a processed antigenic peptide that binds to an **MHC molecule.**

Allele two or more alternative forms of a gene at a particular **locus** that confer alternative characters. The presence of multiple alleles, as in the **MHC**, results in polymorphism.

Allelic exclusion a process that permits expression of only one of the allelic forms of a gene. B and T cells exhibit allelic exclusion of the immunoglobulin and T-cell receptor genes, respectively.

Allergen noninfectious antigens that induce **hypersensitivity** reactions, most commonly IgE-mediated type I reactions.

Allergy a **hypersensitivity** reaction that can involve various deleterious effects such as hay fever, asthma, **serum sickness,** systemic **anaphylaxis,** or contact dermatitis.

Alloantiserum antiserum produced by one member of a species that is specific for the allelic antigens of another individual of the same species.

Allogeneic denoting members of the same species that differ genetically.

Allograft a tissue transplant between **allogeneic** individuals.

Allotype a set of **allotypic determinants** characteristic of some but not all members of a species.

Allotypic determinant an **antigenic determinant** that varies among members of a species. The constant regions of antibodies possess allotypic determinants (see Figure 5-11).

Alpha-feto protein (AFP) see **oncofetal tumor antigen.**

Alternative complement pathway activation of **complement** that is initiated by foreign cell-surface constiutents; involves C3–C9, factors B and D, and properdin; and generates the **membrane-attack complex** (see Figure 17-1).

Anaphylatoxin the complement split products C3a and C5a that mediate **degranulation** of mast cells and basophils, resulting in release of mediators that induce contraction of smooth muscle and increased vascular permeability.

Anaphylaxis an immediate type I hypersensitivity reaction, which is triggered by IgE-mediated mast-cell **degranulation.** Systemic anaphylaxis leads to shock and often is fatal. Localized anaphylaxis involves various types of **atopic** reactions.

Antibody a protein (immunoglobulin), consisting of two identical heavy chains and two identical light chains, that recognizes a particular **epitope** on an antigen and facilitates clearance of that antigen. Membrane-bound antibody is expressed by B cells that have not encountered antigen; secreted antibody is produced by plasma cells.

Antibody-dependent cell-mediated cytotoxicity (ADCC) a cell-mediated reaction in which nonspecific cytotoxic cells that express **Fc receptors** (e.g., NK cells, neutrophils, macrophages) recognize bound antibody on a target cell and subsequently cause lysis of the target cell (see Figure 15-11).

Antigen any substance (usually foreign) that binds specifically to an antibody or a T-cell receptor; often is used as a synonym for **immunogen.**

Antigen-presenting cell (APC) macrophages, dendritic cells, B cells, and other cells that can process and present antigenic peptides in association with **class II MHC molecules.**

Antigenic determinant the site on an antigen that is recognized and bound by a particular antibody or T-cell receptor; also called **epitope.**

Apoptosis morphologic changes associated with programmed cell death including nuclear fragmentation, blebbing, and release of apoptotic bodies, which are phagocytosed (see Figure 3-3). In contrast to **necrosis,** it does not result in damage to surrounding cells.

Atopic pertaining to clinical manifestations of type I (IgE-mediated) hypersensitivity including allergic rhinitis (hay fever), eczema, asthma, and various food allergies.

Autograft tissue grafted from one part of the body to another in the same individual.

Autoimmunity an abnormal immune response against self-antigens.

Autologous derived from the same individual.

Autosomal pertaining to all the chromosomes except the sex chromosomes.

Avidity the functional binding strength between two molecules that (unlike **affinity**) reflects the interaction of all the binding sites.

B cell a lymphocyte that matures in the bone marrow and expresses membrane-bound antibody. Following interaction with antigen, it differentiates into antibody-secreting plasma cells and memory cells.

Basophil a nonphagocytic granulocyte that expresses **Fc receptors** for IgE (see Figure 3-13). Antigen-mediated cross-linkage of bound IgE induces **degranulation,** which releases histamine and other mediators.

BCG (Bacillus Calmette-Guerin) an attenuated form of *Mycobacterium bovis* used as a specific **vaccine** and as an **adjuvant** component.

Bence-Jones protein monoclonal immunoglobulin light chains present (usually as dimers) in the urine of some patients with **multiple myeloma.**

β_2-Microglobulin invariant subunit that associates with the polymorphic α chain to form **class I MHC molecules;** it is not encoded by MHC genes.

Blast cell see **lymphoblast.**

Bursa of Fabricius a primary lymphoid organ in birds where B-cell maturation occurs. The bone marrow is the functional equivalent in mammals.

CAM (cell-adhesion molecule) a family of cell-surface molecules (e.g., ICAM-1, ICAM-2, and VCAM-1) that mediate intercellular adhesion. They belong to the **immunoglobulin superfamily.**

Carcinoembryonic antigen (CEA) see **oncofetal tumor antigen.**

Carcinoma a cancer of epithelial origin.

Carrier an immunogenic molecule containing antigenic determinants recognized by T cells. Conjugation of a carrier to a nonimmunogenic **hapten** renders the hapten immunogenic.

Carrier effect dependence of a secondary immune response to a hapten-carrier conjugate on previous exposure to both the hapten and carrier determinants (see Table 14-3).

CD antigen cell-membrane molecule used to differentiate human leukocyte subpopulations and identified by monoclonal antibody. All monoclonal antibodies that react with the same membrane molecule are grouped into a common cluster of differentiation, or CD (see Table 3-3).

CD3 a polypeptide complex containing five chains: γ, δ, ϵ, ζ, and η, which associate noncovalently with either a $\zeta\zeta$ homodimer or $\zeta\eta$ heterodimer (see Figure 11-7). It is associated with the T-cell receptor and functions in signal transduction.

CD4 a membrane molecule found on those T cells (usually T_H cells) that recognize antigenic peptides associated with a class II MHC molecule.

CD8 a membrane molecule found on those T cells (usually T_C cells) that recognize antigenic peptides associated with a class I MHC molecule.

Cell-mediated immunity host defenses that are mediated by antigen-specific T cells and various nonspecific cells of the immune system. It protects against intracellular bacteria, viruses, and cancer and is responsible for graft rejection. Transfer of primed T cells confers this type of immunity on the recipient. See also **humoral immunity.**

Cell-mediated lympholysis (CML) in vitro lysis of **allogeneic** cells or virus-infected **syngeneic** cells by T cells; serves as an assay for **CTL** activity (see Figure 9-11).

Chemotaxis directional movement of cells in response to the concentration gradient of some substance.

Chimera an animal or tissue composed of elements derived from genetically distinct individuals. The scid-human mouse is a chimera (see Figure 2-1).

Class I MHC molecules membrane heterodimeric proteins that consist of an α chain encoded in the MHC associated noncovalently with β_2-microglobulin (see Figure 9-5). They are expressed by nearly all nucleated cells and function in antigen presentation to $CD8^+$ T cells. The classical class I molecules are H-2 K, D, and L in mice and HLA-A, -B, and -C in humans.

Class II MHC molecules membrane heterodimeric proteins that consist of noncovalently associated α and β chains, both encoded in the MHC (see Figure 9-5). They are expressed by antigen-presenting cells and function in antigen presentation to $CD4^+$ T cells. The classical class II molecules are H-2 IA and IE in mice and HLA-DP, -DQ, and -DR in humans.

Class III MHC molecules various proteins encoded in the MHC but distinct from class I and class II MHC molecules. They include some **complement** components, two steroid 21-hydroxylases, and **tumor necrosis factor α** and **β**.

Class switching see **isotype switching.**

Classical complement pathway complement activation sequence that is initiated by antigen-antibody complexes; involves C1–C9; and generates the **membrane-attack complex** (see Figure 17-1).

Clonal anergy proposed mechanism for induction of immunologic tolerance in which antigen-reactive lymphocytes are present but are functionally inactive.

Clonal deletion proposed mechanism for induction of immunologic tolerance in which the death of self-reactive lymphocytes is induced by their contact with self-antigens.
Clonal selection proposed mechanism in which antigen binds to receptors (membrane antibody or T-cell receptor) on a lymphocyte, thereby stimulating the cell to undergo mitosis and develop into a **clone** of cells with the same antigenic **specificity** as the original parent cell.
Clone cells arising from a single progenitor cell.
Clonotypic pertaining to a unique characteristic of a single clone.
Colony-stimulating factors (CSFs) a group of factors that induce the proliferation and differentiation of hematopoietic cells and some other cells.
Complement a group of serum proteins that participate in an enzymatic cascade, ultimately generating the cytolytic **membrane-attack complex.**
Complementarity-determining region (CDR) see **hypervariable region.**
Concanavalin (Con A) a **lectin** derived from jack beans that is a potent T-cell **mitogen** in many species.
Cogenic denoting individuals that differ genetically at a single genetic locus or region; also called coisogenic.
Constant (C) region The nearly invariant portion of antibody heavy and light chains and of the polypeptide chains of the T-cell receptor.
Coomb's test a diagnostic test used to detect antibody bound to the membrane of red blood cells by the addition of anti-immunoglobulin antibody. It is used to detect the presence of maternal anti-Rh antibodies on fetal red blood cells.
Cortex outer or peripheral layer of an organ.
Cross-reactivity ability of a particular antibody or T-cell receptor to react with two or more antigens that possess a common epitope.
CTL see **cytotoxic T lymphocyte.**
Cyclosporin A (CsA) an immunosuppressive drug commonly used to prevent graft rejection.
Cytokine any of numerous secreted, low-molecular-weight proteins that regulate the intensity and duration of the immune response by exerting a variety of effects on lymphocytes and other immune cells (see Table 13-1).
Cytotoxic having the ability to kill cells.
Cytotoxic T lymphocyte (CTL) an effector T cell (usually $CD8^+$) that can mediate lysis of target cells bearing antigenic peptides associated with an MHC molecule (see Figure 15-5). It usually arises from an antigen-activated **T_C cell** (see Figure 15-1).

D (diversity) gene segment that portion of a rearranged immunoglobulin heavy-chain gene or T-cell receptor gene that is situated between the V and J gene segments and encodes part of the **hypervariable region.** There are multiple D gene segments in germ-line DNA, but gene rearrangement results in only one occurring in each functional rearranged gene.
Degranulation discharge of the contents of cytoplasmic granules by basophils and mast cells following cross-linkage (usually by antigen) of bound IgE (see Figure 18-5). It is characteristic of type I **hypersentivity.**
Delayed-type hypersensitivity (DTH) a type IV hypersensitive response mediated by sensitized **T_{DTH} cells,** which release various **cytokines** (see Figure 15-13). The response generally occurs 2–3 days after T_{DTH} cells interact with antigen and manifests as chronic inflammatory lesions, **granuloma** formation, and skin-test reactivity. It is an important part of host defense against intracellular parasites and bacteria.
Dendritic cell a type of **antigen-presenting cell** that has long membrane processes and is present in the lymph nodes, spleen, thymus, skin, and other tissues.
Desensitization induction of tolerance to an **allergen** or reduction in sensitivity to it by repeated injection of increasing doses of the allergen.
Diapedesis passage of blood cells through an unruptured vessel wall into the surrounding tissue; also called extravasation.
Differentiation antigen a cell-surface marker that is expressed only during a particular developmental stage or by a particular cell lineage.
Domain an independently folded structural unit within a protein. See also **immunoglobulin fold.**

Edema an abnormal accumulation of fluid in intercellular spaces. It often results from failure of the lymphatic system to drain off normal leakage in capillaries.
Effector cell any cell capable of mediating an immune function (e.g., activated T_H cells, CTLs, and plasma cells).
ELISA (enzyme-linked immunosorbent assay) an assay for quantitating either antibody or antigen by use of an enzyme-linked antibody and a substrate that forms a colored reaction product (see Figure 6-4).
Endocytosis a process by which cells ingest extracellular macromolecules by enclosing them in a small portion of the plasma membrane, which invaginates and is pinched off to form an intracellular vesicle containing the ingested material (see Figure 1-3).
Endogenous originating within the organism or cell.
Endosome a small acidic intracellular compartment in which exogenous antigen is degraded (see Figure 10-5).
Endotoxin a lipopolysaccharide (LPS) present in the cell wall of gram-negative bacteria. They are responsible for many of the pathogenic effects associated with these organisms. Some function as **superantigens** (see Table 12-2).
Eosinophil a granulocyte that functions in **antibody-dependent cell-mediated cytotoxicity,** particularly of parasites, by release of cationic proteins contained in its granules and also has some phagocytic ability (see Figure 3-13).
Epitope See **antigenic determinant.**
Epstein-Barr virus (EBV) the causative agent of Burkitt's **lymphoma** and infectious mononucleosis. It can transform human B cells into stable cell lines.
Equilibrium dialysis an experimental technique that can be used to determine the affinity of an antibody for antigen and its valency (see Figure 6-2).
Equivalence a measure of the proportion of antibody to antigen that yields the maximum precipitate in liquids and gels (see Figure 6-4).
Erythema redness of the skin produced in localized inflammatory reactions caused by the movement of erythro-

cytes into tissue spaces when capillary dilation or rupture occurs.

Erythroblastosis fetalis a type II hypersensitivity reaction in which maternal antibodies against fetal Rh antigens cause hemolysis of the erythrocytes of a newborn (see Figure 18-13); also called hemolytic disease of the newborn.

Erythropoiesis the generation of red blood cells.

Exogeneous originating outside the organism or cell.

Exon a continuous segment of DNA that encodes part of a gene product; also called coding sequence.

Exotoxin a toxic protein secreted by gram-positive and gram-negative bacteria. See also **immunotoxin.**

Extravasation see **diapedesis.**

Exudate fluid with a high content of protein, salts, and cellular debris that accumulates extravascularly, usually as a result of **inflammation.**

F(ab′)$_2$ fragment a bivalent antigen-binding fragment of an immunoglobulin that consists of both **light chains** and part of both **heavy chains.** It is obtained by brief pepsin digestion (see Figure 5-3).

Fab fragment a monovalent antigen-binding fragment of an immunoglobulin that consists of one **light chain** and part of one **heavy chain.** It is obtained by brief papain digestion (see Figure 5-3).

Fc fragment a crystallizable, non-antigen-binding fragment of an immunoglobulin that consists of the carboxyl-terminal portions of both **heavy chains,** which possess binding sites for **Fc receptors** and the C1q component of complement. It is obtained by brief papain digestion (see Figure 5-3).

Fc receptor cell-surface receptor specific for the Fc portion of certain classes of immunoglobulin. It is present on lymphocytes, mast cells, macrophages, and other accessory cells.

First-set graft rejection rejection of an **allograft** following first exposure to the alloantigens of the donor. Complete rejection usually occurs within 12–14 days (see Figure 24-1).

Fluorescence antibody an antibody with a **fluorochrome** conjugated to its Fc region that is used to stain cell-surface molecules or tissues, a technique called **immunofluorescence.**

Fluorochrome a fluorescent dye, which can be conjugated with an antibody or other protein. Two common fluorochromes used to tag antibodies are fluorescein isothiocyanate (FITC), which emits a yellow-green color, and rhodamine (Rh), which emits a red color. See also **immunofluorescence.**

Framework region a relatively conserved sequence of amino acids located on either side of the **hypervariable regions** in the variable domains of immunoglobulin heavy and light chains. The framework regions generate the basic β pleated sheet structure of the V_H and V_L domains.

Gamma globulins a group of serum proteins originally characterized by having a greater electrophoretic mobility than other fractions and later shown to contain the immunoglobulins.

Gene locus see **locus.**

Genome the total genetic material contained in the haploid set of chromosomes.

Genotype the combined genetic material inherited from both parents; also, the **alleles** present at one or more specific loci.

Germ line the unmodified genetic material that is transmitted from one generation to the next through the gametes.

Germinal center a region within **lymph nodes** and the **spleen** where B-cell activation, proliferation, and differentiation occurs (see Figure 14-13).

Giant cells large, multinucleated cells, often seen in **granulomas,** that result from fusion of macrophages.

Graft enhancement prolongation of graft survival by preexposure of the recipient to the donor's tissues.

Graft-versus-host disease (GVHD) a reaction that develops when a graft contains **immunocompetent** T cells that recognize and attack the recipient's cells.

Granulocyte any **leukocyte** that contains cytoplasmic granules (**basophil, eosinophil,** and **neutrophil**).

Granuloma a tumor-like mass or nodule of granulation tissue, containing lymphocytes, **giant cells,** modified macrophages (epitheloid cells), and fibroblasts, that arises due to a chronic **inflammation** associated with an infectious disease or the persistence of antigen in tissues.

H-2 complex term for the **MHC** in the mouse.

Haplotype the set of **alleles** of linked genes present on one parental chromosome; commonly used in reference to the MHC genes.

Hapten a low-molecular-weight compound that is not immunogenic by itself but when coupled to a **carrier** can elicit anti-hapten antibodies (see Figure 4-12). Dinitrophenol (DNP) is a common hapten.

Heavy chain the larger polypeptide of an **antibody** molecule composed of one variable domain (V_H) and three or four constant domains (C_H1, C_H2, etc.). There are five major classes of heavy chains in humans, which determine the **isotype** of an antibody (see Table 5-1).

Hemagglutinin an antibody capable of causing agglutination of erythrocytes.

Hematopoiesis formation and development of red and white blood cells.

Hemolytic plaque assay in vitro technique for detecting **plasma cells** based on their ability to lyse antigen-sensitized erythrocytes in the presence of complement, thereby forming visible hemolytic plaques (see Figure 14-3).

Heterologous originating from a different species; see also **xenogeneic.**

High-endothelial venule (HEV) an area of a capillary venule composed of specialized cells with a plump, cuboidal ("high") shape through which lymphocytes migrate to enter various lymphoid organs.

Hinge region portion of immunoglobulin heavy chains between the **Fc** and **Fab** regions. It gives flexibility to the molecule and allows the two antigen-binding sites to function independently.

Histamine one of numerous mediators present the cytoplasmic granules of basophils and mast cells (see Table 18-4). It is released during degranulation and causes increased vascular permeability and contraction of smooth muscle.

Histocompatible denoting individuals whose major histocompatibility antigens, which are encoded by the **MHC**, are identical. Grafts between such individuals are accepted.

HIV (human immunodeficiency virus) a retrovirus that infects human $CD4^+$ T cells and causes **acquired immunodeficiency syndrome** (AIDS).

HLA (human leukocyte antigen) complex term for the **MHC** in humans.

hnRNA (heterogeneous nuclear RNA) the initial product resulting from transcription of DNA, which is processed to form mRNA; also called primary transcript.

Homologous originating from the same species; also refers to similarity in the sequences of DNA or proteins.

HTLV (human T lymphotrophic virus) A retrovirus that infects human $CD4^+$ T cells and causes adult T-cell **leukemia.**

Humoral pertaining to extracellular fluid including the plasma and lymph.

Humoral immunity host defenses that are mediated by **antibody** present in the plasma, lymph, and tissue fluids. It protects against extracellular bacteria and foreign macromolecules. Transfer of antibodies confers this type of immunity on the recipient. See also **cell-mediated immunity.**

Hybridoma a **clone** of hybrid cells formed by fusion of normal lymphocytes with myeloma cells; it retains the properties of the normal cell to produce antibodies or T-cell receptors but exhibits the immortal growth characteristic of myeloma cells (see Figure 2-2). Hybridomas are used to produce **monoclonal antibody.**

Hypersensitivity exaggerated immune response that causes damage to the individual. Immediate hypersensitivity (types I, II, and III) is mediated by antibody, and delayed-type hypersensitivity (type IV) is mediated by **T_{DTH} cells** (see Table 18-1).

Hypervariable region one of three regions within the variable domain of each chain in immunoglobulins and T-cell receptors that exhibits the most sequence variability and contributes the most to the antigen-binding site; also called complementary-determining region (CDR).

Idiotope a single **antigenic determinant** in the variable domains of an antibody or T-cell receptor. Idiotopes are generated by the unique amino acid sequence specific for each antigen (see Figure 5-11).

Idiotype the set of antigenic determinants **(idiotopes)** characterizing each unique antibody or T-cell receptor.

Immune complex a macromolecular complex of antibody bound to antigen, which sometimes includes **complement** components. Deposition of immune complexes in various tissues results in type III **hypersensitivity.**

Immunization the process of producing a state of immunity in a subject. Active immunity may result from inoculation with a specific antigen; passive immunity may result from administration of specific antibodies from an immune individual.

Immunoabsorption removal of antibody or antigen from a sample by adsorption to a solid-phase system to which the complementary antigen or antibody is bound.

Immunocompetent denoting a mature lymphocyte that is capable of recognizing a specific antigen and mediating an immune response.

Immunodeficiency any deficiency in the immune response. It may result from a defect involving phagocytosis, the humoral response, or the cell-mediated response. Combined immunodeficiencies affect both the humoral and cell-mediated immune response (see Table 22-1).

Immunofluorescence technique of staining cells or tissue with **fluorescent antibody** and visualizing the section under a fluorescent microscope (see Figure 6-16).

Immunogen a substance capable of eliciting an immune complex. All immunogens are **antigens,** but some antigens (e.g., **haptens**) are not immunogens.

Immunoglobulin (Ig) see **antibody.**

Immunoglobulin fold characteristic **domain** structure present in immunoglobulins that consists of about 110 amino acids folded into two β pleated sheets, each containing three or four antiparallel β strands, and stabilized by an intrachain disulfide bond forming a loop of about 60 amino acids (see Figure 5-5).

Immunoglobulin superfamily group of proteins that contain immunoglobulin-fold domains, or structurally related domains, including immunoglobulins, T-cell receptors, MHC molecules, and numerous other membrane molecules (see Figure 5-16). The high degree of homology in the amino acid sequences of these proteins suggests a probable ancestral relationship among the genes encoding them.

Immunotoxin an exotoxin or radioisotope conjugated to a monoclonal antibody, which usually is specific for a tumor surface antigen (see Figure 7-10).

In vitro referring to experiments involving living cells or cellular components performed outside the intact organism.

In vivo referring to experiments carrier out in an intact, living organism.

Inflammation a localized tissue response to injury or other trauma characterized by pain, heat, redness, and swelling. The response consists of altered patterns of blood flow, an influx of phagocytic and other immune cells, removal of foreign antigens, and healing of the damaged tissue.

Innate immunity nonspecific host defenses that exist prior to exposure to an antigen and involve anatomic, physiologic, endocytic and phagocytic, and inflammatory mechanisms.

Insulitis cellular infiltration of the pancreatic islets of Langerhans resulting in inflammation and occurring in the early stages of insulin-dependent diabetes mellitus.

Interferon (IFN) several glycoproteins produced and secreted by certain cells that induce an antiviral state in other cells and also help to regulate the immune response. INF-α and INF-β primarily provide antiviral protection, whereas IGN-γ, which is produced by T cells, has numerous effects on various immune-system cells (see Table 13-1).

Interleukin (IL) a group of **cytokines** secreted by leukocytes that primarily affect the growth and differentiation of various hematopoietic and immune-system cells (see Table 13-1).

Internal image a site on an anti-idiotype antibody (Ab-2) that binds to the **paratope** of the antibody (Ab-1) and mimics the **epitope** of the original antigen. Since the internal image stimulates an immune response identical to that induced by the original antigen, it can be substituted for the antigen (see Figure 16-5).

Intron noncoding sequence within a gene, which is transcribed into the primary transcript **(hnRNA)** but is removed during processing and does not appear in mRNA.

Ir (immune response) genes loci within the class II region of the **MHC** that determine T_H-cell responsiveness to a particular antigen.

Isograft graft between genetically identical individuals.

Isotype an antibody class, which is determined by the heavy-chain constant-region sequence. The five human isotypes, designated IgA, IgD, IgE, IgG, and IgM, exhibit structural and functional differences (see Table 5-4). Also refers to the set of **isotypic determinants** that is carried by all members of a species.

Isotype switching conversion of one antibody class **(isotype)** to another resulting from the genetic rearrangement of heavy-chain constant-region genes in B cells; also called class switching.

Isotypic determinant an **antigenic determinant** within the immunoglobulin constant regions that is characteristic of a species (see Figure 5-11).

J chain a polypeptide that joins subunits of polymeric IgA and IgM.

J (joining) gene segment that portion of a rearranged immunoglobulin or T-cell receptor gene that joins the variable region to the constant region and encodes part of the **hypervariable region.** There are multiple J gene segments in germ-line DNA, but gene rearrangement results in only one segment occurring in each functional rearranged gene.

Kaposi's sarcoma a neoplastic lesion characterized by multiple bluish nodules in the skin and hemorrhages; it is common in AIDS patients.

Kappa (κ) chain see **light chain.**

Karyotype the chromosomal constitution of a given cell.

Kinin A group of peptides released during an inflammatory response that act as vasodilators, inducing smooth-muscle contraction and increased vascular permeability.

Kuppfer cell fixed macrophage that lines the blood sinuses in the liver and acts as an **antigen-presenting cell.**

Lambda (λ) chain see **light chain.**

Langerhans cell a type of **dendritic cell** found in the skin that bears Fc receptors and class II MHC molecules and functions as an **antigen-presenting cell.**

Lectin a group of proteins, usually derived from plants, that specifically bind sugars and oligosaccharides present on the membrane glycoproteins of animal cells. Some lectins (e.g., **concanavalin A, phytohemagglutinin,** and **pokeweed mitogen**) are mitogenic.

Leukemia cancer originating in any class of hematopoietic cell that tends to proliferate as single cells within the lymph or blood.

Leukocyte any blood cell that is not an erythrocyte; white blood cell.

Leukopenia reduction in the number of circulating white blood cells.

Leukotriene several mediators of type I **hypersensitivity;** also called slow reactive substance of anaphylaxis (SRS-A). They are formed during degranulation of **mast cells** and **basophils** (see Figure 18-5) and are metabolic products of arachidonic acid.

LFA (leukocyte functional antigen) a family of cell-surface molecules (LFA-1, LFA-2, and LFA-3) that mediate intercellular adhesion. They belong to the integrin family of adhesion molecules.

Ligand any molecule recognized by a **receptor.**

Light chain the smaller polypeptide of an **antibody** molecule composed of one variable domain (V_L) and one constant domain (C_L). There are two major types (**kappa** and **lambda**) of light chains in humans.

Locus the specific chromosomal location of a gene.

LPS (lipopolysaccharide) a group of substances present in the cell wall of gram-negative bacteria that are B-cell mitogens and can induce an inflammatory response; can also function as an **adjuvant.**

Lymph a pale, watery, proteinaceous fluid that is derived from intercellular tissue fluid and circulates in lymphatic vessels.

Lymph node small secondary lymphoid organ that contains lymphocytes, macrophages, and dendritic cells and serves as a site for filtration of foreign antigen and activation and proliferation of lymphocytes. See also **germinal center.**

Lymphoadenopathy enlargement of the **lymph nodes.**

Lymphoblast a cell stage that occurs in lymphocytes after activation and before cell division; it is distinguished by a higher cytoplasm : nucleus ratio than in resting lymphocytes.

Lymphocyte a mononuclear leukocyte that mediates humoral or cell-mediated immunity. See **B cell** and **T cell.**

Lymphokine a **cytokine** produced by activated lymphocytes, especially **T_H cells.**

Lymphokine-activated killer (LAK) cells a heterogeneous population of cytotoxic cells that can be generated in vitro by culturing activated lymphoid cells in the presence of high concentrations of **interleukin** 2 (IL-2).

Lymphoma a cancer of lymphoid cells that tends to proliferate as a solid tumor.

Lymphopoiesis the differentiation of lymphocytes from hematopoietic stem cells.

Lymphotoxin (LT) older term for **tumor necrosis factor β.**

Lysogeny state in which a bacteriophage genome (prophage) is associated with the bacterial host genome in such a way that the viral gene remains unexpressed.

Lysosome a small cytoplasmic vesicle found in many types of cells that contains hydrolytic enzymes, which play an important role in the digestion of material ingested by phagocytosis and **endocytosis.**

Lysozyme an enzyme present in tears, saliva, and mucous secretions that digests mucopeptides in bacterial cells walls and thus functions as a nonspecific antibacterial agent.

Macrophage a large, myeloid cell derived from a **monocyte** that functions in **phagocytosis,** antigen processing and presentation, secretion of cytokines, and **antibody-dependent cell-mediated cytotoxicity.**

Malignant denoting tumors that have the capacity to invade and alter normal tissue.
MALT (mucosal-associated lymphoid tissue) secondary lymphoid tissue located along various mucous membrane surfaces; includes **Peyer's patches,** tonsils, the appendix, and submucosal lymphocytes in intestinal villi.
Marginal zone a diffuse region of the **spleen,** located between the **red pulp** and **white pulp,** that is rich in B cells and contains lymphoid follicles, which can develop into **germinal centers.**
Margination adhesion of leukocytes to vascular endothelium; it occurs normally but is more pronounced in the early stages of **inflammation.**
Mast cell a bone marrow–derived cell present in a variety of tissues that resembles peripheral-blood basophils, bears **Fc receptors** for IgE, and undergoes IgE-mediated **degranulation.**
Medulla the innermost or central region of an organ.
Megakaryocyte a white blood cell that produces **platelets** by cytoplasmic budding.
Membrane-attack complex (MAC) complex of complement components C5–C9, which is formed in the terminal steps of either the **classical** or **alternative complement pathway** and mediates cell lysis by creating a membrane pore in the target cell.
Memory, immunologic the attribute of the immune system mediated by **memory cells** whereby a second encounter with an antigen induces a heightened state of immune reactivity.
Memory cell clonally expanded progeny of T and B cells formed during the **primary response** following initial exposure to an antigen. Memory cells are more easily activated than **naive** lymphocytes and when they encounter antigen in a subsequent exposure, they mediate a faster and greater **secondary response.**
Metastasis the transfer of tumor cells from the primary tumor to a secondary site; a characteristic of all **malignant** tumors.
MHC (major histocompatibility complex) a complex of genes encoding cell-surface molecules that are required for antigen presentation to T cells and for rapid graft rejection. It is called the H-2 complex in the mouse and the HLA complex in humans.
MHC molecules proteins encoded by the major histocompatibility complex and classified as **class I, class II,** and **class III MHC molecules.**
MHC restriction the characteristic of T cells that permits them to recognize antigen only after it is processed and the resulting antigenic peptides are displayed in association with either a **class I** or **class II MHC molecule.**
Migration-inhibition factor (MIF) a **cytokine** that inhibits macrophage movement and is involved in **delayed-type hypersensitivity.**
Minor histocompatibility antigens antigens encoded by genes outside of the **MHC** that contribute to graft rejection.
Mitogen any substance that nonspecifically induces DNA synthesis and cell division, especially of lymphocytes. Common mitogens are **concanavalin A, phytohemagglutinin, LPS, pokeweed mitogen,** and various **superantigens.**
Mixed-lymphocyte reaction (MLR) T-cell proliferation in response to cells expressing **allogenic** MHC molecules; can be used as an assay for class II MHC activity (see Figure 9-12).
Monoclonal derived from a single cell.
Monoclonal antibody homogeneous preparation of antibody molecules, produced by a **hybridoma,** all of which exhibit the same antigenic **specificity.**
Monocyte a mononuclear phagocytic myeloid cell that circulates briefly in the bloodstream before migrating into the tissues where it becomes a **macrophage.**

Naive denoting mature B and T cells that have not encountered antigen; synonymous with unprimed and virgin.
Natural killer (NK) cell a large, granular lymphocyte **(null cell)** that has cytotoxic ability but does not express antigen-binding receptors. It exhibits antibody-independent killer of tumor cells and also can participate in **antibody-dependent cell-mediated cytotoxicity.**
Necrosis morphologic changes associated with death of individual cells or groups of cells, leading to disruption and atrophy of tissue. See also **apoptosis.**
Neoplasia formation of a **neoplasm;** uncontrolled cell proliferation.
Neoplasm any new and abnormal growth; a benign or **malignant** tumor.
Network theory theory proposed by Neils Jerne that the immune system is regulated by a network of **idiotype** and anti-idiotype reactions involving antibodies and T-cell receptors.
Neutrophil a circulating, phagocytic granulocyte involved early in **inflammation** (see Figure 3-13). It expresses **Fc receptors** and can participate in **antibody-dependent cell-mediated cytotoxicity.**
Nude mouse homozygous genetic defect *(nu/nu)* carried by an inbred mouse strain that results in the absence of the thymus and consequently a marked deficiency of T cells and cell-mediated immunity. The mice are hairless (hence, the name) and can accept grafts from other species.
Null cell a small population of peripheral-blood lymphocytes that lack the membrane markers characteristic of B and T cells. **Natural killer cells** are included in this group.

Oncofetal tumor antigen an antigen that is present during fetal development but generally is not expressed in tissues except by tumor cells. Alpha-feto protein (AFP) and carcinoembryonic antigen (CEA) are two examples that have been associated with various cancers (see Table 25-4).
Oncogene a gene encoding a protein capable of inducing cellular **transformation.** Oncogenes derived from viruses are termed v-onc, while their cellular counterparts (**proto-oncogenes**) are denoted c-onc.
Oncogenic causing cancer
Opsonin a substance (e.g., an antibody or C3b) that binds to an antigen and enhances its **phagocytosis.**
Opsonization deposition of **opsonins** on an antigen, thereby promoting a stable, adhesive contact with an appropriate phagocytic cell (see Figure 17-11).
Ouchterlony method a double immunodiffusion technique involving the diffusion of antigen and antibody within

a gel resulting in formation of a visible band of precipitate in the region of **equivalence** (see Figure 6-8).

PALS (periarteriolar lymphoid sheath) see **white pulp.**
Papain proteolytic enzyme used to obtain the **Fab** and **Fc fragments** in the hydrolysis of immunoglobin.
Paratope the site in the **variable (V) domain** of an antibody or T-cell receptor that binds to an **epitope** on an antigen.
Passive cutaneous anaphylaxis (PCA) in vivo technique to determine antigen-specific IgE responsible for type I **hypersensitivity.**
Passive immunity acquired immunity conferred by the transfer of immune products, such as antibody or sensitized T cells, from an immune individual to a nonimmune one.
Pathogen a disease-causing organism.
Pepsin proteolytic enzyme use to obtain **F(ab′)$_2$ fragments** in the hydrolysis of immunoglobulin.
Perforin cytolytic product of **CTLs** that, in the presence of Ca^{2+}, polymerizes to form transmembrane pores in target cells (see Figure 15-8).
Peyer's patches lymphoid nodules located along the small intestine that function to trap antigens from the gastrointestinal tract and provide sites where B and T cells can interact with antigen.
Phagocytosis a process by which certain cells (phagocytes) engulf microorganisms, other ells, and foreign particles (see Figure 3-12).
Phagolysosome product of the fusion of a **lysosome** and a **phagosome.** Ingested material in the phagosome is digested by degradative enzymes of the lysosome (see Figure 3-12).
Phagosome intracellular vacuole containing ingested particulate materials; formed by invagination of the cell membrane during **phagocytosis.**
Phylogeny the evolutionary history of a species.
Phytohemagglutinin (PHA) a plant **lectin** derived from kidney beans that is a potent T-cell **mitogen.**
Pinocytosis a type of **endocytosis** in which a cell ingests extracellular fluid and soluble materials contained within that fluid.
Plaque-forming count (PFC) the number of plaques formed in the in vitro **hemolytic plaque assay,** which detects antibody-forming plasma cells.
Plasma the cell-free, fluid portion of blood, which contains all the clotting factors.
Plasma cell a differentiated antibody-secreting cell derived from an antigen-activated **B cell.**
Plasmacytoma a plasma-cell tumor.
Plasmapheresis a technique in which **plasma** is removed from an individual's blood and the erythrocytes are resuspended in a suitable medium and then returned to the individual.
Platelet a small anuclear membrane-bound cytoplasmic structure derived from **megakaryocytes,** which contains vasoactive substances and clotting factors important in blood coagulation, inflammation, and allergic reactions; also called thrombocyte.
Platelet-activating factor (PAF) a **cytokine** released by basophils and mast cells following **degranulation**. It causes aggregation and lysis of platelets.
Pokeweed mitogen (PWM) a **lectin** derived from pokeweed that acts as a B-cell **mitogen.**
Polyclonal pretaining to many different clones.
Polymorphism presence of multiple **alleles** at a specific locus. The **major histocompatibility complex** is highly polymorphic.
Primary immune response the immune response that is induced by initial exposure to an antigen. It is mediated largely by IgM antibody and sensitized T cells. It develops more slowly and to a lesser extent than a **secondary response.**
Primary lymphoid organ an organ in which lymphocyte precursors mature into antigenically committed, **immunocompetent** cells. In mammals, the bone marrow and thymus are the primary lymphoid organs in which B-cell and T-cell maturation occurs, respectively.
Private specificity antigenic specificity of MHC molecules that is unique to a specific allele of a particular MHC molecule.
Prophylaxis a vaccine or other preventive treatment.
Prostaglandin a group of biologically active lipid derivatives of arachidonic acid. They modulate **inflammation** by inhibiting platelet aggregation, increasing vascular permeability, and inducing smooth-muscle contraction.
Protein A a protein derived from *Staphylococcus aureus* that binds to the Fc region of some IgG molecules. When labeled with a **fluorochrome,** protein A can be used to detect IgG.
Proto-oncogenes genes that in normal cells encode various growth-controlling proteins (see Table 25-1). Under certain conditions, proto-oncogenes are converted into **oncogenes** (see Figure 25-3).
Pseudogene nucleotide sequence that is a stable component of the genome but is incapable of being expressed. They are thought to have been derived by mutation of ancestral active genes.
Public specificity antigenic specificity of MHC molecules that is common to many allelic forms of a particular MHC molecule.
Pyrogen a fever-causing substance released by activated leukocytes.
Pyrogenic pus producing.

Qa antigens class I MHC antigens encoded by a region within the mouse T1a complex.

Radioimmunoassay (RIA) a highly sensitive technique for measuring antigen or antibody that involves competitive binding of radiolabeled antigen or antibody (see Figure 6-13).
Reagin IgE antibody that mediates type I immediate **hypersensitivity** reactions.
Receptor, cell-surface molecule present on the cell membrane that has high **affinity** for a particular **ligand.**
Red pulp portion of the spleen consisting of a network of sinusoids populated by macrophages and erythrocytes. It is the site where old and defective red blood cells are destroyed.

Reticuloendothelial system (RES) collective term for the diffuse system of phagocytic cells associated with the connective tissue throughout most of the body.

Retrovirus a type of RNA virus that uses a reverse transcriptase to produce a DNA copy of its RNA genome.

Rheumatoid factor autoantibody found in the serum of individuals with rheumatoid arthritis and other connective-tissue diseases.

Ricin a potent toxin that is derived from castor beans and can be conjugated to a **monoclonal antibody** to form an immunotoxin (see Figure 7-10).

Sarcoma tumor of supporting or connective tissue.

Second-set graft rejection acute, rapid rejection of an **allograft** in an individual who has received a previous graft from the same donor (see Figure 24-1). The reaction is mediated by **primed** T cells.

Secondary immune response the immune response that is induced following a second exposure to antigen. It occurs more rapidly and is stronger that the **primary immune response.**

Secretory component a protein derived from the poly-Ig receptor that forms part of the secretory IgA and IgM (see Figure 5-14).

Secretory IgA dimeric IgA linked to the **secretory component;** it is present in mucous secretions (see Figure 5-14).

Sensitized lymphocytes effector T cells (e.g., CTLs and T_{DTH} cells) derived from exposure of **naive** T cells to antigen; on subsequent exposure to the same antigen, they rapidly carry out their effector functions.

Serum fluid portion of the blood, which is free of cells and clotting factors.

Serum sickness a type III **hypersensitivity** reaction that develops when antigen is administered intravenously, resulting in the formation and tissue deposition of large amounts of antigen-antibody complexes. It often develops when individuals are immunized with antiserum derived from other species.

Slow reactive substance of anaphylaxis (SRS-A) see **leukotriene.**

Somatic mutation a mechanism by which point mutations are introduced into rearranged immunoglobulin variable-region genes during activation and proliferation of B cells. It contributes significantly to antibody diversity.

Southern blotting a common technique for detecting specific DNA sequences in which restriction-enzyme fragments are separated electrophoretically, then denatured and transferred to another gel, which is incubated with a radioactive probe specific for the sequence of interest (see Figure 2-8).

Specificity, antigenic capacity of antibody and T-cell receptor to recognize and interact with a single, unique **antigenic determinant.**

Spleen secondary lymphoid organ where old erythrocytes are destroyed and blood-borne antigens are trapped and presented to lymphocytes in the **PALS** and **marginal zone.**

Stem cell a cell from which differentiated cells derive.

Superantigen an antigen that can activate all T cells expressing T-cell receptors with a particular V_{β} domain. They function as potent T-cell **mitogens** and may cause food poisoning and other disorders (see Table 12-2).

Syngeneic denoting genetically identical members of the same species.

T cell a lymphocyte that matures in the thymus and expresses a T-cell receptor, CD3, and CD4 or CD8. Several distinct T-cell subpopulations are recognized.

T cytotoxic (T_C) cell generally a $CD8^+$ class I MHC–restricted T cell, which differentiates into a **CTL** following interaction with altered self-cells (e.g., tumor cells, virus-infected cells).

T helper (T_H) cell generally a $CD4^+$ class II MHC–restricted T cell, which plays a central role in both humoral and cell-mediated immunity and secretes numerous cytokines when activated.

T-cell receptor (TCR) antigen-binding molecule expressed on the surface of T cells and associated with **CD3**. It is a heterodimer consisting of either an α and β chain or a γ and δ chain (see Figure 11-2).

T_{DTH} cell generally a $CD4^+$ lymphocyte derived from a T_H cell that mediates **delayed-type hypersensitivity.**

Thy-1 glycoprotein that is the earliest appearing surface marker of the T-cell lineage; also called theta antigen.

Thymocyte developing T cells present in the thymus.

Thymus a primary lymphoid organ, located in the thoracic cavity, where T-cell maturation occurs.

Thymus-dependent antigen an antigen that is dependent on T_H cells in order to induce a humoral immune response.

Thymus-independent antigen an antigen that does not require the presence of T_H cells to introduce a humoral immune response. **LPS**, dextran, and ficoll are examples.

Titer a measure of the relative strength of an antiserum. The titer is the reciprocal of the last dilution of an antiserum capable of mediating some measurable effect such as precipitation or agglutination.

Tolerance state of immunologic unresponsiveness.

Tolerogen substance that can introduce **tolerance.**

Toxoid a toxin that has been altered to eliminate its toxicity but that still can function as an **immunogen.**

Transformation change that a normal cell undergoes as it becomes **malignant**

Tuberculin crude protein fraction isolated from supernatant of *Mycobacterium tuberculosis* cultures. It can be used in a skin test for exposure to *M. tuberculosis.*

Tumor necrosis factors (TNFs) Two related **cytokines** produced by macrophages (TNF-α) and some T cells (TNF-β). Both factors are cytotoxic to tumor cells but not to normal cells; they also exert inflammatory effects on a variety of cells.

Tumor-associated antigens cell-surface proteins that are present on tumor cells and normal cells.

Tumor-specific antigens cell-surface proteins found on tumor cells but not on normal cells.

V (variable) gene segment the 5′ coding portion of rearranged immunoglobulin and T-cell receptor genes. There are multiple V gene segments in germ-line DNA, but gene rearrangement results in only one segment occurring in each functional rearranged gene.

Vaccination intentional administration of a harmless or less harmful form of a pathogen to induce a specific immune response that protects the individual against later exposure to the same pathogen.

Vaccine a preparation of antigenic material used to induce immunity against pathogenic organisms.

Variable (V) domain amino-terminal portion of immunoglobulin and T-cell receptor chains that are highly variable and responsible for the **specificity** of these molecules.

Variola smallpox.

Vasculitis inflammation of the blood vessels.

Virgin see **naive.**

Virulence a measure of the infectious ability of a pathogen.

Western blotting a common technique for detecting a protein in a mixture in which the proteins are separated electrophoretically and then transferred to a polymer sheet, which is flooded with radiolabeled or enzyme-conjugated antibody specific for the protein of interest (see Figure 6-15).

Wheal and flare a reaction characteristic of type I **hypersensitivity** in the skin involving a sharply delineated swell of the skin (wheal) with surrounding redness (flare).

White pulp portion of the spleen that surrounds the arteries, forming a periarteriolar lymphoid sheath (PALS) populated mainly by T cells.

Xenogeneic denoting individuals of different species.

Xenograft graft or tissue transplanted from one species to another.

ANSWERS TO STUDY QUESTIONS

Chapter 1

1. (a) CM. (b) CM. (c) H and CM. (d) H and CM. (e) CM. (f) CM. (g) H. (h) CM. (i) H. (j) H.

2. The secondary immune response involves an amplified population of memory cells. The response is more rapid and achieves higher levels than the primary response.

3. Clonal selection accounts for the amplified number of antigen-reactive memory cells that characterize the secondary response.

4. Only antigen-activated T_H cells express a membrane receptor for IL-2.

5. (a) Both antibody and the T-cell receptors display fine specificity for antigen, and subtle modifications in an antigen prohibit its binding to antibody or the T-cell receptor. The MHC molecules do not possess such fine specificity, and a variety of unrelated peptide antigens can be bound by the same MHC molecule. (b) Antibody is expressed only by cells of the B-cell lineage; the T-cell receptor is expressed by cells of the T-cell lineage; class I MHC molecules are expressed by virtually all nucleated cells; class II MHC molecules are expressed only by specialized cells that function as antigen-presenting cells (e.g., B cells, macrophages, and dendritic cells). (c) Antibody can bind to protein or polysaccharide antigens; the T-cell receptor recognizes only peptides associated with MHC molecules; MHC molecules only bind processed peptides.

6. (a) Macrophages, dendritic cells, and B cells. (b) Class II MHC molecules. (c) T helper cells.

7. They can only recognize antigen that is associated with class I MHC molecules.

8. (a) 13. (b) 19. (c) 6. (d) 12. (e) 2. (f) 18. (g) 8. (h) 15. (i) 4. (j) 14. (k) 7. (1) 9. (m) 17. (n) 5. (o) 3. (p) 10.

Chapter 2

1. (a) the genomic clone contains intervening sequences (introns) that are removed during processing of the primary transcript and therefore do not encode the protein product. (b) DNA must be microinjected into a fertilized egg so that the DNA (transgene) will be passed on to all daughter cells. (c) Primary lymphoid cultures have a finite life span and contain a heterogeneous population of cells.

2.

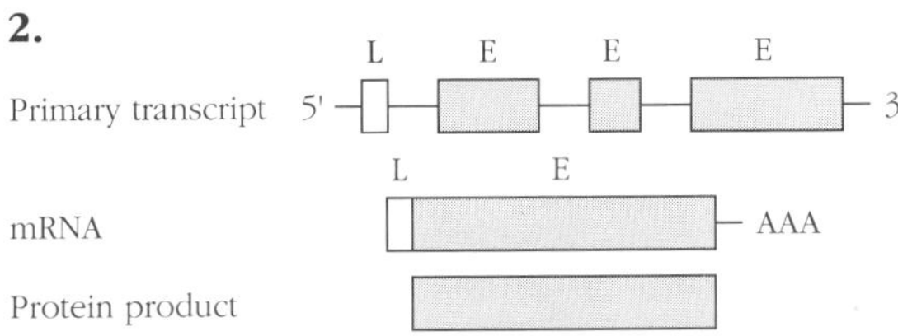

3. Transfected DNA integrates only into a small percentage of cells. If a selectable marker gene also is present, then the small number of transfected cells will grow in the appropriate medium, whereas the much larger number of nontransfected cells will die.

4. The mouse would become a mosaic in which the transgene would have incorporated into some of the somatic cells but not all.

5.

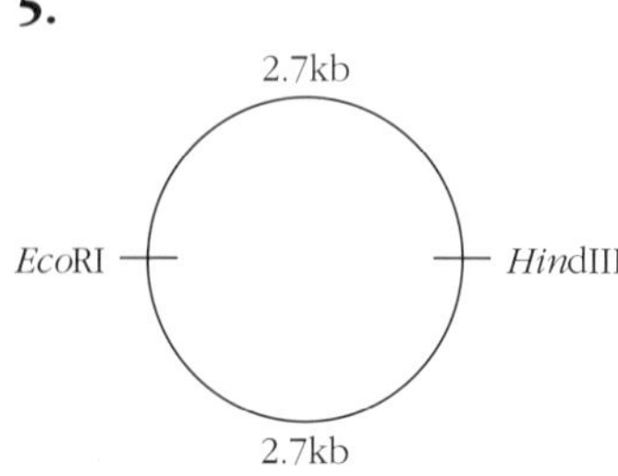

6. Isolate mRNA from activated T cells and transcribe it into cDNA using reverse transcriptase. Insert cDNA into a suitable expression vector, such as plasmid DNA carrying an ampicillin selection gene. Transfer the recombinant plasmid DNA into *E. coli* and grow in the presence of ampicillin to select for bacteria containing the plasmid DNA. Test the bacterial culture supernatent for the presence of IL-2 by seeing if the monoclonal antibody to IL-2 reacts with the culture supernatent. Once a bacterial culture is identified that is secreting IL-2, the cDNA can be cloned.

Chapter 3

1. (a) T_H cells in paracortical areas; B cells in germinal centers within secondary follicles located in the node cortex. (b) T_H cells in paracortical areas. (c) No areas of rapid cell proliferation, since T_H cells are required for B-cell activation. (d) B cells in secondary follicles and germinal centers.

2. Monocyte progenitor cells have receptors for M-CSF; they do not secrete it. If both M-CSF and its receptor were expressed by these cells, then they could autostimulate their own proliferation.

3. The primary lymphoid organs are the bone marrow (bursa of Fabricius in birds) and the thymus. These organs function as sites for B-cell and T-cell maturation, respectively.

4. The secondary lymphoid organs are the spleen, lymph nodes, Peyer's patches, tonsils, adenoids, appendix, and mucosal-associated tissue (MALT). These organs trap antigen and provide sites where lymphocytes can interact with antigen and subsequently undergo clonal expansion.

5. The thymic stroma contains epithelial cells, interdigitating dendritic cells, and macrophages, which form a three-dimensional network. These cells secrete various hormonal factors that are necessary for thymocyte growth and maturation into immunocompetent T cells. Thymic stromal cells also play a role in the positive and negative selection of T cells in the thymus.

6. Antigenic commitment involves random rearrangements of genes encoding the antigen-binding receptors on T cells and B cells. As a result of this process, each mature B or T cell expresses receptors with a single specificity and thus can interact only with antigen of that specificity. Antigen is not involved in antigenic commitment, which takes place in the primary lymphoid organs. Mature, antigenically committed lymphocytes migrate from the primary lymphoid organs to the secondary lymphoid organs where they are exposed to antigen. Those lymphocytes whose specificity corresponds to a particular antigen interact with the antigen. This interaction stimulates proliferation and differentiation of the lymphocyte clone into memory cells and effector cells; that is, they undergo clonal selection. The long-lived memory cells are responsible for immunologic memory.

7. The increased expression of ICAMs on vascular endothelial cells near an inflammatory site facilitates adherence of leukocytes to the blood vessel wall, resulting in increased extravasation of leukocytes in the area.

8. The lethally irradiated mice serve as an assay system for pluripotent stem cells, since only mice injected with bone marrow samples containing pluripotent stem cells will survive. As pluripotent stem cells are successively enriched in a bone marrow sample, the total number of cells that must be injected to restore hematopoiesis decreases.

9. In a neonatal mouse, thymectomy eliminates T-cell maturation, causing the animal to become immunodeficient and eventually to die. In an adult mouse, thymectomy does not have a profound effect because many of the recirculating mature T cells have a long life span and can respond to antigenic challenge by clonal selection.

10. T and B cells in the secondary lymphoid organs could be distinguished by use of fluorescein- and rhodamine-tagged monoclonal antibodies specific for their cell-membrane markers: surface immunoglobulin (antibody) in the case of B cells, and the T-cell receptor or CD3 in the case of T cells.

11. (a) Mouse A might have a defect in the vascular addressins of the cervical lymph nodes, since its lymphocytes are capable of homing to lymph nodes in control animals and in mouse B. (b) Since lymphocytes from mouse B fail to home to cervical lymph nodes in any of the animals, these lymphocytes may lack a homing receptor. (c) To test these hypotheses, you could stain the lymphocytes and cervical lymph nodes with fluorescein monoclonal antibodies specific for homing receptors or vascular addressins. If (a) is correct, then the level of staining of the lymph nodes with antibodies against vascular addressin should be lower in mouse A than in the control mouse, whereas staining of the lymphocytes with antibodies to homing receptor should be comparable. If (b) is correct, then the opposite staining pattern would be expected with mouse B and the control.

Chapter 4

1. (a) True. (b) True. (c) False: A hapten cannot stimulate an immune response unless it is conjugated to a larger protein carrier. However, the hapten can combine with pre-formed antibody specific for the hapten. (d) True. (e) False: A T cell can only recognize peptides that have been processed and presented by MHC molecules. These epitopes tend to be amphipathic and, therefore, often represent internal peptides. (f) True. (g) True. (h) False: Each MHC molecule binds a number of different peptides. It is not yet known what features different peptides must have in common to be able to bind to the same MHC molecule. (i) False: Internal viral proteins can be processed and displayed by MHC molecules and activate T_H or T_C cells. (j) False: Since IA^k and IA^d are encoded by allelic MHC genes and consequently exhibit allelic differences, they would most likely not bind the same hemagglutinin peptide. Thus, a peptide that is immunogenic for a strain expressing IA^k may not be immunogenic for a strain expressing IA^d.

2. (a) The UV-inactivated vaccine would be seen as an exogenous antigen. Exogenous antigens are internalized through phagocytosis or endocytosis and then are processed in the endocytic pathway. The resulting antigenic peptides are presented by class II MHC molecules on the surface of antigen-presenting cells. Since T_C cells are generally class I MHC restricted, they would not be activated by this type of vaccine, although class II MHC–restricted T_H cells might be. (b) Because the attenuated virus replicates within host cells, it is seen as an endogenous antigen. Endogenous antigens are processed within the cytoplasm or endoplasmic reticulum and are presented by class I MHC molecules, which are present on the membrane of most nucleated cells. Therefore, the attenuated virus would be likely to activate T_C cells, which are class I MHC restricted.

3. T-cell responsiveness has been correlated with the amphipathic properties of peptides; that is, peptides with highly amphipathic segments are more likely to stimulate a T-cell response than less-amphipathic peptides. It has been suggested that the hydrophobic residues interact with MHC molecules and the hydrophilic residues interact with the T-cell receptor. Nonetheless, even if a peptide binds to a MHC molecule expressed by a given animal, the peptide will not induce a T-cell response if the animal does not have T cells that recognize the peptide-MHC complex. In other words, the induce a T-cell response a peptide vaccine must possess both an agretope that can bind to the recipient's MHC molecules and an epitope that is recognized by the antigen-binding receptors on some of the recipient's T cells.

4. L cells are not antigen-presenting cells and, therefore, do not express their own class II MHC molecules. The class II MHC genes were transfected into the L cells so that the T-cell response to various peptide-MHC combinations could be assessed without the complication of additional class II MHC molecules. Had the genes been transfected into a macrophage, then other IA or IE MHC molecules would also be expressed by the cell, and these class II MHC molecules might also bind the experimental peptides.

5. See Table 4-4.

Chapter 5

1. (a) True. (b) True. (c) False: Both IgM and IgD have identical V_H and V_L domains and, therefore, have the same specificity for antigen. (d) True. (e) False: Multiple isotypes can appear on the surface of a B cell. The mature B cell expresses both IgM and IgD. Memory B cells can express additional isotypes such as IgG, IgA, or IgE. (f) True. (g) True. (h) False: Both heavy and light chain variable regions contain approximately 110 amino acid residues. (i) False: Secreted IgM is a pentamer. Because of its larger size and valency, it is able to cross-link antigens more effectively than IgG.

2. (a) The molecule would have to possess the following structural features: 2 identical heavy chains and 2 identical light chains (H_2L_2); interchain disulfide bonds joining the heavy chains (H–H) and heavy and light chains (H–L); a series of intrachain domains containing approximately 110 amino acids and stabilized by an intra-domain disulfide bridge of about 60 amino acids; single constant domain in light chains and 3 or 4 constant domains in heavy chain. The amino-terminal domain of both the heavy and light chains should show sequence variation. (b) The antisera to both whole human IgG and human κ chain should cross-react with the new immunoglobulin class, since both of these antisera have antibodies specific for the light chain. The new isotype would be expected to contain either kappa or lambda light chains. (c) Reduce the interchain disulfide bonds of the new isotype with mercaptoethanol and alkylation. Separate the heavy and light chains. Immunize a rabbit with the heavy chain. The rabbit antisera should react with the new isotype but not with any other known isotypes.

3. Advantages of IgG compared with IgM are (1) its ability to cross the placenta and protect the developing fetus; (2) its higher serum concentration, which results in IgG antibodies binding to and neutralizing more antigen molecules and being more effective in antigen clearance; (3) its smaller size, which enables IgG to diffuse more readily into intercellular fluids. The disadvantages of IgG compared with IgM are its lower capacity to (1) agglutinate antigens and (2) activate the complement system, both of which are due to the lower valency of IgG.

4. (a) See Figure 5-4. (b) Draw as a dimer containing α heavy chains. Add J chain and the secretory component (see Figure 5-14a). (c) Draw as a pentamer containing μ heavy chains. The μ heavy chain has 5 domains and no hinge region; the extra C_H domain replaces the hinge. Add J chain. IgM has additional interchain disulfide bonds joining the pentamer subunits to one another and to the J chain (see Figure 5-12e).

5.

Property	Whole IgG	H chain	L chain	Fab	F(ab')$_2$	Fc
Binds antigen	+	Weak +	Weak +	+	+	−
Bivalent antigen binding	+	−	−	−	+	−
Binds to Fc receptors	+	−	−	−	−	+
Fixes complement in presence of antigen	+	−	−	−	−	−
Has V domains	+	+	+	+	+	−
Has C domains	+	+	+	+	+	+

6. (a) Anti-allotype antibodies. (b) Anti-idiotype antibodies. (c) Anti-isotype antibodies. (d) Anti-allotype antibodies. (e) No antibodies will be formed.

7.

	Rabbit antisera to mouse antibody component				
	γ chain	κ chain	IgG Fab fragment	IgG Fc fragment	J chain
Mouse γ chain	Yes	No	Yes	Yes	No
Mouse κ chain	No	Yes	Yes	No	No
Mouse IgM whole	No	Yes	Yes	No	Yes
Mouse IgG-Fc fragment	Yes	No	No	Yes	No

8. The hypervariable regions are located in the V_H and V_L domains. There are three hypervariable regions in each V_H domain, and three in each V_L domain. Residues in the hypervariable regions constitute the major amino acids in the antigen-binding cleft.

9. (a) Immunoglobulin-fold domains contain approximately 110 amino acid residues, which are arranged in two antiparallel β pleated sheets, each composed of three or four β strands separated by short loops of varying lengths. An intra-domain disulfide bond, formed by two conserved cysteine residues about 60 residues apart, stabilizes the domain. (b) See Figure 5-16. The Ig-domain structure is thought to facilitate interactions between the faces of the β pleated sheets; such interactions between nonhomologous domains may allow different members of the immunoglobulin superfamily to bind to each other.

10. The antiserum also contained antibodies to the kappa and lambda light chains. The technician needs to reduce the interchain disulfide bonds with mercaptoethanol and isolate the heavy chain. If the technician immunizes the rabbits with the heavy chains alone, the rabbit antisera will be specific for the IgG isotype.

11. (a) IgA: 3, 6, 10, 11. (b) IgD: 4. (c) IgE: 2, 9. (d) IgG: 5, 12, 13. (e) IgM: 1, 3, 4, 6, 7, 8, 12, 13.

12. (a) Allotypic. (b) Idiotypic. (c) Isotypic.

Chapter 6

1. (a) True. (b) True. (c) False: Papain digestion yields Fab fragments, which are monovalent and, therefore, cannot cross-link antigens. (d) True. (e) True. (f) True. (g) False: It is qualitative but not quantitative. (h) False: Agglutination tests are more sensitive.

2. Coat a microtiter plate with antigens from HIV. Add serum from a patient suspected of being infected with HIV. Incubate the plate, and then wash away unbound antibodies. Add a goat anti-human immunoglobulin reagent that has been conjugated with an enzyme. Incubate the plate and wash away unbound antibody. Add substrate and observe for a colored reaction.

3. (a) Whole bovine serum.
(b)

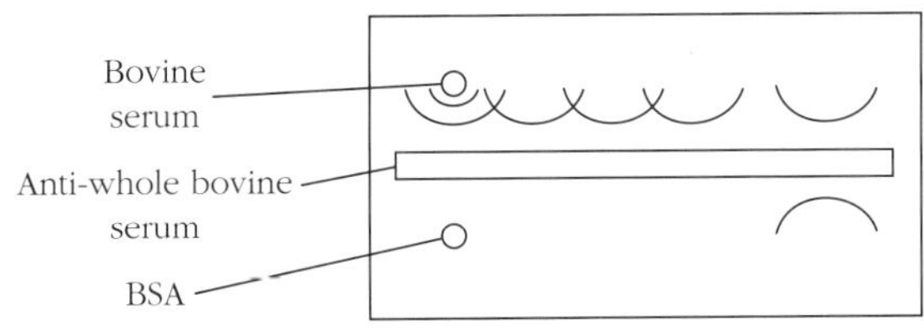

4. Bottle A: H1-C1. Bottle B: H2-C2. Bottle C: H2-C1. Bottle D: H1-C2.

5. ELISA and RIA can both be used to determine the concentration of a hapten.

6. (a) A. (b) D. (c) B. (d) E. (e) F. (f) C.

7. (a) Isolate the heavy chains from the myeloma proteins of known isotype. Immunize rabbits with the isolated heavy chains to obtain antisera specific for each heavy-chain class. Then determine which of these anti-isotype antisera reacts with myeloma protein X. (b) The level of myeloma protein X could be determined by radial immunodiffusion (Mancini method) or by a more sensitive assay such as ELISA.

8. (a) Rocket electrophoresis or Mancini radial immunodiffusion with goat anti-isotype serum specific for IgG. (b) ELISA or RIA with anti-insulin antibody and radioactively labeled or enzyme-linked insulin. (c) RIA with radiolabeled IgE. (d) Immunofluorescence with fluorochrome-labeled antibody to C3. (e) Agglutination test with type-A red blood cells. (f) Ouchterlony double immunodiffusion hamburger extract and antiserum to horsemeat. (g) Immunofluorescence with fluorochrome-labeled antibody to the syphilis spirochete.

9. (a) Antiserum #1 $K_0 = 1 \times 10^5$; antiserum #2 $K_0 = 4.5 \times 10^6$; antiserum #3 $K_0 = 4.5 \times 10^6$. (b) Each antibody has a valence of 2. (c) Antiserum #2. (d) The monoclonal antiserum #2 would be best because it recognizes a single epitope on the hormone and, therefore, would be less likely than the polyclonal antisera to cross-react with other serum proteins.

10. (a) Tube 1 contained $F(ab')_2$ fragments. Because these fragments contain two antigen-binding sites, they can cross-link and eventually agglutinate SRBCs. Activation of complement by IgG requires the presence of the Fc fragment, which is missing from $F(ab')_2$ fragments. (b) Tube 2 contained Fab fragments. Single-valent Fab fragments can bind to SRBCs and inhibit subsequent agglutination by whole anti-SRBC. (c) Tube 3 contained intact antibody. (d) Tube 4 contained Fc fragments. These fragments lack antigen-binding sites and thus cannot mediate any antibody effector functions.

Chapter 7

1. (a) False: An $HGPRT^-$ myeloma cell lacks the enzyme to utilize hypoxanthine. (b) True. (c) True. (d) False: Hypoxanthine allows cell growth by the salvage pathway. (e) False: The unfused revertant would grow in HAT medium making it impossible to select for the hybridomas.

2. Myeloma cells suitable for hybridoma production (1) exhibit immortal growth, enabling the hybridoma to be cultured indefinitely; (2) are Ab^-, ensuring that the hybridoma only secretes antibody characteristic of the plasma-cell fusion partner; and (3) are $HGPRT^-$, ensuring that unfused myeloma cells cannot grow in HAT-selection medium.

3. In the absence of aminopterin, you could not select for the hybridoma because both the fused and unfused cells would grow using the de novo pathway.

4. (a) The hybridoma formed from B-lymphoma cells and human myeloma cells was produced in order to obtain sufficient quantities of the B-lymphoma antibody. This monoclonal antibody (Ab-1) was then used to immunize mice in order to obtain mouse spleen cells primed against the B-lymphoma antibody. When these spleen cells were fused with mouse myeloma cells, hybridomas were produced that secreted antibody against the antibody on B-lymphoma cells. These hybridomas had to be screened to distinguish those that secreted anti-isotype monoclonal antibody from those secreting anti-idiotype monoclonal antibody

(Ab-2), which was desired. (b) To identify hybridomas producing anti-idiotype monoclonal antibody (Ab-2), the mouse hybridoma supernatants could be tested for their ability to bind to the human monoclonal B-lymphoma antibody (Ab-1) and to normal human antibodies. The desired anti-idiotype monoclonal (Ab-2) would only bind to Ab-1 and not to other normal human immunoglobulins.

5. The mouse antibody will (1) be polyclonal and, therefore, recognize many different epitopes on IL-2; (2) have a heterogeneous affinity for IL-2; and (3) consist of more than one isotype. A monoclonal antibody to IL-2 is homogeneous and thus recognizes a single epitope, has a homogeneous affinity for IL-2, and is of a single isotype.

6. If the epitope density on the antigen is very low, a monoclonal antibody may not be able to cross-link antigen molecules, which is necessary for precipitate formation. Because polyclonal antibodies recognize multiple epitopes, they are more likely than monoclonal antibodies to cross-link multiple antigen molecules.

7. Because different antigens can have identical or similar epitopes, a monoclonal antibody to a particular epitope on one antigen may also bind to the same epitope on similar antigens.

8. (a) If the epitope density is low enough, then precipitation in an immunodiffusion assay may not occur. (b) If the monoclonal antibody is specific for a conformational epitope, it may fail to react in a Western-blot assay because the SDS used in this assay may so disrupt the tertiary structure of the antigen that the conformational epitope is destroyed. (c) For the same reason cited in (a) above.

9. (a) Western blot: Electrophorese the HIV antigens, transfer the HIV-antigen bands to a suitable filter, and then flood the filter with either monoclonal A or B; repeat this procedure using the other monoclonal. If both monoclonals react with the same antigen component, then they may be the same. Immunoabsorption: Prepare an immunosorbent column with monoclonal A and one with monoclonal B. Pass a solution of HIV antigens through one of the columns, collect the antigen-depleted effluent, and pass this effluent through the second column. If the second column retains antigen, then the antibodies are different. (b) Sequence both monoclonal antibodies. If the variable regions are the same in monoclonal A and B, then they are the same antibody.

10. (a) Four different antigen-binding sites (indicated in boldface) and 10 different antibody molecules: $\mathbf{H_sL_s}/H_sL_s$, $\mathbf{H_mL_m}/H_mL_m$, $\mathbf{H_sL_m}/H_sL_m$, $\mathbf{H_mL_s}/H_mL_s$, H_sL_s/H_mL_m, H_sL_s/H_sL_m, H_sL_s/H_mL_s, H_mL_m/H_sL_m, H_mL_m/H_mL_s, and H_sL_m/H_mL_s. (b) Two different antigen-binding sites and three different antibody molecules: $\mathbf{H_sL_s}/H_sL_s$, $\mathbf{H_mL_s}/H_mL_s$, and H_sL_s/H_mL_s. (c) One binding site and one antibody molecule: $\mathbf{H_sL_s}/H_sL_s$.

11. Normal cells will not be killed because the immunotoxin lacks the binding polypeptide of the toxin. Thus, if the antibody is degraded, the toxin will be unable to get into cells.

Chapter 8

1. (a) False: V and C are located on separate chromosomes and cannot be brought together during gene rearrangement. (b) True. (c) True. (d) True. (e) True. (f) True.

2. See a–f below.

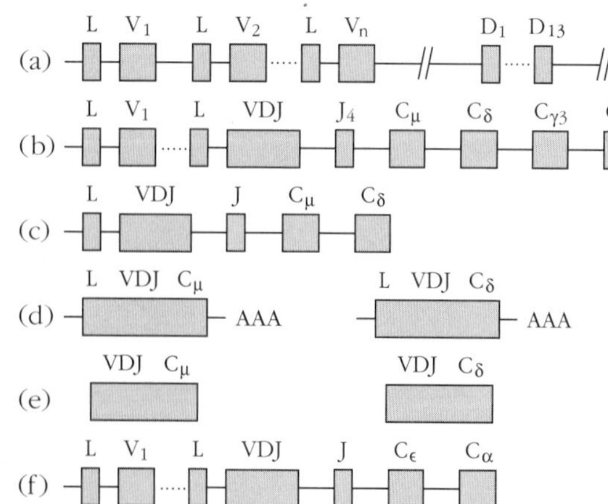

3. Because the recombination signal sequences (RSSs) flanking the V_H and J_H gene segments both contain a 23-bp (2-turn) spacer (see Figure 8-5b). According to the one-turn/two-turn joining rule, signal sequences having a two-turn spacer can only join with signal sequences having a one-turn (12-bp) spacer.

4. Light chains: 500 $V_L \times 4\ J_L = 2 \times 10^3$
Heavy chains: 300 $V_H \times 15\ D_H \times 4\ J_H = 1.8 \times 10^4$
Antibody molecules: $(2 \times 10^3$ LCs$) \times (1.8 \times 10^4$ HCs$)$ $= 3.6 \times 10^7$

5. (a) 1, 2, 3. (b) 3. (c) 3. (d) 5. (e) 2, 3, 4.

6. (a) Progenitor B cell: no cytoplasmic or membrane staining with either reagent. (b) Pre-B cell: anti-μ staining in cytoplasm and on membrane. (c) Immature B cell: anti-μ staining in cytoplasm and on membrane. (d) Mature B cell: anti-μ and anti-δ staining in cytoplasm and on membrane. (e) Plasma cell: anti-μ in cytoplasm; no membrane staining but pentameric IgM is secreted.

7. Somatic mutation contributes to the variability of all three complementarity-determining regions. Additional variability is generated in the CDR3 of both heavy and light chains by junctional flexibility, which occurs during heavy-chain D-J and V-DJ rearrangements and light-chain V-J rearrangements, and by N-nucleotide addition at the heavy-chain D-J and V-DJ joints.

8. (a) R: Productive rearrangement of heavy-chain allele 1 must have occurred since the cell line expresses heavy chains encoded by this allele. (b) G: Allelic exclusion forbids heavy-chain allele 2 from undergoing either productive or nonproductive rearrangement. (c) NP: The κ genes rearrange before the λ genes. Since the cell line expresses λ light chains, both κ alleles must have undergone nonproductive rearrangement, thus permitting λ-gene rearrangement to occur. (d) NP: Same reason as given in (c) above. (e) R: Productive rearrangement of λ-chain allele 1 must have occurred since the cell line expresses λ light chains encoded by this allele. (f) G: Allelic exclusion forbids λ-chain allele 2 from undergoing either productive or nonproductive rearrangement.

9. The κ-chain DNA must have the germ-line configuration because a productive H-chain rearrangement must occur before the κ-chain DNA can begin to rearrange.

10. (a) No. (b) Yes. (c) No. (d) No. (e) Yes.

11. Random addition of N nucleotides at the V-D-J junctions contributes to the diversity within the CDR3 of heavy chains but can result in a nonproductive rearrangement if the nucleotide addition does not preserve the triplet reading frame.

12. (a) Sample B from liver cells. (b) Sample C from pre-B lymphoma cells (both H chain alleles are rearranged). (c) Sample A from IgM-secreting myeloma cells (one H chain allele is rearranged and one L chain allele is rearranged).

13. Joining of variable-region gene segments (V_L-J_L and V_H-D_H-J_H) junctional flexibility, N-nucleotide addition, somatic mutation.

14.

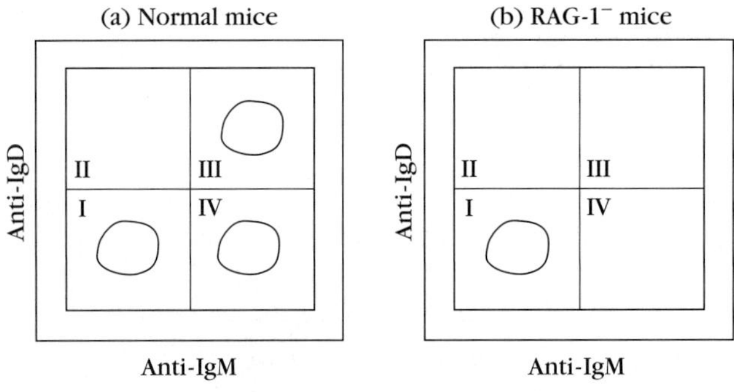

CHAPTER 9

1. (a) True. (b) True.

2. (a) S. (b) both (S and C). (c) S. (d) C. (e) both (S and C). (f) S. (g) C.

3. (a) Strain A. (b) Strain B. (c) Strain A. (d) To introduce strain-A parental alleles at all loci except for the selected MHC. (e) To achieve homozygosity within the MHC: (f) To identify progeny that are homozygous *b/b* within the MHC.

4. Liver cells: Class I K^b, K^k, D^b, D^k, L^k, L^b. Macrophages: Class I K^b, K^k, D^b, D^k, L^b, L^k. Class II $IA\alpha^k\beta^k$, $IA\alpha^b\beta^b$, $IA\alpha^k\beta^b$, $IA\alpha^b\beta^k$, $IE\alpha^k\beta^k$, $IE\alpha^b\beta^b$, $IE\alpha^k\beta^b$, $IE\alpha^b\beta^k$.

5.

	MHC molecules expressed on the membrane of the transfected L cells					
Transfected gene	D^k	D^b	K^k	K^b	IA^k	IA^b
None	+	−	+	−	−	−
K^b	+	−	+	+	−	−
$IA\alpha^b$	+	−	+	−	−	−
$IA\beta^b$	+	−	+	−	−	−
$IA\alpha^b$ and $IA\beta^b$	+	−	+	−	−	+

6. (a) SLJ macrophages express the following MHC molecules: K^s, D^s, L^s, and IA^s. Because of the deletion of the *IEα* locus, IE^s is not expressed by these cells. (b) The transfected cells would express one heterologous IE molecule, $IE\alpha^k\beta^s$ and one homologous IE molecule, $IE\alpha^k\beta^k$, in addition to the molecules listed in (a).

7. See Figures 5-4 and 9-5.

8. The polymorphic residues are clustered in short stretches primarily within the membrane-distal domains of the class I and class II MHC molecules. These regions form the peptide-binding cleft of MHC molecules. MHC polymorphism is thought to arise by gene conversion of short nearly homologous DNA sequences within unexpressed pseudogenes in the MHC to functional class I or class II genes.

9. (a) The proliferation of and IL-2 production by T_H cells is detected in assay 1, and the killing of LCM-infected target cells by cytotoxic T lymphocytes (CTLs) is detected in assay 2. Thus, assay 1 is a class II functional assay, and assay 2 is a class I functional assay. (b) CLass II IA^k molecules are required in assay 1, and class I D^d molecules are required in assay 2. (c) You could transfect L cells with the IA^k gene and determine the response of the transfected cells in assay 1. Similarly, you could transfect a separate sample of L cells with the D^d gene and determine the response of the transfected cells in assay 2. In each case, a positive response would confirm the identity of the MHC molecules required for LCM-specific activity of the spleen cells. As a control in each case, L cells should be transfected with a different class I or class II MHC gene and assayed in the appropriate assay. (d) The immunized spleen cells express both IA^k and D^d molecules. Of the listed strains, only A.TL and BALB/c × B10.A (F_1) express both of these MHC molecules, and thus these are the only strains from which the spleen cells could have been isolated.

10. It is not possible to predict. Since the peptide-binding cleft is identical, both MHC molecules should bind the same peptide. However, the amino acid differences outside the cleft might prevent recognition of the second MHC molecule by the T-cell receptor on the T_C cells.

11. Use monoclonal antibodies specific for each MHC haplotype to determine if both strains express the same set of MHC molecules.

12. If RBCs expressed MHC molecules, then extensive tissue typing would be required before a blood transfusion, and only a few individuals would be acceptable donors for a given individual.

CHAPTER 10

1. (a) Self-MHC restriction is the attribute of T cells that limits their response to antigen associated with self-MHC molecules on the membrane of antigen-presenting cells or target cells. $CD4^+$ T_H cells are class II MHC restricted, and $CD8^+$ T_C cells are class I MHC restricted. (b) Antigen processing involves the degradation of protein antigens into peptides that associate with class I or class II MHC molecules. (c) Endogenous antigens are synthesized within altered self-cells (e.g., virus-infected cells or tumor cells), are processed in the cytosolic pathway, and are presented by class I MHC molecules to $CD8^+$ T_C cells. (d) Exogenous antigens are internalized by antigen-presenting cells, processed in the endocytic pathway, and presented by class II MHC molecules to $CD4^+$ T_H cells.

2. (a) Class I MHC molecules only display peptides derived from endogenous antigens by the cytosolic processing pathway. Since the killed influenza virus cannot replicate in the target cells, no endogenous viral proteins are synthesized. (b) Class II MHC molecules only display peptides produced in the endocytic processing pathway, which is inhibited by chloroquine. Thus, this compound inhibits the response of class II-restricted T cells. (c) Emitine inhibits protein synthesis and thus prevents synthesis of viral proteins in target cells infected with live influenza virus. As a result, class I-restricted T cells do not respond.

3. (a) Chloroquine inhibits the endocytic processing pathway, so that the APCs cannot display peptides derived from native lysozyme. The synthetic lysozyme peptide will exchange with other peptides associated with class II molecules on the APC membrane, so that it will be displayed to the T_H cells and induce their activation. (b) Delay of chloroquine addition provides time for native lysozyme to be degraded in the endocytic pathway.

4. (a) R. (b) R. (c) NR. (d) R. (e) NR. (f) R.

CHAPTER 11

1. (a) False: The distance between CD4 and the TCR is too great for them to coprecipitate; however, CD3 and the TCR are close enough that they will coprecipitate in response to monoclonal anti-CD3. (b) True. (c) True. (d) False: The TCR variable-region genes are located on different chromosomes from the Ig variable-region genes. (e) False: The $\alpha\beta$ and $\gamma\delta$ T-cell receptor each has a single binding site for the antigen-MHC complex.

2. Functional $\alpha\beta$ TCR genes from a T_C clone specific for one hapten on an H-2^d target cell were transfected into another T_C clone specific for a second hapten on an H-2^k target cell. Cytolysis assays revealed that the transfected T_C cells only killed target cells that presented antigen associated with the original MHC restriction element. See Figure 11-9.

3. See Figure 11-2.

4. (a) CD3 is a complex of three dimers containing five different polypeptide chains. It is required for the expression of the T-cell receptor and plays a role in signal transduction across the membrane. CD3 and the T-cell receptor associate to form the TCR-CD3 membrane complex. (b) CD4 and CD8 interact with the membrane-proximal domains of class II and class I MHC molecules, respectively, thereby increasing the avidity of the interaction between T cells and antigen-MHC complexes. CD4 and CD8 also play a role in signal transduction. (c) CD2 and other accessory molecules (LFA-1, CD28, and CD45R) bind to other cell-adhesion molecules on antigen-presenting cells or target cells. The initial contact between a T cell and antigen-presenting cell or target cell probably is mediated by these cell-adhesion molecules. Subsequently, the T-cell receptor interacts with antigen-MHC complexes. These molecules also function in signal transduction.

5. (a) TCR. (b) TCR. (c) Ig. (d) TCR/Ig. (e) TCR. (f) TCR/Ig. (g) Ig.

6. (a) The three assumptions were: 1) That the TCR was an integral membrane protein and was, therefore, transcribed on polyribosomes. They, therefore, isolated the polyribosomal mRNA fraction and eliminated the cytoplasmic mRNA. 2) That subtractive hybridization could be used to subtract the mRNA common to both B and T so that only the unique T-cell mRNA remained unhybridized. 3) That the TCR genes undergo DNA rearrangement and, therefore, can be detected by Southern blotting. (b) If they wanted to identify the IL-4 gene they should perform subtractive hybridization using a T_H clone as an IL-4 producer and a T_c clone as a source of mRNA lacking the message for IL-4. In addition, the gene for IL-4 would not be expected to rearrange, and therefore they could not look for gene rearrangement using Southern blot analysis.

7. (a) cDNA source, 1; mRNA source, 2. (b) cDNA source, 3; mRNA source, 1 or 2. (c) cDNA source, 5; mRNA source, 6. (d) cDNA source, 4; mRNA source, 7. (e) cDNA source, 1, 2, or 3; mRNA source, 8.

8.

	Release of ^{51}Cr from LCM-Infected target cells			
Source of spleen cells from LCM-infected mice	B10.D2 (H-2^d)	B10 (H-2^b)	B10.BR (H-2^k)	F_1 (BALB/c × B10) (H-$2^{b/d}$)
B10.D2 (H-2^d)	+	–	–	+
B10 (H-2^b)	–	+	–	+
BALB/c (H=2^d)	+	–	–	+
BALB/b (H-2^b)	–	+	–	+

CHAPTER 12

1. (a) The immature thymocytes express both CD4 and CD8, whereas the mature CD8$^+$ thymocytes do not express CD4. To distinguish these cells, the thymocytes are double-stained with fluochrome-labeled anti-CD4 and anti-CD8 and analyzed in a FACS. (b) See the table below.

Transgenic mouse	Immature thymocytes	Mature CD8$^+$ thymocytes
H-2^k female	+	+
H-2^k male	+	–
H-2^d female	+	–
H-2^d male	+	–

(c) Because the gene encoding the H-Y antigen is on the Y chromosome, this antigen is not present in females. Thymocytes bearing the transgenic T-cell receptor, which is H-2^k restricted, would undergo positive selection in both male and female H-2^k transgenics. However, subsequent negative selection would eliminate thymocytes bearing the transgenic receptor, which is specific for H-Y antigen, in the male H-2^k transgenics (see Figure 12-8). (d) Because the H-2^d transgenics would not express the appropriate MHC molecules, T-cells bearing the transgenic T-cell receptor would not undergo positive selection.

2. Cyclosporin A blocks production of NF-ATc, one of the transcription factors necessary for proliferation of antigen-activated T_H cells. See Figure 12-14.

3. (a) NF-κB and NF-ATc. (b) IL-2 enhancer.

4.

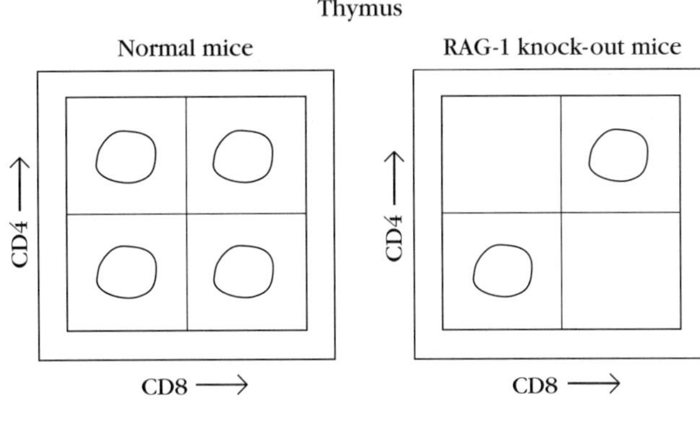

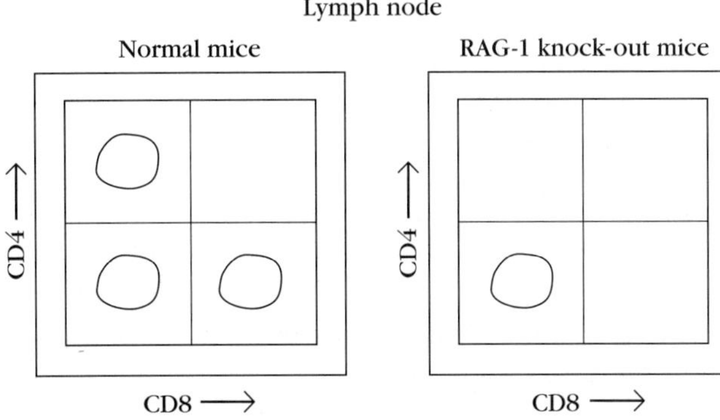

5. (a) Class I K, D, and L molecules and class II IA molecules. (b) Class I molecules only. (c) The H-2^b mice should have both CD4$^+$ and CD8$^+$ T cells because both class I and class II MHC molecules would be present on thymic stromal cells during positive selection. H-2^b mice with knock out of the *IAβ* gene would express no class II molecules; thus these mice would have only CD8$^+$ cells.

6. (a) Thymus donor in experiment A was H-2^d (BALB/c) and in experiment B was H-2^b (C57BL/6). (b) The haplotype of the thymus donor determines the MHC restriction of the T cells in the chimeric mice. Thus, H-2^b target cells were lysed in experiment B in which the thymus donor was H-2^b. (c) The H-2^k target cells were not lysed in either experiment because neither donor thymus expressed H-2^k MHC molecules; thus H-2^k–reactive T cells were not positively selected in the chimeric mice.

7. (a) 70% of thymocytes are expressing the T-cell receptor, the remaining cells are immature thymocytes. (b) No, because some of the CD3$^+$ cells express the γδ TCR instead of αβ. To determine the numer of CD8$^+$ T cells you need fluorescent anti-CD8 antibody.

Chapter 13

1. (a) False: The high-affinity IL-2 receptor comprises three subunits—the α, β, and γ chains—all of which are transmembrane proteins. (b) False: Anti-TAC binds to the 55-kDa α chain of the IL-2 receptor. (c) False: The receptors for some cytokines (IL-4, IL-7, IL-9, and erythropoietin) have only one chain (see Figure 13-6). (d) False: Low levels of the IL-2R β chain are expressed in resting T cells, although expression is increased greatly following activation. The α chain is expressed only by activated T cells. (e) False: The cytoplasmic domains of cytokine receptors appear to be closely associated with intracellular tyrosine kinases but do not themselves possess tyrosine kinase activity. Binding of a cytokine appears to activate these tyrosine kinases, which can then phosphorylate cellular proteins, an essential step in signal transduction.

2. Only antigen-activated T cells will proliferate, because they express the high-affinity IL-2 receptor, whereas resting T cells do not and therefore cannot respond to IL-2.

3. The TNF-α released by activated macrophages during an acute inflammatory response acts on vascular endothelial cells and macrophages inducing secretion of colony-stimulating factors (CSFs). These travel to the bone marrow where they stimulate hematopoiesis.

4. (a) Cell lines that produce high levels of a particular cytokine and cell lines that require a particular cytokine for growth. (b) The high-producing cell lines were important, especially before cloning of the cytokine genes, because they enabled researchers to obtain larger amounts of a particular cytokine. The cytokine-dependent cell lines enable researchers to determine whether a particular cytokine is present in a culture supernatant.

5. Cytokines, growth factors, and hormones are all secreted proteins that bind to receptors on target cells, eliciting various biological effects. Cytokines tend to be produced by a variety of cells, although their production is carefully regulated, and exert their effects on several cell types; most cytokines also act in an autocrine or paracrine fashion. Growth factors, unlike cytokines, are often produced constitutively. Hormones, unlike cytokines, generally act over long distances (endocrine effect) on one or a few types of target cells.

6. (a) γ chain and β chain (low level). (b) α, β, and γ chains. (c) γ chain and β chain (low level); cyclosporin A prevents the gene activation that leads to increased expression of the α and β chains. (d) γ chain and β chain (low level). (e) α, β, and γ chains. (f) β and γ chains.

7. (a) Superantigens bind to class II MHC molecules outside of the normal peptide-binding cleft; unlike normal antigens, they are not internalized and processed by antigen-presenting cells but bind directly to class II molecules. Superantigens also bind to regions of the V_β domain of the T-cell receptor that are not involved in binding normal antigenic peptides. Superantigens exhibit specificity for one or a few V_β domains; thus a given superantigen can activate all T cells that express the V_β domain(s) for which it is specific regardless of the antigenic specificity of thc T cells. (b) A given superantigen can activate 5–25% of T_H cells, leading to excessive production cytokines. The high levels of cytokines are thought to cause the symptoms associated with food poisoning and toxic-shock syndrome.

8. The receptors for IL-3, IL-5, and GM-CSF contain a common β chain, designated KH97. Since this is the signal-transducing chain, each of these cytokines probably induce a similar activation signal.

Chapter 14

1. (a) False: The indirect hemolytic plaque assay detects both IgM- and IgG-secreting plasma cells. (b) True. (c) False: IL-4 increases IgE production by inducing class switching. (d) True. (e) True. (f) True.

2. (a) Heterogeneous; low affinity; IgM. (b) Homogeneous; high affinity; IgG. (c) Heterogeneous; low affinity; IgM. (d) Heterogeneous; low affinity; IgG.

3. (a) Direct hemolytic plaque assay for 1° response (see Figure 14-3a); indirect hemolytic plaque assay for 2° response (see Figure 14-3b). (b) The direct PFC assay gives the number of IgM-secreting plasma cells. Subtract the direct PFCs from the indirect PFCs to obtain the number of IgG-secreting plasma cells. A = 310 IgM-secreting plasma cells and 33-IgG secreting plasma cells; B = 62 IgM-secreting plasma cells and 3998 IgG-secreting plasma cells; C = 366 IgM-secreting plasma cells and 20 IgG secreting plasma cells. (c) Group B illustrates the carrier effect. Only group B received a secondary immunization of both hapten and carrier, and therefore only group B has both memory B cells for DNP and memory T cells for the BSA carrier, allowing class switching from the IgM isotype to the IgG isotype.

4. The signals required for activation of naive B cells are generated by antigen-mediated cross-linkage of mIg molecules, interaction of CD40 and CD40L (contact-dependent help), and IL-1 and IL-4 derived from activated T_H cells. Additional proliferation and differentiation of the activated B cells is provided by IL-2, IL-4, IL-5, IL-6, IFN-γ, and TGF-β.

Chapter 15

1. The monoclonal Antibody to LFA-1 should block formation of the CTL–target-cell conjugate. This should inhibit killing of the target cell and, therefore, should result in diminished ^{51}Cr release in the CML assay.

2.

Population 1	Population 2	Proliferation
C57BL/6 (H-2^b)	CBA (H-2^k)	1 & 2
C57BL/6 (H-2^b)	CBA (H-2^k) mitomycin C-treated	1
C57BL/6 (H-2^b)	F_1 (CBA × C57BL/6)	1
C57BL/6 (H-2^b)	C57L (H-2^b)	Neither

3. (a) CD4$^+$ T_H cells. (b) To demonstrate the identity of the proliferating cells, you could incubate them with fluorescein-labeled anti-CD4 monoclonal antibody and rhodamine-labeled anti-CD8 monoclonal antibody. The proliferating cells will be stained only with the anti-CD4 reagent. (c) As CD4$^+$ T_H cells recognize allogeneic class II MHC molecules on the stimulator cells, they are activated and begin to secrete IL-2, which then autostimulates T_H-cell proliferation. Thus, the extent of proliferation is directly related to the level of IL-2 produced.

4. (a) Neither. (b) Both. (c) CTL. (d) CTL. (e) T_H cell. (f) CTL. (g) T_H cell. (h) CTL. (i) T_H cell. (j) T_H cell. (k) T_H cell. (l) Both. (m) CTL. (n) Both. (o) Both. (p) T_H cell. (q) Neither. (r) CTL.

5.

Source of primed spleen cells	[^{51}Cr] release from LCM-infected target cells			
	B10.D2 (H-2^d)	B10 (H-2^b)	B10.BR (H-2^k)	F_1 (BALB/c × B10) (H-2$^{b/d}$)
B10.D2 (H-2^d)	+	−	−	+
B10 (H-2^b)	−	+	−	+
BALB/c (H-2^d)	+	−	−	+
(BALB/c × B10) (H-2$^{b/d}$)	+	+	−	+

6. To determine T_c activity specific for influenza, perform a CML reaction by incubating spleen cells from the infected mouse with influenza-infected syngeneic target cells. To determine T_H activity, incubate the spleen cells from the infected mouse with syngeneic APCs presenting influenza peptides, and measure IL-2 production.

Chapter 16

1. (a) False: Immature B cells are tolerized more readily. (b) True. (c) False: Antigenic competition will reduce the response to SRBC. (d) True. (e) True. (f) True. (g) False: TEPC-15 is a myeloma-derived antibody specific for phosphorylcholine. It can serve as an antigen to which anti-idiotype antibody can bind. (h) True. (i) False: Deaggregated antigens induce tolerance more readily because they are less able to be internalized and processed by antigen-presenting cells. It is thought that in the absence of a co-stimulatory signal, a state of tolerance is more readily achieved. (j) True. (k) False: Some T-cell tolerance occurs by clonal anergy.

2. Immunize an animal with monoclonal antibody (Ab-1) specific for hepatitis B virus to produce anti-idiotype antibody (Ab-2). Then use the anti-idiotype antibody to immunize other animals. The immunized animals should now be protected against hepatitis B virus.

3. Remove the spleen from the tolerant animal and divide the spleen cells into two aliquots. To remove T cells from one aliquot, add fluorescein-labeled anti-CD3 and then pass the aliquot through a FACS; the remaining cells in this aliquot will include B cells. To remove B cells from the other aliquot, add fluorescein-labeled anti-IgM, which will react with mIgM on B cells, and then pass the aliquot through a FACS; the remaining cells in this aliquot will include T cells. Now culture the B-cell aliquot from the tolerant mouse with syngeneic T cells from a normal mouse, and culture the T-cell aliquot from the tolerant mouse with syngeneic B cells from a normal mouse. Add antigen A to both cell cultures and see if plasma cells to antigen A are produced by performing a hemolytic plaque assay. This procedure should reveal whether the B cells or T cells or both populations are tolerant to antigen A.

4. (a) Paratope: an antigenic determinant within the antigen-binding site of an antibody. (b) Epitope: a site on an antigen that interacts with an antibody or T-cell receptor; also called antigenic determinant. (c) Idiotype: an antigenic determinant within the variable-region of an antibody; each antibody has multiple idiotopes, and the entire set constitutes its idiotype.

5. (a) Both single and double transgenics carried the anti-HEL transgene. Because the transgene is already rearranged, the developing B cells do not rearrange other immunoglobulin H and L chain genes and, therefore, only express the rearranged immunoglobulin encoded by the transgene. (b) Add radiolabeled HEL and see if it binds to the B-cell membrane using autoradiography. To determine the isotype on the membrane antibody (mIg) on these B cells, incubate the cells with fluorochrome-labeled antibodies specific for each isotype (e.g., anti-μ, anti-γ, etc.) and see which fluorescent antibodies stain the B cells. (c) So that the HEL transgene could be induced by adding Zn^{2+} to the mouse's water supply. (d) Isolate B cells and T cells from the transgenic mice using a FACS as described in answer **3**. Mix the transgenic B cells with normal syngeneic T cells, and mix the transgenic T cells with normal syngeneic B cells. Transfer each cell mixture to lethally x-irradiated, syngeneic adoptive-transfer recipients, and challenge the recipients with HEL. Determine if plasma cells secreting anti-HEL are generated by using a hemolytic plaque assay with HEL-conjugated SRBCs.

6. In the Kappler and Marrack experiment, expression of the $V_\beta17a$ TCR was assessed in IE^+ and IE^- mice. In the IE^+ mice the expression of IE on thymic stromal cells resulted in negative selection (clonal deletion) of the self-reactive T cells. In Burkly's experiment IE^- mice were used, and an IE transgene was engineered to an insulin promoter. Therefore, the expression of IE was limited to the pancreatic islet cells, and IE was not expressed in the thymus. As T cells expressing the $V_\beta17a$ TCR matured in the thymus of these mice, they were not exposed to IE on thymic stromal cells, and therefore they were not eliminated by negative selection. When these T cells encountered the IE molecule on a non-antigen-presenting cell (in the absence of a co-stimulatory signal), the T cells entered an anergic state.

7. (a) The T cells would not be MHC restricted. Instead T cells bearing receptors specific for antigen alone or antigen associated with non-self–MHC molecules might also mature. (b) Self-reactive T cells would be released from the thymus, and autoimmunity could develop.

8. (a) When animals were tolerized with high doses of an antigen, the tolerant state could be transferred to syngeneic mice by transferring the tolerant T cells. (b) Inability to identify a unique membrane molecule on the T_s cells distinct from known membrane markers on the $CD8^+$ T_c cells; inability to identify and characterize unique rearranged TCR genes in T_s hybridomas; inability to maintain stable T_s clones capable of mediating suppression; and inability to clone antigen-specific suppressor factors. (c) Absorption of IL-2 by activated T_c cells would deplete the necessary IL-2 from the culture supernatant; antagonistic effects of cytokines produced by different T-cell subpopulations; diversion of the immune response to a different isotype or a different branch of immune activity that was not being monitored and so went undetected.

9. (a) In the H-2^b mice, T cells expressing the transgene will make it through both positive and negative selection in the thymus. In the H-$2^{b/d}$ mice, T cells expressing the transgene will be selected in positive selection but will be eliminated as self-reactive in negative selection. (b) H-$2^{b/d}$ mice were used so that T cells expressing the transgene could make it through positive selection. If H-2^d mice had been used instead, the T cells expressing the transgene would not have matured within the thymus. (c) A CML assay was used in which the CTL cells expressing the transgene were incubated with ^{51}Cr-labeled target cells that expressed L^d molecules.

Chapter 17

1. (a) True. (b) True. (c) True. (d) True. (e) False: Enveloped viruses can be lysed by complement because their outer envelope is derived from the plasma membrane of a host cell. (f) True.

2. Serum IgM is in a planar form in which the complement-binding sites in the Fc region are not accessible. Only after binding to antigen does IgM assume a conformation in which the complement-binding sites are accessible.

3. A C3 deficiency is more serious clinically because it impairs both the classical and alternative pathways. In contrast, with a C1 deficiency, the alternative pathway would still operate.

4. The degraded antibody would be less able both to serve as an opsonin and to initiate complement activation.

5. (a) The initial step in the classical pathway is mediated by immune complexes involving IgG or IgM; the alternative pathway generally is initiated by bacterial cell-wall components. (b) See Figure 17-1. The two pathways differ in the reactions that generate C5 convertase. (c) Both pathways mediate all the biological effects of complement, namely, cell lysis, leukocyte extravasation and chemotaxis, degranulation of mast cells and basophils, clearance of antigen by opsonization and solubization of immune complexes, and viral neutralization.

6. If the C5b67 complex binds to healthy cells, lysis of these innocent-bystander cells may result. This is most likely to occur when C5b67 is formed on immune complexes or other noncellular activating surfaces, since in this case C5b67 cannot anchor into the surface and is released. Binding of S protein, a complement regulatory protein, to released C5b67 prevents its insertion into the membrane of nearby healthy cells.

7. (a) 4. (b) 5. (c) 6. (d) 2. (e) 7. (f) 11. (g) 3. (h) 1. (i) 8. (j) 10. (k) 9. (l) 12.

8. See Figure 17-8. (a) False: C1Inh dissociates $C1qr_2s_2$, thereby inhibiting the classical pathway. (b) True. (c) True. (d) False: C4bBP is a soluble regulatory factor that binds to C4b attached to a surface. This binding induces inactivation of C4b by factor I. (e) False: HRF binds to C5b678, thereby preventing binding of C9 and assembly of poly-C9. (f) True.

9.

	Component knocked out						
	Clq	C4	C3	C5	C6	C9	Factor B
Complement Activation							
Formation of C3 convertase in classical pathway	A	A	NE	NE	NE	NE	NE
Formation of C3 convertase in alternative pathway	NE	NE	A	NE	NE	NE	A
Formation of C5 convertase in classical pathway	A	A	A	NE	NE	NE	NE
Formation of C5 convertase in alternative pathway	NE	NE	A	NE	NE	NE	A
Effector Functions							
C3b-mediated opsonization	D	D	A	NE	NE	NE	D
Neutrophil chemotaxis	D	D	D	D	D	NE	D
Cell lysis	D	D	A	A	A	A	D

CHAPTER 18

1. (a) False: IgE is increased. (b) False: IL-4 increases IgE production. (c) False: IgE is not able to pass through the placenta like IgG. (d) False: Type III hypersensitivity involves immune-complex deposition; mast-cell degranulation plays only a minor role. (e) False: Most pollen allergens contain multiple allergenic components.

2. (a) The complete antibodies would cross-link FcεRI molecules on the membrane of mast cells and basophils, resulting in their activation and degranulation. The released mediators would induce vasodilation, smooth-muscle contraction, and a local wheal and flare reaction. Because the Fab fragment is monovalent, it cannot cross-link FcεRI molecules and thus cannot induce degranulation. However, this type of antireceptor antibody could bind to FcεRI and might thereby block binding of IgE to the receptors. (b) The response induced by complete anti-FcεRI antibodies does not depend on allergen-specific IgE and thus would be similar in allergic and nonallergic mice. Injection of Fab fragments of anti-FcεRI might prevent allergic mice from reacting to an allergen if these fragments block binding of IgE to mast cells and basophils.

3. Engineer chimeric monoclonal antibodies to snake venom that contain mouse variable regions but human heavy- and light-chain constant regions (see Figure 7-11).

4. (a) Type I hypersensitivity: localized atopic reaction resulting from allergen cross-linkage of fixed IgE on skin mast cells inducing degranulation and mediator release. (b) Type III hypersensitivity: immune complexes of antibody and insect antigens form and are deposited locally, causing an Arthus-type reaction resulting from complement activation and complement split products. (c) Type IV hypersensitivity: sensitized T_{DTH} cells release their mediators inducing macrophage accumulation and activation. Tissue damage results from lysosomal enzymes released by the macrophage.

5.

Immunologic event	Type I hypersensitivity	Type II hypersensitivity	Type III hypersensitivity	Type IV hypersensitivity
IgE-mediated degranulation of mast cells	+			
Lysis of antibody-coated blood cells by complement		+		
Tissue destruction in response to poison oak				+
C3a- and C5a-mediated mast-cell degranulation		(some)	+	
Chemotaxis of neutrophils			+	
Chemotaxis of eosinophils	+			
Activation of macrophages by IFN-γ				+
Deposition of antigen-antibody complexes on basement membranes of capillaries			+	
Sudden death due to vascular collapse (shock) shortly after injection or ingestion of antigen	+			

Chapter 19

1. (a) 6. (b) 9. (c) 8. (d) 10. (e) 12. (f) 7. (g) 3. (h) 11. (i) 2. (j) 1. (k) 5. (l) 4.

2. (a) EAE is induced by injecting mice or rats with myelin basic protein in complete Freund's adjuvant. (b) The animals that recover from EAE are now resistant to EAE. If they are given a second injection of myelin basic protein in complete Freund's adjuvant, they no longer develop EAE. (c) If T cells from mice with EAE are transferred to normal syngeneic mice, the mice will develop EAE.

3. A number of viruses have been shown to possess sequences in common with sequences in myelin basic protein (MBP). Since the encephalitogenic peptides of MBP are known, it is possible to test these peptides to see if they bear sequence homology to known viral protein sequences. Computer analysis has revealed a number of viruses that bear sequence homology to MBP. By immunizing rabbits with these viral sequences, it was possible to induce EAE. The studies on the encephalitogenic peptides of MBP also showed that different peptides induced EAE in different strains. Thus the MHC haplotype will determine which cross-reacting viral peptides will be presented and, therefore, will influence the development of EAE.

4. (1) A virus might express an antigenic determinant that cross-reacts with a self-component. (2) A viral infection might induce localized concentrations of IFN-γ. The IFN-γ might then induce inappropriate expression of class II MHC molecules on nonantigen-presenting cells, enabling self-peptides presented together with the class II MHC molecules on these cells to activate T_H cells. (3) A virus may damage a given organ resulting in release of antigens that are normally sequestered from the immune system.

5. (a) So that the IFN-γ transgene would only be expressed by pancreatic beta cells. (b) The mice developed diabetes, and there was a cellular infiltration of lymphocytes and macrophages similar to that seen in insulin-dependent diabetes mellitus. (c) The IFN-γ transgene induced the pancreatic beta cells to express class II MHC molecules. (d) A localized viral infection in the pancreas might result in the localized production of IFN-γ by activated T cells. The IFN-γ might then induce the inappropriate expression of class II MHC molecules by pancreatic beta cells as well as the production of other cytokines such as IL-1 or TNF. If self-peptides are presented by the class II MHC molecules, then IL-1 might provide the necessary co-stimulatory signal to activate T cells against the self-peptides. Alternatively, the TNF might also cause localized cellular damage.

6. Increased expression of IL-2 and the IL-2 receptor on T cells may promote T-cell activation, resulting in production of other cytokines and possibly leading to various effector functions that might cause tissue damage.

7. Anti-CD4 monoclonal antibodies have been used to block T_H activity. Monoclonal antibodies specific for the high-affinity IL-2 receptor have been tried to block activated T_H cells. The association of some autoimmune diseases with restricted T-cell receptor expression has prompted researchers to use monoclonal antibody specific for T-cell receptors carrying particular V_β domains.

Chapter 20

1. (a) True. (b) True. (c) True. (d) True.

2. Attenuated organisms are capable of limited growth within the host cells and are, therefore, processed by the endogenous processing route and presented on the membrane of infected host cells together with class I MHC molecules. These vaccines, therefore, usually can induce a cell-mediated immune response. In addition, because attenuated organisms are capable of limited growth within the host, it is often not necessary to give a second booster with the vaccine. Also, if the attenuated vaccine is able to grow along mucous membranes, then the vaccine will be able to induce the production of secretory IgA.

3. The antitoxin was given to inactivate any toxin that might be produced if *Clostridium tetani* infected the wound. The antitoxin was necessary since the child had not been previously immunized and, therefore, did not have circulating levels of antibody to tetanus toxin or memory B cells specific for tetanus toxin. If the child steps on a rusty nail 3 years later, the child will not be immune and will, therefore, require another dose of antitoxin.

4. The Sabin polio vaccine is attenuated, whereas the Salk vaccine is inactivated. The Sabin vaccine thus has the usual advantages of an attenuated vaccine compared with inactivated vaccines. Moreover, since the Sabin vaccine is capable of limited growth along the gastrointestinal tract, it induces production of secretory IgA.

5. The amphipathic peptides are most likely to represent T-cell epitopes, and the mobile peptides are most likely to represent accessible B-cell epitopes.

6. The MHC molecules of the strain B mice are not able to bind the peptide and present it to T cells. You could test this hypothesis by transfecting the genes encoding the MHC molecules of the strain A and strain B mice into L cells and then incubating the transfected L cells with the peptide to see if they can activate T cells.

7. Pathogens with a short incubation period (e.g., influenza virus) cause disease symptoms before a memory-cell response can be induced. Protection against such pathogens is achieved by repeated reimmunizations to maintain high levels of neutralizing antibody. For pathogens with a longer incubation period (e.g., polio virus), the memory-cell response occurs sufficiently rapidly to prevent development of symptoms, and high levels of neutralizing antibody at the time of infection are unnecessary.

8. The attenuated Sabin vaccine can cause life-threatening infection in individuals, such as children with AIDS, whose immune systems are severely suppressed.

Chapter 21

1. (a) Because the infected target cells expressed H-2^k MHC molecules, but the primed T cells were H-2^b restricted. (b) Because the influenza nucleoprotein is processed by the endogenous processing pathway and the resulting peptides are presented by class I MHC molecules. (c) Probably because the transfected class I D^b molecule is only able to present peptide 365–380 and not peptide 50–63. Alternatively, peptide 50–63 may not be a T-cell epitope. (d) These results suggest that a cocktail of several immunogenic peptides would be more likely to be presented by different MHC haplotypes in humans and would provide the best vaccines for humans.

2. (a) Nonspecific host defenses include ciliated epithelial cells; bactericidal substances in mucous secretions; complement split products activated by the alternative pathway that serve both as opsonins and as chemotactic factors; and phagocytic cells. (b) Specific host defenses include secretory IgA in the mucous secretions; IgG and IgM in the tissue fluids; the classical complement pathway; complement split products; the opsonins (IgM, IgG, and C3b); and phagocytic cells. Cytokines produced during the specific immune response, including IFN-γ, TNF, IL-1, and IL-6, contribute to the overall intensity of the inflammatory response.

3. Humoral antibody peaks within a few days of infection and binds to the influenza HA glycoprotein blocking viral infection of host epithelial cells. However, the antibody is strain specific and therefore its major role is in protecting against re-infection with the same strain of influenza. The cell-mediated response peaks about 8 days after infection and serves to kill virally infected self-cells. The CTL response is necessary to eliminate the virus. Unlike the humoral antibody response, which is strain specific, the CTL response is able to recognize epitopes shared by different influenza subtypes.

4. (a) The fact that the CTL response is cross-reactive means that it might be possible to induce an immune response to several human pandemic subtypes with a single vaccine. However, because the MHC haplotype determines which peptides are presented to the T cells, it will be necessary to identify immunodominant T-cell epitopes for individuals with different MHC haplotypes and then prepare a cocktail of synthetic peptides. (b) The nucleoprotein can serve as a potential vaccine because it will be processed by the endogenous processing pathway and presented together with class I MHC molecules on the membrane of the infected host cell.

5. (a) IA^b. (b) Because antigen-specific, MHC-restricted T_H cells participate in B-cell activation.

6. (a) African trypanosomes are capable of antigenic shifts in the variant surface glycoprotein (VSG). The antigenic shifts are accomplished as gene segments encoding part of the VSG are duplicated and translocated to transcriptionally active expression sites. (b) Plasmodium evades the immune system by continually undergoing maturational changes from sporozoite to merozoite to gametocyte, allowing the organism to continually change its surface molecules. In addition, the intracellular phases of its life cycle reduce the level of immune activation. Finally, the organism is able to slough off its circumsporozoite coat after antibody binds to it. (c) Influenza is able to evade the immune response through frequent antigenic changes in its hemagglutinin and neuraminidase glycoproteins. The antigenic changes are accomplished by the accumulation of small point mutations (antigenic drift) or through genetic reassortment of RNA between influenza virions from humans and animals (antigenic shift).

Chapter 22

1. (a) True. (b) False: X-linked agammaglobulinemia is characterized by a reduction in B cells and an absence of immunoglobulins. (c) False: Phagocytic defects result in recurrent bacterial and fungal infections. (d) True. (e) True. (f) True. (g) True. (h) False: The mice need lymphoid stem cells containing the enzymes that catalyze rearrangement of variable-region gene segments in DNA encoding immunoglobulin and the T-cell receptor. (i) False: These children are usually able to eliminate common encapsulated bacteria with antibody plus complement but are susceptible to viral, protozoan, fungal, and intracellular bacterial pathogens, which are eliminated by the cell-mediated branch of the immune system. (j) False: Humoral immunity also is affected because class II–restricted T_H cells must be activated for an antibody response to occur.

2. (a) Leukocyte-adhesion deficiency results from defective biosynthesis of the β chain of LFA-1, CR3, and CR4, which all contain the same β chain. (b) LFA-1 plays a role in cell adhesion by binding to ICAM-1 expressed on various types of cells. Binding of LFA-1 to ICAM-1 is involved in the interactions between T_H cells and B cells, between CTLs and target cells, and between circulating leukocytes and vascular endothelial cells. (c) No: Formation of T_H-cell/B-cell conjugates is required for B-cell activation. This conjugate formation depends in part on interaction between LFA-1 present on T_H cells and ICAM-1 present on B cells (see Figure 14-13a). Because this interaction is deficient in LAD patients, their ability to produce specific antibody is impaired.

3. (a) The rearranged heavy-chain genes in *scid* mice lack the D and/or J gene segments. (b) According to the model of allelic exclusion discussed in Chapter 8, a productive heavy-chain gene rearrangement must occur before κ-chain genes are rearranged. Since *scid* mice lack productive heavy-chain rearrangement, they do not attempt κ light-chain rearrangement. (c) Yes: The rearranged μ heavy-chain gene would be transcribed to yield a functional μ heavy chain. The presence of the μ heavy chain then would induce rearrangement of the κ-chain gene (see Figure 8-13). (d) The DNA encoding the β chain of the T-cell receptor would undergo defective gene rearrangement in which the D and/or J gene segments are deleted during the joining process.

4. (a) *Scid*-human mice are prepared by implanting portions of human fetal liver, thymus, and lymph nodes into *scid* mice (see Figure 2-1). (b) The fetal liver is used to provide a source of hematopoietic lymphoid stem cells. (c) The human cells are not rejected because the mouse does not have functional immunocompetent B or T cells. (d) Graft-versus-host disease does not develop because as the human T cells mature within the human thymic tissue, they are exposed to mouse MHC molecules and mouse antigens. Therefore, the human T cells become tolerant to the mouse antigens during thymic processing.

Chapter 23

1. (a) False: HIV-2 and SIV are more closely related. (b) False: HIV-1 infects chimpanzees but does not cause immune suppression. (c) True. (d) True. (e) True. (f) False: Some $CD4^-$ cells have been shown to be infected by HIV. (g) False: Patients with advanced AIDS sometimes have no detectable serum antibody to HIV. (h) False: The PCR detects HIV proviral DNA in latently infected cells. (i) True.

2. Soluble CD4 is used to bind to gp120 on the viral envelope and prevent HIV binding to $CD4^+$ cells. The major limitation of this approach is the extremely short serum half-life of soluble CD4. To overcome this limitation, the CD4 gene is engineered with the constant region gene of human IgG1. The CD4-immunoglobulin hybrid, called an immunoadhesin, has a longer serum half-life in the range of that of IgG1 (expected to approach 21 days in humans).

3. No. In the latency period the virus is not replicating, and therefore, the levels of p17 and p24 decline.

4. An increase in the levels of p24 indicates that HIV infection is progressing from the latent phase into lytic infection. Increased levels of p24 can be used to indicate that an HIV-infected individual is progressing into AIDS.

5. Skin-test reactivity is monitored to indicate the functional activity of T_{DTH} cells. As AIDS progresses and $CD4^+$ T cells decline, there is a decline in skin-test reactivity to common antigens.

6. Cell-mediated immunity.

Chapter 24

1. (a) The best possible match is identity in the MHC haplotypes of donor and recipient. (b) There is a 25% chance that siblings will share identical MHC haplotypes. (c) Perform HLA typing using a microcytotoxicity test with monoclonal antibody to class I and class II MHC antigens. In addition, a one-way MLR can be performed using mitomycin C–treated donor lymphocytes as stimulator cells and untreated recipient lymphocytes as responder cells.

2.

Donor	Recipient	Response	Type of rejection
BALB/c	C3H	R	FSR
BALB/c	Rat	R	FSR
BALB/c	Nude mouse	A	
BALB/c	C3H, had previous BALB/c graft	R	SSR
BALB/c	C3H, had previous C57BI/6 graft	R	FSR
BALB/c	BALB/c	A	
BALB/c	F_1 (BALB/c × C3H)	A	
BALB/c	F_1 (C3H × C57BI/6)	R	FSR
F_1 (BALB/c × C3H)	BALB/c	R	FSR
F_1 (BALB/c × C3H)	BALB/c, had previous F_1 graft	R	SSR

3. (a) Graft-versus-host disease (GVHD) develops as donor T cells recognize alloantigens on cells of an immune-suppressed host. The response develops as donor T_H cells are activated in response to recipient peptide-MHC complexes displayed on antigen-presenting cells. Cytokines elaborated by the T_H cell activate a variety of effector cells including NK cells, CTLs, and macrophages, which damage the host tissue. In addition cytokines such as TNF may mediate direct cytolytic damage to the host cells. (b) GVHD develops when the donated organ or tissue contains immunocompetent lymphocytes and when the host is immune suppressed. (c) Monoclonal antibodies to CD3 or to CD4 or to the high-affinity IL-2 receptor could each be tried to deplete T_H cells from the donated organ or tissue. The rationale behind this approach is to diminish T_H-cell activation in response to the alloantigens of the host. THe use of anti-CD3 will deplete all T cells; the use of anti-CD4 will deplete all T_H cells; the use of anti-IL-2R will deplete only the activated T_H cells.

4. (a) Siblings A, C, and E are all potential donors, as they have the same ABO blood type and HLA antigens as the recipient. (b) Sibling A is the best donor as indicated by the low proliferative response in a one-way MLR with the recipient.

Chapter 25

1. (a) False: Cancer cells do not respond to normal regulatory constraints but their rate of cell division is not necessarily any faster than normal cells. (b) True. (c) True. (d) True. (e) False: Some oncogenic retroviruses do not have viral oncogenes. (f) True. (g) False: LAK cells kill a wide variety of tumor cells and are not specific for a single type of tumor.

2. Cells of the pre-B cell lineage have rearranged the heavy-chain genes and express the μ heavy chain in their cytoplasm (see Figure 8-22). You could perform Southern blot analysis with a C_μ probe to see if the heavy-chain genes have rearranged. You could also perform fluorescent antibody staining utilizing methods to stain the cytoplasmic μ heavy chain.

3. (a) Early-stage melanoma cells are functioning as antigen-presenting cells and are processing the antigen by the exogenous pathway and presenting the tetanus toxoid antigen together with the class II MHC DR molecule. (b) Advanced-stage melanoma cells might have a reduction in the expression of class II MHC molecules or they may not be able to internalize and process the antigen by the exogeneous route. (c) Since the paraformaldehyde-fixed early melanoma cells could present processed tetanus toxoid, they must express class II MHC molecules on their surface. (d) Stain the early and advanced melanoma cells with fluorescent monoclonal antibody specific for class II MHC molecules.

4. Because anti-CD3 activates T cells, it is hoped that this agent will enhance the antitumor response. However, the concentration of anti-CD3 is critical, and it is not known whether a particular dose of anti-CD3 will lead to T-cell activation or to unwanted immune suppression.

5. IFN-α, INF-β, and IFN-γ enhance the expression of class I MHC molecules on tumor cells, thereby increasing the CTL response to tumors. IFN-γ also increases the activity of CTLs, macrophages, and NK cells, each of which play a role in the immune response to tumors. TNF-α and TNF-β have direct antitumor activity inducing hemorrhagic necrosis and tumor regression. IL-2 activates LAK and TIL cells, which both have antitumor activity.

CREDITS

Line illustrations rendered by Network Graphics.

Figure 1-2 From N. Sharon and H. Lis, *Scientific American,* Volume 268, January 1993, p. 85. Photograph courtesy of Kazuhiko Fujita.

Figure 1-4 From A. G. Macleod, *Aspects of Acute Inflammation,* Scope Monograph, p. 27. Courtesy of Dorothea Zucker-Franklin. Dept. of Medicine, New York University.

Figure 1-7 From A. S. Rosenthal et al., *Phagocytosis—Past and Future,* Academic Press, 1982, p. 239. Reprinted by permission.

Figure 1-13 From *Immunology: Recognition and Response,* edited by W. E. Paul, W. H. Freeman and Company, 1991, p. 49. Originally from "How T Cells See Antigen," by H. M. Grey et al., *Scientific American,* November 1989, p. 57. Copyright © 1989 by Scientific American Inc. All rights reserved. Micrograph courtesy of Morten H. Nielsen and Ole Werdelin.

Table 2-1 Adapted from Federation of American Societies for Experimental Biology, *Biological Handbooks, Vol. III: Inbred and Genetically Defined Strains of Laboratory Animals,* Pergamon Press Ltd., 1979.

Table 2-3 From J. D. Watson, J. Tooze, and D. T. Kurtz, *Recombinant DNA: A Short Course.* Copyright © 1983 by W. H. Freeman and Company.

Figure 2-8 From J. Darnell, H. Lodish, and D. Baltimore, *Molecular Cell Biology,* 2nd Edition. Copyright © 1990 by Scientific American Books.

Figure 2-9 From J. Darnell, H. Lodish, and D. Baltimore, *Molecular Cell Biology,* 2nd Edition. Copyright © 1990 by Scientific American Books.

Figure 3-2 From M. J. Cline and D. W. Golde, "Cellular Interactions in Hematopoiesis, reprinted by permission from *Nature,* 1979, Volume 277, p. 180. Copyright © 1979 Macmillan Magazines Ltd. Micrograph courtesy of Shirley Quan.

Figure 3-8 From J. R. Goodman, Department of Pediatrics, University of California at San Francisco.

Figure 3-11 From Lennart Nilsson, "Our Immune System: The Wars Within," *National Geographic,* June 1986, p. 718. Copyright Boehringer Ingelheim International. GmpH, Stockholm. Photo by Lennart Nilsson.

Figure 3-14 From A. K. Szakal et al., "Isolated Follicular Dendritic Cells: Cytochemical Volume Antigen Localization, Momarski, SEM, and TEM Morphology," *Journal of Immunology,* Volume 134, 1985, p. 1353. Copyright © 1985 American Association of Immunologists. Reprinted with permission.

Figure 3-15 Adapted from N. K. Jerne, "The Immune System," *Scientific American,* Volume 229, 1973, p. 54. Copyright © 1973 by Scientific American Inc. All rights reserved.

Figure 3-16 From W. van Ewijk, adapted, with permission, from the *Annual Review of Immunology,* Volume 9, p. 591. Copyright © 1991 by Annual Reviews Inc.

Figure 3-17 From M. M. Compton and J. A. Cidlowski, *Trends in Endocrinology and Metabolism,* Volume 3, 1992, p. 17.

Figure 3-19 From W. Bloom and D. W. Fawcett, *Textbook of Histology.*

Figure 3-26a Adapted from A. O. Anderson and N. D. Anderson, "Structure and Physiology of Lymphatic Tissues," in *Cellular Functions in Immunity and Inflamation,* edited by J. J. Oppenheim et al., Elsevier Science Publishing Company, Inc., 1981, p. 39. Reprinted with permission.

Figure 3-26b From S. D. Rosen and I. M. Stoolman, *Vertebrate Lectins,* Van Nostrand Reinhold, 1987.

Figure 3-26c From S. D. Rosen, *Current Opinion in Cell Biology,* Volume 1, 1989, p. 913. Reprinted by permission of Current Science.

Figure 4-2 Adapted from M. Zanetti, E. Sercarz, and J. Salk, *Immunology Today,* Volume 8, 1987, p. 23. Reprinted by permission of Elsevier Science Publishing Company, Inc.

Figure 4-4 Adapted from M. Sela, "Antigenicity: Some Molecular Aspects," *Science,* Volume 166, December 12, 1969, p. 1365. Copyright © 1969 by the American Association for the Advancement of Science.

Figure 4-5 Adapted from M. Z. Atassi, *Immunochemistry* (now *Molecular Immunology*), Volume 12, 1975, p. 423. Copyright © 1975 by Pergamon Press.

Table 4-5 From E. A. Kabat, *Structural Concepts in Immunology and Immunochemistry,* 2nd Edition, Holt, Rinehart and Winston. Copyright © 1976 by E. A. Kabat. Reprinted by permission of the author.

Figure 4-6ab Adapted from W. G. Laver et al., *Cell,* Volume 61, 1990, p. 554. Reprinted by permission of Cell Press.

Table 4-6 From H. Margalit et al., "Prediction of Immunodominant Helper T Cell Antigenic Sites from the Primary Sequence," *The Journal of Immunology,* Volume 138, 1987, p. 2219. Reprinted by permission.

Figure 4-7abc Adapted from D. Benjamin, J. Bersofsky, I. East et al., adapted, with permission, from the *Annual Review of Immunology,* Volume 2, p. 67. Copyright © 1984 by Annual Reviews Inc.

Figure 4-9 From J. Rothbard et al., *Modern Trends in Human Leukemia,* Volume 7, 1987. Reprinted by permission of Springer-Verlag Inc.

Figure 4-10 From H. M. Grey et al., *Scientific American,* Volume 261, November 1989, p. 59. Copyright © 1989 by Scientific American Inc. All rights reserved.

Figure 4-14 From B. Heymer, *Immunology of the Bacterial Cell Envelope,* edited by D. E. S. Stewart-Tull and M. Davis. Copyright © 1985 by John Wiley & Sons, Ltd.

Figure 5-1 Adapted from A. Tiselius and E. A. Kabat, reproduced from the *Journal of Experimental Medicine,* 1939, Volume 69, p. 119, by copyright permission of the Rockefeller University Press.

Figure 5-2a Adapted from R. R. Porter, *Biochemical Journal,* Volume 73, 1959, p. 119. Reprinted by permission of the Biochemical Society.

Figure 5-2b Adapted from J. B. Fleishman, *Archives of Biochemistry Supplement 1,* Academic Press, Inc., 1962, p. 1974.

Tables 5-2 and 5-3 Adapted from I. A. Wilson and R. L. Stanfield, *Current Opinion in Structural Biology,* Volume 3, Number 113, 1993.

Figure 5-5a Adapted from J. Darnell, H. Lodish, and D. Baltimore, *Molecular Cell Biology,* 2nd Edition. Copyright © 1990 by Scientific American Books. Reprinted by permission of W. H. Freeman and Co.

Figure 5-5b Adapted from M. Schiffer et al., reprinted with permission from *Biochemistry,* Volume 12, 1973, p. 4620. Copyright © 1973 by the American Chemical Society.

Figure 5-7b From J. D. Capra and A. B. Edmundson, *The Antibody Combining Site.* Copyright © 1977 by Scientific American Books. Reprinted by permission of W. H. Freeman and Co.

Figure 5-10 abc From R. C. Valentine and N. M. Green, *Journal of Molecular Biology,* Volume 27, 1967, p. 615. Reprinted by permission of Academic Press Inc. (London) Ltd.

Figure 6-5 From J. S. Garvey, N. E. Cremer, and D. H. Sussdorf, *Methods in Immunology,* 3rd Edition. Copyright © 1977 by Addison-Wesley Publishing Company, Inc., Advanced Book Program. Reprinted by permission of the author.

Figure 6-7 From D. M. Weir, (ed.) *Handbook of Experimental Immunology, Volume 1: Immunochemistry,* 4th Edition, 1986. Reprinted by permission of Blackwell Scientific Publications Ltd.

Figure 6-9 From J. S. Garvey, N. E. Cremer, and D. H. Sussdorf, *Methods in Immunology,* 3rd Edition. Copyright © 1977 by Addison-Wesley Publishing Company, Inc., Advanced Book Program. Reprinted by permission of the author.

Figures 6-10 and 6-11 From D. M. Weir, (ed.) *Handbook of Experimental Immunology, Volume 1: Immunochemistry,* 4th Edition, 1986. Reprinted by permission of Blackwell Scientific Publications Ltd.

Figure 6-12 From J. S. Garvey, N. E. Cremer, and D. H. Sussdorf, *Methods in Immunology,* 3rd Edition. Copyright © 1977 by Addison-Wesley Publishing Company, Inc., Advanced Book Program. Reprinted by permission of the author.

Figure 7-2 From R. L. Davidson and P. S. Gerald, *Somatic Cell Genetics,* Volume 2, 1976, p. 165. Reprinted by permission of Plenum Publishing Corporation.

Figure 7-5 From C. Milstein, "Antibody-Secreting Clone," *Scientific American,* Volume 243, October 1980, p. 67. Copyright © 1980 by Scientific American Inc. All rights reserved.

Figure 7-11 Adapted from M. Verhoeyen and L. Reichmann, *BioEssays,* Volume 8, 1988, p. 74. Reprinted by permission of Cambridge University Press.

Figure 7-14 Adapted from R. A. Lerner and A. Tramontano, *Scientific American,* Volume 258, 1988, p. 58. Copyright © 1988 by Scientific American Inc. All rights reserved.

Figure 8-1 Adapted from N. Hozumi and S. Tonegawa, *Proceedings of the National Academy of Science,* Volume 73, 1976, p. 3628.

Figure 8-6 Adapted from F. W. Alt, *Immunology Today,* Volume 13, 1992, p. 306. Elsevier Science Publishing Company, Inc. Reprinted by permission.

Figure 8-7 From K. Okazki et al., *Cell,* Volume 49, 1987, p. 477. Reprinted by permission of Cell Press.

Figure 8-12 Adapted from G. D. Yancopoulos and F. W. Alt, adapted, with permission, from the *Annual Review of Immunology,* Volume 4, 1986, p. 339. Copyright © 1986 by Annual Reviews Inc.

Figure 8-17 Adapted from C. Berek and C. Milstein, *Immunological Review,* Volume 96, 1987, p. 23. Copyright © Munksgaard International Publishers Ltd., Copenhagen, Denmark.

Table 9-6 Adapted from S. Buus et al., *Science,* Volume 235, 1987, p. 1353. Copyright © 1987 by the American Association for the Advancement of Science.

Figure 9-8a Adapted from P. Parham, reprinted with permission from *Nature,* Volume 360, 1992, p. 300. Copyright © 1992 Macmillan Magazines Limited.

Figure 9-8b Adapted from M. L. Silver et al., reprinted with permission from *Nature,* Volume 360, 1992, p. 367. Copyright © 1992 Macmillan Magazines Limited.

Figure 9-8c Adapted from D. R. Madden et al., *Cell,* Volume 70, 1992, p. 1035. Reprinted by permission of Cell Press.

Figure 9-9 Adapted from J. H. Brown et al., reprinted with permission from *Nature,* Volume 364, 1993, p. 33. Copyright © 1993 Macmillan Magazines Limited.

Figure 9-10a From Sodoyer et al., *EMBO Journal,* Volume 3, 1984, p. 879. Published by European Molecular Biology Organization. Reprinted by permission of Oxford University Press.

Figure 9-10b Adapted from P. Parham, reprinted with permission from *Nature,* Volume 342, 1989, p. 617. Copyright © 1989 Macmillan Magazines Limited.

Figure 10-1 Adapted from A. Rosenthal and E. Shevach, *Journal of Experimental Medicine,* Volume 138, 1974, p. 1194, by copyright permission of the Rockefeller University Press.

Table 10-2 Adapted from T. J. Braciale, I. A. Morrison, M. T. Sweester, J. Sambrook et al., *Immunological Reviews,* Volume 98, 1987, p. 95. Copyright © Munksgaard International Publishers Ltd., Copenhagen, Denmark.

Figure 11-4 Adapted from D. Raulet, adapted, with permission, from the *Annual Review of Immunology,* Volume 7, 1989, p. 175; and adapted from M. Davis, with permission, from the *Annual Review of Biochemistry,* Volume 59, 1990, p. 475. Copyright © 1989 and 1990, respectively, by Annual Reviews Inc.

Figure 11-10 From M. Davis and P. J. Bjorkman, reprinted by permission from *Nature,* Volume 334, p. 397. Copyright © 1988 Macmillan Magazines Limited.

Figure 11-13 Adapted from J. McClusky, R. Block, A. Brooks, W. Chen, D. Kanost, and L. Kjer-Nielsen, "The Biology of Antigen Processing and Presentation, 13, in *Antigen Processing and Recognition,* edited by J. McCluskey, CRC Press, Boca Raton, Florida, 1992.

Figure 12-1 Adapted from B. J. Fowlkes and D. M. Pardoll, *Advances in Immunology,* Volume 44, 1989, p. 207. Reprinted by permission of Academic Press.

Table 12-6 Adapted from G. Crabtree, *Science,* Volume 243, 1989, p. 357. Copyright © 1989 by the American Association for the Advancement of Science.

Figure 12-8 From H. von Boehmer and P. Kisielow, "Self-Nonself Discrimination by T Cells," *Science,* Volume 248, June 15, 1990, p. 1370. Copyright © 1990 by the American Association for the Advancement of Science.

Figure 13-6 Adapted from D. Cosman, *Cytokine,* Volume 5, 1993, p. 95. Reprinted by permission of Academic Press.

Figure 13-7 Adapted from T. Kishimoto et al., *Science,* Volume 258, 1992, p. 593. Copyright © 1992 by the American Association for the Advancement of Science.

Figure 13-13 Adapted from "Research News," *Science,* Volume 259, 1993, p. 1693. Copyright © 1993 by the American Association for the Advancement of Science.

Figure 13-14a From L. J. Old, "Tumor Necrosis Factor," *Scientific American,* Volume 258, May 1988, p. 59. Copyright © 1988 by Scientific American Inc. All rights reserved.

Figure 13-14b From B. Beutler, *Hospital Practice,* April 15, 1993, p. 45. Reprinted with permission. Illustration by Hospital Practice.

Table 14-4 Adapted with permission from H. N. Eisen and G. W. Siskind, *Biochemistry,* Volume 3, 1964, p. 966. Copyright © 1964 American Chemical Society.

Figure 14-9 From V. M. Saunders et al., "Characterization of the Physical Interaction Between Antigen-Specific B and T Cells," *The Journal of Immunology,* Volume 137, 1986, p. 2395. Reprinted by permission.

Figure 14-11 From W. J. Poo et al., reprinted from *Nature,* Volume 332, 1988, p. 378. Copyright © 1988 Macmillan Magazines Ltd.

Figure 15-3 Adapted from S. Townsend and J. Allison, *Science,* Volume 259, 1993, p. 368. Copyright © 1993 by the American Association for the Advancement of Science.

Figure 15-4 From J. D. E. Young and Z. A. Cohn, *Scientific American,* January 1988, p. 38. Copyright © 1988 by Scientific American Inc. SEM by Dr. Gilla Kaplan, The Rockefeller University.

Figure 15-5 Adapted, with permission, from P. A. Henkart, *Annual Review of Immunology,* Volume 3, 1985, p. 31. Copyright © 1985 by Annual Reviews Inc.

Figure 15-7 From J. R. Yannelli et al., "Reorientation and Fusion of Cytotoxic T Lymphocyte Granules After Interaction with Target Cells as Determined by High Resolution Cinemicrography," *The Journal of Immunology,* Volume 136, 1986, pp. 377–382. Reprinted by permission.

Figure 15-8a From J. D. E. Young and Z. A. Cohn, *Scientific American,* January 1988, p. 38. Copyright © 1988 by Scientific American Inc.

Figure 15-8b From E. R. Podack and G. Dennert, reprinted from *Nature,* Volume 301, 1983, p. 442. Copyright © 1983 Macmillan Magazines Ltd.

Figure 15-9 Adapted from P. J. Peters et al., *Immunology Today,* Volume 11, 1990, p. 38. Reprinted by permission of Elsevier Science Publishing Company, Inc.

Figure 15-15 Adapted from D. K. Dalton, *Science,* Volume 259, 1993, p. 1739. Copyright © 1993 by the American Association for the Advancement of Science.

Figure 15-17 From J. R. David, *Immunology,* 1970. Courtesy The Upjohn Company.

Figure 16-1 Adapted from C. G. Romball and W. O. Weigle, reproduced from the *Journal of Experimental Medicine,* 1973, Volume 138, p. 1426, by copyright permission of the Rockefeller University Press.

Figure 16-4 Adapted from H. Cozenza, *European Journal of Immunology,* Volume 6, 1976, p. 114. Reprinted by permission.

Figure 16-6 Adapted from S. Hedrick et al., *Proceedings of the National Academy of Science,* Volume 82, 1985, p. 531. Reprinted by permission of the author.

Table 16-6 Adapted from D. A. Nemazee and K. Burki, reprinted from *Nature,* Volume 337, 1989, p. 562. Copyright © 1989 Macmillan Magazines Ltd.

Figure 16-8 Adapted from N. A. Mitchison, *Proceedings of the Royal Society of London,* Volume 161, 1964, p. 275. Reprinted by permission of The Royal Society.

Figure 16-9 From J. Chiller et al., "Kinetic Differences in Unresponsiveness of Thymus and Bone Marrow Cells," *Science,* Volume 171, February 26, 1971, p. 813. Copyright © 1971 by the American Association for the Advancement of Science.

Figure 16-12 Adapted from W. C. Sha et al., reprinted from *Nature,* Volume 336, 1988, p. 73. Copyright © 1988 Macmillan Magazines Ltd.

Figure 17-2a From N. C. Hughes-Jones, "The Classical Pathway," *Immunobiology of the Complement System,* Academic Press, 1986. Originally published in H. R. Knobel et al., *European Journal of Immunology,* Volume 5, 1975, p. 78.

Figure 17-2c From N. C. Hughes-Jones, "The Classical Pathway," *Immunobiology of the Complement System,* Academic Press, 1986. Originally published in J. Tschopp et al., *Proceedings of the National Academy of Science,* Volume 77, 1980, p. 7014.

Table 17-2 From M. K. Pangburn, "The Alternate Pathway," in *Immunology of the Complement System,* Academic Press, 1986.

Figure 17-3 From A. Feinstein, E. Munn, and N. Richardson, *Monographs in Allergy,* Volume 17, 1981, p. 28, S. Karger AG, Basel; and from A. Feinstein, E. Munn, and N. Richardson, *Annals of the New York Academy of Science,* Volume 190, 1981, p. 1104.

Figure 17-7a From E. R. Podack, "Assembly and Functions of the Terminal Components," *Immunobiology of the Complement System,* Academic Press, 1986.

Figure 17-7b From J. Humphrey and R. Dourmashkin, *Advances in Immunology,* Volume 11, 1969, p. 75. Reprinted by permission of Academic Press.

Table 17-8 From N. R. Cooper and G. R. Nemerow, "Complement-Dependent Mechanisms of Virus Neutralization," *Immunology of the Complement System,* Academic Press, 1986.

Table 17-9 Adapted from J. A. Schifferti and D. K. Peters, *Lancet,* Volume 2, 1983, p. 957. Copyright © 1983 by The Lancet Ltd.

Figure 17-10 From R. D. Schreiber et al., "Bacterial Activity of the Alternative Complement Pathway Generated from 11 Isolated Plasma Proteins," reproduced from the *Journal of Experimental Medicine,* Volume 149, 1979, p. 870 by copyright permission of the Rockefeller University Press.

Figure 17-11 From N. R. Cooper and G. R. Nemerow, "Complement-Dependent Mechanisms of Virus Neutralization," *Immunobiology of the Complement System,* Academic Press, 1986, p. 155.

Figure 17-12 From N. R. Cooper and G. R. Nemerow, "Complement-Dependent Mechanisms of Virus Neutralization," *Immunobiology of the Complement System,* Academic Press, 1986, p. 150.

Figure 18-2 From S. Burwen and B. Satir, reproduced from the *Journal of Cell Biology,* Volume 73, 1977, p. 662 by copyright permission of The Rockefeller University Press.

Table 18-5 From F. D. Finkelman et al., *Journal of Immunology,* Volume 141, 1988, p. 2335. Copyright © 1992, The Journal of Immunology.

Figure 18-6 Adapted from T. Ishizaka et al., *International Archives of Allergy and Applied Immunology,* Volume 77, 1985, p. 137. Reprinted by permission of S. Karger AG, Basel.

Figure 18-11 From K. Ishizaka and T. Ishisaka, *Asthma Physiology, Immunopharmacology, and Treatment,* K. F. Austen, L. M. Lichtenstein, eds. Copyright © 1973 Academic Press.

Figure 19-1 From L. V. Crowley, *Introduction to Human Disease,* 2nd Edition. Copyright ©1988 Jones and Bartlett Publishers, Boston. Reprinted by permission.

Figure 19-2 From J. A. Charlesworth and B. A. Pussell, in *Clinical Immunology Illustrated,* edited by J. V. Wells and D. S. Nelson, Williams & Wilkins, 1986, p. 191.

Figure 19-3 From M. A. Atkinson and N. K. Maclaren, "What Causes Diabetes?" *Scientific American,* Volume 263, July 1990, p. 62. Copyright © 1990 by Scientific American Inc. All rights reserved.

Table 19-4 Adapted from M. B. A. Oldstone, *Cell,* Volume 50, 1987, p. 819. Reprinted by permission of Cell Press.

Figure 19-5 From S. B. Abramson and G. Weissmann, "Complement Split Products and the Pathogenesis of SLE," *Hospital Practice,* Volume 23, issue 15, p. 45. Illustration by Albert Miller. Reprinted with permission.

Table 19-5 From D. B. Jones et al., *Immunology Today,* Volume 14, 1993, p. 115. Reprinted by permission of Elsevier Science Publishing Company, Inc.

Figure 19-8 From V. Kumar et al., adapted, with permission, from the *Annual Review of Immunology,* Volume 7, p. 657. Copyright © 1989 by Annual Reviews Inc.

Figure 19-9 From G. Kroemer and G. Wick, *Immunology Today,* Volume 10, 1989, p. 246. Reprinted by permission of Elsevier Science Publishing Company, Inc.

Figure 19-10a Adapted from J. Shizuru and N. Sarvetnik, *TEM,* Vol. 2, 1991, p. 97.

Figure 19-10b From N. Sarvetnick et al., *Cell,* Volume 52, 1988, p. 773. Reprinted by permission of Cell Press.

Figure 19-13 From D. Wofsy, "Treatment of Autoimmune Diseases with Monoclonal Antibodies," *Monoclonal Antibody Therapy, Progress in Allergy,* edited by H. Waldmann, 1988. Reprinted by permission of S. Karger AG, Basel.

Figure 19-14 Adapted from H. Acha-Orbea, I. Steinman, and H. O. McDevitt, "T-cell Receptors in Murine Autoimmune Diseases," adapted, with permission, from *Annual Review of Immunology,* Volume 7, 1989, p. 371. Copyright © 1988 by Annual Reviews Inc. Originally published in *Cell,* Volume 54, 1988, p. 268.

Figure 20-1 From C. A. Mims and D. O. White, *Viral Pathogenesis and Immunology,* Blackwell Scientific Publications, Ltd., 1984.

Figure 20-3 From M. Zanetti, E. Sacarz, and J. Salk, *Immunology Today,* Volume 8, 1987, p. 18. Reprinted by permission of Elsevier Science Publishing Company, Inc.

Table 20-8 From M. Zanetti, E. Sacarz, and J. Salk, *Immunology Today,* Volume 8, 1987, p. 18. Reprinted by permission of Elsevier Science Publishing Company, Inc.

Figure 21-1 From G. Murti, Department of Virology, St. Jude Children's Research Hospital, Memphis, TN.

Figure 21-3 From G. G. Brownlee, *Options for the Control of Influenza,* p. 47, Alan R. Liss. Copyright © 1986 by John Wiley & Sons.

Figure 21-4 From D. C. Wiley et al., reprinted by permission from *Nature,* Volume 289, 1981, p. 373. Copyright © 1981 Macmillan Magazines Ltd.

Table 21-4 Adapted from J. H. Zweerink, B. A. Askonas, D. Millican et al., *European Journal of Immunology,* Volume 7, 1977, p. 630. Reprinted by permission.

Figure 21-6 From M. E. Ward and P. J. Watt, *Journal of Infectious Diseases,* Volume 126, 1972, p. 601. Copyright © 1972. Reprinted by permission of The University of Chicago Press.

Table 21-6 Cited in M. F. Good et al., *Annual Reviews in Immunology,* Volume 6, 1988, p. 663, Copyright © 1988 by Annual Reviews Inc.

Figure 21-7 From T. F. Meyer, modified, with permission, from *The Annual Review of Microbiology,* Volume 44, p. 460. Copyright © 1990 by Annual Reviews Inc.

Figure 21-11 Adapted from M. F. Good et al., *Science,* Volume 235, 1987, p. 1059. Copyright © 1987 by the American Association for the Advancement of Science.

Figure 21-12 Adapted from John Donelson, in *The Biology of Parasitism,* Alan R. Liss. Copyright © 1988 by John Wiley & Sons.

Figure 22-2 From M. E. Conley, reproduced, with permission, from the *Annual Review of Immunology,* Volume 10, 1992, p. 215. Copyright © 1992 by Annual Reviews Inc.

Figure 22-3 From R. J. Schegel et al., reproduced by permission of *Pediatrics,* Volume 45, 1970, p. 926. Copyright © 1970.

Figure 22-4 From F. S. Rosen and R. Kretschmer et al., "Congenital Aplasia of the Thymus Gland," reprinted, by permission of *The New England Journal of Medicine,* Volume 279, 1968, p. 1295.

Table 22-3 From D. C. Anderson et al., *Journal of Infectious Disease,* Volume 152, 1986, p. 668. Copyright © 1986. Reprinted by permission of The University of Chicago Press.

Figure 22-5 Courtesy The Jackson Laboratory, Bar Harbor, ME.

Figure 22-6 From D. D. Manning et al., reproduced from the *Journal of Experimental Medicine,* Volume 138, 1973, p. 488, by copyright permission of the Rockefeller University Press.

Figure 23-2a From R. C. Gallo and L. Montagnier, "The AIDS Epidemic," *Scientific American,* Volume 259, 1988, p. 40. Copyright © 1988 by Scientific American Inc. All rights reserved. Micrograph courtesy of Hans Gelderbloom of the Robert Koch Institute, Berlin.

Figure 23-2b Adapted from B. M. Peterlin and P. A. Luciw, "Molecular Biology of HIV," *AIDS,* 2(suppl 1), 1988, pp. S29–S40. Reprinted by permission of Current Science.

Figure 23-6 Adapted from W. C. Greene, reprinted by permission of *The New England Journal of Medicine,* Volume 324, 1991, p. 308.

Figure 23-10 From H. C. Lane and A. S. Fauci, reproduced, with permission, from the *Annual Review of Immunology,* Volume 3, © 1985 by Annual Reviews Inc.

Figure 23-8 From R. C. Gallo, "HIV—The Cause of AIDS," *Journal of Acquired Immune Deficiency Syndromes,* Volume 1, 1988, p. 521. Reprinted by permission of Raven Press Ltd.

Figure 23-9 Adapted from S. Putney, *Trends in Biochemical Science,* Volume 15, 1992, p. 191. Elsevier Trends Journals.

Figure 23-11a From R. C. Gallo, "HIV—The Cause of AIDS," *Journal of Acquired Immune Deficiency Syndromes,* Volume 1, 1988, p. 533. Reprinted by permission of Raven Press Ltd.

Figure 23-11b From J. N. Weber and R. A. Weiss, *Scientific American,* Volume 259, October 1988, p. 101. Copyright © 1988 by Scientific American Inc. All rights reserved.

Table 24-1 Adapted from A. Svejgaard et al., *The HLA System: An Introductory Survey,* S. Karger AG, Basel, 1979.

Figure 24-3 Adapted from S. P. Cobbold, G. Martin, and H. Waldmann, reprinted by permission from *Nature,* Volume 323, 1986, p. 165. Copyright © 1986 Macmillan Magazines Ltd.

Table 24-3 From J. R. Batchelor and Y. I. Chai, *Progress in Immunology,* Volume 6, 1986, p. 1002. Reprinted by permission of Academic Press.

Figure 24-9 Adapted from S. M. Sabesin and J. W. Williams, "Current Status of Liver Transplantation," *Hospital Practice,* Volume 22, Issue 7, 1987, p. 75. Illustration by Albert Miller. Reprinted with permission.

Figure 24-10 Adapted from T. Moen et al., reprinted, by permission of *The New England Journal of Medicine,* Volume 303, 1980, p. 850.

Figure 25-1 Adapted from J. Darnell, H. Lodish, and D. Baltimore, *Molecular Cell Biology,* 2nd Edition. Copyright © 1990 by Scientific American Books. Reprinted by permission of W. H. Freeman and Company.

Table 25-2 Adapted from H. E. Varmus, with permission, from the *Annual Review of Genetics,* Volume 18, 1984, p. 553. Copyright © 1984 by Annual Reviews Inc.

Table 25-5 From K. M. Hui, *BioEssays,* Volume 11, 1989, p. 23. Reprinted by permission of Cambridge University Press.

Table 25-6 From L. Thompson, *Science,* Volume 258, 1992, p. 744. Copyright © 1992 by the American Association for the Advancement of Science.

Figure 25-11 From L. J. Old, "Tumor Necrosis Factor," *Scientific American,* May 1988, pp. 59–75. Copyright © 1988 by Scientific American Inc. All rights reserved.

Figure 25-13 From J. D. Ellenhorn et al., *Science,* Volume 242, 1988, p. 569. Copyright © 1988 by the American Association for the Advancement of Science.

Color Plate 1 Image provided by the laboratory of Dr. Alexander McPherson. The immunoglobulin structure was determined by Harris et. al., *Nature,* 1992, Volume 360, pp. 369–372. A special thank you to the Academic Computing Graphics and Visual Imaging Lab, University of California, Riverside, for help with the image. The image was generated using the computer program, RIBBONS. The RIBBONS reference is: Carson, M. and Bugg, C. E. (1986). An Algorithm for Ribbon Models of Proteins. *J. Mol. Graph.* Volume 4, pp. 121–122.

Color Plate 2 From K. C. Garcia, P. M. Ronco, P. J. Verroust, Axel T. Brünger, and L. Mario Amzel, *Science,* Volume 257, 1992, p. 502.

Color Plate 3abc From K. C. Garcia, P. M. Ronco, P. J. Verroust, Axel T. Brünger, and L. Mario Amzel, *Science,* Volume 257, 1992, p. 502.

Color Plate 4abc From A. G. Amit, R. A. Mariuza, S. E. V. Phillips, and R. J. Poljak, *Science,* Volume 233, 1986, p. 747.

Color Plate 5 From J. M. Rini, U. Schulze-Gahmen, and I. A. Wilson, *Science,* Volume 255, 1992, p. 959. Photograph courtesy of J. M. Rini, U. Schulze-Gahmen, and I. A. Wilson.

Color Plate 6ab From U. Schulze-Gahmen, J. M. Rini, M. Pique, and I. A. Wilson. *Science,* Volume 255, 1992, p. 959. Photographs courtesy of U. Schulze-Gahmen, J. M. Rini, M. Pique, and I. A. Wilson.

Color Plate 7 From I. A. Wilson and R. L. Stanfield,

Current Opinion in Structural Biology, Volume 3, 1993, p. 113. Photograph courtesy of R. Stanfield and I. A. Wilson.

Color Plate 8ab From G. J. V. H. Nossal, *Scientific American,* September 1993, p. 54. Photograph courtesy of P. M. Colman and W. R. Tulip, Division of Molecular Engineering, CSIRO, Australia.

Color Plate 9ab From R. L. Stanfield, T. M. Feiser, R. A. Lerner, and I. A. Wilson, *Science,* Volume 248, 1990, p. 712. Photographs courtesy of R. Stanfield and I. A. Wilson.

Color Plate 10ab From R. L. Stanfield, T. M. Feiser, R. A. Lerner, and I. A. Wilson, *Science,* Volume 248, 1990, p. 712. Photographs courtesy of R. Stanfield and I. A. Wilson.

Color Plate 11 From M. L. Silver, H. C. Guo, J. L. Strominger, and D. C. Wiley, *Nature,* Volume 360, 1992, p. 367.

Color Plate 12ab From D. H. Fremont, M. Pique, and I. A. Wilson, *Science,* Volume 257, 1992, p. 891. Photographs courtesy of D. H. Fremont, M. Pique, and I. A. Wilson.

Color Plate 13 From M. Matsumura, D. H. Fremont, P. A. Peterson, and I. A. Wilson, *Science,* Volume 257, 1992, p. 927. Photographs courtesy of D. H. Fremont, M. Matsumura, M. Pique, and I. A. Wilson.

Color Plate 14 From J. H. Brown, T. S. Jardetzky, J. C. Gorga, L. J. Stern, R. G. Urban, J. L. Strominger, and D. C. Wiley, *Nature,* Volume 364, 1993, p. 33.

Color Plate 15ab From J. H. Brown, T. S. Jardetzky, J. C. Gorga, L. J. Stern, R. G. Urban, J. L. Strominger, and D. C. Wiley, *Nature,* Volume 364, 1993, p. 33.

Color Plate 16ab From J. H. Brown, T. S. Jardetzky, J. C. Gorga, L. J. Stern, R. G. Urban, J. L. Strominger, and D. C. Wiley, *Nature,* Volume 364, 1993, p. 33.

INDEX